# PARTNERSHIP FOR EXCELLENCE

## Medicine at the University of Toronto and Academic Hospitals

The University of Toronto's Faculty of Medicine is North America's largest medical school and a major health consortium, boasting nine affiliated teaching hospitals and a network of research institutes. It is where insulin was pioneered, stem cells were first discovered, and famous physicians from Vincent Lam to Sheela Basrur began their careers. But despite all its major accomplishments, the faculty's impressive history has never before been comprehensively documented.

In *Partnership for Excellence*, senior medical historian and award-winning author Edward Shorter details the Faculty of Medicine's history from its inception as a small provincial school to its present-day status as an international powerhouse. Deeply researched through front-line interviews and primary sources, it ties the story of the faculty and its teaching hospitals to the general history of medicine over this period. Shorter emphasizes the enormous concentration of intellectual energy in the faculty that has allowed it to become the dominant force in Canadian medicine, home to a legion of medical pioneers and achievements.

EDWARD SHORTER is the Hannah Professor of the History of Medicine in the Faculty of Medicine at the University of Toronto. He is the author of more than twenty books, including *Written in the Flesh: A History of Desire*, shortlisted for the 2005 Governor General's Literary Award for Non-Fiction. He is also a two-time winner of the Royal Society of Canada's Hannah Medal for writing in the history of medicine.

# Partnership for Excellence

*Medicine at the University of Toronto and Academic Hospitals*

EDWARD SHORTER

UNIVERSITY OF TORONTO PRESS
Toronto Buffalo London

Reprinted in paperback 2021

ISBN 978-1-4426-4595-0 (cloth)
ISBN 978-1-4875-4339-6 (paper)

---

**Library and Archives Canada Cataloguing in Publication**

Title: Partnership for excellence : medicine at the University of Toronto and
   academic hospitals / Edward Shorter.

Names: Shorter, Edward, author.

Description: Paperback reprint. Originally published 2013. | Includes
   bibliographical references and index.

Identifiers: Canadiana 20210202122 | ISBN 9781487543396 (softcover)

Subjects: LCSH: University of Toronto. Faculty of Medicine – History. |
   LCSH: Teaching hospitals – Ontario – Toronto – History.

Classification: LCC R749.T74 S56 2021 | DDC 610.71/1713541–dc23

---

University of Toronto Press acknowledges the financial assistance to its
publishing program of the Canada Council for the Arts and the Ontario
Arts Council, an agency of the Government of Ontario.

 **Canada Council** **Conseil des Arts**
**for the Arts** **du Canada**

 ONTARIO ARTS COUNCIL
CONSEIL DES ARTS DE L'ONTARIO
an Ontario government agency
un organisme du gouvernement de l'Ontario

Funded by the   Financé par le
Government  gouvernement    Canadä
of Canada      du Canada

*In overarching respect and admiration for the men and women who people these pages, often renouncing the large incomes they might otherwise have obtained in favour of lives of science, dedication, and public service.*

# Contents

Illustrations follow pages 248 and 520

PARTNERSHIP FOR EXCELLENCE

Medicine at the University of Toronto and Academic Hospitals

# 1  Introduction

This book began life one day when I was lecturing to the medical students. "Stem cells were discovered at the University of Toronto," I said. "What!" They were incredulous and had no idea. This was a group of smart, alert medical students at the University of Toronto (U of T), and they were completely unaware of an important achievement of their faculty.

I realized that the story of medicine in Toronto was a story that needed to be told.

I was trained as a historian, not a physician. But I did go to medical school for two years, after I was already a full professor of history, because I had become interested in the history of medicine and realized that I did not have the knowledge required to study the subject properly. So I enrolled in all the basic medical science courses in the first two years of the medical curriculum and took all the exams – and finished in about the middle of my class.

So my approach in this book is that this is a powerful story and deserves to be told properly. And that means getting into the guts of all the departments and divisions of this sprawling faculty and its nine big research hospitals. (The list of affiliated hospitals appears on p. 746.) Many of these people have made important contributions to the international narrative, such as discovering stem cells. This means telling their stories as they deserve, through interviews and by consulting the archives and libraries in which the record of the past is stored.

Canadian hospital history is a coming field, and a picture of the transfer of resources from the private to the public sector is starting to emerge in many places in this country.[1] But this is not hospital history, even though the teaching hospitals of Toronto are a constant presence on these pages. It is the history of a single faculty in a sole university, which is to say that it is the history of a small group of people and their ideas. Even though such words as "program," "division," and "department" are almost too numerous to index, this book is basically a history of what these pioneers of Canadian medicine thought and how they acted on their ideas. This kind of history has really not been done for medical schools. There are not a great number of histories of medical faculties, and they tend to be written more by favourite sons than by trained historians.[2] So I wish I could say, "Thus, I add to the body of knowledge about faculties." But there is no such body of knowledge, or rather, there is a great deal of knowledge about how these things have evolved elsewhere, but it has not yet been codified. Nobody can say how the evolution of molecular medicine in Toronto conformed to, or departed from, that in other Canadian institutions because no one yet has the sampling of studies that would make the construction of a historiographical tradition possible.[3] Instead, what are featured here are stories, and I shall be at pains to ground them in wider traditions in the pages that follow.

I will state right at the beginning that the faculty and affiliated teaching hospitals of the University of Toronto have become the dominant force in Canadian medicine and an international powerhouse. Why is that? This has happened for two reasons. One is that the University of Toronto is the sole medical school for eight major teaching hospitals. The academic physicians and scientists of these hospitals are all cross-appointed to university departments, and the faculty's students learn and work in the hospitals. This is like a string of locomotives hooked together, and as they pull forward, their force – in terms of bringing large amounts of intellectual energy to important scientific problems – has been enormous. In North American medicine, though there are other brilliant centres, nothing else quite like this exists.

Knox Ritchie, an Irishman, said this about his decision to join the Department of Obstetrics and Gynaecology at Mount Sinai Hospital in 1984: "When you looked at the geography, and the powerhouse Toronto potentially was – it wasn't yet, but it could be, if you looked at these teaching hospitals all sitting opposite each other on Ambulance Alley here. You look at Sick Kids, Toronto General, Mount Sinai. Princess Margaret wasn't there, yet, but it was Sinai that influenced them to come to that site. All of them with research institutes. And you walked up the street, and you had the basic sciences at the University just looking at you … I don't know of any other city in the world where it has that setup … It's unique. It makes Toronto what it is now."[4] So this combination of a major university with its basic sciences and the hospitals with all their brilliance made Toronto distinctive.

Second, the faculty has had a series of unusually gifted leaders to help yoke the locomotives together. This is quite a remarkable story because initially the leaders of the faculty – and this included a number who became world-class scientists – were farm boys from little towns in Ontario. Most were of Scottish Presbyterian stock. The second generation of leaders, who appeared in the 1960s and 1970s, were largely Jewish and of urban origin. This is one of the most remarkable stories in Canadian medicine. But it was these successive generations of leaders that helped outfit the scientists with lab space and funds and, more importantly, inculcated a general research culture in the faculty and the hospitals.

The main theme of this book, as we shall see, is a story of two pivots: a pivot in the life of the faculty from education to research and a pivot in academic vision from the United Kingdom to the United States. These are pivots that happened not just in Toronto but throughout Canadian medicine and constitute one of the major narrative arcs of the twentieth century.

Now many of these stories are real triumphs of the human spirit, models for leaders of the future to reflect upon, and I realize that in telling them I risk jeers of "hagiography!" (Yet the faculty on occasion had feet of clay – particularly in its treatment of women and Jews – and this too will come out.) But one keeps in mind how modest were the material rewards for research those days. The early 1950s were not a profitable time for academic physicians in Toronto. Community doctors earned adequate incomes because they saw paying patients all day. But academic doctors were poorly remunerated for their hospital service and often had a difficult time getting private practices going, despite the prestige of a hospital appointment. It took Barney Berris, who had graduated in 1944, ten years as an academic physician to scrape together enough money to buy a modest bungalow in North York. He said later, "Although I was happy that I was in academic medicine, it was sometimes disconcerting to hear about these doctors' expensive trips, the large homes that they were buying and the private clubs they were joining."[5]

Most of the big stories in Canadian medicine are not well known, these included. Why is that? I asked James Till, the co-discoverer with Ernest McCulloch of stem cells at the University of Toronto in 1960, why he had never written an autobiography. Till, who came from a Saskatchewan farm family, replied, "My father was a very modest man. He's deceased some time ago, but I admired him greatly, and he came from the British tradition that you didn't blow your own horn, that was bad taste. I think I'm still affected by that tradition."[6] As readers will discover, the whole medical faculty at Toronto was once much affected by that tradition.

There is in the Canadian academic character a reserve that comes directly from the United Kingdom, from Oxbridge and Edinburgh, if one will. In British academic life, self-praise has always been considered inappropriate. The British have always had a horror of self-promotion, of trumpeting one's triumphs. There is no doubt that, just as many characteristics of Canadian academic life before the 1970s were derived from the United Kingdom – this may no longer be true – a reluctance to sing one's own praise has been similarly inherited. When Bill Bigelow, the originator of hypothermia (operating at low body temperatures) in heart surgery, set out to tell his story in 1984, he called it "a uniquely Canadian story and there is some unawareness of this on the part of many Canadians ... The powerful United States news media and the large-circulation magazines seriously influence Canadian thinking. They naturally feature the

American component of any medical advance, [while Canadians remain] insufficiently aware of the input of their scientists."[7]

Dean Catharine Whiteside noted this reticence somewhat ruefully in 2006: in the external reviews of many departments, "our academic units are generally regarded as outstanding and often considered not just the best in Canada, but many are recognized among the few top-ranked programs in the world. Nevertheless, I often hear the same message from non-Canadian reviewers and candidates for leadership positions: we are not doing a very good job at communicating our accomplishments. Our education programs are not as well known as they should be. Our researchers and their discoveries are not publicized enough ... In short, we have over achieved and under sold."[8] This book is not an attempt to redress that balance, and the same reticence that restrains my colleagues from boosterism makes me squirm as well at the history of superlatives. There is none of that in here. But I do give credit where it is due, and this is not hagiography.

A big story makes for a long book. Too long? I take the time needed to delve into the lives of these scientists and clinicians, to find out who they were, and to document in detail their accomplishments – so that praise and blame alike will have a factual base. I know that at a certain point some readers may weary of having to navigate, for example, the history of the Department of Anatomy. Yet anatomy was once the queen of the medical sciences! One cannot understand how medicine has pivoted from the study of lesions to biochemistry to molecular genetics without following the rise – and fall – of the Department of Anatomy. The faculty has many departments; they all have their own stories, and all flood into the great narrative river of leadership and research that is medical progress.

Absorbing though it is to bring things up to the present, writing history requires some distance. For this book, the narrative stops around the year 2000, on the threshold of molecular medicine and a new millennium.

The cost of the research for this book was funded by a grant from the Dean's Office. Yet no one has looked over my shoulder and the text, the stories, and the conclusions are entirely of my own choosing. This is in no sense an official history. But it is a compelling history, and those who read the following pages cannot fail to be moved at the difference that medical science has made in the betterment of the lives of Canadians and of people everywhere.

# 2   At the Corner of College and University

For many years Toronto was considered a kind of dull Puritan enclave, of which American poet John Dos Passos said in 1917 to a friend, "So you've been to Toronto – don't you think it's a beastly place? Toronto on a Sunday morning ... I have been there – and I admit, that I loathe it."[1] The city was once considered unpromising and uninspiring, the province of Ontario a sleepy hinterland, in which narrow-mindedness was cradled in the arms of parochialism.

When in March 1909 American educator Abraham Flexner visited Toronto on behalf of the Carnegie Foundation, as part of a continent-wide assessment of the quality of medical schools, he found that "[t]he laboratories are in point of construction and equipment among the best on the continent. Increasing attention has recently been devoted to the cultivation of research." Given his devastating indictments of many other medical schools of the day – isolated from university life, proprietary in nature, and uninterested in research – this was praise indeed. "The school has recently perfected a very intimate relationship with the new Toronto General Hospital," Flexner wrote – this in contrast to many rival faculties that had the most tenuous of hospital connections and little opportunity to teach the medical students at first hand about disease and treatment. Flexner said that the faculty "obtains complete control of the clinical advantages of some 500 beds. Students have free access to all wards, clinical laboratory, [and] dispensary."[2] Clearly in 1909 Toronto worked well, too, classed among the top medical schools of the continent.

A hundred years later Toronto is still among the top medical schools in North America. In terms of enrolment, it is in fact the largest and has been so for decades. In 1950 a somewhat bemused Dean Joseph MacFarlane reported to the faculty, "The school now has the doubtful distinction of being the largest medical undergraduate training centre on the continent."[3]

In understanding how Toronto grew, several themes will appear. One is research. The Faculty of Medicine reached a position of excellence if not size by emphasizing from the get-go science as the underpinning of the art of medicine and, from the 1960s on, by emphasizing research as the expression of the scientific method. Why was research so important? In an interview with a student newspaper in 1987, Fred Lowy, who had become dean of medicine seven years previously, said, "Our primary purpose was to turn out superb health professionals, and ultimately to improve health care for the people of Canada."

Lowy asked rhetorically, "How is this done?" What made an institution first class, he said, "was the quality of its teachers and the quality of its students ... Good students are attracted by good teachers. Students, particularly at the graduate level, contribute tremendously to the intellectual climate." And it was the capacity to conduct world-changing research that attracted good people to a place such as the University of Toronto. Lowy said, "Research is the creation of new knowledge – the conquering of our frontier. That is what makes it challenging. And the brightest people need to be challenged ... There is a spirit of inquiry that prevails in contrast to merely passing on what was known and thought to be true in the past. People who teach in a strong research atmosphere are also preparing students for what is going to be discovered tomorrow, and ultimately this has a positive effect on patient care at the hospital and clinical levels."[4]

Research became the motor of the story. From the very beginning the Faculty of Medicine in Toronto was determinedly based upon science. But only in the 1960s did the enterprise begin to swell with the battalions of investigators and scads of dollars that laboratory research in particular demands. There was a wrenching change from the medicine of yore, dominated by gentleman-scholars who celebrated their achievements in tails at festive annual dinners, to the casual young men and women in running shoes and open-necked shirts of the lab world. "The prospect of the future leaves one alternating between elation and panic," said "Kager" Wightman in 1967, who was head of the Department of Medicine and something of an old boy himself, though a very nice one.[5]

But even though research animates the story, it is not the sole theme. As pointed out earlier, Toronto is a success because it is the only large city in North America to have many teaching hospitals but only one medical school. As a faculty report said in 1993, "No other metropolitan area in North America with a population over two million has only one medical school. The Toronto Academic Health Science Complex has nine fully affiliated teaching hospitals and serves as a major referral centre not only for Ontario but for Canada and North America."[6] "The striking feature of the University of Toronto, Faculty of Medicine," said Wendy Levinson, chair of medicine, in 2004, "is the single medical school in a large and multicultural city. Many cities of comparable size in North America have up to six medical schools competing for patients, trainees and faculty. In contrast, we have a network of multiple strong hospitals ... all sharing the same Faculty of Medicine, Dean and Department structure."[7] (The Department of Medicine means internal medicine and medical specialty disciplines; the Faculty of Medicine is, of course, all the departments together.) The hospitals brought a mix of individual excellences; the university offered top-notch students, trainees, and world-class scientists and clinicians. The faculty would concentrate not just an enormous amount of academic brainpower in these hospitals but a uniquely large and medically interesting patient population as well.

Standing at the corner of College Street and University Avenue today opens in every direction a vast perspective of hospitals and medical buildings that reaches, in fact, far beyond the line of sight to St Michael's Hospital on the east side, Sunnybrook Hospital to the north, and the Centre for Addiction and Mental Health's 27-acre campus to the south; the perspective opens farther north to the large suburban Baycrest, an academic health science centre focused on aging, and west to the Toronto Western Hospital of the University Health Network on Bathurst Street. It is a big scene, in other words. Dean David Naylor said in 2004, "The 'campus' for the Faculty of Medicine includes not only the academic area of the University but also the teaching hospitals and a wide variety of community clinics and agencies."[8] Thousands of clinicians and scientists work in these buildings. There were in 2004, for example, more than 400 full-time and 300 part-time faculty members in the Department of Medicine alone. It is one of the largest health-care complexes in the world.

Does size matter? This is where the hospitals enter the story, contributing their legions of clinicians and investigators at the research foundations to the faculty's core departments. As Eliot Phillipson, chair of medicine, said in 2000, "Good scientists do not like to work in isolation, but rather prefer to be where the action is … Their ultimate success will be determined more by 'the people they talk to,' than by fiscal and physical resources beyond their needs." For this reason Toronto had, in Phillipson's view, a "research environment" comparable to the best in the world.[9] Louis Siminovitch was one of the faculty's top scientists. He had studied in Paris at the Pasteur Institute and introduced molecular biology to the University of Toronto; in short, he was a figure of immense eminence. Siminovitch echoed Phillipson's comments about the importance of having coffee with smart people, telling President David Naylor in 2008, "We have underestimated, or more exactly, not understood the critical importance of collegiality. Naturally having been brought up at the Pasteur and the OCI [Ontario Cancer Institute], I have seen the enormous benefits of appropriate environments, fostered, of course, by leadership at the top."[10] So rubbing shoulders at the corner of College and University was crucial.

The changes that bring this narrative to the corner of College and University were massive. What others accompany the journey to this intersection?

One is the pivot from British to American medical styles. At the beginning, the faculty was massively turned towards the United Kingdom, and many of its barons were of Scottish origin. And a certain British style, now long lost on both sides of the Atlantic, tended to value teaching in small groups, even one-on-one teaching, as the essence of training new physicians. The emphasis was on clinical care. Research, if it existed at all, was decidedly secondary. Contrast this with a hard-charging American style that sees the function of a Faculty of Medicine as generating new knowledge. Toronto shifts from the one to the other. In the early 1950s, Dean Joseph MacFarlane, unsettled by the tsunami of new techniques and treatments engulfing medicine, said, "This school has tried to hold an even balance between the constantly changing and more complicated methods of laboratory investigation, and the system of bedside teaching and theatre clinics with emphasis on the careful taking of history and painstaking physical examination. There are so many human ills that cannot be measured by any laboratory calculation. The student of medicine has much to gain from sound clinicians who still practice the art of medicine."[11] Yes, indeed, the art of medicine. The phrase sounds almost old-fashioned today in the hi-tech blur of international science. Internist Jack Laidlaw likes to talk about "the care of the patient that has the disease," as opposed to the "care of the disease," meaning understanding the factors in the patient's life that might influence the course of the disease.[12] In the fusty, Presbyterian Toronto of yore, the clinicians of the faculty did believe in the tradition of hands-on, personalized care; they believed in the importance of history taking and the clinical examination, as opposed to the interpretation of lab results – and that will emerge on many pages of this history.

One hesitates to introduce an administrative theme this early in the story, and yet it is an important one. One of the seminal events in the life of the faculty and the hospitals was the transition from a part-time to a full-time faculty that occurred during the 1960s and early 1970s at the same time that the medical school underwent a great expansion. Early in the 1960s, most senior clinicians still had private offices and appeared in the hospitals to supervise the residents in public clinics and to teach. The introduction of the Medical Care Act in 1966 changed all this because the federal government paid half of most hospital and physician services, making possible the appointment of clinicians who were full-time in the hospitals. Senior clinicians thus became hospital-based.

The faculty itself remained, however, department-based. One of the characteristics of the Toronto system is the ironclad dominance of the academic department, both in the basic sciences and in clinical medicine. "Institutional autonomy is a strong feature of this medical school," said one outside assessor in 1979.[13] Why is this interesting? Because the alternative is, as Dean Chute put it in 1969 as the faculty was convulsing about its governance, "a structure composed of the basic science departments and several hospitals."[14] A distinctive feature of the Toronto system is the presence of several large and powerful general teaching hospitals – at the outset the Toronto General Hospital (known as "The General" or TGH), the Toronto Western Hospital, and St Michael's Hospital. Under some circumstances, these hospitals could have swallowed the clinical departments, leaving the faculty with only a basic science rump. Yet this didn't happen because of the determination of a series of deans to maintain the university department structure, even in the hospitals. "[Dean Chute] expressed a preference for general Faculty committees rather than committees whose members represent hospitals. The former preserve the concept of a medical school which is primarily an academic community."[15] Chute and his fellow deans appreciated that progress in research is enhanced in the context of an academic community, not in the bustle of the hospital ward.

By the beginning of the twenty-first century, it was the medical faculty that took the lead in enhancing the institutional partnership. Yet the hospitals had by no means been effaced. As Naylor, Peter Singer (head of the Joint Centre for Bioethics), and Lorraine Ferris (an administrative leader in the university's relations with the hospitals) put it in 2004, "The partnership respects the lead roles of the university in education, the hospitals in clinical care, and the overlapping nature of responsibility for research." Like Washington University and the Barnes-Jewish Hospital in St Louis, the U of T had adopted a model in which the university and the hospitals were governed more or less separately, their collaboration codified in a partnership agreement. For full-time clinical faculty, only 7 percent of their earnings came from the university, the rest from practice plans and from the hospitals. What gave the faculty its leverage? Hospital posts required university appointments, and the university facilitated the kind of stability that hospitals and practice plans all required for the smooth operation of a very large "academic health sciences complex."[16]

There is another overarching theme in this story: that of the tension between service and research. It, too, is a constant thread that runs through the history of the faculty's members and through the story of their students as well. For the clinicians of the teaching hospitals, the great tension was between their commitment as clinical teachers – demonstrating methods of examination and clinical findings to their young nestlings – and demands on their time as researchers. This same tension appeared historically in the experience of the students as well, who were in the 1960s and after torn between the desire of the research-oriented faculty to prepare them for careers as investigators and the desire of the community-oriented faculty to make them sensitive to social issues and caring in the face of human distress. Individual students will make their own choices given these options. Yet this tension is very much reflected in the curriculum: whether it is science-based or community-based. Even today it has not been entirely resolved. "This tension is a fundamental part of medical practice which spans generations," said Robert Byrick, former head of anaesthesia. "It will never be resolved because it is so fundamental to medicine. A balance is needed for individual practitioners, and for curriculum and for faculties – therefore this tension is a good experience for students as they need to cope with the challenge throughout their career."[17] This conflict between the demands of science and those of community involvement will persist on many pages of this volume.

In the background of this story are the dramatic changes that swept across medicine and its underlying sciences from the late nineteenth century onwards, changes that accelerated after the Second World War and that are almost overwhelming today with the rapidity of their advance. As William Boyd, professor of pathology in the Faculty of Medicine, said in the eighth edition of his *Textbook of Pathology* in 1970 – worldwide a trusted companion for medical students – "The student should be provided with a stream of knowledge, not a stagnant pool from which to drink. For the picture of disease is changing before our very eyes. Old diseases are passing away as the result of prevention and the assaults of modern therapy, but new ones are continually taking their place, including those that are the result of the well-meant but injudicious use of drugs. The inn that shelters for the night is not the journey's end."[18] Indeed not, and as the present author sits at the keyboard in 2012, in the new century and the new millennium, this account of the history of this distinguished faculty is also just a way station, and the future journey will demand its own authors.

# 3  An Afternoon in October 1903

At the opening ceremonies of the Medical Building in 1903: It was natural that we should endeavour to secure the presence here of some of the leading men of the larger and older institutions of learning ... from the Mother Land.

President James Loudon[1]

## The "New Laboratories"

In 1902 there were still several medical schools in Toronto, which made little sense. Late that year it was finally agreed, after fifteen years of intense wrangling between the two major rivals, that the medical school of Trinity University should be amalgamated into the Faculty of Medicine of the University of Toronto. After the new union was consummated in the summer of 1903, it seemed a good idea to schedule a celebration, together with a ceremony marking completion of the new medical building after two years' construction – the faculty's first building on the university campus since Dean Bulmer Nicol's 1850 medical building was "set in a pine grove on the east bank of Taddle Creek," long since vacated.[2] The celebration was scheduled for 1 October 1903. It was intended to be – and was – a splendid honorary occasion; a number of the big names in the international world of medical science had been summoned to Toronto for the event.

Charles Sherrington, Holt Professor of Physiology at the University of Liverpool, delivered the inaugural address. Students of neuroscience recognize Sherrington as the discoverer of the nervous integration of the body; he accepted the chair of physiology at Oxford ten years later and shared (with E.D. Adrian) the Nobel Prize for physiology/medicine in 1932.

William Henry Welch, the great pathologist, and William Osler, possibly the most famous physician in the Western world at the time, came up from Johns

Hopkins University in Baltimore. Osler was an Ontario boy, born in Bond Head, who had begun his medical career at the Toronto School of Medicine (TSM) after a year in divinity at Trinity College in 1867, forsaking both in 1870 for McGill; he then went on to Europe, the United States, and ultimately became a Regius professor and baronet at Oxford. He was evidently fond of Toronto and had previously attended the opening of the Biology Building in 1889. (He would later throw a special luncheon for all the professors of medicine in the United Kingdom in honour of Duncan Graham, who had in 1919 just become the first full-time professor of medicine in the British Empire.[3])

The great Harvard physiologist Henry Pickering Bowditch (some of whose main contributions were written in German) was invited up from Boston. He did not personally attend but provided a speech, read by a deputy, on a very interesting straw that was blowing in the wind: medicine was becoming a laboratory science. "Whereas thirty years ago Anatomy and Chemistry were the only departments of medicine in which laboratory methods were in use, we have now laboratories of physiology, pathology, pharmacology, hygiene, bacteriology and surgery, while anatomy has greatly extended the scope of laboratory work by including the allied sciences of histology and embryology, and Chemistry has become to a large extent the handmaiden of clinical medicine."[4] A hundred years later, not only would individual departments and divisions have their own laboratories, but individual clinicians as well. In the new millennium after 2000, the pathway from basic science to clinical medicine, which passed via the intermediate stage of "translational research," was thus expected to begin in the laboratory and climb upwards towards usefulness from there.

Lewellys Barker, also born and raised in Ontario – he was a medical graduate of the University of Toronto in 1890 – had come up from Chicago, where he was teaching at Rush Medical College. But Barker, whose parents evidently intended to name him Lewellyn but an *s* was mistaken for an *n*, would shortly forsake Chicago for Hopkins and initiate a brilliant medical career.

There were medical stars from Michigan and McGill, Harvard and the University of Pennsylvania. Oh, it was a splendid afternoon. Osler spoke that evening. On the next day, October 2, all the luminaries received honorary degrees. And that evening Dean Reeve, who was feeling distinctly unwell with a high fever throughout, mustered his forces enough to hold a great dinner.[5]

Richard Andrews Reeve, born in 1842 in Toronto and "of Yorkshire stock," was a medical graduate of Queen's University in 1865. Professor of ophthalmology and otology at the University of Toronto, he was "the first 'Specialist' appointed to the Toronto General Hospital, whose staff he joined in 1872," covering the entire eye, ear, nose, and throat range.[6] He also taught ophthalmology and otology at the Toronto School of Medicine, and when the faculty reopened for business in 1887 he was indeed one of the professors, becoming dean in 1896. It was in 1903 that Reeve orchestrated the union with Trinity Medical College, "in consequence of which," said his eulogist in 1919, "the number of students greatly increased. The harmonizing of the views of these two groups of students required great patience, and much tact."[7]

So on that October afternoon, Dean Reeve, though feeling unwell, could look back on a task well done.

Who else spoke? There was Goldwin Smith, former Regius Professor of History at Oxford, who lived in Toronto and whose orations had adorned Toronto medicine for many of his "fourscore years." Smith delivered a stricture upon medical officiousness. "He admonished them not to prolong the agony of departure when the final summons came to join the innumerable caravan that moves to the pale realms of shade, and quoted with much feeling the words of Kent in Lear:

'Vex not his ghost: Oh, let him pass; he hates him
That would upon the rack of this tough world
Stretch him out longer.'"[8]

Thus it was an auspicious occasion, at a time when the international centre of gravity of medicine was just beginning to tip from German-speaking Europe to the Anglo-Saxon world. Of course the Holocaust would complete this tilt, as the Jewish clinicians and scientists who had been the glory of German medicine were either murdered or driven into emigration. But supremacy in medicine was just beginning to tip westward. It was, after all, at the University of Toronto and not Heidelberg that insulin was discovered in 1921. Yet on that October afternoon in 1903 Lewellys Barker "strongly advocated the view that every medical student should be able to read French and German."[9] Sixty years later he would be thought to have spoken in jest.

The medical building itself, called at the time the "New Laboratories," was a marvel of technology. It was built on the "unit system of laboratory" that Harvard's George Minot – who shared a Nobel Prize in 1934 for curing pernicious anemia with liver extract – had proposed: movable partitions could make the laboratories larger or smaller, accommodating classes of different sizes. In the opening ceremony on October 1, President James Loudon of the university "accepted the care of the buildings from the hands of the Chairman of the Board of Trustees and assured him that the Medical Faculty would use the buildings for the advancement of Medical science in a manner that will enhance the reputation of the University and redound to the benefit of the public."[10]

William Feasby, clinician and historian, describes the "many-windowed structure" of the new medical building. "Its cupolas standing high to match the central tower of the practical sciences building, its façade staring blankly across the main campus towards stately University College, it was indeed an imposing sight. There could be no doubt in anyone's mind that medical training was going to advance in Toronto."[11] (Just as a sad little footnote: many years later, in 1966 when the new Medical Sciences Building was about to be erected on the site of the demolished Medical Building, Dean Hamilton noted scornfully that "the buildings being replaced are without distinction."[12])

President Loudon did touch upon an issue that had agitated the spirits in the past and that would be on people's minds for the next century to come: "There is just one point further to which I wish to refer very briefly, the question of State aid to the teaching of medicine. Old prejudices die hard. The old doctrine of prejudice, of no aid to the students of a lucrative profession, has been reiterated so often since the middle of the last century in Ontario that it may seem almost like heresy to dispute it. But, is the profession after all so very lucrative? (Applause). There are some prizes, it is true; but is the average of wealth in the profession above that of a comfortable living?" The answer was no, he said.[13]

Loudon concluded his talk by pointing out, "We are now entering upon an important forward movement in the work. The federation of Trinity with the University of Toronto is practically assured (applause) and on the strength of this the amalgamated medical faculties begin to-day [October 1] their work in this building. (Loud applause) Medical education through this step enters upon a new and higher stage of development and the future is full of hope (applause)."[14]

The university gymnasium, where the ceremonies were held, echoed with applause on October 1 and 2. But when William Keen, the professor of surgery at Jefferson Medical College in Philadelphia and author of the standard surgical textbook *Keen's System of Surgery*, addressed the special convocation intended for granting the honorary degrees on October 2, there was soon a reflective silence; it was a kind of silence that would echo across the rest of the new century as well. He was discussing the need for government aid to the medical schools. "The profits on the formerly wasted coal tar products [the basis of organic chemistry] alone have more than repaid Germany all her vast grants to her chemical laboratories in which the methods of utilizing this waste were discovered," he said. "And the pre-eminence of Germany in medical research has been maintained by similar expenditures upon her medical schools. Why should not the familiar label 'Made in Germany' be replaced by 'Made in Canada'?"[15] Interestingly, the founders of the faculty did not see German medicine as a model for Canadian. Alexander McPhedran said a few years later that they rejected the "German system" of medical education, which sought to educate well only the elite. "The object aimed at in the reorganization of the faculty was to make it possible ... to train all who are graduated as safe and efficient physicians, able to meet any emergency, medical or surgical, promptly when time is of vital importance to the patient without waiting for the service of an expert, a matter of utmost importance in remote districts."[16]

The year 1903 was a big year. In the spring commencement, ninety-nine medical students graduated. Among the students marching in that procession there were some as yet unheralded stars. William Edward Gallie, later professor of surgery, was in the file. "Gallie has changed – heavens, how he has grown!"

mocked the students' yearbook. Next to a photo of a square-jawed young Gallie funned the editors, "For a young man of Ed's individuality, the search for a vocation was no perplexity, desiring above all things the life of a student ... Gallie has always taken a decided interest in athletics, his prowess in hockey as Barrie's crack cover-point being noteworthy."[17] (Gallie came from Barrie, Ontario.)

Near Gallie in the line of graduates would have been John Gerald FitzGerald, who "enjoys the distinction of being the youngest man in the class." (FitzGerald, born in 1882, was seventeen when he began medicine in 1899.) "We venture to say that his later years will find him enjoying the esteem and confidence of a goodly number of both the sick and well."[18] This prediction was spot on, given that FitzGerald became dean of medicine in 1932 and travelled the world on behalf of the Rockefeller Foundation yet died, as seen later, in tragedy.

In addition to the dean, the post-1887 faculty had the position of secretary, whose job was partly to produce the annual budget. Adam Wright, an obstetrician, was the first, succeeded in 1893 by James Brebner, a non-physician, for a brief year; then in 1894 Alexander Primrose became secretary and would remain so until 1918, just before he assumed the deanship in 1920.

On that October afternoon in 1903, Primrose was thus professor of anatomy and secretary of the faculty. The early deans – William Aikins from 1887 to 1893,[19] Uzziel Ogden from 1893 to 1896, and Richard Andrews Reeve from 1896 to 1908 – would have marched at the head of the commencement procession. Yet all were basically men of the nineteenth century and none a notable figure. Primrose, by contrast, was a person of the future. He would be dean from 1920 to 1932, but even before then he did his utmost to steer the Faculty of Medicine in the direction of science. He was born in Pictou, Nova Scotia, in 1861, into a family with tea-planting interests in India that Primrose was intended to pursue. Yet an accident with a horse intervened. "I was kicked into surgery," he used to say. His broken leg was treated by the surgeon John Stewart of Halifax, a leading light of his day. Said fellow surgeon Robert Harris in a eulogy, "Alexander Primrose's contact with John Stewart opened his eyes to a vision – the world of surgery – which must have been fascinating indeed to any young man in the days when the whole world of medicine was being revolutionized by antisepsis," of which Stewart was a leading apostle.[20]

Like Stewart and many young men in the Maritimes, "Primmy" studied in Edinburgh, where he earned a bachelor of medicine degree in 1886 (an MB was later in Canada rebaptized as an "MD," or doctor of medicine); he interned at Middlesex Hospital in London, qualified MRCS (member of the Royal College of Surgeons) in England in 1888, then in September of that year returned to Canada to take up his new post as assistant demonstrator in anatomy at the University of Toronto, delivering lectures on topographical anatomy "in the brick building on the corner of Gerrard and Sackville Streets," where the teaching facilities of the faculty were situated from 1887 in succession to the Toronto School of Medicine.[21] In 1896 he became professor of anatomy, during which time he apparently initiated the Toronto anatomy teaching tradition of drawing on the blackboard with both hands simultaneously. In 1897 he became associate professor of surgery and was promoted in 1918 to professor of surgery, which post he occupied until his retirement in 1932. He was also secretary of the Faculty Council from 1894 to 1918. Later he would be dean of medicine from 1920 to 1932 – when people tended to call him "Prim" rather than "Primmy" – but in the earlier years he functioned as a behind-the-scenes power broker and historian of the faculty. At his retirement in 1932, President Sir Robert Alexander Falconer, who himself retired that year, said of Primrose, "He has been to me an officer on whom I could lean, a friend to whom I could talk with intimacy, an evenly balanced gentleman – he happened fortunately to be freer from his practice than others and therefore he could do almost the work of a full time Dean and he gave his whole soul to the work."[22]

Why might Primrose be remembered? At his retirement in 1932 the author of the tribute to him in Faculty Council thought it might be that "[t]he great traditions of the Edinburgh School of Medicine which he brought to this university have left an impress for good that is quite inestimable."[23] The impress of Scotland upon the U of T in those years was palpable.

On that October evening in 1903, the ceremonies ended when the faculty entertained over a hundred guests at a sit-down dinner in the university dining hall, and James H. Richardson, "the sole survivor of the faculty of 1853," gave the evening a rather wistful close: "He referred very pathetically to the history of the early days and concluded his interesting reminiscences by thanking God that he had lived to see not only the restoration of the Medical Faculty and the good work it had accomplished in the last seventeen years, but also the final triumph of the unification of Medical teaching in the University."[24]

Oh, really?

### A Glance Backward

The traditional medical school organization was laid down when its sole function was to train undergraduate medical students.[25]

Dean A. Lawrence Chute, 1968

The University of King's College Medical School, the forerunner of the Faculty of Medicine, opened its doors in 1843. It was an intimate little affair. James Richardson, one of the first two medical graduates (the other being a chap named Lyons) later recalled, "During the session of 1843–44, I was the sole regular attendant on Professor [William] Beaumont's lectures [on surgery], delivered in the old Parliament Buildings, and at his kind suggestion I would draw up my chair beside his, in front of the fireplace, while he read his carefully prepared lecture."[26]

The first dean of the medical faculty was William Bulmer Nicol, professor of botany and materia medica in the University of King's College from 1843 until its reconstitution as the University of Toronto in 1849. He and four other King's medical professors in 1844 were the first to be cross-appointed to the Toronto Hospital.[27] Nicol was appointed dean in 1850, administering his office for three years. William Canniff remembered Nicol's "kindly face" among his medical board examiners in 1854, along with "his high ability ... In the diagnosis and prognosis of disease he was almost unequaled, certainly not excelled. In his bearing towards his confreres he was a model; as a professional friend he was the soul of honour."[28]

Growth was rapid. Through the Baldwin Act of 1849, King's College passed from the control of the Anglican Church and became the University of Toronto. Richardson continued, "The prosperity of the Medical department was phenomenal. In 1852–53 no less than sixty students were enrolled as attendants in my class, and the same success attended the other chairs ... The dissecting room – the lecture theatres, were large and commodious – the [anatomical] museum was being built up. Everything was progressing most favourably, when suddenly a blow was struck which annihilated the Medical Faculty, and left the University of Toronto without one for about thirty years."[29]

In 1853 the United Provinces of Canada legislature, on the alleged grounds that popular sentiment opposed "state aid for a lucrative profession," abolished the fledgling medical and law schools as teaching faculties, leaving the university with simply an examining role in those fields for conferring degrees.[30] In reality, the act stemmed from a complex political intrigue, the details of which Richardson explained in his letter to President Loudon but that will be passed over here.[31]

Between the 1850s and 1880s a variety of private medical schools flourished in Toronto.[32] As historian Charles Godfrey shows, at one point in the 1870s and 1880s, there were four: the Toronto School of Medicine, the Trinity Medical School, the Victoria University Medical Department, and the Women's Medical College.[33]

The Toronto School of Medicine itself, the immediate forebear of the faculty and founded by John Rolph, was a pretty punk affair. The reading list for its students included "homeopathic text-books." The University of Toronto gave the exams, and the university would grant an MD degree upon completion of a thesis "upon some Medical Subject," one year after the MB or bachelor of medicine, the basic medical degree in Canada and the United Kingdom.[34]

The very existence of these private medical schools constituted a lobby against re-establishing the university Faculty of Medicine, as one history of the Medical Faculty put it, "on the ground that the State through the University should not engage in the teaching of professional subjects, which, it was also claimed, should also be left to private enterprise." This unusual doctrine did not prevail elsewhere and resulted in "disastrous consequences" for the provision of medical services to the population of Ontario in these bleak years, as diplomas "were sold to candidates who had little or no training, professional or otherwise, and who consequently were unable to pass the required examinations."[35] (One result was the establishment in 1861 of a regulatory board that would, with the advent of Confederation in 1867, become the College of Physicians and Surgeons of Ontario. Medical historians R.D. Gidney and W.P.J. Millar write that the main difference between Canadian and American medical education in these years "was the establishment of superordinate licensing and examining boards with the power to determine standards of medical education and to make these standards the sine qua non of the license to practice."[36])

Among these private medical schools, however, one did stand out for something other than financial recompense to its founders and sometimes public benefit. That was the Women's Medical College, founded in 1883 "to enable women to secure a medical education to prepare them for work in the Foreign Mission Field and elsewhere."[37] The Women's Suffrage Club of Toronto had held a meeting to which various male dignitaries were invited, in the thought that they might lead the effort to found a medical institution for women. The Board of Trustees included, among others, a lawyer, James Beatty, as chair, as well as Mrs James Gooderham (distillery fortune) and Mrs John Harvie. The trustees purchased a house at 227 Sumach Street for $1,400, and the formal opening of the Women's Medical College occurred on 1 October 1883.[38] The faculty included many later stalwarts of the Faculty of Medicine as well as one woman, Augusta Stowe Gullen, the demonstrator of anatomy, who herself had just graduated in 1883 from Trinity Medical College in Toronto (Gullen is known as the first woman to graduate from a Canadian medical school. The daughter of Emily Stowe, the first woman to practice medicine in Canada, Augusta Stowe was married to Trinity classmate John B. Gullen; husband and wife both had practices at 461 Spadina Avenue.) During the first session, three women attended, two of them graduating in 1887. Michael Barrett, the inaugural dean, died in that year, and Alexander McPhedran – later head of medicine in the Faculty of Medicine of the University of Toronto – succeeded him.

From the viewpoint of exams, the college was affiliated with Trinity Medical College. In 1890 the Women's Medical College moved along the street to a larger facility at 291 Sumach and also became connected with the University of Toronto, students having the option of trying the examinations of both institutions. Another women's medical college had been founded in Kingston, Ontario, and in 1895 the Women's Medical College amalgamated with it, becoming the Ontario Medical College for Women.

In 1896 Emma Skinner-Gordon, who had just graduated from the Ontario Medical College for Women, "founded the first outpatient clinic for women, staffed by women doctors," according to the official history of women medical graduates of the U of T, on Sackville Street in connection with the Medical College for Women (the outpatient clinic moved to 18 Seaton Street in 1906).[39] Two years later, in 1898 a dispensary, or clinic, devoted to women and staffed by Jennie Gray and Ida Lynd opened in the basement of the college. This became the nucleus of the Women's College Hospital (see pp. 561–577).

By 1906, a total of 112 women had graduated from the college, "including," as the student yearbook of the University of Toronto said, "23 who are Medical Missionaries in Persia, India, Ceylon, China, Japan, and amongst the Indians in our own North-West Territories." The yearbook further observed, "The College was founded to meet the need for Medical education for women … This movement really owed its origin to the feeling of Professors of the Faculty of Medicine in the University of Toronto that, although women were entitled to medical education, it was not advisable, perhaps not possible – at least, at that time – to give it to them in the University Medical Classes along with men." Yet these delicate male sensibilities evidently crumbled over time. In 1905 a government commission on the reorganization of the University of Toronto stipulated that the university should "provide for the medical education of women," and in 1906 in response to a recommendation of the Royal Commission on the university, the Women's Medical College was absorbed by the Faculty of Medicine of the university.[40] Jennie Smillie was one of the female medical students who had entered the Women's Medical College in 1906 (it was, as stated, officially the Ontario Medical College for Women, yet people continued to call it by its former name). She graduated with the rest of the medical class in 1909 and expressed the keenness with which this pioneering generation of young female physicians approached their mission: "We had girls from three different continents, yet in one respect we were all alike, we were all thirsting for knowledge: that thirst was the tie which bound us together, and we rejoiced in the hope that it would be satiated at this great fount of learning … How proudly we walked the hospitals with our stethoscopes and thermometers!"[41]

Thus the first generation of women physicians entered the world of medical practice. One of these early women medical graduates noted of the alumnae, "Some have become eminent, others have shown good ability, and all have done credit to themselves and honour to the sincerity, ability, and culture of the Dean and Faculty of their Alma Mater."[42]

The time between the end of the first Faculty of Medicine in 1853 and the reconstitution of the second in 1887 was a parlous period in the history of medicine in Ontario. In these years "not more than one in ten of the practitioners of medicine in this Province owed their degree to the University of Toronto," as one observer in the Faculty of Medicine wrote in 1903. Between 1853 and the reestablishment of the faculty in 1887, only 370 students, who had studied in the private medical schools or elsewhere, passed the medical exams of the university (which, as noted, continued to examine but not to teach). In 1881–2, the university senate raised the standard of requirements in the examinations, causing a great reduction in the number of successful candidates. There were fears that the province might run out of physicians, and in 1886 negotiations began to re-establish the university Medical Faculty.[43]

Not only from the viewpoint of medical practice but from that of science as well were these private medical schools handicapped because they couldn't afford "microscopes and laboratory equipment for chemistry and physiology experiments," as historian Marianne Fedunkiw puts it: "Not having equipment for the emerging laboratory loosened schools' competitive grip on students. This, coupled with growing interest in the science of medicine brought back by graduates studying in Germany, led to the general feeling that Canadian medical schools were falling behind."[44] Primrose noted in an unpublished 1904 review meant for the president's eyes, "The schools were unable to train the students in the sciences because ... they were unable to provide the extensive equipment and the necessary staff ... required in modern scientific laboratories for efficient teaching. The only reasonable solution for the problem seemed to be the establishment of a teaching faculty in Medicine in the provincial university."[45]

In Ontario, the University Federation Act of 1887 brought the Medical Faculty of the University of Toronto back to life. The university would assimilate the private Toronto School of Medicine on the condition that "the new medical school would not be a financial drain on the slender resources of the university."[46] Primrose said, "The undergraduate class at once began with some two hundred and fifty students, and once more the University was in full control of medical teaching."[47]

In 1887 the medical students ferried back and forth between the university buildings, where the basic sciences of biology, chemistry, and physiology were taught, and the former building of the Toronto School of Medicine, located on Gerrard Street some distance away, opposite the pre-1913 Toronto General Hospital, "where anatomy and the clinical subjects were taught."[48]

William Thomas Aikins was the first dean of the refounded faculty. He was born in 1827 on a farm near Cookstown, Ontario, to a Northern Irish family who had come to Ontario via the United States. He attended John Rolph's Toronto School of Medicine from 1847 to 1849, then sought further training in surgery at the renowned Jefferson Medical College in Philadelphia, receiving an MD in 1850.[49] Aikins then returned to Toronto as John Rolph's partner in private practice. At Rolph's school from the early 1850s, Aikins lectured in anatomy and became a kind of general factotum and leading figure in the vicissitudes of Toronto medicine in the subsequent years. He agitated for the refoundation of the Faculty of Medicine and, having retired from his post at the Toronto General Hospital in 1880, in 1887 became the first dean of the new Faculty of Medicine. (He then lost the reelection in 1893.)[50] According to his biographer Charles Harris, Aikins was the product of a stern Calvinist upbringing. "His alleged lack of humour, like his beard, was a concession to Victorianism ... When he died in 1897 it was said of him, 'He put a watch on the door of his lips, his words were few and seasoned with grace.'"[51] This is a reminder of the Scottish Presbyterian ethic in which this faculty, and many of its early figures, had marinated.[52]

Under Aikins, rapid changes began in undergraduate medical education. Charles Godfrey, an Aikins biographer, writes, "While microscopy had been taught in a superficial manner [at the Toronto School of Medicine], now first year students learned the use of the instrument. Instruction in physiology and chemistry, previously lectured in a theoretical manner, was now taught in a laboratory and the students were required to perform experiments." Students were encouraged to relate this knowledge to pathology. The anatomists of the faculty imported into the dissecting room the methods used in Britain. "Clinical instruction doubled over the first three years and included more teaching in pathology and demonstrations of biopsies and their relation to the sick patient."[53] This was the beginning of the changes over which Abraham Flexner was to wax enthusiastic in 1910: "The laboratories and equipment [are] among the best on the continent."[54]

The hallmark of the faculty's refoundation in 1887 was science. Two years later the Biological Building was opened, and at the inauguration ceremony, as university historian Martin Friedland points out, all agreed that "the future of medicine lay in science."[55] The great science of the day was physiology, the term itself a kind of global description of the patient antemortem. Medical historian Pauline Mazumdar says of the understanding of "physiology" in those days, "In the hospital it explained the condition of the patient; in the school, [physiology explained] the anatomy [of] the cadaver."[56]

Ramsay Wright, though not a physician, was among the scientific fixtures of the faculty.[57] He held the chair of biology and physiology from 1887 to 1892, and when in 1892 Wright's student Archibald B. Macallum became professor of physiology, Wright continued to profess biology until 1912. An influential figure through external contacts such as Osler and Newell Martin, Wright also steered Toronto – and through his students a good deal of North American medicine – "towards the research ideal," as Gidney and Millar put it.[58] On that October afternoon in 1903, Osler referred especially to "the great work which Professor Ramsay Wright had done for the cause of scientific Medical education in Ontario."[59]

Macallum himself was a farm boy from eastern Ontario who turned into "a man of striking appearance and forceful personality, slender but over six feet in height, with a beard, moustache, and a leonine head."[60] He studied as an undergraduate at Toronto and later received a PhD from the newly founded Johns Hopkins University in 1888; there he was a student of the Englishman Henry Newell Martin, the first physiologist at Hopkins. Macallum also obtained an MB from the University of Toronto in 1890. At the refoundation of the faculty, Macallum became the instructor in physiology, a subject that he had already begun in 1885 to teach to the students of the Toronto School of Medicine. He later wrote, "In Canada the advancement of the science [of physiology] began in 1885 when the writer, a student of Henry Newell Martin introduced in the teaching of medical students the modernized type of physiology, all under the influence of R. Ramsay Wright, an outstanding exponent of Biology in the University of Toronto."[61]

Macallum was primus inter pares of a small group of Wright's former students who drilled the spirit of science into medical undergraduates. Others included James McMurrich, the chair of anatomy, and John J. Mackenzie, the professor of pathology. "Both of them," pathological chemist John Bereford Leathes observes, "like Macallum [were] biologists before, as an after-thought they had studied medicine; a nucleus was formed for the band of Scots whose fighting leader was Macallum." Leathes continues, "On the clinical side they could count on the enlightened support of Alexander McPhedran, professor of medicine, and of Irving Cameron, professor of surgery, and in a few years this company completely transformed the medical school, gave it new ideals and built it on a sound foundation of biological science."[62]

In 1889 the new Biological Building was built on campus as a facility of the Faculty of Arts, although medical students attended the lectures in physiology. In 1891 the Museum Wing was added to the Biological Building, and on the top floor the medical students unofficially were instructed on dissections.[63] This led to public embarrassment for the university when the building's residential neighbours objected to human dissections – specifically contrary to the official agreement of its uses. Dean Walter Geikie of Trinity Medical School, which did not receive government grants for its facilities, also complained to the provincial government. The deception was apparent from the medical faculty's claim in its promotional recruitment advertisements of 1889 to 1892 that "[t]eaching of Anatomy [takes place] in the lecture room, dissection room ... of the Medical College." President Wilson admitted privately to Chancellor Blake that "Dr. Geikie's statement could not be contradicted, so I said nothing about it."[64] Vice Chancellor Mulock mounted a spirited defence of the broad public interest while personally absorbing responsibility for the misunderstanding. The *Calendar* of the university for 1892–3 could then openly declare, "In the new Biological Building every facility is now provided for practical training in Biology and Physiology. The advantages of the well equipped Faculty of Arts are now available for the students in the Faculty of Medicine. The results cannot fail to elevate the standard of medical education in Ontario."[65]

Laboratory facilities for the students were available by the mid-1890s at the Toronto General Hospital: "The Faculty has in the General Hospital a laboratory for clinical pathology and chemistry, which has been furnished with microscopes and all apparatus required for the examination of all pathological fluids and specimens."[66] Lectures and demonstrations for the first- and second-year students took place at the university "and in the Anatomical Department in the west wing of the Biological Building." Third- and fourth-year lectures and demos took place in the TSM building of the Faculty of Medicine "on the corner of Gerrard and

Sackville streets, opposite the Toronto General Hospital."[67] Happy memories of the old Gerrard Street building were few. "The ancient pile looked dingy, smelled horribly and was ventilated like a tomb," said the med students.[68]

How demanding the first-year meds found the lectures! Fresh from high school in their little Ontario towns, they encountered Alexander Primrose lecturing in 1902 in anatomy:

"Our first lecture – Anatomy, how shall I describe it? How vast and deep the subject seemed to our verdant minds! Dr Primrose left no doubt as to the importance of the osseous structure, and exhorted us not to forget the skin and superficial fascia. His drawings on the board were to us productions of a Raphael or Rembrandt. The display of color in the drawings, picturing each muscle, nerve or artery in a new hue was lavishly chameleonic, for hardly was our sketch finished when it vanished to be replaced by another of still more gaudy iridescence. Could it be that we had to worry and scratch our heads about the Torcular Herophyli or the Sustentaculum Tali? We had never heard the family physician say anything about these."[69]

The faculty was turning into a scientific heavyweight. Edward Gallie, later professor of surgery who began his studies at U of T in 1899, said, "Most of the teachers were on a fulltime basis and were members of departments in the Arts Faculty. A.B. Macallum and Ramsay Wright were outstanding. In Anatomy Alexander Primrose held full sway, and I never think of those days without thinking what a superb lecturer and demonstrator he was ... It was this development that made it impossible for Trinity to compete with our School."[70] Trinity's merger with the faculty in 1903 was thus ineluctable.

Under the four-year program then in force, the class that graduated in 1903 had enrolled in 1899. The student yearbook sighed expansively, with tongue in cheek, "The Fall of 1899 was a memorable one. It saw the advent of an epoch in the history of the Medical Faculty ... Dr. Primrose looked aghast as one after the other of the long line filed in, and each declared his intention of enlisting under the glorious red, white and black [the colours of the faculty]. Never before had such a throng found its way to the Biolog [Biological Building; the new Medical Building had not yet been built]."[71]

**The Way Ahead**

In those sunny days before the First World War, everything smacked of progress and growth. In 1906 control of the university was transferred from the provincial government to a Board of Governors. In 1907 Robert Falconer, a deeply literate Nova Scotia Presbyterian cleric educated at Edinburgh, became president, and wide horizons beckoned.

But there was one problem: financing a modern Faculty of Medicine on income derived almost solely from student tuition. "The only source of [operating] income of the Faculty of Medicine," said Primrose in 1905, "is from the fees received from students for tuition." And although that might be adequate for the paltry salaries the professors received (most lived from the income of their private practices), it was inadequate to finance research. "The Faculty of Medicine of the State Institution cannot advance as it should do if there were no relief forthcoming from the Provincial Government. It is felt that the members of the Faculty of Medicine of the Provincial University have done perhaps more than their duty in paying such large amounts for equipment in the past and it is desirable that a rearrangement of the financial relations of the Faculty to the University should be made." Everywhere else in the Atlantic community, Primrose said, "the provision of research laboratories" was the wave of the future. It was similarly essential in Ontario "if this country is to keep abreast of the advances made in scientific medicine elsewhere." Surgery, for example, required research laboratories. "But [as well] research laboratories should be provided in such Departments as Pathology and Bacteriology, Physiology, Anatomy and Public Health ... It is quite impossible with the present state of our finances to carry on research work to the extent reasonably to be expected from the Faculty of Medicine of the State University."[72]

This, too, was a theme that would echo down the halls of ivy across the next hundred years.

# 4 Getting Going

In the first third of the twentieth century, Canadians, as a colonial people, had a model before them of all that was excellent and wonderful – and that model was not the United States. It was England and – for the large contingent of physicians born here but with Scottish blood in them – Scotland. (One observer called attention in 1923, amid laughter, to "the dangers of having too many Scotsmen on the University faculty."[1]) When in 1934 President Cody wished to conjure up a model polity, it was not to "our Canadian democracy" that he referred but to "our British democracy."[2]

The faculty emulated the British model. After clinicians received the bachelor of medicine (MB) degree in Toronto, those with academic aspirations would almost certainly train a year or two further, in the hospitals of London, Oxford, and Cambridge. Of the class that graduated in 1905, four years later, one-third had already done postgraduate work in England or Europe.[3] And when departments wished to make truly stellar professorial appointments that would garner them more international visibility, it was not – as later – to the United States that they reached but to the United Kingdom. (Similarly, when UK institutions wished to appoint the best of the international ranch, they often reached to Canada, or as in the case of William Osler, who left Johns Hopkins for Oxford, to the Canadian-born.) It is wonderful that in 1909, when the Toronto General Hospital (TGH) wished to acknowledge the contributions of its ex-interns ("house staff") who had moved on in life, it summoned them back to an annual dinner and awarded the scientifically most promising of them a "gold-headed cane." "It is expected that the cane will be made in London, England, and will be patterned after the celebrated gold-headed cane of medical history, which is now in the possession of the Royal College of Physicians of London, England."[4] The story is either cringe-inducing, as evidence of colonial toadery, or endearing, as a sign of a powerful transatlantic connection from which these young Canadian physicians drew strength and knowledge. One recalls, however, that the traffic went two ways. It wasn't just a bunch of grateful colonials waving Union Jacks and gawking at Westminster. Plenty of Brits were happy to come to Toronto for their "BTA" qualification (been to America). British-born Barrie Fairley, who joined the Department of Anesthesia at the Toronto General Hospital in 1955, said, "Toronto at that time was a tremendously attractive medical centre for a young British doctor to visit or work. In the UK we had all been brought up on textbooks by such authors as Best and Taylor (Physiology), Grant (Anatomy), and Boyd (Pathology) and the overall quality of medicine was extremely high."[5]

In any event, it is impossible to understand the unfolding story without knowing the Mother Country is clucking in the background.

## Hospitals

Just as the Faculty of Medicine was rising on campus, the hospitals themselves were in the whirlwind of change from hospices to therapeutic institutions. Toronto belonged to a much bigger picture of change in the nature of general hospitals all across Atlantic civilization. Previously, hospitals had been the last refuge of those who had no other place to go, the terminally ill who had no families, the aged, and the destitute. They had been refuges, not treatment centres. Such were the changes that swept over surgery in the 1880s and after, as the new principles of antiseptic and aseptic surgery made major operations possible, that hospitals rapidly became places where the sick could be cured. The progress in drug therapeutics was somewhat less dramatic but perceptible: a flood of analgesics and anesthetics reached the marketplace that promised the relief of pain and sedation for the distressed. Hospital birth became sought out instead of home birth because anesthesia eased the pain of labour – and quick surgical interventions could save the baby's life in case of a complication. Finally, there were big changes in the clinical investigation with the introduction of the ophthalmoscope and the blood pressure cuff late in the century and the X-ray in 1896.

Toronto was not resistant to these trends. As TGH superintendent John Nelson Elliott Brown pointed out in 1905, "Up to within a comparatively recent period the services of the hospital were sought for by those only who, as the result of poverty, or accident, were unable to receive medical aid under other auspices. The popular sentiment, therefore, toward the hospital, was one of timidity rather than of confidence." Under such circumstances, few save the desperate sought out hospital care. "Today," Brown continued, "all this is changed. Owing to the remarkable advance in all departments of medical science, and also to the wider dissemination of general knowledge, the popular attitude toward the hospital has undergone a great transformation. In contrast with former time hospital aid is now sought for by rich and poor alike, not only for the graver, but for many of the minor ailments."[6]

Superintendent Brown emphasized the research role of the hospitals as well as healing. The hospital must "do all in its power to add to the general stock of medical knowledge. Inasmuch as humanity generally is benefited by such additions, it may be said that [research] is scarcely less important than [treatment]. In order that a hospital may fulfill this part of its functions, it cannot be too strongly emphasized that its requirements will be much greater than if it confined itself solely to the routine care of the sick."[7] Here sounds strongly a note that will accompany this book throughout: research as a shared mission of hospitals and faculty.

### Primrose

In 1920 Alexander Primrose succeeded Charles K. Clarke as dean of the faculty. Because the deanship was then still a part-time job, he continued as professor of surgery. A native of Pictou, Nova Scotia, born into a family of Scottish origin, Primrose studied medicine at the historic University of Edinburgh (birthplace of modern medicine late in the eighteenth century), earning an MB in 1886. He interned at the Middlesex Hospital in London, migrating to Canada in 1889. He was professor of anatomy in Toronto from 1892 to 1906, followed by tenure as associate professor, then professor of clinical surgery until his retirement at the end of 1931. During the First World War he served alongside Duncan Graham and J.J. Mackenzie with the University of Toronto Base Hospital at Salonika in Greece. He was on staff at both TGH and the Hospital for Sick Children. As secretary of the faculty from 1894 to 1918, he belonged to that core group of clinicians and academics who constituted the institutional memory of the faculty.

As dean, Primrose radiated good will and optimism. In his Christmas message in 1926 he said, "The immediate future is full of promise for further development. In the Faculty of Medicine we have received large bequests of money which have enabled us to plan expansion on a scale hitherto impossible."[8] He reflected pride in the faculty and believed, not necessarily incorrectly, that "[t]he student graduating from the University of Toronto possesses qualifications unsurpassed in English speaking countries."[9]

### Medicine

The Department of Medicine is the soul of a teaching hospital. Referred to often as "internal medicine," the Department of Medicine embraces the diagnosis and pharmaceutical treatment of just about everything that can go wrong with the body, except the organs of reproduction and the head and neck. From the very beginning in 1887, Toronto had professors of medicine and the teaching hospitals had dedicated Departments of Medicine.

The first important lecturer on clinical medicine was Alexander McPhedran. He was born in 1847 in Halton County, Ontario, where he completed his high school education and taught for some years in the public schools. In 1873 he enrolled in the Toronto School of Medicine, was said to have a brilliant course as a student, and graduated with a MB in 1876. He received an appointment in 1885 at the Hospital for Sick Children and later at St Michael's Hospital and TGH. In 1887, at the refounding of the faculty, McPhedran was a lecturer on clinical medicine; he became associate professor in 1898. In 1900 Graham died and McPhedran succeeded him as professor and head of the Department of Medicine, stepping down in 1919. As Dean FitzGerald said on the occasion of McPhedran's passing in 1935, "[He] was a great physician and one of the most distinguished clinician teachers of his time. There can be little doubt that he exercised a greater influence than any other on the minds of the students of his day. He was clear, sharp and incisive. His clinical lectures were models of lucidity and comprehensiveness ... No former student of Professor McPhedran will ever cease to be grateful to him for the part he played in their professional training."[10] McPhedran railed against the tiny sums available to the Department of Medicine to encourage clinical investigation and created a small fund with this purpose in view. "After his retirement the Board of Governors of the University supplemented this fund and established the Alexander McPhedran Research Fellowship in Clinical Medicine."[11]

### The Eaton Gift, and Duncan Graham Becomes Professor of Medicine

The professors were all practicing physicians until Duncan Graham became the first full-time professor of medicine in 1919 and Clarence L. Starr the first full-time professor of surgery in 1921.

Flash back for a moment to 1903, the year in which Edward Gallie, later professor of surgery, graduated from medical school. He recalled a system of clinical training that was virtually nonexistent: a total of seventeen internships for the entire city, no postgraduate training in any specialty, mobs of medical students surging in and out of operating rooms, searching for shards of surgical learning and spreading microbes in great clouds. It was at this point that Joseph Flavelle, the packing-house magnate, became chairman of the Board of Trustees of the Toronto General Hospital and resolved to change things. Flavelle decided, first, in Gallie's words, "that a new General Hospital must be built somewhere in the neighbourhood of the University, and that it must be closely linked with the University for teaching purposes and for scientific investigations; second, that henceforth the character of services rendered or work accomplished should form the only basis for claims to appointment or promotion on the staff."[12] The new Toronto General Hospital was relocated to College Street in 1913 and the stage set for reform.

The reorganization that Flavelle desired was somewhat delayed owing to circumstances, but in 1919 a gift from the Eaton family created the faculty's first full-time professorship, and Duncan Graham – whatever ill might be said about his medical ideas or his personal style – is entitled to enormous credit for remedying the catastrophic situation that Gallie encountered upon graduating in 1903. How did this happen?

When Alexander McPhedran retired as professor of medicine in 1919, William Goldie, an internist, is said to have taken up the torch to have the professorship of medicine become a "full-time" position (a concept then all the rage in North American medicine), meaning that academic clinicians should have salaries rather than living from the fees of their clinical practices, in order to devote themselves to teaching and research. (Full-timers would also not be permitted to accept fees by way of moonlighting.) Goldie, born in Ayr, Ontario, in 1873, the son of a flour miller, had graduated as silver medalist in medicine at the University of Toronto in 1896 and taught in the Department of Pathology and Bacteriology before joining the Department of Medicine. He became physician-in-charge of infectious diseases at the children's hospital, until retiring from the post in 1911 after a reorganization. From 1913 to 1919 Goldie directed the outpatient service of the Toronto General Hospital (with time out for overseas duty in 1918–19). Goldie was among the most influential members of the faculty in these early days, and Edward Gallie remembers that "the man to whom we owe eternal gratitude, not only for amalgamation [with Trinity] but also for the most important organizational advances that have been made since that time, is William Goldie," who used the question-and-answer method in teaching. "His method was new, and to some of us, such as John Oille, quite thrilling." "Without doubt he was the father of our present School."[13]

Thus, at the end of the First World War, Goldie found himself contemplating the deficient organization of the Department of Medicine. When the chair of medicine became vacant, Goldie apparently persuaded President Sir Robert Falconer that the position should be full time. Then it became necessary to drum up a full-time salary. Having convinced the president, Goldie had to find the means to accomplish his idea. According to one source, "Fortunately, two of [Goldie's] patients were Sir John Eaton ... and his wife Flora, a former nurse." Eaton apparently turned the funds over to Goldie, saying, "Here's the money. You do what you like with it."[14]

In 1918 while in England, Goldie set out to find someone suitable, meeting young Duncan Graham, a U of T medical graduate in 1905 and at the time at the No. 4 General Hospital in Basingstoke. Given his background in laboratory medicine, Graham was a bit of a surprising choice, yet he had demonstrated administrative competency at the Basingstoke hospital and argued for "the basic sciences as the basis of good medical practice." Here the model was Johns Hopkins University, where the system of medical education that Osler had helped install was based on a thorough knowledge of physiology and pathology and on "the teaching hospital [as] an integral part of the university with full time professors," as Graham's eulogist put it. "In looking for a new Professor of Medicine at Toronto, the University was influenced by this new type of medical education in which the professor would be primarily a teacher and not a busy consultant."[15]

Thus, Goldie wrote to Eaton of Graham, "He is not only respected but liked even though he is an exacting task-master." Indeed. At the personal level, Graham was not the most endearing of men. Said Helen "Nell" Farquharson, Ray Farquharson's daughter, who had known Graham in the latter days of his career, "Duncan Graham frightened people. He was very severe, very autocratic ... Most staff people, I think, were a bit intimidated by him." Unlike his cousin the bulky surgeon Roscoe Graham, Duncan "was sort of a little person, but rather gruff, and his word was law." In reviewing a book about Graham, one of his students, Arthur Squires, who seems on the whole rather well disposed to his former professor, nonetheless describes Graham as "ruthless."[16]

Graham may have elicited this sense of unease in people because he was something of a racist and quite uninhibited about displaying it. In 1923 at a meeting of the Faculty Council, "Professor Graham asked if some steps could be taken to exclude coloured students from the medical course, owing to the difficulty in providing for their clinical instruction." The faculty did not vote on the matter.[17] (For Graham's attitudes towards Jews, see chapter 22.)

Duncan Graham was born near Ivan in Ontario in 1882 and may have owed some of his less winning characteristics to an unforgiving father in childhood. As his eulogist comments, "His mother died while he was fairly young and I am sure residents have often wondered whether his father pounced on young Duncan for a wrong observation or an illogical conclusion in the same way that Professor Graham would demolish the feeble arguments of a resident presenting a patient at rounds."

As mentioned, Graham graduated in medicine at the University of Toronto in 1905, then worked as a bacteriologist for the Ontario Board of Health; in 1906 he was placed in charge of the Pathological Laboratories at TGH. He also spent two years as a pathologist and physician to the Pittsburgh Sanatorium in Pittsburgh, Pennsylvania. This was followed by two years at London, Dresden, Heidelberg, and Vienna. He returned to Canada in 1911 as a lecturer in bacteriology at U of T, then returned to Berlin in 1913 for graduate work in internal medicine, forced to return, however, because of the outbreak of war. He went overseas in 1915, first to England, then to France, then to Salonika with the University of Toronto medical unit. He finished the war at Basingstoke, where Goldie encountered him.

Osler, now Regius Professor of Medicine at Oxford, got wind of Toronto's interest in Graham as a candidate for the professorship of medicine and took an active interest in the appointment, convening in 1918 a big dinner for Graham at Oxford and inviting "15 or 20 of the outstanding medical scientists and other scientists ... This was a tremendous event that allowed Professor Graham to build up associations with outstanding [researchers] in England who later provided training posts for Dr. Graham's residents." Osler encouraged Graham to accept the post, and it was possibly through Osler that Graham insisted "that the Professor of Medicine be the Physician-in-Chief as well. This was not the model in the English schools but was at Hopkins."[18] Graham, who already had studied extensively in the United States and on the Continent, was therefore not Anglophiliac in his thinking about medical training, not an adept of the English emphasis on close teaching rapport, but rather a fan of the American system – as manifest at Hopkins – that saw science as the basis of medical practice and the university teaching hospital as its locus.

In many ways, Hopkins had been the model for the new Toronto General Hospital; its image as a research university had guided the 1906 Royal Commission on the University of Toronto, and indeed Osler in 1906 had been invited to be president of U of T. Michael Bliss observes, "Hopkins was also the model for the full-time movement, which the Rockefeller people were pressing on everyone else, and that was almost certainly in the minds of the Torontonians and the Eatons by 1918."[19] So despite the many ways in which the faculty remained an appendage of London and Edinburgh, Graham was bent upon importing the Hopkins model and doing so with a relentlessness that changed forever teaching and research in internal medicine in Toronto.

In April 1919 Falconer announced that Graham would become the head of the medical clinic at TGH, effective 1 July 1919. Graham was not pleased at what he found. In scientific terms the Department of Medicine was somnolent. A 1920 report stated baldly, "Members of the Staff have devoted the greater portion of their available time to a thorough clinical and laboratory investigation of the patients on the Wards ... and to teaching the large number of Students. Little or no time has been available for pure research."[20] Graham proceeded to chop away the dead wood, dismissing 40 percent of the existing staff and causing "a heated debate in the press and legislature."[21]

At this point the aforementioned Eaton gift came in handy. Sir John and Lady Eaton, who had acquired their fortune from the department store named after the Eaton family, decided in 1919 to make a charitable gift to the Faculty of Medicine of $25,000 per year for a period of twenty years. Of the $25,000, $5,000 was to go to pediatrics, a subunit of medicine; of the $20,000 to medicine, $10,000 would support the Eaton professor's salary. As Duncan Graham told university president Sidney Smith in 1946 (as the university struggled to reconstitute the paper trail of these events, hopeful of further grants – the original correspondence had all been discarded), "It was agreed that the rest of the fund should be used chiefly in the payment of salaries to promising young men joining the staff of the Department in order that they might devote their whole time for a few years to hospital work, teaching and research."[22] Interestingly, only in 1932 was the chair of medicine designated by the Board of Governors "the Sir John and Lady Eaton Chair of Medicine."[23]

Kager Wightman, later professor of medicine, had his own take on the Eaton grant: "The purpose of this gift was to provide the same kind of single-minded devotion to the development of the Department and its scientific basis as had the earlier establishment of full-time professorships in the Departments of Pathology, Physiology etc. An effort was then made to recruit physicians who combined clinical skills with sufficient scientific training and experience to be able to interpret the advances of science to students and practitioners of medicine."[24] The emphasis here was not on research but on clinical care and medical education.

Just as a footnote: an agreement in 1946 between Lady Eaton and the Board of Governors placed the choice of incumbent of the chair in the hands of a committee of five members, two of whom were to be nominated by the Eaton Company, a perquisite that the university would later deny to other benefactors of named chairs.[25]

The Eaton grant greatly improved the laboratory situation at TGH. Graham later told Sidney Smith, "In 1919 the Department of Medicine had no laboratory facilities in the University or in the Toronto General Hospital for clinical research, and in the first ten years was dependent upon other departments in the University for laboratory facilities. After the establishment of three small medical laboratories on the medical wards of the hospital and [later new animal facilities in the Banting Institute] the clinical research programme of the department expanded. Until 1931 the budget of the department was more than adequate to meet its needs."[26] Perhaps in his enthusiasm to impress President Smith with the generosity of the Eatons, Graham neglected to mention a second grant of $20,000 that he and fellow internist John Oille had obtained from Mrs A.R. Clarke in 1921 "for the purpose of establishing a better Laboratory service in the Medical Wards of the Hospital." Two six-bed wards were closed to make room for the new laboratories.[27]

Before Graham's arrival at TGH in 1919, there had been four independent medical services under the direction of scientifically undistinguished but socially quite considerable figures such as – to use their wartime ranks – General John Taylor Fotheringham, Colonel Graham Chambers, and Major William Brown Thistle. In September 1919 Graham retired them all involuntarily and brought in his own crew. The former chieftains were really quite grumpy about this and sued.[28]

Graham later explained how he had reorganized the medical services of "The General": "Four clinicians were appointed as Ward Supervisors, and patients were segregated according to types of disease. Five clinicians specially qualified in laboratory methods ... were appointed, and they devoted eight hours a day to necessary examinations of patients. The Outpatient Department was placed under clinicians specially qualified in general medicine. The majority of teachers in Clinical Medicine are in private practice, but have charge of a certain number of patients in the hospital and teach without salary from four to nine hours a week."[29] In the large public wards of TGH, care was free for the patients and the doctors worked without honoraria, making a living from the fees they received from the patients in the private pavilion and from their private practices. At that point the General had 193 medical teaching beds, with 21 teachers and 250 students.

In 1921 the university decided to expand the full-time system. The small honoraria for clinical services were no longer to be paid to members of the Department of Medicine, or to other departments, "with the purpose of devoting part of the money to salaries for such of the staff in the Clinical Departments as are not dependent for their living upon private practice and are giving all or nearly all their time to the work of the University."[30] This was the beginning of what were later called practice plans, donating a percentage of billings to a department fund for teaching and research.

These events permit one to place Graham's tenure in perspective. He reorganized the Department of Medicine into a unified service capable of being science-driven. But he himself was not a scholarly giant. He bought into a number of the colossally wrong-headed ideas of his epoch, such as the notion that sites of "focal infection" in the gums or the bowel (always infected!) might produce symptoms of distant disease. "If focal infection is the primary cause of ill-health," Graham wrote in 1931, "and all foci of infection have been found and can be eradicated, one may expect that the patient's health will improve, and a cure or a marked amelioration of symptoms result."[31] This advice led to an orgy of sacrificial offerings of wisdom teeth and tonsils.

With the Eaton money, Graham brought on board a whole cohort of young physicians who would provide the scientific steel of the Department of Medicine and would be known as "Clinicians to the Toronto General Hospital." Goldie headed one of the divisions of the service, a post that he held until his retirement in 1928.[32]

Among the new recruits was Walter R. Campbell, born in 1890 in Port Robinson, Ontario, and a matriculant of St Catharines Collegiate Institute. He had earned a BA in sciences at U of T in 1911 and in 1912–13 trained in biochemistry under Macallum. As a medical student he was a member of the Society for Experimental Medicine, and when he graduated with an MB in 1915 he was keen to do scientific work.[33] Campbell was the uncle of obstetrician Jim Goodwin, and Goodwin recalled, "He was an absolutely brilliant man. The medical students used to call him 'Dynamite' because he was a very boring lecturer, but that was the only thing that was boring about him." (The 1947 Daffydil, the medical students' annual music-hall production, saluted Campbell thus: "Oh Dynamite your accents sweet are never loud and strong. / So we're going to help conclude them with this therapeutic song; / So if we call you 'Mumbles' it's because you've got a fault, / We think you ruined your vocal cords with iodized salt."[34])

Goodwin's father died early, and Walter Campbell took Jim Goodwin under his wing, especially after Goodwin fell ill for a time. "Walter would come over and sit by my bed and tell me stories about the old days. He had treated diabetic mothers before insulin. It was a matter of keeping them alive – the babies would die like flies, and the mothers would die, too, they could die, and he was telling me how you would balance dietary input and exercise, to see them through this sort of thing. This was before insulin."[35]

Graham also brought Andrew Almon Fletcher into the Department of Medicine. Born in 1913 in Kingston, Ontario, in a university professor's family (his father held the chair of Latin at Queen's), Fletcher took one year of arts at the University of Toronto, then transferred into the five-year medicine program. He was president of his fifth-year class, graduating in 1913, and chose as his motto, "Story! God bless you! I have none to tell you, sir."[36] But shortly he would, just as Campbell, be part of the insulin story.

The Eaton grant, and then the Rockefeller grant just afterwards which created a full-time professor of surgery, banished with a stroke the educational chaos Gallie had encountered upon graduation in 1903. Gallie said, "These gentlemen [Starr in surgery, Graham in medicine, and Alan Brown in pediatrics] "began the gradual building up of their staffs and the promotion of education and research which has led to the wonderful prominence that this hospital [the Hospital for Sick Children] now occupies among the children's hospitals of the world."[37]

## Surgery

In the late nineteenth century internationally, surgery replaced anatomical pathology as the queen of the medical sciences, the specialty leading the scientific advances. Surgeons, unlike physicians, had always been able to do useful things, such as limb amputations, managing haemorrhoids, and setting fractures. But with the discovery of the principle of surgical cleanliness (antisepsis and asepsis) and of anesthetics, surgery opened the way to the body's major cavities: abdomen, chest, and cranium. A royal road was trod upon that outdistanced all other specialties in delivering benefits to humankind. This happened ineluctably in Toronto as elsewhere.

The Department of Surgery was founded in 1887 by the dean of the faculty, William T. Aikins, who as professor of surgery directed surgical affairs for the next ten years.[38] At Aikins's death in 1897, Irving Heward Cameron, who had been professor of "clinical surgery" at the beginning of the department's history, became chair. Cameron was the son of a chief justice of the Court of Common Pleas of Ontario. He began as a law student, then took his MB in 1874 from the Toronto School of Medicine.[39] He achieved the fellowship of the Royal College of Surgeons in England before returning to Toronto. In England he "adopted Listerism, recently promulgated," as his biographer puts it. It is positive that he was an early adept of antiseptic principles in surgery. Less promisingly, "he remained an exponent of Lister's methods [spraying the operative field with phenol] long after others had been converted to asepticism." In Toronto,

Cameron was a student of Aikins, and after the refoundation of the faculty, in 1892 Cameron became professor of clinical surgery.[40] In a world of increasingly aseptic surgery (keeping microbes from reaching the wound) Cameron did not use gloves. "Yet the kindly healing of his operative wounds," said his eulogist, "and his own freedom from infections were ample evidence of the efficiency of the antiseptic method."[41]

The stamp of Britain upon him, Cameron's main contribution to the reorganization of the Toronto General Hospital that began in 1906 was to suggest changing its name to "The Toronto Royal Infirmary and University Hospital."[42] "Never operate," he counseled, "just to see what is inside," excluding the exploratory laparotomy.

In those days a different concept of the doctor-patient relationship prevailed. According to Cameron's eulogist C.W. Harris, "The story is told that the late Mr Timothy Eaton had fallen and injured his hip. Mr. Cameron [as he preferred to be addressed] was called in and during the course of his examination caused the patient pain; the latter understandably used his uninjured limb to violently push the doctor away. Mr Cameron went to the bottom of the room, picked up his hat and gloves, bowed and left the room."[43] A colleague then attended Mr Eaton. Cameron headed the department until his retirement in 1920.

Contemporaries would have ranked highly a third early surgeon, F.N.G. Starr. Frederic Newton Gisborne Starr, a Toronto School of Medicine graduate in 1889, joined the Faculty of Medicine in 1891 as a demonstrator in surgery after postgraduate study in England, Germany, and France. In 1923 he became professor of clinical surgery, retiring ten years later, for a total of over forty years of service. Starr much embodied the old school of medical instruction. On the occasion of his retirement in 1933 a colleague said, "He was more interested in teaching the craft as a master to apprentice than as a clinical or didactic lecturer. To the small groups of senior students, house surgeons and personal assistants about him, he was a teacher of the very highest order."[44]

One sees here coming alive a principle of medical education quite distinctive to Toronto and borrowed from the United Kingdom: the apprenticeship system of instruction in which small groups of trainees cluster about the master for one-on-one teaching. It was a tradition in which the master teachers were quite indifferent to research, and excellence in training was the desideratum. The system was dislodged with some difficulty by the wholesale rush to research in the 1960s.

One more name is important: George A. Peters, at the Hospital for Sick Children, in July 1899 made the first contribution of the Department of Surgery to the international scientific literature when he successfully transplanted the ureters into the rectum of a two-year-old child who had both an ectopic bladder and a procident rectum. "The occurrence of both in one subject makes the sufferer's life so unutterably miserable, and renders him so repulsive to his friends, that life without relief is well-nigh intolerable." Peters devised a method of giving the infant some control over urination by finding a route for the transplantation of the ureters into the rectum outside the peritoneum (the incising of this protective layer of the abdomen, in those pre-antibiotic days, often led to catastrophic infections). "If thus converting the rectum into a cloaca," Peters wrote, "the patient can hold his urine even from one to three or five hours, he is surely in a much better position to take his part in life than he could possibly be with the best apology for a bladder that can be expected to result from any flap operation."[45] (A flap operation means raising a layer of tissue.) Gallie later wrote, "I saw some of these patients several years after their operations, completely changed from a condition of abject misery to one of comparatively happy childhood. They had gradually developed control of the rectum so that the urine could be retained for several hours, without mishap."[46] This initiated a long tradition of transplantation surgery in Toronto.

Peters himself, as so many of his colleagues, was shaped in the soil of small-town Ontario. Born in 1859 in Eramosa, he received an MB in 1886, a year before the refoundation of the faculty. He then studied in England and became the first Toronto surgeon to become "FRCS Eng." (Fellow of the Royal College of Surgeons of England).[47] He joined the Department of Surgery in 1892, serving until his early death in 1907. The procedure he perfected became known as the Lenden-Peters operation. Peters was also appointed to the General and enjoyed there a "brilliant career" in a wide variety of surgical treatments, among them the surgical removal of both lobes of the thyroid for exophthalmic goiter (which the Mayo brothers initiated and Peters introduced to Canada in 1904[48]); he also perfected in 1898 the making of easily removable plaster-of-Paris casts.[49]

Gallie remembered of Peters, "As a clinical teacher he was superb. One day he called me over to a child with a distended abdomen and asked me to put my stethoscope on the lower half of the abdomen and tell him what I heard. I listened for a while, expecting to hear intestinal gurgling, but before long became aware of the loud beating of the heart. Then he suggested that I listen for breath sounds and sure enough they were quite audible. This was 'Peters' sign' for general peritonitis."[50]

Peters died at age forty-seven of "angina pectoris," likely to have been a heart attack. Gallie said, "Even when he knew the end was approaching he dictated to his stenographer a description of the radiating pains of this dread disease as exemplified in his own case, and pointed out where they differed from the ordinarily accepted ideas. That is the kind of man he was."[51]

Around the time of the First World War, the organization of surgery at the Toronto General Hospital had become highly fragmented. In 1920 there were four different surgical services with 150 beds. There was a laboratory consisting of "a small room off two of the Surgical wards in which facilities are available for testing urine and making blood counts." If one wanted to do surgical research – which meant animal work – one needed go over to the Pathology Building.[52]

Yet change was coming. A donation from the Rockefeller Foundation announced on New Year's Day 1920 resulted in the appointment of a full-time professor of surgery. The Rockefeller Foundation envisioned the gift explicitly as a reward for Canada's participation in the First World War. The letter of transmittal said, "The Canadian people are our near neighbors. They are closely bound to us by ties of race, language and international friendship; and they have without stint sacrificed themselves, their youth and their resources, to the end that democracy might be saved and extended."[53] The grant served as a counterweight to the full-time professor of medicine, whom the Eatons had funded. In 1920 several Rockefeller executives undertook a tour of Canadian medical schools and found, "The most satisfactory school is the University of Toronto with McGill a close second."[54] In fact, McGill and Toronto received $1 million apiece from Rockefeller and among the uses to which Toronto put the money was the full-time professorship of surgery.

The faculty struck a committee, headed by Primrose, to consider the allocation among departments of the Rockefeller grant. In a working paper of 16 February 1920, the committee outlined the future organization of the Department of Surgery, recommending, "that there be one Head of the Department of Surgery … The Head of the Department shall have full control of the administration of the entire department in the University, hospitals and surgical laboratories [the Hospital for Sick Children, the Toronto Western Hospital, and St Michael's also had departments of surgery and some laboratories]. The Head of the Department should be in charge of surgical wards, out door and emergency departments of the Toronto General Hospital. This will necessitate doing away with separate surgical services and the establishment of a single surgical service in this hospital. All patients admitted to the public ward beds in the Hospital will be under the direct charge of the Head of the Department," who would also be the surgeon-in-chief at the Toronto General Hospital. "He shall have absolute control of matters in connection with teaching in all Hospitals granting privileges to the University." He would also have control of hiring. This coming professor might operate on some private patients, but only at TGH and for no more than three hours a day. "His mornings from nine to one must be devoted to his duties as Head of the Department."[55] The report could not have been clearer: the disorganization of the old system must be replaced by a Duncan Graham–style titan.

Two weeks later, on 1 March 1920, the committee recommended to the Faculty Council that in medicine, surgery, and obstetrics and gynecology, a single full-time head should be appointed who would organize undergraduate teaching effectively and provide "a system of training for the junior members of the staff which will in the course of a few years result in the production of well trained specialists who … may be chosen to fill senior positions on teaching staffs in this University or elsewhere." In each hospital there would be but a single service in surgery, medicine, and obstetrics-gynecology, led by a single powerful figure who "will be chief and in control."[56] This was a system that had proved itself admirably at Johns Hopkins University and now would show equal merit at Toronto.

Who might be competent to fill such a post in surgery? Of these early figures, the only one to graduate from Toronto was Clarence L. Starr. Born in 1868, he finished his studies at U of T with an MB in 1890, then trained at the Hospital for Ruptured and Crippled Children in New York. In New York, he earned an MD from Bellevue Hospital Medical School, "from which," his eulogist tells, "his father had graduated twenty-five years before." Clarence Starr then studied in England and Germany, returning to Toronto in 1893 to begin practice. In 1894 he received a staff appointment at the Hospital for Sick Children. "Here he laid the foundation for the development of orthopaedic surgery." But the next year he left for the General and worked as first assistant to I.H. Cameron until 1911, when he found himself again back at the children's hospital, but this time as surgeon-in-chief. He served in England during the war, then upon his recall to Canada in 1918 was involved in organizing veterans hospitals. "It was largely as a result of his high qualities as an organizer and administrator of surgical services that he was appointed in 1921, Professor of Surgery in the University of Toronto and Surgeon-in-Chief at the Toronto General Hospital." At the General, as Cameron's successor, he reorganized the Department of Surgery.[57] His salary and other departmental expenses were paid by the annual $50,000 interest from the $1 million Rockefeller grant.[58]

As the new professor of surgery, Clarence Starr proceeded to clean house as Duncan Graham had done in medicine. Said a hostile account of events in 1921 in the medical press, "The general plan of reorganization ... was that already adopted by the Department of Medicine, namely, one so-called 'full-time' professor endowed with very large powers of his staff, the policy of teaching and the care of patients in the wards and out-patient department of the General Hospital." The plan, the article said, had been conceived during absence on military duty of Professor Cameron. "The new professor of surgery, Clarence L. Starr, immediately set to work to reorganize his department, with the final result that ... in Sept 1921 four men (all well-known surgeons long in the service of the hospital and the university), received notice of their retirement." They were Herbert A. Bruce, James A. Roberts, John McCollum, and Andrew Moorhead. "Two men over the statutory age-limit, the late Dr. [George Arthur] Bingham and the Dean of the Faculty, Dr. Primrose were retained."[59] (There followed a big protest on the part of those in medicine and surgery who had been let go, which I shall not follow in detail.[60]) Cameron, who had been in the Department of Surgery since 1887, was thus rather unceremoniously booted out.

Dean Primrose was beside himself with pleasure at the new Department of Surgery: "The existing organization has attracted widespread attention, many prominent teachers from abroad have visited our clinics and laboratories for the purpose of learning our methods and have been most favourably impressed.

Eulogistic references have appeared in the medical press in England."[61] Clearly, this was the acme of praise. But the reorganization of medicine and surgery into departments with a powerful full-time head was not received everywhere with applause, certainly not by the physicians who were discontinued as not up to speed. They protested and in October 1922 the provincial legislature set up a special committee to hold hearings on the changes. On 12 Jan. 1923, Starr testified "that when he first took office there were seven services not co-ordinated and since then there had been two reorganizations." Starr said, "I have no doubt that the present unit system is the best." He said there were staff conferences twice a month, "and each division knew the work of the other division." This was the system he had learned at the children's hospital.[62]

Powerful letters from respected authorities in favour of the changes were weighed in the balance. On 30 January, a letter of Alexander McPhedran, the former professor of medicine and clinical medicine from 1898 to 1918, was read out: under the old system graduate instruction was impossible and the best people were lost to the United States for further training. It would be, he said, as though "the department stores should stock each floor with every variety of goods under an independent head; in fact, establish as many stores as floors." George Young, a member of the Department of Medicine for the previous thirteen years, added, in the words of the newspaper reporter, that "the present system provides the staff with better facilities for teaching medicine and gives a unity which was sadly lacking before ... Looking back, he could not see how an effective reorganization could have been accomplished without the services of some one who could give his full time to the work."[63] (The special committee issued a begrudging report that was not further acted upon,[64] and the reforms in medicine and surgery remained in place.)

Starr himself continued in office until his death in 1929. It is interesting to see what the faculty considered to be his greatest honour. To be sure, in 1926 he had served as temporary chief surgeon at the Peter Bent Brigham Hospital in Boston, substituting for Harvey Cushing, the great American neurosurgeon. Yet for the faculty the crowning summit of his career, as things were then conceived, lay in England. "Just before his death he received what he looked upon as the highest and most flattering honour of his career, when he was proposed by the governors of St Bartholomew's Hospital in London for appointment to the temporary post of Director of the Department of Surgery,"[65] briefly to replace the incumbent, George Gask, whose name has not survived in the annals of surgery. But this was Toronto in the 1920s: it was a British colony.

## Blood Transfusion

From the Hospital for Sick Children (HSC) came an early scientific triumph. Lawrence Bruce Robertson, a junior assistant surgeon at HSC, helped popularize the practice of blood transfusion. Born in Toronto in 1885 into a prosperous

Scottish merchant family, Robertson was educated at Upper Canada College and graduated in arts in 1907 from U of T. Two years later he became a medical graduate, interning at the Hospital for Sick Children, of which his uncle, publisher John Ross Robertson, was board chairman. (On graduation Lawrence Robertson chose as his motto for the yearbook, "The deepest rivers flow with least sound."[66]) In 1910 he trained in pediatric and orthopedic surgery at Bellevue Hospital in New York, learning there, evidently from Edward Lindeman, the concept of blood transfusion, and was evidently further instructed in the technique at the Boston Children's Hospital. By 1913 he was back at the HSC in Toronto as an assistant surgeon, introducing blood transfusion.[67] In 1914 he and Alan Brown wrote an article in the *Canadian Medical Association Journal* on the transfusion of blood in "infants and young children," followed by several further.[68]

At the outbreak of war he stepped forward, as did so many academic physicians, for military service. It was in 1915, as he was serving as a captain in the Canadian Army Medical Corps, that he introduced blood transfusion to British military physicians. For soldiers in shock, saline solution was already being widely administered, but, Robertson said in 1916, "The introduction of whole fresh blood into the circulation at once not only helps to restore the depleted bulk of circulating fluid, but provides the patients with [a replacement for lost blood]." Was compatibility a problem? "The milder degrees of incompatibility between the donor's blood and that of the recipient result usually in a slight chill and a rise in temperature ... These symptoms are not uncommon even between familial bloods, and should occasion no alarm."[69] Blood transfusion saved the lives of thousands of men. One wounded British officer told Robertson in 1917 of his post-operative progress, "I owe most of all to your handling of my amputations and transfusion at the CCS [Casualty Clearing Station]."[70]

In the army Robertson had also attempted partial exchange transfusion – called "exsanguination-transfusion" – on two soldiers with carbon monoxide poisoning. Back at HSC in 1921, Robertson applied this treatment to "haemorrhagic disease of the newly born" (later called erythroblastosis fetalis): "In a few cases horse serum or human blood injected subcutaneously may be used successfully, but to ensure a cure blood transfusion is beyond any question the best and most reliable procedure." At the children's hospital they used a syringe cannula. In this population, Robertson felt that ascertaining the blood group was secondary. In a series of forty cases, thirty-six had survived.[71] (William Mustard resumed this approach again at HSC in 1948, see p. 102.) In 1921 Robertson also pioneered blood transfusion for severely burned children.[72] In a twelve-month period between 1922 and 1923, a total of 516 transfusions were undertaken at HSC. "The results show brilliant success," said G. Kerr Cross, a laboratory physician in Alan Brown's Department of Paediatrics.[73] Robertson died tragically in 1923 at age thirty-seven of pneumonia following influenza.

## Gallie

A page was turned when Clarence Starr died on Christmas Day 1928. William Gallie, the great figure in the history of surgery in Toronto, now strides front and centre. In 1929 Gallie succeeded Starr as professor of surgery. Among Gallie's achievements were bringing St Michael's Hospital and Toronto Western Hospital into the university training program and creating the "Gallie Course." As one of his students put it, "When he became Professor of Surgery in 1929 … the University hospital facilities, supplemented by the resources of the Departments of Physiology, Anatomy and Pathology, were organized into an integrated whole for the purpose of training surgeons … This was the first organized plan for the systematic training of surgeons in Canada. His pupils have made it known as the Gallie Course in Surgery."[74]

Gallie, who was called "W.E," started out as an orthopedic surgeon, the first subspecialty in Toronto to split off from general surgery, and with his appointment in 1906 as a resident at the Hospital for Sick Children, he continued Starr's work.

Gallie was born in Barrie, Ontario, in 1883, his father the owner of a lumber mill. As a youngster he was an avid athlete and played hockey for Barrie teams – and later for the Meds. He graduated in medicine from the faculty in 1903, as his students Robert Harris and Robert Janes point out, "the youngest member of his class." While a student, Gallie played on the U of T hockey team – and coached varsity in intercollegiate matches before the war. (In 1910 he upgraded his MB degree to an MD.) After interning at the Hospital for Sick Children and the Toronto General Hospital, he spent a year at the Hospital for Ruptured and Crippled Children in New York. When he entered the Hospital for Sick Children, or HSC, his chief was Clarence Starr, the only other surgeon on staff. In these years, there weren't so many surgeons at TGH either, and the staff at each hospital often went back and forth, often holding simultaneous appointments. Thus Gallie progressed at HSC from junior surgeon to associate surgeon until in 1921 he succeeded Starr as surgeon-in-chief at HSC when Starr became surgeon-in-chief at TGH and professor of surgery at the university. After Gallie took over from Starr in 1929, he remained at both posts until he retired in 1947.

Starr and Gallie worked hard at expanding the surgery staff at both hospitals with promising young residents. Said Dean Joseph MacFarlane in 1959 at Gallie's death, "[At TGH Gallie] quickly recognized the need for a rational system of resident training and education for young Canadians who wished to meet the ever increasing challenge of surgery and of the various specialties which were rapidly developing within the parent discipline."[75]

By all accounts this was a tight little band of brothers, men knit together by the common challenge of building the discipline of surgery in these exciting early years when everything remained to be discovered. Gallie's students happily called themselves "Gallie slaves."[76] Starr recruited, for example, David

Edwin Robertson, who graduated with an MB from Toronto in 1907, three years after Gallie. Gallie and Robertson became fast friends, writing together in 1919 one of the earliest papers on bone metabolism and transplantation, a matter of great interest in treating the casualties of the war.[77] In 1936 Robertson and two companions became "trapped by the collapse of the shaft in the lower levels of a gold mine at Moose River in Nova Scotia." As Janes and Harris tell the story, "[Gallie's] frantic rush across one-third of the continent was followed by ten days of desperate efforts and agonized suspense. By good fortune that bordered on the miraculous two were finally brought out alive. One of them was 'D.E.R [David Edwin Robertson].'"

Gallie's reputation spread during the First World War as a result of his bone-grafting operations at the Davisville Military Hospital. Resting upon animal experimentation, this research gave rise to Gallie and Arthur LeMesurier's concept of "living sutures," or transplantation of the fascia (the tissue that wraps the muscles and other body organs) "into strips and sheets and other shapes which facilitated its use in the repair of defects." They published a preliminary report in 1921,[78] then in 1922 elaborated "the free transplantation of fascia and tendon": "It is obviously more rational to use as ligaments, tendons, or sutures, material which we know will live and retain its normal characteristics."[79] "In these forms," say Harris and Janes, "the fascia survived and became a part of the tissue into which it had been transplanted." These sutures were used for the repair of injured ligaments and to repair failed previous hernia operations. (Gallie said the idea had occurred to him "after absently watching someone darn a hole in a pair of socks with a cross-stitch."[80]) In 1923, two years after the introduction of the procedure, they reported great success in reuniting portions of the abdominal wall in patients –typically wounded veterans – whose previous hernia repairs had failed. "If these principles are followed, we believe we have at our command a method of dealing with doubtful and difficult hernias which will give general satisfaction and considerably widen the field to which surgical treatment is applicable."[81] This became known as the "Gallie operation."

**The Gallie Course**

In 1931 the Royal College of Surgeons of Canada was established, beginning a program of fellowship examinations in surgery. In that same year Gallie organized the first systematic training program in Canada for surgeons to help them pass their examinations. The larger significance of the Royal College exams was that, as Bigelow said, "It involved persuading the surgeons in charge of hospital surgery divisions at the university that it was no longer their privilege to appoint their own residents."[82] The training of surgeons was to be standardized as had been done in England. The immediate significance is that it made William Gallie the central figure in the history of surgical training in Canada.

The Gallie Course was originally conceived as a small, elite program. Gallie wrote in June 1932, "This year has seen the establishment in this school of a definite plan for the postgraduate training for surgeons. Hitherto it has been impossible for a graduate to receive adequate training here in general surgery and he has been forced to seek it in hospitals abroad." But now the Boards of Trustees of the general and children's hospitals had approved a three-year course "which it is hoped will place the teaching of surgery in this school on a high level. In this plan the Toronto General Hospital offers to graduates of approved medical schools who have served one year as rotating interns … two appointments of three years' and one of two years' duration which are arranged as follows."

He described the three-year program, which was to become the standard for training surgeons in Toronto:

- First year: six months' medicine and six months' pathology
- Second year: one year as senior house surgeon on a general surgical division
- Third year: one of the following options: (a) six months as house surgeon at HSC plus six months in a genitourinary department; (b) six months at HSC plus six months' neurosurgery at TGH; (c) six months' neurosurgery at TGH (this latter option evidently for those uninterested in pediatrics).[83]

"This plan has been in operation now for a full year [NB it was founded 1930–1]. It at once became very popular with our interns." Seventeen had applied for the three spots.

Gallie said the program had two choice features:

First, these house surgeons are no longer treated as chance wayfarers through the wards of the hospital, but are accepted as apprentices to the art of surgery and are so treated by the attending staff. Second, when they accept their appointments they automatically enter the course for the postgraduate degree master of surgery and they undertake to pursue the course of study in anatomy and physiology and in surgery and pathology required for that degree. During the past year these house surgeons spent two evenings a week in the dissecting room and one afternoon with an instructor in physiology, so that they will be prepared for the primary examination for the master's degree and the diploma of fellowship in the Royal College of Surgeons of Canada or England, as they may choose.[84]

The Gallie program thus offered an intensive training program for trainees in surgery ("house surgeons") and a method of keeping them up to date on advances in science – the extra study in anatomy and physiology – to propel surgery away from its historical origins as a handicraft, alongside cabinetmaking and leather-tanning, that trained recruits through apprenticeships.

Then a kind of layering began, with the elite on top and the journeyman surgeons bound for nonacademic careers on the bottom. In the 1934–5 session,

Gallie said that originally enrolment in the master of surgery course was required for all surgical "interns" (meaning residents). Yet the department had to give this up because most interns, "owing to the pressure of work at the hospital, have been unable to take advantage of the opportunity provided by the Departments of Anatomy and Physiology to prepare for the primary examination. To get over this difficulty, we are now giving preference in the appointment of surgical internes to men who have already passed the 'Primary' examination for the MS [master of surgery] or for Fellowship in one of the Royal Colleges, and as a result almost all of our internes have obtained one of the diplomas before coming into Surgery [i.e., into the Gallie Course]."[85] This would be a surgical elite.

By the late 1930s there were clear levels. In 1938 Gallie described postgraduate training in surgery; one notes how small the number of core enrollees was. "In Surgery one must recognize three pretty distinct groups among the graduates: first, the ordinary Bachelor or Doctor of Medicine who has learned the fundamentals and is qualified to enter general practice ... ; second, the master surgeon who has had several years of special training in Anatomy, Physiology, Pathology and Medicine, and a thorough apprenticeship in hospitals as assistant to a group of hospital surgeons; third, the very small group who because of their ability, enthusiasm and devotion to work are likely to be leaders and may be expected to become actual contributors to the science. It is in the development of groups II and III that this department has found the greatest enjoyment in the last decade."[86]

Thus began the training program for surgeons that would soon people the academic surgical departments of Canada and many American centres as well.

### Gordon Murray

The overwhelming scientific figure in the Department of Surgery before the Second World War was not, however, Gallie but Gordon Murray, who pioneered the clinical uses of heparin before the war and heart surgery after the war. He was not a product of the Gallie program. Born in Oxford County, Ontario, in 1894 of a Scottish immigrant father, Murray was a real farm boy and later in life even returned to work the family farm. He attended high school in Stratford, Ontario, then enlisted in 1915. He evidently experienced great horrors in the trenches. Bigelow said later, "All four Murray brothers joined up – three were old enough for overseas duty, one was killed and Gordon, who experienced Ypres, Somme and Vimy Ridge, was blown up and buried [in the dirt of a shell explosion] with major wounds. It is said that the site in which he was buried was taken by the Germans, then recaptured before he was disinterred and discovered to be alive."[87]

Murray earned his MB from Toronto in 1921 at age twenty-seven, typical of so many of the men in this cohort of returning, battle-scarred veterans. As a medical student he was anything but an antisocial recluse, having served, for example, as secretary of the Daffydil committee.[88] Once graduated, he apprenticed with a physician in Stratford, performing "fix it up" operations on the kitchen table when needed, which gave him the idea that he would like to be a surgeon. Murray spent a few months at the Mayo Clinic in Rochester, Minnesota, as a junior assistant pathologist, then left for England.

In London, Murray trained for the next six years, first as resident medical officer at the West End Hospital in 1922, then as house surgeon at Hampstead General Hospital and several other facilities. By 1926, according to historian Shelley McKellar, he had "performed over two hundred major operations during his various rotations." He passed the demanding fellowship examination of the Royal College of Surgeons in England on the first attempt; 76 of the 110 who tried it failed. Having acquired a comprehensive knowledge of anatomy in London, "[h]e saw how American surgeons, unsure of their anatomy, wasted time and lacked confidence. In contrast, Murray's mastery of anatomy and his extensive operating experience in London hospitals made him a skilful and confident surgeon." Murray's London experience also made him a determined Anglophile – he was later known to wear spats.[89]

On returning to Toronto, Clarence Starr offered him a one-year surgical residency at TGH; because it didn't start for another half year, in 1927 Murray spent some time in New York as house surgeon at New York Hospital under Eugene Pool, who introduced him to experimental research, trying new techniques first on animals. "Murray was delighted," says McKellar, "by the American enthusiasm for experimentation and innovation." He also worked at the Hospital for Ruptured and Crippled Children. Later in 1927 Murray returned to the General in Toronto and from 1929 on was senior surgeon in the hospital and associate professor of surgery in the university.

At the Toronto General Hospital Murray came into his own. McKellar writes, "Starr recognized Murray as a good fit with the new philosophy and direction of the Department of Surgery. Murray's surgical apprenticeships, teaching experience, and interest in research corresponded well with the faculty's growing orientation towards medical science ... Starr sought to replace the older, 'scientifically untrained' practitioners in the department with surgeon-scientists such as Murray – younger, more scientifically trained surgeons, who alongside their private practices were oriented towards surgical research and clinical instruction."[90] This, then, was the background of the heparin story.[91]

In the early 1930s Charles Best interested Murray in bringing heparin, an anticoagulant that Best and others were developing (see pp. 65–66, into the clinic. Goodness knows, the surgeons were ready for it, given that pulmonary emboli (blood clots in large arteries supplying blood to the lungs) were almost universally fatal and the various thrombi of the circulatory system equally devastating. Patients with pulmonary emboli would, in Bigelow's terms, become "extremely breathless, blue, and sometimes in shock." Pre-heparin the only

Banting was back to Toronto the following spring, with a keen interest in the subject but little experience in laboratory investigation.[109] He was knocking on the door of a Department of Physiology with a long and distinguished history. It has been seen how Archibald Macallum, who founded an independent chair of physiology in 1891, had pioneered the study of physiology in North America. Macleod himself, as Mladen Vranic notes, "was one of the world's leading physiologists, with a particular reputation in the field of carbohydrate metabolism." It was a department, in Vranic's words, "not only well-equipped to carry out the necessary experiments which led to the discovery of insulin, but one willing to gamble on an idea."[110]

"[Banting] arrived about the middle of May, 1921," Macleod later wrote. "I found that Dr. Banting had only a superficial text-book knowledge of the work that had been done on the effects of pancreatic extracts in diabetes."[111] Macleod suggested various approaches, assisted on the first experimental operation, and was involved with the research for nearly a month before leaving for Scotland in mid-June. According to historian Michael Bliss, who has written the definitive history of the discovery of insulin, "the widely held belief that Macleod set Banting and Best to work and then immediately left town for his holidays is not true."[112] During one of the early meetings, Macleod introduced Banting to his two student assistants, Charles Best and Clark Noble, both fourth-year students in the Honours Physiology and Biochemistry course planning to do the master's program with him the next year. Noble later confirmed that the two tossed a coin to see who would work with Banting first; Best won and ended up spending nearly the whole summer on the project.[113] Most of Best's accounts of the discovery omit the coin-tossing incident,[114] and his son and biographer Henry calls it a myth.[115] Best was then twenty-two, just finishing his undergraduate degree with an undergraduate's knowledge of diabetes from Professor Macleod's lectures. His aunt had died in a diabetic coma in 1918 – merely three years previously – so he had a certain personal involvement in the subject. Banting described the working conditions in the small room they had been assigned in the Medical Building during the summer heat, "The place where we were operating was not fit to be called an operating room. Aseptic work had not been done in it for some years. The floor could not be scrubbed properly or the water would go through on the laboratories below … There were dirty windows above the unsterilizable wooden operating table. The operating linen consisted of towels with holes in them."[116]

On July 30 the duo had encouraging results. Some of the pancreatic extract they had prepared lowered blood sugar in one diabetic animal, dog no. 410, as did subsequent injections into two other dogs.[117] On August 9, Banting and Best reported to Macleod that "they had obtained a fall in blood sugar following injections of extracts made from degenerated pancreas." Macleod wrote back encouragingly on the twenty-third, suggesting further experiments "in order that there may be no possibility of mistake … [I]f you can prove to the satisfaction of everyone that these extracts can really have the power to reduce the blood sugar in pancreatic diabetes, you will have achieved a very great deal."[118] Macleod did supply useful guidance, and Best, referring to their first interesting results, said to Macleod, "We followed your directions in preparing the extract."[119] Yet by the time Macleod's reply arrived on September 6, Banting and Best had already implemented several of his earlier suggestions.[120] His claim to have guided them during these crucial summer months must therefore be skeptically assessed.

The research picked up steam during the fall of 1921, yet it did not always go smoothly. Soon after Macleod's return to Toronto, he clashed with Banting, who threatened to "apply to the Rockefeller Institute or the Mayo Clinic"[121] if his demands for a salary and improved working conditions were not met. A day or two later, Macleod "apparently relented," giving the researchers a separate room, offering a part-time lab boy to look after the dogs, and "having the physiology operating-room floor tarred so it could be cleaned properly." Macleod also arranged to have them paid for the summer's work,[122] but as Banting later remarked with some bitterness, Macleod never gave him "an appointment in the Department of Physiology." He was able to remain in Toronto only because Velyien Henderson offered him a temporary post in the pharmacology department to help him make ends meet.[123]

At this point Macleod suggested to Banting and Best that they publish their preliminary results. He helped them edit a draft. "When finally the manuscript was ready," said Macleod, "Banting asked me if I wished my name to appear along with his and Best's, and my reply was that I thanked them but could not do so since it was their work and 'I did not wish to fly under borrowed colours.'"[124] This statement contradicts the widely held belief that Macleod took undue credit for the work done in his lab but would have done nothing to counter Banting's growing resentment as Macleod's polished presentations of the research outshone his own halting attempts, first at the university's Physiological Journal Club on November 16 and more dramatically before the December 30 session of the American Physiological Society at Yale. Bliss noted, "About this time Banting began telling his friends that Professor Macleod was stealing his research."[125]

The dog research belonged to Banting and Best alone, and in the fall of 1921 they prepared a paper on their intravenous injections of extract from dog's pancreas that showed the pancreatic substance "invariably exercises a reducing influence upon the percentage sugar of the blood and the amount of sugar excreted in the urine." The paper was published in February 1922, the first public documentation of the research.[126]

In the meantime Banting moved to extracts from fetal calf pancreas and asked Macleod to invite James B. Collip to help him on the technical side, especially with the preparation of pure extracts. Collip, then twenty-nine, was an experienced researcher who had been promoted to professor of biochemistry at the University of Alberta in 1920 and just arrived in Toronto on sabbatical with a temporary appointment in the Department of Biochemistry.[127] (Historian Alison

Li calls Collip "a member of the first generation of medical researchers to obtain a PhD at a Canadian university and then to pursue a successful research career within the country."[128])

Macleod suggested that the three young men (all were under thirty!) put the pancreatic extracts into living rabbits that had experimentally been rendered diabetic in order to observe the effects on the rabbits' blood sugar. "Within a day or so, Dr. Collip reported that he had tried this and found the blood sugar to be lowered, thus confirming the effectiveness of the extract and making further development of its production for clinical purposes very much more simple since normal rabbits could be used to test its potency instead of depancreated dogs."[129] (Unlike previous researchers, Collip precipitated the insulin out of the pancreas extract with a solution of alcohol, largely freeing it from contaminants: insulin is insoluble in pure alcohol, which previous researchers who also had isolated pancreatic extracts never discovered.)

Word about "isletin," as the researchers were still calling the extract ("insulin" was coined only in April 1922) spread rapidly within the Toronto medical community. In December Banting and Best had a meeting with Walter Campbell, Duncan Graham, and Almon Fletcher from the General.[130] Campbell was already involved with diabetes research, and *Epistaxis* poetized of him in 1921, "C is for Campbell, who dickers with urine. / And says diabetes the nation will ruin."[131] So the meeting came very propitiously for him.

It was now January 1922 and time to try the pancreatic preparation in diabetic patients. After "repeated solicitations" from Banting, Macleod persuaded Duncan Graham to let him and Best try their extract on a case of diabetes in the Toronto General Hospital.[132] On 11 January they administered it to a lad under the clinical care of Walter Campbell. Charles Best tells the story from here: Best had gone to the slaughterhouse and removed the pancreas from a big steer, from which they extracted an insulin solution. "We tested it on diabetic dogs and it was very potent. Then Fred and I gave large doses to each other … The first patient to receive insulin was a very severely diabetic boy, aged 14, Leonard Thompson. The houseman, Ed [Edward S.] Jeffrey on the diabetic ward, gave the injection. Leonard's blood sugar decreased and the first trial was considered a success."[133]

Best's assessment, however, was overly optimistic. Impurities in the extract caused abscesses at the site of injection, and although Thompson was close to death, his doctors decided not to continue the treatment. Now under pressure to prepare a purified extract quickly, Collip refused to give the successful formula to Banting and Best, and a violent confrontation ensued in late January 1922. No contemporary references to the fight have survived. According to Bliss, Clark Noble drew a cartoon of the incident, "unfortunately now lost, of Banting sitting on Collip, choking him; he captioned it 'The Discovery of Insulin.'"[134] Subsequent accounts by Banting and Best indicate their suspicion that Collip intended to patent it himself "and was only prevented from doing so by Professors Macleod, [Connaught Laboratories director Andrew] Hunter, and

Henderson."[135] In a 1940 memoir, Banting described his reaction to Collip's refusal: "He made as if to go. I grabbed him with one hand by the overcoat where it met in front and almost lifting him I sat him down hard on the chair. I do not remember all that was said but I remember telling him that it was a good job he was so much smaller – otherwise I would 'knock hell out of him.'"[136]

Best claimed in a 1954 account that "Banting was thoroughly angry and Collip was fortunate not to be seriously hurt … I can remember restraining Banting with all the force at my command."[137] Best's son Henry provided a more graphic description matching the vanished Noble cartoon: "Banting jumped [Collip] and tried to throttle him. Best pulled them apart, prompting him to say later, 'I may have helped to save millions of diabetic lives, but I know of one life I saved for certain – Bert Collip's.'"[138] Macleod's anodyne comment was, "As a result of Collip's researches a non-irritating highly potent preparation of insulin was supplied to the Medical clinic and was used in the cases reported in the Canadian Medical [Association] Journal [*CMAJ*] in March."[139]

The appearance of the article in the *CMAJ* caused a local sensation. The front page of the *Toronto Daily Star* for March 22 ran the story under the banner headline "Toronto Doctors on Track of Diabetes Cure."[140] There had been a previous scientific report on the dog research in February in the *Journal of Laboratory and Clinical Medicine*, but the public was indifferent to dog research. The main announcement of the discovery to the international medical world, however, was given by Macleod at the May 3 meeting of the Association of American Physicians in Washington, DC. Banting and Best were not present.[141]

Yet there was a problem. When Collip attempted to make large amounts of insulin at the University of Toronto's Antitoxin Laboratories, his batches lacked potency. Then he started having trouble duplicating his original formula even in the lab. The result of this failure was "an insulin famine in Toronto during the spring of 1922" as the whole research team searched frantically to recover the secret, which they eventually did by mid-May.[142] In the meantime Macleod, concerned that someone else would discover and patent their own process, recommended that the Toronto group take out a patent of its own. Because physicians were barred by the Hippocratic oath from profiting from their discoveries – a lost world! – the two nonmedical members of the team, Best and Collip, patented their process of isolating the pancreatic secretion, then transferred the rights to the Board of Governors of the University of Toronto. The purpose of this move was not to prevent others from making the extract but to ensure that no one else could set up a profitable monopoly.

The Toronto group resumed production of insulin after rediscovering the method but could not make nearly enough to meet the demand. They needed outside help. At the recommendation of the research team and J. Gerald FitzGerald of the Connaught Laboratories, the Board of Governors set up an agreement between the University of Toronto and the Eli Lilly Company in Indianapolis, Indiana.[143] The Lilly Company made crucial changes in the production procedure, and the Connaught Labs, in producing their own insulin, just adapted these. Proceeds from the patent license fuelled medical research in Toronto for decades to come.

It was the Department of Medicine at the General that helped move insulin from test tube to bedside. In June 1922 Graham "organized a diabetic clinic on the second floor of the Pavilion" under Campbell, Fletcher, and Goldie.[144] The hospital established a "Metabolic Kitchen" for diabetes and other metabolic conditions as well, the staff of which grew from one dietitian in 1922 to seven in 1931.[145] The Rockefeller Foundation donated $10,000 for its support in 1923.[146] In 1925 Macleod and Campbell published a monograph on the underlying science of insulin and its use in the treatment of diabetes. The preface contained epochal news: "Since it became available, insulin has proved to be of inestimable value in the treatment of diabetes ... By its use combined with intelligent regulation of the diet, the efficiency and the sense of well-being of the patient can be restored practically to normal and life again made reasonably tolerable."[147] On the basis of this kitchen, in 1937 Campbell said, "[D]iabetes is a controllable disorder of metabolism" and described the stringent daily diet required, initiating the dietetics of diabetes.[148]

The clinical results of the use of insulin were among the most dramatic in the history of medicine. Bill Bigelow, a young surgeon, recalled routine scenes several decades after the discovery of insulin: "Patients who were brought into the emergency ward, unconscious in diabetic coma, [and] when they were injected with insulin they awakened dramatically, snatched from death's door."[149]

The historic drama that Michael Bliss recounts – of young lives saved by the availability of insulin – is deeply moving.[150] But lending piquancy is the personal misunderstandings that alienated the investigators from one another. Hoping to settle the matter of credit once and for all, Colonel Albert Gooderham, chairman of the university's Insulin Committee, wrote to Macleod, Banting, and Best on 16 September 1922 – Collip had by this time returned to Alberta – asking each of them for a typewritten statement of their understanding of the discovery. The resulting accounts, though "invaluable sources" to Bliss and subsequent historians, proved impossible to reconcile, and no comprehensive version was ever prepared.[151]

Macleod's response of 20 September provided the longest account, emphasizing his "position with regard to the most unfortunate misunderstandings which have arisen concerning questions of priority ... To Dr. Banting and Mr. Best is ... due full credit for showing that extracts of foetal pancreas have a beneficial effect on experimental diabetes." Banting and Best had offered Macleod the option of putting his name on their original paper but he declined, as many laboratory chiefs would not have done (the practice was standard of head of a laboratory including one's name on a paper whether one had contributed to it or not). "By this step I made it perfectly evident that I considered the full credit for this investigation to be Banting and Best's. This is surely what counts in questions of priority."[152]

In a 1923 addendum, a wounded Macleod expostulated of Banting's continuing protests, "I consider this a most unjust, ungracious and unreasonable attitude. With regard to Dr. Banting being allowed even to start the experiments there are, I imagine, very few directors of laboratories that would have been willing to allow an outside person the free use of whatever animal material was available at the time, of the only operating room and its appliances that the department possessed, of the services of the animal caretaker, of anaesthetics and other surgical necessities, of the chemical apparatus and reagents necessary in the analysis." Moreover, Macleod had made Charles Best available, who was being paid as a research fellow, and paid various salaries and expenses.

Macleod also explained essentially why the research of the Department of Physiology in decades ahead would be dedicated heavily to insulin and pancreatic endocrinology: "The present status of our knowledge of Insulin depends practically entirely on work which has been done in this Department with the collaboration of the Medical Clinic and the Connaught Laboratories. Through concentrated effort, for the co-ordination of which I have been responsible, we have given to Science in little more than one year a practically completed piece of research work – we have proved the value of Insulin."[153]

Banting and Macleod were jointly awarded a Nobel Prize in 1923. An enraged Banting threatened to turn down the prize before being calmed down by Colonel Gooderham, then immediately sent a telegram to Best giving him "equal share in the discovery … hurt that he is not so acknowledged by the Nobel trustees." Macleod, upon hearing this news, shared half of his with Collip.[154] But history is fickle. In the eyes of the public, Banting and Best have retained the historic priority and Macleod has been unjustly forgotten – though in 1926 he authored the book that remained the standard text for decades, *Carbohydrate Metabolism and Insulin*.[155] Yet as Michael Bliss has shown, the discovery was made in an entirely collaborative way. Macleod's name is preserved in a medical auditorium in the faculty named after him. The names Banting and Best are reflected in several buildings of the faculty, in a department of research scientists named after them, and in the memory of a grateful world that the terrible scourge of diabetes had at least been tamed if not banished.

In May 1922, the Board of Governors of the university constituted a Special Committee on Diabetes, later called the Insulin Committee, to administer the several patents arising from the discovery, including the later patent for protamine zinc insulin, and to disburse the royalties for medical research. The final royalty payments arrived in October 1956, and in 1957 the Insulin Committee Trust Fund, by then worth around $3 million, recommended that the funds be "confirmed for the purposes of the Banting and Best Department of Medical Research." This gets ahead of the story a bit but is worth noting here, a member of the committee said, as "the first example of a university undertaking to administer a university invention for the public good."[156] (This is not exactly true, considering the University of Minnesota granted the thyroxine patent to Squibb in 1919.)

Out of insulin came a number of benefits for the University of Toronto. One was the establishment of the Banting Research Foundation, incorporated in July 1925. The background was this: Early in 1923 President Falconer approached the chancellor, Sir William Mulock, asking if the latter might be willing to raise funds for a foundation to honour Banting and to fund medical research now that the benefits of such research for the public welfare were so apparent. Mulock, a former president of U of T and veteran fundraiser from World War I, convened a dinner at the York Club, from which emerged commitments of almost $1 million. In July 1925 a campaign to raise further funds was then launched and the foundation was duly incorporated. An organizing committee recommended a constitution to the Board of Governors and the Alumni Association, and a Board of Trustees for the foundation was organized. In addition to monies from the initial fundraising campaign, the foundation lived over the years from bequests, such as that of $600,000 in 1948 from the estate of Miss Kate E. Taylor.[157]

This development is significant because "from 1926 to 1938 the Banting Research Foundation was virtually the only organization in Canada which offered financial support for Medical Research throughout the country."[158] It is hard to imagine by what a slender thread medical research hung in those days and what large benefits flowed from so little money.

### FitzGerald, Connaught Labs, and the School of Hygiene

*Origins*

The teaching of hygiene and public health goes right back to the refoundation of the faculty in 1887. William Oldright had graduated from the Toronto School of Medicine in 1865, lectured on hygiene there, and was forty-five as he acquired the chair of "hygiene and sanitary science" in 1887 in the newly founded faculty.[159] He came on staff as well at St Michael's Hospital as an associate professor of surgery. (Something of a polymath, Oldright also began lecturing in 1869 on Spanish and Italian in the Faculty of Arts.) At his retirement in 1910, he was praised for his enterprise "in establishing a practical and theoretical course leading to a diploma in Public Health."[160]

By 1903 U of T had a Department of Preventive Medicine, chaired by Charles Sheard, and a Department of Sanitary Science, chaired by Oldright. Sheard, born in Toronto in 1857, was unlike most of the farm boys who became academics before the Second World War; he originated from the upper crust of Toronto. His father was a future mayor of the city, and he himself attended exclusive Upper Canada College and graduated from Trinity Medical School in 1878. He trained further in Europe; acquired his membership in the Royal College of Surgeons of

England; and taught histology, physiology, and clinical medicine at Trinity from 1880 until it joined the Faculty of Medicine in 1903. From 1893 to 1910 he was the city's medical officer of health, where he worked diligently on behalf of testing the milk and water for bacteria and improving the water and sewage systems. In general, Sheard led a rather upper-middle-class lifestyle with a house on Jarvis Street in the days when that was a fashionable address. Historian Heather MacDougall's judgment is that "Sheard's career represented the transition from doctors as 'professional gentlemen' to research scientists." Sheard was known for "diffusing European knowledge among Canadian practitioners." Later involved in politics, he was not exactly focused on academic life, yet it was he who founded the Department of Preventive Medicine.[161]

Oldright stepped down from the chair of hygiene and sanitary science in 1910, succeeded by John Andrew Amyot, an 1891 medical graduate of the University of Toronto and a key figure in the history of public health in Ontario. (In 1910 Amyot also became director of the Provincial Board of Health Laboratory.) Sheard resigned in 1911 from the chair of preventive medicine, and in future years the title Department of Hygiene and Preventive Medicine became used as well as Department of Hygiene.[162]

In 1904 the faculty created a postgraduate Diploma of Public Health program (as it was initially called) to train physicians as medical officers of health for Ontario's local Boards of Health. It attracted no graduates until 1911, however, when an experienced health officer obtained the diploma by examination without taking any courses. The first applicant actually trained by the university was Robert Defries, who began the program in the 1912–13 session and earned his diploma in 1914.[163] Donald T. Fraser, a major scientific figure in the early days of the School of Hygiene, said in 1945, "As far as I am aware this department in the Faculty of Medicine is the first to provide for formal and regular graduate instruction to physicians." Since then, "some 400 physicians have successfully completed their courses of study."[164]

### FitzGerald and the Connaught Antitoxin Laboratories

Although the history of hygiene and public health at the University of Toronto antedate the appearance of John Gerald ("Gerry") FitzGerald, his name is inextricably connected with the development of vaccines in Toronto – the finest work of the School of Hygiene and the Connaught Laboratories. FitzGerald was born in Drayton, Ontario, in 1882 and apprenticed in his father's drugstore. His mother seems to have had some kind of chronic illness, possibly depression, and his father descended into a grief-stricken depression upon her death in 1907.[165] FitzGerald may thus have inherited from both of them the melancholia that dogged him in his later years. He had, in any event, an early tropism towards psychiatry, and after graduating in medicine from U of T in 1903, he served on the staff of a private mental hospital in Toronto run by Campbell

Meyers (who in 1906 organized the psychiatry service at the Toronto General Hospital – see pp. 367–369).

FitzGerald spent the next several years kicking about the asylum world, first at the Buffalo State Hospital, whose superintendent, Arthur Hurd, recommended that he proceed to Hopkins, where his brother, Henry Hurd, was professor of psychiatry. FitzGerald landed a staff post at the Sheppard-Pratt Hospital, a private asylum outside of Baltimore. Clarence B. Farrar, professor of psychiatry in Toronto who knew FitzGerald in those Baltimore years, recalled jolly evenings at the staff table, "where good-natured pleasantries at the expense of one or another of the group were routine, and FitzGerald was likely to be the gayest at the table." After a year, FitzGerald returned to Toronto, taking a post as pathologist at the provincial mental hospital from 1907 to 1908.[166]

Yet his interest shifted from psychiatry to bacteriology, possibly because the one seemed a dead end – a "funereal science" as someone put it[167] – whereas bacteriology appeared to hold the promise of the future. Between 1909 and 1911 he became a lecturer in bacteriology at the University of Toronto.

Married in 1910 to the heiress of a foundry fortune, he and his new bride, Edna Leonard of London, Ontario, were able to summer in Europe. FitzGerald spent the time as a research student at the Pasteur Institutes in Paris and Brussels, "establishing," in the words of medical historian Chris Rutty, "close friendships with Emile Roux, director of the Institute in Paris, as well as other European leaders in the field.[168] This "working honeymoon" marked the beginning of "an extraordinarily intense three-year period" during which FitzGerald repeatedly shuttled back and forth across North America and Europe. In the summer of 1911 he visited the Institute of Pathology in Freiburg and made a quick "side trip to London and the Lister Institute" before travelling 7,000 miles to take up a two-year appointment as an associate professor of bacteriology at the Hearst Laboratory in Berkeley, California. Within eighteen months he had visited four major labs in four different countries. In the spring of 1912, he again hurtled eastward for another working holiday, this time studying the latest advances in the treatment of diphtheria with William Park, director of the New York City Department of Health.

When FitzGerald returned to Toronto following his second year in California, he was eager to apply what he had learned. In 1913 he was invited by Amyot to assist in producing Canada's first indigenous rabies vaccine at the provincial lab during the summer, then take up an appointment as an associate professor in the Department of Hygiene.[169] In all of these venues FitzGerald learned, as his friend Farrar put it, "about the preparations of sera and vaccines for the treatment and prevention of certain infectious diseases."

Farrar continued, "One of his immediate concerns was the alarming death toll of diphtheria among children. The necessary antitoxin was not made in Canada."[170] As of 1913, FitzGerald's grandson James explained, Canada was "one of the few remaining Western nations that still depend[ed] on other countries to supply its preventive medicines." Because few families could afford the prohibitive cost of imported American antitoxin, diphtheria remained the leading killer of children under fourteen, with death rates from the asphyxiating throat inflammation of up to 12 percent in the first decade of the century.[171] In a 2004 interview, James added, "[M]y grandfather thought this was appalling, and he just said 'I can make this medicine myself here, because I now have the expertise' – and he was the only man in Canada really who had it at that point."[172]

Encouraged by his success with the rabies vaccine, FitzGerald "boldly proposed to the University of Toronto that he manufacture a safe, effective Canadian-made antitoxin for diphtheria, and distribute it free or at cost ... to boards of health across Canada."[173] The university's Board of Governors was uneasy about linking their academic mission to the commercial production of a drug and unwilling to fund a laboratory for FitzGerald. So with $3,000 from his wife's inheritance, in December 1913 he built a small stable at 145 Barton Avenue, fitted it out with lab equipment, bought four aging horses "bound for the glue factory for about $5 each and hired a technician." The horses – named "Crestfallen," "Surprise," "Fireman," and "JHC" – were injected on 1 February 1 1914 with diphtheria toxin;[174] in March, after their immune systems produced antitoxin, the serum was harvested and the antitoxin extracted. The same month, the Ontario Board of Health agreed to purchase it for 35¢ per thousand units (representing a 10¢ profit margin for the lab), and the first batch was sold on 31 March at one-fifth the going commercial price.

In April 1914, just before the outbreak of war, the Board of Governors approved the Antitoxin Laboratory as part of the Department of Hygiene, and on 1 May the lab, stuffed into the basement of the Medical Building, opened for business.[175] Private investors in Toronto sprang to FitzGerald's assistance, including Colonel Albert Gooderham, commanding officer of the Royal Grenadiers, an officer of the Canadian Red Cross, and member of the Board of Governors of the University of Toronto. As the antitoxin was distributed in Ontario, the death rate from diphtheria fell from 31 per 100,000 cases in 1903 to 12 in 1918. "Deaths from diphtheria are preventable," said FitzGerald, "and delay in the administration of antitoxin is one of the most important reasons why deaths continue as a result of this disease."[176]

In 1915 Colonel Gooderham offered to the university a 57-acre farm on Dufferin Street (north of what was then Toronto), where FitzGerald was able to construct more extensive laboratories and mass-produce diphtheria and tetanus antitoxins that he sold to the provinces of Canada, which distributed them free to the population. During the war there was a huge demand for tetanus antitoxin for the armed forces. Gooderham asked only that the farm be named after the Duke of Connaught, who had been the governor general of Canada, so in 1917 the facility was renamed the Connaught Antitoxin Laboratories. Laboratory insiders, however, always referred to it as "The Farm." In July 1920 the

Connaught Labs became an independent unit within the university, reporting directly to a "Connaught Committee" appointed by the Board of Governors; in 1923 the committee approved shortening the name to "Connaught Laboratories" to reflect the facility's expansion into research and the preparation of insulin and other products.[177]

Amid the horrors of the Great War, Canada had achieved a significant public health triumph: In contrast to past conflicts, where eight soldiers died of disease for each one killed in battle, the proportion dropped to one in twenty. The Connaught Labs contributed in no small measure to this reversal, producing one-fifth of all the serums used by Britain and her allies.[178] Close on the heels of this advance came a second triumph for Toronto with the discovery of insulin in 1921–2. These were momentous developments.

### The School of Hygiene

Meanwhile, on the academic side, hygiene was a gathering concept. After completing his course work for the Diploma in Public Health (DPH) in the 1913–14 academic year – but before sitting the exam – Defries became a demonstrator in hygiene, FitzGerald teaching the course. This was the beginning of a twenty-seven-year partnership and also marked the start of public health education in Ontario and beyond: the second graduating class included John W.S. McCullough, the chief officer of health for the province, and A. Grant Fleming, who became a professor of preventive medicine at McGill in the 1920s.[179]

Following the creation of a federal Department of Health in 1919, Amyot was made the first deputy minister of health. He turned over his academic duties at the University of Toronto to FitzGerald, who was then promoted to the first full professorship in the Department of Hygiene and Preventive Medicine. FitzGerald proceeded to appoint Defries and other Connaught staff members to the teaching staff – thereby formally linking the university department with the lab[180] – and to upgrade both undergraduate and postgraduate instruction in public health, transforming the DPH from an apprenticeship program to a comprehensive full-year curriculum. In 1924 he pushed through a regulation mandating a field course in preventive medicine for all medical undergraduates.[181]

In May 1924 the Rockefeller Foundation gave the university $650,000 for a School of Hygiene ($400,000 for a building, $250,000 for the endowment).[182] This donation constituted the Rockefeller Foundation's second big gift to the Faculty of Medicine; the first, of $1 million, was conveyed in 1920–1.[183] "Over the next two years, a stately red-brick, four-storey School of Hygiene [was constructed] on the southern edge of the University of Toronto campus adjacent to the twin-towered medical school, at 150 College Street."[184] It was formally opened on 8 June 1927, with a ceremony in Convocation Hall, following which the assembled dignitaries proceeded to tour the new facility with FitzGerald leading the way, "flanked by his wife and sister, the Bantings, and the Bests."[185] Toronto's

School of Hygiene was to be one of three in North America being funded by the International Health Board of the Rockefeller Foundation, the others (called "Schools of Public Health") at Johns Hopkins University and at Harvard.

In 1924 FitzGerald became director of the School of Hygiene, which, like the Connaught Laboratories, was not part of the Faculty of Medicine but reported directly to the president and the Board of Governors. The Connaught Labs were adjoined to the new school, and the antitoxin and insulin units merged "to constitute a public-service section of the School." The Connaught Laboratories Research Fund was also to contribute to the endowment.[186]

Among FitzGerald's leadership team in both institutions were Robert Defries and Donald Fraser. Both became significant figures in the history of Toronto medicine.

Robert Davies Defries was thirty-eight years old when the School of Hygiene opened in 1927; he firmly established himself as FitzGerald's right-hand man. A native of Toronto and 1911 medical graduate, he was awarded an MD the following year for postgraduate work in biochemistry under Macallum before, as seen earlier, becoming the first applicant for the DPH course. His first public health appointment outside the Faculty of Medicine was as assistant bacteriologist to the Ontario Board of Health in 1913–14; then in February 1915 FitzGerald asked him to head up tetanus antitoxin production for the army at the Department of Hygiene's Antitoxin Laboratory (housed at the time in the medical school's basement). In 1916 Defries was named assistant director of the lab and the following year became associate director at the newly established Connaught Antitoxin Laboratories north of the city. He remained in that position until 1940 when he succeeded FitzGerald as the second director of both Connaught and the School of Hygiene until his retirement in 1955.[187]

Defries was instrumental in the research and production of numerous vaccines and other products and in the wartime expansion of Connaught and the School of Hygiene. During the Second World War, antitoxin production required the purchase of more than 1,100 horses, housed in temporary buildings at the Farm and in Hamilton. To accommodate the school's research and production of penicillin and blood products for the war effort, he persuaded the Board of Governors to purchase the former Knox College building on Spadina Crescent. (This facility became known as the Spadina Division.)[188] Like his predecessor FitzGerald, Defries was involved in numerous scientific and health organizations, including the U of T's Insulin Committee, the Dominion Council of Health, and the Canadian Public Health Association (editing the latter's journal for more than thirty-five years). Following the war, he oversaw the Connaught Labs' production and supply of nearly all of the polio virus used in the 1954 field trials of the Salk poliomyelitis vaccine in both Canada and the United States. For this achievement, as well as for his "distinguished leadership in the development of preventive medicine and public health throughout Canada," Defries was honoured with a Lasker Award in 1955.[189]

Defries's life was shaped by the early death of his father and the influence of his stern and pious mother, who "relentlessly pushed both her sons to become ascetic, self-sacrificing doctors."[190] The earnest "Bobby" took these lessons to heart, his entry in *Torontonensis* describing him as "one who will never spare himself if he can be of help to others."[191] An evangelical Presbyterian, he entered the public health field with the intention of becoming a medical missionary but was persuaded by FitzGerald to devote himself instead to developing the discipline in Toronto and Canada.[192] He nevertheless remained a staunch supporter of Bloor Street Presbyterian (later United) Church and of medical missionary activities,[193] and he never married, living with his widowed mother until her death in 1942.[194]

Donald Thomas Fraser, thirty-nine as of 1927, was the son of William H. Fraser, long-time head of the departments of Spanish and Italian at the university. Donald obtained a degree in arts, then graduated in medicine in 1915. After service in the war, he joined the Connaught Labs in 1918 and became a lecturer in the Department of Hygiene and Preventive Medicine two years later, obtaining his DPH in 1921. His scientific contributions included developing a mouse assay for insulin; he was, as his eulogist put it, "the first to publish on this subject."[195] Fraser was among the Canadian leaders in the war against diphtheria in the middle decades of the twentieth century and cut an international profile in the rising field of immunology. A trial led by Fraser in 1943 established the effectiveness of tetanus toxoid with the typhoid element added (TAB T) and the workability of the recall schedule (a recall dose should coincide with "the entry of troops into the combat zone").[196]

At the School of Hygiene, Fraser assumed much of the responsibility for the text of FitzGerald's textbook, *An Introduction to the Practice of Preventive Medicine* (which Mosby of St Louis published in 1922), and helped plan the expansion of the school building in the early 1930s. By 1933 he was not only a full professor but the de facto head of the department as FitzGerald's other responsibilities multiplied. He also distinguished himself as a mentor: as colleague Donald A. Scott later remarked, "'Ask Fraser' was a common solution to any baffling problem facing researchers or students in the School of Hygiene Building."[197] Following FitzGerald's death in 1940 Fraser officially became the head of the Department of Hygiene and Preventive Medicine as well as the associate director of both the School of Hygiene and the Connaught Laboratories;[198] he remained in that position until his death during an official visit to Santiago, Chile, in July 1954.[199]

In addition to his scientific accomplishments, Fraser excelled at combining research with a humanistic focus and remained part of the larger university community. The Frasers lived in an exclusive little enclave of Toronto called Wychwood Park along with numerous other university figures. At the time of his death in 1954, Dean MacFarlane summed up that broadly learned quality that had clung to Fraser throughout his career (and that characterized his son, pediatrician Donald Fraser, as well): "He had what another bacteriologist, Dr Hans Zinsser, has described as 'a type of learning that cannot be acquired by study alone, but represents the ripening of gifted minds that are attracted by everything about them worthy of interest.'"[200]

When the new School of Hygiene opened its doors in 1927 with FitzGerald as director, it consisted of three departments: Hygiene and Preventive Medicine (which continued as a joint department of the school and the Faculty of Medicine); Epidemiology and Biometrics; and Physiological Hygiene. The Department of Hygiene and Preventive Medicine was the largest of the three, with twelve part-time faculty members, including FitzGerald as professor and Defries and Fraser as associate professors.

The Department of Epidemiology and Biometrics was established in 1924 and until the early 1930s was largely a three-person operation, with Defries as head, assisted by Neil McKinnon and Mary Ross. The department also included two part-time instructors from the provincial health department: John W.S. McCullough, the chief officer of health for Ontario, who taught public health administration, and Albert Berry, a demonstrator in public health engineering.[201]

McKinnon, thirty-three in 1927, had graduated from U of T in 1921, selecting for the university yearbook the motto, "I am in earnest; I will not equivocate; I will not excuse; I will not retreat a single inch, and I will be heard."[202] Of tough Highland Scots ancestry (and a speaker of Gaelic),[203] McKinnon was known for his strong opinions and forceful manner. Although not always popular or easy to get along with, he established a reputation, in the words of historian Paul A. Bator, as "one of the unique characters in the School of Hygiene," gaining respect "as a serious teacher who constantly challenged his students to give evidence for their views and who presented them with issues of philosophy and humanism." By 1930 he had become an assistant professor at the school and was head of its Department of Epidemiology from 1944 until his retirement in 1962.[204] In the summer of 1932 he was also appointed as director of the Connaught farm and relocated with his family to a house on the property, becoming as well one of FitzGerald's closest confidants during his troubled last years.[205]

Mary Ross, another original member of the department, was a nonphysician who spent five months at the Johns Hopkins School of Public Health studying epidemiology before beginning her responsibilities at the School of Hygiene. She assisted McKinnon in conducting a major field study of diphtheria toxoid in 1927 (detailed later) and prepared a statistical analysis of mortality from the disease in Ontario between 1880 and 1925 for her 1928 MA thesis at the school. In 1934 she earned her PhD for further work on the decline in mortality and morbidity from diphtheria and other diseases in the province.[206] Defries, McKinnon, and Ross emphasized "the imaginative use of statistics in the planning and direction of health services" in instructing DPH students, and they put this policy into practice by upgrading the collection of vital statistics in Canada, particularly in the classification of causes of stillbirth and morbidity. Their work resulted in the creation of a new death registration certificate by the Dominion Bureau of Statistics.[207]

The Department of Physiological Hygiene, the third original academic unit, benefited from the international renown of Charles H. Best, who headed the department between 1927 and 1941. Although not formally connected with the Faculty of Medicine's Department of Physiology, the two were closely linked, especially after Best succeeded Macleod as professor of physiology in 1929, becoming at age thirty (and only four years after obtaining his medical degree) one of the youngest departmental chairs in the history of the faculty. Yet such was the magnitude of the insulin discovery that he was instantly lionized.

After becoming professor of physiology in the faculty, Best resigned his administrative responsibilities as an assistant director at Connaught but remained a research member in addition to his position at the School of Hygiene.[208] For the next thirty-five years he was closely involved with both the Department of Physiology and Connaught, beginning by assembling a heparin team just after assuming the chair (see p. 65). Following Fred Banting's death in an airplane crash in February 1941, Best was appointed head of the faculty's Banting and Best Department of Medical Research in addition to continuing as head of physiology. He gave up his position in the school at that point[209] but remained an honorary consultant to the Connaught Labs.

In his later years, Best was plagued by depressive illness (having apparently a family history), beginning with a possible bout in the 1950s, then a distinct episode in 1963, followed by a severe depressive experience the following year. He was obliged by illness to step down as chair of physiology in 1965. In 1978, Best became critically ill just after hearing of the death of his older son, Sandy, and died shortly thereafter.[210] Said his eulogist at the Faculty Council at the time of his death, "Dr. Best was a man of action, a realistic, hard taskmaster, but also a kind man. A genuine understanding of human misery was an outstanding trait of his personality."[211]

*Connaught between the Wars*

In the years to come, the Connaught Laboratories contributed to public health by developing a variety of vaccines and other drugs. The usefulness of liver in the regeneration of hemoglobin in pernicious anemia had been noted in 1926 by George Minot and William P. Murphy at Harvard.[212] Minot suffered from diabetes and had been treated with insulin at the Toronto General Hospital, so he told Charles Best of their findings, and Best asked Earle W. McHenry at the Connaught Labs to develop a liver extract for clinical use. By 1929 McHenry had devised a suitably purified oral extract, by 1931 an extract for intramuscular injection. Defries later said that McHenry's success was "the result of the high degree of purification which he obtained." Working together with Ray Farquharson at the General, they established the efficacy of the extract in a trial of more than sixty patients with pernicious anemia, publishing in the *Canadian Medical Association Journal* in 1933. "Liver extract prepared for intramuscular administration … has been found safe, dependable, and effective when used in adequate dosage," they concluded.[213]

The clinical story of heparin at the General has been told. The physiological story transpired at the labs. Here is how heparin developed: In 1916 Jay McLean at Johns Hopkins University extracted from dog liver a substance that delayed the coagulation of the blood, named "heparin" two years later by William Henry Howell and Luther Emmett Holt at Hopkins, who isolated it.[214] But the substance was impure and could be produced only in small amounts. In 1929 David A. Scott and Arthur F. Charles at Connaught embarked upon an effort to overcome these roadblocks, learning that heparin could be derived from beef liver with an alkaline aqueous extraction. Several further technical steps were required, and by 1933 they had devised a method capable of extracting heparin from large lots of beef liver, with a yield of about 1,000 units per pound, indeed doubling this return by letting the raw liver sit for a day ("autolyse") before extraction. After 1935 they used only beef lung, also a source of heparin, because it was cheaper.

The crude heparin extract they came up with in 1934 was not usable clinically, but by 1936 Scott and Charles succeeded in purifying the crystalline pure sodium salt that, as has been shown, surgeon Gordon Murray immediately employed in operations on blood vessels. The preparation of the extract created such foul odor that in 1937 heparin extraction was shifted from the Hygiene Building on College Street to the Connaught farm, which processed about 400 pounds of beef liver a day.[215] In 1938 Best and his younger colleague in the Department of Physiology Donald Solandt showed how heparin could prevent the formation of thrombi in the coronary vessels of dogs. "The availability of a potent solution of heparin which can safely be administered to human patients … makes necessary a consideration of the possibility of clinical application of these findings," they wrote.[216] The following year Solandt and Best experimentally produced cardiac mural thrombosis in dogs, demonstrating that heparin would prevent the formation of such thrombi.[217]

Scott and Albert Fisher at the laboratories determined that adding zinc to protamine insulin increased the miscibility of the insulin (Best had obtained some protamine insulin from Hans Christian Hagedorn in Denmark; protamine prolonged the action of the insulin). The laboratories began distribution of protamine zinc insulin in 1936, and the TGH insulin team of Robert B. Kerr (then a junior staffer), Campbell, and Fletcher, together with Best, reported on its use in diabetes ("gives promise of being an important contribution to the restoration of a more physiological state in the diabetic patient").[218] In 1938 Kerr and Best demonstrated experimentally that the duration of action of protamine insulin was much longer than with regular insulin, permitting the maintenance of low blood sugar without a "hypoglycemic reaction."[219]

In the years between 1919 and 1939 the laboratories developed – in addition to the diphtheria toxoid (discussed on p. 68) – a long list of antitoxins, toxoids, and vaccines, a detailed discussion of which would range too far afield; among the most important were scarlet fever streptococcus toxin (the "Dick Test," 1924) and antitoxin (1930); staphylococcus toxoid and antitoxin (1934–5); tetanus toxoid (which P.A.T. Sneath began in 1927, following the discovery of tetanus toxoid at the Pasteur Institute); and Nelles Silverthorne's preparation of a practicable pertussis (whooping cough) vaccine in 1936.[220] Of the pertussis vaccine, Alan Brown, professor of pediatrics, said, in the words of a journalist, "Results obtained with whooping cough vaccine perfected in conjunction with the Connaught laboratories indicate that 98 percent of the children inoculated are rendered immune, so that 'the universal use of this vaccine will result in the saving of many lives.'"[221] These accomplishments, poorly remembered today, all took place on FitzGerald's watch.

### FitzGerald and the School of Hygiene to 1940

An important feature of the School of Hygiene during FitzGerald's tenure was the familial (if paternalistic and hierarchical) spirit he sought to instil in his senior staff. He established a special "officers' mess" for the scientists (the male ones only!) where he always sat in a chair reserved for him at the head table.[222] "Tea was also served in the late afternoon" to this inner circle as a further venue for collegial discussion, "a tradition carried on by FitzGerald's successor," Defries. Yet these gatherings were evidently quieter affairs than those FitzGerald enjoyed during his early psychiatric sojourn in Baltimore – no longer the source of jocularity at the staff table, "he detested noise and loud laughter or singing."[223]

He was also a proponent of healthful living, mandating regular physical checkups for the entire staff and maintaining a full cafeteria at the school under the direction of a trained dietician. He also ran "a mandatory program of recreational sports, including an annual golf tournament and regular games of deck tennis on the windy roof of the School of Hygiene." The scientific staff were also keen on running around the track at Hart House (the university's athletic centre, at the time also restricted to men) and swimming as many lengths of its pool "as time allow[ed]." In 1930 an annual competition was launched for the "FitzGerald Cup, a silver, foot-tall trophy with the names of the annual winners carved into plaques." FitzGerald and Best, the keenest athletes in the group, were the only two-time winners.[224]

The Department of Hygiene and Preventive Medicine remained the largest department in the School of Hygiene throughout FitzGerald's tenure, becoming the "launching pad for a number of lifelong careers at the School."[225] Frieda Fraser, Donald Fraser's sister and a physician and scientist in her own right, completed her MB at Toronto in 1925 and joined the staff of the department in 1927 as a demonstrator in hygiene. Her work on scarlet fever streptococcus toxin and antitoxin between 1927 and 1936 was important, although active immunization against the disease was eventually rendered unnecessary with the introduction of the sulfonamides in the mid-1930s and penicillin in the 1940s.[226] She eventually rose to the rank of full professor, moving from the department to the school's Department of Microbiology in 1956.[227] Other departmental "alumni" included Milton Brown, appointed as a demonstrator in 1931, who became the third head of the department in 1956, and Frank Wishart, who lectured on immunology and later took over direction of the building's immunization clinic.[228] Like Fraser, he became a professor in the microbiology department in 1955.[229]

By 1930, the building of the school, as the university division of the Connaught Laboratories, needed to be enlarged to accommodate both its academic mission and its rapidly growing insulin and liver extract production. Seizing the initiative, FitzGerald personally contacted F.F. Russell of the Rockefeller Foundation to seek support. The foundation agreed on the condition that the additional costs be shared by Connaught's research fund and an increase in the annual grant to the labs from the Province of Ontario. The following April the deal was finalized, with Connaught (and the province) putting up $350,000 and the Rockefeller Foundation providing an additional $600,000, thereby increasing the total grant to the School of Hygiene to $1,250,000.[230]

In autumn 1932 the northern wing of the Hygiene Building (later called the FitzGerald Building) was completed, and the Department of Hygiene had space for its rapidly growing graduate program, which was attracting young physicians from many parts of Canada who then returned home with their diplomas in public health to spread modern concepts.[231] In 1930 the department established the school's first sub-department, "Chemistry in Relation to Hygiene" – a parallel to the faculty's big departments of pathological chemistry and biochemistry – under the leadership of chemist Peter J. Moloney, another of FitzGerald's key recruits.

Born in 1891, Moloney completed an MA in chemistry at U of T in 1915 and joined the staff of Connaught Laboratories in September 1919. He assisted in the purification of insulin in the early 1920s and received his PhD in 1924 for a dissertation based on this experience. Moloney was one of the first scientists without a medical degree recruited to Connaught and the School of Hygiene, and as historian Paul Bator pointed out, "His contributions revealed the growing importance of non-medical specialists in public health."[232] During his lengthy career – which extended for nearly two decades past his official retirement in 1961 – Moloney went on to become one of the founders of the discipline of immunochemistry.[233] (For improving methods of producing heparin at Connaught he received a Gairdner Award in 1967.)

Chief among Moloney's early achievements was his involvement in introducing diphtheria toxoid, a denatured and safer version of the diphtheria antitoxin, which had been discovered in 1923 by Gaston Ramon at the Pasteur Institute in Paris. The following year, FitzGerald visited Ramon in Paris,[234] where he "became so impressed by the new toxoid that he immediately called Dr. Peter J. Moloney at Connaught ... and asked him to drop everything"[235] and begin duplicating Ramon's methods. In 1925 Moloney became the first scientist in North America to prepare the toxoid and in addition made a critical contribution to its safe use by developing a skin test to identify children who would react adversely to the new vaccine.[236]

In results published in 1931, McKinnon and Mary Ross from the school's Department of Epidemiology and Statistics, along with F.S. Burke from the Toronto health department, conducted a field trial of the new toxoid on 30,000 schoolchildren. In the absence of immunization, the 16,829 high-risk children who received it would have had an estimated 222 cases of diphtheria. Given the toxoid, the actual number of cases was twenty-three. There were no deaths. "This is a reduction of approximately 90 percent," the authors concluded.[237] The toxoid had virtually banished diphtheria, the once-feared childhood killer, in Toronto and wherever else it was given, usually in combination with pertussis and tetanus vaccines.

The conquest of diphtheria represented another major scientific advance for FitzGerald and his colleagues, as their field trials "made history by statistically demonstrating for the first time the value of a non-living vaccine in preventing a specific disease."[238] Yet because the findings were initially reported mainly in the *Canadian Journal of Public Health* rather than in the international literature, this breakthrough was not widely known for some time. In addition, the British authorities, who had a much more cautious approach to preventive medicine, remained unconvinced and failed to launch a decisive vaccination campaign until 1941.[239] The Americans got the message much more quickly. According to James FitzGerald, "Toronto and Hamilton were the first cities in the world to be diphtheria-free – like wiped out, eradicated. So that's one of the big feathers in their hat. And that's why people started taking notice, and Rockefeller started sending people here. And Toronto became the international hub. This is what Canadians don't know, is that we became the lighthouse School [of Public Health, or Public Hygiene] in the world ... They were doing a lot of firsts."[240]

The 1930s were years of great activity for FitzGerald. Between 1930 and 1936 he served on the Health Organization of the League of Nations, travelling to Geneva to attend its semiannual congresses; in May 1931 he was selected as one of the six scientific directors of the Rockefeller Foundation's International Health Division, becoming the first Canadian named to the position; and at U of T, he received his "third major appointment within the space of months" upon becoming dean of the Faculty of Medicine, effective January 1932. (During this era the deanship was still a part-time post held in connection with some other headship; FitzGerald also remained director of the School of Hygiene.) According to his grandson James, the decanal appointment was "seen as a clear endorsement of Gerry's vision, a recognition by the faculty and university of the growing importance of hygiene and preventive medicine in the medical curricula."[241] FitzGerald was also close to the Rockefeller Foundation, serving them in various capacities.

*Eclipse*

In the fall of 1936, FitzGerald stepped down from the deanship and took a leave of absence from the university in order to undertake a nine-month project for the Rockefeller Foundation, "touring eighty-five medical schools in twenty-seven countries in North America and Europe" to investigate the "state of undergraduate teaching in preventive medicine."[242] When he returned to Toronto the following June, "[c]olleagues were quietly shocked by his haggard appearance; in the space of a nine-month trip living out of a suitcase, he seems to have aged twenty years."[243] The graduating class photos for the School of Hygiene confirm his rapid decline: in the 1937–8 picture his hair has "turn[ed] completely white in one year."[244] The official explanation of FitzGerald's subsequent breakdown was thus "overwork." The poor man had merely collapsed from the strain. But the story is more malignant.

Already in 1932, as he began his first tour as dean, was there a hint of depressive ideation? In accepting the office he told the Faculty Council, "[N]o one, I am sure, can be more deeply conscious of the shortcomings and inadequacies of your newly appointed Dean than I am."[245] A reflexive kind of self-deprecation is often appropriate for such ceremonial occasions, but still.

According to his grandson James, Gerry FitzGerald was troubled with insomnia and migraine headaches from 1932 on; during the summer of 1938 he spent nearly two months in a London hospital with a haemorrhaging duodenal ulcer. He sailed home at the end of September, determined to resume his work, but after a final brief effort of rallying himself to escort Governor General John Buchan around the Connaught Labs on 23 November, he collapsed in his office and was hospitalized in the grips of a psychotic depression.[246] "I mark that as the moment when he really fell apart," James said.[247]

In February 1939 he made his first suicide attempt, with Nembutal tablets (the barbiturate pentobarbital), falling into a coma but recovering. His old friend Farrar arranged for his admission to the Retreat in Hartford, Connecticut, a private and very expensive psychiatric hospital, though owing to his high professional standing, FitzGerald was charged the charity ward rate of $17.50 per week[248]). McKinnon took him down, FitzGerald, reluctant to go, begging him, "Don't let them, don't take me, don't take me." At Hartford he had fifty-seven insulin shock treatments. FitzGerald wrote in a letter to Farrar, "I am a disgrace to my family ... I should be taken outside and shot." Though not a religious man, he asked for a Catholic priest, saying that he had committed an unpardonable sin for which "the penalty is death."

In April 1940, "Gerry returned to Toronto and tried to resume work. But on June 16, 1940, in a state of paranoia he told his wife that the University of Toronto was out to get him." He overdosed with Nembutal a second time and was admitted to

Toronto General Hospital, under the care of Ray Farquharson. "On June 20, 1940, as my grandfather lay recovering from the toxic drug overdose ... a nurse placed a tray of food on his lap. When she withdrew, he grasped the knife and ... felt for the femoral artery in his thigh, and stabbed his flesh again and again. In less than five minutes, John Gerald FitzGerald was dead. He was 57."[249]

The details of this story were known to only a handful of insiders.[250] "Imagine the shock," said James. "Dean of Medicine kills himself in TGH." A wider circle was aware, however, that he had committed suicide, although the story never reached the public press. His hospital chart disappeared. Such was the stigma attached to suicide that people froze when they heard FitzGerald's name. James describes the memorial service for his grandfather held on the stage of Convocation Hall, the university's main lecture hall. "When people were invited to view the body, only a single soul – an elderly caretaker who had worked for my grandfather for years – shuffled up to the stage and gazed at his face. My grandmother suppressed a cry of anguish. No one else came forward."

A vast silence settled upon the memory of John Gerald FitzGerald and upon many of the triumphs that the School of Hygiene had achieved in the early decades. "Almost eradicated," said James in an interview. "It's almost as if that unpardonable sin ... had caused this amnesia, or wiping out this great achievement. But I'm saying, 'Wait a minute. Just look at the achievement. Forget the suicide for a second.'" From the historical viewpoint of this author, what is interesting is the fact that all of this has slumbered in semiforgetfulness because of the suicide. To this thought, James FitzGerald replied, "I believe so."

There is an interesting historical lesson here for those who write histories of faculties of medicine. The facts, the achievements and journal articles, do not speak for themselves. History edits things in strange ways. It was the personal hell of one man, who happened to be the director of the School of Hygiene and the dean of the faculty, that caused this story of the vaccines that triumphed over infectious disease almost to be lost. The old School of Hygiene was dissolved in 1975. But this tradition of progress in health has come to life again with the foundation in 2008 of the Dalla Lana School of Public Health in the Faculty of Medicine. As Dean Catharine Whiteside noted in 2008, "The Dalla Lana School builds on the Faculty's pioneering work in public health as well as the ongoing tradition of excellence, and it will help our modern world tackle new challenges faced by health care systems internationally."[251]

### From 1887 to 1932

In January 1932 retiring dean Alexander Primrose looked back on the past forty or so years of the history of the faculty he had joined in 1888. Although the faculty had been refounded a year previously, it was in 1887 still located in the single building in the east end of Toronto that had been home to the Toronto School of Medicine. Since then, he said, "The laboratory equipment has gradually increased until at present we have a series of buildings in which the various departments are adequately housed." First came the so-called "Medical Building" that he dated from 1902 but was really ready for occupancy only in 1903. Then came the Pathology Building on the grounds of the Toronto General Hospital in 1911. There followed the Anatomy Building just after World War I and the School of Hygiene in 1927, "made possible by the munificent gifts from the Rockefeller Foundation." It was, he said, "a far cry" from "the small brick building ... to the series of fine laboratory buildings and hospitals which now constitute the teaching quarters of the Faculty of Medicine of the University of Toronto."[252] Yet there was more to come.

## An Appendix to the Chapter: Further Eaton Gifts

The Department of Medicine later had some difficulty reconstituting the story of the Eaton gifts because the files had vanished and memories started to fade. In 1969 Kager Wightman, the professor of medicine, told Dean Chute, "Professor Graham tells me that the original donation was merely to support a full-time Professor and Department Head – at first more or less on a quinquennial basis. After about three years (1922?) the University at the urging of Sir Robert Falconer, set up the Sir John and Lady Eaton Professorship as a named Chair in recognition of the generosity of the family ... This really means that John David Eaton may have something to say about what their money is used for." Wightman said that Graham was "positively contemptuous about my (our) lack of knowledge of the history of the situation."[253] It is unclear how the Eaton Chair was financed in the 1920s and early 1930s.

In 1937 the Eaton gift was renewed in the amount of $25,000 per year for five years. This attracted wide notice, including an editorial in the *Globe and Mail* that saluted the public benefits of support for science: "Because of such gifts the Department of Medicine of the University of Toronto has become noted throughout the world for its research work and its assistance to research workers ... If the scourges to which humanity is heir are to be overcome, there remains to be done a vast amount of research work ... By virtue of these contributions in money, other now baffling diseases [aside from diabetes] will be understood and mastered. In what better way can citizens who can afford to do so benefit the human race?"[254]

When in 1944 the Eaton gift was renewed, William Goldie – who had retired from teaching in 1928 – was again the liaison between the family and the faculty. In July 1944 he sent President Henry John Cody a cheque for $125,000 the Eatons had given him and wondered what the best way might be for the family to endow a permanent chair in medicine. Would there have to be a change in provincial budget arrangements? He reminded Cody that not only had the department been "efficient" in making medical discoveries but "has also materially contributed to the War effort, for the men trained by the Medical Department have shown distinguished leadership in the Army, Navy and Air Force."[255]

In 1946 the Eaton Company gave the university a further $375,000. This and the 1944 cheque were intended to establish a $500,000 Endowment Fund for the Sir John and Lady Eaton Chair of Medicine, which would produce an annual interest payment of around $15,000 for the Department of Medicine. Meanwhile, unspent portions of past grants had accumulated in the Endowment Fund. This unexpended balance was used for salaries of members of the Department of Medicine returning from military service. In consequence, Graham told Smith, the expenditures of the Department of Medicine were greater than the revenue from the Endowment fund and the department would need "to increase very substantially the University grant to the Department to maintain a pre-war basis of work."[256] Today, these do not seem like large sums but at the time they were considerable. The Eaton family stands historically as the first great benefactor of the Faculty of Medicine. Many other benefactors were to follow.

# 5  Big Deeds

After the Second World War, academic medicine in Toronto made several very large strides with worldwide implications. These steps occurred in the areas of neurological surgery, heart surgery, the victory over polio, and – the great medical watchword in the 1990s and after – the discovery of stem cells at the University of Toronto.

## Teaching Hospitals

In the background of these strides were the teaching hospitals of Toronto. Just after the war there were three of them, though numerous others later joined the story.

The queen bee of Toronto medicine is the Toronto General Hospital. Established in 1812, it was the oldest and largest general hospital in English Canada and in 1945 had around 1,200 beds. By the time this story picks up, it had moved from its site on Gerrard Street in Toronto's east end (where it began in 1855) to its College Street site in 1913. It expanded from there to include tall towers in the entire block that runs south and east from the intersection of College Street (a major east–west avenue) and University Avenue (a major north–south route). Toronto General Hospital, or just "the General," was the original teaching hospital of the faculty, and all the early generations of medical students learned on its wards. The General dominated academic medicine in Toronto, and its great barons did so in a rather lordly way. As obstetrician Jim Goodwin later said, "Immediately after the [Second World] War, the place was called the House of Lords, and nothing else mattered. The General was just the place. And the surgeons were very lofty, just arrogant as they could be, and I will not mention names, but they just were."[1]

The wards themselves were divided into two categories: the single rooms for "private patients," whom clinicians admitted on a fee-for-service basis, and the open public wards in the main College Building consisting of long rows of beds, where patients paid no fees, physicians received no honoraria, and medical students received hands-on instruction. In a tit-for-tat, clinicians lived off the income from their private patients whom they saw on "the Pavilion" in the General and in their offices in the Medical Arts Building. In exchange, mainly for the recognition and whatever pleasure the involvement in teaching and research brought, they ranked as members of the Faculty of Medicine and had university appointments as junior or senior lecturer or, the very few, as "Professor." (For readers unfamiliar with Toronto topography, the hospitals of "University Row," on University Avenue, are at the absolute heart of town. The university campus, with its Faculty of Medicine buildings, is slightly to the north and west, and the Medical Arts Building, at the corner of St George and Bloor Streets, is just north and west of the campus. The Medical Arts Building was erected in 1928 in a cooperative effort of 200 physicians and surgeons headed by Alexander Primrose.[2])

The second teaching hospital of the faculty in 1945 was St Michael's Hospital in the east end on Queen Street. A Catholic hospital, it was founded in 1892 by the Sisters of St Joseph and had over 600 beds. Care at all of these teaching hospitals was excellent, but St Michael's in particular had a historic reputation of great kindness to the patients. By the end of the Second World War the nuns were fading from the scene as nurses, yet the caring climate of the hospital lingered on and even at the present writing remains a distinguishing characteristic of the hospital.

The Toronto Western Hospital, on Bathurst Street in the west end, was the third teaching hospital. Established in 1896, it had around 500 beds. Originally conceived by the local doctors who founded it as a community hospital, the Western's ambitious board saw to it that by 1945 clinicians in most of the services had faculty appointments, thus making their departments "teaching departments" for medical students, interns, and residents. For example, at the Western, the Department of Medicine became a teaching department in 1936 with the appointment of Herbert K. Detweiler, fifty at the time and a U of T medical graduate in 1914, as physician-in-chief of the hospital. Duncan Graham, then the head of the university's Department of Medicine, later said, "In 1936 Toronto Western Hospital reorganized its Medical Service and provided facilities for the scientific study of patients. A teaching staff, the majority of whom had received training at the Toronto General Hospital, was appointed. In order that the staff might be able to devote more time to hospital work, the Western Hospital agreed to remunerate the Physician-in-Chief and one junior member of the staff."[3] This process, multiplied many times over for the various departments of the city's hospitals, ensured that Toronto's medical graduates received proper clinical training at the university's teaching hospitals.

The Hospital for Sick Children – always called "the Children's Hospital" or by its initials "HSC," never "Sick Kids" – was a fourth teaching hospital at the end of the war. Established in 1875 and with over 400 beds at the close of the

First World War, it was a pediatric hospital, not a general hospital, and will be considered in chapter 10.

These events were part of tremendous post-war growth of health care in Toronto and in Canada. "The last ten years have seen a remarkable expansion in the hospital and medical research facilities of Toronto," said President Sidney Smith in 1955. "Since 1944 the Hospital for Sick Children, Sunnybrook Hospital [a veterans hospital] and Mount Sinai Hospital [a Jewish hospital] have been erected; substantial additions have been made to the Toronto Western Hospital, St Michael's Hospital ... The long-awaited building at the Toronto General Hospital is under way; the Cancer Treatment and Research Institute is being erected."[4]

The motor driving these various hospitals to join the Faculty of Medicine as "teaching hospitals" was in part the prestige that the distinction conveyed, in part the university's own desperate need for more teaching beds. As average class sizes in the first clinical year began to top 150 after the First World War, the General simply did not have enough beds to avoid patients being swarmed by the scads of students keen to acquire the skills of physical examination and history taking. The teachers were quite sensitive to the question of how much the patients could bear, so the continual addition of clinical units to the category "teaching department" in these three hospitals, and in others, relieved the pressure of numbers. Ray Farquharson, who in 1947 had just become the Eaton Professor and head of the Department of Medicine, told his colleagues in 1949 that the department could now expand teaching to the Wellesley Hospital, a community hospital in the east end that had just been annexed by the General Hospital, thus increasing the number of clinical groups in the second year from twelve to sixteen and in the third year from twelve to fifteen. Now there would be only ten students in a group. But the large incoming class of demobilized veterans would make the groups as large as before, "and the problem of providing close critical supervision of each student's work will actually become more difficult. The student must learn by working under guidance; relatively little can be told him in lectures; he must take histories and examine patients and discuss his findings with trained teachers till he acquires skill and confidence and understanding." All this will be more difficult in coming years, Farquharson said.[5] Ultimately, the New Mount Sinai Hospital, Women's College Hospital, and Sunnybrook Hospital would all affiliate with the faculty as general teaching hospitals. In each case there was a momentary sigh of relief as the medical students were accommodated, the residents found services where they could train, and the pool of researchers (and the patient population upon whom they drew) was enlarged.

**Neurosurgery**

In the beginning Toronto had two sites of neurosurgery, the Toronto General Hospital and the Hospital for Sick Children. Even though the participants dash back and forth, it is simpler to tell the stories separately.

*McKenzie*

Neurosurgery as a discipline was established in North America early in the twentieth century, and in Toronto even before 1914 nonacademic surgeons conducted operations for brain tumours in places such as the Grace Hospital.[6] Considered mildly courageous, they were part and parcel of general surgery.

The history of academic neurosurgery in Toronto began in 1924 when Kenneth McKenzie was appointed to the surgical staff of the Toronto General Hospital. McKenzie was born in 1892, the son of a busy practitioner in rural Ontario. His parents sent him in 1905 to a private school, St Andrew's College, in the chic Rosedale district of Toronto, where McKenzie played rugby, cricket, and – as McKenzie's biographer, fellow neurosurgeon Tom Morley, points out – "really shone in wrestling and, to a lesser extent, in boxing." Indeed, in his second year at U of T, McKenzie became the intercollegiate wrestling champion in his class (125-pound class), called "'Rubber' McKenzie because of his agility in the ring." He received a medical degree from the University of Toronto in 1914, beginning his postgraduate training in the Department of Pathology. Weeks after the First World War broke out in August 1914, McKenzie joined the Royal Army Medical Corps and served in France with a field ambulance unit. In 1917 he transferred to the Canadian Army Medical Corps (CAMC) and joined the medical officers of the Davisville Military Hospital in Toronto.

After the war's end, he bought a general medical practice in Toronto, working as well at the Christie Street Hospital for veterans (established 1920 as the Dominion Orthopaedic Hospital, with 875 beds for veterans). At this point – apparently following a conversation with Clarence Starr[7] – surgery began to interest him. As neurosurgeon Harry Botterell tells the story, "He was, with great persistence, trying to persuade Clarence L. Starr, the Professor of Surgery, to help him to become a surgeon. He took a correspondence course from England and then went to England to try the primary examinations of the Royal College of Surgeons, passing in physiology and failing in anatomy."

At this point, quite fortuitously, McKenzie learned that Toronto had awarded Harvey Cushing, the American founder of neurosurgery, the Charles Mickle Fellowship, which was accompanied by an award of $1,000. "McKenzie learned of the award from the newspapers, and of the fact that Cushing had asked Clarence Starr to send a man to Boston to train as a neurosurgeon and to whom he would contribute the $1,000 from the Mickle Fellowship." McKenzie – who, according to Botterell, had a total of $2 in his pocket at that point – asked Starr if he, McKenzie, might not go down to Boston and study with Cushing for a year. The McKenzie family, now penniless, rented out their house in Toronto; Mrs McKenzie took the three children to live with her family in Chatham, and McKenzie found himself training in Boston in neurosurgery with the world authority.

On returning to Toronto in 1923, McKenzie served a residency year in surgery with Starr at the General, apparently selectively being given neurological cases for operation. After the completion of this residency year, neurosurgery began as an independent service at the General – and in Canada – in 1924.[8] (Neurosurgeon Wilder Penfield came from New York to Montreal only in 1928.)

As McKenzie came on staff, Dean Primrose noted, "While we may deplore the multiplication of specialties, yet it is an obvious fact that remarkable advances in recent times in the surgery of the nervous system demand very special training in order that the surgeon may be able to carry out with skill and judgment the difficult technique required in ... lesions of the brain and spinal cord."[9] Yet despite this decanal endorsement, McKenzie at first was a bit of a black sheep. Clarence Starr was slow to accept specialties in surgery, just as Duncan Graham opposed them in medicine, and only slowly did the Department of Surgery cotton to the subspecialty of neurosurgery. Morley said, "It was years before the neurosurgeon was given his own OR [operating room]. Meanwhile he had to be satisfied with the use of an OR at the end of the day, when the nursing staff was tired; to wait until the room had been cleaned after preceding cases; and to find an assistant from among the house or nursing staff and an anesthetist who were prepared to delay their own departures home, often for many hours." Morley writes, "McKenzie survived the difficult years, protecting himself from overt anger and despair, by withdrawing into his shell."[10]

Then in the 1930s McKenzie began to come into his own. A Division of Neurosurgery was formed in 1929–30 with him in charge (see p. 79). He won his first student in 1930, when William Keith became his first full-year neurosurgery resident. Only in 1936 did "KG," as his residents called him to one another, get a dedicated operating room for neurosurgery. Then the keen young surgeons desiring training in the neurosurgical specialty became more frequent. A neurosurgical group began to grow.[11] In 1936, in the context of Gallie's new program for training surgeons, E. Harry Botterell signed on as a resident in neurosurgery under McKenzie. And in 1940 William ("Bill") Mustard, of whom one shall read later in connection with cardiovascular surgery, stepped up as McKenzie's only assistant. McKenzie's pleasure at this small coup was brief, given that Mustard shortly decided to enlist.

Down in Operating Room D "all by his lonesome," as Don Wilson said, McKenzie developed his own style as a neurosurgeon. Said one of his residents later, "Being educated under [Harvey] Cushing, he had learned many things, not the least of which was patience and great gentleness in the handling of the special tissues with which he worked. Until McKenzie came on the scene, it was generally thought that there was at least some virtue in speed in operations but McKenzie showed us that with proper anaesthesia and plenty of donor blood there was no need for hurry ... During these long hours, he never seemed to weary or lose his patience or control, even in the face of the most critical and terrifying situations."[12]

Charles Drake – who learned his lessons well and went on to become a brilliant aneurysm surgeon at the University of Western Ontario (surgery on sacs formed by dilatations in the walls of arteries) – recalls the following memories as a resident on McKenzie's service: "As a surgeon he was superb, a master nearly unequaled in his time. I was privileged to watch the best of that day later in the United States and in the UK and Europe – few were his equal. His touch on the brain whether with his forefinger searching for a soft spot overlying a deep glioma [a tumour of glial cells] or with the forceps or retractor was gentle and there followed beautiful technical precision." "He called the acoustic neuromas [tumour of the acoustic nerve] the queen of brain tumors. They were all huge in those days and … he had one of the lowest morbidities of the time." "The two things he loved to do because the patients had such good outcomes were a chronic subdural hematoma [bleeding in the narrow space between the layers that line the brain] and a benign spinal cord tumour before the patient had become paraplegic."[13] Many of the other patients had terrible outcomes, and McKenzie was weighted down by the constant deaths. Indeed, he was often subject to bouts of depression.

McKenzie is known for several innovations. Among the earliest problems the budding specialty of neurosurgery took on was spasmodic torticollis, or jerking of the neck. McKenzie recalled his first case in 1923 while he was a resident with Cushing: "The patient, an intelligent woman with a pleasing personality, was dreadfully incapacitated by constant spasmodic jerkings of the head to the left and backwards." McKenzie suggested to Cushing a certain approach to the roots of the spinal nerves that he published the following year. The procedure turned out to be a failure, although it became known as "the McKenzie operation," "or the McKenzie-Dandy operation," after the Johns Hopkins neurosurgeon Walter Dandy who in 1930 described a similar operation. Over the next thirty years, however, McKenzie kept at it, refining his approach in the course of treating eighteen cases. In 1955 he published his revised and much more successful technique, which involved paralyzing one of the sternomastoid muscles and dividing several of the cervical motor nerves intradurally (in this case beneath the covering of the spinal cord). McKenzie said of the revised approach, "Satisfactory results have been obtained in 10 out of 12 patients by radical surgery. When one considers the hopeless pre-operative condition of these patients the results are indeed gratifying."[14]

McKenzie is also remembered in the history of neurosurgery for his demonstration in 1932, as Morley puts it, of "the advantage of dividing the vestibular component of the acoustic nerve to relieve Ménière syndrome [hearing loss, tinnitus, and vertigo from inner-ear disease]."[15] In the 1930s McKenzie finally started receiving international recognition, becoming in 1936 president of the Cushing Society (American Association of Neurological Surgeons). Subject to periodic depression and, in Findlay's analysis, somewhat demoralized by all the deaths that then haunted neurosurgery, he retired in 1952 at age sixty.[16]

An unhappy footnote in McKenzie's memory is his involvement in the partial destruction of the frontal lobes of the brain for treatment of mental disease in an operation known as leucotomy or lobotomy, depending on how it was done. The operation was introduced by Portuguese neurologist Egas Moniz in a monograph in 1936, and it quickly attained great currency in the absence of other means of quieting the agitation of severely disturbed patients. Lobotomy came to a quick end in the early 1950s with the introduction of the first anti-psychotic drugs. McKenzie and Lorne Proctor at the Toronto Western Hospital made Toronto a centre of leucotomy, describing in 1946 a series of twenty-seven cases: "A special instrument is passed through the frontal lobe to the orbital plate. The instrument is then opened, closed, rotated and again opened, then closed and withdrawn. This procedure is repeated on the other side. The dura is closed ... The scalp is closed with a double layer of fine silk." They claimed that 85 percent of their often severely ill patients were "improved or recovered." "In our opinion, this neuro-surgical procedure offers a valuable addition to our therapeutic armamentarium in the treatment of what previously would have been considered hopelessly ill mental patients."[17]

In 1945 Clarence Farrar, the professor of psychiatry, said, "We are favour-ably impressed with the value of this neurosurgical therapeutic procedure in the treatment of our chronically mentally ill patients."[18] Many of the operations were conducted at the Toronto General Hospital and supported by a grant from the Rockefeller Foundation. Of course one is always wiser in hindsight, but it does look like lobotomy, in view of the permanent brain damage it inflicted, represented a significant failure of clinical judgment, certainly on the part of the psychiatrists who referred the patients, as well on McKenzie's part for acceding to the requests.

Neurosurgeon Thomas Morley asks, "Why is it important for us to remem-ber McKenzie? Hardly for his surgical innovations and dexterity alone." Rather, says Morley, it is in the words of Hippocrates "to honor and emulate as far as we are able our teachers and our teachers' teachers to keep the memory of their example a permanent part of our professional heritage." McKenzie's contribu-tion to the great neurosurgical tradition in Toronto was thus: as a model of "diligence, his detached empathy toward his patients, his self-discipline, and equanimity ... are the necessary basics on which every career in clinical medi-cine must be built."[19]

A hospital "division," meaning the basic subunits into which departments are divided, grew up about McKenzie. Gallie said in 1930, "Through the suc-cessful efforts of Dr. Kenneth McKenzie neurological surgery has advanced so rapidly that it has become necessary to create a separate division for this branch of surgery and to release Dr. McKenzie from all other duties in order that he may take charge of it ... one of the outstanding advances made at the hospital during the past few years."[20]

Technology raced ahead alongside neurosurgery. In the 1937–8 session, the Department of Medical Research in the Banting Institute built an electroenceph-alograph machine (EEG), and McKenzie had it installed "in a room adjacent to the neuro-surgical operating room." Gallie said, "It is hoped that this apparatus will prove of value in the definite localization of brain tumours. Having the apparatus close to the operating room will make it possible for the surgeon to apply electrodes directly to the surface of the brain."[21] In 1945 Douglas C. Eaglesham, who had trained at the Montreal Neurological Institute, was appointed as Toronto's first neuroradiologist. His successor in 1948, Delbert Wollin, had similarly trained at the Montreal Neurological Institute, as had his successor in 1959, George Wortzman. (The lesson of this story is that Toronto often fed from the strengths of McGill, though the relationship went the other way as well. In pediatric neuroradiology Toronto was a world leader and owed nothing to McGill – see pp. 88–89 and 270–271.)

*Botterell*

McKenzie students began to spring up. Among his earliest was Edmund Henry Botterell, known universally as "Harry." Harry Botterell was born in Vancouver in 1906 and graduated in medicine in 1930 from the University of Manitoba, where he trained in general surgery and in medicine at the Montreal General Hospital. In 1932 he moved to Toronto and served as a tutor in the Department of Physiology under Charles Best; then, owing to a fortuitous vacancy among the surgical trainees, he moved across College Street in 1933 to begin training in neurosurgery. (He was McKenzie's chief resident from 1936 to 1937.) One day in 1934, according to biographer Max Findlay, Botterell bumped into McKenzie at a lunch at Hart House, the university's campus centre, "and McKenzie, having learned of Botterell's qualities, suggested that Botterell join him in neurosurgery." McKenzie then immediately sent Botterell off on the grand tour that characterized the training of the elite young surgeons: In 1934–5 he served as an intern in neurology and neurosurgery at the prestigious National Hospital for Nervous Diseases in Queen Square, London, "where," says Tasker, "he came to know the amazing constellation of neurological figures of the time."[22] The following year found Botterell at Yale in a research fellowship in the new Department of Neurophysiology under John Fulton. In 1936 he returned to Toronto, now attending neurosurgeon, to continue his career with McKenzie. (Bill Keith was actually McKenzie's first resident, and his career at HSC is followed later.)

Botterell became interested in the care of patients with spinal lesions. As early as 1936, before completing his residency, he began to work with spinal cases and saw that nurses, orderlies, physical therapists, and doctors must provide a coordinated effort in the treatment of these patients, whose previous prognoses had been so hopeless. The orthopedic surgeon Robert I. Harris brought back from England a tidal drainage apparatus for Botterell to irrigate the bladder and reduce infections in these patients.[23] According to Findlay, "Professor Gallie, a generous man dedicated to supporting his young staff with new practices, made a point of sending to Botterell any of his spinal fracture patients who had associated spinal cord injuries. One of the first was a young man who was paralysed from a football injury. Botterell took on this patient, who had only a trace of cord function left, and tried carefully to prevent bladder infection … The result was dramatic. At a time when such patients usually died from sepsis this patient made a remarkable recovery."[24] Botterell operated with similar success in two more patients, then decided upon a lifelong interest in the care of paraplegic patients.

In 1940 Botterell enlisted in the Royal Canadian Army Medical Corps and was sent to the Canadian No. 1 Neurological Hospital in Basingstoke, England, which was redesignated the Neurological and Plastic Surgery Hospital in 1943. There, Botterell soon became chief neurosurgical officer. Wounded soldiers and civilians received state-of-the-art care. According to John Russell Silver, historian of the treatment of spinal injuries, "Their policy was to perform suprapubic catheterization [inserting a catheter into the bladder above the pubic bone] to control the bladder during transportation of the wounded; and management of the bowels by enemas on alternate days. Patients were turned every two to three hours day and night and wet beds were changed immediately to prevent the development of pressure sores … They were conservative in their neurosurgical procedures on the cord for pain and believed that their treatment programme was a model, which other nations followed."[25]

In 1945, Botterell was recalled by the army in order to organize a Neurosurgical Unit at the Christie Street Military Hospital.[26] Upon his return he found, says Findlay, "many of the spinal cord-injury patients from the war, some who had gone through his service at Basingstoke, 'lying around rotting' at the Christie Street Department of Veteran Affairs Hospital in Toronto." He resolved to "remain in the army long enough to assist in the plight of these pitiable patients, and straighten out in particular the problem of the young veteran paraplegic patients." Botterell needed a full-time physician to take over an institution that he organized in January 1945 for their care, Lyndhurst Lodge near the intersection of St Clair and Bathurst Streets. McKenzie pointed him towards the internist Albin Jousse, who had aided the short-staffed McKenzie during the war and was just about to take a post in Sudbury. Botterell talked Jousse out of Sudbury and, says Findlay, "in 1945 Jousse was appointed Medical Director to the first hospital dedicated to the rehabilitation of spinal cord injured patients in North America." Jousse later told Findlay, "It became clear to us that we were not saving them for much of a life to look forward to: to send these young fellows home to live in bed, or get pressure sores and die, or have recurrent urologic infections that the local doctor might not know how to treat. You had to educate them and get them in wheelchairs and get them active … to make them self-sufficient so that they could live independently with a vocation … in society as productive citizens."[27]

"Lyndhurst Lodge," says Silver, "was the first institution of its kind in North America. The programmes provided individuals with the knowledge they needed to manage their own care when they returned to the community. By 1946 many veterans had purchased cars with newly designed hand controls. They used their wheelchairs to go to restaurants, barbershops and a local cinema."[28] "Dr Botterell was a no-nonsense man, I suppose one might say he was a bit rough," according to one former patient, "but he knew what he was doing, and every paraplegic owes their life to him."[29]

By 1946 Botterell – together with urologist Carl Aberhart, plastic surgeon Stuart Gordon, and Jousse – was achieving such "dramatic results," as Dean Gallie put it, "that the programme has been extended to Workmen's Compensation cases and to civilian patients. Their contribution is of the highest practical importance."[30] Botterell's student Tom Morley later said that Botterell had "removed spinal cord trauma from the list of causes of death."[31]

In 1952 Botterell succeeded McKenzie as head of the Division of Neurosurgery at the Toronto General Hospital. It was here that he and William Lougheed pursued his second great research theme: the treatment of cerebral vascular disease, mainly aneurysms and subarachnoid haemorrhage (the arachnoid is one of the layers that envelop the brain), then treated conservatively with bed rest. Hyland and Richardson's work on the neurological side of these brain haemorrhages had interested Botterell, and he pursued his belief "that direct neck clipping [of the aneurysm] was going to become the optimal method of treatment," despite his own initial poor results (58 percent mortality up to 1953). Botterell persuaded, in the words of his neurosurgical colleague Fred Gentili, "young bright anaesthetists Drs Stuart Vandewater and Brian Marshall to take an interest in neuroanaesthesia and he recruited Del Wollin in neuroradiology to develop the techniques to image aneurysms." He also encouraged "a bright young nurse, Jessie Young, to take charge of that field by the boast that he was going to develop the best (damn) neurosurgical unit in the world."[32]

Bill Lougheed was then Botterell's resident, and Botterell encouraged Lougheed to pursue in Boston the interest in hypothermia, or operating once the patient's body temperature had been lowered, that Lougheed had already developed (see pp. 83–84). With all the pieces in place, in 1956 Botterell and colleagues reported their results in twenty-two patients who had experienced direct surgical clipping of ruptured "berry" aneurysms under conditions of hypothermia between May 1954 and April 1955. Of nineteen survivors, sixteen were considered excellent or good. (The paper also introduced a scale from one to five for judging operative risk that later became known as the "Botterell scale.")[33] Gentili comments, "The timing of this paper was very important because, coming at a time when there was hesitancy and uncertainty in aneurysm surgery, it encouraged others to be more aggressive and to operate directly on aneurysms with or without hypothermia." The paper established Botterell as "a major force" in neurosurgery.[34] (This new technique of clipping aneurysms was a big deal: when former Botterell student Ross Fleming clipped his first aneurysm as a staffer, Botterell somehow heard of it and called Fleming's wife to "let her know how pleased and proud he was."[35])

Under Botterell's aegis, in 1958 a "New Unit" for neurosurgery was opened on the twelfth floor of the Urquhart Wing of the TGH, marking the definitive take-off of neurological surgery in Toronto. "A tall, imposing individual, with a rich, forceful, and commanding voice," said Findlay of Botterell, "he had more than most the presence of a neurosurgeon ... He was by nature impatient, and according to some, sometimes difficult to assist in the operating room. At least one of his residents took to putting folded newspapers into his socks when assisting Dr Botterell, in order to protect his vulnerable shins in the event that the Chief felt he was not concentrating on his task sufficiently."[36] In 1962 Botterell left Toronto to become the dean of medicine at Queen's University.

### Botterell's Chief Residents

Just after the war, McKenzie and Botterell established a structured program for training neurosurgeons. McKenzie soon stepped down, and the baton was passed to a generation of Botterell's students. Botterell had eight chief residents, and in their careers one can read the progress of neurosurgery in English Canada in the 1950s and 1960s. (Of course, the other part of the story would be Wilder Penfield and his students at McGill University; Botterell's students Bruce Hendrick and Harold Hoffman are discussed later under neurosurgery at HSC.)

William Horsey, Botterell's first chief resident, finished training in neurosurgery in 1954 and returned to St Michael's Hospital, where he had interned, to establish their neurosurgery program. Horsey and fellow resident William Lougheed were men of slight stature, and Botterell, "a tall man made even taller by his imposing and dominating demeanor, towered above them," as Max Findlay recalls. "The sight of this group on the wards, and the occasional difficulty the residents had in assisting Dr Botterell with their heads in his direct line of vision, sometimes had comic overtones." At St Michael's, Horsey "became a notable spinal surgeon," in Findlay's terms, "and in Toronto kept that aspect of surgery firmly in the realm of neurosurgery."[37]

William Lougheed, Botterell's second chief resident – a 1947 medical graduate of U of T – finished neurosurgical training in 1955, following a McLaughlin Fellowship in Europe and the United States. While a fellow in the neurosurgical service at the Massachusetts General Hospital in 1953, Lougheed was, with Hannibal Hamlin and William H. Sweet, in on a first: in a fifty-year-old widow, they removed an occluded segment of the left internal carotid artery and, suturing the ends together, created an "anastomosis."[38] This was "one of the world's first surgical corrections of carotid stenosis," said Findlay, but they reported it only in 1958 and didn't get the priority.[39]

Then there was hypothermia, a technique that cardiac surgeon Bill Bigelow had pioneered. Lougheed had previously discussed the procedure with Bigelow (who wanted Lougheed to become a cardiovascular surgeon[40]). In 1955 in Boston, Lougheed and D.S. Kahn introduced hypothermia into neurosurgery while stopping the circulation in cerebral vascular surgery.[41] Two such firsts for a junior fellow are not bad.

In Toronto, Lougheed initiated hypothermia in neurovascular surgery at the General in 1954. The first Toronto publication on hypothermia in this area was issued in 1956, together with Botterell, anaesthetist Stuart Vandewater, and neurophysiologist John W. Scott, on the management of the team's first twenty-two patients with ruptured intracranial aneurysms.[42] Aneurysms tend to rupture during surgery, and in repairing them it is often necessary to interrupt the cerebral circulation by clipping the carotid or vertebral arteries supplying blood to the brain. Yet prolonged stoppage can cause brain damage. The logic was that hypothermia lessened the damage to the brain during the interruption of blood flow. It was Lougheed who worked up the technique. Hypothermia was induced in the following way: First the patient was given a cocktail of phenothiazine agents plus Demerol. As the preliminaries were underway, "the patient is in the hypothermic bath on the operating table and his legs, groins and lower abdomen are covered with crushed ice." Then "the bath is filled with ice water covering the legs and trunk to about the nipple line," the patient's rectal temperature being monitored continuously. The results of the operation were good: of twenty-two patients operated on for berry aneurysms, there were only three deaths. This was thought an improvement over the previous seven deaths in nineteen patients. Yet there was no control group, and it is unclear, given other changes in procedure and selection, how these patients would have done in the absence of hypothermia.[43] Findlay says, "This paper ... was the world's first description of hypothermia and temporary cerebral circulatory arrest for aneurysm surgery."[44]

Further accounts of Lougheed's career in the 1960s and 1970s are found at p. 388.

In 1956 J. Ross Fleming, who graduated from Toronto in medicine in 1947, finished training as Botterell's next chief resident, then embarked upon the kind of grand tour of European centres that Botterell himself had undertaken: neurology at Queen Square, stereotactic surgery (a three-dimensional technique for locating areas precisely in the brain) on the Continent. He joined colleagues Bill Keith and Bruce Hendrick at the Toronto Western Hospital later that year, then became head of the division in 1965 after they went over to the Hospital for Sick Children.

In 1957 Robert Hetherington, a Rhodes Scholar and U of T graduate in 1950, served as Botterell's chief resident, decamping then for Queen's University, where he inaugurated neurosurgery.

Last in this series of Botterell students pioneering neurosurgery was Ronald Tasker, who finished his medical studies in 1952 as one of its two silver medalists. (The other was John Evans, who went on to become president of the university. The gold medalist was Marguerite "Peggy" Hill, later physician-in-chief at Women's College Hospital. "Not a bad triumvirate!" according to current president David Naylor.[45]) When Tasker began training in medicine, he was "bewildered by the high death rate of hospitalized patients on the medical floors," and switched to surgery, which he completed in 1959. With a McLaughlin Fellowship, he spent a year in neurophysiological research at the University of Wisconsin, then a second in Europe studying stereotactic surgery, which opened the door for him to thalamotomy in the treatment of movement disorders (the thalamus in the base of the brain is a relay station to the cerebral cortex for sensory impulses). No sooner was he back in Toronto than he was appointed a Markle fellow for 1961–6, permitting him to do research alongside his clinical work at the General. Tasker became an international authority on using electrodes to situate the exact site at which to operate in surgery, for example, for Parkinson's disease. Tasker also helped advance radiofrequency-lesioning in pain control and is considered one of the pioneers of "stereotactic and functional" neurosurgery.[46]

Despite this list of glittering residents, it was rather Thomas P. Morley, who had trained in neurosurgery in Manchester with Sir Geoffrey Jefferson, who would succeed Botterell in 1962 as head of the Division of Neurosurgery at the General; he became head of the university department two years later. Born in Manchester in 1920, Morley had studied medicine at Oxford (taking his degree in 1943) and had come over to Sunnybrook Hospital, then a veterans hospital, in 1954. Morley's field was cancer surgery, but it was as a surgical leader rather than a cancer specialist that the next generation of neurosurgeons trained under him.

In 1957 the Division of Neurosurgery of the Toronto General Hospital came up out of the basement in Operating Room D to a brand-new neurosurgical unit that was then "officially" opened in November 1958 with the hosting of a meeting in Toronto of the American Academy of Neurosurgery.

### Neurosurgery at the Hospital for Sick Children

The sick child in need of an operation for a spreading brain cancer or a haemorrhaging vessel has a poignancy all its own. And whereas the technical side of the story can be folded into the main narrative of neurosurgery, the emotional side cannot.

*Bill Keith*

In 1929 Gallie "conceived the idea that [the Hospital for Sick Children] needed a full-time neurosurgeon," as Harold Hoffman put it, and asked William Keith to prepare himself for such a post.[47] In 1933 Keith initiated pediatric neurosurgery in Toronto. Born in 1902, Keith grew up in Toronto and earned a Toronto medical degree in 1927 (excelling in rugby and winning the silver medal). He interned at the Toronto General Hospital, where, according to his biographer

Robin Humphreys, William Gallie "encouraged Keith to pursue further ed-ucation in the neurological sciences." On a fellowship, Keith studied at the University of Chicago with Roy Grinker in neurology and Percival Bailey in neurosurgery, returning thereupon to Toronto for a year to work with McKen-zie. In 1931 Keith clerked at the National Hospital at Queen Square on the neu-rology service. "He subsequently became chief resident in Surgery at HSC, and upon joining the staff in 1933 was expected to be equally facile in general and orthopaedic surgery as well as neurosurgery." Three years later, in 1936, Keith started the neurosurgery service at the Toronto Western Hospital as well. There was tension with Alan Brown, the powerful professor of pediatrics at the chil-dren's hospital. "They argued," says Robin Humphreys, "over which patients Keith would operate on and where he was to park his car."[48]

These years were the fear-filled epoch of neurological survey. "[Keith] re-called operating in 1961 on an aneurysm in a three year old girl and having ex-posed it asked his resident if 'you remember I told you I wasn't afraid of these things anymore?' When the resident nodded in the affirmative Keith replied, 'Well, that was a lie!'"[49]

Keith had strong basic science as well as clinical interests, and as early as 1935, under the supervision of Eric Linell in neuropathology, he and Joseph Albert Sullivan of the Department of Otolaryngology at St Michael's attracted campus attention for their studies of nerve regeneration.[50] Keith joined the Canadian armed forces in 1942, saw action in France and Germany, then in 1945 was re-called by HSC, needed more urgently there and at the Toronto Western Hospi-tal to train young neurosurgeons than at the front.[51]

On the scientific side, according to Fleming, "[Keith] was an early propo-nent of lumbo-peritoneal shunting for hydrocephalus, which he introduced [to HSC] in 1948." His student Harold Hoffman recalls, "He had to work at a fre-netic pace, since he was the only neurosurgeon at the Hospital for Sick Children and the Toronto Western Hospital until he was joined by Dr. Ross Fleming at the Toronto Western Hospital in 1954 and Dr. E. Bruce Hendrick at The Hospital for Sick Children in 1955."[52] Ross Fleming said that at HSC Keith was "[c]hief of what is widely recognized as one of the world's outstanding paediatric neuro-surgical units."[53]

*The Three "H's"*

In the 1950s, there were two young neurosurgeons who joined HSC under Keith. Both their last names began with "H," and there was a third "H" who came a bit later, giving rise to the appellation "the three H's." The older of the two was Bruce Hendrick, "a rare Torontonian who was actually born in the city in which he still practices."[54] In the history of pediatric neurosurgery in Toronto it was not so much Keith who built up the service – many operations on children con-tinued to be conducted at TGH on his watch – but Hendrick.

Hendrick graduated from U of T in medicine in 1946 but achieved the bulk of his training in Boston in a two-year fellowship at the Children's Medical Center and Peter Bent Brigham Hospital. After a travelling fellowship abroad, Hendrick returned to Toronto in 1955 to begin neurosurgery under Keith at HSC and the Toronto Western Hospital (TWH). But his heart was clearly at the children's hospital. Hoffman recalls, "Many a resident [might] find himself suddenly caught in the crossfire of a water pistol fight between Bruce and his patients. It was a serious business on Friday afternoons, when nurses, parents and child life therapists joined the patients to develop strategies for these sessions. The children wore green garbage bags; 'Uncle Bruce' took the soakings in his OR scrub suit."[55]

On Keith's retirement in 1964, Hendrick became neurosurgeon-in-chief at HSC and thus, says Findlay, "the first full-time paediatric neurosurgeon in the world."[56] His principal achievement was training the following generation of pediatric neurosurgeons.

The other young pediatric neurosurgeon at HSC, the second "H," was Harold Hoffman, who was, as his student James Rutka points out, "in his day … arguably the most famous paediatric neurosurgeon in the world." Hoffman earned a medical degree from U of T in 1956 and travelled to various neurosurgical centres in Europe and the United Kingdom with the aid of a McLaughlin Fellowship. This trip included studying with Murray Falconer at the Maudsley Hospital in London, where Hoffman acquired an abiding interest in the surgery of epilepsy; in 1964 Hoffman returned to Toronto to join the HSC neurosurgical staff. This was the year when the thirty-two-bed specialized pediatric neurosurgery unit was opened on Ward 5G of the Gerrard Wing. For years, Hoffman and Hendrick were the only two neurosurgeons in the hospital, and, to get on with research, they alternated weeks on call.

Humphreys recalled the surgeons' lounge at the children's hospital, "which almost took on a country club atmosphere. A Hospital attendant waited on tables and served hot, fresh coffee and doughnuts on sparkling china … Characteristically, the residents sat about the perimeter of the room perhaps analyzing their role models most of whom were then world prominent."

Hoffman published so widely that he became, as Rutka says, "an authority on virtually every topic in paediatric neurosurgery." In 1968, for example, Hoffman began a databank on hydrocephalus (an accumulation of cerebrospinal fluid within the skull), then expanded it to spina bifida (a defective closure of the vertebrae through which the spinal cord might protrude) and brain tumours; the bank was supported financially by Mr David Bloom, CEO of Shoppers Drug Mart. The divisional newsletter noted in 2000, "We have reached the point where this division has shown its international primacy in the analysis of hydrocephalus shunting techniques, the associated infection risks and alternative therapies."[57]

But Hoffman's fame in the public eye dates to 1993, when Hira and Nida Jamal were born in Pakistan as conjoined twins, joined at the head. The government of

Pakistan donated $100,000 for what the *Toronto Star* termed "a global search for a doctor who would take on the challenge. The hunt ended at Toronto's Hospital for Sick Children, where Hoffman and his team separated the Jamal twins in a harrowing 16-hour procedure that involved detaching brain matter and blood vessels one by one. One of the twins, Nida, failed to survive. The other, Hira, "came out of the surgery healthy and alert."[58] Rutka assisted at the operation and remembers, "At one critical juncture in the case, a blood vessel which joined the twins had let loose and was bleeding profusely. Harold quickly hooked the vessel with his index finger and clipped it with his other hand. In answering questions about this Harold simply stated, 'One doesn't think about what one is going to do, one just does it."[59]

The third "H" in the neurosurgical division of the Hospital for Sick Children was Robin Humphreys, a U of T medical graduate in 1962, who joined the staff in 1970 and inaugurated with surgeon Ian Munro the craniofacial program. Their student Jim Rutka recalled, "As all three neurosurgeons' last names began with the letter 'H', they became known endearingly as the '3 H's.'" (Humphreys, modest to a fault, claims that "[t]he ladies of the Women's Auxiliary dubbed them, 'He, Ho and Hum!'") Rutka noted, "Collectively, they co-authored most of the definitive works on paediatric neurosurgery."[60]

*Derek Harwood-Nash*

The story of neurosurgery has a sort of footnote though not really a footnote because Derek Harwood-Nash was probably the best-known neuroradiologist in the world – but, nonetheless, not a surgeon. Harwood-Nash was born in Bulawayo, Rhodesia, in 1936 and studied medicine at the University of Cape Town. Alan Hudson, who later became president of The Toronto Hospital (TTH) following the merger of TGH and the Western in 1986, was a classmate; both graduated together in 1960 and both interned in surgery under, among others, the famous pioneer of heart transplantation Christiaan Barnard. Hudson's fiancée was living in Toronto, and in 1963 the two pals travelled to Canada to let Alan spend some time with her. Hendrick astutely gave both of them fellowships in neurosurgery at HSC working, according to Harwood-Nash's biographer Michael Huckman, on a project on pediatric head injuries. (Humphreys calls the publication that eventuated from this "a benchmark in children's head injury analysis."[61]) Harwood-Nash stayed on to train in surgery in Toronto, doing a one-year residency in neurosurgery at TGH and another year in orthopedics at Sunnybrook. Yet at the encouragement of George Wortzman at the General, Harwood-Nash became increasingly interested in neuroradiology and from 1964 to 1967 embarked upon a three-year residency in the Toronto program under Brian Holmes. In January 1968 Harwood-Nash joined HSC as a staff radiologist and director of neuroradiology. In 1976 he and colleague Charles Fitz published their magisterial *Neuroradiology in Infants and*

*Children*, "giving birth to the specialty of pediatric neuroradiology and making Toronto its capital."[62] The Hospital for Sick Children, says Huckman, "soon became the Mecca to which men and women from all over the world flocked to be trained in his section. He taught his fellows to perform neurodiagnostic procedures with safety and meticulous radiographic technique in the most fragile of human creatures."[63]

## Heart Surgery

All three of the techniques required for open-heart surgery originated in Toronto: Murray introduced anticoagulation; Bill Mustard and Lawrie Chute achieved the first survival in a canine cardiac bypass; and Bill Bigelow introduced body temperature control using hypothermia. "The origin of these separate factors within a single university is of interest," deadpans heart surgeon Bernard Goldman.[64]

Thus the story begins in the 1930s as Gordon Murray introduced heparin into vascular surgery. And it was Murray who led the new wave of post-war innovation. He began, actually, in 1936, with Frederick R. Wilkinson and Ross Mackenzie, in experimental animal work replacing the mitral valve in a closed-heart operation that involved punching through the apex of the auricle. (The mitral valve prevents backflow from the left ventricle into the left atrium.)[65] In 1937 Murray, Best, and others reported on the physiological effects of administering heparin in seventy-six patients post-operatively: it lengthened the clotting time.[66] The first clinical application of heparin – an important one – was Charles Best and Donald Solandt's demonstration in 1939 that administering heparin in a heart attack would help localize the damage and prevent the clot from extending: "We would like to … point out that the administration of heparin early in an attack of coronary thrombosis, even before the actual vascular thrombosis, is not necessarily contra-indicated."[67] The comment is a triumph of indirection and understatement.

In 1941 Murray reported on the over 400 surgical patients who had received heparin, with famous results in the treatment of pulmonary embolism in particular: "When pulmonary embolism has occurred and the patient has survived long enough to have heparin administered intravenously, there has been striking clinical improvement": forty-four of forty-six patients had suffered "no further attacks of embolism and showed rapid clinical improvement."[68] (As noted, Duncan Graham remained suspicious of heparin and refused it admission to the medical wards of the Toronto General Hospital until after the Second World War.[69])

In 1946 Murray took a big stride upon the stage of cardiac surgery as the first to perform successfully in the commonwealth the operation for oxygen-starved babies ("blue babies") that Alfred Blalock and Helen Taussig had introduced in 1945 at Johns Hopkins University; the operation targeted a pediatric cardiac malformation called the "tetralogy of Fallot," in which the surgeon performs an anastomosis, or joins, a branch of the aorta to one of the pulmonary arteries.[70] This is not open-heart surgery because the infant's heart is not actually penetrated, yet it is risky enough, and the brilliant operation opened up cardiac surgery for both infants and adults. (Blalock was probably willing to risk it only because the sulfa drugs – and soon penicillin–were available to control the infections that had doomed so many of the dogs on which these experiments had previously been performed.) By December 1947 Murray had performed the operation sixty times, with a mortality of 11 percent.[71] In that year Murray also succeeded in the partial closure of atrial septal and ventricle septal defects (holes in the heart's interior walls) using, as Baird says, "fascia lata sutures passed in and out of the beating heart."[72]

In 1947 as well Murray described under the term "paradoxical systole" the experimental surgical creation and excision of those parts of the muscle of the heart that had been damaged, or infarcted, in a heart attack, opening an approach to the damaged myocardium that would later be of importance. Cardiac surgeon Rudolph Matas – who was sitting in the audience next to Alfred Blalock as Murray was presenting his paper in an American Surgical Association meeting at Hot Springs, Virginia – said to Blalock, "This work may be epoch-making." Typically, Murray declared in the paper, "This work was done without University or other assistance, apart from limited laboratory facilities in the Banting Institute."[73] (Murray and Ray Heimbecker revived this approach in 1967.[74])

At the same time that Murray was immersed in heart operations, he applied his remarkable surgical virtuosity and active mind to the problem of kidney failure and pioneered the mechanical kidney! Murray was preceded – possibly even inspired – in these efforts by William Thalhimer, then at the Manhattan Convalescent Serum Laboratory, who later became a visiting fellow in Toronto, profiting from the work of Best and Donald Solandt on "experimental exchange transfusion." In 1938 Thalhimer jury-rigged an artificial kidney that was never used clinically. Technically, it is a first. In Toronto, Thalhimer worked at a lab in the School of Hygiene, just across University Avenue from the Banting Institute where Murray laboured; in 1938 he published an article with Solandt and Best on "experimental exchange transfusion." It is inconceivable that Murray did not know of this work.[75]

Beginning in 1933 Murray had undertaken animal experiments to clear the blood of acute toxemia. "It seemed possible that if the patient could be protected from death from toxemia in such conditions, after a time there would be sufficient recovery in a number of cases so that the affected kidneys might resume function," he wrote in 1947. He actually attached the renal dialysis machine he had constructed to a patient who had been given up for lost, and she survived. It was a twenty-six-year-old woman who had stopped passing urine for nine days after an attempt at induced abortion, thus poisoning her kidneys. "She was comatose, was having mild uremic convulsions, was greatly edematous, and was not passing urine. She was seen by the internists, the gynecologists and the genitourologists, all of whom agreed that the case was utterly hopeless." Murray hitched her up to his dialysing device by passing a catheter into the inferior vena cava on the right side and another into the femoral vein on the left. She was dialysed over a period of days. "The clinical improvement of the patient was striking. She was comatose at the beginning of each of these runs, and at the end the delirium and coma had disappeared." A day after the last dialysis "there was an enormous secretion of 4000 cc of urine." She made an uninterrupted recovery and left the hospital well.[76] At the end of 1949 he reported in the *British Medical Journal* that about half of the patients were surviving, those who succumbed having chronic kidney disease whom even "purification of the blood" was unable to keep from relapsing into a uremic state.[77]

In 1952 Murray carried out a successful kidney transplantation, a subject then of active interest in international scholarship, but this must have been one of the very first. Of the four patients on whom he attempted kidney transplants, only the fourth, twenty-six-year-old Dorothy Pezze, survived. As Shelley McKellar tells the story, "She had suffered chronic kidney disease for fifteen years and had no chance of survival without a new kidney. Pezze wanted the experimental surgery and understood the risks." She underwent the transplant operation on 2 May 1952 and apparently lived on for years, although Murray did not follow her up. In 1990 Joseph E. Murray at Peter Bent Brigham Hospital in Boston won the Nobel Prize for kidney transplantation, having done, it must be said, a much more thorough job of working up the science than did Gordon Murray.[78]

Triumph followed triumph. In October 1955 Murray successfully transplanted the aortic valve of a young man dying of heart failure. "The first patient was one with marked aortic regurgitation," he reported, "with typical findings, with a very large heart going into failure." They harvested an aortic valve segment postmortem from another young patient. "It was very gratifying, on removal of all the clamps, to see the effect of this valve in the thoracic aorta." Following the operation the patient's heart decreased greatly in size, and, eight months later, he seemed perfectly well.[79]

Murray's operation was the first valve replacement. Ray Heimbecker, who had just joined the Department of Surgery, assisted and the day before had harvested the valve. Heimbecker described the operation:

The aorta was finally clamped off. This had to be done gradually and gently in order to avoid a sudden severe strain on the ailing heart. This huge artery was then divided, and the new valve was transplanted into place. Forty minutes later, the clamps were gradually released. The transplanted leaflets began to open and close with each heart beat. Our excited fingers could feel the vigorous throb as the fragile leaflets closed and opened with each contraction. As I placed my hand on the heart muscle, it too had dramatically changed to a much quieter and more peaceful contraction ... The aorta was now carrying a smooth, sustained flow of blood, where before it had struggled, expanding and collapsing with every beat. In a few days [the patient] was back with his jubilant family. The world's first heart valve transplant had been a thrilling success.[80]

Astonishingly, Murray kept the operation secret from his colleagues, who did not learn about it until Murray described it a year later in what Baird called "an obscure Italian journal."[81] All the while, Murray's own behaviour was becoming increasingly odd. He seemed paranoid and would hang towels over the windows of the operating room so that others could not look in and "steal his ideas." He emphasized in his papers that all the work had been done by him alone, implying that he owed nothing to his surgical colleagues. In the 1953–4 session he resigned from the Department of Surgery and hived himself off in a private research institute he had founded in 1949.[82] His colleague Bill Bigelow says, "Murray was a loner, and suspicious ... He had a fear of plagiarism and a strong desire to be sure he received the recognition he felt he deserved."[83]

Embittered at being passed over as departmental chair in favour of Robert Janes,[84] in collegial relations Murray became increasingly remote, even bizarre. One day he and Barney Berris were having lunch and, said Berris, "out of the blue he asked me, 'Do you brush your teeth?'"

"Of course," Berris replied.
"Why do you?"
"Because the dentist tells me it prevents cavities."
"Well," said Murray, "I've looked up the literature and as far as I can tell, there is no real evidence that it does."
"Do you brush your teeth?" Berris asked.
"No, I don't," Murray said.[85]

Murray lost his hospital privileges for falsifying a report about spinal surgery. His last days in the faculty brought a tragic and unproductive end to a career that had contributed probably more to medical science – certainly to surgery – than any other single Canadian.

### Bill Bigelow

"Who led the charge towards specialization in cardiac surgery here in Toronto?" an interviewer asked cardiac surgeon Donald Wilson.
WILSON: "I think Bill Bigelow. I think Gordon Murray did it, but Bill is the one who really made it."[86]

Brilliant though Murray was, he did not give rise to the Toronto school of cardiovascular surgery, though he may have pointed the way to the heart as the future of surgery. The originator of the Toronto school was Bill Bigelow, the first surgical scientist in the department.

Wilfred Gordon Bigelow was born in 1913 in Brandon, Manitoba, into a medical family that generations past had emigrated from the American colonies in 1761 to Nova Scotia. Of his youth he said, "My fine mother instilled a strong Scottish Presbyterian accent to our Sundays. Sitting in a cool prairie church in the winter, with a fresh and very itchy suit of all-wool long underwear, gave me a sense of humility and kinship with those early Christian martyrs."[87]

His physician father advised him to attend the University of Toronto. Bigelow graduated with an arts degree in the Biological and Medical Sciences program in 1935, going on directly to medical school. He received his MD in 1938, having played interfaculty hockey and served as president of the 3T8 class[88] while a med student.[89] Bigelow then trained in surgery at the General in the Gallie program and enlisted in the Canadian Army Medical Corps as a military surgeon from 1941 to 1945. While in England, he acquired an active interest in vascular surgery. He later said, "I was appalled at the amputation of an arm or leg whose main artery had been severed, when the limb itself was still functional." His curiosity remained intellectual, yet his interests became known in the Department of Surgery, and after Bigelow had returned to Toronto, Gallie asked him, "How would you like to be a vascular surgeon? I can arrange to have you work with this fellow Blalock at Johns Hopkins, then you can come back on the staff at the Toronto General Hospital."[90]

In 1946–7 Murray spent a fellowship year at Johns Hopkins, where Alfred Blalock was just doing the first "blue baby" heart surgery. In 1947 he returned to Ward C in the General, the cardiopulmonary and vascular centre (which was shared with orthopedics), just as Shenstone retired and Janes was appointed professor of surgery. Bigelow was eight years older than Murray and not a student of his, though Murray's reputation antedated Bigelow's. Historian Shelley McKellar calls the relationship between them "competitive" and "distant," although Bigelow was the number-two man on Murray's surgical service on Ward C.[91] Among the earlier procedures Bigelow undertook was the first closed mitral valvotomy ("commissurotomy") in Toronto, and the second in Canada, which he did at Sunnybrook Hospital in the early 1950s. (Only later did he undertake the operation at TGH.)[92]

Ruth Mather, the medical secretary of cardiologist Sidney Carlen (who had an office on College Street and was the father of TWH neurologist Peter Carlen), recalled Bigelow from the days of these operations on the mitral valve: "On one occasion, Dr Bigelow came to our office for this discussion [of a patient proposed for a commissurotomy]. He entered the room quietly and stood before my desk. He was a tall, handsome man with a Scottish complexion and an almost boyish smile. In fact, he had a college-boy look even though he was in his early forties. He was dressed in casual tweeds and his manner was also casual." She recalled him as "unostentatious," never announced by secretaries. He would usually exchange a few words with her. "I rose to greet him and he extended his hand to me. It was a big, strong, masculine hand, freckled by the summer sun. I was astonished. Somehow I had expected the surgeon's hand to be thin and delicate. This was the hand that worked miracles!"[93] For Sidney Carlen's patients, they were no less than miracles.

*Bigelow the Mover*

Bigelow had a wider vision than did Murray. In 1955 he proposed that a cardiovascular service, including surgery and cardiology, be set up at TGH, just as the volume of heart surgery was soaring: "In the brief period of heart surgery over one thousand heart operations have been performed [at TGH]. It is one of the commonest operations in the hospital." Bigelow wanted Ray Heimbecker as a "full time surgical staff man" and Ramsay Gunton, a cardiologist, "appointed to the position of full time physician from the Department of Medicine." Such a service was all the more needed because at present the patients were being neither adequately worked up nor followed. Also, "[s]uch a service will make it possible to set up a post-graduate training scheme in cardiology, peripheral vascular disease, and cardiovascular surgery. Such a scheme is timely in Canada." The "senior internes" were doing so much cardiovascular work that they would be incompetent for general surgery. "In effect Ward C [Bigelow's ward] will become essentially a cardiovascular service whether or not it is designated as such by name."[94] This laid out a vision for the first training program in cardiovascular surgery in English Canada. Unfortunately, it came to nothing.

Bigelow was like a battle tank. In 1956 he got the service moved from the basement of the Banting Institute where the animal work was done to the 8th floor pavilion, where there was space not only for clinical investigation but for offices and "a common meeting ground with the cardiologists."[95] In April of that year he succeeded in opening a cardiovascular investigative unit at the General set up to undertake angiocardiograms, heart catheterizations, aortograms, and arteriograms. It was run by a joint committee of cardiologists and surgeons. Before this, there had been no facilities at the General for investigating cardiovascular cases, the big hospital lagging behind the Western and the Wellesley. Next, Bigelow agitated for a heart operating room (H-OR) in the pavilion. "Failing that C.O.R. [chest operating room] must be used for all pump operations, public and private. That means clearing the patients out of the four bed female room on Ward C to find adequate room for nursing, chemist, electrocardiogram, etc to create an intensive therapy unit. It will require *specialized* nursing care." Against the resistance of the chest surgeons and of Fred Kergin, head of the Department of Surgery, Bigelow forced open a cardiovascular space at the big hospital (and persuaded a former patient, John McFayden, to donate a cardiac catheterization lab – "Bigelow's Bungalow," which was a small add-on behind the Dunlap building – to the Toronto General Hospital).[96] At Bigelow's request, in 1958 the hospital set up a dedicated cardiovascular surgical unit covering two floors of a wing and including the segregation of cardiac patients (see p. 98).[97]

## Bigelow the Scientist

Bigelow is known for three scientific accomplishments and one technical improvement. It was not Bigelow who introduced surgery for the leaflets of the mitral valve that had become stuck together following an illness such as rheumatic fever. Yet in 1951 he began applying a straightforward technical procedure for it that involved making an incision in the atrium, then freeing up with the surgeon's finger the calcified leaflets of the valve. He reported on it in general terms in October 1952 and gave a precise account of his first sixty-five patients in 1953.[98] It was his first surgical innovation and was widely imitated.

As for the three scientific accomplishments, one was performing open-heart surgery under conditions of hypothermia. Going back to the Second World War, it had been the area of vascular surgery that interested Bigelow. At the Casualty Clearing Station in Normandy during the landings, it pained him "to see amputations carried out in otherwise good limbs because of vascular insufficiency." Later, while he was watching Blalock operate at Hopkins, "The idea of general hypothermia with interruption of the circulation occurred to me … and although there was very little evidence that surgery would progress much beyond the shunting procedure for tetralogy of Fallot, nevertheless the hypothermia concept was the first stimulus to consider cardiac surgery as an eventual goal."[99]

Back in Toronto, he had organized a little laboratory at the Banting Institute and began experimenting with open-heart surgery on dogs after first cooling them, using for example a fan blowing across a couple of blocks of ice or electric cooling blankets. By April 1950 they had cooled a total of 176 dogs, performing experimental heart surgery on most of them. "It has been possible at a body temperate of 20 [degrees] C to exclude the heart from the circulation for periods of 15 minutes with survival. In some of the animals during the period of exclusion the heart has been opened and then sutured."[100] This was among the earliest instances of open-heart surgery – on dogs – and came on the heels of Bill Mustard's experimental open-heart surgery at HSC in 1949 (see pp. 104–105). Human open-heart surgery began in 1952 with F. John Lewis of Minneapolis using Bigelow's hypothermia to close an atrial septal defect under conditions of "inflow stasis."[101] (An atrioseptal defect, or ASD, is a hole in the septum between the two atria of the heart that fails to close spontaneously.) Nonetheless, Bigelow's work established the principle that it might be applicable to humans if the dogs' hearts could be stopped and incised successfully.

Bigelow's first operation using hypothermia was on a patient referred by McKenzie with a large pituitary tumour. Griff Pearson, Bigelow's resident and research assistant, cooled the patient. The patient died and Bigelow was upset. "But this is the big league," he said.[102]

In 1954 Bigelow, Bill Mustard, and John Evans reported twenty-one patients operated on for various cardiac lesions under hypothermia and arrest of the circulation (but not bypass – the hypothermia itself reduced the body's need for oxygen). They were not the first to use hypothermia in experimental intracardiac surgery, but they specified practical techniques for employing it in humans. They introduced unprecedentedly low temperatures and made the technique applicable, with a pacemaker available to restart the stalled heart. They also used the new phenothiazine agents that served as a "lytic cocktail" to aid further in lowering temperature. They concluded, "Hypothermia would appear to be a physiologic approach to some of our problems in cardiac surgery … The dangers of lowering body temperature below the present safe levels may be reduced."[103]

Whatever the real virtues of hypothermia, it gave surgeons courage to attempt surgery on the heart. It is said that after John Lewis heard Bigelow speak on hypothermia in 1950, he returned to Minneapolis "to perform the world's first successful ASD [repair] in 1952 with this new technique." Bigelow did his first in 1953.[104] Surgeons later would bypass the heart with a heart-lung pump, and in 1990 surgeons at St Michael's Hospital established that the heart did not have to be cooled for open-heart surgery "on pump."[105] Yet hypothermia marked the beginning of a procedure that initiated the great era of cardiac bypass surgery.

Bigelow's second achievement was the cardiac pacemaker. The discovery was quite accidental:

> One morning … as I entered the laboratory, an anesthetized dog was already being cooled in refrigeration blankets with ice bags … Just as we were about to begin [the] tests, the heart unexpectedly stopped and lay quietly in standstill. Cardiac massage did not restart it. In some frustration and desperation, since the experiment would have to be postponed, I gave the left ventricle a good poke with the forceps I was holding. There was an immediate and strong contraction that involved all chambers – and then it returned to standstill. I did it again with the same result … I poked it regularly every second. It resembled a normal beating heart. The technician/anesthetist said, 'Hey, I am getting a blood pressure here.' Not only were these real contractions that I induced, but the heart was forcibly expelling blood into the circulation.[106]

The investigators now reasoned that "perhaps an electrical impulse had the same effect as a poke." They enlisted Jack Hopps at the National Research Council in Ottawa to help them build a pacemaking device and began to use it on animals the hearts of which failed to restart after hypothermia surgery. They discovered that applying a "defibrillating shock" to the heart through two electrodes – one on the sino-atrial node area, the other on the chest – restarted the heart in four animals. "In two experiments the artificial pacemaker was used for ten to 15 minutes, and when it was discontinued the heart returned to standstill. In the other two animals following electrical control of the heart beat for ten and 30 minutes, normal spontaneous heart beats returned." The authors concluded, "Should such a technic prove worthwhile, its extension to other clinical conditions with cardiac arrest might be considered."[107] The following year, 1951, Bigelow and his research fellow John C. Callaghan described experimental results in dogs and rabbits of "an electrical artificial pacemaker." Their conclusion that "[i]t is possible to create good expulsive beats of the heart by applying electrical impulses" represented a milestone in the history of cardiac treatment.[108] Yet the device was too large to be practical, and other researchers elsewhere would devise the implantable pacemaker.

In the years ahead Bigelow performed a number of other innovative procedures that, though not necessarily world firsts as the previous two, testify to the ingenuity and vitality of the cardiovascular surgery program in Toronto.

These innovations had a great impact on the world of cardiac surgery. By October 1957, Bigelow had received over 12,000 requests for reprints; "60 to 70% of the requests come from Europe and Britain." He had received sixty-one invitations to speak on hypothermia alone, six of them from Europe and Great Britain, of which he accepted two. He lamented, "The University of Toronto and the Toronto General Hospital did not capitalize on the hypothermia concept by early clinical application. Part of the reason for this was the lack of investigative facilities which would have provided the surgical teams with congenital heart material for operation."[109] So he had at TGH a tough row to hoe (and excited some envy as well; the cardiovascular surgeons, nine in number by 1965, were only 7 percent of the hospital's surgical staff, but from 1956 to 1965 they had thirty percent of the surgery publications).[110]

In 1955 Bill Bigelow recruited Ray Heimbecker to the Department of Surgery. Heimbecker, the first full-time staff appointment at the General to the cardiovascular service, arrived just in time to assist Gordon Murray in the aforementioned aortic valve transplant and regarded Murray rather than Bigelow as his teacher. Heimbecker had come east from Calgary, Alberta, where he was born in 1922 and earned a BA from the University of Saskatchewan in 1944. He gained his MD from the University of Toronto in 1947, going on to train in surgery at the University of Toronto and at Johns Hopkins University. He qualified for his fellowship from the Royal College of Surgeons in 1955.

After joining the Department of Surgery on a fellowship from the Ontario Heart Foundation, Heimbecker worked in "the dingy windowless lab in the subbasement of the Banting Institute" on a heart-lung machine. The work was often scorned by fellow surgeons. "Ray. You're wasting your time." "Ray, get out of your ivory tower," helpful colleagues said.[111] The investigation of bypass techniques was happening in other centres as well. Bill Mustard had just operated at HSC on bypass using a monkey's lung as an oxygenator. Canadian Pipe and Steel Fabricators in Toronto then manufactured his design.

On 12 January 1958 Heimbecker, Bigelow, James Key, and Don Wilson performed Canada's first adult open-heart surgery on "the pump." (In 1957 there had already been several open-heart operations elsewhere in Canada with other forms of ventilation;[112] see the later section on William Mustard for pediatric open-heart surgery.) They repaired a large atrial septal defect in a twenty-five-year-old woman from northern Ontario. "The operating room was electric that day – indeed the whole hospital became electric," Heimbecker said. "Much to our delight the operation proceeded beautifully. The pump run was no longer than about twenty-five minutes and the defect was closed without a patch for the tissues were very lax. I also had to supervise the operation of the heart-lung machine, for I was in fact the chief perfusionist! ... So I would scrub and un-scrub throughout the procedure. It was thrilling to see inside the living human heart."[113] Said Heimbecker later, "It looks quite primitive by today's standards, but it saved quite a few lives."[114] (James Key himself, an Edinburgh graduate in 1939, helped pioneer microsurgery techniques under Bigelow at a time when few centres were offering the necessary laboratory facilities.[115])

There was close collaboration with the cardiologists. In 1958 Heimbecker also undertook the first left-heart catheterization in Canada, with Ramsay Gunton, estimating the insufficiency of the mitral valve and measuring "regurgitant flow" back into the left atrium.[116]

In the spring of 1958 a separate cardiovascular surgery unit was planned for TGH, the first in Canada. (It actually opened only in 1961, on the ninth floor of the Private Patients' Pavilion.) Occupying the eighth and ninth floors of the Private Patients' Pavilion, there were two big operating rooms, a smaller room for pacemakers, and an adjacent cardiovascular intensive care unit. Baird recalled, "The staff then consisted of Bill Bigelow, James Key, Ray Heimbecker, and myself."[117] Another cardiovascular service was also planned for the Toronto Western Hospital that year under Don Wilson. In 1960 Bigelow founded "the first resident training program in cardiovascular surgery in Canada."[118]

In 1962, after extensive experimental research, a team headed by Heimbecker conducted the world's first total replacement of a whole heart valve, inserting an aortic valve taken from a cadaver into a patient whose mitral valve was failing. The operation was conducted "under bypass" with a heart-lung machine. Although the patient died a month after the operation of an infection, at autopsy the donor valve was found "to be completely normal, in good position and functioning well."[119]

The Toronto Western Hospital also shone in cardiovascular surgery in the 1960s, and it is there that Ron Baird first enters the story. He was born at the Western in 1930 and earned an MD from the University of Toronto in 1954. As a final-year student he vividly recalled watching Gordon Murray operate, and according to cardiac surgeon and historian Bernard Goldman, "at a party to celebrate the end of final exams, his clinic group watched a television program in black and white on a tiny screen in which C Walton Lillehei [in 1954 at the University of Minnesota] described the first closure of a ventricular septal defect using his bold technique of cross circulation from mother to child." Baird trained in surgery with Bill Bigelow, working as well in the famous lab in the basement of the Banting Institute where so many young surgeons put in time doing basic science, in Baird's case the mechanism of hibernation, analogizing from hypothermia to the life of the groundhog. Goldman continues, "Ron … returned from a year as a Graham Travelling Fellow … with an interest in valve repair. Bill Bigelow gave him the opportunity of performing all aortic valve replacements at TGH."[120]

As a resident, Baird assisted Bigelow, Wilson, and Heimbecker in five or six aortic valve replacements in the late 1950s, then, as a staff surgeon himself, performed two in 1960–1. In 1964 Baird left TGH to work with Wilson at the Western. In 1968 Baird proposed an important modification to the technique that McGill surgeon Arthur Vineberg had first suggested in 1946 of increasing the blood supply to the heart muscle by attaching the nearby internal mammary artery to the coronary vessels.[121] (In 1946 Vineberg operated on dogs, in 1950 on humans.) Baird's modification, as he said, "encourage[d] high initial flow rates and sustained patency."[122] The Vineberg procedure launched cardiac surgery in Canada in general, and the procedure came to an end only with the advent of coronary artery bypass surgery in the 1970s.

The next step was transplanting replacements for failing hearts. A new era in cardiac surgery began on 3 December 1967 as Christiaan Barnard and his team in Cape Town, South Africa, performed the first human heart transplant.[123] In Toronto, an unidentified heart surgeon confirmed that researchers at the Banting Institute were conducting experimental transplant procedures on dogs, but there were "no immediate plans … to attempt a human heart transplant."[124] This attitude changed within a few months as new heart transplant programs began springing up "seemingly overnight."[125] In May 1968, William R. Drucker, Chair of Surgery, suggested to the cardiovascular surgeons that "in view of the recent publicity and world-wide interest in the subject of heart transplantation, I feel it behooves all centres with a sincere interest in the development of cardiac surgery to devote attention to this problem … The past record of the cardiovascular service in this University is such that I believe we are expected to demonstrate leadership in this terribly complex new area of surgery." He said he had asked Bigelow to take responsibility for organizing a heart transplantation program.[126]

Bigelow began the work-up. He sent Bernie Goldman on a McLaughlin Fellowship to Houston to observe Denton Cooley and Michael DeBakey doing open-heart operations. Alan Trimble was sent to Jackson, Mississippi, to learn the technique of doing primate transplants. The whole spirit of operating rapidly that had been developed in Houston on stilled hearts under bypass (under "anoxia") suffused the fledging program in Toronto.[127] Goldman said, "Everything was flaccid, everything was still – it was boom, boom, and you're out." These young surgeons prided themselves on the same rapidity. Goldman continued, "As they say, more people were killed outside of Houston than ever died in Houston, because surgeons would say, 'oh, that looks so simple,' and then after an hour of futzing around, the patient wouldn't come off the pump. Al Trimble could do it – it was this directness of surgery that Cooley had introduced."[128]

Yet despite these preparations the program did not go as planned. The first Toronto transplant was performed at the Toronto Western Hospital on 6 October 1968 by Don Wilson and Ron Baird, followed by a second later the same month.[129] The sole transplant done by Bigelow's team at the General in 1968 ended in the patient's death. Reporting on the first five Toronto procedures at a symposium in June 1969, the surgeons described the program as "a co-operative effort" despite being carried out in three separate hospitals.[130] But in Baird's recollection the early heart transplant program was instead "fraught with inter-hospital competition and acrimony."[131]

The one bright spot in this discouraging story was cardiac surgeon Clare Baker's record at St. Michael's Hospital. Baker undertook his first heart transplant (Toronto's fourth) in November 1968 and went on to perform four more with only one fatality. He "recorded the second longest survivor in the world (Perrin Johnston, seven years survival) despite a demonstrable lack of enthusiasm for this venture from Dr. Bigelow and a direct order from the then professor of surgery, William Drucker, not to proceed with the transplant."[132]

Baker had graduated in medicine from the University of Toronto in 1946 and interned in Toronto but found it impossible to enter a residency program because all slots were occupied by returning veterans. After a residency in the sanatorium at Prince Albert, he obtained three years of general surgical training in The Hague and then in thoracic surgery at Utrecht. But upon returning to Toronto to fellow at St Michael's in 1951–2, he had some difficulties with Robert Janes and Fred Kergin, the chiefs of surgery at the Toronto General Hospital. So Baker spent a year at Hopkins learning cardiac surgery under Alfred Blalock before joining the staff at St Michael's. There he organized a cardiac catheterization laboratory.

In 1958 Baker began an open-heart surgery program with the purchase of a Mayo-Gibbon pump oxygenator. He tried to persuade the Avro company (of the Canadian aerospace concept "the Avro Arrow") to develop a pump, yet the downtown department refused to collaborate.

Baker and colleagues tell the story from here:

Clare Baker had a unique relationship with the colourful chief coroner of Ontario, Dr Smirlie Lawson, a fraternity brother, who instructed all pathologists on call to notify Baker prior to any postmortem examinations. Baker carried a sterile instrument bundle in his car trunk so as to harvest aorta and femoral arteries, which were then freeze-dried … Throughout his career, Baker had to work independent of the university program but was supported by the sisters who ran the hospital. Indeed, he brought dogs from the Banting Institute to St. Michael's in order to train anaesthetists and nurses in open-heart surgery with perfusion using a 'Rube Goldberg' assembled pump ... The project was halted rather abruptly when a dead canine was returned and left outside the Banting Institute doors on a hot summer Friday evening.[133]

St Michael's then developed its own animal facility. Though St Michael's had no formal connection with the U of T training program, cardiac surgery there thrived anyway and residents and fellows turned up, keen for a chance to sharpen their skills and work with a great teacher.

"Baker became widely known for his success with open-heart surgery in Jehovah's Witnesses and indeed performed major operations on 147 such patients with only a single death after double valve replacement. He performed over two hundred open mitral [valve] operations without a single mortality."[134]

Why the heart transplant patients at St Michael's had survived is unknown. Goldman said they "got lucky." Cyclosporine was not yet available, and organ transplants were often doomed because the body's immune rejection of the foreign organ could not be suppressed (heart valves are different in that they do not have a blood supply of their own). Lasting successes came only post-cyclosporine – at the University of Western Ontario – after Ray Heimbecker left Toronto to become professor of surgery at UWO in 1973. In 1983, Tirone David and Chris Feindel at the Western resumed cardiac transplantation in Toronto. Baird lamented, "In general, heart transplantation has never flourished in Canada both due to a lack of available donors and improving success with other therapies for heart failure."[135] This ended the great string of innovations in Toronto cardiac surgery of the 1950s and 1960s. Baird became hospital division head at TWH in 1972, then returned to TGH as head of cardiovascular surgery. He became university chair for cardiovascular surgery in 1977.

Even the participants themselves were awestruck at the progress they had made in two decades. James Key talked of "signposts towards surgical treatment which simply did not exist prior to the 1950s. It is rather wonderful to be able to look back on the early days when we operated on patients with mitral disease who very often were in severe failure with bilateral pleural effusions, when our operative mortality in certain groups was in the region of 20–30%, and to think that now we are rather upset if we have one to two cases in 100 who die as a result of surgery."[136]

Was there anything distinctively Canadian about these achievements that placed Canada in the international forefront of cardiac surgery? A theme of this book has been a distinctive Canadian willingness for medical leaders to shun the posture of "the titan" and work peaceably together. Bigelow felt this was the key to the take-off of heart surgery in Toronto: "These men and most of their contemporaries de-emphasized the cult of personality and converted the teacher back to perpetual student. This eliminated the academic hierarchy (Herr Geheimrat) typical of European countries, where excessive authority in the past has often strangled creative work."[137] The Toronto cardiac surgeons actually liked one another and were buddies.

*Hypothermia: A Rather Deflating Footnote*

For all its virtue in inaugurating the world chapter on open-heart surgery, hypothermia turned out to be unnecessary. This was established at St Michael's Hospital (SMH). Tomas Salerno came to St Michael's on Baker's watch in 1984, Samuel Lichtenstein in 1986. When Bernie Langer became professor of surgery, attitudes towards St Michael's warmed; the hospital became drawn into the university training program in heart surgery when Salerno became chair of the university division of cardiovascular surgery in 1987.

Salerno and Lichtenstein, assisted by Arthur Slutsky, introduced warm-heart surgery, or "continuous normothermic myocardial protection with oxygenated warm blood cardioplegia." "Recently, the authors have developed a technique … in which cardiac arrest is maintained using warm blood with potassium. This approach is currently the myocardial protection of choice of the cardiac surgeons at St Michael's Hospital in Toronto, and has been applied with great success in well over 200 patients."[138] Baker and colleagues said, "This created a stir in a city and university whose history was based on hypothermia."[139]

Shortly after Salerno and Lichtenstein undertook "normothermic" coronary bypass surgery, a randomized trial by the "Warm Heart Investigators" of 1,732 heart-surgery patients found normothermic even superior to hypothermic heart surgery. Based at Sunnybrook Hospital, and led by Slutsky, the investigators included David Naylor as the study epidemiologist, Lichtenstein himself as the SMH site director, and a large number of other participants, who found that "warm heart surgery may be preferable to hypothermic techniques for isolated coronary bypass surgery."[140]

This golden era in cardiac surgery came to a provisional end at St Michael's in 1988 when a patient died, after numerous previous cancellations, while awaiting bypass surgery; a provincial kerfuffle resulted. Lichtenstein and Salerno left. A happy by-product of the episode, however, was the creation of the Cardiac Care Network of Ontario, which established rules for access and nurse coordinators to supervise placement on waiting lists.[141]

*Mustard at HSC*

William T. Mustard, one of the international founders of pediatric heart surgery, was a bit of a wild card. On one occasion, after a tense operation, when his residents had begun closing the chest, "Mustard eased the pressure on the operating room staff by dropping to his knees and crawling out of the theatre on all fours. Outside, in the corridor, John Law, the administrator of the hospital, was escorting two VIPs on a tour of the building as the surgeon crawled toward them. 'May I present our Chief of Cardiovascular Surgery,' said the dignified Mr Law. The surgeon waved a paw and said, 'If you live a dog's life you might as well behave like one', and kept on crawling."[142]

Born in Clinton, Ontario, in 1914, Mustard was a year younger than Bigelow. Both of Mustard's parents were teachers, and his colleague George Trusler noted that he "was said to be exceptionally bright, reading widely." He attended the University of Toronto Schools, then entered medical school, which, Trusler said, "he literally coasted through ... applying his energies to theatrical skit nights where his wit and sense of humour allowed him to write and play in most of the [Daffydil] productions." Mustard was active in sports too, and later in life at scholarly meetings he was known to spend most of the time in the hotel pool. Graduating in 1937, Mustard interned in 1937–8 at the General, spent another year at the Hospital for Sick Children, then went in 1939 to the New York Orthopedic Hospital. In July 1940 he entered the Gallie program in surgery at the General, just as the war began. Thus in September 1941 he enlisted in the Canadian Army Medical Corps, taking overseas with him a supply of heparin. At the field surgical unit, "he inserted the vitellium tubes [a glass tube introduced in the First World War for reconstructing blood vessels] and administered heparin to soldiers with severely damaged leg arteries in an attempt to save their limbs. This was probably the first time a prosthetic material was used in the human cardiovascular system and he was awarded an MBE."[143]

After the war Mustard served two residencies, the first at HSC from July 1945 to January 1946, the second at the New York Orthopedic Hospital from January to December 1946. In the 1948–9 session, Mustard spent three months with the great cardiovascular surgeon Clarence Crafoord in Stockholm, who in 1944 was first to repair a coarctation, or stricture, of the aorta. "At about this time," Segall says in his history of Canadian cardiology, "Dr. John Keith became chief of cardiology at the Sick Children's Hospital. Presently, the need for a surgeon who would specialize, full-time in paediatric cardiovascular surgery made itself felt. Dr. Mustard accepted this new challenge."[144]

In 1947 Mustard entered for the first time the world of heart surgery in children, describing his own efforts to close surgically a defect called "patent ductus arteriosus" that Robert Gross of Boston first repaired surgically in 1938. The ductus is a normal fetal structure – usually closing spontaneously after birth – that shunts blood from the left pulmonary artery to the descending aorta (without being oxygenated in the lungs, unnecessary in the fetus). A ductus that fails to close, remaining "patent," is a danger to the child, in Mustard's terms, because "the increased load on the heart may lead to eventual failure and the diminished systemic circulation to underdevelopment." The eddying blood also lends itself to the growth of bacteria-laden "vegetations" within the heart, causing fatal subacute bacterial endarteritis. Around

1940 Toronto surgeon David E. Robertson (MB in 1907) attempted a number of "very bloody and difficult" ductus operations with uncertain outcome.[145] Other surgeons had already described a successful technique. Mustard implemented it with good results at the Hospital for Sick Children.[146] He was thus not the first surgeon to perform it but offered a careful guide, at a time when penicillin was just becoming available and perspectives for the operation brightened. The pulmonary artery and aorta are of course outside of the heart and this is not intracardiac surgery.

There was a parenthesis. In October 1948 Mustard and John Fraser took up again a torch first lit at the Hospital for Sick Children in 1921 by Lawrence Bruce Robertson: the replacement of an infant's entire blood volume, or exsanguination, in erythroblastosis fetalis (blood group incompatibility between mother and fetus leading to accelerated destruction of red cells): Mustard and Fraser found it superior to repeated transfusions.[147]

In cardiac surgery, the next step for Mustard was a giant one. In 1949 he and A. Lawrence ("Lawrie") Chute, later dean of medicine, initiated open-heart surgery on bypass support by beginning a long series of operations on animals in order to get the procedure right so that it could be some day used on humans. This counts as the world's first open-heart bypass surgery, even though it was on dogs. Others had attempted compromises, but the HSC group was first to take the returning venous blood, pass it through an oxygenator, and return it to the body on the arterial side. The circulation is thus continued outside the body: "The entire circulation of the animal is maintained," said the investigators, "yet the heart is empty of blood."[148] The main problem was oxygenating the blood – in bypassing the lungs while the heart was stopped. "It was our experience that the amount of heparin required, the lack of filtering, and the relatively ineffectual oxygenation secured caused our experimental animals to die for reasons of bleeding, emboli and anoxia." They therefore abandoned artificial oxygenators and tried using the lung of another animal just removed at autopsy and kept alive in a solution: "In Experiment 3 of our second series, we were able to bypass the heart successfully for 17 minutes using a lung which had been removed 2 and a half hours previously." The dog survived in perfectly normal condition for more than two months before being sacrificed.

"We never did get a picture of that dog," said Mustard. "We should have had one like Banting and Best of the first insulin dog. I think ours was the first dog in the world to survive having its heart opened."[149]

The researchers also continued to work with artificial oxygenators and finally began to achieve a modicum of success. In 1950 they reported at the Royal College of Physicians and Surgeons meeting in Ottawa, "In our second experimental series, which consisted of 45 operations, we have had ten survivals." They had successfully undertaken all manner of operations upon these dogs: "We have performed valvulotomies on the pulmonic valve through the pulmonary artery and we have opened the right ventricle to visualize the interventricular septum." The paper was published in 1951.[150] (Technically, this was not the world's first heart-lung machine because the lung was biological, not mechanical. John Gibbon at the University of Pennsylvania Medical School in Philadelphia built the first heart-lung machine in 1939.[151]) The next step, clearly, would be undertaking these open-heart operations in humans.

The next step failed. In 1951 Mustard operated on a sixteen-month-old child with the "tetralogy of Fallot." There were operative difficulties, the ventricular septal defect was not repaired, and the patient died.[152]

In 1952 the Mustard team, which included Chute and John Keith among others, attempted bypass operations on seven infants who had transposition of the great vessels. This is much more complex than the operation for tetralogy of Fallot, for it involves the repair of vessels entering and leaving the heart and lung on the wrong side. They used a monkey's lung as an oxygenator. None survived, although proof of concept was the preservation of life in these infants for brief periods. "The important thing," observed the *Toronto Daily Star* in June 1952, "is that the machine worked, and the fact it kept these eight [*sic*] infants alive at all while their own hearts were stopped holds out tremendous promise for the future when used in cases where there is some hope."[153] Mustard reported the work in 1954. "We feel that this application of an extracorporeal circulation could be undertaken in less hopeless cases," the team concluded optimistically. Sheer technical innovativeness in undertaking the procedure made Mustard's name internationally.[154]

In 1953 he began having successes. His colleague George Trusler said, "It was in 1953 that he had his first surviving patient, the first in Canada surviving a congenital repair on cardiopulmonary bypass."[155] By 1955 they had undertaken 480 cardiovascular operations of all kinds, with a mortality of about 25 percent.[156]

Still, open-heart operations remained challenging. By 1957, of the twenty-one humans Mustard had put "on the pump" since 1951, three were "alive and well." These were not unencouraging results, considering that these were desperate cases and that Mustard was learning from past failures, his techniques improving all the time. Mustard said, "Our results at present lead us to explore cautiously the possibility of operation on better risk patients."[157]

In 1964 Mustard devised a simplified operation for the transposition of the great vessels, replacing the septum between the atria with a baffle of pericardium.[158] (This became known as the "Mustard operation.") "The operation was greeted with much enthusiasm," said Trusler, "being relatively simple, easily reproducible, with good early results. For the next thirteen years [until his retirement] Mustard lived with increasing fame and Sick Children's enjoyed a wonderful reputation with patients coming from all over the globe. He built a five-foot-high inflatable see-through plastic model of the atrial chambers of the heart with the Mustard baffle in place and he would take residents and visitors on a walk through the model in his own inimitable style … and he would finally pronounce the whole procedure 'baffling.'"[159]

"All of these new procedures carried a relatively high surgical mortality when they were first introduced," said John Keith, head of cardiology at the children's hospital, who introduced pediatric cardiac catheterization and angiocardiography to Canada just after the Second World War. "The mortality has fallen to relatively low levels. But one would shudder to have to go through it a second time."[160]

### Polio Vaccine

The Connaught Laboratories received attention in the previous chapter because of their development of important vaccines before the Second World War. Yet after the war there was one more big one: they made a major contribution to the polio vaccine.

Historian Christopher Rutty tells the story. In Boston in 1949 John Enders figured out how to grow the polio virus in test tubes with tissues other than from the nervous system. The problem was learning how to grow the virus in amounts sufficient for research. In 1947, Andrew Rhodes, a Scottish medical microbiologist with an international reputation for his groundbreaking 1940 textbook on virology, had come to Connaught. His initial work was epidemiological, and in 1950 he identified an association between the Coxsackie and the poliomyelitis viruses.[161] Rhodes became part of an "elite research team" – including Raymond Parker, an experimental cytologist, and John F. Morgan, a biochemist – that Robert Defries, the director of the laboratories, had put together for the development of a polio vaccine.[162] In research funded by the Canada Life Assurance Company and the National Foundation for Infantile Paralysis in the United States, Rhodes began growing in 1951 the virus in test tubes along the lines Enders had suggested.

Between 1947 and 1949, Morgan and Helen Morton at Connaught, under the supervision of Parker, had developed a synthetic nutrient base called "Medium 199." In the fall of 1951 Morgan gave a member of Rhodes's team, Arthur Franklin, some "199" to see if it might better grow the poliovirus. Rutty said, "To Franklin's surprise it worked incredibly well and was particularly effective for cultivating the poliovirus in monkey kidney cells." Medium 199 solved a big problem for Jonas Salk, originator of the inactivated polio vaccine.

Salk was confident that an inactivated vaccine could prevent polio in humans as it seemed to in monkeys. However, it was not yet safe for human trial, nor could he make enough for the millions who were clamouring for protection from the dreaded crippler. Connaught solved both problems. Medium 199 provided a chemically pure culture base, which encouraged the National Foundation for Infantile Paralysis [NFIP] in New York to finance a major pilot project at Connaught to cultivate the poliovirus in large quantities. In 1952, this effort led to the 'Toronto Method,' developed by Leone N. Farrell, who held a PhD in biochemistry (1933) from the University of Toronto. It involved culturing the poliovirus in a solution of '199' and monkey kidney cells using large Povitsky bottles incubated on a special rocking machine.[163]

In 1952 the availability of "199" prompted Salk to undertake a clinical trial of his vaccine. In July 1953, on the threshold of a polio epidemic, the NFIP asked Defries to provide quantities of poliovirus fluids sufficient for a national field trial of Salk's vaccine. Rutty noted, "Through the fall and winter of 1953–54 large bottles full of each of the three poliovirus types were sent in station wagons to Parke, Davis in Detroit and Eli Lilly in Indianapolis, for inactivation and processing. In total Connaught produced some 3,000 litres of poliovirus fluids for the trial."

The rest of the story is well known. In 1954, almost two million children were given either the vaccine or the innocuous "199" as a placebo. The results of the trial were announced on 12 April 1955 and caused an international sensation. In September 1955 Hart van Riper, the medical director of the NFIP, told the members of the Canadian Public Health Association, "The record stands clear that in 1955 you successfully manufactured nearly 2,000,000 cc. of a safe and effective poliomyelitis vaccine and promptly administered two 1 cc. doses of it to almost 1,000,000 Canadian children without mishap or suspicion that the vaccine might have induced any case of ... poliomyelitis."[164] This Canadian public health triumph is legendary, but the Toronto contribution to it was, before Rutty's work, not widely known.[165]

Rhodes briefly left Connaught in 1951 for a post as virologist at the Hospital for Sick Children and in 1953 served as the founding director of the Research Institute at HSC. In 1956 he returned to campus as director of the School of Hygiene and head of its Department of Microbiology. He was probably Canada's premier virologist.

## Stem Cells

Seen from the first decades of the twenty-first century, the major contribution of Faculty of Medicine scientists to the world narrative was undoubtedly stem cells, for today the therapeutic applications of stem cells seem legion, offering dramatic breakthroughs in a host of diseases. The discovery of stems cells occurred in the Department of Medical Biophysics of the faculty, founded in July 1958 (though research had begun the year previously) and housed at the Ontario Cancer Institute (OCI), then on Sherbourne Street and including a cancer hospital called the Princess Margaret Hospital[166]. The discoverers were Ernest McCulloch and James Till.

The discovery was the capstone of the assembling of scientific talent at the OCI from places as diverse as Paris, New Haven, and Saskatoon and concentrating these researchers in the same department, called medical biophysics, where, side by side, they could work together. Arthur Ham headed the department, a member of the faculty since 1932 and headquartered in the Department of Anatomy as the chief histologist. Yet even though Ham prepared an enormous textbook on histology, his main scientific interest was cancer: How do tumours arise? In the Department of Anatomy in the 1950s he headed a crack team studying carcinogenesis. It was Ham who assembled the rest of the team at OCI.

Ham's right-hand man, in a sense, was the virologist and geneticist Louis ("Lou") Siminovitch. Siminovitch, thirty-eight in 1958, was a Montreal PhD in biochemistry who had worked at the Pasteur Institute just after the Second World War with François Jacob, André Lwoff, and Jacques Monod, who all won Nobel Prizes in 1965. In 1953 he had joined the Connaught Laboratories and was firmly planted in the mainstream of research on somatic cell biology (as opposed to molecular biology – the study of the DNA of cells and its workings). It was Siminovitch who brought somatic cell biology to the University of Toronto. But by the late 1950s he was increasingly distracted by administration (a matter that interested Ham little), and had become more of an enabler than an active bench scientist. Yet he was a sure judge of science and of talent, and he helped assemble the staff of the Department of Medical Biophysics.

Siminovitch brought with him from the Pasteur Institute an incandescent commitment to science. He recalled working in Paris with the later Nobelists: "There were no research applications in the Paris lab, no reports and no meetings – obviously in stark contrast to today's culture. Science was the order of the day. I cannot recall any disputes other than those concerned with science, or any arguments about credit. Sounds utopian – and it was!" (Siminovitch was disarmingly frank about why he drifted into the role of enabler at OCI: the Nobel Prize winners he had known were "the crème de la crème. I came to the conclusion that there was a level of science achievement that I would likely never reach."[167])

Also coming over from the anatomy department was Arthur Axelrad, thirty-five in 1958. He had been educated at McGill as an MD and held a PhD in anatomy, receiving both degrees in 1954. He had been a member of the Department of Anatomy at U of T since 1956 and had done pioneering work there in carcinogenesis.

One member of the Department of Medical Biophysics was central in the stem cell story: Ernest McCulloch. "Bun," or "Bunny," McCulloch (as a childhood nickname had somewhat improbably survived) was born in Toronto in 1926, earning an MD in 1948, then training in hematology, with a special interest in plasma proteins, at the Lister Institute of London. He joined the Department of Medicine at Sunnybrook in 1952 and, at age thirty-one in 1957, was in at the ground floor in the Division of Biological Research at the Ontario Cancer Institute. A year later, he was a founding member of the Department of Medical Biophysics. Until 1967 McCulloch was cross-appointed at the General and the OCI. When McCulloch arrived at OCI he was keen, as he later put it, "to study the function of bone marrow by transplanting marrow cells into irradiated hosts and needed the institute's facilities to irradiate mice."[168] Thus, except for Ham, this crack research was conducted by relatively young men in their thirties. (Further details of McCulloch's life are found in chapter 13.)

Harold Johns, head of the OCI's Physics Division, insisted that members of the Biological Research Division of the Cancer Institute who wanted to employ radiation must collaborate with a physicist. (McCulloch later said, "Harold Johns' reputation was built on accurate measurement of radiation and he wasn't going to have any damn doctor ruining his reputation by misusing his machine."[169]) A likely volunteer was the young biophysicist James Till.

Till was born in Lloydminster, Saskatchewan, in 1931 and graduated with a bachelor's degree from the University of Saskatchewan in 1952. He went on to take a master's degree with Harold Johns and became inspired. "What needed to be better researched," he said later in an interview, "was the biological effects of radiation – what was it that was killing cancer cells."[170] The only PhD program going at the time in radiation biology was Yale's, so in the fall of 1954 Till and fellow student Gordon Whitmore went down to New Haven, Connecticut. Till earned a PhD in biophysics at Yale in 1957, taking a number of microbiology courses as part of the program.

At Yale, he had become interested in individual cells growing in cell culture: How many cells were capable of forming colonies after receiving various radiation doses ("survival curve")? Till thought he might pursue this after graduating if he could find someone to work with, and he discovered that one of the world experts was Lou Siminovitch, who was just being hired at the Ontario Cancer Institute in Toronto. And his old mentor Harold Johns was going to OCI as well! So Till and Whitmore were both hired as postdocs at OCI just before it opened. They spent the year out at the Connaught "Farm" working with Siminovitch on mouse "L" cells. The first paper to come out of this work was published in 1957 in the *Proceedings of the National Academy of Sciences*.[171]

In the fall of 1957 Till, Whitmore, and Siminovitch came down from the Farm to the brand-new OCI building on Sherbourne Street, still so empty they didn't even have distilled water. None of the new staff, with the exception of the physicists who had been students of Johns, knew the others very well. So Arthur Ham, who did not like going out in the evening, had some get-togethers in his home. Here Till met McCulloch.

Till was interested in what McCulloch wanted to do: "study total body irradiation of mice." McCulloch wanted to study this because he and pediatrician John Darte had done some bone marrow transplants on children with leukemia, "in an effort to enhance their survival, which was dismal at the time. Those transplants failed."[172] So McCulloch wanted to carry out some experiments irradiating mice. He needed a volunteer physicist to help him, and Till said, "I'll volunteer." He volunteered because he remembered how McCulloch had described his own interests during those get-togethers at the Ham home. "But even more, how interesting a person I had found him to be. He was clearly – to me – not a conventional doc."

They were also different in social terms. McCulloch was a graduate of Upper Canada College. Till's father had been a farmer in Alberta. "McCulloch was the rumpled stocky foil to Till's tall and trim elegance," said an obituary of McCulloch in 2011. Yet they became close friends and remained so. Said McCulloch later, "One of the things I'm happiest about is that even now, all these years later, we're very good friends."[173]

So McCulloch and Till went to work in McCulloch's lab, irradiating mice to kill their bone marrow cells, then transplanting the mice with various numbers of healthy new marrow cells. To their great surprise, the transplanted cells formed little bumps, or colonies, on the spleen. The colonies were formed from a single cell, "so they were clones. They weren't formed from a cluster of cells." Till continued, "We didn't think of them as stem cells, initially. We wondered, but we were careful to call them 'colony forming units [CFUs] … We knew they were single cells from [graduate student] Andy Becker's work."

The other interesting thing about the colonies was that some of them "contained more than one kind of blood-forming cell," Till later said in an interview. McCulloch, as a hematologist, was familiar with the long-standing debate about whether mature blood cells, such as red cells and white cells, "each had a separate progenitor, or whether there was a common progenitor for more than one of these mature cells types."

The answer from the McCulloch-Till research was a common progenitor. That progenitor was a stem cell. The classic paper was published in 1961.[174]

At this point Lou Siminovitch enters the story. The next step was to ask a genetic question: Do the cells in the colonies "breed true"? "If you transplant cells from individual colonies, do you get more colonies?" (Remember that Till and McCulloch are still calling the stem cells "CFUs" at this point.) So they transplanted the colonies into irradiated mice, and they got new colonies containing the same mix of cells as in the old colonies, as well as the CFUs (stem cells) in the new colonies. "You could get new colony forming units from a colony, which is the crucial finding. So they can self-renew. That was the term that was used." They key paper showing clonal cells was lead-authored by Becker in 1963.[175] The counterpart key paper giving a functional definition of stem cells for the first time was lead-authored by Siminovitch, also in 1963.[176] This was the first paper to use the term "stem cells," said Till retrospectively (although by 1962 the dean, Lawrie Chute, was using the phrase "stem cells" in describing their work[177]).

The term "stem cells" had been around, Till said, "since the beginning of the 1900s – or before, when the term was used to describe a fertilized egg that becomes an organism. But the research on it had been entirely observational, and mostly speculative. People looked in the microscope at sections of tissue and tried to track what cells came from where. But they couldn't. If there were progenitor cells there, they weren't recognizable by any of the standard light microscopy and staining techniques." Till and McCulloch had revolutionized the literature by "experimental studies on the function of stems cells. We didn't care what they looked like."

What Till and McCulloch did and did not do: they didn't isolate the stem cells. They did not see under the microscope any cells they identified as stem cells. That came later from other investigators. "We just took marrow transplanted into mice. Some of the stem cells migrated to the spleen, which is a blood-forming organ in the mouse, and produced these colonies. So we detected the stem cells by virtue of the progeny they produced."

Their contribution lay as well in one important technical detail: they varied the number of marrow cells they transplanted into the irradiated mice from 10,000 (a small number) to a million. "Most people had just been giving a million or more."

Would a million have been too many? "Oh, yes. If that had not been the design, it would not have been possible to see individual spleen colonies. They would have all overlapped, and you would just have seen a regenerating spleen."

But other investigators had seen bumps on the spleen too. Why didn't they interpret the bumps correctly? Till said, "What they didn't have was a background in microbiology. They had to have prepared minds that made them think about clonality. The point of view that came from microbiology that I have been describing, a colony makes you think, 'what's the cell origin of that, and was it an individual cell?'" At Yale, Till had been trained in microbiology, and McCulloch as a hematologist was an experienced hand at cell cultures. So they knew to ask the right questions. It is remarkable that Harold Johns and Arthur Ham had brought together exactly the right mix of "prepared minds," in Louis Pasteur's term, at OCI to make this epochal discovery.

The stem cell research was one of the Ontario Cancer Institute's greatest contributions to science. McCulloch said later, "The stem cell paradigm, as applied to both normal and malignant populations, was a unifying force for the OCI. The discovery and implementation of the paradigm remains one of the institution's major contributions to cell biology and cancer research."[178] The whole concept of stem cells emerged from Toronto. Robert Phillips, deputy director of the Ontario Institute for Cancer Research, said, "The pair had laid down, right from the beginning, the properties that stem cells must possess. Stem cells have the potential to develop into all cell types, including skin cells, heart cells and blood cells, and are capable of renewing themselves. With their regenerative capabilities, they offer new ways to treat diseases, from diabetes to heart disease."[179] They also laid the foundation for bone marrow transplantation in leukemia, to let the bone marrow transplants renew the blood. Long before the importance of stem cells loomed on the scientific radar, their existence was established in the Faculty of Medicine.

But the story didn't move on from here. Science was plunging into molecular biology, and at that point one couldn't study the DNA of stem cells because no one could identify them in the colonies. So after an initial burst of scientific interest, the discovery languished for a long time. It was only in 2005 that Till and McCulloch won a Lasker Award. The further stem cell story is told in chapter 28.

### Goodbye to the 1950s

In 1955 Dean Joseph MacFarlane, in a talk to the businesspeople of the Empire Club in Toronto, summed up what a difference science at the University of Toronto, and elsewhere, had made for people's health. Since 1900, life expectancy for boys, he said, had increased by more than eighteen years, for girls twenty-one. "Diabetes and pernicious anemia are under control. The common infections that were the major causes of illness in the early part of the century can for the most part be controlled, if not eradicated." Preventive medicine had made the great childhood killers typhoid and diphtheria "almost forgotten diseases in this generation of Canadians." People now understood the basic mechanisms of these diseases as well as their active treatment by drugs. "No longer is lobar pneumonia the winter scourge of the Canadian community. It is rare indeed to hear of death or even prolonged illness from blood poisoning." The surgeons now had access to the organs of the body's major cavities – brain and central nervous system, and chest and heart – thanks to advances in anesthesia and blood transfusion. "This golden age of medicine in the first half of the twentieth century is contemporaneous with the new concept and organization of medical schools. Who will say they are otherwise unrelated?"[180]

# 6  Surgery

Surgeons are really doctors who also know how to operate.[1]

Richard Reznick, Chair, Department of Surgery, 2005

**Professors of Surgery and Heads of the Department of Surgery:**

William T. Aikins, 1887–97
Irving Howard Cameron, 1897–1920
Clarence Leslie Starr, 1921–9
William Edward Gallie, 1929–47
Robert M. Janes, 1947–57
Frederick Gordon Kergin, 1957–66
William Richard Drucker, 1966–72
Donald Richard Wilson, 1972–82
Bernard Langer, 1982–92
John H. Wedge, 1992–2002
Richard K. Reznick, 2002–10
David Latter, acting chair, 2010–11
James Rutka, 2011–present

It was in the 1960s that surgery pivoted from the United Kingdom to the United States; in the 1980s, under the leadership of Bernard Langer, it pivoted from teaching to research. The story is a dramatic one.

Few today can recall how it once was. Back in the days of surgery without antibiotics – the 1930s – Fred Dewar, later head of orthopedic surgery at the Toronto General Hospital, recalled the infections he saw as an intern at the General. "Some of them, if it really got severe, they would die … This was the time of severe streptococcal abscesses of children's ears, septic arthritis in the hips, fused hips. One patient, I remember, had an operation for a hernia and he was dead in 48 hours from streptococcal peritonitis. It is hard to believe these things occurred, but this was part and parcel of surgery, fingernail infections, boils, abscesses, they were all over the place."[2]

The 1930s were just a step away from the days when antisepsis and asepsis were still new and the surgeon scarcely a cut above other craftsmen; surgeon and carpenter alike were once trained in apprenticeships. In 1892 the faculty received a letter, addressed to the "Superintendent of the University," from Mr A.H. Gerry, in Randolph, Nebraska: "I am advised by Dr A Eddy, a Physician here, to go to your institute and take a term of lectures in Surgery. Please enform [sic] me what would be expected of me to enter that Part of your institute. I have been doktering horses in this vicinity for several years and Castrating and such work and I do not claim to do any thing except by experience. Hoping to hear from you."[3]

By the 1930s surgery was established as a specialty the equal of if not superior to medicine – because surgeons could actually make patients better, whereas the Department of Medicine was still in the slough of therapeutic despond that only the antibiotics would end. By the 1930s, the Department of Surgery at the University of Toronto was prestigious indeed.

I will peel back the surgery story layer by layer, starting with teaching.

## Teaching in the Department of Surgery

From the get-go the surgeons felt themselves mobbed by undergraduates who were for the most part unteachable and uninterested. In 1934 Gallie complained that the many students lacked opportunity to examine the patients. "There is a limit to the amount of handling by students that sick people can stand and that limit has long since been reached."[4]

How much surgery should they teach the undergraduates? There was a range between teaching them very little and "training all students in the principles of technique." The rule was no knife on the skin of the abdomen unless you had postgraduate training. This was a definite retreat from the old notion that the training of "physicians and surgeons" produced doctors who would be equally competent at removing a gall bladder on a farmhouse kitchen table at night and diagnosing strep throat. Gallie said in 1939, "We are definitely committed to the idea that surgery has grown to such proportions that no man should engage in it unless he has taken several years of postgraduate training as a house-surgeon in a service in which he is gradually stepped up from the position of a second assistant to that of a surgeon performing the various operations under the critical eye of his teacher." So the undergraduates are taught principles and methods of examination and diagnosis plus "just enough of the technique of the surgery of everyday office and visiting practice ... to stimulate the student's interest in his work."[5]

After the war the question of how to teach surgery to undergraduates again surfaced. In 1952 Robert Janes, head of the department, said, "The great problem is to sort from the vast amount of material what may be regarded as fundamental knowledge." Undergraduates felt overwhelmed. "Because of the shift of emphasis from the teaching of technique to the teaching of the diagnosis of surgical conditions, the indications for surgical therapy, and the benefits that may be expected from surgery, the graduate of today possesses much more useful knowledge than graduates before him. Unfortunately, many probably feel that they have been taught little of what they regard as surgery."[6] It was pointless to teach surgical techniques – knife on the skin – to undergraduates, but at least as family doctors out in the community, they would know when it was appropriate and what might be expected from it.

On the whole then, in the early days the undergraduates came second. As Bernard Langer, who later became professor of surgery, put it, "The priority activities were excellence in clinical practice and postgraduate teaching. Undergraduate teaching was secondary to most but there were outstanding teachers such as Bruce Tovee."

In the William Drucker years, from 1966 to 1972, undergraduate teaching received more emphasis. Drucker was, said Langer, "a passionate teacher who encouraged and inspired young staff to take teaching more seriously."

Don Wilson as chair in 1972–82 "recognized that academic physicians had not been trained to teach and that the university should prepare them better. He invited speakers from the Faculty of Education to rounds and made available seminars on teaching principles for young staff. This was a seminal contribution." What emerges from the archives, supplementing Langer's analysis, is that Wilson thought it pointless to teach family doctors the rudiments of surgery. When at a meeting of the Long-Range Planning Committee in May 1974 Wilson was asked to comment on the division of responsibility between the general surgeon and the family practitioner, he said, in the secretary's paraphrase, "At present there is no need for the family practitioner to do surgical work except in minor cases or emergencies … Regarding surgical training necessary for a family practitioner, [Wilson] defined this as the ability to recognize surgical problems and know what the surgeon has to offer."[7]

The years after Wilson saw a greater emphasis on teaching skills in both undergraduate and postgraduate education. For all his emphasis on research, Langer himself, during his own tenure from 1982 to 1992, was a great advocate of improving the teaching of residents. He encouraged surgical residents, such as Richard Reznick, a 1977 McGill graduate, to seek formal training in education and sent him off to complete a master's degree in surgical education at the University of Southern Illinois, after which Reznick returned to U of T as a colorectal surgeon and head in 1987 of the department's undergraduate education committee. Langer hired a full-time nonphysician educator (Robert Cohen) to provide in-house guidance in education; Langer made excellence in teaching an acceptable criterion for promotion alongside research. In the 1989–90 session he said, "Teaching as an academic endeavour is now accepted as an important criterion for academic promotion ... In 1990 the promotions of several members of the Department were announced, based largely on the sustained excellence of teaching by these surgeons." A stream of surgeons who had completed MAs in education began to flow.[8] Making educational achievements a criterion for promotion, begun in the Department of Surgery, was later adopted by all other departments. Still, it was under Langer and his "Surgeon-Scientist" program that research in surgery took a great leap forward.

John Wedge took the chair in 1992, and together with Zane Cohen he established in 1998 the surgical skills laboratory at Mount Sinai Hospital, where the 210 third-year students might develop their talents in one-week sessions over the academic year.[9] In this, they were aided by Reznick, who, said Langer, "was on his way to becoming a leader in medical education" and was made vice president of education at TGH.[10] The Department of Surgery took great advantage of the simulation technology for both postgraduate and undergraduate instruction. "The simulator," said Reznick in 2008, "will have haptic feedback – it will provide a realistic sense of touch during palpation of tissues and it will bleed when incised."[11] This was a far cry from the hordes of disoriented undergraduates milling about the operating rooms in Gallie's day.

*Towards a Coordinated University Program in Surgery: The Gallie Course*

The great problem that has dogged the faculty throughout its history has been converting the disparate hospital departments into a unified university program of teaching and research. It is tedious to describe such an effort as "unification" or "coordination," yet the outcome is of great importance because it is only when forged into a single powerful university department that these isolated hospital entities may be hooked together as locomotives. This hooking-together occurred sooner or later for all the departments in the faculty. But it occurred earlier for surgery, which is one reason why the Department of Surgery in Toronto has been such a hugely successful enterprise.

Early in his tenure in the 1930s, Gallie tried to organize a university program in surgery, so that training in one hospital would not be vastly different from that in another, trainees could rotate, rounds would be held in common, and all the other forms of cooperation would occur that made a university program something more than an aggregate of hospital programs. "For a number of years," Gallie said in 1938, "it has been the hope of the Department of Surgery that the Surgical Divisions in the University Hospitals might be established on such a basis that the teaching could be conducted in a similar way in each. This hope has now been realized and it has become possible to distribute the students ... to the Toronto General Hospital, Saint Michael's Hospital and the Toronto Western Hospital in proportion to the number of surgical beds." Each surgical division had approximately eighty beds. TGH had three such divisions, St Michael's two, and the Western one. "The time-table is so arranged that every student has part of his surgical training in each of the three general hospitals." In the fifth year, all students rotated through a number of clinics at the children's hospital.[12]

Right after becoming professor of surgery, in the 1930–1 session, Gallie organized a systematic training program in surgery, the first in Canada.[13] To get into the very selective Gallie Course after a rotating internship was not easy. One had to spend a year tutoring in anatomy and physiology, then pass the primary examinations of the Royal College of Surgeons of Canada or of England, the latter of which meant going to England to take them. "Many of the candidates take a year off to prepare for it," said Gallie, "during which, through the kindly co-operation of the Departments of Anatomy and Physiology, they act as demonstrators in those departments and are granted an honorarium sufficient to cover their expenses." Then in the first year of the Gallie Course the residents spent six months in medicine, six months in pathology; in the second year they undertook general surgery, "in which the student acts as senior house-surgeon on one of the divisions"; in the final year the candidate served six months each in two of the three choices of urology, neurosurgery, or pediatric surgery. He was then qualified to attempt the final examination of the master's degree in surgery. But "he" was the wrong pronoun, for in the 1938–9 session, as Gallie was writing those words, Jessie Gray, a woman, successfully passed the qualifying exam for the master's. By 1939, thirty young men were said to have completed it or to be still in training.[14] Gallie emphasized rotating among the various hospitals during the three-year Gallie Course.[15]

Wasn't this a long time to spend in training? "It may be objected," wrote Gallie, "that this scheme, which calls for at least four years of post-graduate work, delays too long a young man's entrance into practice. To this there is only the one answer, that competence in surgery cannot be acquired in a shorter time. When this University grants a candidate the degree of Master of Surgery it is not simply awarding him a degree which can be obtained by any clever student by a process of examinations. It is guaranteeing that the candidate has been adequately trained and is, in all truth, a master of his craft."[16]

During the war the Gallie Course was abolished.[17] Surgery staff were shipping out constantly to war zones, and any systematic training program was out of the question. The department struggled to give candidates a minimum of preparation for wartime surgery and offered refresher courses in specific subjects – such as "as opening and closing the head, opening and closing the chest," as Gallie volunteered in 1941 to the director of military medical services in Ottawa. Gallie had in mind not lectures or clinics, "but rather a scheme by which individual officers would be attached for a period to a hospital service and given an opportunity to take active part in the work." He added, "As you may well imagine, an opportunity to render such a service as this would be welcomed by all old A.M.C. [Army Medical Corps] officers."[18]

World War II soldered the surgeons together into a kind of club; many of the later surgical leaders had been comrades-in-arms. Langer recalled, "Many of the young surgeons at TGH volunteered for service and distinguished themselves in England and in the war zones in Italy and Europe. These included: Fred Kergin [later chief of surgery at TGH and Department chair]; Joe MacFarlane [later dean of medicine]; Bruce Tovee [later head of general surgery]; Harry Botterell [head of neurosurgery, TGH]; Charles Robson [head of urology]; Ted Dewar [head of orthopedics]; Bob Mustard [chief of surgery, TGH]; Bill Mustard [head of cardiac surgery, HSC]; and many others."[19] The wartime shared experience may have been part of the secret of Toronto's success, bonding the comrades-at-arms so that they collaborated agreeably after the war rather than squabbling like prima donnas.

Though victory was not yet in sight in Europe, it was in sight in the Department of Surgery as in June 1944 Gallie asked how the department might cope with postgraduate training for the mass of young army surgeons returning from the war: "Each hospital will increase its staff of senior interns and ... an intern service will be provided at Christie Street Hospital and at Weston Sanitarium. We shall now revert to the programme of three years or more of training in surgery, disrupted by the war." He noted, "The interns will henceforth be viewed as post-graduate students proceeding to the exam for the diploma of Fellowship in the Royal College of Surgeons and for the Master of Surgery degree."[20] The Gallie Course was thus restored.

*Roscoe Graham and His Generation*

A whole generation of forward-looking surgeons thrived in Toronto between the wars. Roscoe Graham is remembered for pioneering surgery on the stomach and pancreas. Born in Lobo, Ontario, in 1890, the son of a country physician, Graham finished medical school in Toronto in 1910; he was elected president of the Medical At-Home Committee (a major social activity of the undergraduates).[21] After an internship at St Michael's Hospital, he travelled widely in Europe, training in surgery at St Bartholomew's Hospital in London and in some of the great centres on the Continent. During the war he served with the Canadian Army Medical Corps at the No. IV General Hospital in London. He returned in July 1919 to join the surgical staff of the Toronto General Hospital, where, as director of the first surgical division, he specialized in abdominal operations. Said his eulogist, "He was one of the first men in Canada to use iodine in the preparation of patients for the operation of partial thyroidectomy. His method of closure of perforated peptic ulcer was accepted widely throughout North America."[22]

In 1929 Graham successfully resected an islet cell tumour – a first – although, bafflingly, it was the internists caring for her who wrote the paper and Graham's name was not on it (though the piece did mention Graham as the surgeon and quoted from his notes).[23]

In 1938 Graham pointed out that surgery on uncomplicated duodenal ulcers was actually not necessary; one had only to deal with their complications such as perforation. Conservative about abdominal surgery, he pointed out that a rather austere lifestyle was preferable (but in those days a duodenal ulcer was indeed analogous to a sentence to a penal colony): "The patients must continue throughout their lives to be moderate in the expenditure of energy, both mental and physical, must continuously abstain from the use of alcohol and tobacco … No surgical procedure yet devised is more than a physiologic make-shift, which is no substitute for the self-discipline of a carefully-controlled life."[24] An internationally distinguished investigator, in 1932 Graham became the youngest surgeon ever elected to fellowship in the American Surgical Association. In the days when perforated ulcers were common, the "Graham patching technique" was widely adopted.

"[Graham's] manner and speech exuded energy," said his former student Barney Berris, "and he moved and spoke quickly and purposefully. He conducted a series of classes in which the chief resident in surgery would present findings from a patient's history and physical examination. At appropriate intervals, Dr. Graham would stop the presentation and with the help of the students would try to analyze the symptoms and findings that would serve to formulate a list of possible diagnoses. When the presentation and discussion were completed we would have arrived at a diagnosis we considered to be correct."

"At that point," Berris continued, "the chief resident went to the door and the man who was the attendant in the adjacent students' lounge entered wearing white gloves and carrying a silver tray on which there was a sealed envelope. Dr. Graham then picked up the envelope, tore it open and read, 'The correct diagnosis is ——.'"

"He then strode from the room without another word. If the deduced diagnosis was correct, there was no further discussion. If it was wrong, we spent the first few minutes of the next lecture analyzing the faults in our reasoning."[25]

For his technical capabilities, Graham acquired a huge reputation. The story Bigelow tells is about Edsel Ford, of the Ford family in Detroit, who needed surgery for a stomach tumour. He supposedly searched the world to find the absolutely top-notch surgeon. "He could have crooked his finger at any surgeon in the world," Bigelow said. "Instead, he invited Dr Roscoe Graham of Toronto General, who went to the Ford Hospital in Detroit and operated on Mr Ford."[26]

Graham is remembered as a large jolly man, in contrast to his cousin Duncan Graham, the first Eaton Professor of Medicine and something of a sour apple. Helen "Nell" Farquharson, Ray Farquharson's daughter, remembered, "Roscoe was big, he could have marched down the wards in the hospitals in England

– and he did – with nurses trailing behind him. He was the doctor's doctor. Everyone went to him about surgery. He had a very good sense of humour." Staff often brought their families to the Toronto General Hospital on Sundays. "You'd meet Roscoe Graham, and he'd go, 'oh, there's something wrong with your nose' – and we'd be terrified, 'but I can fix it.' And he'd go tweak [laughter]. He had little gifts like this. But he died young. It turned out he'd had diabetes for many years."

Was it undiagnosed? "Oh no, he was treating himself. He had a cottage up on a lake, and in the winter he skied. And the day he died, he said to his wife, 'Well, I guess this will be the last run of the day,' and it was. He died at the foot of the hill."[27] It was in 1948. He was fifty-eight.

Together with Robert Mustard, Harold Wookey founded cancer surgery of the head and neck in Toronto. Wookey was born in 1889 at Mandeville, British West Indies, and attended high school at Jarvis Collegiate in Toronto. Bill Bigelow recalled him, along with Robert Janes and Norman Shenstone, as one of the giants of the department, "great teachers, skilled surgeons, and exemplary family men."[28] In 1951 Wookey, together with Mustard and radiotherapist Clifford Ash, described the treatment of oral cancer with a combination of radiation therapy and surgery. It was, they noted, primarily a male disease and found "in those who habitually chew tobacco," in one of the earliest reports linking tobacco and cancer.[29] Wookey went on to become surgeon-in-chief at the Toronto General Hospital.

Looking back on these years with Robert Harris, Roscoe Graham, Robert Janes, and other surgical colleagues, Bigelow said, "It was an environment pervaded with curiosity, open-mindedness, and a concept of humility … which I believe is important for an understanding of research."[30]

*Gallie at the End of His Career*

In 1947 Gallie and his old collaborator Arthur LeMesurier at the Hospital for Sick Children proposed an operation for the repair of recurrent dislocations of the shoulder joint using the "living suture" technique that he had pioneered decades previously.[31] It was a kind of last hurrah: he retired that year. At the height of his powers, Gallie acquired a large international reputation, which did not go to his head. Offered the chair of surgery at a famous British university, he declined, saying, "If I'm as good as they say, I must remember that I'm a Canadian and Canada is entitled to everything that I can give."[32]

Four years later, in 1951, Gallie persuaded his friend Sam McLaughlin, the president of General Motors Canada, to establish the Robert Samuel McLaughlin Foundation. The story goes that on one of their Atlantic salmon fishing trips in New Brunswick, Gallie seemed a bit out of sorts. What was the problem? As Don Wilson tells the tale, "Dr Gallie was getting pretty fed up because he had a good training course here and then he would send them to, say the States or somewhere else for an extra year, and they would be of a stature that they were offered a job, so they would stay at Mayo's or wherever they'd been sent."

So Gallie told McLaughlin, "I'm training these guys and they don't come home." McLaughlin said, "Well, what do you need?" Gallie said, "I need some money that will pay for them while they're away, and their wives, and that they will come back to Toronto where the University must promise them a job and the hospital appointment must be settled."[33]

In 1952 the McLaughlin Fellowships were introduced for all Canadian medical schools to give trainees experience abroad. Gallie and a lawyer at the National Trust administered the fellowships. "I think it's probably one of the best things that ever happened in Canada," said Wilson.

In his retirement, in 1955 Gallie visited old friends in London and Edinburgh, leaving a memoir that captures the poignancy of an older generation of Toronto surgeons being left behind as science in surgery raced forward. Here he is in Edinburgh at the Royal Infirmary. Things began well: "I got the impression that the equipment of the operating rooms is not [as] complete as ours, and that the ritual of operating room technique, ie sterility of onlookers' gowns, operating room shoes, toweling of the operative incisions, is not observed as extensively as in our hospitals, or in the United States. But the traditional mastery of the anatomy of the human body … was as apparent as ever and the technical skill of the operators was beautiful."

However, trouble lay ahead. "The ward rounds, with the presentation of cases by the young staff-men (registrars) upset me a bit because of their glib use of the scientific language of the physicist, the biochemist, and the physiologist. Half the time I didn't know what they were talking about in their references to acid-base, water-balance, Ph, radio-active sulphur and phosphorus, and so on … So, I just kept quiet and veiled my ignorance as well as I could by nodding approval and encouragement." But there was comfort over cocktails: "The senior surgeons didn't know any more about all this scientific jargon than I did, and they continued to make their diagnoses and ultimate decisions on the time-honoured examination of the patient as a whole, rather than on the analysis of his various body-fluids." One really does glimpse here some kind of spirit of Old England, or at least understand why the Canadians were attracted to what they imagined it was.

Yet there is more. Gallie progressed on to London and to a conversation with Sir James Paterson-Ross, professor of surgery at St Bartholomew's Hospital (Bart's). Here science again reared its head. "He recognized the same difficulty as I have observed, that the present method of obtaining expert advice and direction on research problems, which involve physics, biochemistry and physiology, is difficult. He thinks, as I do, that the hiring of young scientists, on a full-time basis, to do the researches, results in collecting a group of second class investigators who, after a few years of work, have failed to produce anything and are then out of a job. I think he is troubled by the tendency of so-called full-time professoriates in Surgery to justify their existence by the amount of research that is done in the department." This was an unwitting malediction indeed for the coming rush of the Department of Surgery at the University of Toronto into the world of science.[34] Gallie glimpsed ahead the pivot from English-style teaching to American-style research.

In 1955 Gallie stood on the cusp of a new world of basic science as the platform of clinical medicine. Throughout the faculty the feeling grew that medicine was in fact, or should be, much more of a science than an art. James Goodwin, later an obstetrician at Women's College Hospital, recalled,

> There were two stages [in the evolution] of clinical education: the first from 1910 with the Flexner Report to 1949/50 emphasizing the teacher and the mentor – 'characters' who were great clinicians, strong practitioners who didn't mind being memorable (unforgettable), and some who were exacting and tough with medical students and interns and residents – who distanced themselves from basic science. Then there developed the stage of the full-time clinical scientists with a background in laboratory work … who became enamoured of evidence-based medicine, odds ratios and the Cochrane trials – and who seemed to downplay clinical expertise and were not concerned with becoming memorable clinical teachers. You may think this is a trifle brutal but I think this does apply to a certain extent to all clinical departments.[35]

*Janes*

As the war concluded, the returning veterans of the Royal Canadian Army Medical Corps virtually overwhelmed the Department of Surgery with demands for further training. The department doubled the positions at the teaching hospitals, staging special night courses for the returning military physicians in anatomy, physiology, and surgery. This was the first time the department had offered such "systematic instruction" in these subjects.[36] The war thus created a huge demand for postgraduate instruction as physicians who had been rushed through medical school to fill wartime needs began returning. Gallie said in 1944 that over 500 of "our own young graduates who have gone overseas with only an eight months' internship … will now be returning with the hope that they may be able to pick up the threads of their education where they were broken by enlistment." A survey had shown that a great number would "seek such postgraduate training."[37] This set the stage for the chairmanship of Robert Janes.

In 1947 Robert M. Janes became chair of the Department of Surgery, besting Gordon Murray, whose scientific achievements, according to Shelley McKellar, would otherwise have made him the natural candidate.[38] Born on a farm near Watford, Ontario, in 1894, Janes graduated from Watford High School in 1911 and finished his medical studies in 1916, acclaimed by his classmates for his "congeniality." He immediately enlisted for the duration of the war, then trained at HSC, at Bart's in London, and at the Toronto General Hospital. In 1923 he joined the surgical staff of the General. Janes made his reputation partly in general surgery, with a technique for parotidectomy that spared the facial nerve, but mainly in chest surgery, specifically in the surgery of tuberculosis.[39] He and Norman Shenstone are above all known for a simple device, the lung tourniquet they invented in 1929, that made the resection of a lobe of the lung, or even an entire lung, "relatively simple and safe" as Fred Kergin said in a eulogy of Janes. Shenstone and Janes presented their "tourniquet" for constricting the stump, or hilum, of the lung at a conference in 1930. Those were the days when, as Kergin put it, "surgeons held their breath during dissection of the hilum."[40] The tourniquet was designed to control haemorrhage during the operation, protect the stump of the removed lung from developing a fistula, and reduce mortality. (The dean mentioned their "remarkable results" in his Annual Report of 1930.[41])

Swiss surgeon André Naef said, "The tourniquet constriction of the hilum at the time allowed a fairly speedy resection, prevented spilling of copious sputum [infected matter] and simplified hemostasis by suture-ligature." Howard Lilienthal of Mount Sinai Hospital in New York City, who pioneered lobectomy (the removal of the lobe of a lung, in which the tourniquet proved invaluable), said, "Any lobectomy lasting longer than 45 minutes would almost certainly result in the loss of the patient. Patients desperately asked to be operated and even threatened suicide if refused the chance of operation [despite an almost 50 percent mortality]." Lilienthal continued, "To refuse to operate on a wretched patient otherwise incurable, merely because the statistics may be unfavorable, seems hardly fair. To have been the instrument of restoring one of these doomed patients to blooming health after years of revolting illness and risk of fatal hemorrhage is the richest reward surgery can offer."[42]

It was the Shenstone-Janes tourniquet that made Toronto a centre for thoracic surgery. Janes's student Fred Kergin commented at Janes's death in 1966, "Surgeons throughout the world were attempting to evolve a technique for lung resection to alleviate the suffering of patients affected by bronchiectasis [dilatation of the bronchi accompanied by expectoration of pus], chronic lung abscess or tumour. The methods in vogue were crude and associated with a mortality rate of about 50% and prolonged morbidity. This opened the door; from that time on progress in lung surgery was rapid."[43] In the 1945–6 session, Janes replaced his teacher Norman Shenstone as "senior surgeon at the General Hospital" and was set to ascend to the professorship of surgery in 1947.

Kergin recalled Janes as "the surgeon's surgeon – a tall distinguished presence, confident and imperturbable in the operating room, gentle in his skilled handling of tissue, and a master of sharp dissection with scalpel and scissors."[44] From the get-go Janes attempted to "weld the four university hospitals into a great teaching unit," rotating rounds among them.[45] In scientific terms, he practiced surgery as an art. Said his student Robert Delaney, "Dr Janes felt that the science of surgery was easier to teach than the art and that, to a large extent, the art must wait upon experience." He advocated between the science and the art "a happy marriage."[46]

Norman Shenstone was born in Brantford, Ontario, in 1881, into the family of a one-time president of the Massey Harris Company. After graduating with a bachelor's degree from U of T in 1901, Shenstone studied medicine at Columbia University (MD in 1905), then served as house staff at the New York Hospital and St Mary's Hospital. Thereupon he trained also in Britain. After returning to Toronto in 1909, he was appointed to Irving Cameron's service and, said his eulogist W.G.", "was one of the brilliant trio who served under [Cameron] at the Toronto General Hospital – C.L. Starr, Norman Shenstone, and W.E. Gallie."

After the war Shenstone rejoined the staff of the General, and in 1920 he became chief of one of the surgical services; he signed on as well as senior surgeon at the Dominion Orthopaedic Hospital for veterans on Christie Street (a hospital of the Department of Soldiers Civil Re-establishment).[47] "He was dedicated to looking after those who were ill," said another eulogist. "He made certain that either he or his associate saw every patient at least once a day and made it a point to know of the progress of every patient who was critically ill upon his service. Not infrequently at the end of rounds he would send for the relatives of a patient who was critically ill ... to inform them of the situation."[48] This is not to say that the surgeons of today are indifferent to their patients' welfare! But in glimpsing these men, one sees the English tradition of dedicated teaching and meticulous clinical attentiveness.

*Research Becomes a Theme*

As the Gallie Course was restored in 1945, interest in scientific research gathered in the Department of Surgery. Indeed, it had begun to quicken even in the early 1940s yet was interrupted by the war. In the session of 1940–1, a surgical follow-up clinic was established at the General under Charles B. Parker: "At intervals after their discharge these patients are recalled to a special follow up clinic; the surgeon who operated and the students will see them and record the findings on the history. In this way, both students and teachers will acquire a more accurate knowledge of the results of treatment and the records will be made infinitely more valuable to those who wish to make use of them for the more exhaustive study of groups of cases."[49]

In the 1945–6 session, laboratory training in one of the basic sciences was added to the Gallie Course: "In order that the foundation for surgical practice may be broadened, it has been arranged that from time to time students who have been selected for surgical training will spend a year in the lab of one of the fundamental medical sciences. This has already been in practice in respect to Anatomy and Pathology but it will now be extended to include Pharmacology, Physiology, and Pathological Chemistry. These basic medical sciences are becoming of ever increasing importance to surgery and it is hoped that an introduction to the experimental method may later have a beneficial effect on the attitude of the clinical surgeon to scientific investigation."[50]

After the war the custom began of fellowing for a year of research in the basic sciences as a precondition of an academic appointment. In 1949 Janes said, "Nearly all prospective appointees now spend one year as fellows in one of the basic science departments ... In many instances these men engage in a research problem with a member of the surgical staff in close association with the head of the department to which they are attached ... Those who continue the training in surgery are able to apply this year in a basic science to the requirements for the Fellowship in the Royal College of Surgeons of Canada."[51]

In the 1950–1 session the department organized a Division of Research, directed by the head of the department. "In most instances young men come with problems which they would like to pursue. If the project seems reasonable, facilities are provided. The Department is fortunate in having the friendly cooperation of the basic departments whose heads are always willing to render advice and assistance."[52] These early efforts dispel the notion that little research was done before the advent of the "Surgeon-Scientist" program in 1984. Yet it would be fair to say that a culture of research had not yet formed.

Still, it was forming. Some surgical faculty had received research training elsewhere, and as these men returned after the war they established research laboratories in their new areas of interest. Looking back, Bernie Langer mentioned as keen researchers Bigelow in cardiac surgery, hypothermia, and pacemaker; Murray in heparin and renal dialysis; Botterell in hypothermia for brain surgery; and Bill Mustard in innovative operations for polio in children and corrective procedures for congenital heart disease. And the next generation recruited in the 1950s and 1960s included people such as Bob Salter, Bill Lindsay, Bill Lougheed, Ron Tasker, Griff Pearson, Bill Kerr, and Ray Heimbecker.[53] So the stage was set.

*Further Integration*

Under Janes, the integration of the surgery training programs in the four big teaching hospitals got serious. MacFarlane as dean was keen on furthering cooperation among the hospitals. He said in December 1947 on the subject of selecting residents for the training programs, "I have talked this matter over with the Professor of Surgery and it is hoped that after the first of July we will receive most of our new internes from a joint selection board with representatives from all the teaching hospitals." He added, "So far as surgery is concerned the program is already underway and they have agreed that they will refer applications to a Joint Committee of the teaching hospitals. The group will be considered as a whole."[54]

In June 1948 Janes described an attempt to forge the university hospitals "into a great teaching unit. Ward rounds have been conducted by the head of the department one week each month at St Michael's and the Toronto Western Hospital in addition to the regular rounds at the General Hospital." He noted, "Postgraduate teaching is occupying an increasingly important place. The four university hospitals are functioning as a unit in this scheme so that the men may be rotated freely between the various hospitals ... The Department of Veterans Affairs hospitals at Christie Street and Sunnybrook have joined the scheme this year and the head of the Department [Janes himself] has assumed responsibility for providing these hospitals with a constant flow of residents of a high caliber."[55] In the 1948–9 session Janes started making monthly surgical rounds with Keith Welsh, who had just been appointed surgeon-in-chief at St Michael's, and with Robert Laird, who likewise had just become surgeon-in-chief at the Western.[56] The hospitals participating in the Gallie Course had now expanded to include Sunnybrook and the Toronto Hospital for Tuberculosis, where final-year students spent two days watching Kergin operate for lung tuberculosis and Robert I. Harris operate for bone and joint tuberculosis.[57]

Then came the next step in integration. By 1950 a special committee of the chiefs-of-surgery and the heads of divisions in the six participating hospitals had been struck to select the trainees and to organize their rotation according to academic program. Janes said of the residents, "The majority serve in more than one hospital. This tends to broaden their outlook and to emphasize the university character of the training."[58]

## Kergin

In 1957 Frederick Kergin succeeded Robert Janes as professor of surgery. Fred Kergin was one of the giants in the history of the Department of Surgery. He was born at Port Simpson in British Columbia in 1907, the youngest son of a doctor's family, and grew up in Prince Rupert. He entered the University of Toronto at age sixteen, graduating from the Biology and Medical Sciences ("B and M") program in 1927 and from medicine in 1930. In med school he was a big rugby player and participated readily in campus athletic organizations. In 1931 he became a Rhodes Scholar, spending the next two years at Oxford earning a master's degree in physiology and anatomy and graduating with first-class honours – as indeed he had graduated with honours from the "B and M" program in Toronto. In 1934 he began the four-year Gallie Course in surgery at the Toronto General Hospital, obtaining the fellowship of the Royal College of Surgeons of England in 1935 and that of the Royal College of Physicians and Surgeons of Canada in 1939. But already in 1937 he was appointed to the surgical staff of the General Hospital, as his eulogists put it, "an illustrious surgical division which was staffed at that time by Norman Shenstone, Gordon Murray and Robert Janes."[59]

It was Kergin who, as chief resident, oversaw in the late 1930s the introduction of the wondrous sulfa drugs, the predecessors of such antibiotics as penicillin, in the Department of Surgery. Kergin summoned Fred Dewar, who was just an intern, into the emergency room: "Come and look at this patient."

Dewar said, "He was a big, black gentleman with lovely white teeth with an arm that was as big around as a leg. He had a flaming temperature, he was right out of his mind, and he was going to die of streptococcal septicemia."

Kergin told Dewar to give him Prontosil, the trade name of the precursor sulfa drug of which sulfanilamide is an active metabolite. "I can remember it distinctly because I put it in a syringe, jammed the needle into his hip muscles, and squirted with all my might, and the syringe came off the needle and turned me into what looked like as though I had measles ... But almost every doctor in the Department of Surgery came to see that patient because he got well."[60]

Like so many of his generation, Kergin joined the RCAMC at the outset of hostilities in 1939 and served for the duration. In 1945 he returned to the General and became head of the Ward "B" service, simultaneously serving as a surgical consultant at the Toronto Hospital for Tuberculosis (located outside the city in rural Weston). In the 1949–50 session Kergin replaced Harold Wookey as head of the second Division of Surgery at the General.[61]

Tuberculosis rather than cancer was still the main enemy of the chest surgeon. As Kergin's student F. Griffith ("Griff") Pearson notes, "This was during the era when the surgical treatment of pulmonary tuberculosis was at its peak." With his craggy countenance, "Dr Kergin may have presented a slightly forbidding image to many of us," as Pearson and Ron Baird said, "but it was soon evident that he was utterly devoted to the support of his individual trainees, and the attainment of the highest possible quality of surgical practice among his graduates."[62] Griff Pearson recalls Kergin as "a remarkable man. A visionary, good to work for. But I don't think he had a real sense of humor."[63]

Kergin is known for having proposed the "ear oximeter" as the first means of monitoring the patient's blood gases during an operation.[64] In the absence of such a device, as Bigelow put it, "[o]xygen saturation could be as low as 75 per cent with the surgeon and anaesthetist smiling cheerfully and blissfully unaware of any danger to vital organs such as the brain. In those days, the patient's family, or his cronies who hung around the local garage ... would often observe, 'Joe hasn't been quite the same since his surgery in the city.'" It was, said Bigelow, an "acceptable aftermath" in the days when the only way to discern oxygen saturation was to see how blue the blood was.[65]

According to Pearson, "[Kergin] was spending two days of every week in the operating rooms of the Weston Sanatarium [Toronto Hospital for Tuberculosis], wrestling with some of the most tedious and difficult cases in thoracic surgery. The Kergin thoracoplasty, which spares the intercostal [rib] muscle bundles, is among his original contributions."[66] The advent of the new antimicrobial drugs after the Second World War made it possible to treat pulmonary tuberculosis by

just removing the diseased sections of lung (resection) rather than surgically removing some ribs to collapse the lung (thoracoplasty), and in 1954 Kergin urged
the field, on the basis of his experience at the Toronto Hospital for Tuberculosis,
to move from thoracoplasty to resection.[67]

To residents, Kergin was perceived, said Pearson, as "a stern authority, spare
with smiles and chuckles, and an unforgiving taskmaster for the tardy or care-
less." Yet he was forgiving of his residents' mistakes. Pearson said, "When I was
Dr. Kergin's chief resident, I experienced the haunting trauma of 'losing a patient' in the operating room as a result of uncontrollable hemorrhage that I, the
surgeon, had initiated." Pearson told Kergin, who replied, "Griff, you did the
best you knew how to for this man. I have experienced every complication described in surgery, including most of the fatal ones. You will experience many
more yourself before you are through. Accept that."[68]

In 1957 Kergin became professor and head of the university Department of
Surgery, where he greatly expanded the surgical program and introduced "the
concept of interhospital coordinating committees in the various surgical specialties." These committees became the germ seed of the divisions, the formation of which was a crucial step in forging the individual hospital departments
into a unified university Department of Surgery. Kergin was instrumental in
integrating Sunnybrook Hospital into the faculty and after 1966 also helped in
the Dean's Office with the undergraduate curriculum.[69] Kergin is considered
among the pioneers of thoracic surgery in Canada; owing to his tenacity, thoracic surgery in Toronto remained a separate field rather than being folded into
cardiac surgery as at many other institutions.

By the late 1950s the master of surgery degree had become moribund, and
people stopped referring officially to the Gallie Course, though its basic outlines
remained in place. Kergin in fact forbade the use of the term. Under Kergin,
postgraduate training in surgery had become excellent. In the 1961–2 session, for
example, there were seventy-four residents in the graduate training program.
For 1955–61 the Royal College pass rate for the sixty-one candidates trained in
the Department of Surgery of the University of Toronto was 74 percent on the
first attempt, and another three people passed on the second or third attempt,
giving a total pass rate of 79 percent. Of the sixty-one, forty-five were medical
graduates of U of T: their pass rate was 87 percent. Kergin noted, "When it is
remembered that the passing rate for the entire group trying this examination
is in the neighbourhood of 30 per cent, the results quoted appear reasonably
satisfactory."[70]

Under Kergin's leadership, by 1961 there were five divisions in the Department of Surgery: cardiovascular surgery, neurosurgery, orthopedic surgery,
plastic surgery, and urology.[71] The stories of these individual divisions are
told in the following chapter. These five divisions were to be found, in varying combinations, in all the teaching hospitals. But the flagship hospital was
the General, and the renovations of the early 1960s created a physical space for

the department that left its head almost euphoric: "The entire surgical wing of the College Street Building, representing the old public wards so familiar to generations of students, has been renovated into modern teaching wards. The transformation is truly remarkable."[72] Only the lab space in the Banting Institute remained "grossly inadequate." Under the new chair William Drucker in the 1967–8 session, the transition from the old public and private wards to the new system of beds in "teaching units" that included all patients in each service was effected.[73]

*Drucker and Team*

In 1966 William Drucker, an American from what is now Case Western Reserve University in Cleveland, who earned his medical degree from Johns Hopkins University in 1946, succeeded Kergin as professor of surgery; Kergin became associate dean "with special responsibility for the development of Sunnybrook Hospital into a modern teaching hospital."[74] Drucker, a specialist in surgical metabolism and on haemorrhagic shock, stayed in Toronto only six years before accepting a post at the University of Virginia.

Bernie Langer puts the Drucker years in perspective: "Bill Drucker was the first (and last) chair of surgery to be recruited from outside the University of Toronto. There may have been several reasons for this including: (1) The need to modernize the undergraduate medical curriculum – Bill was from a very progressive school and much involved in undergraduate education; (2) the need to create a larger emphasis on surgical research – he had an excellent reputation as a scientist; and (3) the need to initiate a practice plan in surgery – most progressive surgical departments in the USA had practice plans in place which gave chairs control over faculty members and redirected significant funds to both the department chairs and the dean of medicine."

The pluses of the Drucker years? Langer said, "Bill was a great teacher especially at the undergrad level and inspired many of our residents to a career in research. His strength was not in clinical practice and because of that he did not have the respect of many senior leaders in the department. [The primary criteria for surgeons were still clinical excellence and graduate teaching.]Some powerful components of the chair's job were taken out of his hands – Bob Mustard was made 'director of surgery' and was in charge of the postgraduate training program and also ran the department of surgery at TGH even though Bill was nominally the chief."

On Drucker's watch the Divisions of General Surgery and Thoracic Surgery came into being (see chapter 7), and the committee of surgeons-in-chief created after the war to admit residents and coordinate their schedules became a full executive committee of the department.

But there was a hook. Langer continued, "Bill Drucker's major problem was his ill-conceived effort to introduce a practice plan and 'full-time' academic system in surgery. His proposal was a top-down system where the chair had the control of the funds – a plan that was doomed from the start and eventually led to his frustration, disappointment and departure after six years. He did not get much credit here but I believe that he shook up the department by proposing these new ideas; he inspired some people (me included) to think differently about what the department should be and made it easier to make the changes that he desired twelve years later."[75]

Under Drucker, as mentioned, the department acquired its first director of postgraduate training, Robert A. Mustard (not to be confused with the pediatric cardiovascular surgeon William Mustard – his cousin – or the laboratory investigator Fraser Mustard). Robert Mustard, born 1913 in Toronto, was a big jock during medical school, from which he graduated in 1938 to begin surgical training that was interrupted by the war. In 1949 he joined the surgical staff of TGH and became widely respected as "a surgeon's surgeon." He was said, somewhat tongue in cheek, to "hold the unofficial world record for number of emergency tracheostomies (single-year and career)." In a whimsical note colleague John Bohnen added, "He is probably the only faculty member in the department who could actually pass the Royal College POS [Principles of Surgery] Exam on a day's notice."[76]

In 1969 Owen Gray succeeded Mustard in charge of the residency program. Yet Owen Gray looms much larger in the history of surgery in Toronto than this glancing reference would suggest. In 1966 he was head of general surgery at Toronto Western Hospital, and in 1970 he was appointed professor and associate chairman of the university Department of Surgery. Gray was born in Edmonton in 1922, attended high school at Ridley College, and studied medicine at Toronto, where he was considered a "great athlete," graduating in 1944. He continued this interest in sports and was at some point "the pro" at Jasper. "In later years," said his eulogist, "he was a keen curler and a very ardent golfer."[77] (It is evident from these pages that a balanced attitude towards athletics conduces to health and success, not to academic failure!)

Integration progressed on its tippy-toes. In the 1969–70 session, an interhospital coordinating committee for research was established under Walter Zingg.[78] As well, by 1970–1, the divisional system was firmly in place in surgery. Drucker said, "Each of the surgical specialties has now developed a university orientation with an interhospital co-ordinating committee." And St Joseph's Hospital and the Toronto East General Hospital were brought into the residency program.[79] These administrative changes mark the way to the formation of unified university departments.

Finally, under Drucker younger members of the department began enrolling in PhD programs in order to perfect their research abilities. There had always been a kind of Wanderjahr, or year of visiting other centres after completing the Gallie Course. Bernard Langer said, "It used to be: Go to the UK, go to Britain and visit the centres there, maybe go to the Continent, or go to the United

States, visit a number of centres, pick up all the new stuff that they were doing, and bring it back."[80]

Yet what was happening with these newly minted surgeons was different: they weren't going off to learn surgical techniques but to learn basic science. As Drucker said in 1970, "In recognition that clinicians are frequently compromised in their conduct of research because they lack formal instruction in investigative work, an increasing number of young faculty members have undertaken additional education of one to three years' duration. Support for these years has been proved in the past almost exclusively … by the McLaughlin Foundation." At that time nine young surgeons who had completed their residencies were "working with experienced investigators in other universities."[81] By 1971 the department had inhabited its research space in the new Medical Sciences Building; some of the young clinician-investigators who had spent the last few years working with basic scientists at other medical schools were starting to return to Toronto, and a new research culture was beginning to take hold.[82]

### Pearson at the General

From 1978 to 1989 Griff Pearson was hospital surgeon-in-chief at the General, the captain of an unruly crew indeed. When he took the helm in 1978, he found the spirit of cooperation wanting. Only three of seven divisions had developed group practice arrangements (neurosurgery, 1965; thoracic surgery, 1967; general surgery, 1970). Moreover, the scrambling for fees among the other surgeons was unseemly and unproductive. Pearson noted in a later review, "In the remaining Divisions most income was generated from medical fees and there was inappropriate individual competition within Divisions for resources which impacted on individual income. This system interfered with the essential commitments of time and interest necessary for the conduct of educational and research programmes."[83]

Nor, despite Drucker's changes, was there much of a spirit of departmental unity ("lack of departmental focus" was the administrative phrase). A review in 1983 found "a high level of divisional autonomy … a general lack of any sense of mutual purpose relating to the Department of Surgery as a whole." The heads of the hospital divisions did not meet regularly, hired without consultation, and had autonomy over their divisional budgets. Battered by funding cutbacks and a declining image of medicine "in the public eye," many surgeons hedged "a negative and paranoid attitude," especially towards the hospital administration. Nor were the surgeons at the General highly inclined to cooperate with other hospital departments ("independence and skepticism").[84]

But as is known, when the going gets tough, the tough get going, and Pearson's stewardship of this big hospital department over the next decade was an important moment in the history of the Toronto General Hospital, even though Bernie Langer took over much of the day-to-day administration. He set up a regular schedule of departmental meetings for divisional heads. He drove the establishment of group practices forward so that, five years later, only the plastic surgeons had not yet set one up. Previously, the divisional heads had stayed on forever, from the time of their appointment until their retirement. Pearson set up search committees for them, requiring formal reviews of their leadership every five years, and he brought in new division heads for four of the divisions. He brought in oversight of new appointments and a departmental finance committee to deal with the funds from the new practice plans. Orthopedic surgery at the General and at Mount Sinai were amalgamated under the head of Allan Gross at Mount Sinai. Orthopedic research surged forward.

In 1979 Pearson brought in cardiovascular surgeon Hugh Scully, later president of the Canadian Medical Association, to run the educational programs of the department, organizing the popular Saturday morning seminars for the residents. In 1981 Pearson established a nineteen-bed surgical intensive care unit (SICU); the neurosurgeons acquired an eight-bed ICU. As the province cut down on residency slots, merging programs and divisions became the order of the day, and under Pearson five of the General's surgery divisions either increased collaboration or amalgamated with Sinai.[85]

The story of Pearson's stewardship of this single hospital department for a decade is not so important in itself, but it illustrates the role of leadership in a time of change. Everything seemed up in the air for the surgeons: their livelihood, their research, and their institutional loyalties, whether to the university (as the deans wished them to sign their articles), to the department (as Pearson wished), or to the division (as they themselves were inclined). Pearson, the son of the Toronto optometrist, stepped in and led them forward.

*Donald Wilson*

In 1972 William Drucker stepped down and Donald R. Wilson became chair of surgery, while remaining surgeon-in-chief at the Western; this was the first time in the Department of Surgery that the professorship had been separated from the post of surgeon-in-chief at the General. Among the pioneer generation of cardiac surgeons, Wilson was, like anatomist Jim Thompson and many others who became medical leaders in Toronto, a Westerner. He was born in Saskatoon in 1917 and attended university there. His mother and father sat down with him and asked, "What would you like to be?"

Wilson said, "Well, I'd like to play basketball." There was a complete silence after he said this, and then his mother said, "Are you going to be a doctor or a preacher?" Wilson said, "If those are my two choices, I'm going to be a doctor" (Wilson laughs).[86]

Wilson earned a BA from the University of Saskatchewan in 1939 and started his premedical studies in Saskatchewan, where he was president of his class. But Saskatchewan in those days didn't offer clinical subjects, so Wilson, along with ten of his class of twenty-four, came east to Toronto. He graduated with an MD with the April class of 1942 (in the hurry-up of the war, there were two that year). Unsurprisingly, the tall and lanky Wilson played intramural basketball for the Toronto Meds.

Wilson served in Europe, then with the war's end returned to Toronto and tried to be admitted to one of the six annual slots in the Gallie Course, beating out the competition probably, in his view, because "I'd been in the Army." He completed training in surgery in 1951, then, as was customary in the Gallie Course, spent a year touring European centres, where he learned how famous Murray and Bigelow had become. Back in Toronto, he joined the surgical staff at St Joseph's Hospital, Queensway General, and the Mississauga Hospital before coming to the Western, where he became chief surgeon.

Wilson had little taste for research – it was technique that impassioned him – and the Western, otherwise a secondary centre, was his first choice. Bob Laird, head of surgery at the Western, said to Wilson, "If the General's going to have a cardiac unit, I'm going to have a cardiac unit." Wilson went to "Uncle Bill" Bigelow and "told him I'd had this offer, and because I was more interested in teaching and things like that rather than the research side of things, I think Uncle Bill supported my move."

Wilson's tenure as professor of surgery saw stronger efforts to pull the department together as a university department. "When I took over," Wilson later said, "we had X number divisions of surgery, we didn't have a Department. If you asked somebody where they worked they could name the hospital. If you said, 'What's your relationship with the university?' 'I don't know.'" Wilson continued, "So my approach was to get these people to see the University was number one on their list and that their hospital was close behind." He asked members to start signing articles with their university affiliation. "I was ashamed that a lot of us didn't know people in the other teaching hospitals, so we arranged that the rounds were held in different hospitals around the city." People would come early and chat over breakfast. Wilson had some leverage, the ability to confer prestigious university appointments upon hospital people, which would further increase their solidarity.

Wilson wanted them to realize "that they were part of a very powerful teaching organization, and they'd better stand up and do their thing. The idea was to say, 'Look, you're part of the University, this is your responsibility, and if you have any trouble let me know.' I think people were ashamed they didn't know what was going on in their own university, and I think that they became aware that to be part of the University was a worthwhile thing."[87]

Wilson's tenure as professor is also remembered as a human relations triumph because Wilson himself was the kindly judicious clinician incarnate. An external review in 1981 said, "There was an overwhelming feeling of admiration, respect and gratitude towards [Wilson]. It was felt that he had been the right man at the right time and that he had ... drawn the department together as a unit. He had established confidence and communication. He had healed wounds and cleared up misunderstandings and had succeeded in presenting the new Chairman [Langer] with an extremely favourable and solid ground to build on."[88]

One less solid piece of ground, however, was research, which the external reviewers found underdeveloped: "There is now an urgent need for an increase in scholarly activities in the Department of Surgery."

### Bernard Langer and the Surgical Scientist Program

It is the feeling of the Committee that there is a very evident change in culture in the Department of Surgery. In times past junior faculty … felt that in order to establish themselves as surgeons and as members of the department their first obligation was to develop a large practice and be considered an "operator." This single route to peer approval has interfered with the development of surgical science in the department."[89]

External reviewers, 1991

In 1978 the McLaughlin Chair of Surgery was created and in 1982 Bernard Langer, universally known as Bernie, succeeded Wilson as its incumbent. If Wilson had loosened the dominance of the General Hospital over academic appointments by remaining at the Western, Langer broke it entirely by not being surgeon-in-chief anywhere: running the Department of Surgery, with its hundred-plus full-time staff, was more than a full-time job.[90] Langer's lasting memorial, not just to the University of Toronto but to all of Canadian academic medicine, was the Surgical Scientist Program.

Langer was born in 1932 near the intersection of College and Bathurst Streets, then the heart of the Jewish community. His parents had immigrated from Poland to Canada in 1910. He went to Harbord Collegiate, then decided "at the very last minute," as he said in an interview, to study medicine because he figured that actuarial science – his first love – was too isolating a career for someone who would rather "have a lot to do with people than lock myself up in a building, pushing numbers." He had intended to become a family physician but in his final year became fascinated by surgery and applied for the program.

Langer recalls, "When I was interviewing with Bob Janes for the Gallie Course, he was skeptical that I could manage the rigors of a surgical residency because I had married at the end of the second medical year. I reminded him that I had also been captain of the University Toronto swim team and water polo teams as well as being class president and had graduated with the Gold Medal, so the residency should not be a problem. He was convinced and I was accepted for training."

After completing his residency, Langer did not go to England. He spent 1962–3 in the Department of Surgery at the Peter Bent Brigham Hospital in Boston. At the Brigham, Langer studied with surgeon Francis Moore, who, Langer said, "wanted to be the first one to transplant a liver in a human. The Peter Bent Brigham Hospital had done the first kidney transplants, so they had background and expertise in transplantation. Joe Murray, a urologist, had done the first kidneys, for which he eventually received the Nobel Prize, and Franny Moore was keen to follow suit. A good part of his energy in the lab was devoted to figuring out how to transplant a liver in a dog and keep the dog alive." So Langer became part of the dog ICU team "trying to keep these dogs alive that Franny was transplanting during the day."

After seven years of training, including the aforementioned year split between M.D. Anderson Hospital in Houston and the Brigham, in 1963 Langer joined the Department of Surgery at the General. He almost didn't join it. Langer explains, "Anti-Semitism was common in those days and there was an unofficial quota on Jews admitted to study medicine. There had never been a Jew appointed as a full attending surgical staff at TGH until my appointment. In truth, no one at the General ever considered appointing me until I was offered a job at the Sick Children's Hospital – and I then approached Fred Kergin to ask for a job. To his great credit, and I am sure over the objections of some, he offered me a position. That marked a watershed and after that the barriers were down and appointments were made on merit alone."[91]

When Langer returned to Toronto, he got some funding from the Ontario Cancer Treatment and Research Foundation "to do liver transplants in dogs." Yet Langer immediately recognized his lack of research training. In the Gallie Course he had spent an obligatory year taking cortisol samples from monkeys with brain lesions for a neurosurgeon. "I recognized at that time that my research training was not the kind of research training that was going to turn me into a scientist." While at the animal facilities in the Banting Building, Langer bumped into pathologist Jan Steiner (who later became an associate dean), "really a brilliant guy, a very stimulating guy … So what research I learned in terms of methodology and research type thinking, I learned from Steiner."

When Langer was at the Brigham, he realized what superb clinical training young surgeons in Toronto had received. "I thought I had been far better trained than their chief residents." But the problem in Toronto was research: "Research was an integral part of their overall practice [in Boston]," whereas "[a]t the clinical conferences at the Toronto General … surgeons talked about their experience, and others talked about their experience, and their opinions, and then decisions were made. At the Brigham, when they had a clinical problem, they talked about the research that had been done on this problem." He noted, "I learned that the Brigham was a better academic place than Toronto, because it had integrated research, including research thinking and research training, into their overall surgical activities, and that was something that I thought we had to do."[92]

Back in Toronto, Langer came to realize that some of the surgical research was not up to snuff "because [the surgeons] had had no training in the fundamentals of surgical scientific research, and there were others who did what they called research, which was descriptive work and retrospective reviews, observational research, if you want to call it research. There was a lot of that – and some of that was pretty bad. I think that gave surgical research a bad name, and the basic scientists were much more disciplined and had to face pretty critical review in journals when they published; some of them had contempt for surgical research, which could get published even though it was pretty bad."[93]

In 1984 Langer created the Surgical Scientist Program. The concept he originally fashioned for Toronto was the "clinician-scientist," already very familiar in the literature. Langer said that, "A clinician scientist is an individual who has completed a program of clinical training sufficient to practice independently as a specialist and also completed a program of training in science sufficient to function independently as a scientist." The clinician-scientist was thus neither a basic scientist in a clinical department nor "a clinician who has had some exposure to research and collaborates in a minor fashion with basic or clinical scientists."[94] The clinician-scientist was a free-standing investigator and a free-standing clinician.

The program arose for several practical reasons. One was Langer's impatience with constantly having to send people away to learn how to do research elsewhere: Wayne Johnston had an interest in vascular surgery research and had to go to England to learn how to do it. Hepatobiliary surgeon Robert Stone had to go down to New Jersey to learn methods of measuring liver function from an internist. "I did not want Toronto to always be sending people elsewhere to learn what's new and how to do it. I wanted people to be coming to Toronto to learn what's new and how to do it."[95]

To be sure, there were some excellent surgical research laboratories in Toronto: Langer mentioned Griff Pearson's lab in lung surgery, Allan Gross's lab on knee transplantation, Bob Salter's lab in orthopedics, Dick Weisel in cardiac surgery, and Ron Tasker and Charles Tator in neurosurgery. "But there were also other orthopedic surgeons who were doing 'my last 20 years of spinal cases' research. It was obligatory for anybody who wanted to get into some programs to first do a year of research ... So there were people who were coming into the program, using up research money, who had no intention of ever doing research."[96]

There was also unevenness across the divisions of surgery in attitudes towards research: "In some it was frankly discouraged, in others encouraged to varying degrees." Only neurosurgery, under the direction of Alan Hudson, "set a consistent high standard for selection of both trainees and supervisors." Some of the trainees were gung-ho; others regarded "the obligatory [research] year as the price of admission to the clinical residency." Most spent only the one year doing research. Nor with the exception of neurosurgery did any of the divisions have a "long range strategy ... The result was that much of the training was wasted, at significant cost in time and resources." The research wheels were grinding, in other words, but knowledge was not being cranked out.

What to do? Langer sat down with some of the people in the department who were "very committed to research. Steve Strasberg [general surgeon at the Western] was one of them. Charles Tator [neurosurgeon at Sunnybrook] was another." Langer had recruited Rudolph Falk into the general surgery division at TGH and thereafter sent him to the Karolinska Institute in Stockholm for a year of research. "The idea was to bring him back and provide research support for the transplant program." So the four of them sat down, "and I asked them to help me design a program for surgical research training." Langer wanted to restrict the program to a few people, who would commit to a minimum of two years' training in a postgraduate degree program. "They wouldn't just be parked in somebody's lab like I was: 'you're going to be the pair of hands that does this project that we've invented.'"

Langer gathered about him a cohort of enthusiastic young surgeons keen on doing science that also included Ori Rotstein, later chief of surgery at St Michael's, who worked in Strasberg's lab at the Western; thoracic surgeon Bob Ginsberg; vascular surgeons Wayne Johnston and Paul Walker; and Bryce Taylor, director of surgical postgraduate training and later associate chair of the department. Langer was swimming against a strong clinical tradition in the department. Rotstein later said, "The big issue at the time was that Toronto's department was so clinically driven that there's kind of a town/gown, rat/human mentality, and if you were a researcher doing basic research, you weren't a surgeon. And Steve [Strasberg] would probably say the same thing. He came up with a lot of frustration during the early years of his career, over the fact that he was perceived more as a rat surgeon than he was a people surgeon. I think Steve was kind of the prototype, but Bernie supported him, and said, 'Look, this is the surgeon of the future, we're going to be scientists and surgeons.'"[97]

Langer decided to initiate a separate academic training track called "Surgical Scientist Program at the University of Toronto." It would enroll a small number of promising residents and give them sufficient training "that they could eventually function as independent clinician investigators." The guidance of the program lay with the departmental Research Committee, under Steve Strasberg, Charles Tator, and Ori Rotstein, with assistance from Bryce Taylor, the director of the department's clinical training program. Although candidates could enter the program at any time, most did only after their first two years of clinical work. They had to commit to a minimum of two years' research training and to register for a university degree at the School of Graduate Studies, through either a basic science department or the Institute of Medical Science. The supervisor him- or herself was required to be a member of the graduate school and to have an "active, funded, productive research laboratory." The department guaranteed the resident's salary, which turned out to be a wise investment given that, Langer explained, "good selection led to success in external competition for fellowship support funds." Another major source of the funds was the practice plan that Langer introduced to the department at the same time. The

Surgical Scientist Program thus brought the Department of Surgery into the Institute of Medical Science.

The only division that bought into the program immediately in 1984 was the general surgery division with three of its trainees. "Well, that wasn't too hard because I was head of the division," said Langer. "The orthopods didn't want any part of it, and nobody else did." But then the program started to catch on slowly because, said Langer, "[o]ther people saw that (a) the only way they could get any money out of the department was to have people in the Surgical Scientist Program, and (b) the young research people in those other divisions wanted it, so that they could train people in the program."

Under Steve Strasberg, the inaugural director, the popularity of the program grew and by the eighth year about one-third of the residents in surgery from some divisions had enrolled in the Surgical Scientist Program (SSP). In neurosurgery, participation was mandatory (but neurosurgery had already begun its own mini surgical scientist training program before the department began its own).

The SSP flourished under the umbrella of the Institute of Medical Science, a division of the School of Graduate Studies, especially under nephrologist Mel Silverman's direction. Langer said, "When Mel became head of IMS, it was love at first sight. Mel and I had the most wonderful working relationship. He encouraged it and he fostered it, and in fact the Surgical Scientist Program became the jewel in the crown of IMS." He continued, "In the whole Institute of Medical Science, there is no other program that graduates a higher percentage of people … than the Surgical Scientist Program – it's in the range of 80 percent of people who register for a degree eventually are granted their degree, which is just unheard of in basic science."[98]

By the 1988–9 session, the program numbered thirteen trainees, ten in master's courses and three in PhD degree courses. "Thirty-two members of the Department are designated as Supervisors … the criteria being that they have appointments in the School of Graduate Studies, are actively engaged in research, and have sufficient research funds and spaces for trainees."[99] By 1996 participation in the Surgical Scientist Program had grown to forty-four. The cost of funding was $1.5 million a year, half from peer-review agencies, the rest from resident salaries and from faculty and hospital funds. Fully half of the enrollees had switched to PhD programs and would be "double-doctors." Langer concluded that, "in spite of the length of clinical training in surgery, some residents are prepared to commit an additional period of time, which now averages about three years during their residency, to research training." Langer felt that the SSP "has substantially changed the culture in the surgical training program," yoking bright young minds to scientific progress.[100]

In 1994 the Council of the Royal College of Physicians and Surgeons of Canada – spurred on by Langer, Bob Volpé, and Mel Silverman – adopted its own Clinician Investigator Program for Canada as a whole.[101] By the new century, physician-scientist programs anchored medical research in the United States and Canada.[102] Toronto's was among the first.

Under Ori Rotstein, who succeeded Strasberg in 1990–1 as program director, and under Reznick as department head, the Surgical Scientist Program blossomed further. In these years Rotstein emerged as a force majeure on behalf of research, becoming in the 1994–5 session director of research as well as director of the SSP. Rotstein, a 1977 U of T graduate, would later become director of the Institute of Medical Science, then surgeon-in-chief at St Michael's Hospital.

"What distinguishes us," Reznick said in 2002, "is the staggering success of our visionary Surgeon Scientist Program." Reznick said this differentiated U of T "from many if not all other institutions in North America." Under Ori Rotstein's leadership at this time, thirty-four residents were "engaged in serious study and serve as a model for North America."[103]

*Langer as Chair of Surgery*

To deepen its involvement in science, the department began appointing non-surgeon scientists. In 1986 Langer engaged Geoff Fernie, a mechanical engineer with a background in rehabilitation (his thesis was on bedsores) as the first full professor of surgery who was not a surgeon. Trained in England, in 1973 Fernie established the Amputee Research Program at the West Park Hospital in Toronto to train Canadian prosthetists and orthotists. Fernie had designed "the first battery operated portable patient lift" (SturdyLift) and began working with the Department of Surgery to learn at first hand the problems of patients needing mechanical assistance. By the time of his cross-appointment to surgery, Fernie was vice president for research at the Toronto Rehabilitation Institute (see also chapter 23).[104]

Bringing nonsurgeon scientists on board, not as employees in somebody's lab but as colleagues, was innovative. Said Ori Rotstein, "The old idea was that if you were a surgeon and a scientist you basically ran the group and you hired PhDs to work for you. When you recruited somebody, you didn't recruit them as faculty, you recruited them as a member of your lab as a research associate. That changed to saying, 'Okay, what we're going to do is hire world-class scientists to be our colleagues, and not to work for us anymore.'"

Rotstein himself took the initiative in implementing this concept. The results? "It's unbelievable!" he said. "If you look at our grant funding everybody goes up and these guys are getting awards and they've got great students." He mentioned his own collaboration with Andras Kapus, or the collaboration between Richard Weisel and Ren-Ki Li in cardiac surgery, or Shaf Keshavjee and Mingyao Liu in thoracic surgery. "If you look across our department, the building of bridges occurred through the change of environment from one where we were the boss of those guys to where we were partners with them."[105]

What were the achievements of the Langer years? He later said,

The introduction of the practice plan was probably the most important thing that I accomplished during my term as chairman – even greater than the SSP (without it, the SSP would not have been possible) The fiasco during the Drucker years related to the failed attempt to introduce a 'full time' system on the American style with central financial control. It had a polarizing effect, alienating many older surgeons who were largely practice oriented, and many younger surgeons who were more progressive but had been disappointed by the failure. One of Don Wilson's most important contributions as the next chair was to heal the wounds from that era and build a sense of community across the whole department. But research was not his priority and except for the initiatives taken by individual division heads, the department as a whole was marking time.

Langer continued, "When I was appointed I was given a strong mandate to develop a practice plan and to upgrade the performance of the department in research as my top priorities. The SSP was the major initiative at the training level and provided us with our own farm system for developing our own future faculty – we now attract the best and the brightest from other Canadian schools who seek an academic career." Langer listed some of the other initiatives he introduced to improve the visibility and credibility of surgeon-investigators, including the publication of an annual report, increasing the awards to faculty and residents for research and teaching accomplishments, rewarding committed teachers and researchers with higher salaries, recruiting new staff based on academic potential, not just clinical prowess, and finally, "[a]ppointment of people to leadership positions based on academic credentials."

Other changes of Langer's influenced the culture of the Department of Surgery. There was a formal recognition of the status of surgical divisions (see chapter 7). Langer said,

Until 1982, the divisions each had an interhospital coordinating committee (IHCC) of which the division head was chair. Their internal organization was self determined and they reported to the department chair through the division head, who was appointed by the chairman at his pleasure. The heads of divisions in hospitals were appointed by the respective surgeons in chief without consultation. I changed the status of university division heads from Chair of IHCC to Chairman of the Division of XXXXX at the University of Toronto. This may seem a trifle but its effect was profound. Our Divisional Chairs had new status at their international meetings (equivalent to department chairs) and it opened the possibility of obtaining funding for endowed divisional chairs through the University (we now have several: orthopedics, neurosurgery, general surgery, pediatric general surgery, vascular, thoracic, and urology). The Divisional Chairs became members of the new Senior Advisory Committee and participated in policy development and were part of a new search process for hospital division heads.

A second cultural change affected "process and accountability in leadership appointments." Before 1982 surgeons-in-chief were appointed by hospital boards with participation of the department chair but with no fixed term or review. Hospital division heads were appointed by surgeons-in-chief – same terms. University division heads were appointed by the department chair – same terms. Only the university chairs were appointed (by the dean) after a formal review and open search and for a term of five years – renewable once after a formal five-year review of the department. As a result I inherited a number of division heads and surgeons in chief who had been in place for well over 10 years, some over 20 years. That situation had not only inhibited change, but had discouraged bright young people with leadership potential from staying in our department long term."

Langer changed this antiquated system in several ways:

> I introduced a new system of appointment and review that required all leadership positions in our department: surgeon-in-chief, university Division Chair, hospital division head, department director of Postgraduate or Undergraduate Education or Research to require an open search, an appointment for 5 years, a 5-year review including a possibility for one more 5-year appointments and then a new search (at which the incumbent could be a candidate). I got the agreement and support of all the hospitals and was able to obtain the resignation of all the overdue leaders within two years of bringing in the new policy.
>
> The result has been dramatic – we now have a collection of young, bright, energetic, committed, accomplished leaders in all positions in our department. Not only do we have a farm system in our SSP for recruitment to our faculty, we have a farm system in our junior faculty leaders for our senior positions in the future. As an example – we have a group of internal candidates for the vacant chair of surgery that would be the envy of any medical school anywhere.

No longer was recruitment solely in the hands of the all-powerful surgeon-in-chief (SIC). "Before 1982," said Langer,

> a surgeon was appointed to a hospital by the surgeon-in-chef with an informal consultation with the department chair – and that appointment was virtually for life. Because we were trying to create a new department based on academic excellence, I insisted that every surgeon that was proposed for recruitment in any hospital be vetted by the university Division Chair and meet academic standards for research or education training, and fit into the hospital and divisional priorities. Before I would approve such an appointment, a Memorandum of Agreement would have to be signed by the candidate, the division chair, the SIC and the hospital CEO. This Memorandum of Agreement outlined the responsibilities and performance expectations of the candidate and also the commitments in space, time and funding by the department and the hospital. The initial appointment was for a 3-year term at which time

a formal review would take place and if the candidate did not meet expectations the appointment could be terminated. This process focused the minds of those who were recruiting and led to a marked improvement in the quality of our recruits.

Langer attempted to coordinate the offer of services among hospitals, where serious competition remained in clinical care, especially among the high-profile services.

> For example trauma was being managed at every hospital with no coordination, hospitals were competing for pre-eminence in transplantation (3 doing hearts, 5 kidneys, 2 planning livers). We had a department planning process with the objective of consolidating some services to provide better clinical care and to facilitate the basic research needed to develop these programs as academic programs. A retreat was then held which hospital CEOs and representatives from the Dean's office and the provincial Ministry of Health attended. Recommendations for consolidation of trauma services and transplantation were approved. With the agreement of the Ministry of Health, committees were set up in trauma and transplantation, prerequisites were developed for the facilities required for Level 1 trauma centers and for an integrated multiorgan transplantation center. Hospitals were invited to submit proposals and many did. The result of this unique process was the designation of Sunnybrook and St Mikes as the two Level 1 trauma centers for the Greater Toronto Area and of TGH as the site of the new multiorgan transplant center. These are now among the leading clinical care and research units of their kind in North America.

Thus, a powerful slate of changes. "Not all the proposals worked out so well. I could not get the orthopedic and plastic surgeons to consolidate their hand surgery and research in any one institution. As a result we are still working away in competition and the leading Hand and Upper Limb unit in Canada is in London, Ontario. This exercise taught me the importance of working closely with hospital CEOs, and after its completion I arranged to have meetings every six months with each hospital CEO, and with my Associate Chair and the hospital SIC to discuss plans and review problems."[106]

In retrospect, Langer emerges as one of the great "builders" of the faculty in the late twentieth century. He turned the huge Department of Surgery into a scientific powerhouse and adopted programs such as the SSP that became a model for the entire faculty, having a multiplier effect far beyond its importance in surgery as such. An important question for a volume such as this is how to make further Bernie Langers spring up, to provide leadership for future generations.

### Wedge and Reznick

The tenures of the department heads who followed Langer are too recent to be properly evaluated in historical context. But a couple of remarks are appropriate. In July 1992 John H. Wedge succeeded Langer as the McLaughlin Chair of

Surgery and head of the department. In 1995 he became as well surgeon-in-chief of the Hospital for Sick Children. Wedge, who had graduated with an MD from the University of Saskatchewan in 1969, had trained in pediatric orthopedic surgery in the United States before coming to Canada. As he completed his ten-year term as chair in 2002, the University of Toronto Department of Surgery had become among the most distinguished in the world. Dean David Naylor had this to say at Wedge's retirement dinner: "A few weeks ago, two external reviewers came to appraise the Department of Surgery. These distinguished surgical leaders, one from Harvard and the other from McGill, later wrote to say that our Department was unequivocally number 1 in Canada and among the top ten in the world. I promptly wrote to John Wedge, repeating this high praise, and seeking to direct some of it his way. The one-sentence response came back within a few minutes. According to John, the success of the Department simply reflected the talent and commitment of the faculty and staff and the legacy of those leaders who had gone before him."[107]

In 2002, Richard Reznick succeeded Wedge as McLaughlin Chair and head of the department; he stepped down in 2010 to become dean of medicine at Queen's University. Mindful of the perils of writing contemporary history, nonetheless one might say a couple of things about the Reznick era.

Reznick had his own background in surgical education and boosted the department's pedagogic efforts. Under Wedge, he organized a fellowship program in medical education as part of the Surgical Scientist Program, and by 1994 two surgeons had received master's degrees and several others were in the pipeline. Moreover, in the 1993–4 session the department added the new post of director of core surgical education to oversee the first two years of the residency.[108] (And in the 2006–7 session Reznick initiated a "Scholarship in Surgery" program in which surgical trainees pursue an MBA degree.[109])

For all his enthusiasm for education, Reznick never believed that a surgical residency was anything other than hard work. On one occasion he expressed dismay about a European tendency to limit the time commitment in a program. "We cannot train surgeons in a 40-hour per week time frame … Disciplines that require a high degree of technical competence are fundamentally different from specialties that don't have that added need. Surgeons are really doctors who also know how to operate."[110]

Even though Reznick was grounded in medical education, as chair of the department he put the research pedal down hard. "Landmark discoveries should be our driver," he said on taking office. To be sure, by the time Reznick became head, a piece of this road had already been covered: the number of endowed chairs was up from four to twenty. The department employed forty basic scientists, and new research funding streamed in from federal, provincial, and private agencies. "We can't be shy in our goals," said Reznick.[111] By 2008 the Department of Surgery had appointed over forty nonclinician scientists. "Our total research funding continues to exceed that of even many of the Universities in Canada, over $30,000,000 this year," he said.[112]

Plans for the new Clinical Services Building of the Toronto General Hospital, University Health Network, at the corner of University Avenue and Gerrard Street had been laid long before its opening on 1 July 2003. Yet it was on Reznick's watch that the department's physical cadre changed: twenty-two new operating rooms replaced the space in the Bell Wing built in the 1950s. Adopted especially for "minimally invasive surgery," the operating rooms represented, as Martin McKneally put it, "perhaps the best in North America" and had been constructed under "the visionary surgical leadership of Alan Hudson."[113]

In the 2006–7 session Reznick looked back in triumph over a record of success: the department had grown from 90 full-time faculty in 1974 to 220 in 2007, in addition to numerous part-timers and adjunct staff and 25 research scientists. In the previous five years, fifty new surgeons and scientists had been added. The department had successfully negotiated thirty-one practice plans across the various divisions in the different teaching hospitals; additional alternative funding plan monies were about to arrive, 30 percent of which were earmarked for teaching and research. Eleven residency programs were currently training "in excess of 200 future surgeons." And 175 surgeons from fifteen countries were in the fellowship program.[114] Of the eleven programs in the Department of Surgery, six were "direct entry programs": cardiac surgery, general surgery, neurosurgery, orthopedic surgery, plastic surgery, and urology. And there were five "subspecialty surgical programs": thoracic surgery, vascular surgery, pediatric general surgery, colorectal surgery, and general surgery oncology.[115]

Behind these numbers were the surgeons themselves. Reznick continued, "The feature that has been most powerful is the incredible talent within the Department. The surgical expertise is astounding. Images of Andrew Pierre performing a lung transplant, Loch McDonald clipping a cerebral aneurysm, Pippi Salle correcting a complex urogenital malformation, Mike McKee restoring function after a complex fracture, Rob Zeldin removing a lung, Vern Campbell doing a fem-tib bypass, Mark Peterson doing his first endovascular repair, Brent Graham re-implanting a severed digit, John Semple restoring form and function after cancer, Calvin Law doing a trisegmentectomy ... these are the enduring images."[116]

In the background of these events in the Department of Surgery lay the ever greater predominance of the hospitals and their research institutes. The hospitals had the money as the faculty grew increasingly unable to fund such enterprises as the Surgical Scientist Program. Noted two external assessors in 2007, "The [university] department's research interests are not always aligned with those of the hospital research institutes. Departmental representation on these research institute committees is something lacking ... A challenge is the reduction of the surgery operating budget by the University of Toronto. Hospitals are increasingly supporting the academic mission, leaving the impression that the University of Toronto has been 'let off the hook.'" Nonetheless, the reviewers found that the "stature of the department remains extraordinary as the leading

Canadian University Department of Surgery and amongst the top 10 internationally."[117] An external review in 2004–5 found that the department had "a higher citation factor than the Mayo Clinic."[118]

In the spring of 2007, Reznick reinforced the policy – initiated by the Memorandum of Agreement of 1984 – of making all future staff appointments the object of mandatory searches, meaning the end of "recruitment by convenience," hiring somebody because he or she seems like a "natural fit." (As Langer put it, it "ended the hiring of the resident standing across the table when a colleague died.") "Opening the playing field widely," Reznick said, "will lessen the chance that we become overly parochial and insular." The department had already made several appointments from abroad that would not have happened in the absence of searches. "Bringing in new ideas, new ways of doing things, new technical approaches, new cultures, will only serve to enrich this Department as it realistically strives to be amongst the very best departments in the world."[119] This kind of talk was very new for Toronto, but so was the ambition of a big department like the Department of Surgery to be among the best in the world.

Combined with intense ambition, Reznick had a vision of surgery that valorized the majesty of the discipline: "We have a lot to teach our future colleagues … We know more about trauma, critical illness, cancer, cardiovascular physiology, wound healing, and nutrition than most. There is a closeness to our relationships with patients that is unrivaled in most other domains of medicine. Last, but certainly not least, a surgeon's job is the most exciting and gratifying of any of the medical professions."[120]

# 7 The Surgical Subspecialties

When I was chair from 1982 to 1992 the emphasis was on the need to recruit people who had training in research and education, in addition to being able to look after patients – so that we would have a department that excelled in all three areas.[1]

Bernard Langer, 2010

The story of the subspecialties began when William Gallie took office as professor of surgery in 1930 and implemented a number of changes. The three surgery wards of the General had been undifferentiated. Thus one change was organizing the department by subspecialty. In June 1930 Gallie wrote, "During this year an experiment has been tried of placing all the fractures under the care of a small group of surgeons." Composed of Roy Hindley Thomas from the Emergency Department and one representative from each of the surgical divisions, the group took on the subspecialty of fractures. "The result has been the arousing of greater interest in fractures, the establishment of the first surgical follow up clinic in the hospital and, it is to be hoped, the more successful treatment of patients. The principle of concentrating certain types of patients for a time under small groups of surgeons will be extended wherever possible." Also, the surgeons had learned how weak their follow-up system was. "This defect in our methods will be gradually remedied by the establishment of other follow up clinics in the Outpatient Department."[2] By 1932–3 there was a fracture ward, "whereby fracture cases are segregated in one ward and are treated by a special group of surgeons."[3]

Simultaneously three specialized clinics were set up, one for plastic surgery under Stuart Douglas Gordon, one for rectal surgery under Joseph MacFarlane, who became dean after the Second World War, and one for varicose veins and ulcers of the leg under Robert M. Janes, who was later professor of surgery. Gallie added, "Two new follow-up clinics have also been established for the study of the late results of the treatment of goiter and of the surgical diseases of the stomach ... in addition to one previously established for ... results of the surgical and radiological treatment of cancer of the mouth conducted by Dr [Harold] Wookey in association with Dr [Gordon] Richards of the Radiological Department."[4] Wookey and Janes were older surgeons, born in 1889 and 1894 respectively. MacFarlane and Gordon were younger and clearly leaders. It was the best and the brightest whom Gallie was selecting for these new specialized services.

Specialization in surgery sharpened when Robert Janes became chair in 1947. The wards at the General were reorganized: Ward A was general surgery plus neurosurgery; Ward B was general surgery, head and neck, and plastic surgery; and Ward C was orthopedic and, soon, cardiac.[5]

This kind of specialization had a distinctive role in the life of the faculty. In 1990, when much seemed endangered from prolonged and relentless budget cuts, Dean John Dirks told A. Richard Ten Cate, the vice provost of medical sciences, "Many of these sub-specialty programs are unique nationally and Toronto has an obligation to take advantage of this centre's abundant clinical resources and to sustain these highly acclaimed and essential programs ... The Faculty of Medicine's national reputation rests heavily on it."[6] Readers from elsewhere may smile wryly at these lines. Yet Toronto did intend to lead the nation in surgical subspecialization.

The Second World War, with the military's unremitting demand for physicians and surgeons for the treatment of combat casualties, increased the trend towards specialization. Specialist training in radiology, neurology, anaesthesia, and ophthalmology, among other disciplines, all received big boosts. But the army pushed no specialty as much towards subspecialization as surgery. Not only was there a rush towards the kinds of surgery needed in combat, but the Department of Surgery at the University of Toronto stepped up its offering of refresher courses for general surgeons and educated military surgeons in quick courses for the needed subspecialties. As Gallie said in 1945, "From time to time well-trained surgeons were sent to us for short reviews on special subjects such as thoracic operative technique, neurosurgical technique and so on. They were given temporary staff appointments." One special course, for example, concerned "the technique of external pin fixation in the treatment of fractures." Fifty officers took the course under Robert I. Harris, later head of orthopedic surgery. "[The courses] were of great value in establishing a new method of fracture treatment on a sound basis."[7] In this way the starting gun was sounded for the great sprints that orthopedic surgery and other subspecialties experienced after the war.

## Division of General Surgery

When a patient with a massively bleeding ulcer come to the ER: The colorectal surgeon is away at a national meeting. The HPB [hepato-pancreatic-biliary] has exceeded his mandated work hours for the past 24 hours and is home. The breast surgeon doesn't do emergency laparotomies. The minimally invasive surgeon did only two open ulcer operations during her residency training. And the surgical oncologist restricts his practice to melanoma and sarcoma.[8]

> Richard Reznick, head of Surgery, on the "deepening shortage of general surgeons" that had taken place in many North American centres but not yet in Toronto, 2009

Bernard Langer, head of general surgery in the 1970s, later waxed thoughtful about how the rise of the subspecialties had affected general surgery because all the surgeons in the department had once considered themselves general surgeons:

> The evolution of the specialties is an interesting story and occurred as the result of increasing knowledge about disease and the development of new therapies requiring special training. In the beginning there was surgery in general (or General Surgery). As subspecialties developed, those pieces were carved off general surgery and it became more narrowly defined. Each of these excisions was accompanied by some pain and sometimes quite a bit of opposition. When I was a resident, general surgeons looked after most of the fractures, and I did so in practice for the first five years. When Griff Pearson set out to develop a separate division of thoracic surgery at TGH there was a lot of resistance by other general surgeons.
>
> This phenomenon was common everywhere, since every subspecialty that split from general surgery took a component of their practice and general surgeons did not want to end up as "residual surgeons" – looking after what was left after the good stuff was gone. There is literature over three decades lamenting about the "future of general surgery.
>
> When I became head of General Surgery at TGH [in 1972], I recognized that we had to subspecialize further in order to develop the expertise, volume of practice and critical mass of subspecialists to provide tertiary clinical care and to be at the leading edge in teaching and research. This was accomplished by specific training and recruitment of people to form the nucleus of subspecialized programs within our division of general surgery. I had developed the interest in hepatic, pancreatic and biliary (HPB) surgery and brought back others to expand that field (Bob Stone, Bryce Taylor, Paul Greig). Wayne Johnston and Paul Walker were recruited to develop vascular surgery, and eventually split off to form their own division with our support. Zane Cohen and Robin Mcleod were trained or recruited to develop colorectal surgery, and Lorne Rotstein and Ulo Ambus to develop surgical oncology. Each of these programs grew into University of Toronto collaborative programs and became the leading academic and clinical programs in Canada. As an example, the HPB program has trained academic HPB surgeons for 13 of the 16 medical schools in Canada and many others elsewhere in the USA and Europe.

The footprint left by general surgery, and by Langer himself, was very large. General surgery may thus be considered the first subspecialty, even though Bruce Tovee founded the division at Toronto General Hospital only in 1958.

Tovee became the chair of the university interhospital coordinating committee (IHCC) in General Surgery when these committees were established in 1967. He later reported of their first meeting in November 1967, "We felt that it was important to recognize that General Surgery is really the 'mother' of all other specialties and made up the roots from which the tree of surgery branched."[9]

Tovee himself came from Hamilton and enrolled in medicine in Toronto in 1932. He was known to have financed his medical studies "by playing the piano on a local radio station"; elected to a number of leadership roles in his class, he graduated silver medalist in 1938. Tovee completed his training in surgery at the General during the war, after which Gallie sent him for a year to Chicago to study gastric physiology with Lester Dragstedt. He also spent a year in Edinburgh and returned to Toronto in 1947. In 1972 and nearing retirement, Tovee stepped down from both the hospital and the university divisions of general surgery, believing, as his eulogist and student Bernard Langer said, "that it was important to turn these leadership positions over periodically to allow for the promotion of younger people and the development of new ideas." Langer continued, "No student, intern, resident, or colleague ... was safe from that questioning, probing mind." At the end of the year he typically would give a summary for the final-year medical students facing their qualifying exams of "Everything You Need to Know about Surgery," a format that was adopted in other disciplines and became known as "The Tovee Lectures."[10]

In 1963 Bernie Langer returned from the Peter Bent Brigham Hospital in Boston as a staff general surgeon at the TGH with a new interest (but no training) in liver transplantation. He worked for three years in the laboratory on an animal model of auxiliary liver transplantation and developed his clinical interest in liver surgery by assuming responsibility for the patients with chronic liver disease and portal hypertension (high blood pressure, often caused by alcoholism, in the "portal" venous system that drains from the stomach to the liver). Langer later said, "My entire training in portal hypertension surgery consisted in watching Jim Key, one of the cardiovascular surgeons, do a portacaval shunt and then having him help me do one."[11] This interest in liver surgery led to the development of a large clinical practice in pancreatic and biliary tract surgery as well and to the recruitment of Robert Stone, Bryce Taylor, and later others, creating the aforementioned program in hepatic, pancreatic, and biliary (HPB) surgery.

In 1972 Langer succeeded Tovee as head of general surgery at TGH. He recruited Gary Levy, a hepatologist, to lead the medical and research side of the liver transplant program, and on 31 October 1985, with Paul Greig and Bryce Taylor, Levy carried out the first of the two transplants his team was to achieve that year.

"We went to the lab," said Langer, "and we did a whole series of pig transplants. The pig is a model that's more similar to the human as far as anatomy is concerned, so we were pretty well geared up." When it came time to do the first transplant, Leonard Makowka flew back to scrub in. Makowka had trained with Langer at the General but then had gone to Pittsburgh to work with Tom Starzl. Starzl had done the first successful human liver transplants at the University of Colorado. Said Langer, "He gave us a degree of comfort; he was now an expert, he had done a lot of them in Pittsburgh, so he coached us through the first operation." The operation, which began at 8:00 p.m. on 31 October 1985 and finished the next morning at 9:00, attracted so much attention that at one point no fewer than twenty-two medical staff were in the operating room. Robert Ginsberg, "freshly scrubbed and gowned," walked in and announced, "There are too many people in here. Anyone who isn't absolutely necessary must leave." No one left.

The patient, unintentionally overtreated with immunosuppressive drugs, died of a post-operative infection, but "his liver was actually in very good shape at the time he died," said Langer. The Hospital for Sick Children joined the program when the first pediatric liver transplant was done on 9 October 1986. By 1988 TGH had a transplant ward. Toronto thus acquired "one of the leading liver transplant programs in North America." Steve Strasberg from Mount Sinai and Ric Superina from HSC had joined Langer, Greig, and Taylor from TGH on the transplant team by the 1987–8 session.

It was the second such program in the province, following that of the University of Western Ontario. But, as Langer pointed out, "[t]his University had something to offer that is not available in London [Ontario], ie a broad range of first class research associated with the program." The program grew under Levy's leadership to be the largest in Canada and one of the most academically productive in the world. Langer said of the full scope of Levy's accomplishments, "[i]t is huge."

The second subspecialty area of general surgery was colorectal surgery, led by Zane Cohen, who developed an interest in inflammatory bowel disease and introduced the operation of continent ileostomy (a surgical opening into the ileum that maintains continence of feces) to Canada. He also started a familial colon cancer registry which became the foundation for a colon cancer genetics program currently housed at the Mount Sinai Hospital. With Robin McLeod he started a fellowship training program in colorectal surgery in Toronto, which became the first such program recognized by the Royal College of Physicians and Surgeons of Canada in 1990. Cohen and McLeod moved to Mount Sinai Hospital in 1990 when Cohen became chief of surgery there, and in 1999 he was appointed the chair of the University of Toronto Division of General Surgery.

The third subspecialty area was vascular surgery, developed with the recruitment of Wayne Johnston and subsequently Paul Walker. Johnston was interested in noninvasive imaging of vessels and, with his collaborator Richard Cobbold in the Department of Biomedical Engineering, became a world leader in research in this area.

In 1988–9 Bryce Taylor, a U of T medical graduate, replaced Langer as head of the university Division of General Surgery; he also headed the hospital division at the General when the new gastrointestinal transplantation unit for liver and pancreas opened in the fall of 1989. In the 1990–1 session, laparoscopic chole-cystectomy (gall bladder removal via a small incision and specialized camera) came to North America from Europe and was actively promoted by the in-strument manufacturers. To ensure that surgeons already in practice had ad-equate training, Steve Strasberg, with other members of the division, organized a hands-on refresher course in the subject.[12] By 1992, most of the university di-vision's ten hospital divisions were carrying out laparoscopic appendectomies, bowel resections, and other procedures.[13] In January 1999, an external assessor found that, under Taylor, the general surgery program "ranks among the top ten on the continent."[14]

## Division of Orthopaedic Surgery

Because of its ancient and worthy history, orthopaedic surgery is of interest to all devo-tees of medicine. Standing in its midst … is that interesting, but oftentimes tragic and pathetic figure, the cripple. It is with strange, even indignant, feelings that the student notes the attitude of society toward that forlorn figure down through the ages and it is with great satisfaction that one considers the care that is his to-day.[15]

Melvin S. Henderson, Section of Orthopedic Surgery, the Mayo Clinic, Rochester, Minnesota, delivering the Donald C. Balfour Lecture in Toronto, April 1936. Henderson and Balfour graduated together from U of T in 1906.

Spurred by the introduction of the X-ray machine in 1896, in June 1899 orthope-dic surgery made its first eruption in Toronto: at the Hospital for Sick Children with the foundation of the pediatric orthopedic department. Said the hospital's annual report in 1900, "No other department is so enthusiastically spoken of or excites such sympathy as that which removes deformities and aids those unfor-tunately afflicted with club feet, bow-legs, knock-knees, flat feet, infantile pa-ralysis, spinal disease, etc."[16]

Orthopedics became the oldest subspecialty of the Department of Surgery. In 1903 Clarence Starr was the associate professor of clinical surgery in charge of orthopedics at the General.[17] The division itself was founded in the 1939–40 ses-sion by Robert Inkerman Harris. Harris was born in Toronto in 1889, graduated from North Bay High School, and received his medical degree from Toronto in 1915. He began his career in surgery at the Hospital for Sick Children, moving over to Roscoe Graham's service at the General in 1929–30. Having had tubercu-losis himself as a child, he developed a special interest in the disease and estab-lished a "roof ward" at the Christie Street Hospital to let veterans benefit from heliotherapy (such was the paucity then of effective treatments for TB). "Most of them lived," said his biographer, "to take part in a 1934 'Re-union of the Sun Worshippers.'" Harris came on staff at the Toronto Hospital for Consumptives in Weston, which had been established in 1904.[18]

In 1939, as noted, Gallie made Harris inaugural chief of the orthopedic surgery division, a consolation prize for not making Harris chief of the Ward B service (Harold Wookey won out).[19] Gallie commented, "At the General Hospital the outstanding change in the Department of Surgery has been the organization of an orthopaedic service." They didn't need this in the past, he said, "as many of the junior members of the staff had been trained under the late Professor CL Starr and the present head of the department [Gallie]. It has been becoming increasingly evident, however, that if we are to maintain our position in competition with the other great hospitals of Great Britain and the United States, we must concentrate the patients in the hands of men who are specially qualified to take care of them."[20] The war interrupted events. Yet post-war Toronto became among the few centres in North America that started to attract surgeons interested in orthopedics.

In 1951 under university rules, Harris was obliged to retire as university head of service (though he stayed on as chief at Sunnybrook), and Frederick P. Dewar, Harrris's first resident, succeeded him. Only at that point did a real orthopedics training program get going, based on the orthopedic patients at the Toronto General Hospital, the Hospital for Sick Children (under Bill Mustard), and Sunnybrook. Interestingly, the Western and St Michael's both passed up the opportunity to have orthopedic divisions because, as Dewar put it, "They were dedicated to the original principle of general surgical teaching." St Joseph's Hospital and the East General Hospital joined the postgraduate orthopedic training program. So the young program could accept five or six trainees a year.[21] (Then eventually Paul McGoey did initiate an orthopedics program at St Michael's Hospital.)

Dewar was born in Saskatoon in 1911, his father a bank manager. But he grew up in Orangeville, Ontario, whence his father and mother originated, and the family had moved back to Ontario after various misadventures. He got through medical school owing to a cheque for $500 that his Aunt Lil sent him every year, plus the slightly worn suits of one of his wealthy clothes-horse cousins. After graduating from U of T in 1936, he served as senior house surgeon to Roscoe Graham. During his wartime service in England, he became a Fellow of the Royal College of Surgeons of England and finished his training at the Hospital for Ruptured and Crippled Children (later called the Hospital for Special Surgery) in New York. In 1947 he joined the Division of Orthopedic Surgery at the General under Harris, having as a special research interest scoliosis, a sideways deviation in the normally straight spine. Dewar was noted for an early successful use of the Küntscher nail for the intramedullary fixation of "high-energy" femoral fractures (a chilling phrase, signifying terrible fractures), a technique that decreased the duration of the hospital stay from 120 to 25 days. The spine unit in the division is named after him.

Dewar was said to have done well in the department partly because, "quiet and reserved" himself, he had a brilliant wife, Lucy Dewar. Wilson said, "Ted

Dewar married a very vivacious, outgoing lady who was open and readily approached by anybody that needed help, and she and Ted really were the soul of the Dewar club. It was a team effort for them."[22]

Among young surgeons serving under Dewar was Ian MacNab, born in India in 1921 into the family of a Scottish shipbuilder living there. He finished medicine at the University of Birmingham in 1943, then, after the war, completed his surgical training at the Royal National Orthopaedic Hospital in London, with a special interest in low-back disability. Robert I. Harris brought him to the Banting Institute in Toronto in 1950 to study the origins of low-back pain. Although he was internationally known as a spinal surgeon, his interests were quite eclectic, and he was awarded the Hunterian Lectureship of the Royal College of Surgeons of England for his work on the rotator cuff, the muscles of the shoulder joint.[23]

W. Robert Harris figured also among this generation. He was a surgeon who, Cosbie says, "took a keen interest in amputations and especially in the production of new and better types of artificial limbs" – for which the returning veterans created an especially poignant demand. What gave a special boost to orthopedic surgery in these years was antibiotics. "Open reduction of fractures and the use of plastic and metal prostheses were now free from the haunting fear of sepsis," said Cosbie.[24]

Dewar launched a university Division of Orthopaedic Surgery in 1951 by heading an interhospital coordinating committee (IHCC) on the subject, the forerunner of a division. The heads of the hospital Divisions of Orthopaedic Surgery had started meeting unofficially and then received official status, with Dewar named as chair. This was the template on which the other surgical divisions were organized.[25] Dewar later said, "This system grew because Toronto was like that. It's a multi-hospital University and we still have ... the biggest number of hospitals with totally separate staffs in any orthopedic training program I have ever heard of." He then continued, on the subject of Toronto's distinctiveness, "Most big cities in the world have several universities. This is the only city of its size in the world that I know of – 4 million people around [1973] – that has only one medical school. It's completely unique."[26]

Dewar remained head of the university division and chief of the hospital division at the General until 1976, initiating the postgraduate training program in orthopedics that would become world-renowned.[27] In 1973 Dewar said, "The most pleasant thing that happened to me, was the enthusiasm of all the orthopedic surgeons in Toronto to make it the best training program in the world, and it took us about 15 years before we were even beginning to be recognized and suddenly, one of our visiting professors came out and made a statement in Great Britain, that we were now amongst the leading orthopedic schools in North America."[28]

Yet medical leader though he may have been, Dewar was not attuned to research, and in the 1960s the faculty was beginning to press the research button.

In 1967, Melvin Glimcher, chief of the Orthopedic Service of the Massachusetts General Hospital, visited the Toronto division. He judged that, in teaching, schools are going to "require physician-scholars who are capable of integrating the basic sciences and the clinical aspects of disease … This is new for us." Indeed it was. Orthopedics was not used to undertaking basic research as the platform for solving clinical problems. "There has been a long tradition in Internal Medicine for excellence in teaching based on pathophysiology, for the training of physician-scholars and the commitment of such departments to fundamental research, but this has not generally been true for either general surgery or the surgical specialties, all of which now face the same critical situation." Orthopedic surgery is expanding so rapidly it's turning into "[o]rthopedics," he said, "since it now undoubtedly lies somewhere between internal medicine and surgery, concerning itself more and more with fundamental problems of the musculoskeletal system rather than simply with the technical and surgical aspects of these diseases."[29]

Still, orthopedics in Toronto made some important clinical contributions. At the children's hospital, Walter P. Bobechko was known as an advocate of early fusion of the vertebrae in young children with progressive spinal curvature.[30] Said one eulogist, "At a time when most children with Perthes disease [necrosis of the head of the femur followed by recalcification] were spending months in plaster casts with consequent knee stiffness, he developed the Toronto brace that allowed movement of the knees, improved mobility, and removal of the brace for physical therapy."[31] Bobechko is, however, best known for an implantable electric muscle stimulator to correct scoliosis. This research began at HSC in 1974, reached a provisional end in Toronto in the late 1980s,[32] and then was perfected with Bobechko's move to Texas. Of this work of Bobechko and others, *Time* magazine said in 1982 that the patients were delighted because they could just be like other children. Indeed, some flaunted their hardware. According to Bobechko, "The kids take the transmitters to school and say, 'See, I'm the bionic woman.'"[33]

Born in Toronto in 1932, Bobechko was educated at Parkdale Collegiate and earned a medical degree from U of T in 1957, then trained at the General and HSC and at the Mayo Clinic. With a McLaughlin Travelling Fellowship, he spent 1964 at a Russian institute and in Goteborg in Sweden. "Wally" Bobechko was chief orthopedic surgeon at HSC from 1977 to 1987, when he joined a surgical institute in Texas. Said his eulogist, "His surgical techniques were spread around the world by the fellows he trained."[34]

Among the other leading lights of the division was David MacIntosh, who specialized in knee injuries (he developed in 1958 the knee-joint prosthesis named after him[35]). In 1972 MacIntosh led a team that described "pivot shift," a clinical diagnostic sign of instability in the anterior cruciate ligament of the knee joint, causing tears in the lateral meniscus in the floor of the knee.[36] MacIntosh developed in 1976 an operation for the repair of these injuries.[37] A medical graduate of Dalhousie University in 1939, MacIntosh ran the sports medicine clinic at the University of Toronto's student centre Hart House from 1951 to 1958; the David L. MacIntosh Sports Medicine Clinic at the university's Athletic Centre is believed to be the oldest dedicated sports medicine facility in the world. (In 1977 orthopedic surgeon John P. Kostuik at the General reported a widely used adaptation of the MacIntosh procedure.[38] "The use of these techniques," Kostuik said, "has served to rehabilitate many young athletes and working people who would otherwise have had severe residual restrictions of function." Kostuik later played a role in transplant surgery in Toronto; see p. 157.)

Generations of athletes – and not only athletes – have MacIntosh's colleague Robert W. Jackson to thank for the introduction in North America of arthroscopic surgery on the knee. Toronto-born in 1932, Jackson graduated in medicine from the U of T in 1956. After a year of research on fractures of the tibia, he trained in general surgery in Toronto, then in the next several years studied orthopedics at several international centres, including Boston, Bristol, and the Royal National Orthopaedic Hospital in London. It was, however, a Markle scholarship that made it possible for Jackson to travel in 1964 to Japan for study with the originator of arthroscopy, Masaki Watanabe. They exchanged lessons, Jackson learning arthroscopy, which means using an endoscope to examine the interior of a joint, in exchange for teaching Watanabe English. Later, in 1964, Jackson served as physician for the Canadian Olympic team at the summer games in Tokyo, applying the lessons he had learned from Watanabe. The following year Jackson returned to Toronto and "began to practice arthroscopy using the Watanabe no. 21 arthroscope," as he later said. He was then joined by a colleague from Tokyo to improve the technique and in 1968 he gave the first instructional course on arthroscopy at the annual meeting of the American Academy of Orthopedic Surgeons.[39]

One biographer writes, "Jackson's particular genius was to recognize a wider application for the procedure than Watanabe ever did. Jackson returned home to his new position as team doctor for the Toronto Argonauts of the Canadian Football League. In 1967 he performed the first arthroscopic procedure on an Argonaut." The introduction of fibre optics in the 1970s facilitated arthroscopy, and by 1980 this variety of "needle with an eye" operation had become mainstream.[40] In 1976, together with David J. Dandy, Jackson published the standard textbook, *Arthroscopy of the Knee*.[41] From 1976 to 1985 Jackson was chief of orthopedics at the Toronto Western Hospital, then from 1985 to 1992 chief of surgery at the Orthopaedic and Arthritic Hospital. In 1992 he moved to Baylor University in Dallas. In recognition of his international importance, in 1994 *Sports Illustrated* named him "one of the 40 most influential individuals in sports, the only physician on their list."[42]

The division thus had this galaxy of international stars. Yet foremost of them was Robert Salter. In 1976 when Robert Harris succeeded Dewar as chief of the Division of Orthopaedic Surgery at TGH, Salter became the university professor of orthopedic surgery.

Salter, whom Reznick called in 2003 "one of Canada's most famous sur-geons,"[43] was without any doubt the division's great international luminosity. He spent his career at the Hospital for Sick Children.

Born in Stratford, Ontario, in 1924, Salter earned his MD at the U of T in 1947. He spent two years serving at the Grenfell Medical Mission in Newfoundland and Labrador, then trained in surgery at the Hospital for Sick Children under William Mustard. In 1954, Salter travelled to London on a McLaughlin Fellow-ship, where he studied with orthopedic leader Sir Reginald Watson-Jones. Col-league John Wedge tells this story: "Watson-Jones was known for his dictum that immobilization for fractures should be complete, rigid, enforced, and pro-longed. Bob's intuition told him that this dogma was false, much to the ire of his supervisor."[44]

Armed with this intuition, Salter joined the Division of Orthopaedic Surgery of HSC in 1955 and two years later became chief of the hospital division. He as-cended in 1966 to the university chair of surgery as well as becoming chief surgeon of HSC. Among his many innovations, three deserve special mention: the Salter osteotomy, proposed in 1960, to repair congenital hip dislocation (innominate bone osteotomy, which involves redirecting the acetabulum, or bony socket for the head of the femur, to make it stable during weight bearing);[45] the Salter-Harris classification of injuries to the epiphyseal plate (which regulates bone growth in children) in 1963;[46] and the revolutionary concept – epochal in its impact on the treatment of cartilage injuries in children and adults – of "continuous passive motion" in 1979. Salter's *Textbook of Disorders and Injuries of the Musculoskeletal Sys-tem: An Introduction to Orthopaedics* (1970), in its third edition at this writing, has sold 195,000 copies worldwide and been translated into six languages.[47] In 1969 Salter won a Gairdner Award and was inducted into the Canadian Medical Hall of Fame in 1995. In the late 1960s, he founded the first clinical fellowship program in pediatric orthopedics in North America at the children's hospital. Animated by a desire to get more residents to undertake research, Salter famously formulated the steps of the "cycle of surgical research," which remain as valid today as when he proposed them in 1980.[48] Devoutly observant, Salter once said that he himself was inspired to undertake basic research, in his case fifty years' worth, by the phi-losophy of St Luke the Physician: "Unto whomsoever much has been given, of that person shall much be required."[49]

Then there was Allan Gross and knee transplantation. In 1975 a team led by Gross at Mount Sinai published the results for eight patients of two years of work in knee transplantation: harvesting the weight-bearing parts of cadaver allograft knees and transplanting them into patients in need of replacements owing mainly to trauma (results in osteoarthritis were less brilliant).[50] Gross had graduated in medicine from U of T in 1962. By 1985 he and his team had per-formed the operation, transplanting fresh osteochondral fragment allografts, in one hundred patients. The success rate in patients with traumatic injury to the articular surface was 75 percent. Reoperations were minimal for grafts in place longer than five years because revascularization of the joint was complete "and the allograft has been completely incorporated into the patient's metaphyseal bone."[51] Gross's "knee replacement" operation made headlines. (Gross was also the team doctor for the Toronto Blue Jays.)

In the 1980s and after, great organizational changes swept over orthopedics. In 1982 the orthopedic units of the Toronto General and Mount Sinai Hospitals merged, under Sinai's Allan Gross. Fast-lane research rushed to the forefront. Immunology was by 1986 the "major thrust" at Mount Sinai, whereas TGH emphasized biomechanics. A transplant program thrived under John P. Kostuik, who would shortly become head of the combined hospital division.[52] In the 1988–9 session it was decided to shift all orthopedics except the spinal unit to the Toronto Western Hospital, as part of the division of labour that merged the two hospitals into The Toronto Hospital. Mount Sinai would concentrate on musculoskeletal oncology and tertiary joint replacement.[53] At the same time the A.J. Latner Chair of Orthopaedic Surgery was created, the first named chair in this field in Canada, with Gross, the head of the university division, as the first incumbent in 1992.[54] In 1994 a "combined Tri-Hospital Orthopedic Unit" was formed among Mount Sinai, the Toronto Hospital, and Women's College Hospital, with Gross as its head.[55] Shortly thereafter, neurosurgeon Michael Fehlings became head of the combined Orthopaedic/Neurosurgery Spinal Unit at the Toronto Hospital.[56] These were enormous changes that brought the oldest surgical division of the faculty abreast of modern science and up to speed on the functional division of labour among hospitals that the provincial paymasters so badly wished.

### Division of Cardiovascular Surgery

The Division remains the most academically productive cardiac surgical unit in the world.[57]

Richard Weisel, Chair, Division of Cardiac Surgery, 2008

As seen in chapter 5, in 1960 a Division of Cardiovascular Surgery was created with Bigelow at its head. In 1977 Ronald Baird succeeded him. Yet the existence of this division meant relatively little because the five different cardiac surgery programs in Toronto had little interest in cooperating. "It was an amiable group," said Don Wilson, "but everybody did their own thing. There was sort of a meeting once or twice a year in which residents were assigned. But there were very few meetings of cardiac people, [who] related more to the cardiologists than they did to the other people. That was, like neurology and neurosurgeons; so they developed their own little teams all over." Formal organization did not get beyond, "Uncle Bill [Bigelow], I'm looking for a new man."

The back story was soaring demand for cardiovascular surgery as the prolongation of life finally became a realistic prospect for people with heart disease.

Bypass surgery swamped the existing arrangements. In 1973 Charles Hollenberg noted "increasing pressure on our existing cardiology services" as a result of coronary bypass operations that increased diagnostic need and of the introduction of cardiac catheterization and new cardiac drugs.[58]

New hands came on board. Baird was the first new surgeon recruited at TGH as a specifically designated "cardiovascular" surgeon.[59] Born in 1930 in Toronto, he graduated in medicine from U of T in 1954 and earned his fellowship in 1959. In 1964 he left the General for the cardiovascular surgery division of the Western under Donald Wilson, then in 1972 returned to the General as director of surgical research at the university and at the hospital. Baird had a keen interest in valve repair; yet he also introduced a wide range of procedures, such as, in Bernard Goldman's words, "the technique of hypothermic total circulatory arrest for repair of aneurysms of the [aortic] arch and descending thoracic aorta" in 1982.[60]

In the 1980s, coronary artery bypass surgery became routine. The faculty produced several videos illustrating medical procedures, and Dean Lowy described the video about bypass: "One lawyer who before surgery was barely able to cross a room without severe angina, now runs five miles a day only eight months after his bypass ... Another patient, a carpenter, forced to quit work because of his heart problems, is back on the job six months postoperatively ... A biochemist of 59 who was barely able to climb the stairs before surgery is now back skiing, playing tennis and yachting actively."[61] Baird said, "[B]ypass surgery is now considered no more hazardous than many other operations, such as gallbladder removal, for some patients." In 1981, some 2,400 Toronto patients received bypass operations, an average of 98 percent surviving. Goldman, then a cardiovascular surgeon at TGH (and later founder of cardiovascular surgery at Sunnybrook), said that in 1982–3 the "mortality rate for coronary bypass procedures was only 0.9 per cent or one in a hundred" – down from 30 percent in the 1970s.[62]

For adults, Toronto had two important centres of cardiovascular surgery (St Michael's and Sunnybrook were not big research players): the General, where Baird's staff included Goldman, Richard Weisel, and Lynda Mickleborough (a 1973 McGill graduate and one of the few women in this kind of surgery); and the Toronto Western Hospital, where cardiovascular surgery was headed by Tirone David, who graduated in medicine from Paraná University in Brazil in 1968, trained at the Cleveland Clinic, and moved in 1975 to Toronto. The founder of cardiovascular surgery at the Western was Donald Wilson, by the early 1980s now a full professor and chief of surgery there.

The pacemaker story has a further Toronto chapter. In 1970 Goldman organized with Bigelow a pacemaker follow-up clinic. In that same year, the nuclear cardiac pacemaker was introduced in Paris. About the size of a small cigarette package, it promised a much longer life than the conventional battery-powered pacemaker.[63] In October 1973 Goldman implanted Canada's first nuclear pacemaker at TGH and became director of the hospital's Pacemaker Centre. The patient still lives at the present writing.

There was no cardiovascular surgery without cardiology, and care of both went back to Bill Bigelow in the mid-1950s. In 1956 the General Hospital opened a Cardiovascular Investigation Unit in a concrete-block extension called "Bigelow's Bungalow" as "a joint medical and surgical unit."[64] Yet its resources were limited, and the waiting lists of desperate patients awaiting heart-valve replacements in these early days of open-heart surgery grew ever longer. As Bigelow tried to add on physiologists and more imaging apparatus, and meet the other demands of the new cardiovascular science, space became ever more inadequate.

In 1962 this unit was significantly expanded. In an opening ceremony on 19 January Bigelow expressed a vision of the future: "I think the Toronto General Hospital should take on a major responsibility as a postgraduate training centre of Canada ... It is not enough to teach a postgraduate student how to diagnose and treat disease skillfully. Postgraduate training is not complete unless he comes in contact with research."[65] Research became the watchword.

In 1964 the campus was abuzz with talk about expanding research laboratory space, so tight had facilities become. Bigelow made a claim for space in the proposed "new Toronto General Hospital Clinical Building." (The TGH Clinical Services Building did not in fact open until 2003.) "The section of Cardiology of the Department of Medicine and the Division of Cardiovascular Surgery in the Department of Surgery are so intimately involved in any clinical research area that it was considered that this be a single submission [requesting space]." The waiting times justified a cardiovascular unit. "[At present] a patient destined for open heart surgery [has] to await three months for his admission to hospital for investigation, following which he is booked for surgery which cannot be done at this time, and will involve a two to three month wait again before surgery is available. Many of the valvular lesions and practically all of the aortic valve surgery cannot wait this long. This requires an urgent admission for investigation." But, said Bigelow, when the patient is admitted, the catheterization is often delayed several days. Yet if the cardiovascular division had its own beds, on its own unit, all could be done with much greater dispatch.[66]

Ever since Bigelow, cardiologists and cardiovascular surgeons had aspired to a centre for heart research. In 1990–1 it was finally created, centred at the General.[67] This facility underwent a great clinical and research expansion, culminating in October 1997 in the opening of the Peter Munk Cardiac Centre (PMCC). It aspired, as the *Toronto Star* reported, "[to] bring together all the cardiac services, staff and patients currently dispersed throughout the Hospital ... The Centre will enable the Hospital to implement what is now being called The Toronto Hospital Cardiac System ... patterned after one used at the Oxford Heart Centre in England, reduc[ing] a patient's length of stay in intensive care by half for routine open-heart surgery." The article continued, "The Centre is being funded by a $25 million capital campaign, 'From the Heart.' ... Peter Munk has made the lead donation of $5 million; the Hospital will contribute $6 million and the remainder will be raised from donations from the community."[68] In 2003 the PMCC moved to its new home in the General's Clinical Sciences Building. (On the collaboration between the cardiologists and cardiac surgeons in this centre see chapter 9.)

In cardiovascular surgery, integration among the divisions of the teaching hospitals was slow. Not until 1987–8 did Goldman, appointed division director of postgraduate education, start to organize city-wide clinical and research conferences.[69]

In terms of teaching, cardiac surgery became a "base specialty" in the 1994–5 session, accepting medical school graduates into a six-year program leading to the fellowship in the "specialty" of cardiac surgery. The first two years of the program were spent in core surgery. "The following four years," the department explained, "include one year of academic enrichment, which may be a stepping stone to Clinician-Scientist Program for academically inclined residents who wish to undertake an MSc or PhD during their cardiac training." The Royal College of Physicians and Surgeons approved the program in the spring of 1995.[70]

In 1981 the divisions of cardiac and vascular surgery separated, the latter headed by Baird's former resident Wayne Johnston, who became in the 1992–3 session the inaugural holder of the Fraser Elliott Chair in Vascular Surgery; Johnston was known for a long series of 681 percutaneous transluminal dilations (TLDs), in which a balloon catheter dilates and clears an occluded peripheral artery, performed at the Toronto General Hospital between 1978 and 1984; this research established TLD as a safe alternative to surgery.[71]

In the 1987–8 session, Tomas ("Tom") Salerno, a McGill graduate of 1971, replaced Baird as head of the university division, while Baird stayed on for one more year as head of the hospital division at TGH. Then in 1988–9 Tirone David succeeded Baird as leader of the hospital division at the same time that cardiac surgery was shifted from the Western to the General. The huge transfer of resources between the two large teaching hospitals was now more or less complete: neurosurgery and musculoskeletal work were entirely at the Western, cardiac surgery entirely at the General.

The members of the division devised several important innovations. In the 1983–4 session, Lynda Mickleborough proposed the technique of "mapping" the left ventricle with a kind of balloon to determine the source of irregular heartbeats.[72] Then Mickleborough went one step farther and used the electrodes on the balloon to deliver electric shocks to the diseased heart muscle that was causing ventricular arrhythmias. The scar created in the endometrium by the balloon was tidier than the original scar and reduced the chances of further heart attacks. The balloon was threaded through the mitral valve into the left ventricle and was considered closed-heart surgery, less dangerous than a ventriculotomy. By 1989 Mickleborough had successfully employed the technique, called balloon electric shock ablation (BESA), in six patients, who became free of arrhythmia.[73] In 1994 Mickleborough and colleagues determined that removing the scar tissue restored the geometry of the left ventricle and gave best results: "Aneurysm repair with a tailored scar excision and linear closure is associated with low operative mortality ... and long-term survival even in patients with advanced left ventricular dysfunction and mitral regurgitation."[74]

In the 1980s Richard Weisel led research on "myocardial protection and donor heart (lung) preservation." Weisel was one of the main surgeon-scientists in the division and was called "one of the most prolific cardiovascular surgeons in the world."[75] In the 1980s and 1990s a substantial interest arose in protecting the myocardium with drugs during surgical interventions. Weisel, an American, was born in 1943 and majored in philosophy at Yale. In 1969 he completed medical school in Milwaukee at Marquette University, where his father chaired the cardiac surgery department. Weisel trained in cardiac surgery at Boston University Medical Center and came to Toronto in 1976 for further work, joining the TGH staff in 1978. As head of the division, "he emphasizes how important it is for young surgeons to 'keep their skis together' by pulling their clinical work towards their research."[76] In 1989 he became a professor in the Department of Surgery, director of surgical research for the university, and associate director of the centre for cardiovascular research at the General (headed by Michael Sole); in 1998, as stated, he was made head of the Division of Cardiovascular Surgery.

Increasingly, members of the Department of Surgery became involved with basic scientists in investigating such issues as the repair of the myocardium after a heart attack or episode of heart failure: How to restore those damaged heart muscle cells, or cardiac myocytes? In 1996 Ren-Ke Li at the Division of Experimental Therapeutics of the Toronto General Hospital Research Institute, working together with Weisel and others in the cardiovascular division, proposed experimentally implanting healthy mouse muscle cells into scarred heart muscles in order to prevent heart failure. They found that "the transplanted cardiomyocytes formed cardiac tissue in the myocardial scar, limited scar expansion, and improved heart function compared with findings in the control hearts."[77] Three years later, by 1999, it was clear that "BMCs [bone marrow cells] should be considered as an alternative transplant-cell source to repair the damaged myocardium." Further animal work found that when treated with the agent 5-azacytidine, transplantation of the bone marrow cells "into the scar of the failing heart improved contractile function and all transplanted BMCs induced angiogenesis."[78] By 2006 their research had progressed to the point of demonstrating in animal models that in a heart attack "c-kit receptor" cells derived from bone marrow initiate angiogenesis and help restore the damaged cardiac muscle. (This partially explains why elderly patients with bone marrow senescence experience poor cardiac repair and progress eventually to congestive heart failure.) The authors concluded, "Transplantation of bone marrow cells prepared from young allogenic donors may significantly enhance cardiac repair."[79]

In 1997, Christopher Feindel's team elaborated a technique for preservation of hearts for transplantation.[80] Feindel, a McGill medical graduate (1976) who had trained in cardiovascular and thoracic surgery at U of T from 1981 to 1984, became director of heart transplantation in 1985. In 2008, Feindel brought to Toronto the transcatheter implantation of aortic valves for aortic stenosis, first perfected in France by Alain Cribier in 2002. The transfemoral version of this procedure had been aided by Sam Lichtenstein, once on staff at St Michael's Hospital, after his move to Vancouver. Lichtenstein flew back to scrub in with Feindel for the first Toronto procedure. Once symptoms developed, these patients had suffered a two-year mortality of over 50 percent; they now saw their risk reduced to around 10 to 14 percent.[81]

The work of Tirone David with artificial replacement valves became internationally celebrated. He and Chris Feindel had resurrected heart transplantation in 1983, once cyclosporine became available.[82] (Ray Heimbecker, after going to the University of Western Ontario, performed the first "modern" heart transplant in Canada in 1981.) In 1988, David proposed aortic valve replacement with stentless porcine aortic bioprostheses (called "SPVs").[83] This technique was introduced clinically in 1991 and became known as "the Toronto valve."[84] There followed David's replacement together with Chris Feindel of the aortic root with a Dacron graft (1992)[85] and the reconstruction of the aortic valve (1995).[86] Tirone David is also known for pioneering surgical techniques including complex ventricular resections. He is probably the most renowned cardiac surgeon for many of these procedures worldwide.

As technology galloped on, drug eluting stents began to replace coronary bypass, which was diminishing by 2008. Weisel said, "Cardiac surgeons have developed catheter skills and embraced transvascular approaches to a variety of cardiac and vascular diseases. Our recent recruits are performing procedures we did not imagine ten years ago and their case mix is dramatically different. Hybrid procedures were first introduced at the Hospital for Sick Children and are now common at all of our institutions ... The new era in cardiac surgery promises to be very exciting."[87]

### Division of Cardiovascular Surgery (Division of Cardiac Surgery) at HSC

In the post-Mustard era, the history of cardiovascular surgery at the Hospital for Sick Children is essentially bound up with two clinicians: George A. Trusler and William G. Williams. Trusler was born in 1926 in Toronto, finished his medical studies at U of T in 1949, and trained in medicine and pathology for the next six years. It was only in January 1955 that he started preparing for surgery under Janes. During this period he spent a research year with Bigelow at a time when Bigelow was shifting from general surgery to cardiovascular. At Bigelow's request, the hospital created the post of resident in cardiovascular surgery, and Trusler became the first. Six months later, Mustard asked Trusler to come over to HSC. "For this purpose," said Trusler later, "I spent six months on a McLaughlin Travelling Fellowship in the United States." Then in 1958 he became a resident in general pediatric surgery and pediatric cardiovascular surgery at HSC.[88] When Mustard retired in 1976, Trusler was appointed chief of the service. Trusler contributed notably to the complexities of managing septal defects in children.[89]

William G. Williams succeeded Trusler in 1988–9 and for a while Trusler and Williams were the only members of the division. Bill Williams grew up in Toronto in a medical family (his father was an orthopedic surgeon at St Joseph's Hospital) but went to medical school at the University of Western Ontario, finishing his studies in 1964. Williams trained in cardiovascular and thoracic surgery in Toronto, specializing in the congenital defects that are the essence of the field. In 1987 he and co-investigators, including cardiologist Douglas Wigle and Trusler, established that "a generous transaortic myectomy" (excising a portion of the heart muscle) greatly improved patients with hypertrophic obstructive cardiomyopathy, an enlargement of the cardiac ventricles of mysterious origin.[90] In 1992–3 he became the university chair of cardiac surgery. Williams presided over the inception in 1991–2 of a multidisciplinary cardiac transplantation program, as well as the expansion of the existing Extracorporeal-Membrane Oxygenation Support (ECMO) Program in neonatal pulmonary disease.[91]

In July 2001, Glen Van Arsdell became head of the Division of Cardiovascular Surgery. A graduate of Loma Linda University in California, Van Arsdell joined the surgical staff of the hospital in 1996.[92] By 2008 faculty in the Division of Cardiac Surgery at the children's hospital had increased from two members in 1983 to six. Their research ran the gamut from basic science to the translation of basic findings into clinical results, in the form of articles that now put the term "inoperable" in quotation marks.

## Division of Thoracic Surgery

Griff Pearson recognized that folding thoracic surgery into cardiac surgery gave insufficient attention to the particular problems of thoracic surgery, and that by concentrating the scholarship, research, and clinical training on thoracic surgery exclusively, he could strengthen and develop the specialty – which is exactly what he did.[93]

Martin McKneally, 2009

Some fields are driven by the advent of new therapies, others by new technologies. It was the bronchoscope, introduced in the United States in 1904, that opened the door for chest surgery. Yet later on, chest surgery was often swallowed up in the larger cardiovascular sea. By the 1970s, the dominant service in most centres was "cardiothoracic surgery," with pulmonary cases receiving little attention. With non-cardiac thoracic surgery declining elsewhere, Toronto became the main training centre for the specialty on the continent.[94]

In Toronto, thoracic surgery maintained its independence from cardiovascular surgery largely because of the distinction of its founding figures. Norman

Shenstone, introduced in chapter 6, was born in Toronto in 1886. He earned an MD from Columbia University in 1905 and thereupon returned to Toronto in 1909 to join the Department of Surgery. He is the seminal figure in the history of thoracic surgery in Toronto, founding the "Sub-department of Thoracic Surgery." Shenstone and his student Robert Janes became virtual household names in the world of lung surgery in 1932 when they published a technique for dealing with the pus-filled lung at its removal, for example, in tuberculosis (see p. 123).[95]

Among the Toronto chest surgeons, Harold Wookey, also encountered in a previous chapter, played a big role. Wookey trained in surgery in England and became known in 1942 for restoring esophageal continuity in cancer operations with a skin flap.[96] In 1948 he authored an overview of the reconstruction of the cancerous lower pharynx and esophagus that was widely cited.[97]

F. Griffith ("Griff") Pearson, later head of the division, said, "When I completed my internship at TGH in 1950, Norman Shenstone, Robert Janes, Frederick Kergin, and Norman Delarue were the staff members responsible for thoracic surgery in a large division of general surgery."[98] Shenstone, Janes, and Kergin went on to become leaders in the department.

Norman Delarue figures in the story for work he did in 1949 while training at Washington University of St Louis under surgeon Evarts Graham. He and Graham described a kind of cancer that is common in smokers, "alveolar cell carcinoma of the lung," calling it a specific entity of "epithelial" origin carrying an unfavourable prognosis; their article did not mention smoking as a cause.[99] The smoking and lung cancer link was discovered by others. Back in Toronto, Delarue published research suggesting that the lung cancer epidemic could be halted through smoking cessation.[100] (Delarue, who graduated in medicine in 1939, had been a big athlete and president of his fourth-year class; he was apparently not a smoker, and Graham, a heavy smoker, is said to have been unconvinced by the early findings of his fellow.) In the 1950s and 1960s Delarue was among the earliest physicians to "promote the antismoking gospel," as Douglas Waugh, executive director of the Association of Canadian Medical Colleges (and himself a former "heavy smoker"), said. "He ... joined a small but growing minority of health care professionals who did not believe the conventional wisdom that smoking was a harmless way to relax." In doing so, he made himself something of an object of fun in the faculty. Robin Humphreys recalls of his own education, "While I was at medical school [MD in 1962], a senior thoracic surgeon was regarded as almost anomalous by my classmates, at least one-half of whom were smokers, because of his strident views on the evils of cigarette smoking."[101] Did Delarue vaunt his forward-looking advocacy? Waugh said, "In typical Canadian fashion, Norm Delarue was modest about his role in the antismoking movement."[102]

In the early 1950s a crisis loomed in thoracic surgery "in the face of a dramatic reduction in the surgery of tuberculosis and pulmonary sepsis." Yet the situation soon turned about, owing to "a relentless increase in the prevalence of lung cancer."[103] In the midst of this historic, tragic pivot from one killer to another, Stuart Vandewater arrived in 1952 on Ward B of the Toronto General Hospital, the chest ward headed by Kergin ("Fearless Fred," as the residents called him). Surgery for cancer was leaping into the foreground. Kergin and Delarue used new tomography techniques to locate the bronchogenic carcinomas, which they asked the head-and-neck surgeons to confirm by bronchoscopy; surgery was also required for the "parotid tumours, cancer of the tongue, pharynx and larynx requiring major block dissections, mandibulectomies and laryngectomies," that Harold Wookey and Robert Mustard undertook. "The surgery was lengthy and radical (eg lung cancer surgery usually included mediastinal [the area between the sternum and the spinal column] lymph node dissection). Surgery for oropharyngeal and tracheal cancer was radical, with great skin-flap rotations, and this was the early era of oesophagectomies. We used lots of blood, then dextran [a plasma volume expander] when that ran out."[104] These resembled almost battlefield operating conditions as the great smoking epidemic pushed cancerous patients into the Ward B service.

The Division of Thoracic Surgery dated from 1967, when the first resident was taken on. In 1968 Drucker, who had succeeded Kergin as university chairman, formally established the separate thoracic division. Because cardiovascular surgery was already functioning as a separate division, "this early, chance establishment of separate and autonomous divisions of thoracic and cardiovascular surgery created an exceptional opportunity for the development of thoracic surgery in Toronto."[105]

The circumstances of organizing the new division were these: Griff Pearson was Kergin's student. Pearson was born in Toronto in 1926, his father an optometrist. He attended the University of Toronto Schools, where he was inspired by his science teacher and became enthusiastic about botany and zoology. Pearson told the teacher he had decided to become a science teacher. "That's fine," said the teacher, "but I recommend you go into medicine."[106]

Pearson followed this advice and enrolled in medicine in 1944, graduating five years later. After a junior rotating internship at the General, Pearson worked for a general-practice surgeon in Port Colbourne, Ontario, then returned to train in surgery under Bigelow, where he spent 1951–2 as Bigelow's research fellow studying hypothermia in groundhogs. For Pearson, "[Bigelow's] laboratory was an introduction to the scientific method in practical terms."[107] After this scientific interlude, Pearson again went out into the world to make money, as a general practitioner in Wawa, Ontario. Three years later, in 1955, Pearson returned to surgical training. "I really liked the North Country," said Pearson later in an interview, "But Dr Fred Kergin approached me with a job offer … Because of [his administrative duties], he had to cut back on his thoracic surgery practice. He needed another thoracic surgeon who could also do general surgery. He offered me the job of chief resident for all of the surgical services and I took it."[108] Pearson wrote his fellowship in 1959.

In 1959–60 Pearson obtained a travelling fellowship and visited a number of centres in Europe and Britain, where he learned "there are many ways to skin the same cat ... Homespun myths are dispelled, and open-mindedness is enhanced. Bowel can be anastomosed [joined] with one layer of sutures as well as three." Pearson spent six months of his travels with Ronald Belsey, the well-known thoracic surgeon in Bristol, England, who had introduced a new technique for operating on the esophagus, for which organ "the prevalence of surgical mismanagement and misadventure was, to use one of Belsey's favorite adjectives, appalling."

After seven years of general surgery on Ward B, in 1967 Delarue and Pearson asked Kergin for permission to restrict their practices to thoracic surgery, "so we don't have to send residents to England for training."[109] (Pearson had apparently arranged with Belsey in Bristol a senior house officer slot reserved for U of T thoracic trainees.[110])

Essential to a division was an interhospital coordinating committee (IHCC), and Kergin, who was big on outreach, encouraged the development. It was actually under Drucker, the new chair, that the coordinating committee was set up in the 1966–7 session with Pearson as head.[111] In 1967 as well, the little thoracic group agreed on a group practice plan, among the few members of the department willing at the time to do so. Pearson said in an interview that the cardiovascular surgeons opposed the new division on the grounds that they didn't wish to surrender a part of their practice.[112] By 1979 the Royal College of Physicians and Surgeons had created a certificate of special competence in thoracic surgery.[113]

With the wind of the IHCC behind them, Pearson and team encouraged the development of thoracic programs at St Joseph's Hospital, Sunnybrook, St Michael's, and the East General Hospital: "Our IHCC was a meeting place for all these people." Kergin's student Robert Ginsberg went from the residency program to the Toronto Western Hospital. "He was ready to reach out to other institutions. This was the beginning of the Lung Cancer Study Group. This was an extension of Kergin's idea." The Lung Cancer Study Group arose in 1977 in response to a request for proposals from the National Institutes of Health to study adjuvants in the surgical treatment of primary lung cancer. Although a number of other centres participated, Toronto contributed, Pearson said, about half the total patients because Ginsberg "had developed such a good relationship with all of the other teaching hospitals." Harvard has numerous teaching hospitals as well, "but they don't work together," he explained. Cooperation among the Toronto hospitals "was an accomplishment of Ginsberg's."[114]

In these years mediastinoscopy – inserting an endoscope through an incision in the suprasternal notch permitting inspection and biopsy of the tissue of the mediastinum – was coming in. Eric Carlens in Stockholm had initiated it in 1959, and it became possible to stage lung cancers. Kergin, who "foresaw the need for endoscopy in general thoracic surgery," told Pearson to take responsibility for introducing it to Toronto. Until then, Pearson said, "Surgeons had done pneumonectomy for all cancers without staging them … The thinking was that you treat all cancers with radical surgery that takes out everything in the vicinity." So Pearson became the first in North America to describe the use of the mediastinoscope in staging; he began in 1960 and published on it in 1963.[115] "The open-and-close rate [discovery that the cancer was inoperable] had been as high as 30 to 40 percent," Pearson said. After the introduction of mediastinoscopy, the cancer turned out to be inoperable only in 7 percent. As Clarence Crafoord, the Swedish chest surgeon, pointed out at the meeting in 1965 at which Pearson gave his follow-up paper, "There are a great many of those [lung cancer] patients in whom we feel, when we open them, that once they are opened we should continue and do something more radical for them. I think in a great many of those patients we do them more harm for the rest of their lives than if we had not touched them."[116]

Thus Pearson's introduction in Canada and the United States in 1963 of a technique already commonly used in Europe was an important step forward. Two years later, in 1965, Pearson said of a series of sixty-seven cases seen at the Toronto General Hospital, "It appears reasonable to consider mediastinoscopy as the last step in the preoperative assessment of all patients with presumably operable bronchial carcinoma … In some patients it will be shown that resection is not technically possible, and useless thoracotomy will be avoided." In others, the appropriate treatment will appear clearer. "It is concluded that the operation is safe, relatively simple, and decidedly useful, both for the assessment of operability and resectability in bronchial carcinoma and for establishing a tissue diagnosis in certain intrathoracic lesions."[117]

Pearson also pioneered in trachea replacement. How many rings could be taken out? "We tried replacing trachea with intercostal muscle [muscle between the ribs]. That didn't work. Then someone suggested Marlex mesh. I started doing studies in dogs. In 1963 we had the first patient, a fifteen-year-old girl with a tumour of the trachea. We replaced it with Marlex mesh. She did extremely well." He continued, "By 1968 it appeared you could do much more than take out a few rings." They learned, Pearson said, they could remove half of the trachea.

Intubation, especially with positive pressure machines, caused stricture, or narrowing from scars, in the trachea in about 20 percent of the extubated patients, imperiling breathing. "The number of people who needed repairs was horrendous … Removing those subintubation strictures gave me a great deal of satisfaction. I originated subglottal resection with preservation of the recurrent laryngeal nerve [that innervates the larynx] that many Europeans call 'the Pearson operation.'"

Pearson innovated other procedures as well. "Esophageal surgery was a no-man's land," Pearson said. Assisted by Bernie Langer and Robert D. Henderson, Pearson set to lengthening the esophagus with procedures he had learned from Leigh Collis in Birmingham and Belsey in Bristol and then modified.[118] Pearson said in a 1971 paper, "The optimal correction of peptic stricture with acquired short esophagus should restore normal swallowing and prevent further gastro-esophageal reflux." In the discussion Pearson said to Belsey, who was present at the meeting, "I would like this audience to know that I am indebted to you, Mr. Belsey, for most of my approaches to the management of esophageal disease, which I learned as your resident."[119] This procedure also became known as the "Pearson operation."

Finally, together with Barrie Fairley, in 1958 Pearson became a co-founder of the Respiratory Failure Unit (see chapter 9). Pearson's stewardship of the division was in some ways more significant than his later tenure as head of the Department of Surgery, for it was as its chief that he brought the Division of Thoracic Surgery to world renown. Joel Cooper, who led the surgical team that later performed the world's first successful lung transplant, said of Pearson's role, "I am personally indebted to him for focusing our group in Toronto on the goal of successful human lung transplantation."[120] Pearson's many contributions to the specialty were acknowledged by the American Association for Thoracic Surgery in 2004 with its first Lifetime Achievement Award.[121]

*Lung Transplantation: The Jewel in the Crown*

The path to lung transplantation had not been an easy one. Pearson had begun experimenting on dogs as early as 1963. J.M. (Bill) Nelems, who came to the general surgery division in 1969, had led the first Toronto transplant attempt (and thirty-ninth worldwide) in 1977. Like all the others, it failed.[122] Said Joel Cooper of this experience, "We performed a right lung transplantation for a ventilator-dependent victim of burns." "The patient died in the third postoperative week" as the bronchial anastomosis dehisced (separation of the layers of a surgical wound). They did more research and discovered that the use of steroids was a mistake. They also discovered "that the new immunosuppressant, cyclosporine, caused no adverse effects on bronchial healing."[123]

Then Nelems moved to British Columbia, and Cooper, "with his limitless energy and persistence," entered the picture. Cooper, who graduated in medicine from Harvard in 1964, was lured away from the Massachusetts General Hospital to the general surgery division of the Toronto General Hospital in 1972. His arrival in Toronto meant for Pearson "five happy years" of collaboration in solving the lung transplantation problem. Cooper replaced Nelems as the "designated transplant guy" in the surgical team of eight. The arrival of cyclosporine changed the picture because they were able to suppress the attempts of the body's immune system to fight off the foreign transplanted lung.

On 24 August 1982, they tried again. They did first a right lung transplantation, then nineteen days later on the same patient a left lung transplantation. Pearson harvested the donor lungs; Cooper and G. Alexander Patterson inserted them. "But it was a team effort, absolutely, and ... remarkably well-coordinated," said Pearson.[124] The patient, James Franzen, a thirty-one-year-old nurseryman from Georgia with Paraquat poisoning, survived three months, ultimately to expire of a stroke after a trachea-innominate artery fistula.[125] The autopsy, however, confirmed that "had it not been for the Paraquat itself," the procedure would have succeeded.[126] "It had a huge impact," said Pearson. "We had people coming from all over the globe."[127]

The Paraquat case initiated a formal lung transplant program. In November 1983 Tom Hall, a fifty-eight-year-old Toronto man, was transplanted, in what would become hailed as the world's first successful single-lung transplant. Discharged from hospital six weeks after surgery, he returned to work six months later. "No previous lung transplant recipient had returned to a normal life," noted the hospital as they celebrated the triumph.[128] By 1987 they had five long-term survivors.[129]

In 1986 Joel Cooper conducted the world's first double-lung transplant after perfecting the technique by operating on puppies.[130] It was on Ann Harrison, who had emphysema; she survived another fifteen years, dying in 2001 of a brain aneurysm at fifty-six. Cooper, by now in St Louis, said on the occasion of her death, "Ann began a new era, one that has brought immense relief to emphysema patients. Having received this gift, she became a den mother for so many other patients." He shows a picture of her in every lecture that he gives on transplantation. "I still marvel when someone so close to death is returned to a vigorous life," he said.[131]

Alas, the "golden period" in the history of the thoracic division ended here, at least as far as Pearson was concerned, for Cooper went to Washington University in St Louis in 1988 and persuaded Patterson to come down three years later. Ginsberg, who had founded a second thoracic surgery division at Mount Sinai Hospital in 1984, departed for Memorial Sloan-Kettering in 1991, and Pearson retired in 1999.

But of course that was not the end of the story. In 1997 a team of lung transplant surgeons led by Thomas R.J. Todd, a 1969 Queen's University graduate, introduced in the treatment of emphysema patients who had received single-lung transplants the reduction of lung volume (in the other lung) as a way of improving overall lung function.[132] The concept caught on and started to become an alternative to lung transplants in chronic obstructive pulmonary disease (COPD). The value of volume reduction was demonstrated in a randomly controlled trial in several Canadian teaching hospitals, led by Roger Goldstein at the West Park Healthcare Centre in Toronto and including Todd and Shafique Keshavjee in the TGH Lung Volume Reduction Surgery Clinic.[133] (Joel Cooper had described the technique of lung volume reduction after his move to the Barnes Hospital in St Louis, the teaching hospital of Washington University.[134])

In the 1994–5 session Todd became chair of the university Division of Thoracic Surgery. Two years later, Shaf Keshavjee became director of the lung transplantation program. A decade later, he himself would head the division. (In 2010 he was also named surgeon-in-chief.)

Keshavjee, a surgeon-scientist, is one of Toronto's great success stories. He was twelve when he moved with his family from Kenya. He finished his medical studies at U of T in 1985 and was strongly attracted to surgery, though not necessarily to chest. In an epiphany, as a second-year medical student he was driving over a bridge on Mount Pleasant Avenue and heard a radio news bulletin saying that Joel Cooper and his team had just achieved the world's first successful lung transplant at the Toronto General Hospital.

"I thought, wow, that's cool," he later told a medical journalist. He trained in surgery under the giants who strode the surgical wards of TGH in the 1980s. But then the Toronto lung transplant program came virtually to an end as the giants mostly left for lucrative American posts. It was Keshavjee who revived it. "Despite offers to go to the U.S., he stayed, hoping to rebuild Toronto's reputation."[135]

The vulnerable point in lung transplantation was waiting for a donor lung; in the meantime the pulmonary hypertension would be worsening, threatening a fatal outcome. To forestall this eventuality, Novalung, a German firm, invented a miniature bypass machine, about the size of a CD case, sitting outside the body attached to blood vessels in the leg, with one end plugged into the venous return, the other to the arterial outflow, delivering oxygenated blood to the body. (The artificial lung contained a membrane that oxygenated the blood.) On 2 December 2006, a twenty-member team at TGH led by Keshavjee attached a Novalung to a patient – a twenty-one-year-old mother of fraternal twins and a baby of fourteen months – for the first time in North America. Said Keshavjee later, "This young woman came to TGH and was found to be so ill that she was admitted to our intensive care unit on the same day. She needed to have a lung transplant urgently and the wait for donor lungs can be between three to five months." In fact, she needed wait only a day. After the operation she said, "I'm so glad to be alive and I'm so glad that I can go home to my children."[136]

Meanwhile Keshavjee and his team continue working on the problem of making more lungs available for transplant. The Toronto XVIVO Lung Perfusion System, which maintains and restores harvested lungs for several hours, shows promise in early trials and could potentially double the number of transplants at TGH.[137] The University of Toronto remains the world leader in lung transplantation. Most cases are best outcomes. For the Department of Surgery, this is a great point of pride.

## Division of Plastic Surgery

The history of modern plastic surgery is intimately related in general to the two recent major wars ... and in particular to the advent of explosive bullets and other missiles.

William K. Lindsay, 1989

During the First World War, the British Army established a Jaw and Face Unit in Sidcup, Kent, to deal with the consequences of high explosives. Among the

Commonwealth surgeons invited to participate was E. Fulton Risdon, of St Thomas, Ontario, who had earned a previous dental degree in 1907 and was a medical graduate of the University of Toronto in 1914. On his return from England, Risdon became the first plastic surgeon in Toronto and, according to William Lindsay, in Canada as well. He was known for fixating the ramus of the mandible with "the Risdon wire." Risdon had an appointment at the Toronto Western Hospital and an especially ample practice.

Many Toronto surgeons had an interest in reparative operations, and Harold Wookey's reconstruction of the neck after cancer surgery,[138] Arthur LeMesurier's repair of cleft palate,[139] and J. Harold Couch's operations on the injured and infected hand[140] could qualify them as plastic surgeons even though they were members of other divisions.

The history of plastic surgery in the faculty goes back to a special clinic set up in the session 1932–3 at TGH under Stuart Douglas Gordon.[141] Gordon, born in Fernie, British Columbia in 1902, was an honours matriculant at Markham High School in Ontario, subsequently graduating in medicine at U of T in 1926. "Impersonates the ladies – on Daffydil night," said *Torontonensis*, adding somewhat delphically, "His pugilistic career was short and thrilling."[142] Gordon trained in surgery and was licensed in Ontario in 1929. Gallie, seeing the need for a surgical specialty in plastics, sent Gordon and Alfred Farmer to England for further training. Upon their return in 1932, Gordon practiced plastic surgery at Toronto General Hospital and Farmer at the Hospital for Sick Children. Gordon led the special military Unit for Plastic and Reconstructive Surgery established in 1941 at Basingstoke in Hampshire. According to William K. Lindsay, author of a history of plastic surgery in Toronto, "In 1942 the Royal Canadian Air Force established the Plastic Surgery and Jaw Injury Unit at East Grinstead, Sussex, attached to the Queen Victoria Hospital, where modern plastic surgery is said to have begun."[143] It was headed by A. Ross Tilley, who later established a burn unit at Sunnybrook Hospital. "Many patients, including Battle of Britain casualties, received major reconstructive surgery at these two Canadian units." In 1943 Farmer, as consultant to the Royal Canadian Air Force, recommended the formation of a Plastic Surgery Unit at the Toronto Veterans Affairs Hospital at Sunnybrook.

Gordon was recalled in 1944 to organize a similar unit for veterans at Christie Street.[144] He became a professor of surgery at the University of Toronto with a specialty in plastic surgery and in 1958 established the division at the General and at Sunnybrook. According to Lindsay, the training program in plastic surgery after the war was shared with McGill University, and residents spent a year in each city. Soon, however, each centre developed its own program.

At the children's hospital, the focus of plastic surgery has been the face, lip, and palate. Plastic surgery began as a discipline of its own at HSC in 1954 when Lindsay established a Cleft Lip and Palate Research and Treatment Centre. Lindsay, who grew up in Vancouver, "spent two years at UBC, then came east to civilization and bought himself a lab coat," as the yearbook noted in 1945 when he graduated in medicine from U of T.[145] As a pediatric plastic surgeon, he chaired the medical advisory committee of the Ontario Society for Crippled Children in the days when so many were crippled by polio.

Sometime after 1956, Egil Harvold joined the team of cleft palate surgeons. Harvold, then forty-one, an orthodontist of Norwegian origin appointed in the Faculty of Dentistry, is seen as one of the founders of surgery for cleft lip and palate. After training in Norway, he was professor of orthodontics at Michigan State University, then came to the Faculty of Dentistry in Toronto in 1956, consulting as well to the children's hospital. In the 1988–9 session, Ronald Zuker was appointed medical director of the Cleft Lip and Palate Program.[146] (More on Zuker will be discussed later.)

Out of this initiative grew the division's craniofacial program, begun in 1972 when Lindsay appointed Ian Munro to staff. Munro brought with him the radical new approaches of French cleft lip and palate surgery, especially those of Paul Tessier in Paris. In 1986 Jeffrey Posnick succeeded Munro, who went to Dallas; Posnick made the craniofacial program autonomous from the cleft lip and palate work. In 1987 Posnick began the craniofacial program registry. John Phillips, a student of Munro's, became medical director of the program in 1992. Both the cleft lip and palate program and the craniofacial program are coordinated through the Facial Treatment and Research Centre.

In 1965 Lindsay succeeded Gordon as chair of the IHCC for plastic surgery. Under his leadership, a generation of plastic surgeons grew up who established the specialty at hospitals across Canada.

The stage was now set for the arrival of one of the major international figures in the Toronto story. In 1978 Ralph Manktelow became hospital division chair of plastic surgery at the General, succeeding Donald C. Robertson, who had headed the division for many years. (Only in the 1985–6 session did Manktelow succeed Lindsay as chair of the university division.) The division was now being led by the person who, in Pearson's terms, "developed a team capability for microvascular surgery which is unequalled anywhere else in the country."[147] Manktelow, a U of T graduate in 1964 (and world champion rower), pioneered muscle transplantation. In 1976 his work on finger flexion – published in 1978[148] – was said to be the first muscle transplant in North America. In 1979 he was appointed head of plastic surgery at the General and for many years led the university division.

The plastic surgeons at the General did little cosmetic surgery but concentrated on burn management, at least until 1984 when the Wellesley Hospital became the home of a regional burn unit, and Walter J. Peters left the General to run it.

In early January 1984 Manktelow made history in Canada by carrying out the first successful "living joint transplant," removing the second joint from one of the toes of nineteen-year-old Kingston resident Steve Bujacz and transplanting it to his index finger. The operation had already been done successfully elsewhere, but this was the first Canadian essay of a procedure that would dramatically affect patients with traumatic joint injuries or those with disabling joint diseases unsuited for standard artificial joints. The microvascular surgery had been conducted with the aid of Canada's first ceiling, track-mounted microscope, donated by the McLaughlin Foundation.[149]

One of the big stories in plastic surgery in Toronto involved a collaboration between Ronald Zuker and Manktelow. Zuker, a U of T graduate who obtained his fellowship in 1976, had travelled to Japan on a McLaughlin Fellowship to study techniques of microsurgery with investigators already practised in transplanting tissues from one part of the body to another. In 1978 he returned to Toronto, joining the Division of Plastic Surgery of the children's hospital. He became head of the division the following year. When Manktelow moved to TGH in 1979, the way was clear for an innovative collaboration with Zuker in microvascular surgery in what became known as the Facial Paralysis Program, a collaboration between HSC, for operations on children to restore the mobility of their faces, and TGH, for similar operations on adults. Children with Möbius Syndrome are unable to smile, a terrible stigmatizing condition that isolates them from the happiness of childhood. In the 1982–3 session Zuker and Manktelow "performed the first successful muscle transplantation to correct facial paralysis in Canada."[150]

By 1989 Zuker and Manktelow had achieved "a smile for the Möbius Syndrome Patient," successfully transplanting facial muscles in seven patients to achieve "facial animation."[151] They had advanced to various paralyses involving the entire face. "Because more meaning is communicated by facial expression than by speech itself," they wrote, "it is the loss of facial expression that is most disturbing to the facial paralysis patient. This expressive communication comes from the forehead, eyebrows, eyes, mouth and cheeks."[152] At that point Manktelow and Zuker had just begun to reconstruct the lower face, moving later to the upper face.

Zuker and Manktelow innovated in other kinds of operations. Zuker, for example, performed advanced surgery on children with disfiguring vascular malformations.[153]

Other members of the division made notable scientific contributions. Building on the work at HSC in the 1960s of Hugh Thomson, who used a new high-speed pigment injection machine, in 1973 Robert A. Newton, a 1958 McGill graduate who had trained in plastic surgery at the General, described an operation for removing a hemangioma called port wine stain with a kind of surgical tattooing[154] – this problem was later managed with an argon laser. In 1988 Susan MacKinnon, who had trained in plastic surgery at U of T, participated with Alan Hudson in the world's first nerve transplant. She had trained in surgery at Queen's, spending a fellowship year in plastics at U of T in 1980, and another fellowship in neurosurgery in 1981, before departing to the United States. She returned to Toronto in 1988 for the historic procedure.[155]

By 1992 the division was filled with collaborative enterprises: a head-and-neck program at TGH with otolaryngology and general surgery, a hand program with orthopedic surgery, and an adult/child program in maxillo-craniofacial surgery with HSC and Sunnybrook.[156] In 1993 the hand program, now shifted to the Toronto Western Hospital, officially opened under Vaughan Bowen.[157]

Peter Neligan became chair of the TGH division and the university division in 1996, and by the time Dimitri Anastakis succeeded him in 2006, it was the largest division of plastic surgery in North America.[158]

## Division of Urology

As the Canadian population continues to age, demand has increased on those services that are provided by the Division of Urology.[159]

Urology began in Toronto in 1914 with the establishment at the General of a "Genito-Urinary Clinic," directed by W. Warner Jones.[160] Jones, a U of T medical graduate in 1896, had trained at St Peters Hospital for Stone in London, becoming a Fellow of the Royal College of Surgeons before the First World War. Jones established the "subdepartment of urology" at TGH in 1919 and headed it until 1933, when Robin Pearse succeeded him, at which time urology was referred to as a hospital "department." At Jones's retirement in 1938, Dean Gallie lauded its growth "from a very small beginning to a great and most important department." By the end of the Second World War the urology subdepartment had fifty beds and a large outpatient service.[161]

Robin Pearse, born in 1886, joined the subdepartment at TGH in 1919; he had studied medicine in England (MB in 1909) and trained in surgery there, becoming licensed in Ontario in 1914. He served as the inaugural president of the Canadian Urology Association, founded in 1945. On Pearse's watch, the division participated in several important therapeutic innovations, introducing heparin in the prevention of thrombosis in the 1933–4 session[162] and – of capital importance – being the entry portal into Toronto of the new sulfa drugs of the mid-1930s. In 1938 David Mitchell published a preliminary report on sulfanilamide "as a urinary antiseptic."[163] Then, working with Philip Greey in the Department of Bacteriology and Gordon R. Hall and Colin C. Lucas of the Department of Medical Research, Mitchell studied sulfanilamide in detail in the treatment of urinary tract infections, publishing on the work in 1939; this was the "miracle drug's" world introduction into urology.[164] Similarly, research that Mitchell published in 1939 together with pediatrician Pearl Summerfeldt, a 1923 U of T graduate, represented the introduction of sulfanilamide in the treatment of urinary tract infections in children.[165]

From 1945–6 until 1948–9 James C. McClelland succeeded Pearse as head of the Division of Urology; then in 1949 David Mitchell began his leadership of the division, which would endure until 1966. Mitchell grew up in Oshawa, Ontario, and earned his medical degree at U of T in 1927. He trained in surgery in England, taking the fellowship of the Royal College of Physicians and Surgeons of Canada and the Royal College of Surgeons of England. Under Mitchell, urology in Toronto witnessed a number of landmarks including the organization of a dialysis service in 1958 and the beginning of peritoneal dialysis in 1962 and of chronic hemodialysis in 1965.[166] In 1965 urologic surgeon William K. Kerr, who was cross-appointed to the Banting Institute and the Ontario Cancer Institute, established a relationship between smoking and bladder cancer, a finding that made it into *Time* magazine: "Men who were using cigarettes excreted in their urine abnormally large amounts of an ortho-aminophenol known to be capable of causing cancer. Going off cigarettes reversed the effect. The researchers' conclusion: inhaling smoke into the lungs, a practice that would seem to have no bearing on cancer of the bladder, is directly related to that disease through the complex chemistry of human metabolism."[167]

In these years, the urology divisions were integrated into the various hospitals to form an effective teaching unit. The process began in the 1948–9 session with joint monthly rounds among members of the three teaching hospitals: the General, St Michael's, and the Western.[168]

In 1966 Charles J. Robson succeeded Mitchell as head of the hospital division at the General and in 1971 also became chair of the university division. British-born but educated in Toronto at Upper Canada College, he graduated from the University of Toronto in the April class of 1942. The yearbook noted of his student career, "'Church' came to Medicine via UCC and a mining camp at Timmins. Shows a keen interest in his studies as well as being a party boy. Was Fraternity President in 1939, and director of entertainment for his class. "Interested in obstetrics, motorboats and skiing."[169] Despite this auspicious beginning, Robson nonetheless joined the surgical staff of TGH in 1949. In 1956–7 he founded the Division of Urology at the Hospital for Sick Children,[170] then between 1966 and 1982 led the urology division at the General. He was, as his biographer says, "particularly noted for his work associated with spinal cord injuries, fractures of the pelvis, paediatric urology, and radical surgery for cancer of the kidney and the prostate."[171] Kidney transplantation began in 1967 during Robson's chairmanship, and the establishment of the Metro Organ Retrieval and Exchange program, chaired by Michael A. Robinette of TGH, doubled the number of kidney transplants.[172]

In 1982 Andrew Bruce continued the Anglophiliac orientation of the Division of Urology, succeeding Robson as chair. Bruce graduated with an MB from the University of Aberdeen in 1947; his Canadian career included heading the urology division at Queen's and at McGill; he was recruited to Toronto in 1982 as professor of urology and head of the university and TGH divisions. While at Queen's, Bruce was senior (last mentioned) author in 1976 of the first report on the use of the Bacillus Calmette-Guérin (BCG) vaccine in superficial bladder cancer.[173] Shortly after arriving in Toronto, Bruce mandated the opening of a new Urology Research Laboratory, said to be "one of the few such centres of its kind in North America."[174] Bruce brought in "an established, active and very productive research programme in the fields of prostatic cancer and urinary tract infection," as well as two PhD investigators.[175] A big event in the life of the division occurred in the 1987–8 session with the opening of the E.C. Bovey Lithotripter Unit at the Wellesley Hospital, directed by Michael Jewett, offering quick relief to the agonies of kidney stones.[176]

By the end of the 1980s, renal transplants had become a major priority of the division, and more than sixty were performed at TGH in the 1988–9 session, in close cooperation with the division of nephrology and the Multiple Organ Transplant program.[177] (The work of Vincent Colapinto at St Michael's Hospital on dialysis and transplantation is discussed in chapter 25.)

In the 1990s and after, under Michael Jewett and Sender Herschorn as division chairs, the urology division moved strongly, along with the rest of the Department of Surgery, towards basic science. They hired Marc Mittelman, a microbiologist recruited from the University of Tennessee, who would work alongside the division's twenty-three surgeons as their first PhD research scientist; he simultaneously directed the newly established Centre of Infection and Biomaterials research laboratory at The Toronto Hospital.[178]

Joao L. Pippi Salle, in the Division of Urology at the Hospital for Sick Children, came to Toronto from McGill in 2003. It was at McGill that he perfected a major contribution to pediatric surgery, lengthening the urethra with an anterior bladder wall flap as a remedy for neurogenic incontinence or exstrophy (the turning inside out of the bladder), which became known as the "Pippi Salle procedure."[179] (He devised it while a staff surgeon at the Hospital de Clinicas de Porto Alegre in Brazil, where, as a pediatric surgeon, he was completing research for a PhD.) He brought several members of the original team with him to the children's hospital in Toronto, a marker of the opening of Toronto urology from the United Kingdom to the wide world.

## Division of Anatomy

Before the 1999–2000 session, the division was the Department of Anatomy (see chapter 15). On July 1, 1999, the Department of Anatomy became a division of the Department of Surgery with Michael Wiley as chair and seven faculty members brought along. Histologist David Cormack, who had authored the ninth edition of *Ham's Histology*, left the department in retirement. Anne Agur and Ming Lee supervised the release of the latest edition of *Grant's Atlas*. Freed by the new problem-based curriculum from the need to teach gross anatomy to generations of medical students, the division started experimenting with multimedia forms of supporting anatomy education.[180] In one multimedia stroke the microscope was abolished from the histology education of medical undergraduates. From 2004–5 on, the Internet would deliver "high resolution annotated scans of microscope sections … allowing a student's computer to emulate a microscope. This approach will eliminate the classic histology 'microscope lab' from the medical timetable," said Wiley.[181] The traditionalist is dumbfounded:

the "mike," for generations of medical students an icon of learning, gone! The division had a scientific triumph in 1994, when Cindi Morshead and co-workers discovered the existence of neural stem cells (on her work, see also chapter 15).[182]

## Multi-Organ Transplant Unit

The program began, as this book has shown, with kidney transplantation in the late 1960s. In 1976 the Multiple Organ Retrieval and Exchange program (MORE program) was initiated to ensure a supply of organs for transplantation. After Langer became chair of the Department of Surgery in 1982, he arranged for a planning retreat to deal with the duplication of transplant and other programs which were starting up all over the city: surgeons were trying to get a liver transplant program going at TGH (it began in 1985); there were cardiac programs starting at the Western, the General, and St Michael's. Said Langer in an interview, "There were kidney programs at the Western, St. Michael's, the General, Sunnybrook, and I think the Wellesley. There was a lung transplant program that they were just gearing up at the General. So there was this competitive work going on all over the place."[183] The department concluded that transplantation should be consolidated in fewer academic units.

Recommendations in 1985 proposed that a multi-organ transplantation unit be developed within the Faculty of Medicine and four of its teaching hospitals – the General, the Western, St Michael's, and the children's hospital. Said a medical journalist in 1985, "According to Joel Cooper … in addition to having considerable dramatic appeal to a surgeon, organ transplantation is also of great interest to the pathologist, immunologist, histologist and hematologist … This type of team effort generates an aura of excitement in academic circles."

As of the fall of 1985, Tirone David at TWH had done "three successful cardiac transplants." Cooper had done two lungs, as well as two combined heart/ lung transplants. Cooper said in 1985, "Transplants can be broken into two groups: those that are more or less routinely established – heart, kidney, liver, cornea and bone – and those that are still experimental in nature –lung, heart/ lung, pancreas and small bowel."[184]

The liver transplant program became the core of the new multi-organ scheme, with Langer as interim head. The faculty Multi-Organ Transplantation Programme (MOTP) executive committee met for the first time in July 1989 and agreed on funding (the faculty would pay for the immunologists in the program, the Departments of Medicine and Surgery and the hospitals for the rest[185]). After an extensive search, in 1993 Gary Levy, who was already running the liver transplant unit, succeeded Langer as the first appointed head of both the TGH and the university programs. Langer said, "We pushed to turn it into the multi-organ transplant program because we wanted to get the scientists into the same laboratory environment, and we wanted to get a nursing unit at the General Hospital in which all the transplant patients would be together.

Because the problems of immunosuppression, drug use and infection … are so similar, we felt that a group that were transplant specialists would do better than separate groups that were primarily organ specialists." But it would be the cardiac surgeons who came in and did heart transplants, the thoracic surgeons who performed the lung transplants, and so forth. (Kidney transplants were done by both urologists and general surgeons.) The common feature was the ward and the nursing staff. Langer said, "We've got something better than Franny [Francis Moore, the chair of surgery at the Peter Bent Brigham Hospital in Boston] ever had. Franny had a surgical lab, and in another building were the medical labs, and in another building there were the molecular biology labs, and they didn't talk much. We have a transplantation lab, where we have molecular biologists, and infectious disease specialists, pathologists and surgeons, and internists all working together."[186]

The path to the Multi-Organ Transplantation Unit involved a number of steps. In 1972 a tissue typing lab was organized by Judy Wade. Said Wade in 1985, "There is a proven clinical need. With so many trained, talented people in surgery and basic research, it will take very little to make our program world class."[187] In 1986 Imperial Oil made a substantial material donation to support the liver transplant program – for adults at TGH, for children at HSC.[188]

By 1990 the city's transplant programs were consolidated at the Toronto Hospital site, together with a combined nursing unit. Liver and lung transplants began increasing rapidly. Said Langer, "This site consolidation brings together a wide range of experts from the various organ transplant programmes, and the unique multi-organ transplant group thus created will form a world-class organization."[189] In 1989 the Faculty Council decided to make the MOTP a "priority program," one of the "priority extra-departmental units" (EDUs) of the faculty.

In May 1990 the Multi-Organ Transplant Unit opened, under Langer. Mary Wolfe received the first transplant on 4 May, a multi-organ procedure. She received "a new liver and a new lung in the same-eight hour operation." Mrs Wolfe had been suffering from multi-organ failure because of pulmonary hypertension. Said a medical journalist, "These diseases left Mrs Wolfe feeling fatigued, nauseated, bloated and short of breath. In order to breathe, she needed a constant supply of oxygen pumped through a tube in her nose … The day before her transplant, Mrs Wolfe's condition was so poor she was hospitalized in her hometown of Orangeville, Ont." At 2:00 the next morning her husband received a call "saying that organs were available and Mary should come to The Toronto Hospital as soon as possible for a transplant."

Said Mrs Wolfe later, "I always said, if I got to the table, everything would be OK. I was only worried that the call wouldn't come." Three weeks after the successful operation, she was home. "My friends just can't believe it," she said. "They all call me a 'Miracle Lady.'"[190]

In the unit, said a TTH spokesperson, "Cardiac and renal transplantation specialists from The Western have joined with renal, liver and lung transplantation specialists from The General to produce a new team." There are as well six transplant coordinators: "Three renal coordinators and one each handling heart, lung and liver transplants ... Although these coordinators have been part of the transplant programs for many years, they did not work as a team until the creation of the Multi Organ Unit." There was also a central organ transplant office. Paul Greig was clinical director of liver transplantation. Gary Levy, director of gastrointestinal transplantation, said, "I see a day when the people who are involved in this area will be called transplantologists."[191]

By 1997 there were four hospitals participating in solid organ transplantation: The Toronto Hospital for heart, lung, liver, kidney, kidney/pancreas, and cornea; St Michael's Hospital for kidney; HSC for heart, lung, liver, kidney, and bone marrow; and Mount Sinai Hospital as the bone bank. In 1996 there had been around 90 adult and child liver transplants, 35 lung transplants, 180 kidney transplants, 10 kidney/pancreas transplants, and around 600 bone grafts. Kidney/pancreas was a new program just added in 1995 by Mark Cattral.[192] (In 1999 Atul Humar was recruited to the University of Toronto to begin a program in transplantation infectious disease, in which he was joined by his wife Deepali Kumar.) The Hospital for Sick Children also had its own transplantation program, known as the Paediatric Academic Multi-Organ Transplant Program (PAMOT). In 2002 Levy headed an international study showing that a new type of monitoring of cyclosporine improved results in liver transplants.[193] By 2005, the Multi-Organ Transplant Program employed an academic staff of thirty-eight, in addition to forty-two fellows.[194]

When the MOTP was assessed in 1997, Dean Aberman praised Levy as a "charismatic" leader and gave the deanery's ultimate accolade: "MOTP members consider themselves to be under the University umbrella, rather than that of their individual hospitals."[195] A 2002 review recommended the formation of a "Transplant Institute that is recognized internationally as 'top shelf' across the board."[196] In 2007 an external review of the transplant program seconded the recommendation that it be elevated to institute status within the faculty, and the following year the Faculty Council approved a University of Toronto Transplantation Institute, to be headed by Levy.[197]

In addition to its great humanitarian contribution, the history of the multi-organ transplantation program at the University of Toronto marked the intimate collaboration between the basic and the clinical sciences: immunology was essential to transplantation, suppressing the body's immune response and matching the donors. And pathology played a fundamental role in assessing organ quality. It was, in a sense, Dean Gallie's dream of surgery based on medical science come true.

# 8 Medicine

This department, because of its talents and sheer size, dominates the Faculty at all levels.[1]

Faculty Self-Study, 1983

## Professors of Medicine and Heads of the Department of Medicine

Duncan A. Graham, 1919–47
Ray F. Farquharson, 1947–60
Keith J.R. Wightman, 1960–70
Charles H. Hollenberg, 1970–81
Gerard N. Burrow, 1981–8
Kenneth Shumak (acting chair), 1988–9
Arnold Aberman, 1989–92
Eliot Phillipson, 1992–2004
Wendy Levinson, 2004–present

Under the leadership of Duncan Graham, the Department of Medicine rested for many years on the laurels of insulin, which the department had introduced clinically. As people looked back on the pre-Hollenberg years before 1970, there was a rather reluctant acknowledgment that all was not as it might have been.

Yet there were a few research stirrings, perhaps not in heft comparable to the department's sheer size, yet advances nonetheless. And in the world of science they were reminders that the colleagues were still players.

In the 1938–9 session the new sulfa drugs – the first "wonder drugs" – arrived in the department: Graham had requested a supply of sulfapyridine (M&B 693, or "Dagenan") from the firm May and Baker. The department was thus "first in Canada to use this drug in the treatment of pneumonia." They confirmed the finding that "the drug is effective for all types of pneumococcal pneumonia" and published the work in the *Canadian Medical Association Journal* in 1939.[2]

What difference did Dagenan make? Surgeon Frederick Dewar recalled, "Prior to its use, Ward I used to be lined with dozens and dozens of oxygen tents in which dozens of patients were lying with high, dreadful fevers, and many of them dying, because the mortality for pneumonia in those days was extremely high every winter. When we had Dagenan, we had the problem of getting the pills down the patients who never wanted to take them." So the doctors would grind the pills up and give them through a nasogastric tube. "Very soon you very seldom saw an oxygen tent on the ward any more; there were not orderlies carrying buckets of ice all night and all day keeping these tents cool, or people trundling around great tanks of oxygen. It changed the whole picture of the treatment of pneumonia and lung infections."[3]

The arrival of effective medications, including not just the antibiotics but a cornucopia of other agents, transformed the nature of internal medicine and of medical practice in general. Cardiologist John Oille later said, "Pneumonia, the kind one used to see 20 years ago, is almost a curiosity. The danger of a fatal epidemic of influenza such as occurred in 1918 and 1919 has, I think, completely passed. The deaths in the 'flu' epidemic were almost all due to pneumonia caused by secondary invaders, common organisms such as streptococci, pneumococci, staphylococci, etc, all of which respond more or less easily to the modern antibiotics."[4]

Being able to heal infections with antibiotics, and meliorate many other conditions with the new pharmacopoeia, meant that medicine began to deliver the same level of therapeutic benefits as surgery. Much after the initiation of these events, "Kager" Wightman, head of medicine in the 1960s, wrote, "It has been difficult to overcome the traditional view that a hospital is primarily a surgeon's workshop, and to establish the fact that developments in the past thirty years have brought to the physician [internist] powers of definitive therapy which now match his long recognized diagnostic and prognostic skill. The laboratory and the clinical investigation unit are the physician's workshops, and more and more of his patients require study and treatment in hospital as a result of the increasing complexity of medical therapy and investigation."[5] So the new therapeutics ushered in a new era in internal medicine.

### A Page Is Turned

In 1947, Duncan Graham retired from the Eaton Chair. At the medical convocation that year Lady Eaton "sat upon the platform," as the *Toronto Daily Star* recorded the event, "with university officials and prominent medical men and smiled at each graduate as he or she came forward to receive the degree of doctor of medicine." Eight graduates of the class of 1897 were also on hand to have the degree "doctor of medicine" conferred upon them (because, of course, in the early years the initial degree they received was an MB, or bachelor of medicine, rather than the MD). Yet despite the magnificence of the commencement ceremony in 1947, the underlying story for the Department of Medicine was not a happy one. Under Graham, the department had stagnated. The rather brutal judgment of Barney Berris, later head of medicine at Mount Sinai, was that, "During his tenure, the development of the department remained in a static state and did not keep up with the advances in diagnosis, treatment and research that were taking place in medicine. The University of Toronto Department of Medicine was not recognized either nationally or internationally as an important teaching or research centre. There were only two full-time staff doctors in the department: Dr. Farquharson and Dr. Wightman. They were excellent clinicians and teachers, but were given no time or support to do research."[6]

With the advent of Ray Farquharson as chair of medicine in 1947, a page was turned. Berris continued, "Dr Farquharson was the first chair to understand the need for modernization. He began to appoint full-time staff who had completed all their training in their subspecialties and in research, and he supported those doing research with funds and research space." Berris said that Farquharson also ended the exclusion of Jews from the university's Department of Medicine.[7] Farquharson thus emerges as a seminal figure in the history of the faculty.

*Ray Farquharson*

Farquharson, the son of a Presbyterian minister, was the epitome of his generation of academic physicians with their roots in the farms and small towns of Ontario. Born at the "Manse" in Claude, Ontario, in 1897, he attended school in Durham and Harbord Collegiate in Toronto, entering medicine at U of T in 1917. The yearbook noted, "Believes in hard work and short hours. Ancestry 'Scotch' but he has never tasted it."[8] Farquharson served briefly at the end of the war as a gunner in the Canadian Field Artillery, then graduated in 1922. He thereupon trained in the Department of Medicine, finishing as a resident fellow in 1927 in time to spend a year at Harvard working with Joseph Aub at the Massachusetts General Hospital, "on the famed Ward 4" (as Jack Laidlaw, author of a biography of Farquharson, points out), "the first clinical investigation unit in North America."[9]

In 1928 Farquharson, or "Farky" as he was known, became a "demonstrator" in the Department of Medicine, becoming head of therapeutics in 1934 (remaining there until serving as a wing commander during the Second World War). In 1945 the Department of Veterans Affairs made a large commitment to upgrading Christie Street Hospital, a dilapidated veterans hospital founded in 1920; it also created Sunnybrook, as the second veterans facility. Christie Street received two rather remarkable appointments: Joseph ("Mac") MacFarlane as head of surgery and Farquharson as head of medicine. Neither stayed long. In

1946 MacFarlane became dean of medicine and in 1947 Farquharson became the Eaton Professor of Medicine. His colleague Waring Gerald Cosbie remarked of Ray Farquharson in these years, "He had soon established himself as an idealistic teacher and open-minded clinician through the readiness with which he discussed problems of diagnosis and treatment with interns, residents and Fellows of the department. From him they learned the primary value of clinical observation."[10]

If Duncan Graham achieved scientific prominence for anything, it was because of collaborating with his student Ray Farquharson. In 1930 the two clinicians offered convincing evidence for the efficacy of liver treatment for subacute combined degeneration (SCD) of the spinal cord, the neurological condition associated with pernicious anemia. The active principle of liver extract, vitamin B12, was not yet discovered at that point.[11] B12 treatment later became the standard remedy for SCD. (In 1933 Farquharson, together with Earle W. McHenry from the Connaught Labs and a researcher at the Montreal General Hospital, confirmed that liver extract in the treatment of pernicious anemia, first described by George Minot and William Murphy in Boston in 1926,[12] could be given in an intramuscular extract that McHenry had developed to increase the potency of the treatment.[13]) Don Cowan remarks of this research, "It is clear that the Department of Medicine in Toronto was up to date therapeutically and were quick to adopt the knowledge and therapy put forth by Minot and Murphy in the treatment of pernicious anemia. Although the original work wasn't done here, Toronto was quick to join and add to the leading edge, and Farky played a role. It must have been a very exciting time, to see patients with a previously fatal disease – pernicious indeed – make such a dramatic recovery."[14]

In these years Farquharson also founded an outpatient hematology clinic in the old Mulock Building of TGH, with its beautiful ceramic ceiling. Says Cowan, "It was known as the PA [Pernicious Anemia] Clinic because of the large number of patients with that disorder who came through. It spanned the days from when PA was treated by having the patient eat raw liver, through the days of liver injections, and, finally, Vitamin B12 injections. It was staffed by some of the greats of Toronto medicine, such as Farky, Kager Wightman, Arthur Squires, and neurologist Herbert Hyland, who was likely there because of the disabling neurological manifestations of PA."[15]

In 1931 Farquharson and Duncan Graham sparked North American interest in Simmonds' disease (pituitary cachexia) with a study of three cases, characterized by shrunken hearts, pallid waxy skin, emaciation, and loss of body hair.[16] Morris Simmonds of Hamburg first described the atrophy of the anterior lobe of the pituitary gland in 1914, and the pituitary collapse named after him surfaced in the 1940s and 1950s in discussions of anorexia nervosa: clinicians simply could not believe that young women were voluntarily refusing food and thought they must have Simmonds' disease. Intrigued by the similarities between Simmonds' disease and anorexia nervosa, in 1938 Farquharson and

Herbert Hyland definitively described anorexia nervosa as a mental disorder in its own right and not a disorder of an endocrine gland.[17] The Farquharson work differentiating anorexia from Simmonds' disease was a landmark and typical of Farquharson's relentlessly curious approach to clinical investigation. In 1966 they published a classic follow-up study.[18] Nell Farquharson, Ray Farquharson's daughter, said, "The patients stopped being anorexics because they didn't want to hurt his feelings."[19]

But Farquharson's impact on medicine went beyond psychiatry. Laidlaw said, "He was responsible for the dawn of the full-time clinical investigator in his department and medical school."

Ray Farquharson appears again later in the story, but it's worth noting here that, in Laidlaw's words, "He was responsible for one of the first research wards in Canada, later called the Farquharson Investigation Unit," of which Laidlaw in 1956 was the first director. As a member of the Canadian Society for Clinical Investigation, Farquharson penned in 1958 a report (the "Farquharson Report") that advocated establishing in Canada a research council for medicine, resulting in the formation in 1960 of the Medical Research Council– which Farquharson chaired – the first infusion of federal funds into Canadian medical research.

Veterans of the faculty comment on Farky's "remarkable physical presence." Said Jack Laidlaw, "He had broad shoulders and a strong voice and a wisp of a smile on his face."[20] There was a gentlemanly mannerliness and absence of self-importance about Farquharson that, if not somehow very Canadian, were characteristic of educated men and women in those years. An anecdote from Bill Goldberg, a resident of Farquharson's and later physician-in-chief at St Joseph's Hospital in Hamilton, states, "I remember when Patient A, one of Canada's most distinguished medical scientists, was in hospital with a myocardial infarction, and I was called to his room because he had become impacted and was in great stress. He was very disturbed about this as was his wife … I phoned Dr. Farquharson because of all the concern and he stated that he had not really paid attention to the whole problem of Patient A, he had been so concerned with his blood and his heart that he forgot to provide him with an adequate laxative. I told him that I would of course disimpact him [manually]; however, Dr. Farquharson said since he made the error, he would come down and do this rather unpleasant job. It indicated to me the greatness of Dr. Farquharson on this small point that he would come all the way down on a weekend at night to correct what he thought had been an error in his management."[21]

These were the days of internal medicine looking at "the patient as a person," as the expression from the 1920s went, not treating patients as a sack of enzymes but as distinctive individuals. Hippocrates had said, "It is far more important to know what sort of person has a disease than to know what sort of disease a person has." This tradition was very much alive in the Department of Medicine wards. Farquharson probably went one step beyond, looking after troubled influential citizens who did not want it known they were in psychiatric care and, above all, troubled fellow physicians. His daughter Nell remembers the constant presence of the phone on the dinner table. "Every night if my father was home one of us would go upstairs and bring down a phone. We had a jack there, and the phone was placed on the table ... So someone would ring in, and one of us would answer. We'd make up names for the people, some of them were patients, like I remember one was 'the dying swans' – 'oh, the dying swans are back,' and we'd give him the phone." Many of these callers were troubled with psychiatric disorders.

The family had an enclosed sun porch, and on Sunday afternoons Farquharson would receive those patients who required confidential consultations, closing the doors to the living room to keep the children from overhearing. "They were people who were depressed, people who were on drugs, and people who were on alcohol ... Some of the wealthy people were chronic. They had bipolar disorder, some of them. He'd hand them over to one of his junior staff, who needed the money, and say 'charge them anything you want.' As far as we were concerned, he didn't charge any health care worker, hardly any people in the education field, and yet these were the type of people who came to see him." Because of Farquharson's refusal to charge, Nell said the family in those days before the Second World War was chronically short of money.[22]

It is interesting that in the last days of his illness, Gerry FitzGerald was hospitalized not in the Toronto Psychiatric Hospital (where he would have had no privacy) but on the medical wards of the General, where Ray Farquharson attended him. Jack Laidlaw once dined with the Farquharson family. "During dinner he took calls of at least 15 minutes in length from two patients who I knew had illnesses with major psychological components."[23]

As head of medicine, Farquharson departed sharply from the autocratic style of Duncan Graham, introducing collegiality into decision-making in the form of a kitchen cabinet. Nell Farquharson recalls that it was not so much a formal executive committee as "little groups of consultants ... If my father was going to move, do a major shuffle, he wouldn't just have it all in his own head, he'd have a group of people who were knowledgeable in that area." Laidlaw was among Farky's trusted advisers, as were cardiologist Alexander McKelvey, a 1943 medical graduate of the U of T, and Trevor Owen, who graduated in 1918 and was in charge of the medical outpatient department (where he propounded the psychosocial elements of patients' "dis-ease"). Nell Farquharson said, "They had a department meeting once a month and Trevor Owen always came here afterwards, and they'd sit in the [sunroom] and they'd talk. My mother would say, 'okay, it's staff meeting night, who's going to make the hot chocolate.' Whoever happened to be home had the job of giving them a tray with some biscuits and hot chocolate."

Farquharson died of a heart attack in Ottawa in 1965 at a meeting of the Medical Research Council, of which he was the inaugural president. Nell recalled, "He went out with the guys after and went to bed, got the pain, and refused to

– or decided not to – call anyone until morning, cause they needed their sleep. So by the time he called [G. Malcolm] Brown from Queen's, and he got him to the hospital, he was dead within three or four hours."[24]

Few today remember Ray Farquharson, though those who do treasure their recollections. Yet one thing must be said, not just about Farquharson but about that whole generation of clinicians in the Department of Medicine: they saw their main mission as preparing students to be doctors. They did not see themselves first and foremost as researchers or scientists. The emphasis was on care of the whole patient, or what a later generation might call "the biopsychosocial model." In 1953 Farquharson said, "Increasing emphasis continues to be placed on consideration of the patient as a whole – his constitution and heredity, emotions, personality and environment – in diagnosis and treatment of disorders from which he suffers."[25]

Grounded in bedside learning, Farquharson was suspicious of medical fads. In 1958 he said, "It is easy to be critical of the ideas of our predecessors and to wonder how they ever believed what they did. It is equally easy to be complacent about our own situation and fail to appreciate how difficult it is for all, and especially for the young, to distinguish truth from fashion. No one ever succeeds completely in the attempt. A new idea, not necessarily true, often gains credence on presumably scientific evidence; it may be pushed much too far and in error dominate customary treatment for many years ... We are still the victims of fashions which take a firm hold on us and of the tendency for uniformity in ideas of all kinds."[26] These sentiments have not lost their wisdom.

Admirable though Farquharson's humane attitudes to patient care might have been – and praiseworthy the personal example he set as an investigator – he did little to encourage research. Berris, who had returned to Toronto from a high-science environment at the University of Minnesota, was appalled at what he found when he joined the Department of Medicine in Toronto in 1951: "Standards of residency training and patient care in Toronto were of a lower quality. Residents were not required to be involved in research. The staff were not keeping up with new methods of investigation and treatment of disease. If research studies were being carried out, they were not communicated to the clinical staff." Berris had performed numerous liver biopsies in Minneapolis and knew them to be important diagnostic aides. When he proposed that he might undertake some in Toronto, the suggestion was batted aside on the grounds that "liver biopsies didn't add anything to the diagnosis or treatment of liver disease." Berris said, "Unfortunately, it appeared that the Department of Medicine at that time did not have an investigative mindset." This condition endured until Wightman became professor of medicine in 1960 and "began appointing full-time staff who were trained to do research and established research programs at the Toronto General." Farquharson, Berris noted, had been able to beat the bias against Jews but not against research.[27]

Yet led by service demand, the Department of Medicine in the Farquharson years grew greatly. In 1961 it was noted, "A comparison of the Department of Medicine ten years ago and today reveals that the teaching staff has increased from 42 to 107 ... 3 new University full-time posts have been created and 18 full-time posts supported by granting bodies or by arrangement with the teaching hospitals. The number of Fellows in the department has gone from 12 to 36."[28] Thus, despite the relative disinterest in research, these were not exactly years of stagnation.

In 1960 Kager Wightman succeeded Farquharson as Eaton Professor and chair of the Department of Medicine. It was Wightman who led the dramatic expansion of the department in the 1960s. "While Kager was chair," said Berris, "the University Department of Medicine grew rapidly and acquired a completely new look. All the teaching hospitals were adding new staff based entirely on their qualifications. Many had received their training outside of Canada and a number were Jewish men and women."[29] Kager Wightman thus emerges as the second great leadership figure in the history of the department and of the faculty.

*"Kager"*

Of the leaders of the faculty is those golden years – when money was becoming plentiful and growth incessant – "Kager" Wightman was perhaps the most beloved of all the figures looked back upon with such fondness. Keith John Roy Wightman was born in Sandwich, Ontario, in 1914, his father a schoolteacher. But Wightman grew up in Peterborough, where his father served first as principal of one of the schools and then as superintendent of schools and, finally, director of education. Other than being very kind, people remember immediately of Wightman that he was very bright, and he graduated from high school at sixteen. But, being too young for medicine, he did another year of high school. He had As, but some Bs and Cs; "I wouldn't get into medical school nowadays with the grades I had," he later said.[30]

Wightman graduated from medical school at the University of Toronto in 1937 as the gold medalist; with an Ellen Mickle Fellowship he was able to spend a year in Cambridge, studying research techniques with Sir Alan Drury. In 1938 he returned to Toronto, where he trained in medicine and earned his Royal College Fellowship in 1942. Wightman served in the war, then came on staff in 1946 at the General as a demonstrator in the Department of Medicine. In 1950 he succeeded Robert Kerr as professor of therapeutics,[31] and for the next seven years he led the Department of Therapeutics. In 1960 he was named the Sir John and Lady Eaton Professor of Medicine; he was simultaneously physician-in-chief at the Toronto General Hospital and held this post for ten years, until becoming in 1970 associate dean and director of the Division of Postgraduate Medical

Education. In 1974 he took up the post of medical director of the Ontario Cancer Treatment and Research Foundation, which he held until his retirement. He died in 1978 of metastatic carcinoma of the colon.

Of Wightman's tenure as Eaton Professor, colleague John M. Finlay said, "He was instrumental in developing within this Department [of Medicine] a climate conducive to the growth of clinical investigation which led to an extraordinary flowering of research ability when resources became available for the recruitment of young investigators."[32] Wightman extended the teaching program of the department to the New Mount Sinai Hospital, Women's College Hospital, and Sunnybrook Hospital, which in these years were becoming teaching hospitals of the university. According to Charles Hollenberg, it was Wightman who first appointed the "specialty co-ordinators" that became the basis of the powerful division system in the Department of Medicine.[33]

Throughout his tenure, Wightman pressed for full-time appointments. Why were they necessary? Partly, he said, it was the complexity of research today: "Productive research requires at least 50 percent of one's time in the laboratory, so it is necessary to have full-time appointments to carry out all these assignments." But also, "[t]he modern teaching hospital attracts patients whose problems require considerable time to elucidate. The attempt to close the gap between new science and its application in medicine [later called translational research] requires time devoted to developmental research. In addition to all this there is a need to improve the documentation of patients, to review series of cases with similar disease, to study in an orderly fashion the response to various drugs (new and old), as well as to carry on research in education and teaching."[34] These lines sketch out a comprehensive picture of the Department of Medicine as it was to come: reflective patient care based on the latest science, plus a personal commitment to leading-edge lab research, plus, finally, inquiry about how best to teach and instruct. In the next decades all this was to happen, but not in the same person!

As for Kager as a physician, in Finlay's view, "Unquestionably he was at his best as a diagnostician and as a clinical teacher. At the bedside he demonstrated repeatedly the excellence of his clinical skills and showed an intuitive awareness of the importance of psychological factors in illness." Wightman became known as "the specialist's specialist" and was widely sought in consultation, particularly in cases of serious illness among colleagues' families. Finlay said, "Despite the fact that Kager Wightman was one of the most brilliant men of his era at the University of Toronto, he was profoundly modest. He was slow to take credit for himself, quick to praise and quick to encourage the abilities of others. His soft and quiet demeanour often distinguished a great sense of humour, one which was completely without malice and ... often directed towards himself."[35] (On the subject of Wightman's unassuming side, it was said that once when he stopped to help at the scene of an accident, "the bystanders looked at him skeptically and continued to rush around calling loudly for a doctor."[36])

"Individuals were important to him," said Cowan. "As we made rounds through the Toronto General, he was forever helping cleaning ladies with their buckets over the bumps onto elevators. As he sat talking with a sick patient ... he gave that patient his undivided attention as if he or she had the only important problem in the world at that moment." Cowan asked Wightman to see one of his own patients in consultation and told the patient "that I would be bringing the professor to examine her and give his opinion. Later that day I brought Kager to the bedside. At that precise moment the patient needed to go to the bathroom. He was quickly on his hands and knees to get her slippers from under the bed, helped her on with her gown and when she returned he quietly, efficiently and thoroughly evaluated the situation ... As we started away, she spoke to Kager, told him how much better she felt about things and then said, 'You know that there's a big professor coming to see me later this afternoon.'"[37]

Cowan said of Wightman simply, "He had a superior intellect." Charles Hollenberg, who followed Wightman as the Eaton Professor, said, "Kager had an unusual and extraordinary intellect." His contemporaries clearly wondered at the quality of his mind, and Ernest Maltby, one of the senior clinicians at the General, declared, "He is the most brilliant student we've had in Toronto." The story goes that, when he sat for his oral fellowship exams in Toronto, as Don Cowan relates the story told by others, "He impressed the examiners so that they began to show him unsolved problems from the wards." Just after returning to Toronto from the war, he was placed in charge of the course on physical diagnosis for second-year medical students, and in 1950–1 he revised the *Patient Examination Outline and History Taking*, first published in 1942 by the University of Toronto Press and known to generations of medical students and residents as "the Green Book"; it was emblematic of Wightman's teaching and in 1977 was in its fourth edition.[38]

But for all his qualities, Kager Wightman was not a crackerjack administrator. Nell Farquharson said, "He was very bright, but I would call him rather a weak person. Because he was criticized for something or other, we all went to the auditorium, and he stood up and said he didn't think he had the confidence of the department, and he was going to retire. So having started as my father's successor, he didn't last very long."[39]

In the Toronto tradition of the attentive personal care of patients, Wightman was sensitive to the conflict between psychological effectiveness at the bedside and the new technologies spilling into medical practice. In 1960, in his last year as head of the Department of Therapeutics, he said, "This department faces increasing problems in attempting to keep in focus an ever-growing complexity of scientific methods of investigation and treatment of patients ... At the same time, one is aware of the need for an increasing emphasis on the humanistic aspects of treatment and an increasing respect for what [the treatments] accomplish for the patient. The aim ... is to inculcate a critical attitude with respect to treatments, and one which is sympathetic toward patients. This is a thing which can only be truly attained when one begins to accept the responsibility for the care of individual patients, but at least an initial bias in this direction can be inculcated in the students."[40]

It is unknown what Wightman would say today about the notion of "evidence-based medicine," but it would have fit poorly with his concept of therapeutics as an art that differed subtly from patient to patient just as paintings differ. "The scientific aspects of treatment are multiplying so rapidly as to eclipse any interest in the so-called art," he said in 1959. "This latter is difficult to define, ranging in various minds from refinements of the bedside manner to the rational approaches of psychotherapy ... There is an 'art' in the manipulation of quite potent and dangerous agents, in the sense that one learns to make correct decisions which cannot always be explained on rational grounds."[41] Veteran clinicians today will understand immediately what he was talking about, those who trained in Toronto all the more because they trained in that tradition.

In common with the rest of the Department of Medicine in those days, Wightman did not have a keen interest in research. In fact, he had little interest. He disliked writing. Don Cowan remembered, "Kager was probably brighter than all of them, but he didn't have a research record, and this is why I think that he won't be remembered in the same way. Research in the department probably didn't flourish as much as it should have." Wightman began to realize they were separate functions, saying in 1969, "As science has developed so markedly and as the techniques of biologic research have become so complex, it is more and more difficult to combine clinical research with clinical acumen and good clinical teaching."

Why were so many good clinicians leaving the department for the peripheral community hospitals? Wightman asked in 1969. It wasn't just the pull of these "new, well-appointed" facilities, he said. They were also being pushed from the department, partly by new teaching arrangements and other dislocations but also by "the emphasis on research" that had begun to appear in the divisions. This emphasis he regarded with distaste.[42] The department for him existed to turn out first-class clinicians; research was not a matter of indifference, but it did not have the same white-hot urgency as later under Hollenberg and Phillipson.

When in 1969 the Independent Planning Committee, a group of top-level faculty and hospital executives, assessed the Department of Medicine, the judgment was damning: "The Department, while historically the main centre of research in the faculty, has, however, not enjoyed the reputation as a leading research centre. The proliferation of knowledge in medical science demands that the Department step up its research activities significantly ... Scientific medicine must match the pace of clinical medicine." How to remedy this? Committed full-time clinician-researchers were needed. The clinician who dabbled in research was finished. "In former years, the newly qualified internist establishing himself as a practicing consultant was, if academically inclined, attracted to the teaching hospital where he could develop his skills while acquiring a personal

reputation and following ... The older patterns of recruiting the part-time clinical teacher have now been broken. Increased numbers of full-time teachers are
needed" to teach, administer, and research.[43] The Independent Planning Committee thus struck the closing bell of the old regime in medicine with its British-
inspired one-on-one system of dedicated teaching.

*Keen Young Researchers*

The 1950s saw several new departures in research. Interdisciplinarity increased.
In the late 1940s and early 1950s much of the research of the Department of
Pathological Chemistry occurred in conjunction with the staff of the newly established Clinical Investigation Unit at Sunnybrook under James Dauphinee.
Objects of study included, for example, the treatment of rheumatoid arthritis
with ACTH and cortisone, both of which had just become available in synthetic
forms. Allan Gornall of pathological chemistry, thirty-six at the time, whose
background was in clinical chemistry, was in charge of the new Steroid Hormone Research Laboratory that opened in autumn 1949.[44]

As Ray Farquharson and Kager Wightman were shaping the Department of
Medicine into its new post–Duncan Graham form, a number of keen young
investigators came on board who basically fashioned medicine at U of T as a
fast-lane group of researchers. One of them was John Coleman Laidlaw, known
universally as Jack, who grew up in Toronto rather than the tiny Ontario towns
that disgorged so many of his colleagues. Laidlaw attended the elite University
of Toronto Schools (UTS). His father was an official at the university, and there
was no history of practicing medicine in the family.

At UTS, Laidlaw said in an interview, "We had a kind of Mr Chips teacher
called Tommy Porter. In grade 8 he of all things gave us a talk on health and
the body. And I was just enormously fascinated, and at the end of the series of
lectures I went up and said, 'Dr Porter, I thought that was just terrific.' Well, he
said, 'my boy, I'd like you to be a doctor some day.'"[45]

Laidlaw earned an arts degree in the "B and M" course at the university
in 1942, leading to medicine. "It was an eight year course," he said, "a lot of
science. Really, four heavy science years before you ever got into medicine."
But because of the war, they did it in six, and Laidlaw graduated in medicine
in 1944. After a year's internship, he taught as a demonstrator in the Department of Biochemistry. The next few years he spent away from Toronto: first
as a lecturer in biochemistry at the University of London, where he earned
a PhD in 1950, then, after a year's residency in Toronto, from 1951 to 1954 as
a research fellow and instructor at Harvard. In 1954 Laidlaw returned to the
Department of Medicine in Toronto, succeeding Walter Campbell as director
of the Metabolism Laboratory in the Banting Institute.[46] (Campbell retired
in June 1953 from teaching on the public wards of the General.[47]) Between
1953 and 1958 Laidlaw was also a Markle Scholar, a remarkable fellowship

that supplemented the salary of young researchers for five years to encourage them to investigate whatever they chose (neurologist John Wherrett and Charles Hollenberg were later to join this select group). In 1956 Laidlaw established the Clinical Investigation Unit at the Toronto General Hospital, which marks the de facto founding of the Division of Endocrinology in the Department of Medicine. (Laidlaw gave up this unit in 1958, then resumed its direction in 1966.)

Under Laidlaw's direction this investigative unit became highly productive, discovering, for example, two new types of hypertension: hypertension simulating primary aldosteronism caused by renal artery occlusion[48] and a hereditary hypertension owing to increased aldosterone and with decreased plasma renin (not Conn's syndrome) and relieved by glucocorticoids.[49] (Aldosterone is a hormone secreted by the adrenal cortex that helps regulate fluid balance.) Edmund Yendt, a 1948 Toronto graduate and assistant director of the unit, was equally active, with internationally recognized studies of patients with disorders of calcium and phosphorus metabolism. While at Hopkins in 1954 as a McLaughlin Fellow, Yendt had helped document the role of renal artery stenosis in hypertension and its relief through nephrectomy.[50] Yendt is also remembered eponymously for Yendt-Gagne Syndrome, normocalcemic hyperparathyroidism, also described in 1968.[51] In 1968 Yendt accepted the chair of medicine at Queen's University – one of a number of Toronto Department of Medicine nestlings who became heads of medicine across Canada.

In 1967 Laidlaw became the founding director of the Institute of Medical Science, established initially within the Faculty of Medicine but reporting to the School of Graduate Studies, with a mandate to train academic physicians across the clinical departments in basic and clinical research in the context of MSc and PhD programs.

### The Wightman Watch

Wightman, not the best administrator by any stretch, struggled with the growing size and complexity of the Department of Medicine. In the 1961–2 session he hired an executive assistant (internist Duncan Gordon, who graduated in 1955) to help sort out problems of "communication" in this large department. Wightman regularly raged against "the thoughtless accumulation of administrative detail which has been allowed to occur" as he struggled to run a department that, by the mid-1960s, numbered 265 staff including fellows.[52]

By the mid-1960s the pace had become frenetic. All the teaching hospitals were growing. Wightman saw renovations, construction, and expansion on every front! "In seeking new men" we must have balance, he said. "The Department cannot be made up entirely of research men nor can it consist solely of pragmatic practitioners." Emotionally, he felt closer to the old guard of clinicians who saw themselves as teachers and healers. Politically, he was being tugged in the direction of organizing a research department by a young guard whom the research bug had bitten.[53]

On another occasion, Wightman noted that planning for the Department of Medicine was "incredibly complex." Communication "has reached a new dimension, which threatens to bring all ordinary work to a standstill! ... The prospect of the future leaves one alternating between elation and panic."[54]

Yet things got worse. It was the late 1960s and the beginning of the student revolt in which many of the medical students began demanding "parity" in decision-making and freedom from the strict supervision of their elders. These stirrings necessitated many meetings and much heartburn. In the 1967–8 session Wightman moaned, "This year will undoubtedly be remembered as 'The Year of the Committee' ... The process has been time-consuming, fatiguing and instructive. So far, not many final decisions have been made, and there are those who begin to be weary of the democratic process and are calling for more 'leadership.'"[55]

Irritated at the student revolt in the teaching hospitals, veteran clinicians began draining out of the system and accepting posts in community hospitals without a student presence. Wightman sighed in 1969, "These hospitals have already taken some of our staff, but this year an unprecedented number of resignations has occurred. While we are accustomed to experiencing a drain from other universities, this growing demand from community hospitals is new." The clinicians receiving these appointments were, of course, to be congratulated. "However, one feels there is still an element of discontent and dissatisfaction in their going." The student revolt, he said, was not the only factor, and there was further stress in the new curriculum, resentment about the hiring of new full-time staff [more than one hundred were hired on his watch[56]] and the new emphasis on research. "All these have contributed to an air of headlong and unpredictable change in the University. In spite of great efforts to increase the mechanisms of communication and participation in the issues, there is widespread distrust and suspicion." Wightman, who had spent the last several years up to his neck in committees, said, "There is a good deal of discontent with the function of committees. Think-ins and teach-ins are very popular."[57] Indeed. Older readers may recall the students of the late 1960s, the bearded young men, the tie-dyed T-shirts, the calls for "revolution." The Department of Medicine was leaching out its talent.

Faced with complexities on every front, Wightman brought more hands into the wheelhouse. In the 1966–7 session Joseph R. Hilliard, a 1952 Toronto graduate who had just returned to Toronto from the University of Alberta, agreed to supervise the postgraduate training program in medicine. (Under Hilliard the number of trainees grew rapidly; there were more than 180 by 1969.[58]) In 1967–8 Wightman effectively separated, on an interim basis, the positions of physician-in-chief at TGH from university chair of medicine: "The complexity of the operation [in the Department of Medicine] has led to a decision to appoint a Director of the Department of Medicine at the Toronto General Hospital who will in effect carry out the functions of the Physician-in-Chief there, so that the Departmental Chairman will be relieved of these responsibilities."[59]

Late in 1968 it was apparent that a change in leadership was coming in the Department of Medicine. Wightman decided to vacate the Eaton Chair and agreed to become director of the Division of Postgraduate Medical Education in the Dean's Office, a post that assured him greater tranquillity.[60] "In many ways this marks the end of an era," he said after reaching the decision to retire. "A new Department Head is to be appointed, a new curriculum is being introduced, and many changes in the pattern of University and departmental administration appear imminent … In some ways the function and importance of the Department is being eroded."[61]

On 4 February 1969, John Hamilton, the vice president of Health Sciences, told Dean Chute that the Eaton Advisory Committee should be convoked to approve Wightman's successor.[62] The following day Wightman explained to President Claude Bissell why he was stepping down from the Eaton Chair: because he had had enough. The department had grown from 124 in 1960 to 317 in 1969, spread out over eight teaching hospitals. Also, "[i]n the past year I have felt that the undergraduate students have been less appreciative of my teachings efforts, and I feel less confident in my relationships with the postgraduates also." Last year, he said, the Toronto General Hospital had requested the appointment of "some sort of deputy to act as Physician-in-Chief, the implication being that the present arrangement was unsatisfactory." A note of weariness infused the letter. Wightman looked forward to the relative peace of the dean's corridor.[63]

That Wightman became weary of the burdens of office towards the end should not, however, obscure the solidity of the legacy he left to Hollenberg. And, according to Don Cowan, this was Hollenberg's view of the Wightman legacy: first, Wightman accumulated a large budget, which gave Hollenberg "the flexibility to make new and important appointments without difficulty." Second, Wightman brought about a big increase in the number of teaching beds, especially at Sunnybrook and the Toronto East General. Third, Wightman developed, in Cowan's words, "a postgraduate teaching base and residency establishment." Cowan continued, "Charlie pointed out that this meant that he (Charlie) had beds, budget, and residents which provided all he needed for further developments. It also allowed Charles to make research appointments." Cowan's own summation of the Wightman years was thus: "Wightman may well have been the last of the Professors who excelled at the bedside in the Oslerian fashion – patient care and teaching."[64]

On 31 March 1969, Dean Chute wrote John David Eaton that Wightman's successor was to be chosen and that the search committee "would welcome your views and advice in this most important matter." Chute told Eaton that "Dr John Hamilton, Vice President Health Sciences and I would be happy to discuss these matters with you personally if you so desired."[65]

In the search for his successor, Wightman showed his finest colours. His successor was Charles Hollenberg, who was Jewish. Wightman was not a bigot and Hollenberg's widow Michelle ("Mimi") later said in an interview, "Wightman was like Jack Laidlaw: you could be green, pink or blue."

So after Hollenberg accepted the chair, Wightman said to him, "You know, Charles, I really think you should belong to a club, because you've got to have a place to take people out."

Charles replied, "What do you think I should join?" Wightman said, "I think you should join the University Club." Charles said, "That would be fine, Kager. Is it restricted?" (Mimi noted, "Now has Kager Wightman ever been turned down by anything?")

Kager said to Charles, "Yeah, you have to be a graduate of a university." Charles said to Kager, "Kager, you don't understand what I mean. Do they take Jews?" Mimi said, "I think Kager nearly had a coronary. He'd never been asked that before. He said, 'I'll have to check.' So he checked, and he came back and he said, 'They'd be very happy to have you as a member.'"[66]

### Charles Hollenberg

Donald Cowan (in 2009): "Personally I believe the break came from the point of view of research in the Department of Medicine with Charlie."
Interviewer: "'Cause he brought that McGill ethos?"
Cowan: "Because he brought that McGill ethos, exactly."[67]

There have been many distinguished clinicians and scientists in the Department of Medicine but few legends. Charles Hollenberg, who became chair of medicine in 1970, was a legend. The Hollenberg era, which even today old hands look back on with awe and fondness, marked the take-off of research in the Department of Medicine. To be sure, individual internists had always been engaged in research, almost as a private pursuit of personal interests. But under Hollenberg things got serious. His successor Eliot Phillipson later said that Hollenberg "more than anyone else began [the department's] transformation into a department of research intensity. By the end of his tenure in 1981, the Department had an impressive cadre of members who were trained both in clinical medicine and in research."[68] Said site visitors to the department in 1979, "It is the impression of the team that Dr. Hollenberg has emerged as the strongest chairman within the University of Toronto, Faculty of Medicine."[69]

Hollenberg was part of the cohort of physicians who came to Toronto from McGill after the FLQ (Quebec Liberation Front, separatist) troubles in Quebec in 1970. This cohort also included Arnie Aberman, Fred Lowy, and Aubie Angel. Although several of them in interviews denied that the anti-Semitism that seemed to lurk just beneath the surface of Quebec nationalism mattered, it is interesting that all were Jews.

Hollenberg was also the first major figure whose training abroad had been entirely in the United States, not the United Kingdom. He was born in Winnipeg into a distinguished medical family and received his entire education at the University of Manitoba, earning his medical degree in 1955. He trained in internal medicine at McGill and the New England Medical Center, which is a teaching hospital of Tufts University, earning his fellowship in the Royal College of Physicians and Surgeons in 1959. In 1960 he became a Markle Scholar, one of a select group of Canadians who won this award of an American foundation. In 1960 he joined the McGill Department of Medicine.

At McGill Douglas Cameron, the professor of medicine, was Hollenberg's mentor. Mimi Hollenberg said of Cameron, "He was one of the toughest guys in the whole world, and he loved my husband. Loved him. He was one of his boys." Hollenberg reciprocated these sentiments at the Royal Victoria Hospital and the Montreal General Hospital, said Mimi. "He loved his colleagues at the Vic too. And it's a funny way to put it, but Charles was going places, as a professional." It was then, supposedly after being passed over as chair at McGill, that at age thirty-nine Hollenberg came to Toronto as chair of medicine and chief physician at the Toronto General Hospital.

Why Toronto?

"Charles would have been offered jobs anywhere. This was the best and the biggest job, one of the biggest in North America," Mimi said.[70]

The appointment almost didn't go through, however. How the search committee and the hospital board dealt with the question of Hollenberg's Jewishness has never become publicly known, but Hollenberg was offered the Eaton Chair.

Hollenberg's tenure as professor of medicine is discussed later. He stepped down from the chair in 1981 to become the Charles H. Best Professor in the Best Institute, then served as vice provost of health sciences from 1983 to 1989; he became president and chief executive officer of the Ontario Cancer Treatment and Research Foundation in 1991, reshaping the organization as Cancer Care Ontario; he was its president and chief executive officer from 1997 to 1999. (Hollenberg also led the Banting and Best Diabetes Centre from 1981 to 1993.)

At the time of his death from cancer in 2003, Hollenberg was said to be "retired," but it was from illness: the man was a dynamo of energy and never retired from anything. In scientific terms, his research was in fat metabolism and diabetes, but he was primarily a medical leader, and he led well because he enjoyed it hugely. "If you're going to succeed in medicine," he said, "you've got to enjoy the work that you're doing, you've got to enjoy your teaching, you've got to enjoy looking after patients, you've got to enjoy bringing along very good young students, and not worry terribly much about the other factors that impinge upon the practice of medicine these days."[71]

John Evans, a medical colleague and later president of the University of Toronto, said of his friend Hollenberg, "There is a directness in his manner, there is a sense of purpose that is apparent to everybody, and he is straight as a die.

There is no waffling on the issues, there is no politics, it's achieving the goal and having everybody understand it. And this is why he was so successful in building the premier Department of Medicine in Canada – pulling together people, giving them a common sense of direction, and supporting them where they needed support in order to achieve it. He was really a remarkable chair of Medicine in Toronto."[72]

Hollenberg's conception for the Department of Medicine was "link[ing] the bedside to the bench," as his successor Eliot Phillipson put it in a eulogy. The clinician-scientists that Hollenberg recruited generated large amounts of new knowledge. But they also were, as Phillipson pointed out, "fundamental to development of the Department's medical subspecialty training programs."[73] Hollenberg thus became the leading figure in the remarkable growth of subspecialties in medicine that are glimpsed in the next chapter.

Hollenberg saw to it that funds for much of this research were generated by the academic practice plans, or group billings within each hospital division. Said Barney Berris, "While Kager had been able to obtain a decent budget to support research, Charles anticipated a rapid increase in the volume of research and he introduced a staff practice plan in which incomes were pooled. After the doctors' salaries were paid, a portion of the money was retained to support departmental research … Charles added immeasurably to the continuing development of the department as a centre for research."[74]

*Hollenberg's Watch*

Unlike the fragile Wightman, stress was a term apparently not in Hollenberg's vocabulary. He moved ahead on a number of fronts.

Budget cuts imposed by the province were threatening to savage the number of residents and shrink the subspecialty programs. What to do? Make the house staff more responsible. Hollenberg said in 1972, "Any overall reduction in the size of our total programme will inevitably require us to place more clinical responsibility in the hands of Internes and Junior Residents and thus we must maintain our efforts to strengthen the Clinical Clerkship programme so that our Internes are prepared during their Clerkship to assume greater patient responsibility."[75] Hard times meant moving responsibility downward.

After the plush 1960s, Hollenberg had to confront a series of financial stringencies that would continue almost up to the new century. He began to reach the conclusion that some kind of practice plan, already in effect at Sunnybrook, might be the only way to finance teaching and research. Future growth in staff, he wrote in 1971, "must be borne, in considerable measure, by revenue derived directly or indirectly from patient care. An effective way of dealing with this problem would be to establish hospital based group practices."[76]

Hollenberg drove forward like an express train on the group practice plan, incurring the ill will of some colleagues. He said, "A Faculty committee, chaired by Dr. W[illiam] Horsey, has been studying this problem ... and will propose controls over remuneration that are much more rigorous than any that have heretofore been suggested ... Increasingly it appears that Hospital-based group practices provide the teachers, the Hospitals, the University and Government with an equitable, sensible and accountable solution to this most difficult problem." Preconditions of success, he said, were that all the members of a hospital department must be included, and the government must be convinced that department size reflects need, so that one didn't get "a bureaucratic judgment arrived at under some supposedly universally applicable formula."[77] The practice plan thus made it possible to accept sharp cuts and at the same time to move forward with research and education.

Here is a footnote: How much difference did practice plan revenues make in the larger scheme of things? In 2003, of the $38 million the department committed to academic programs, $19 million came from the practice plans, $11 million came from the university, and $8 million from the hospitals, research institutes, and foundations. Thus fully half of total academic support derived from the practice plans of the department. Two outside reviewers noted, "[These] are very substantial contributions that compare well with major institutions in the US."[78]

Second, Hollenberg had to confront the same mushrooming of subspecialties that is described in chapter 7 for the Department of Surgery. He gave Abraham ("Abe") Rapoport the file, asking him to define better the "specialty programmes" of the department.[79] Rapoport, born in Toronto in 1926, had graduated in medicine from U of T in 1949, trained in endocrinology at the Postgraduate Medical School in London and at the University of Michigan, then returned to Toronto in 1957 to direct the Department of Biochemistry at the Toronto Western Hospital, where he later became physician-in-chief; Rapoport was also cross-appointed to the Department of Medicine.

Hollenberg pushed the department forward on the research front, making of research not just a desirable pastime but an activity that must infiltrate every root and branch of the department's being. He created a research committee. And in a series of meetings in the 1972–3 session, this committee formulated research objectives for the department:

(1) "High": Research in the Department of Medicine must "compare favorably with work being done anywhere else in the world."
(2) "Broad": "Each subspecialty ... should aim to develop a spectrum of research ranging from the investigation of basic problems (by investigators in this department, or by an interface with a basic department) through to the testing of the clinical significance of new findings."
(3) "Parsimonious": Research must be coordinated among the teaching hospitals so that there is no overlap.
(4) "Deep" in its penetration of departmental life: "Research should filter through the whole department and affect undergraduate teaching, postgraduate training and clinical practice."[80]

Even though Wightman had avidly encouraged research, this went way beyond Wightman: every division was to be world-class.

In 1978, at a meeting of the science policy committee of the faculty, Hollenberg offered a look at the new centrality of research in the department. The key individuals were the university division coordinators, who oversaw the collective hospital divisions of a given subspecialty (for more on this, see the next chapter). Of the 150 full-time staff in the department, "about 100 spend a majority of their time on research." In the recruitment of full-time staff, Hollenberg said research was the main criterion: "Normally the individual being considered for full-time status must be prepared to undertake a major research responsibility, in excess of 50% … If after three years an individual's output in term of research activity is considered unsatisfactory, the full-time status may be changed to part-time which means that his salary is dropped below the minimum level … and he is encouraged to develop another aspect of his career." (Much later, this policy was modified: In 2005 it was determined in the Clinical Faculty Policy that at the three-year review, appointments "may be terminated only for cause."[81])

As for research coordination across the various teaching hospitals, Hollenberg said that the Department of Medicine had experienced varying success. In chest disease this had worked. "By comparison, efforts to co-ordinate research in Cardiology have been less successful. A strong division exists at the Toronto General Hospital, for example, but this has tended to overshadow programmes at other hospitals … It is undesirable to have a concentration of strength in one hospital only." Within the hospitals, success in recruiting interns and residents into research had been mixed: "This appears to be a general problem across Canada," Hollenberg said. Exposure to research should start "by encouraging students to complete a degree before entry [into medical school]."

Of considerable interest, finally, was Hollenberg's opinion in 1978 that the dean should intervene more strongly in setting research directions. "It is essential for the Dean to have the capability, with proper advice, of introducing new research developments in selected areas." The dean needed a research advisory committee and at this point didn't have one, showing that research in the faculty was being driven at the department level, not the decanal. (That would begin under Dean Fred Lowy in the 1980s.)[82]

In the background, the role of the professor of medicine itself was shifting. Still an enormously influential position, under Duncan Graham or even Ray Farquharson, the Eaton Professor commanded respect in the classroom and the clinic. But Hollenberg could see that the chair of medicine was becoming more of a bureaucrat than a leader, with 13 specialty programs to organize and 155 full-time staff, spread across nine teaching hospitals. In 1975 Hollenberg mentioned this to the long-range planning committee: "He was of the opinion that the primary responsibility of the Professor of Medicine was to set the standards of education, patient care and service, and to provide a mechanism to ensure that the standards are met." It was a tough job but somebody had to do it: In the mid-1970s the Department of Medicine received a fifth of the total faculty budget and "generated approximately 36% of the research funds."[83] Medicine and surgery were clearly the heavy hitters of the Faculty of Medicine.

In retrospect, Hollenberg's leadership of the Department of Medicine represented a crucial period in the history of this flagship group. Not only were all hands brought on deck for the research mission, but the mission became funded with the practice plans. Individual projects were financed with grants. Yet all the rest of the superstructure for organizing research and bringing the somewhat resistant residents on board – sending them elsewhere for training and the like – was funded through the practice plans. As an act of generosity, it was somewhat involuntary on the part of the individual clinicians and feasible only through the driving force of iron-willed leadership. It was thus under Hollenberg that the massive pivot from the United Kingdom to the United States, and from teaching to research, began to gain momentum.

### Gerard Burrow

I have attempted to have the department function as a single entity.[84]

Gerard Burrow, 1985

In 1981 Hollenberg stepped down from the Eaton Chair to become the Charles H. Best Professor of Medical Research. He was succeeded by Gerard N. Burrow, the first American to hold the chair. Hitherto, almost all important events in the history of the Department of Medicine had somehow been associated with the British Isles: Duncan Graham, who had been asked to serve while actually living in London, Ray Farquharson, who had been made a member of the Order of the British Empire in 1946, and so forth. One suspects that Anglophiliac honours and invitations had not been showered upon Hollenberg only because of the residual anti-Semitism that still lingered in some of the vaults of British medicine. But Burrow was 100 percent American and owed nothing to Britain or its colonies. He was hired entirely on merit and on his particular American research-oriented coloration.

Burrow was born in 1933 in Boston, educated at Brown University, and studied medicine at Yale, earning a medical degree in 1958. He trained at Yale and passed his US boards in internal medicine in 1965. Thereafter he was taken on staff as an endocrinologist in the Department of Medicine at Yale until coming to Toronto in 1975 as a member of the department at the General. In 1981, as stated, he became the Eaton Professor and physician-in-chief at TGH. Burrow had been abroad once to teach – not in the United Kingdom but in France.

Burrow had several not inconsiderable administrative accomplishments.

In 1982 he introduced the notion of "areas of concentration" as a way of "concentrating different strengths in different hospitals."[85] This was the beginning of long-range planning in the Department of Medicine, and Burrow struck a Planning Committee to take responsibility.[86]

In 1983 he brought order to the numerous divisions of the department, sprawling as they did across the nine teaching hospitals, by giving the university coordinators of a division much more power, not only to distribute the residents about the teaching hospitals but to control appointments and to sign off on research grant applications. And he introduced the plan of naming the coordinators the department division directors ("DDDs").[87] This was a major accomplishment in strengthening the authority of the Department of Medicine against the hospitals.

To further knit things together, he introduced departmental grand rounds, to "give an opportunity for the entire department to be exposed to the outstanding teachers in each hospital."[88]

Yet the faculty was by no means in full control of the hospital departments and divisions. In 1985 the reviewers deplored the independence of the hospital departments, which failed to communicate either with one another or with the departmental chair: "The attending staff in all teaching hospitals identify more with their hospital rather than their University Department." (A rather indignant ad hoc group of department members responding to Lowy's request for feedback to the review and headed by Don Cowan – who was deputy chair of the department and chief physician at Sunnybrook – protested that Burrow had exerted a good deal more leadership than people thought.[89])

Burrow attempted to bring greater clarity to the practice plans, which at that point were controlled by the chief physicians of the hospitals and were kept "shrouded in an air of mystery," as the external reviewers said in 1985. The division directors had a good deal of input, culminating in a large "think in," as the expression went, at the end of the process. Cowan said, "This was perhaps the first large scale Clinical Department planning endeavour in our Faculty."[90]

In postgraduate education, Burrow introduced the carefully controlled examination system (Objective Structured Clinical Exams, OSCE) for resident evaluation, under the direction of Kenneth Robb. These spread to other departments and came to characterize postgraduate training in general.

In the 1986–7 session, Burrow prepared the hospital Department of Medicine at TGH for a coming merger with the department at the Toronto Western Hospital. (Aberman was the first combined chief of medicine as the operational merger occurred in 1989.) Burrow noted, "The realization that we could not continue to meet our commitments with constantly diminishing resources has resulted in a decision to become a focused, highly academic Department of Medicine. We will continue to deliver exemplary patient care but will choose those areas in which we can excel. The merger of the two hospitals offers even more opportunity to put together focused academic programs." He continued, "With its history and resources, the mission of the Department of Medicine is to educate physicians to be leaders in their chosen fields."[91]

In 1987 Burrow played an instrumental role in founding the new Centre for Cardiovascular Research in the Max Bell Research Centre of the Toronto

General Hospital, committing $2.5 million in faculty funds and a number of faculty salaries to make this new centre possible (see p. 221).[92]

The following year, in 1988, Burrow accepted a post as dean of the School of Medicine at the University of California in San Diego and was gone. "I think Toronto is the most exciting, livable city in all of North America," he said, rather wistfully, in a last interview.[93]

He was supplanted for a year by hematologist Ken Shumak, who led the department on an acting basis until Arnie Aberman was appointed Eaton Professor in 1989.

### Arnie Aberman

Arnold Aberman, universally known as Arnie, will be remembered more as dean of the Faculty of Medicine than as the Eaton Professor. He became dean of the faculty in 1992 and served for seven years of great change in the life of the medical school. Yet his tenure as head of the Department of Medicine is interesting at this point.

Born in 1943, Aberman grew up in Montreal and, after first earning an undergraduate degree in science, studied medicine at McGill. He graduated with an MD in 1967, after student days filled with campus politics (he was vice president of the McGill University Students' Society). Training in medicine, he was a house officer for two years at the Royal Victoria Hospital, then finished in the subspecialty of chest medicine in New York at the Albert Einstein College of Medicine – and its university hospital – where he was chief medical resident. From 1971 to 1973 he fellowed in pulmonary medicine at the University of California in San Francisco and at the Shock Research Unit of the University of Southern California School of Medicine in Los Angeles. In 1973 Aberman joined the Department of Medicine of the University of Toronto.

His rise was meteoric. In 1973 he began as co-director of the intensive care unit of Mount Sinai Hospital. In 1977, at age thirty-four, he became physician-in-chief at Mount Sinai – to the knowledge of the present author the youngest physician-in-chief in the modern history of the faculty. In 1989 he became physician-in-chief at the Toronto General Hospital and simultaneously Eaton Professor of Medicine. In December 1992, at age forty-eight, Aberman became dean of medicine and in 1994 vice provost for Relations with Health Care Institutions.

In March 1991, to devote his entire energies to being the university chair of medicine, Aberman stepped down as chief of medicine of The Toronto Hospital (TTH); on his recommendation, Michael Baker, who was the head of hematology, was appointed chief of medicine. This move raised a question as to the Eaton Chair – did it belong to the chief of medicine at The Toronto Hospital or to the university chair? The Eaton family had a very close relationship to both institutions. Investigation into the history of the establishment of the Eaton

Chair determined that the Eaton donation was to the university – and hence the Eaton Chair remained with the department chair.[94]

Aberman effected some big changes. As physician-in-chief at Mount Sinai Hospital (MSH), he grew the department from four to thirty-eight full-time members. As professor of medicine he amalgamated the departments of medicine of the faculty's six teaching hospitals into a single integrated university department with a single central budget. He merged all twelve divisions of The Toronto Hospital's Department of Medicine in a similar manner, "replacing," as he said, "the dual leadership with a single leadership for each division." (Previously, each hospital had its own head for each division.) "In essence," as Eliot Phillipson put it, "Aberman merged the Department of Medicine within The Toronto Hospital and its subspecialty divisions within the Hospital into single functional units."[95] Aberman also lined up the members of the Department of Medicine on behalf of a new and more profitable practice plan that produced $50 million annually, "of which," Aberman said, " a good whack went to teaching and research."

Aberman made salary in the department more dependent on function that on reputation. Lou Siminovitch was a kibitzer: "Arnie said, 'What counts in how we run this department is how we pay people, and whether we pay people for what they do and not just for their names.' And he went through every single person in the department and made his pay related to function. That was new."[96]

Aberman had a reputation for an agile mind and high energy levels. Berris, who had been chief of medicine at MSH, said, "Arnie seemed to work constantly and it was not unusual for me to receive phone calls from him at eleven or twelve o'clock at night to tell me about a new idea he had."[97] Aberman was known for incessant telephoning. Nell Farquharson recalled, "He was a real jumping jack. You could pass his door, he had two phones to his ears and he was talking alternately to two people at the same time."[98]

But when he talked, people listened.

## Eliot Phillipson

When Arnie Aberman stepped down from the Eaton Chair in 1992 to become dean, Eliot Phillipson was appointed chair of medicine, remaining in office until 2004. Born in Edmonton, Alberta, in 1939, Phillipson graduated in medicine from the University of Alberta in 1963, earning his fellowship in 1968. In 1971 Charles Hollenberg recruited him for Toronto, and Phillipson joined the respiratory division, becoming director in 1983. From 1987 to 1997 Phillipson followed Aberman as physician-in-chief at Mount Sinai Hospital and then again followed Arnie Aberman in 1993 in the university chair of medicine. (Phillipson served in both positions from 1993 to 1997, the first time in the history of the university department that the chair simultaneously served as physician-in-chief in a hospital other than the Toronto General Hospital – or The Toronto Hospital.) He confessed to being highly ambitious: once when he was being interviewed for a fellowship, the chairman of the Medical Research Council, Malcolm Brown, asked him, "Tell us, Dr. Phillipson, where would you like to be ten years from now?" Phillipson replied, "Dr Brown, I would like to be on the other side of this table."[99]

Phillipson's twelve years as professor of medicine were extraordinarily productive. On his watch the annual research budget of the Department of Medicine doubled from $30 million to $60 million. He borrowed the concept of the Clinician Scientist Training Program from the Department of Surgery and implemented several other such "job descriptions."

For the residents as a whole, Phillipson initiated the Core Training Program to make uniform the training experience and ensure academic control of it. The largest postgraduate program in the faculty – with 160 trainees at any given time – it had been hospital-based until the early 1990s and was viewed, Phillipson said, "as 'belonging' to the hospital." But it was lacking in diversity of experience. Also, it "made the postgraduate training experience vulnerable to the service needs of the hospital, rather than being driven by the educational needs of the trainees." Today, said Phillipson in 2001, the Core Training Program is "centrally organized and peripherally delivered." Each trainee has a standard three-year curriculum with flexibility in choosing rotations. Yet assessment is evaluated centrally.[100] The Core Training Program attracted applicants from across Canada: by the late 1990s, 43 percent of the first-year residents (PGY1s) were from other universities.[101]

For the brighter lights, in 1993 Phillipson created the Clinician Scientist Training Program, modelled on the template of the Surgical Scientist Program in the Department of Surgery. Jack Laidlaw put this in perspective: "To train young clinicians, you needed two things, you needed the Institute of Medical Science, and you needed the chairmen of the clinical departments pushing young residents to get involved, and that's what Phillipson did in Medicine and Langer in Surgery."[102] In the Department of Medicine, Kathy Siminovitch was the first director of the Clinician Scientist Training Program, followed in 1997 by Cathy Whiteside, who previously had been graduate coordinator of the Institute of Medical Science. The basic features of the program were, as in surgery, enrolment in a course of study leading to a PhD and a guarantee of salary support during the training period. Phillipson said in 1997 that the Clinician Scientist Training Program was conceived to answer the problem of "inadequate research training" for clinicians, "as a result of which they find themselves unable to compete with PhD scientists for research grants, as the cutting edge of science moves beyond their level of training and expertise." Phillipson continued, "Until the past decade the research training of clinician-scientists generally consisted of 1–3 years in a research laboratory (usually following the completion of clinical training) in which the quality of supervision and the rigor of the scientific experience were variable and at times deficient. There is broad agreement that this model is no longer tenable in the present era of science" and that clinician-scientists must get training as rigorous as that of basic scientists. "The most effective approach to ensuring such structure and rigor is through a formal graduate program (generally a PhD) that requires the trainee to master the discipline technically, methodologically, and conceptually."[103]

As of 1997, trainees were required to enter a formal graduate program. Phillipson said that the department would guarantee funding for two years, expecting that they will be able to "capture" outside grants for the third and fourth years. He wanted ten students a year to come into the program, about one-quarter of the class in internal medicine. Thus each of the eighteen subspecialty divisions would have "an average of about one new clinician-scientist trainee every two years." He wanted to train them "in all three domains of scientific inquiry: basic cellular and molecular biology, integrative animal and human biological, and clinical evaluative sciences and epidemiology."[104] By 2000 the program had enrolled twenty-seven trainees, twenty-three at the doctoral level and four at the master's level.[105]

Of the Clinician Scientist Training Program, Wendy Levinson, who followed Phillipson in the Eaton Chair, said that "the total cost for one physician per year of training is approximately $75,000"; training typically lasted for four or five years for a PhD or two years for a master's degree. "It is clearly expensive," she noted, "but well worth it!" By 2006, of the thirty-nine graduates, twenty-nine had become faculty members in the Department of Medicine and another six had joined other medical faculties in North America. Levinson said, "In short these training programs are the pipeline for our young, talented faculty ... They represent the future."[106]

By 1997 the new scientific ambitions of the Department of Medicine were giving it a cross-Canada, indeed an international, allure. For the nationwide resident-matching program, the Canadian Resident Matching Service (CaRMS), almost 300 graduating Canadian medical students applied for the forty available slots in the Toronto Department of Medicine.[107] For the period 1991–7, ten members of the Department of Medicine were elected to the prestigious American Society for Clinical Investigation, "a figure that is unmatched by any other Department of Medicine in Canada," as Phillipson pointed out.[108] This is evidence that the new research strategy was paying off.

Encouraged by the success of the Clinician Scientist Training Program, in the mid-1990s Phillipson created a similar program for those who wanted graduate work in medical education. Thus arose the Clinician Educator Training Program, to give the department professional internist-educators. Other such labels followed. The creation of functions of such specificity gave rise to the concept of "job description," and in 1997 it became official: the department created "job descriptions" that permit a better accounting of the academic functions of department members: "clinician-teacher, clinician-educator, clinician-investigator, clinician-scientist, or PhD scientist."[109] The breakdown of the 110 full-time faculty hired between 1993 and 1998 by job description was: clinician-teacher (48); clinician-scientist (25); clinician-investigator (18); clinician-educator (14); research (PhD) scientist (5). Of the 404 full-time faculty in the Department of Medicine in 1998, 47 percent were "predominantly researchers." Said Phillipson, "Clinician-scientists (many of whom were involved in basic science) were expected to devote 75% of their time to research, whereas clinician-investigators (who were involved in clinical science) were expected to devote only 50% of their time to research."[110]

A Master Teacher Program was introduced in 2002, ending with a master of education degree.[111] This splintering of the classic image of the academic physician – the thoughtful healer caught for the camera with a pipe in his mouth and wearing a three-piece suit – really does take one a long way from the world of Duncan Graham.

The hallmark of the Toronto style was cooperation and collegiality. The Department of Medicine under Phillipson embodied this kind of leadership style. When two external reviewers assessed the department in 2003, they commented on the uniqueness of the divisional system, the details of which are discussed in the next chapter. No other academic system in North America had anything comparable, they said. Harvard, for example, had multiple teaching hospitals, each with its own residency program and "no overall chair of the Department of Medicine, and there are no overarching division chiefs across all sites." This was true of many other US departments of medicine: no overarching divisional chiefs. One could imagine a situation in which the grand barons of the hospitals repudiated the authority of the university department and divisional chairs. But it was part of the genius of the Toronto system – part of the explanation why it "worked" – that this almost never happened.

Eliot Phillipson's reply to the reviewers' comment showed how sensitive the faculty was to this possible complication involving the hospitals. He said that the opposite scenario would be "a model in which a committee of Physicians-in-Chief would effectively replace the Chair. The disadvantage of this model is that it would represent a return to decentralized governance in which there would be a risk that academic priorities (such as standards for postgraduate education ...) would essentially be determined by each hospital, and could be driven unduly and distorted by clinical needs. Such an arrangement would also disenfranchise members of the Department who are not members of a hospital Department of Medicine, including most of those in Emergency Medicine ... and many of the PhD scientists." This scenario would have undone more than fifty years of evolution in hospital-faculty relations. Yet it never happened. As chapter 12 shows, the predominance of the faculty over the hospitals continued apace.

Interestingly, the new force field in the Department of Medicine was not a conflict between the department chair and the hospital physicians-in-chief. Phillipson said the latter had lost too much power. The real tension was "between the Chair and Physicians-in-Chief, on the one hand, and the hospital research institute directors on the other. This problem (which is not unique to the Department of Medicine) again emphasizes the importance of ensuring that the Toronto Academic Health Sciences Centre functions as a cooperative and interdependent network."[112]

## Coda

The size and complexity of the Department of Medicine can be numbing. What personal satisfaction could individual clinicians and researchers find within such a huge organization? In 1997 Phillipson answered with an eloquence that really embraces all academic medicine: "For the majority of members of the Department, the tie that binds them to teaching hospitals and to the University has little to do with equipment (or remuneration), and everything to do with the excitement, satisfaction, and prestige of academic medicine." People had to choose at some point, he said, between the financial benefits of community practice versus "the intrinsic personal satisfaction derived by the teacher when the student finally grasps the concept, understands the physical finding, or formulates an appropriate differential diagnosis: the surge of excitement and exhilaration felt by the scientist when a new piece of knowledge is revealed for the first time (and the P values are significant!); and the sense of pride and prestige felt by the educator, investigator, and scientist when their academic contributions are recognized by teaching and research awards, by invitations to speak at international meetings, and by academic promotion."[113] It is interesting that, despite almost universal societal deference to the title "Doctor," the title that academic physicians most embrace is "Professor."

In 1997 Phillipson attended the annual meeting of the Association of Professors of Medicine. What he witnessed gladdened his heart about his home university: "The most compelling and potentially most serious impact of managed care on academic Internal Medicine in the United States has been on the ability of Departments of Medicine to sustain basic research programs. Simply put, because the driving force in the managed care system is competition based on price, there is little room in the system for additional expenses for education, and even less for research, particularly basic scientific research ... As I listened to these debates ... the [concept] that all teaching in the University of Toronto must be rooted in, built upon, and delivered in the context of research took on added significance."[114]

## The Department of Therapeutics

The main object of the course in Medicine is treatment.[115]

The Department of Therapeutics was virtually a division of the Department of Medicine, as well as a seedbed for leadership. Most medical schools at the dawn of the twentieth century had departments of "materia medica," the old-fashioned name for what evolved into pharmacology and internal medicine. In Toronto, what was called elsewhere materia medica began in 1887 with the refoundation of the faculty in the chair of pharmacology and therapeutics. The post never really had an administrative structure of its own but huddled in the shadow of the Department of Medicine. In time it was, in fact, folded into the Department of Medicine. Yet "Therapeutics" deserves a few words because the holders of the chair envisioned a special closeness in the doctor-patient relationship.

In 1887 the professor of pharmacology and therapeutics was James D. Thorburn, a graduate of the old Toronto School of Medicine who went on to collect a postgraduate MD at the University of Edinburgh. In these years "materia medica," the study of medicinal plants, and "therapeutics" were taught separately, the former situated in the first curricular year, the latter in the clinical years. This was a source of some unhappiness among the med students, who found plant studies uncompelling (because there was no exam). As they said in a letter to the student newspaper, the *Varsity*, in February 1891, they simply didn't bother to attend the materia medica lectures. Animated perhaps by a series of talks the Franco-American neurologist Edouard Séguin had given on campus in 1890, the meds wanted materia medica and therapeutics integrated into a sole course, to make the entire subject more digestible.[116]

In 1892 James M. MacCallum succeeded Thorburn in the chair of pharmacology and therapeutics. MacCallum, born in 1863, graduated in 1886 from the Medical Department of Victoria University, in Toronto. He acquired the Licentiate of the Apothecaries' Society (LSA) of London. After laying down his professorship of therapeutics in 1908, he became an associate professor of pathology and otology. Neither Thorburn nor MacCallum had any visibility as a scientific figure.

In the 1908–9 session, therapeutics and pharmacology were split because the university was finally able to fund a professorship in pharmacology.[117] The chair of therapeutics went in 1908 to Robert D. Rudolf, a Nova Scotian who grew up in England and had a medical degree from Edinburgh (1889) and membership in the Royal College of Physicians of London. Rudolf had joined the faculty in 1900 as a demonstrator in clinical medicine.[118] A chair of pharmacology was created in 1909 for Velyien Ewart Henderson, a distinguished figure in the history of the faculty (see p. 436).

Rudolf stayed on as professor of therapeutics until retiring in 1934. When Duncan Graham came in as professor of medicine in 1919, he reorganized the Department of Therapeutics, adding William V. Watson and Edward C. Cole.[119] The therapeutics courses were said to flourish in popularity among the undergraduates, who, according to Rudolf, "seem to realize more and more that after all the main object of the course in Medicine is treatment."[120]

A page was turned in 1934 when Ray Farquharson became professor of therapeutics. For Graham, appointing a member of the Department of Medicine to the therapeutics chair made "possible the inauguration of a combined course of instruction in Medicine and Therapeutics."[121] The president's report for 1934 said of therapeutics, "While this remains a separate chair, the holder will work in close co-operation with the departments of medicine and pharmacology."[122] Therapeutics was now essentially a subspecialty program within medicine and never again changed this status.

In 1934 physical therapy became a subdepartment of therapeutics, as did anesthesia. Although these stories are told elsewhere (in chapters 23 and 20 respectively), it is worth remarking here that physical therapy was taught robustly to the medical students in the context of therapeutics. Dean Gallie in the late 1930s said that under William J. Gardiner in the Department of Therapeutics, "[t]he teaching of Physiotherapy has been established on a scientific basis and each student is given an opportunity to acquire both theoretical and practical training in the essentials."[123] By the 1951–2 session, the teaching of physical and occupational therapy to nonmedical students had been spun off to another department, and the offering of physical and rehabilitation medicine to medical students and trainees would proceed under the title physiatry.

By the beginning of the Second World War, the Department of Therapeutics had become a kind of forcing ground for future faculty leaders: Wightman had just finished his residency and was on staff, along with surgeon Robert A. Mustard and internist Arthur Squires.[124] In 1953–4 Ernest J. ("Bun") McCulloch, studying leukemia, worked as a research fellow of the National Cancer Institute in the department, collaborating with Charles Bardawill in the hematology division at St Michael's.[125] McCulloch and James Till would shortly discover stem cells. Farquharson was gathering the coming elite about him.

Before the Second World War, therapeutics had been an unpromising field because so few specific treatments were available. This changed dramatically after the war. As historian W.G. Cosbie points out, "The advent of the specific therapy of the sulphonamides and antibiotics gave new importance to the subdepartment of Therapeutics."[126]

In the 1947–8 session Robert B. Kerr succeeded Farquharson as head of therapeutics, and in 1950 Wightman, who would be the last major figure as professor of therapeutics, succeeded Kerr. Wightman, like many physicians, was reeling from the introduction of the new drugs and saw in them a threat to medicine's humanistic mission. He said in 1951, "As the scientific aspects of therapy advance, they impose ever increasing demands on the practitioner ... The preoccupation with minutiae of various types of specific therapy which is engendered ... has a tendency to obscure the humanistic values which are implicated in the treatment of a patient as an individual ... Under these circumstances the teaching of therapeutics becomes a matter of greater and greater difficulty ... It therefore devolves upon the Department of Therapeutics to act as a clearing house, as it were ... above all to give [the students] an opportunity of learning to apply to individual patients the principles which they have been taught."[127] As an affirmation of the values of humanism against those of technology in the teaching of medicine, the statement is exquisite.

In the late 1950s and early 1960s, the pharmacological cornucopia widened increasingly. Ever more new drugs appeared on the market, bewildering and swamping clinicians who had been accustomed in their pharmaceutical armamentarium to a handful of painkillers, alkaloids with physiological effects, and vaccines. "The students have tremendous difficulty in orienting themselves [in therapeutics]," Wightman noted.[128] Said Dean MacFarlane in 1960, "The doctor himself, rather breathless at the pace, has little time to think of what the future holds for him. He is constantly being provided with ... new drugs which may result from the sometimes difficult association of the entrepreneur with the research scientists ... If he is wise he holds fast to the truth that he must still assess the patient's individual needs in the midst of this ever-changing world ... and hope to have the wisdom and training to give the patient the sort of advice to which an ill, disturbed or injured human is entitled in the light of present-day knowledge."[129]

Helping the clinician apply this pharmaceutical avalanche wisely at the bedside was becoming increasingly the job of the Department of Therapeutics. Wightman said in 1958 this should be the department's message for the medical students: "The teaching of therapeutics is a matter of ever increasing difficulty since the number of agents available continues to grow, and more diseases are becoming amenable to some kind of treatment, be it curative or palliative ... Above all it is necessary to emphasize the personal aspect of the relations between patients and physician and the factors which must be kept in mind apart from the purely scientific aspects of treatment. Thus the subject becomes something more than an extension of pharmacology."[130]

The Toronto faculty prided themselves on good bedside medicine, and the pharmacological avalanche threatened to bury this tradition by making, as Wightman feared, clinical medicine an extension of pharmacology. As head of medicine he warned in 1962, "There is still a need of giving students a sense of proportion in the treatments and investigations they order for individual patients. The bewildering increase in new drugs still continues, and information as to their value is hard to come by."[131] Wightman feared, not unreasonably, that the students would become awash in the sea of pharma.

After Wightman in his turn became head of medicine, following Farquharson, there was a hiatus of several years, then in 1963 cardiologist Ramsay Gunton became the professor of therapeutics. When in 1966 he stepped down to become head of medicine at the University of Western Ontario, no further incumbent was appointed. The chair was folded into the Department of Medicine. Yet Gunton left on a poignant note: even though the concept of "therapeutics" as a discipline was outmoded, there was something of value here, he said. "Organizing committees of new medical schools are not creating separate Departments of Therapeutics and only a few remain in older schools." Should this department be merged with medicine or pharmacology? No, he said. To be sure, the emergence of clinical pharmacology as a separate, new discipline had "put Therapeutics in an uncomfortable squeeze between it and Medicine. But Therapeutics is not just the acquisition of knowledge about the drug ... Therapeutics is the art and science of treatment."[132] This was precisely Wightman's concept: therapeutics was more the study of the doctor-patient relationship than of therapeutic agents.

To be sure, the study of the art of treatment in the future would belong to family medicine and not languish in complete oblivion. Yet the specialists looked down on family medicine, and with the disappearance of the Department of Therapeutics, in the future no one would instruct them in the art of treatment.

# 9   The Medical Subspecialties

This is one of the challenges in our department – how to take advantage of our depth and breadth but align us so that we are pulling in the same direction.[1]

Wendy Levinson, Eaton Professor of Medicine, 2009

The Department of Medicine is only one of many departments. Yet in size and influence "internal medicine" overpowers all others except surgery. The professor of medicine is probably the single most influential clinician in the faculty. In the training of physicians, it is always the internists who do the heavy lifting. Yet the difference between 1900 and, say, 1990 is dramatic. In 1900 the leaders of medicine were distinguished "doctors." By 1990 they were distinguished "professors." In 1900 specialists learned their skills in hospitals. By 1990 they were still learning them in hospitals, but in the context of academic divisions and departments.

In March 1998 Phillipson mused about the transformation of postgraduate medical training, which, he said, had gone from a hospital to a university model. Historically, "postgraduate medical training was very much an apprenticeship, during which the trainee learned the skills of the discipline by participating in the provision of patient care. In this model there was little pretense about 'education.' Postgraduate trainees were generally based in, lived in, and paid by hospitals; hence the terms house staff, house officers, and residents. Many of the hospitals had no particular connection with a medical school or affiliation with a university." Yet in recent decades this model has changed radically: In 1970 the Royal College of Physicians and Surgeons vested authority for postgraduate training programs "in universities, not in hospitals," and all trainees have to be registered in the University Postgraduate Medical Education Office. Also, all postgraduate teachers must hold a university appointment. Finally, the Royal College insists that the program be weighted on the side of education rather than service, "a concept clearly based on the concept of trainees as students, as opposed to service providers."[2] Thus the passage of medicine from art to science and from hospital to university.

What gives the story unity is the relentless forward drive of technology. Dean Joseph MacFarlane said in 1955, "The increased demand for special postgraduate training, both in the basic sciences and in the clinical fields, is a reflection of the tremendous increase in medical knowledge and the diversity of techniques, and the recognition of the fact that only by long years of application can one perfect his knowledge and skill in certain special fields."[3] With each significant technical innovation, a new subspecialty emerged: cardiac catheterization helped boost cardiology, renal micropuncture launched nephrology, and arterial blood gas analysis promoted respirology. This process led, as Phillipson observed, to "the emergence of modern-day clinical science ... physicians who were not only trained broadly in Internal Medicine, but had also acquired highly specialized research skills." Phillipson saw "the transformation of clinical medicine to a science-based enterprise" as having begun with the Flexner Report of 1910 and culminating with the creation of the National Institutes of Health in the United States in the 1950s and the Medical Research Council of Canada.[4] Thus, the rise of the subspecialties in medicine mirrors the march of medical progress.

At the University of Toronto, the subspecialty story in the Department of Medicine goes back to the mid-1960s when this huge department was literally being torn apart by countervailing forces: some of the big subspecialties wanted to leave and become departments in their own right, other fields, not yet specialties, were burrowing into the core of medicine itself and threatening to drain away its patients.

In 1967 Wightman bemoaned all the subspecialties wanting to leave: psychiatry in the general hospitals, then part of the Department of Medicine, wanted a separate department (there was a separate mental-hospital-based Department of Psychiatry); hematology wanted to join pathology. "The neurologists are urging that theirs is a special science, with its own basic disciplines, its own vocabulary, and very special qualifications on the part of its practitioners such as to justify a separate department. Similar arguments could be adduced for at least fifteen other divisions." Wightman feared the effect on undergraduate teaching. He said they were appointing "co-ordinators" for some of these fields, "such as haematology, neurology, cardiology, and rheumatology – where the size of the operation [permits] a mechanism which will foster its development and yet allow for its integration into the whole fabric." These coordinators were the forerunners of the university division heads, though initially they limited themselves to resident training and not research. Wightman said the department was becoming virtually a mini medical school: "If this sort of thing is to work, it must be carried to the point where the department is virtually converted into a miniature faculty, with an organization of corresponding complexity. It is quite difficult to superimpose this upon the arrangements at the separate teaching hospitals, which have their own aspirations and problems, and desire to maintain a degree of autonomy."[5]

"On the other hand," Wightman continued, "the Department is also in danger of attrition from the 'general' side." The family doctors were all setting up clinics "which would afford students an opportunity to see the nature of general practice." These clinics had developed under the aegis of the Department of Medicine. "However, we are already beginning to hear that they should be separate departments."[6] Wightman was unsuccessful in his efforts to persuade the family physicians to remain in a "division" of their own. Yet he did staunch separatism among the bigger subspecialties by turning them into divisions with wide-ranging autonomy, and in Toronto they remain divisions of medicine to this day, at a time when many such subspecialties (e.g., neurology, dermatology) elsewhere have long since constituted departments of their own.

The coordinator system did not catch on at once. In 1969 Wightman commented, "The co-ordinators who were appointed two or three years ago to supervise activities in such fields as haematology, rheumatology, neurology, cardiology, etc, have had various degrees of success ... They have encountered various degrees of resistance to regimentation on the part of the staff of the teaching hospitals."[7] Yet the advantages from the viewpoint of senior administrators were apparent: central faculty control over these mushrooming subspecialties, making teaching uniform, and preventing duplication of research. The frondeurs who protested had no chance.

Under Hollenberg the system of coordinators was honed. In 1980 a team of assessors was able to report, "As a mechanism of gaining cohesion through the specialties, a system of co-ordinators has been established within the Department. There are two chief-coordinators, one for general medicine and one for the specialties. For each specialty, a co-ordinator is named who has the responsibility for the development of education and communication within the particular specialty." The system functioned as a "clear communication channel." (Under Burrow, the hospital coordinators became "division directors" with expanded functions; see previous chapter.) The coordinators' functions were limited in these years to residency training. The assessors wondered if the role of the coordinators "might not be extended to include the planning and development of research and other academic functions." Dean Brian Holmes noted in the margin beside this comment, "On reflection, I think we should encourage the naming of subspecialty chiefs or chairmen – perhaps the latter."[8] This casual notation was thus the birth of the department division directors (DDDs) several years later.

When external assessors looked at the department in 1986, they found the politics of the divisions precarious. Who had more power, the division directors or the hospital physicians-in-chief? It was, at this point, definitely the latter. "There is a power imbalance," the assessors said, "between the vertical structures of the Department's matrix (the committee of Physicians-in-Chief) and its horizontal structure (the committee of divisional coordinators and directors). Most of the power with regard to policy and decision making and virtually all of the financial control is in the hands of the Physicians-in-Chief."[9]

Yet the vertical-horizontal matrix was a work in progress, and power was drifting slowly but ineluctably away from the hospitals and towards the head of the university department. Under Burrow the coordinators all became the DDDs. These were university posts, not hospital posts. Then under Wendy Levinson the DDDs became directly constrained to work in a collaborative rather than a competitive manner. Each DDD had an executive committee, including the division heads of the individual hospital divisions, the training program directors, and so forth. Levinson said in 2007, "During my tenure as Chair of Medicine, I have asked the DDDs to ensure that the recruitment of new faculty members is collaborative, rather than competitive, between the Hospitals." The executive committee must discuss all new appointments to see which hospital fits best. "This discussion allows the DDD to plan recruitment to the most appropriate location in the city."[10] These were important posts, and international searches were conducted for them, which definitely had not been the old U of T way. In other words, the taming of the hospitals, once so proud of their institutional autonomy, was complete.

In the administrative hierarchy of these large flagship departments, the department heads as such functioned as the generals, who marshalled the forces in a great order of battle. But the actual units that got done the work of teaching and research – and were directly responsible for medical progress – were the subspecialties, deployed on this vast field as "divisions." It is not possible to tell the story of all of them, but some accomplishments may at least be mentioned. (The narrative of the Division of Hematology and Oncology will be found in chapter 13 on cancer care; the Division of Neurology is in chapter 14. On the role of Ricky Kanee Schachter in the Division of Dermatology, and the move of the division to Women's College Hospital in 1983–4, see pp. 574–575.)

## Division of Cardiology

Without doubt the recent advances in the correction of congenital and acquired heart lesions will be claimed by the surgical side, but the recognition, diagnosis and advice as to suitable treatment of the particular case is due largely to the persistent application of new methods of examination by the medical staff members over a broad front, and this element should be more adequately recognized.[11]

Walter R. Campbell, 1963

Cardiology is among the first subspecialties of internal medicine, and its history in the University of Toronto goes back to around 1912, when John Oille joined the staff.

Oille was among the beloved senior figures in the history of the faculty. *Epistaxis*, the student satirical handout for the annual skit night Daffydil, alphabetized him thus in 1921: "O is for Oille, the dread of the shirkers; / But great admiration he has for the workers. / You answer his question, he'll ask you the 'why.' / You simply can't fool him, so please do not try."[12]

John Oille was born of a Quaker family in 1878 on a farm near the village of Sparta in Elgin County and attended the local village public school before progressing to high school in the Collegiate Institute at St Thomas. After graduating, he taught in public school for five years before commencing medical studies at the U of T, where he graduated in 1903, said to be "one of the clever men of this year's class. [He won the gold medal.] ... Not only so, but his modesty and unassuming manner have deservedly made him one of the most popular members of his year."[13] Indeed he later became one of the most esteemed among his colleagues in medicine. After interning at the General, Oille took up general practice at Byng Inlet, a lumbering settlement on Georgian Bay. Then, having become interested in diseases of the heart, he spent 1911 in London at the Brompton Chest Hospital at a time when Sir James Mackenzie, the founder of modern British cardiology, was in his prime and (as Hugh Segall observes) "Thomas Lewis, at University College, was at the beginning of his distinguished career as a pioneer in electrocardiology," a subject then in its infancy. Oille brought electrocardiology back to Toronto around 1912, securing a junior appointment in the Department of Medicine at TGH. In 1915, he published an article on endocarditis with Duncan Graham and Herbert Detweiler, the first of a number of contributions that would make Oille the "senior cardiologist" in Canada by the 1940s and the second president of the Canadian Heart Association.[14] In Toronto, he is considered "the first cardiologist on the University staff" and "one of the most dynamic teachers the Faculty ever had."[15] He retired in 1944 but returned to duty later to help reform the curriculum (see chapter 27).

Andrew R. Gordon might have been considered a co-founder of cardiology in Toronto, had he not died in 1916 at an early age. A U of T graduate in 1890, Gordon studied for a year in Edinburgh and London, then entered practice. He enjoyed great success as a family physician, yet in 1913 decided to train further in internal medicine and spent another year abroad, "perfecting himself particularly in disease of the heart, to which special work he proposed to devote his life." Alas, fate intervened. He went to war in May 1915, then was invalided home. In the spring of 1916 he fell from a horse and died in December that year of his injuries.[16]

Among the earliest electrocardiographers was Ross Alex Jamieson, born in Mount Forrest in 1883. After graduating from high school there, in the fall of 1903 he entered arts in Toronto at Trinity College, then began medical studies and received his degree in 1910. After interning at the Hospital for Sick Children, in 1914–15 he trained at several institutions in New York, among them the Hospital of the Rockefeller Institute, working with Alfred E. Cohn, one of the pioneers of modern cardiology. He stepped forward in World War I, then joined the Toronto General Hospital in 1919. In 1921 he bought his own electrocardiograph and doubtless kept it in his office in the Medical Arts Building on St George Street.[17]

A whole generation of notable cardiologists flourished in Toronto between the wars. A third member of the triad beside Oille and Jamieson, who all would attend meetings together, was John Hepburn. In Segall's recollection, Hepburn "was somewhat taller than the others and walked with a military gait [he had been in the war]. As the trio approached, he was noticed first. His rather florid complexion and wiry constitution gave one the impression of a man with considerable physical and mental reserves."[18] A Scotsman, Hepburn was born in Glasgow in 1888 and went to high school in the Orkney Islands, where his father was the principal. He began medical studies in Edinburgh but gave it up after the second year and came to Canada in 1909 to resume in Toronto, graduating with an MB in 1921 after many adventures. He was wounded in the war at Lens in 1917. He chose as his motto for the class yearbook, "Here was a Caesar; when comes such another? Never, Never."[19] After working for a year with Macleod while Banting and Best were busy with insulin, he trained at TGH and was singled out for promotion by Duncan Graham, who appointed him to the teaching staff in 1923, "just two years after his graduation," as Hepburn's eulogist noted. "Dr Hepburn quickly acquired a great reputation for his clear, incisive and highly informative teaching, his penetrating wit, his intensely practical knowledge of medicine and his excellence as a physician."[20]

Hepburn took part in early studies of insulin, "frequently taking blood from patients for blood sugar determinations at one or two hour intervals day and night." In 1926 Hepburn and Jamieson reported the importance of electrocardiograph (ECG) findings in determining prognosis; previous studies had concerned mainly the arrhythmias, where prognosis was not difficult to establish. ECG, they said, foretold prognosis when the T-waves were negative in any of the three leads then in use. Also, "[s]igns of bundle-branch block would appear to be the most serious electrocardiographic abnormality." Finally, "low voltage … is a prognostic sign of serious import."[21] In 1935 Hepburn and Harold Rykert described, in a much-cited article, the distinctive electrocardiographic abnormalities in left ventricular hypertrophy secondary to hypertension.[22]

Hepburn, like many of the Scotsmen on the faculty, had a reputation for acerbic humour. This anecdote comes from 1934:

Hepburn: "What is the cause of cancer?"
Student: "I – I – did know – but I've forgotten."
Hepburn: "What a pity! The only man that ever knew the cause of cancer – and he's forgotten it!"[23]

Barney Berris remembered that Hepburn was "very tough and direct and demanded perfection, which was sometimes difficult to obtain." But Hepburn did help Berris get his private practice started. Berris found Hepburn, distinguished though he might have been, as somehow typical of the closed-mindedness of the Department of Medicine before the 1960s. During a staff discussion of a patient hemolyzing his blood during an episode of pneumonia, Berris volunteered, "I saw a similar case when I was in Minneapolis."

Hepburn, who was the ward chief, interrupted and said, "We are not interested in what you saw in Minneapolis. If you like, you can go to the record room and see what our experience has been with cases like this in Toronto."[24]

A younger generation then came on line. Harold E. Rykert, from Dundas, Ontario, got his medical degree in 1928 and was summoned by Duncan Graham to join the department. As mentioned, in 1935 Rykert and Hepburn collaborated in an important ECG study. In 1946 Rykert authored an early contribution on penicillin dosing in subacute bacterial endocarditis, a crippling disease; penicillin had just become available to the civilian population. "In the majority of cases ... a daily dosage of 200,000 units of penicillin for a period of 28 days is considered an adequate course of treatment."[25] Of this research Graham said, "Prior to the discovery of penicillin no form of treatment cured this disease and over 95 per cent of patients died in from one to three years ... Our results, which are in agreement with those obtained in the United States and Great Britain, show that the infection can be arrested in about 50 per cent of the cases."[26]

William Greenwood is remembered for having resolved around 1948 the dispute between Gordon Murray and Graham over heparin. Murray, of course, thought it safe and effective given that he had introduced it clinically; Graham thought it dangerous, and, as historian Shelley McKellar points out, "prevented Murray from administering heparin treatment to any patient on his medical wards."[27] Greenwood reviewed all the patients with an arterial embolus at the General between 1938 and 1948: of the 310 patients, in those who had been heparinized after an embolus in the femoral artery, only 13 percent developed gangrene as a complication; of those receiving Graham's standard "medical treatment," 42 percent developed gangrene. Murray and heparin were vindicated. Greenwood later told Bill Bigelow, "After I presented this study to the staff, there was no more argument about how a femoral embolus should be treated."[28] Greenwood himself was born in 1913, attended Ridley College (a private boarding school) in St Catharines, graduated in Biological and Medical Sciences from Trinity College in 1934, and finished his medical degree in 1937.

Ramsay Gunton's main interest was hemodynamics, or patterns of blood flow through the heart, and he is recalled for having pioneered left heart catheterization in Canada to determine the degree of mitral insufficiency. The first major publication of this work was in 1962.[29] He is also remembered at the General, rather tongue-in-cheek, for "Gunton's sign" to describe the grossly enlarged hearts seen in x-rays of early cardiac patients. Bigelow said on "Gunton's sign," "If your heart is as big as your head, you're in trouble."[30] Gunton was born in Lexington, Kentucky, but studied medicine in Canada, graduating with an MD from the University of Western Ontario in 1945. He interned at the Montreal General Hospital, where his primary interest changed from surgery to cardiology. He was a Rhodes Scholar and received a doctoral degree from Oxford in 1949, trained in cardiology in Toronto, then joined the Division of Cardiology at the General in 1953.

Space was desperately short. The TGH cardiologists performed cardiac catheterization in the radiology department of the Wellesley from 1946 until a patient donation and the support of the Ontario Heart Foundation made it possible to open a new cardiovascular unit in 1956 in "Bigelow's Bungalow" (see pp. 94–95).

The year 1956 thus marks the beginning of the actual division of cardiology. The Ontario Heart Foundation funded a full-time appointment for Gunton and paid the salaries of technicians whom staffers had previously often funded from their own pockets. This marked the opening of the "cardiovascular research laboratory," funded as well by donations from John McFayden and John Frame of Toronto and by a National Health Grant. The laboratory was shared by the Departments of Medicine and Surgery. January 1962 saw the formal opening of an expanded version of TGH's cardiovascular unit, of which Douglas Wigle became director in 1964. The opening occurred at the same time the Royal College initiated a fellowship for cardiovascular and thoracic surgery.[31]

Simultaneously in 1962 the Toronto cardiologists scored a big first: Robert L. MacMillan and Kenneth W.G. Brown opened the first coronary intensive care unit in the world.[32] MacMillan, the senior of the two, was born in Toronto in 1917 into a medical family; his father was an anesthetist at the Wellesley Hospital and his mother a nurse. MacMillan attended high school in Switzerland and the University of Toronto Schools, and he and his brother, in the words of journalist Sandra Martin, "were both burly and very athletic and were known as Big Beef and Little Beef."[33] He attended Trinity College at the University of Toronto, then studied medicine, graduating in 1941. After service in the war, he took postgraduate studies in London and Oxford and upon returning to Toronto held a fellowship in pathology. He then trained in medicine at the General, becoming a Fellow of the Royal College in 1948. (Noted Canadian author Margaret MacMillan is his daughter.)

Brown, too, hailed from Toronto, born in 1923 and a medical graduate of U of T in 1946. He took all of his postgraduate training in Toronto. His father was a pharmacist, and medical matters such as heart disease were often the subject of dinner table conversation.

"When the unit opened on March 12, 1962," said MacMillan's eulogist, "four patients were attached to improvised electro-cardiogram machines to record every beat of their hearts. Nurses became expert at recognizing complications and instituting life-saving procedures while waiting for doctors to arrive. After a year, this team approach and quick interventions to adjust or restart heartbeat rhythm had reduced the death rate by 10 per cent." Douglas Wigle said that the significance of the coronary unit was "huge."[34] When Brown and MacMillan admitted their first patient to the new coronary care unit, Brown said, "We did not know what to expect from this approach but it appears now that this type of care has made some definite improvement in the mortality figures for this dread disease."[35]

In 1966 Gunton left for the University of Western Ontario, but the investigation of cardiac disease had been well launched. Said Greenwood, "It is very unusual for our surgeons to be presented with a case of valvular disease or other types of acquired or congenital heart disease in which the diagnosis is not substantially correct."[36] In 1966 Greenwood became director of the division.

By the 1970s, the cardiology division had acquired an imposing reputation in Canada and beyond. For their seven postgraduate positions in 1974, the division received twenty-six applications – sixteen of them from outside Ontario. Scientifically, bridging basic and clinical research was very much on, hampered only by a lack of space.[37]

In 1972 E. Douglas Wigle succeeded Greenwood as division director. Wigle, one of the major scientific figures in the division, was born in Windsor in 1928 and educated at the University of Toronto, receiving his MD in 1953 and his fellowship in the Royal College in 1958. His cardiology career at the General began in 1959 as a McLaughlin fellow in cardiology. He remained at TGH, becoming professor of medicine in 1972 and at the same time division director. Wigle pioneered the study of hypertrophic cardiomyopathy, "as common as cystic fibrosis and ... the most common cause of sudden death during athletic endeavour in young people."[38] Under Wigle's leadership interventional cardiology blossomed in the division.

What did not blossom in the division – or blossomed late – was any sense of belonging to a campus community as opposed to a hospital affiliation. In September 1979 Gunton, now at the University of Western Ontario, was asked to review the division. He found, "There is no sense of identity with or loyalty to a University division of Cardiology. Cohesion is sought by scheduling of two types of inter-hospital conferences or seminars, but these are academic, not administrative vehicles. Administrative union when it occurs, takes the form of the annual 'dog fight' among directors for residents."[39]

In 1986 Peter R. McLaughlin (a U of T medical graduate in 1970) took the baton as division director from Wigle, who had served for fourteen years. Under McLaughlin there were major changes. The year he took office a cardiovascular planning committee was struck to consider the future of cardiology and cardiovascular surgery at The Toronto Hospital. In May 1987 the Faculty Research Committee approved the plan of the cardiovascular planning committee: Michael Sole, director of the university Division of Cardiology, told them "that the concept of a Cardiovascular Research Centre was not new, but that previous proposals in the later 1970s for co-ordinating activities in the cardiovascular area were unsuccessful ... The current proposal was triggered in part by the re-organization of cardiology at The Toronto Hospital following the merger of the Toronto General Hospital and the Toronto Western Hospital, and a fund-raising campaign being launched by The Toronto Hospital in which cardiovascular research has been identified as a priority."[40] The financing fell into place in November 1987 when Vickery Stoughton, president of The Toronto Hospital, appeared at a meeting of the Research Program Advisory Committee and pledged $10 million from the generation fund for the centre. Dean Burrow committed $2.5 million under his jurisdiction, in addition to the salaries contributed by the university.[41] The centre opened in March 1989 with Sole as the director and cardiac surgeon Richard Weisel as associate director. Sole, excited at the prospect, told Peter McLaughlin, chair of the executive committee of the new centre, "Peter, the development of a Centre for Cardiovascular Research has been my dream for the past decade."[42]

In 1999 Michael Sole expanded the original Centre for Cardiovascular Research with a joint donation of $13 million from the Heart & Stroke Foundation of Ontario and the family of Richard Lewar, into the Heart and Stroke Richard Lewar Centre of Excellence for cardiovascular research at the University of Toronto, with offices in the FitzGerald Building. He was succeeded by Peter Liu. The director of the centre reported to the dean of the Faculty of Medicine. The centre intended to bring cardiovascular research at the university together, introducing, as some called it, the Age of Molecular Cardiology.

Simultaneously the spotlight returned to cardiovascular care at the University Health Network, where the hearts of many were set upon a full-blown heart institute, concentrating resources from cardiology, nursing, cardiovascular surgery, and other disciplines. The organizers noted the many contributions to knowledge that previous cardiac researchers at U of T had made. Yet "despite these very considerable successes, research in the cardiovascular sciences at the University of Toronto falls short of its potential – its whole is less than the sum of its parts." In the 1960s and 1970s the faculty had been able to recruit "many gifted investigators, providing a broad base of expertise for our health sciences center. However, the lack of structure for interdisciplinary communication and coordination often led to a myriad of individual projects, uncoordinated with each other – resulting in lost opportunity." The authors said that basic scientists were hived off in the Medical Sciences Building, remote from the clinic. "This fractured an important interface – that between those in applied research and those doing basic work." But now the structure of knowledge had changed. "New times call for new approaches. The explosion of knowledge in the cardiovascular sciences makes it a formidable task for individual investigators ... to cope with the resulting flood of literature." Clearly, the time for a heart centre had come.[43]

In 1997 Peter Munk donated $6 million to the Toronto General Hospital for the creation of a cardiac centre, to be named after him. Munk followed this donation in 2006 with $37 million, the largest gift ever made to a Canadian medical institution, to help support the Peter Munk Cardiac Centre.

## Division of Respirology (Respiratory Medicine)

The background of the founding of a respiratory division was a polio epidemic in Ontario in the 1950s, creating a need to ventilate the many young victims suffering respiratory paralysis. This was the beginning of the concept of "critical care" in Canada.[44] "One afternoon in 1957," said anesthetist Barrie Fairley, "Richard Chambers – a British-trained neurologist – came to talk to me about setting up a different arrangement for managing paralysed patients with diseases such as Guillain Barré syndrome or poliomyelitis." The routine had previously been to put the patient in an "iron lung" and to manage their aspirated saliva with ENT (ear, nose, and throat) surgery that would try to clear the airway by bronchoscopy. "The mortality was horrendous," Fairley said.

Chambers had trained at Queen Square and was familiar with "intermittent positive pressure respiration" that an anesthetist had introduced there (inflating the lungs with positive pressure rather than lowering the air pressure around the body – as the iron lung did). Chambers and Fairley agreed to establish a service at the General employing this principle of intermittent positive pressure ventilation, staffed by a full-time team of specialized nurses and physicians. They used a ventilator tube inserted through a tracheostomy rather than reducing the air pressure around the body. The service was organized in 1958. Colin Woolf, a respirologist, and Hugh Barber, an ENT surgeon, agreed to come on board. The hospital wanted a senior member of the Department of Medicine in charge of the show and appointed Bill Oille chair of the "Poliomyelitis Committee," although Oille had little to do with the actual operation of the unit.[45]

Farquharson, under whose aegis as head of medicine this development was taking place, opined that the service "has greatly improved the treatment of patients with respiratory paralysis from various neurological disorders ... serious traumatic injuries of the chest, with barbiturate and other types of poisoning, tetanus, etc."[46] In 1959 the four members of the unit said that, of twenty-one patients to date, sixteen have left hospital "and returned to their usual occupations"; three others have left hospital for further investigation. "Even in patients apparently dying, the institution of adequate ventilation by the methods described usually leads to striking improvement and eventual return to a normal life. Accordingly," the article concluded, "we have had to revise our criteria of 'hopelessness' in such cases."[47] This was an encouraging note.

Colin Woolf, among the central figures in the new unit, began directing the Tri-hospital Respiratory Service in 1963. He had earned his medical degree in 1947 at the University of Cape Town in South Africa and trained at the Brompton Hospital in London and the chest service of Bellevue Hospital in New York before coming to the General in 1955 as a research associate of the Ontario Heart Foundation. When he first suggested starting a program for pulmonary function, Farquharson told him, "We don't need a laboratory for this. I can get as much information as I need about a patient's pulmonary function by walking up the back stairs with him."[48] After Woolf was finally appointed to staff, he was among the organizers of the respiratory unit, marking the birth in 1958 of the Division of Respirology. Griff Pearson was a consultant.

In 1967 the Joint Hospitals Committee agreed to the Ontario Health Services Commission's proposal that this would be the regional "respiratory failure unit."[49] It later became the "respiratory care unit" under anesthetist Arthur Scott and chest surgeon Joel Cooper, who helped develop a membrane oxygenator to support respiration during surgery for pulmonary embolism or lung transplantation.[50]

The division remained, however, rather anemic. When the Division of Respirology responded in the 1972–3 session to a survey ("Petch committee"), Eliot Phillipson, writing on behalf of the group, said, "No respirology research at 5 teaching hospitals (SBH, WH, WCH, SMH, and PMH)." (He might also have added New Mount Sinai Hospital to the list.) "The respirology group was rather discouraged when this research survey was conducted. Some excellent research was in progress in the Medical Science Building, but there was little communication between investigators." The report continued, "It has been proposed that a respirology group be formed to coordinate and promote interdisciplinary research, and to recruit additional personnel ... Also, we need to avoid duplication of research. We have a number of labs capable of conducting research in pulmonary mechanics," but nothing on lung metabolism, such as on surfactant (a chemical secreted into the lung alveoli that makes lung tissue more elastic).[51] In 1973 Hollenberg, now head of medicine, drove this inadequacy home by calling the respiratory disease program "one of the weakest programs that the Department operates."[52]

These deficiencies were remedied with new leadership. Although Colin Woolf remained the legacy figure in respirology (he was in director of the Tri-Hospital Respiratory Service), Anthony Rebuck became division coordinator. Then in 1979 Michael A. Hutcheon at the Wellesley Hospital took the baton as coordinator of the faculty respirology division. He chaired the Respirology Committee, the main responsibility of which was postgraduate training. Shortly thereafter in 1979, a site assessor from the University of Manitoba gave the division significantly better marks. Of research, he said of the Toronto General Hospital, mentioning Rebuck, Noe Zamel, and Elliot Phillipson, "This is probably about as good a set-up as presently exists in Canada." He waxed ecstatic about the service at the Sinai: "This hospital's major asset ... is its ICU and the presence there of Doctor Aberman, a splendid teacher. This unit could probably function as an alternative to the Toronto General Hospital unit in so far as training is concerned."[53]

In 1983, Eliot Phillipson, an Alberta graduate in 1963 and later professor and head of the Department of Medicine, was appointed division director of the university Division of Respirology. Phillipson sorts out the competencies: "I continued in this role until 1989, when Arthur Slutsky succeeded me, who was followed several years later by Greg Downey. Colin Woolf had served as the coordinator for the respiratory training program until the time of my appointment, when the position of coordinator was subsumed by the new position of division director. Colin continued to serve as head of the Respiratory Division within the Toronto General. In 1986 Colin stepped down from this position, and I was appointed division head at TGH, but in 1987 I moved to Mount Sinai as physician-in-chief. Michael Hutcheon, who headed the division at the Wellesley Hospital, was recruited to TGH to succeed me as head of the Division."[54] It was thus Woolf who moved the fourteen-bed pulmonary unit from the College Wing to the tenth floor of the Norman Urquhart East Building, where they could consult closely on lung transplants.

Phillipson was also keen on boosting research in the division and on liaising with the Respiratory Service at the Hospital for Sick Children to make possible a smooth transition of their fibrocystic patients (an overgrowth of fibrous tissue into cystic spaces in the lung) once they reached the age of eighteen and could no longer be cared for in a children's hospital. "Post polio syndrome" was still an issue in Toronto, and Phillipson boosted "positive pressure" ventilation in the pulmonary unit.[55]

Further services were added to what became in 1994 the Division of Respiratory Medicine. By 1986–7 an ambulatory asthma and occupational lung disease clinic was being run by the British-trained researcher Susan Tarlo. Janet Maurer, a Minnesota graduate (1976) directed the transplant program; Eliot Phillipson and T. Douglas Bradley were studying respiratory sleep disorders, together with Harvey Moldofsky, a notable sleep researcher, at the Western. Important science began to flow from the pulmonary unit (which by 1988–9 was being called the Respiratory Therapy Department).

In 1985 Bradley joined the division, focusing on the relationship between sleep apnea, or transient cessation of breathing during sleep, and cardiovascular disease. A 1978 medical graduate of the University of Alberta, Bradley trained in medicine in Toronto, then fellowed at Toronto and McGill on the relationship between sleep apnea and respiratory muscle physiology. He directed the Sleep Research Laboratory at the Toronto Rehabilitation Institute and the Centre for Sleep Medicine and Circadian Biology at the university. In 1989 Bradley and colleagues reported that nasal continuous positive airway pressure relieved sleep apnea and improved cardiac function in congestive heart failure.[56] He also pioneered the study of the relationship between sleep apnea and congestive heart failure, among other cardiac conditions.[57]

Arthur Slutsky picked up on the work of Griff Pearson on respirator-induced injuries by demonstrating the pathogenesis of ventilator-induced lung injury. He initiated a clinical trial published in 1999 in the *Journal of the American Medical Association* showing that high frequency oscillation (HFO) – "a subtype of high-frequency ventilation that provides pressure oscillations around a relatively constant mean airway pressure, delivering very small tidal volumes at high respiratory rates" – offers superior lung protection.[58] In 2000 Slutsky became vice president of research at St Michael's Hospital yet continued with his scientific work, and in 2002 his group determined the mechanism in the lung epithelium of injurious ventilation: an increase in the expression of tumour necrosis factor-alpha and of interleukin-6.[59] Although technical-sounding, this work held out the promise of less lung injury during ventilation.

### Division of Endocrinology

In 1933 Robert Cleghorn joined the Department of Medicine, thus founding endocrine research in Toronto. Cleghorn was born in Cambridge, Massachusetts, in 1904. He studied medicine at the University of Toronto – where he was a big athletic manager and sports writer – graduating in 1928. After a rotating internship at the General, he went to Aberdeen, Scotland, where he earned a doctor of science degree in 1932, also working as an assistant in the Department of Physiology under Macleod. He returned to Toronto as a demonstrator in the Department of Medicine and, after military service, in 1946 definitively left Toronto for McGill, making a great name for himself in the budding field of psychosomatic medicine. As Cleghorn was appointed at U of T in 1933, the dean noted, "He is interested in a study of the relationship between disturbances of the endocrine glands and the development of nervous disorders."[60]

The time was propitious for such a study because the hormones of the adrenal cortex were just being isolated and identified by various labs including the Connaught. In 1937 Cleghorn composed an initial report on the treatment of adrenalectomized dogs with an adrenal extract.[61] In 1938–9 the Ciba company in Basel sent Cleghorn and colleagues a sample of the synthetic adrenal cortical hormone, desoxycorticosterone. Cleghorn treated nine Addisonian patients with it, with indifferent results. He wrote in 1940, quite presciently, "We anticipate that the chemist will yet place at the disposal of the clinician chemical substances which will permit even fuller substitution therapy than so far has obtained in the treatment of Addison's disease."[62] This was the beginning of endocrine research in Toronto.

After Cleghorn's departure, endocrine interests in Toronto resumed in autumn 1949 with the erection of "a newly equipped laboratory for the study of steroid chemistry and its clinical application," directed by Allan Gornall, a Nova Scotian born in 1914 who, after a bachelor's degree at Mount Allison University, earned a PhD in pathological chemistry, or clinical chemistry, in Toronto in 1941. After service in the navy, in 1946 Gornall became a lecturer in the Department of Pathological Chemistry, with particular interest in endocrines. As the new lab, supported by the National Research Council, was announced, Gornall was on leave from the university on a Nuffield Fellowship, working with Guy F. Marrian, professor of biochemistry at Edinburgh, who intended to visit Toronto "to guide the work." Dean MacFarlane commented, "This laboratory will be devoted to the study ... of fundamental and clinical problems in the realm of endocrinology and it is hoped that it will serve a very useful purpose, not only as a research laboratory, but also as a source of stimulus and information for all those who are interested in the endocrine field."[63] Gornall worked closely with clinicians in the Department of Medicine and should probably be considered the founder of clinical interest in the endocrine system, even though he was not medically trained.

In 1950 an isotope laboratory was created in the Banting Building to serve TGH under James Dauphinee.[64] By the 1950–1 session, internists Almon Fletcher and Dauphinee began research with Gornall on adrenocorticotrophic hormone (ACTH), which had just been isolated and synthesized. Interest in endocrines was flaring. But the seminal figure in the Division of Endocrinology was Jack Laidlaw, who was introduced in the previous chapter. In 1949, while still at the Department of Biochemistry of University College London, he had published an article in *Nature* which showed that thyroxine rather than a thyroxine-containing peptide was the circulating thyroid hormone.[65] In the early 1950s, while serving as director of the metabolic unit at the Peter Bent Brigham Hospital in Boston under George Thorn, Laidlaw and Thorn had published a series of articles on the adrenocorticoid steroids (the steroid hormones, such as cortisol, manufactured by the core tissue of the adrenal gland).

"That was the very beginning of the cortisone-ACTH era," Laidlaw said in an interview. "We were giving cortisone-ACTH for practically every disease that required some new therapy that you could think of. Oh, there was enormous ferment." Thorn, said Laidlaw, was "appointed to his chair at age 32. Can you imagine?"[66]

After Laidlaw returned to Toronto, in 1956 he set up a metabolic unit, or clinical investigation unit, at the General, on the model of Ward 4 of the Massachusetts General Hospital. This was the de facto founding of the Division of Endocrinology. "We ended up in the basement in Ward G, an eight-bed unit, with our own nurses, and our own dietitian and so on." They measured urinary sodium, "collecting 24-hour urines, and we had put the patients on a constant diet so we knew that the sodium intake was the same every day. And we noticed on certain days there was sodium retention. Well, one of my fellows said, 'Don't you realize, those are the Stanley cup nights?'" The stress of watching the hockey game was causing aldosterone release which in turn caused sodium retention.[67]

From 1953 to 1958, Laidlaw was a Markle Scholar in medical science, which gave him time and funds for research. The first publication to come from his work in Toronto, with pediatrician Donald Fraser, concerned the treatment of hypophosphatasia – a genetic deficiency of alkaline phosphatase – with cortisone, in 1956 in the *Lancet*.[68] In 1960 he, Edmund Yendt, and Gornall discovered that hypertension simulating primary aldosteronism came in reality from occlusion of the renal artery.[69] In 1966 he, Donald Sutherland, and two other investigators discovered there was a subpopulation of genetically determined hypertensives with low serum potassium that responded to the administration of the artificial steroid dexamethasone.[70] In 1970 Laidlaw became head of the Division of Endocrinology and Metabolism at the General.

In touch with Toronto's long tradition of diabetes research, in the late 1970s Bernard Zinman at TGH joined Walter Zingg, then a surgeon at the Hospital for Sick Children (and after 1978 director of the Institute of Biomedical Engineering), and A. Michael Albisser, a PhD in biomedical engineering, in developing an artificial pancreas.[71] From 1993 to 2000 Zinman directed the Banting and Best Diabetes Centre, and in 2000 he became director of the Leadership Sinai Centre for Diabetes. In 1983 Zinman commenced leadership of the Diabetes Control and Complications Trial, the largest diabetes study ever conducted in type 1 diabetes. Funded by the National Institute of Diabetes and Digestive and Kidney Diseases of NIH, the study randomized 1,441 patients with insulin-dependent diabetes mellitus to intensive or conventional therapy and treated them for a mean of 6.5 years. The study found that continuous insulin therapy greatly reduced serious complications of diabetes.[72] This had a worldwide impact on the management of the disease. (On the work of Edmund Yendt in the division see chapter 8.)

Calvin Ezrin was among the earliest scholars of Jewish origin to come on staff in the Department of Medicine. Ezrin, born in Toronto in 1926, received his medical degree from U of T in 1949 and trained in internal medicine and pathology at the General. He became a research associate in the Division of Neuropathology of the pathology department in 1953, then joined the Department of Medicine in 1959 (leaving the faculty in 1977 for UCLA). In 1954 Ezrin and William D. Wilson distinguished among three types of chromophil (easily stainable) cells in the anterior pituitary gland, a significant contribution to understanding the working of that organ.[73] Ezrin led "the first group to show that the intractable diarrhoea without ulceration was due to gastric stimulation caused by the gastrin-like hormone produced by a [non-beta] type of islet cell tumour."[74] (Islet cells, of course, are in the pancreas and secrete insulin.)

A triumph for the division issued in 1960: MacAllister Johnston's work, with others, on radioiodine in the treatment of hyperthyroidism. Johnston began the research in 1950 and published the definitive report with Robert Volpé as first author on New Year's Eve in 1960.[75] The use of radioactive iodine in treatment of hyperthyroidism goes back to researchers in 1942 who they got their I-130 isotopes from cyclotrons "usually at great cost, and frequently in such form as to require considerable chemical manipulation before they could be used." The TGH group, by contrast, was first to use I-131 from a nuclear reactor.[76]

In the 1960 work on radioactive treatments of hyperthyroid, Robert Volpé was a key figure. Bob Volpé was born in Toronto in 1926, and after Harbord Collegiate – and wartime service – he studied medicine at U of T, graduating in 1950. He trained as an internist, completed a fellowship in pathology, and was an endocrine research fellow from 1955 to 1957. He served as director of the Endocrine Division of the Wellesley Hospital from 1965 to 1974, thereafter being chief physician. From 1987 to 1992 he directed the university's endocrine division. In 1972 he argued for Graves' disease as an immune disorder and said, "Such an explanation might also explain the close association among Hashimoto's disease, Graves' disease, and pernicious anemia. These disorders tend to occur in the same patients and their families. The appearance of these diseases may depend on two variables: the extent of the inherited defect in immunologic surveillance ... and the chance mutation of the appropriate clone."[77] (When asked by an interviewer why he didn't move up to molecular genetics in studying thyroid disorder, Volpé said about himself and collaborator Paul Walfish, "I didn't think we were 'big time'; others did better work. I stayed with the immunology because it was a relatively small effort in terms of fiscal resources and I could encompass it. The Canadian MRC was always my sponsor, and you always had to think of how much they would give ... and how much they would spend on thyroid disease."[78] This is an interesting comment on the difficulties in those days of doing big research in a small country.

The endocrinologists at Mount Sinai Hospital were among the most active research groups. Paul Walfish became a leader in international thyroidology, pioneering techniques for the early detection of thyroid cancers. Walfish, a 1958 medical graduate of the University of Toronto, specialized in medicine, then, after receiving a McLaughlin Foundation Fellowship, studied endocrinology for a year at Harvard. He joined the staff of Mount Sinai Hospital in 1964 and in 1976 led a team that proposed a schematic flow diagram for hyper- and hypofunctioning thyroid nodules. The chart – incorporating radioisotope scintiscanning, echography by B-mode ultrasonography, aspiration of the nodule with needles of various sizes, and cytologic examination of the aspirate – became widely adopted in the management of thyroid lesions.[79]

The later evolution of the division under Dan Drucker and then, after 2001, George Fantus takes the story too far afield here, given that it is bound up with the development of molecular medicine. It is, however, of interest to note that Laidlaw and Volpé were very much barons of the faculty and involved in decisions discussed in later chapters.

On balance, the division was among the academic stalwarts of the faculty. Two site visitors commented in April 1979, "The University of Toronto Training Program in Endocrinology is, undoubtedly, currently unmatched in breadth and depth anywhere in the country. It surely compares favourably with any centre on this continent and has the potential to be pre-eminent in North America."[80]

### Division of Gastroenterology

Gastroenterology is among the oldest subspecialties of internal medicine. As early as 1915, the Toronto General Hospital had a gastrointestinal (GI) department, headed by Frederic Whitney Rolph,[81] a 1905 U of T graduate born in 1880 in Markham, Ontario; Rolph had first taken an arts degree at Trinity University (Trinity College). What predisposed him to the study of gastroenterology is unknown, but he counts as the founder of the subspecialty in Toronto. In 1932, the GI clinic at the General became one of the hospital's "follow-up clinics," and the patients were deemed of sufficient interest to merit several scholarly papers.[82]

After the Second World War, there was as yet no division of gastroenterology. Yet several internists at the General had begun to specialize in research in the subject, such as Ernest J. Maltby, studying diseases of the biliary tract. Maltby was born in 1898 in Iberville, Quebec; he moved to Toronto in 1912 and graduated from Humberside Collegiate in 1917. He served overseas with a heavy artillery unit, was wounded, and "got a Blighty," meaning that he was invalided home, in 1918.[83] Maltby graduated in medicine in 1924, won his fellowship in the Royal College, and came on staff at the General, where GI medicine was among the areas he studied. Likewise his younger colleague Jonathan C. Sinclair, born in 1908, qualified with the Royal College as an internist (after finishing a medical degree in 1933); in the mid-1930s Sinclair was a research fellow in the Department of Therapeutics, and in the Department of Medicine he worked in gastroenterology; liver disease became his main interest.

Youngest of the gastroenterologists at the General was John M. Finlay, who obtained his medical degree from U of T in 1947, became a Fellow of the Royal College and a clinical instructor of the faculty at the General. By the 1954–5 session, Farquharson was listing a section on "gastroenterology" in the research part of the annual report of the Department of Medicine.[84]

The gastroenterologists in the Department of Medicine had a long-standing curiosity about fat absorption, going back to Wightman himself, who had a big interest in gastrointestinal medicine.[85] Caroline Hetenyi at Women's College Hospital, who graduated in medicine in Budapest in 1947 but passed her Royal College fellowship in Canada, continued this tradition.

The Toronto Western Hospital also developed as a centre of GI research, and here the central figure was John R. Bingham, who earned his medical degree in Manitoba in 1940 and after military service won his Royal College fellowship. He worked further at the Massachusetts General Hospital and in 1950, together with Franz Ingelfinger (later editor of the *New England Journal of Medicine*) and Reginald Smithwick, was senior author of a paper on sympathectomy (cutting part of the nerve supply) and the gastrointestinal tract.[86] Bingham had a strong interest in gastrointestinal motility, which he pursued after a donation from Elsie Watt made possible the establishment of a GI research centre at the Western in the 1962–3 session.

It was in 1968 that one of the major figures in Canadian gastroenterology came to the University of Toronto: Khursheed N. Jeejeebhoy ("Jeej"). Born in Rangoon, in what was then Burma, in 1935, Jeejeebhoy graduated in medicine in Madras, India, in 1959; he passed his fellowship from the Royal College of

Physicians of London in 1961, gaining a PhD in clinical gastroenterology in 1963. He tutored in gastroenterology in London at the Royal Postgraduate Medical School from 1961 to 1963, returned to India in the area of radiation therapy, then immigrated to Canada and in 1968 joined the University of Toronto as an assistant professor. He had an appointment in the Department of Nutrition but in 1975 became a professor of gastroenterology in the Department of Medicine. In 1990 Jeejeebhoy joined the staff of St Michael's Hospital.

Jeejeebhoy modified total parenteral nutrition (TPN), a technique originated experimentally in dogs by Stanley Dudrick in Houston in 1966;[87] TPN means receiving all of one's nourishment from a tube surgically implanted into one of the major vessels and brought back to the surface of the skin just under the clavicle. Jeejeebhoy conceived this innovation in 1970 – two years after Dudrick's first human interventions – when he saw a patient named J.E.T., a thirty-six-year-old housewife who had developed severe abdominal pain and underwent surgery. All did not go well, and she was left with only a stomach, duodenum, and descending colon, unable to absorb food from the gut or to digest it in the absence of small and large bowel and gallbladder. Her weight dropped from 140 to 113 pounds and she was "profoundly malnourished." Yet she could be nourished by injecting nutrients into her veins, and on 6 October 1970, Jeejeebhoy at the Division of Gastroenterology and the Banting and Best Department of Medical Research set her up with a series of bottles containing casein, glucose lipid emulsion, and other ingredients that flowed into her bloodstream using a pneumatic pressure system. Jeejeebhoy adopted Dudrick's term "total parenteral nutrition." "Currently," he wrote in 1973, "after 23 months on home alimentation (32 months total), she is a clinically healthy, active mother of three children, capable of most normal domestic and social functions."[88] Jeejeebhoy's daughter Shireen described this story in *Lifeliner*, published in 1973.

Bernie Langer, who headed the general surgery division of the Department of Surgery, was in on these events. It was Langer who operated on Mrs J.E.T. after she had lost her small bowel, and he remembers that Jeejeebhoy "was trying to keep her alive on TPN, and he was doing very well, but he had to send her home. So I [Langer] developed a delivery system to provide her with the TPN at home. I went to Neurosurgery and took one of the shunt tubes that were used for patients with hydrocephalus and adapted it, and put it in one of her neck veins and down into her [vena] cava, and she went home on TPN, and she lived with no small bowel at all for something like seven years."[89] TPN thus revolutionized the care of patients who had suffered catastrophic abdominal damage.

Yet with the exception of a couple of bright spots such as this, the gastrointestinal division did not shine in scientific terms. Gastroenterologist Gordon Forstner at the Western, a 1958 U of T graduate who was interested in basic research, told the Petch committee in 1973 that the GI division had "little hospital-based research" except at the Toronto General Hospital. Gastroenterologist Nicholas Diamant at the Western, who worked on esophageal motor function, had no basic researcher in the Department of Physiology with whom to collaborate. Forstner noted, "Virtually all gastrointestinal research takes place at the Medical Sciences Building and is well divorced from the gastrointestinal wards."[90]

Things had changed little by the time of a site visit in 1979. To be sure, the stars such as Jeejeebhoy and Diamant were praised. But "[l]ike many other GI units in Canada and the United States, trainees that have entered the training program have shown little desire to do research." And indeed research in Toronto was even less than "in many of the gastrointestinal centres in the United States and Great Britain."[91]

It was the hepatology unit, founded in 1974 at the General,[92] and the liver transplant service that permitted the division to expand scientifically. In 1987–8 the gastrointestinal division at the General formally divided its attending system into a hepatic service and a hollow gut service. "In this way, a great degree of organization has been implemented in the unit and a formal hepatic service has been initiated." A major clinic is the Home Parenteral Nutrition Clinic. "The other major clinic is the hepatic transplant clinic which is a joint clinic run between physicians and surgeons." "The major special development during the current year [1987–8]," a report said, "has been the development of an active hepatic transplant program [begun in 1985] which is a joint medical/surgical program involving a surgical team led by Dr. Langer and the medical team which is led by Dr. Gary Levy and Dr. [Laurence M.] Blendis. This program has become extremely active and has transplanted 31 patients."[93] (On the surgical side of the liver transplant program, see chapter 7.)

Hepatologist E. Jenny L. Heathcote, a member of the team, made major contributions to research on the genetics of hepatitis[94] and also in 2003 co-authored a popular patients' guide, *Living with Hepatitis C: Everything You Need to Know*.

### Division of Infectious Diseases

In a hospital staffed overwhelmingly with physicians whose origins lay in rural Ontario, it would be fair to say that tropical diseases and parasitology were not major concerns. But Michael Lenczner was born in Italy, trained there and in France and Romania, and in 1939 became consulting physician to several hospitals in Bombay, India. It was in India that he fought during the war on the medical staff of the Royal Army and remained until immigrating to Canada in 1952. In 1966 he founded the Clinic for Tropical Diseases at the Toronto General Hospital. Charles Hollenberg said in a eulogy, "He rapidly became Canada's leading authority in the clinical aspects of parasitic diseases … In the late '50's and early '60's, when he was struggling to establish the Tropical Medicine Clinic at the Toronto General, few members of the profession were aware of the impact that worldwide travel would have on the incidence of tropical disease in Canada. Michael Lenczner not only foresaw this problem but also had the strength of personality to force a development in this field at a time when few other members of the medical community were prepared to support him." Hollenberg called the General Hospital's Clinic for Tropical and Parasitic Disease "one of the outstanding units of its kind in the western world."[95]

Not only because of foreign travel but because of immuno-suppressed patients in the transplant and tumour areas, the division was needed.[96] The infectious disease division was founded as a fully integrated bi-hospital division between the General and the Sinai in 1973 with double directors: John Angus Smith, director of microbiology at the Sinai and Michael Bach at the General. Simultaneously with the founding of the division, a two-year subspecialty training program was introduced, the only one in Ontario, based at the General and the Sinai. Residents cross-trained in microbiology.

All members of the new bi-hospital division were simultaneously appointed in infectious diseases and microbiology. When Smith left for Vancouver in 1977 (and Bach went elsewhere as well), Hillar Vellend, a 1968 U of T graduate and associate professor of medicine and medical microbiology at Mount Sinai Hospital, became acting head and in the following year full-time head of the Division of Infectious Diseases. In 1983 Vellend became the inaugural department division director (DDD), according to the system that Gerard Burrow had established for the Department of Medicine as a whole.[97]

In 1976 Jay Keystone replaced the late Lenczner as director of the Tropical Disease Unit, turning it in a more academic direction. (This unit then became integrated into the Division of Infectious Diseases.)[98]

In the 1984–5 session the division set up an AIDS screening clinic.[99] It was at that time that Donald Low became chair of the Department of Microbiology at Mount Sinai and a member of the infectious disease divisions of both hospitals, helping to bridge microbiology and infectious diseases. Women's College Hospital's affiliation with the division followed shortly, so that infectious diseases became a tri-hospital service and the major Ontario referral centre for AIDS.[100] By the late 1980s the infectious disease divisions of the General and the Sinai were fully integrated under Vellend: the HIV clinic – bolstered by large amounts of provincial funding – directed by Jay Scott and Irving Salit, the tropical diseases unit by Keystone.

When Vellend resigned from the positions as tri-hospital head and DDD in 1988, Salit succeeded him, first as acting head, then in 1991 as full-time head of the tri-hospital division. In 1998 James L. Brunton took on both positions and remained in this dual role until 2006 when Conrad Liles moved from the University of Washington in Seattle, where he worked on cytokines in infection, to become director of the Division of Infectious Diseases.[101]

The McLaughlin-Rotman Centre for Global Health also formed part of the division. The unit was housed in the McLaughlin Centre for Molecular Medicine, on the tenth floor of the MaRS building[102] on College Street, with Kain serving as director. Peter Singer and Abdullah Daar, from medicine and surgery respectively, soon affiliated with it and initiated an international study of infectious disease and bioethics funded by the Medical Research Council.[103]

Thus, life flooded back into the study of infectious diseases. Anita Rachlis, gold medalist from U of T in the class of 1972, was trained in the Toronto infectious diseases program and subsequently mentored by Barney Berris at Mount Sinai as his chief resident. She joined the Department of Medicine at Sunnybrook after earning her Royal College fellowship in 1976. According to Don Cowan, head of medicine at Sunnybrook, "Many of the staff, in all departments had to be persuaded that we needed an ID specialist. These views changed quickly, and within the first year Anita was run off her feet as the various services sought her advice. With the advent of AIDS she ran a large AIDS service at Sunnybrook."[104]

## Division of Nephrology

The Division of Nephrology had its origin in dialysis, which initially was entrusted to the Department of Therapeutics. But in 1966–7 therapeutics became a division of the Department of Medicine, receiving responsibility for the kidney dialysis unit at TGH, just as the facilities for chronic dialysis were being expanded.[105] Then the therapeutics division was discontinued and in 1970 the nephrology division created.[106] By 1973 it had become a "tri-hospital" service, meaning the Toronto General, the Mount Sinai, and Women's College Hospitals.

The new division was soon overwhelmed by dialysis service and had a low scientific profile. The nephrology portion of a Department of Medicine report in 1972–3 deplored the lack of an immunologist in the division and the "lack of coordination of research development within the Division … There are currently no Nephrologists trained in the area of Immunology, the area where most renal disease probably originates. Although there is a larger transplant program in Toronto involving four hospitals (TGH, TWH, SMH, SCH [HSC]), there has been no collaboration and little research coming out of this program. This is to a large degree due to the absence of immunological development." Clinical duties overwhelmed research. "Priorities: We must increase the number of Nephrologists with a major commitment to research," the nephrologists said.[107]

This lack was soon remedied. In 1977 a team at the Toronto Western Hospital led by nephrologist Dimitrios Oreopoulos, and including nephrologist George A. de Veber (whose daughter Gabrielle became a pediatric neurologist and founded the pediatric stroke registry at HSC, see p. 268), simplified and popularized peritoneal dialysis as an alternative to hemodialysis.[108] In peritoneal dialysis (PD) a catheter is surgically implanted in the abdomen and the patient's peritoneum functions as a membrane across which fluids and dissolved substances such as urea are exchanged from the blood; when done at night the procedure is called automatic peritoneal dialysis, during the day continuous ambulatory peritoneal dialysis (CAPD) . Oreopoulos later pointed out that automatic PD is less risky than continuous ambulatory PD "because of the fewer connections it requires and because changes are made in an environment that offers more control of infections."[109] Stephen Vas was a co-author of the paper. Precisely because of the risk of peritonitis, peritoneal dialysis remains less common than hemodialysis, yet these discoveries represented immense contributions.

Oreopoulos earned his medical degree from the University of Athens in 1960 (and a subsequent PhD at the University of Belfast), coming to Canada in 1969; he simplified the technique with use of a single catheter rather than multiple risky perforations in the abdominal wall. He was also the first doctor to treat children with PD.

Stephen Vas (pronounced "Vash"), a microbiologist, is remembered for his 1981 description of "Vas-Peritonitis" (during CAPD).[110] He graduated with an MD from the University of Budapest in 1950, earned a PhD in 1956, and fled Hungary in the same year for Vienna. Vas ended temporarily at McGill, where he became chair of the microbiology department; in 1977 he moved to Toronto as chief of microbiology at TWH.

Governance in nephrology as of the late 1970s was assured by the Nephrology Coordinating Committee (NCC), chaired by the division coordinator with a representative (a division director) from each teaching hospital. A big responsibility was postgraduate education, but the committee endeavoured to coordinate recruitment as well. In terms of coordinating divisional programs across teaching hospitals, the major – and most forward-looking – function of the NCC was the central assignment of patients for dialysis. "On a monthly basis," said Douglas Wilson, the division head in nephrology in 1979, "we assess the number of openings on dialysis programs at the various hospitals and although almost all are usually full, there is the potential to transfer patients or at least refer transient dialysis to units that have space."[111]

In transplantation, city-wide tissue typing and organ procurement occurred through the Metro Organ Retrieval and Exchange Program (MORE).

Procedures such as renal biopsies were performed by the urologists, of whom the nephrology fellows complained bitterly, "It would seem almost as if the aim of the Toronto General Hospital Nephrology Program was *NOT* to teach how to do renal biopsies." Of the hospitals with nephrology programs, the Western won honours as "best organized." Said site assessor Mortimer Levy from McGill University of the Western, "There are clear distinctions in the division of labour between those nephrologists engaged in peritoneal dialysis, hemodialysis and transplantation, and medical nephrology. This is in my opinion a far superior system to that employed at the Toronto General Hospital where everybody does a little bit of everything."[112] This judgment is unsurprising in view of the historic role of the Western in the development of nephrology.

Kidney transplantation raced ahead in Toronto, aided by the MORE Program. At the Toronto Western Hospital, Carl Cardella pioneered the use of rabbit anti-thymocyte serum treatment and the successful transplantation of high-risk patients who had circulating antibodies levels that generally precluded transplantation at the time. Cardella was instrumental in establishing cardiac transplantation at the Toronto Western Hospital in the mid-1980s.[113] In 1983 the nephrology division said, "We carried out 52 kidney transplants in 1982 (a 44% increase) and we are following approximately 170 transplant patients, including our first patient, who celebrated the 15th anniversary of his transplant and continues to feel well ... The overall success rate of kidney transplantation is now slightly above 80%."[114] It was, of course, the urological surgeons who conducted the transplants, but the nephrologists who cared for the patients and followed them.

In 1984 Melvin Silverman – known everywhere as "Mel" – succeeded Douglas Wilson as head of the division. Silverman was part of a cohort of physicians who left McGill in the early 1970s for Toronto, including Charles Hollenberg and Aubie Angel. Born in Montreal in 1940, he earned a bachelor's degree in science from McGill in 1960 and an MD in 1964. After training, he served as an associate research scientist in the Department of Medicine of New York University from 1966 to 1968, then received his fellowship from the Royal College in 1969. Silverman joined the medicine staff of the Montreal General Hospital and the teaching staff of McGill from 1970 to 1971, then left for the Division of Nephrology at the Toronto General Hospital. From 1984 to 1990 he directed the tri-hospital nephrology service, and from 1987 he was the director of the MRC [Medical Research Council] Group in membrane biology at U of T. Given that he also held an appointment as professor of physics, Silverman's interests in nephrology spanned the entire range from basic through translational to clinical research. (The membrane biology group included nephrologists Catharine Whiteside and Karl Skorecki and biochemist Reinhart Reithmeier and was a major research initiative in nephrology.)

In its new quarters in the Gerrard Wing of the General, the dialysis program, under Stan Fenton, now brought together all modes of treating end-stage renal failure, including centre and home dialysis and transplantation. The Centre Hemodialysis program could accommodate up to 66 patients, the Centre Peritoneal Dialysis program 22 patients and another 139 on home dialysis.[115] The transplantation program under Phil Halloran, part of the Multiple Organ Retrieval and Exchange Program of the Toronto General Hospital, averaged around one new transplant per week, with a one-year graft survival rate of 85 percent, said to be the best of any centre in North America. "A major technological improvement in the Transplant Programme took place in October 1984 with the purchase of a creatinine analyzer dedicated for the sole use of the Nephrology Division. [Creatinine is excreted into the urine and its measurement is a direct reflection of kidney function.] With the cooperation of Clinical Biochemistry, this machine is having an enormous impact on our ability to better monitor transplant recipients on an out-patient basis."[116]

In the mid-1980s, the transplant program in lung, heart-lung, liver, and kidney went into high gear. "These transplants have advanced from the stage where they are considered research, to the point where they are now recognized as life-saving operations, " said a TGH report. Small intestine and bone marrow were still considered "research-oriented operations." "The expansion of the Multiple Organ Retrieval Exchange Programme also ties in with the transplant programme." The report continued on the subject of renal dialysis and transplantation, "It is now more probably true than ever before that all clinical activities are highly integrated between the Toronto General Hospital, Mount Sinai Hospital, and Women's College Hospital revolving around the chronic dialysis and transplant programmes focused at the TGH." In the fall of 1985 the 500th renal transplant was performed at TGH.[117]

Growth in the renal division was rapid. In the 1987–8 session, they introduced a renal diagnostic unit under Daniel Cattran, a 1966 U of T graduate, in order to do research on ambulatory patients. In the following year, 1988–9, the renal programs of the TGH and TWH merged. By 1992 renal transplantation was limited to the General and St Michael's and remained at the latter hospital mainly because administrators protested vigorously at attempts to concentrate all kidney transplantation at the General.[118] (In the renal area, St Michael's also had an international reputation in fluid and electrolyte physiology. Mitchell L. Halperin, Marc B. Goldstein, and Kamel S. Kamel were among the most revered clinician teachers and mentors in the faculty. Kamel's *Fluid, Electrolyte and Acid-Base Physiology*, the standard textbook first published in 1988, was in the fourth edition by 2010.[119])

The end-stage renal dialysis program was now following almost 700 patients. The nephrologists divided the Inpatient Renal Unit at the General into an acute care unit and a Renal Rehabilitation Unit, the latter being the first in Canada.[120]

By the beginning of the new century, the division had expanded from its original focus on dialysis to include the entire range of renal disorders from molecular to clinical: Catharine Whiteside's lab focused on the cellular mechanisms of diabetic glomerulopathy; Judith Miller ran an integrative physiology lab; Dan Cattran was in charge of clinical trials on cyclosporine; Phil Marsden's lab studied vascular biology; Norm Rosenblum and Sue Quaggin worked on development of the kidney.[121] In an outreach effort, in 2006 John Dirks, a prominent nephrologist who had come to the faculty in 1987 as dean of medicine from the University of British Columbia (and since 1993 was director of the Gairdner Foundation), created World Kidney Day, an international awareness event focusing on such ailments as high blood pressure and diabetes.

### Division of Rheumatology

The central figure in the history of rheumatology at the University of Toronto is James Wallace Graham, and in 1947 he founded the rheumatology division at the General.

Graham was the virtual founder of rheumatology in Canada. Born in Sudbury in 1906, the son of a Presbyterian minister, he was, as his eulogist said, "reared in an atmosphere of spiritual values and a British background of education and achievement." He graduated in dentistry from U of T in 1928, then began a course of medical study that he finished in 1933. "He was a well-known campus figure as a star Varsity athlete on the Track and Harrier Teams." (Graham would live to see the three-mile interfaculty record, which he had set in 1927, broken by Bruce Kidd in 1961.) After two years as an intern at the General, he studied in the teaching hospitals of London, England, and qualified in 1936 as a member of the Royal College of Physicians. Back in Toronto later that year, he joined the Department of Medicine at the General and continued the research with Almon Fletcher that he had begun in England on focal infection and on managing the long-term vascular damage of diabetes.[122] (Fletcher, for all his service to the cause of diabetes, seems to have bought into Duncan Graham's line that diet could improve the "abnormalities" in the colon that, he believed, caused arthritis.[123])

Wallace Graham tried to overturn this doctrine, correcting the then widespread belief that arthritis was due to "focal infection," especially of the gums.[124] During the war, in command of a special unit for rheumatic fever and arthritis at St Thomas, Ontario, his concern for patients with arthritis intensified. His wife, K.M. Graham, later recalled "his real concern for some of the [arthritic] patients he was seeing who had been lying in bed at home, sometimes for years, receiving little medical attention. There was a negative feeling in the air that not much could be done for them. I remember him saying, 'Somebody has to do something about this.' Having been brought up in a manse, his good Presbyterian conscience bothered him."[125]

After the war Graham joined a rheumatic unit at Sunnybrook Hospital and began training young internists in rheumatology. Here Graham inspired the field. When Hugh Smythe was later asked why he had chosen rheumatology, he said, "The short answer is Sunnybrook." A team of brilliant clinicians there created "the best post-graduate learning environment I have experienced ... At Sunnybrook, there was a 90-bed ward for patients, plus a 12-bed clinical investigation unit where metabolic balance studies could be performed. The treatment model was that of the sanitarium; patients with active disease would be kept in hospital until their disease was under control."[126] Thus did Graham create the forcing ground of Canadian rheumatology. He then continued his teaching at the General, dying in December 1962, a month before the unit at the Wellesley Hospital opened under the direction of Metro Alexander Ogryzlo.

In research going back to 1940, Graham and Fletcher proposed gold therapy in rheumatoid arthritis.[127] In 1953 Graham expanded the Toronto tradition of interest in fibrositis (long in medical discussion) into a "fibrositis syndrome."[128] With his close friend Philip Hench at the Mayo Clinic, "Wally" Graham was among the first to introduce cortisone in the treatment of arthritis (a treatment that Hench pioneered). As well in 1953, he was first to suggest intravenous colchicine in the treatment of gout.[129] Notable for Toronto is that "[h]e was ... the main influence which led Mr J.A. Gairdner to establish the Gairdner Foundation to encourage medical research"[130] – and to initiate the Gairdner Awards. Around 1947 Graham founded the Division of Rheumatology at the TGH.[131]

Graham's eulogist reports that "British recognition came in 1956 when he was elected Fellow of the Royal College of Physicians [FRCP]" of London. He was already member. Wally Graham belonged to the last generation of Canadian physicians for whom an English FRCP represented the summit of recognition. In a great half-turn, academic medicine in Toronto would soon pivot from looking across the Atlantic to looking southwards.

Rheumatology thrilled in those years to the discovery of the endocrine hormones, as cortisone seemed to open up the whole question of arthritis; several hormonal approaches to lupus were also attempted. In 1950 Graham and Metro Ogryzlo described the effectiveness of adrenocorticotropic hormone (ACTH) in the treatment of Reiter's syndrome, a symptom complex of arthritis, urethritis, conjunctivitis, and diarrhea.[132] In December 1956, Ogryzlo said the "LE (Lupus Erythematosus) cell reaction," an unusual degeneration of white cells seen in vitro in the presence of the "LE factor,"[133] was to be found in a number of diseases such as rheumatoid arthritis, not just lupus; and Hugh Smythe and Ogryzlo were internationally known for their careful application in 1957 of the concept as a diagnostic marker.[134] (Smythe was also team physician for the Toronto Maple Leafs.) Later, Smythe was to become a kind of apostle of the diagnosis "fibromyalgia."[135]

"Met" Ogryzlo himself, director of the Toronto Rheumatic Disease Unit at the Wellesley, was said to be Canada's most distinguished rheumatologist. Born in Dauphin, Manitoba, Ogryzlo graduated with an MD with the gold medal from the University of Manitoba in 1938. After serving as a medical officer with the Royal Canadian Air Force, he trained at the Toronto General Hospital, in 1948 becoming chief medical resident. He joined the staff of the hospital in 1952, also directing from 1955 to 1966 the Clinical Investigation Unit at Sunnybrook Hospital. In 1963 he became director of the University of Toronto Rheumatic Disease Unit. Almon Fletcher at Sunnybrook, one of the pioneering insulin scholars, wrote to Kager Wightman at that time, "Dr. Ogryzlo was, I think, the first student of the arthritic disease in Canada to subject the rheumatic disease to careful laboratory study and he has continued to carry on with his investigations for nearly twenty years. He introduced the use of [the] electric densitometer in the estimations of the plasma proteins," contributing in 1960 to the *American Journal of Medicine* an important paper on the serum proteins. "I would think he was the first to recognize that the L. E. Phenomenon may be observed in a number of diseases although it reaches its highest titres in Lupus Erythematosis."[136]

Wallace Graham was the director of a Rheumatic Diseases Unit set up at the Queen Elizabeth Hospital in 1960, with Ogryzlo and Hugh Smythe as consultants in rheumatology and John Crawford a consultant in physical medicine. The Canadian Arthritis and Rheumatism Society had given the university a block grant, funding twenty-four beds at this chronic-care hospital, along with space for physiotherapy and occupational therapy. The great majority of the patients had rheumatoid arthritis, and most came from the General. In assessing the "reasonably satisfactory" results, Graham quoted from rheumatologist Edward Lowman: "Much can be done to better the plight of the rheumatoid cripple and many such disabled persons can be salvaged, and thus maintained to lead more productive lives of independence, usefulness and personal dignity."[137]

In 1966 the Division of Rheumatology was transferred from TGH to the Wellesley Hospital. Said Ogryzlo's colleagues in a memorial observance at the Faculty Council, "As university co-ordinator of rheumatology he promoted the development of rheumatic disease unit divisions at three other teaching hospitals in Toronto." Further, "[he] recognized early in his career that the complex needs of the arthritic patient were not being met in any teaching hospital in Canada, and he saw that a radical revision in traditional concepts was required. [In the program that he developed] arthritic patients could be removed from the competition with the more acutely ill and yet be provided with a program of 'total care.'" The unit he headed at the Wellesley was such a unit.[138] The Wellesley harboured the "core" division of rheumatology, including the four key figures in the program: Ogryzlo, Smythe, Murray B. Urowitz, and Edward C. Keystone. They worked closely with Charles Godfrey, the head of the physical medicine and rehabilitation department. With the closing of the Wellesley Hospital in the late 1990s, the unit moved to the Toronto Western Hospital.

The academic rheumatologists in Toronto wanted a rheumatology institute. Did external reviewers in 1977 think that a good idea? Not at all, and the reasons give interesting insight into the cross-currents that beset academic medicine. The reviewers offered an intellectual objection: "The viability of an institute is to a large extent dependent on one or two individuals in its hierarchy and when these are no longer there, the impetus which it developed is lost with subsequent inertia." They also suggested a rather self-interested political argument – they were, of course, all from other universities – against a rheumatology institute in Toronto: "An institute such as the one proposed will undoubtedly swallow the lion's share of the monies available for ... rheumatology ... to the detriment of the development of rheumatology across the whole of Canada. It may, so to speak, become an albatross around the neck of rheumatology in general."[139] The comment is significant because it shows that the growth of medicine's footprint at the University of Toronto did not occur in a political vacuum.

### Division of General Internal Medicine

There is a reason why general internal medicine was among the last subspecialties of medicine to be founded, rather than the first (as in the case of general surgery). Eliot Phillipson says, "The subspecialties evolved when technology became available that required special expertise: the cardiac catheter, arterial blood gas analysis, endoscopy, hemodialysis, so you had to have people that were scientifically and technologically trained. That doesn't mean that they were any less 'humanistic,' but certainly the flavor in the subspecialty divisions was focused very much on the science underlying the specialty, and on research."

And general internal medicine? "General internal medicine had its focus on patients, and even the research that they undertook was not based on technology. It was on clinical outcomes, it was on population health, it was on errors in treating patients … more focused on the clinical aspects of whatever the question was."

What was the demand for these specialist "generalists"? In urban areas, said Phillipson, they would care for and manage "the very complex patients, patients with multiple illnesses, that needed someone to sort out, over and above what the family physician could do." In smaller communities that couldn't afford a cardiologist or nephrologist, "the general internist would be the consultant, the secondary line of investigation." Family physicians in small towns offered primary care, "but the internist would decide whether the problem could be taken care of locally or whether the patient had to be referred to a tertiary centre."[140]

All this, however, was realized somewhat later. In the 1960s and 1970s the general internist became something of an "endangered species" in the community. But in academic settings, "general internal medicine" became central to the department's core training program in medicine. Thus, in the early 1970s Joe Hilliard directed the residency program in "general internal medicine," meaning the department's basic training program.[141] At some point the Toronto General Hospital developed a general internal medicine division within its hospital Department of Medicine; a hospital report mentions it in 1985.[142] Joe Hilliard was director. And in 1985–6 the hospital added clinical epidemiology to its general internal medicine division, bringing epidemiologist Allan Detsky into the spotlight.[143]

Detsky, a Harvard medical graduate in 1978, trained in medicine at the Massachusetts General Hospital and after 1981 at the Toronto General Hospital. Before becoming director of the hospital Division of General Internal Medicine in 1987, he was on staff in the Department of Health Administration of the faculty from 1980 to 1985 and a member of the Department of Medicine. In these years Detsky was the chief scientific figure in the clinical epidemiology program and sparked a number of important papers.[144] With a PhD in economics from the Massachusetts Institute of Technology, he also had a lively interest in health economics and policy and held a cross-appointment in the Department of Health Policy, Management, and Evaluation of the faculty. From 1997 to 2009 Detsky served as chief physician at Mount Sinai.

Just as a footnote, clinical epidemiology surged strongly on campus in the mid-1980s, and in 1985 Dean Lowy struck a task force on it under John Evans that involved a number of faculty heavyweights such as Gerard Burrow and Bernie Langer. A formal program sprang up at the faculty level in "close relationship" with the Division of General Internal Medicine.[145]

As stated, in 1987 Detsky replaced Hilliard as hospital division director, and in 1988 he became founding director of the university Division of General Internal Medicine.

When Phillipson became acting chair of medicine in 1992, he further enhanced the teaching role of the general internists in the department's clinical teaching units (CTUs), of which there were four, with around twenty-five to thirty-five beds apiece, in each of the five major teaching hospitals. For the most part, these units accommodated medical patients referred from the emergency department who did not require care in subspecialty units such as the Coronary Care Unit or the Respiratory Failure Unit. It was in the CTUs that all residents in internal medicine received a considerable portion of their first three years of training, and clinical clerks received the bulk of their teaching in internal medicine. A fourth general internal medicine year was added to the three-year core training program for those who decided not to push on to the two-year subspecialty programs in cardiology and the other established fields.

An important figure in the development of the CTUs was Herbert Ho Ping Kong, chief of medicine at the Western. A Chinese Jamaican by birth, Ho Ping Kong was a medical graduate of the University of the West Indies in 1965. He had trained in London, England, then was attracted to McGill, where in 1981 he founded the Division of General Internal Medicine at the Royal Victoria Hospital. He was recruited to Toronto in 1984. In 2008 he and Rodrigo Cavalcanti established the Centre for Excellence in Education and Practice (CEEP) in general internal medicine at the Western, which was named in his honour two years later at its official "opening." Ho Ping Kong had a reputation as one of the faculty's great clinical teachers, and when he once received an award, he insisted, in the words of a journalist, that "the evening was not only about him, but rather represented a call to all doctors, young and old, specialist and generalist, to seek the good in others, help those less fortunate, heal the sick and 'not let even insurmountable difficulties stand in the way of good and heroic deeds. There is no greater joy than being your brothers' and sisters' keepers.'"[146] (Ho Ping Kong might well have had in mind the heroic deeds of Department of Physiology member Jacob Markowitz in a Japanese prisoner-of-war camp during the Second World War – see chapter 16.)

Thus the clinical teaching units acquired a central role in general internal medicine. No less scientific than their colleagues in other subspecialties, the general internists had a slightly different mission. Phillipson said, "Obviously part of their role was not simply to teach the medicine and the science, but the practice and the art of medicine." The division "became very quickly, by far, unequivocally, the strongest research general internal medicine division in the country."[147]

Stepping back a pace, the creation of the Division of General Internal Medicine gave the pendulum a farther push in its swing back from technology towards better communication with patients. Phillipson said, "It was an impetus to balancing the pendulum between the science and the art of medicine." He continued, "On the Clinical Teaching Units there was a sensitivity to the fact that the students not only had to learn how to pick up a heart murmur, they were also evaluated on their ability to interact with patients and with colleagues, and to work with the other health professionals. In other words, there was an attempt to bring medicine into a more balanced position between the scientific surge of the '60s and '70s, driven appropriately by technology, and [concern about] the entire patient."[148]

Having a hospital exclusively for children has also given excellent opportunity for studying infantile diseases. These, as every mother and every nurse knows, are so sudden, so fluctuating, and so mysterious, and often so rapid in their fatality, that a large section of the medical profession in all parts of the world give special attention to the diseases of childhood.[1]

John Ross Robertson, 1906

**Professors of Paediatrics/Physicians – Paediatricians-in-Chief, HSC**

Allan MacKenzie Baines, 1913–19
Alan Brown, 1919–51
Andrew Lawrence Chute, 1951–66
Harry Bain, 1966–76
David Carver, 1976–86
Robert Haslam, 1986–96
Hugh O'Brodovich, 1996–2006
Denis Daneman, 2006–present

**Emergence of the Department of Paediatrics**

The first children's hospital in Canada was founded in 1875 by a group of philanthropic women, a "Ladies' Committee" led by Elizabeth McMaster.[2] Located in a rented house in downtown Toronto, the six-bed Hospital for Sick Children was a charitable institution dedicated to caring for the poor. Initially the Ladies' Committee managed the institution, but in 1878 a five-man Board of Trustees was added, allowing the hospital to incorporate and to purchase property.

Although members of the Ladies' Committee continued to serve the hospital until May 1899, they were gradually supplanted by the board, especially after *Toronto Telegram* publisher John Ross Robertson became its chair in 1891.

Between 1883 and his death in 1918, Robertson was HSC's leading benefactor. In addition to appealing for public donations in the hospital's annual reports and in the *Telegram*, his personal contributions totaled some $500,000. He oversaw in 1883 the establishment of the Lakeside Home for Little Children, a summer convalescent retreat on the Toronto Islands, the creation of a milk pasteurization plant in 1909, and most significantly, the construction in 1891 of an impressive new four-story, 320-bed hospital at the corner of College and Elizabeth Streets. At the request of the Toronto City Council, the name inscribed over the main entrance reads "Victoria Hospital for Sick Children," in honour of Queen Victoria's Jubilee in 1887, for which the city had made a $20,000 contribution,[3] but this name was never officially adopted and eventually fell into disuse. (A 1915 appeal, for instance, cited "the incorporated name" as "The Hospital for Sick Children."[4])

Between 1875 and 1891, HSC moved five times to keep up with the growing demand for beds, but the College Street facility was the first specifically designed as a children's hospital. With its greatly expanded capacity, the hospital became "a Provincial Charity … Every sick child whose parents are citizens of Ontario is entitled to exactly the same privileges and has the same claim upon the Hospital as the child who lives within the shadows of its walls."[5]

HSC was organized in an era when children's hospitals were just springing up in the big cities. Toronto's, however, was to become world-famous because of not just the quality of the care but the quality of the science conducted there. From the very beginning there was a recognition that science was the basis of competent pediatric care. Robertson and the Board of Trustees were quick to recognize this, and the important professors in the faculty virtually all had cross-appointments at the children's hospital.

The Faculty of Medicine was involved with the hospital from the time of the refounding in 1887 onwards. As of 1887, several of the professors, including H.H. Wright and James Thorburn, were listed among its "consulting medical officers."[6] In 1892, Alexander McPhedran and James M. MacCallum were cross-appointed as physicians. Irving Cameron and George Peters were surgeons, Richard Reeve served as the consulting ophthalmologist, and James Caven was the consulting pathologist.[7]

From the beginning it was deemed important for physicians in training to hear about diseases of children. By 1894 medical students were receiving some instruction at HSC,[8] and as early as 1899 Henry Thomas Machell initiated instruction in pediatrics at the university. Born in 1850 in Aurora, Ontario, he graduated from the Toronto School of Medicine in 1873. He then trained for seven years in Paris, Edinburgh, and St Thomas's Hospital in London, collecting a series of British qualifications, and at Bellevue Hospital in New York. In 1900

he became associate professor of pediatrics within the Department of Medicine[9]
– of which pediatrics remained a subspecialty for decades.

It was, however, Allen MacKenzie who became in 1913 the first physician-
in-chief at HSC, thus in fact founding the Department of Paediatrics (at first, a
"subdepartment" of medicine). Born in 1853, he attended the prep school Upper
Canada College, where he was said to be "a fine cricketer, of international form
and reputation in all three branches of the game."[10] He graduated in 1878 from
Trinity Medical College, then qualified in England as a Licentiate of the Royal
College of Physicians, "where he remained for nearly four years doing much of
his work in St. Thomas' Hospital."[11] He joined the faculty in 1903 with the amalgamation of Trinity, as associate professor of pediatrics. Machell and Baines lectured at the university and worked at HSC. Baines retired as chief in 1919 at the
rank of "Professor of Paediatrics" and at the time of his death in 1922 had been
associated with the hospital for thirty years.[12]

Soon, the hospital began appointing resident physicians from among the
graduating class to serve for a year. "The opportunity," it was said in 1904, "thus
afforded for obtaining a practical knowledge of this very important department
of medical practice is unsurpassed." Among the four residents selected for
1903–4 was William Gallie.[13]

Just as the Departments of Medicine and Surgery at the General were undergoing convulsions, similar events began at HSC in 1911, as Clarence L. Starr,
newly appointed as surgeon-in-chief, merged the general surgical and orthopedic services and let a number of staff go.[14] As Gallie recalled these events many
years later, staffing then began afresh, especially with the appointment of Alan
Brown as physician-in-chief. "These gentlemen then began the gradual building up of their staffs and the promotion of education and research which has led
to the wonderful prominence that this hospital now occupies among the children's hospitals of the world."[15]

**The Alan Brown Era**

In 1919 Alan Brown became chief physician at HSC, and therewith head of the
Department of Paediatrics, a unit that he was to build into one of the most distinguished pediatric units in the world. Born 1885 in Guelph, Ontario, of Scottish parents and raised in Toronto, Brown earned a Toronto medical degree in
1909 and with it a silver medal. To his classmates he was known as "Buster," an
appellation that soon faded. He was president of the University Rugby Club
and held several offices in campus athletics.[16] He interned at HSC, then trained
for three years at the Babies' Hospital in New York City, "under two small men,
who were nevertheless the paediatric giants of their time in North America,"
Brown's biographer Allison Kingsmill relates.[17] They were Emmett Holt and
Abraham Jacobi, who jointly might be considered the fathers of American pediatrics. Then it was on to study at Children's Hospital of Berlin and elsewhere

in Europe, returning to Toronto in 1914 as Canada's first professionally trained – not self-taught – pediatrician. After a start-up collision with his predecessor Allen Baines, in 1915 he joined the staff of HSC.[18]

Brown told John Ross Robertson, the chairman of the board, who appointed him assistant physician, "that if he were in charge of the infant ward he would reduce the [infant mortality] rate by 50 percent." In 1920 the boast was fulfilled: infant mortality fell from 155 per 1,000 admissions to 88. "This accomplishment," said Brown's eulogist, pediatrician J. Harry Ebbs, "marked the beginning of Alan Brown's career as a pioneer in pediatrics."[19]

Like many senior clinicians, Brown did not suffer fools gladly. *Epistaxis* reports the following exchange with a student in 1926:

> Brown: "What is whey?"
> Burton Williscroft (who came from Owen Sound and would return there to practice): "Well ... It's mostly water."
> Brown: "Say, you're so sharp you'll cut yourself."[20]

Brown's autocratic personality did not sit well with everyone, certainly not with his biographer Kingsmill, who subtitled her study "Portrait of a Tyrant." Barney Berris, whose commonest reaction to his former professors was adulation, said cautiously of Brown, "Although he taught us a great deal of paediatrics, he was not universally loved."[21]

Under Brown, in 1920 pediatrics at HSC was a "Sub-department of Medicine," with one head and eight assistants, attending to 150 beds. As for university commitments, a decanal committee pointed out in that year: "The Head of the Medical Service devotes half of his time to the teaching of Paediatrics and to Hospital work. He receives no salary" for supervising the teaching of almost 170 students.[22]

Around this time, a closer relationship between the hospital and the university began to emerge: "The University of Toronto has come to a full realization of the value of the tuitional side of hospital work" and began providing funding for a number of faculty members "to place a greater portion of their time at the disposal of the hospital. Though the Hospital for Sick Children ... retains its full independence from any measure of outside control, a method of close co-operation with the University has been evolved, from which may be safely foretold gratifying results in the near future."[23] Under this arrangement, "[t] wo chemists appointed by the University devote their whole time to this work of the Department."[24] In 1920, the hospital's educational function was further enhanced with an expanded lecture theatre provided by a donation from John D. Rockefeller "for development of the medical school ... The Hospital for Sick Children is admittedly one of the greatest institutions in the world and, in order that in every way the whole province may derive full advantage from the work it accomplishes, it has amplified the unexcelled facilities it has always extended to the doctors of the future."[25]

On the science side, in 1920 Brown recruited Angelia M. Courtney from Radcliffe College, Harvard, as director of the hospital's new Chemical Research Laboratories. "This is a vitally important factor in solving the manifold problems of child nutrition," he reported.[26] The same year he brought Gladys Boyd on staff as "Fellow in Paediatrics,"[27] who would help to introduce insulin in 1922. (Boyd, who earned her medical degree in 1918, headed the endocrine service at HSC from 1921 to 1950 and was an international authority on childhood nephritis.)

In June 1922 a small group under Brown's chairmanship created the Society for the Study of Diseases of Children (later, the Canadian Paediatric Society). At the society's first annual scientific meeting, held in Montreal in June 1923, Boyd gave the first account of "childhood diabetes treated with insulin. She reported 20 cases of diabetes treated in 1922 with insulin ... over a period of eight months," concluding that "'[i]nsulin will probably not cure but arrests the course of the disease.'"[28]

Among Brown's main accomplishments is placing the study of pediatric nutrition on a scientific basis. His dedication to proper infant nutrition hallmarked him. Satirized *Epistaxis*, "G is for Grandma, Alan's foe / What's best for kids she ought to know. / You can't tell her; she raised her brood / On Allenbury's Patent Food." The Department of Paediatrics under Brown was organized around nutrition research. Brown was also very enthusiastic about genetics: "H is for Heredity, / Be careful whom you wed, says he. / Be sure and search her family tree / For blemish or infirmity."[29]

In 1936 Brown said that their emphasis on "prevention of disease" is paying off.

> The severe degrees of malnutrition which were formerly frequently seen have now become a rarity. Very few cases of rickets [vitamin D deficiency] and scurvy [vitamin C deficiency] are now encountered. Formerly rickets accounted for many severe bone deformities requiring months of surgical treatment for their correction. The level of health of the children admitted to the hospital is higher than that encountered ten years ago ... In September 1931, the mortality rate was 39 per cent. This had dropped in September 1933, to 32 per cent, and in September 1935, to the low figure of 16 per cent. This remarkable improvement in the infant mortality rate is due not only to the improved methods of treatment but to the infants being in better physical condition on admission to the hospital.[30]

In 1942 Alan Moncrieff at the Hospital for Sick Children on Great Ormond Street in London said, "The paediatricians of this country, taking a great deal of their ammunition from the work of Professor Alan Brown and his colleagues in Toronto, have ... driven a wedge well into public consciousness [about the distinctiveness of pediatric medicine]."[31] For all his faults, Brown at HSC helped to put pediatrics on the map.

Brown initiated a one-month postgraduate program in pediatrics in July 1923. This was the beginning of systematic training in pediatrics in Toronto, but the announcement contained one sentence suggesting that Brown was not entirely a beacon of progress: instruction would consist, among other things, of "conditions arising following focal infection, such as heart disease." The theory here was that "focal infections," such as diseased teeth, infected tonsils, or constipation ("intestinal toxemia") caused far-distant lesions in the body, and in the name of focal infection many unnecessary surgical and dental interventions were undertaken. Mental hospitals routinely had dental labs. The doctrine was later exploded as nonsense but Brown – as well as Duncan Graham – propagated it for years in Toronto.[32]

Under Brown, there was progress in the treatment of tetanus. Between 1924 and 1929, fifteen cases were admitted to HSC "with only two recoveries." In the past seven years, he said in 1937, there had been twenty-four cases with thirteen recoveries. "In other words, if a child develops tetanus to-day his chance of being saved is many times that of a few years ago. Similar results are being obtained with influenzal meningitis": 1919–29, one recovery in seventy cases admitted to hospital; 1930–6, ten recoveries in thirty-six cases. The incidence of rickets was reduced from 121 cases in 1920 to 4 cases in 1936.[33]

Progress in the treatment of infectious diseases continued. In 1938 Brown commented on the extraordinary success of the whooping cough vaccine developed at the Connaught Labs: "The results obtained with this vaccine have been so striking that the routine use of whooping-cough vaccine for the immunization of children against this dread disease is now advocated by practically all paediatricians in Ontario." In 1936 there had been "no less than 29 deaths in the Province from whooping-cough. As the results with this vaccine indicate that 98 per cent of the children inoculated are rendered immune, the universal use of this vaccine will be the means of saving the lives of many little children." Also, as a result of the Connaught Labs' serum for influenza meningitis, "in the last 50 cases at the Hospital for Sick Children, 12 recovered and are now perfectly normal." Previously, the disease had been invariably fatal.[34] These were stunning results of global significance.

The 1930s saw other scientific achievements at HSC. There was the "Pablum" story, created jointly by Frederick Fitzgerald Tisdall and Theodore G.H. Drake, under the aegis of Alan Brown.

Drake was the older of the two, born in Webbwood, Ontario, in 1891, and a 1914 medical graduate of U of T (where he played rugby and chose as his motto for the yearbook, "And death in ambush lay in every pill"[35]). He trained at HSC, spent two years at Harvard, then in 1929 came on staff full-time at HSC. Tisdall, who graduated from U of T in 1916, stemmed from Clinton, Ontario; as an undergraduate tennis star, he was said to have "many scalps hanging from his tennis belt."[36] He joined HSC in 1921 and in 1928 succeeded Angelia Courtney as director of the hospital's research laboratories.[37]

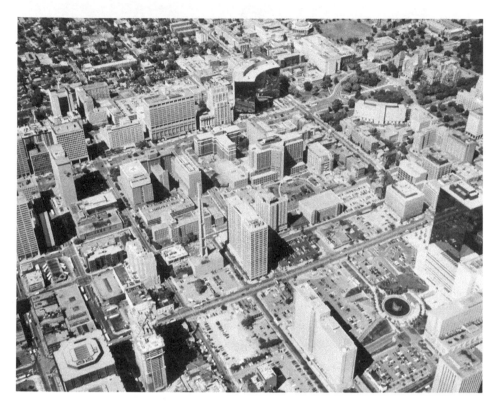

1. The Corner of College and University, 1980s

The emerging Toronto Academic Health Sciences Complex that persuaded Irish peri-natologist Knox Ritchie to join the Faculty of Medicine in 1984. "It's unique. It makes Toronto what it is now." TGH dominates the centre of the photograph, with the Hospital for Sick Children just to its left (rooftop heliport marked with a red cross on white) and Mount Sinai across the street on University Avenue. The southern portion of the University of Toronto campus, including the Medical Sciences Building, appears at the upper right.

UHN, Toronto General Hospital Aerial View, ca. 1980, RG 1.

Department of Public Affairs and Communications fonds, TH 2.4.429.

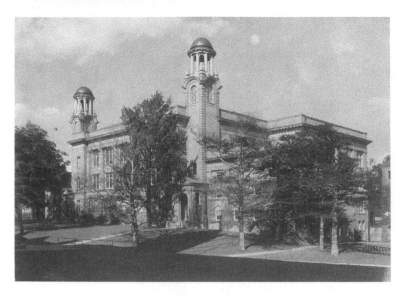

2. The "New Laboratories" of the Faculty of Medicine

Officially opened on 1 October 1903, the new medical building boasted the latest technology of the day. It was built on the "unit system of laboratory" proposed by Harvard's George Minot, with moveable partitions that allowed its rooms to be made larger or smaller to accommodate classes of varying sizes.

University of Toronto, Department of University Extension and Publicity; UTA A1965-0004/007.

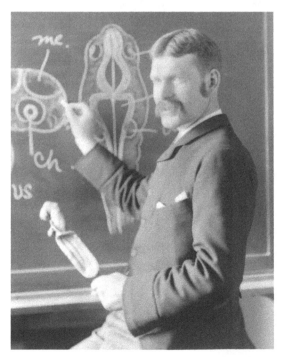

3. Ramsay Wright, 1880s

Scottish zoologist Robert Ramsay Wright was one of the first nonphysicians in the early years of the faculty. As professor of biology between 1887 and 1912, he was instrumental in steering medical education in Toronto and across North America towards basic science and research. University of Toronto, Department of University Extension and Publicity; UTA A1965-004/16 (19), Digital image no. 2001-77-38 MS.

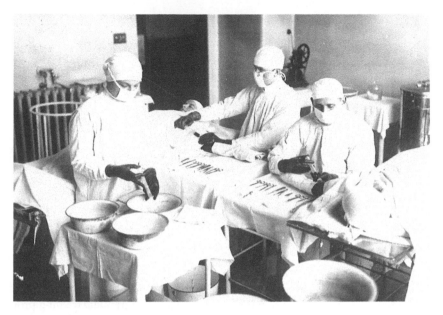

4. Exsanguination-transfusion, ca. 1918

Surgeon Lawrence Bruce Robertson pioneered blood transfusion and exchange procedures ("exsanguination-transfusion") at the Hospital for Sick Children and saved thousands of wounded soldiers by introducing blood transfusion to British military physicians during the First World War.

HSC Archives.

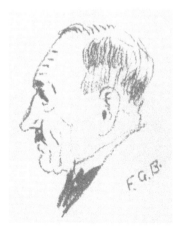

5. Duncan Graham, Professor of Medicine, 1919–47

In 1919 Duncan Graham became the first full-time professor of medicine in the British Empire, thanks to the philanthropy of the Eaton family. During his tenure the Department of Medicine developed a systematic undergraduate training program and the beginnings of postgraduate medical specialization. Drawing by Sir Frederick Banting, whose initial dislike of the dour chief eventually mellowed into friendship.

Reproduced courtesy of Associated Medical Services, Inc., from Robert B. Kerr and Douglas Waugh, *Duncan Graham, Medical Reformer and Educator* (Toronto: Hannah Institute/Dundurn Press, 1989; Canadian Medical Lives, no. 1.), 14.

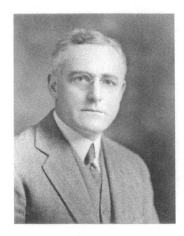

6. William E. Gallie, Professor of Surgery, 1929–47

Gallie was responsible for a number of surgical innovations involving bone grafting and the use of "living sutures" in hernia repair. His chief claim to fame, however, was the creation of the "Gallie Course," Canada's first organized postgraduate training program in surgery.

HMP (Provenance unknown).

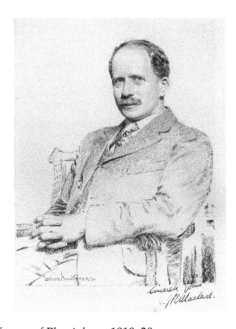

7. J.J.R. Macleod, Professor of Physiology, 1918–28

John James Rickard Macleod was an authority on carbohydrate metabolism before the discovery of insulin and wrote a classic text on *Carbohydrate Metabolism and Insulin* in 1926, as well as being awarded the 1923 Nobel Prize along with Banting. Yet Macleod's role in the historic discovery has been unjustly overlooked in the public imagination in favour of Banting and Best. Photograph of a drawing by Joshua Smith, 1924.

Thomas Fisher Rare Book Library, University of Toronto, The Discovery and Early Development of Insulin (online collection), P10076; from MS COLL 241 (Charles H. Best papers), box 52, folder 61.

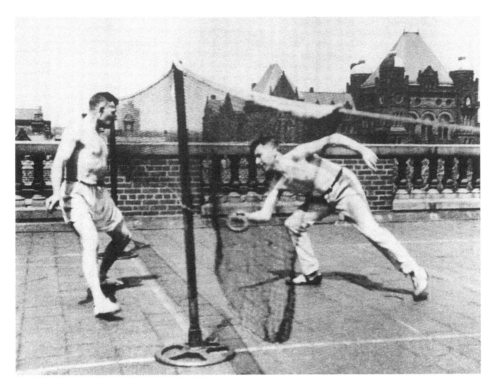

8. John Gerald FitzGerald and the School of Hygiene, 1930s

An advocate of healthy living, FitzGerald organized a mandatory sports program at the School of Hygiene, including tennis matches on the school roof. He appears here on the right, with future deputy health minister Donald Cameron. The Ontario Legislature building is visible in the background.

Sanofi Pasteur Archives, Toronto; reproduced in Paul A. Bator with Andrew J. Rhodes, *Within Reach of Everyone: A History of the University of Toronto School of Hygiene and the Connaught Laboratories*, vol. 1, *1927 to 1955* (Ottawa: Canadian Public Health Association, 1990), 47.

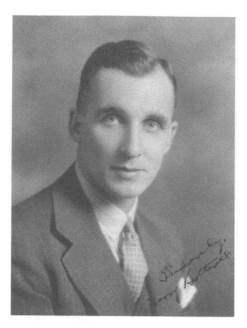

9. Pioneers of Neurosurgery: Harry Botterell

Edmund Henry Botterell became interested in caring for patients with spinal lesions during his residency in the 1930s and quickly recognized the need for coordinated treatment and rehabilitation. In January 1945 he revolutionized the management of spinal cord injuries among young veterans with the creation of Lyndhurst Lodge, the first specialized rehabilitation facility in North America. University of Toronto, Department of Surgery; UTA A1989-0030/004 (11).

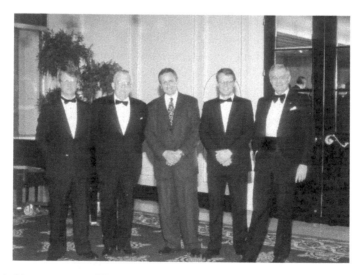

10. Pediatric Neurosurgery: The "Three H's" and "Two Jims" at a Professional Reception, 1997

Neurosurgery at the Hospital for Sick Children was pioneered during the 1950s by E. Bruce Hendrick and Harold Hoffman (second and third from left), followed in 1970 by Robin Humphreys, "the third H" (far right). Their successors James Drake (at left) and James Rutka (second from right) moved neurosurgery at the hospital toward neuroscience and translational research. Courtesy of Dr. Robin Humphreys.

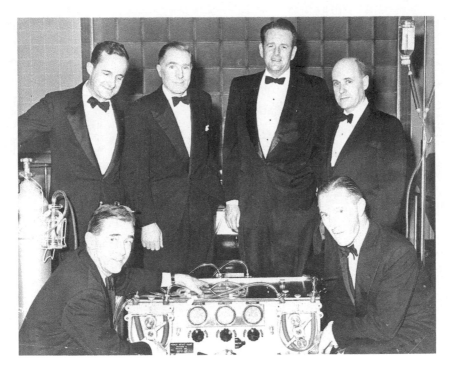

11. Pioneers of Heart Surgery: Evolving Cardiovascular Facilities at TGH, January 1962

Division chief Wilfred G. (Bill) Bigelow and his colleague James A. Key kneel beside a new commercially produced heart pump at the official opening of the hospital's expanded CV unit. Sharing in the celebration are TGH heart surgeon Raymond Heimbecker; Frederick Kergin, head of the Department of Surgery; and two distinguished guests: pioneer heart surgeons Henry Swan from Denver and Edouard Gagnon from Montreal. In March the same year the cardiologists opened the world's first coronary intensive care unit at TGH. Courtesy of Pixie Bigelow Currie.

Photograph by Bill Cole, originally published in W.G. Bigelow, *Cold Hearts: The Story of Hypothermia and the Pacemaker in Heart Surgery* (Toronto: McClelland and Stewart, 1984), fig. 9, 127.

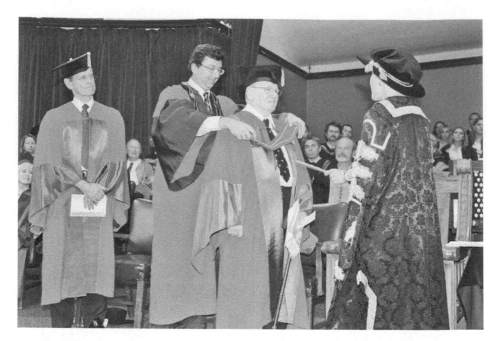

12. The Discovery of Stem Cells in 1961: Ernest McCulloch and James Till

By the beginning of the twenty-first century the chief international contribution of medicine in Toronto was undoubtedly the discovery of stem cells, with their limitless therapeutic applications. The two researchers eventually received numerous awards for this discovery, including honorary degrees at a June 2004 convocation at the University of Toronto. President David Naylor (centre) "hoods" McCulloch as Till (left) looks on.

Lisa Sakulensky photography.

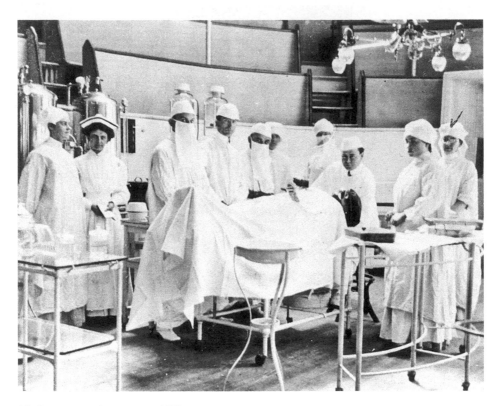

13. Surgery in Toronto ca. 1900

The beginning of scientific medical education in the late nineteenth century was paralleled by the rise of the hospitals themselves as therapeutic institutions. By 1900, the operating room at the Toronto General Hospital was equipped with anesthetics, and the principles of aseptic surgery were evident in drapes, gowns, and (long!) masks.

UHN, The Operating Room at the Toronto General Hospital, ca. 1900s, Acc. 0081, unprocessed collection.

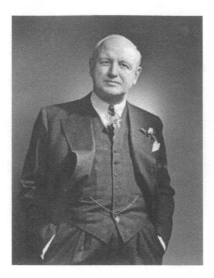

14. Roscoe R. Graham, a Pioneer of Surgery on the Stomach and Pancreas between the Wars

"He could have marched down the wards in the hospitals in England – and he did – with nurses trailing behind him," said hematologist Helen "Nell" Farquharson. But in contrast to his stern cousin Duncan, Roscoe Graham combined a commanding presence with a "very good sense of humour" and invited staff members' families to visit him at the hospital on Sundays.

HMP; Portrait by Karsh.

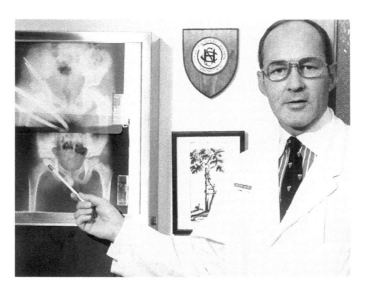

15. Orthopaedic Surgery: Robert B. Salter

The faculty's Division of Orthopaedic Surgery boasted numerous international stars, the most eminent being Bob Salter of the Hospital for Sick Children. Among his many innovations was the innominate osteotomy which he is demonstrating here, developed in 1960 to repair congenital dislocation of the hip, and the revolutionary concept of "continuous passive motion" rather than immobilization in the treatment of soft tissue injuries.

HSC Archives.

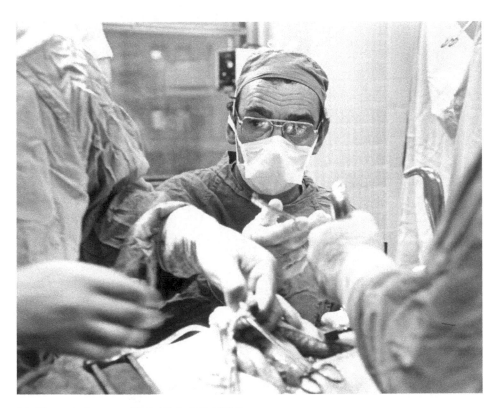

16. Thoracic Surgery: F. Griffith ("Griff") Pearson

Toronto's pre-eminence in thoracic surgery began with a succession of distinguished surgeons and the creation in 1968 of a free-standing division (separate from the cardiovascular service) helmed by Griff Pearson. In addition to his pioneering work in tracheal and esophageal surgery, Pearson was instrumental in establishing the world's first successful lung transplantation program at the Toronto General Hospital in the 1980s.

UHN, Dr Griff Pearson, removal of kidneys, donor for lung transplantation, RG 1, Department of Public Affairs and Communications fonds, TH 2.4.246.

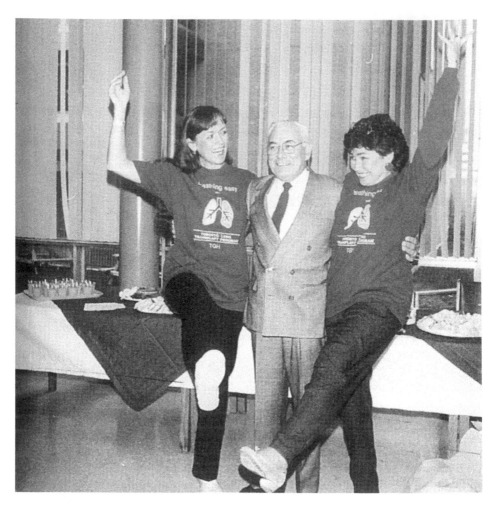

17. Lung Transplantation, a Toronto Triumph

The Toronto Lung Transplant Group led by Joel Cooper performed the world's first single-lung transplant with long-term survival at the Toronto General Hospital in November 1983. Three years later the team carried out the first double-lung transplant. The recipients of these landmark procedures thrived, becoming ambassadors for the transplant program: Tom Hall, the first single-lung recipient, is flanked by Monica Assenheimer, the second, and Ann Harrison, the first double-lung recipient.

Reproduced from Thomas R.J. Todd, *Breathless: A Transplant Surgeon's Journal* (Renfrew, ON: General Store Publishing House, [2007]), 143, fig. 10.

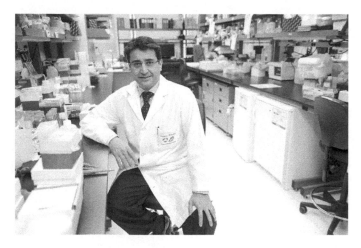

18. Lung Transplantation, the Next Generation: Shaf Keshavjee at TGH, 2010

A surgical resident during the first golden age of lung transplantation at the General, Shaf Keshavjee chose to stay in Toronto and rebuild the program as its original members were recruited elsewhere or retired. Since becoming head of the transplant program in 1997, Keshavjee has pioneered the use of an artificial lung and developed a system to preserve and repair donor lungs for transplantation.

Carlos Osorio/GetStock.com.

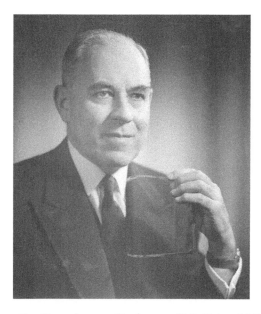

19. Post-war Changes: Ray Farquharson, Professor of Medicine, 1947–60

In 1947 Duncan Graham retired as head of a Department of Medicine that had not kept pace with advances in treatment and research. According to Barney Berris, later head of medicine at Mount Sinai, "Dr Farquharson was the first chair to understand the need for modernization," expanding the full-time staff and supporting research. Farquharson also ended the exclusion of Jews from the department in 1951 by threatening to resign unless Berris was given an appointment.

HMP (Provenance unknown).

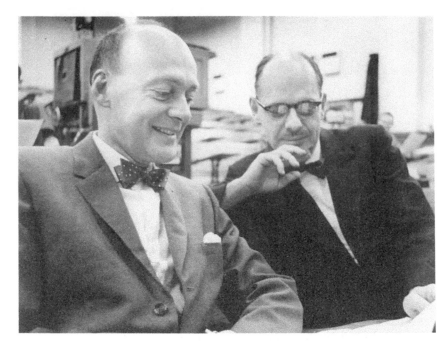

20. 1960s Expansion: K.J.R. Wightman, Professor of Medicine 1960–70

Farquharson's successor Keith John Roy ("Kager") Wightman (right) led the dramatic expansion of the Department of Medicine in the 1960s, developing postgraduate and residency education and increasing teaching hospital beds, especially at the Sunnybrook and East General Hospitals. With him is John Drennan Hamilton, dean of the faculty during the first half of Wightman's tenure and vice president of health sciences during the second.

HMP, donated by Dr Donald Cowan; photograph by Bob Lansdale of Jack Marshall & Co.

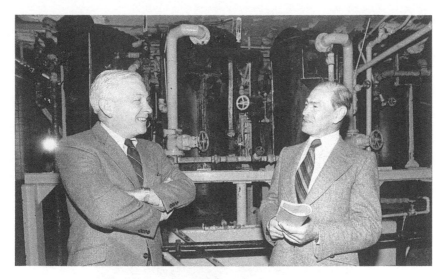

21. 1970s Transformation: Charles Hollenberg, Professor of Medicine, 1970–81

Hollenberg's appointment to the Eaton Professorship in 1970 marked the beginning of a seismic shift in the culture of the Faculty of Medicine: from rural Scots Protestants and an emphasis on the British model of clinical teaching to urban Jews, American influences, and a focus on research. Hollenberg went on to reshape the Ontario Cancer Treatment and Research Foundation into Cancer Care Ontario in the 1990s, after serving as second head of the Banting and Best Diabetes Centre between 1981 and 1993. He is seen here with the centre's inaugural director, Edward A. Sellers, a close personal friend of Charles Best.

Strategic Communications Department, University of Toronto; photograph by Steve Behal.

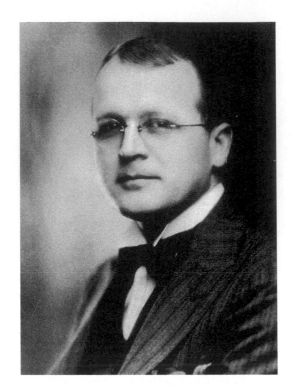

22. Alan Brown, Chief of Paediatrics, 1919–51

Canada's first professionally trained pediatrician joined the staff of the Hospital for Sick Children in 1915 and by 1920 had succeeded in reducing its infant mortality rate by 50 percent. Although his autocratic style made him more feared than loved by staff and students, Brown was instrumental in establishing the discipline of pediatrics in Canada and transforming HSC into a world-class children's research and treatment facility.

HSC Archives.

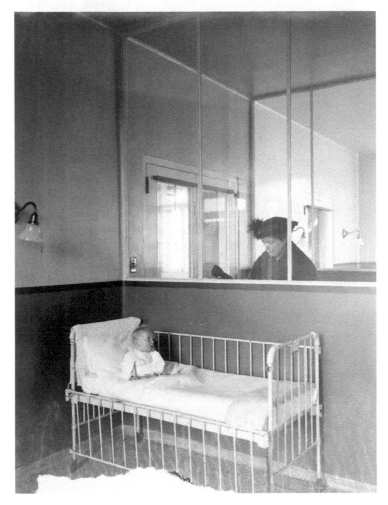

23. Pediatric Care in 1915: Babies' Isolation Ward at the Hospital for Sick Children

Modelled on the infant wards at the Pasteur Hospital in Paris, the facility featured individual glass cubicles to permit isolation and prevent cross-infection. Visiting hours were strictly limited and parents were barred from the cubicles.

HSC Archives.

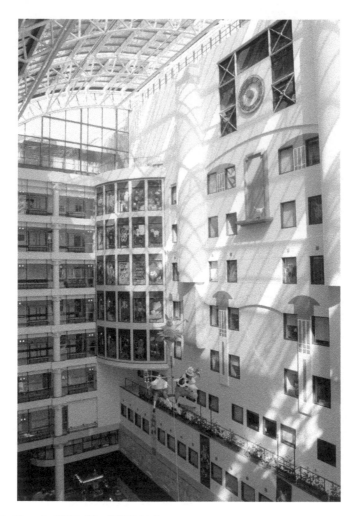

24. Pediatric Care in 1993: The HSC Atrium

The new eight-story wing of the Hospital for Sick Children, opened in 1993, again provided individual suites for the young patients but now included daybeds for parents as
well. Its glass-topped atrium lent a cheery and playful atmosphere to the hospital with
trees, fountains, and an overhead mobile of larger-than-life animals on a trapeze.

HSC Archives.

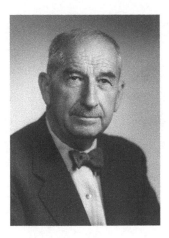

25. Joseph Arthur MacFarlane, Dean of the Faculty of Medicine, 1946–61

The post-war shift of the faculty towards scientific research was driven by many factors, including eager veterans, medical breakthroughs, and large increases in funding. Yet the research wave was also driven by a series of deans, beginning with Joseph MacFarlane.

University of Toronto. Department of Information Services; UTA A1978-0041/14 (5).

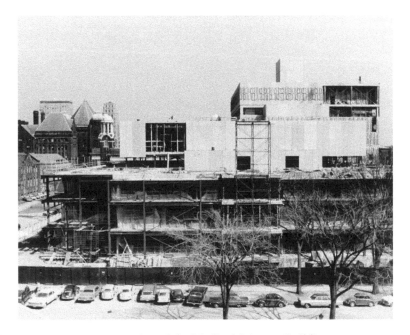

26. 1960s Expansion: Construction of the Medical Sciences Building

The new Medical Sciences Building, completed in 1969, resulted from an agreement between the university and the provincial government to increase the size of the medical class in return for expanded facilities. One casualty of the new construction was the 1903 Medical Building – one of its towers still visible at this point – which was demolished in 1966 to make way for the J.J.R. Macleod Auditorium.

UTA A1972-0045/002 (156), Digital image no. 2007-33-3MS.

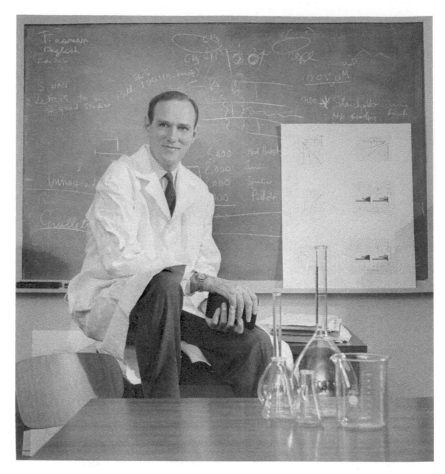

27. Biochemist George Connell, Advocate of Research, 1966

As head of biochemistry between 1965 and 1977, Connell oversaw a major expansion of the department and began some of the first collaborations with the emerging hospital Research Institutes, as well as assuming leadership roles in basic science and planning policy. Following a term as president of the University of Western Ontario, Connell returned to U of T in 1984 and aggressively pursued the goal of transforming the Faculty of Medicine into a great research faculty.

UTA B1998-0033/009P (721012-1), Digital image no. 2006-19-1MS.

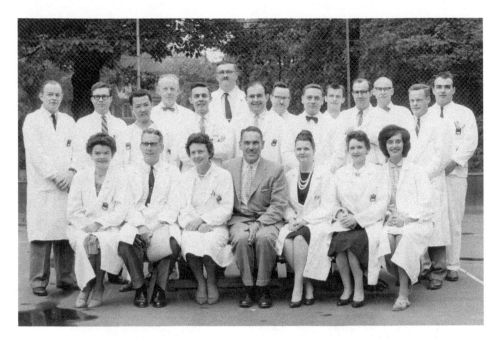

28. Staff of the Princess Margaret Hospital, 1959

In addition to the research staff of the Ontario Cancer Institute, its clinical wing, called the Princess Margaret Hospital, had several important figures, including medical oncologist Harold Warwick, radiation oncologist Vera Peters and radiotherapist/chief physician Clifford Ash (seated second, third, and fourth in the front row, respectively). Radiation oncologist Walter D. ("Bill") Rider is standing at the far left, and the towering figure in the middle of the back row is pediatric radiation oncologist John Darte. Peters proved the most eminent of this group, becoming the first female physician in the faculty to achieve international distinction.

HMP (Provenance unknown).

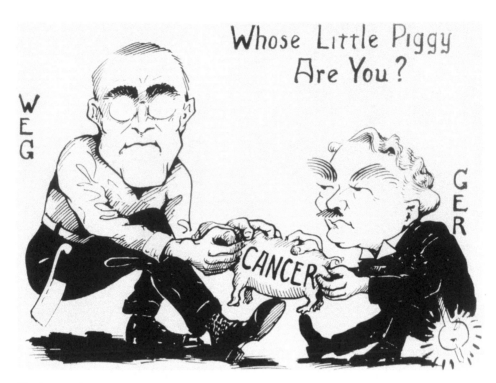

29. Cancer Treatment in Toronto: Surgery vs. Radiotherapy

Until 1995, when the Ontario Cancer Institute joined the other hospitals on University Avenue, cancer treatment in Toronto took place in two separate spheres. As illustrated in this cartoon (regrettably unidentified) cancer surgery in the 1930s and 1940s took place in the big teaching hospitals under the leadership of W.E. Gallie, while medical and radiotherapeutic approaches were carried out at OCI and its predecessor the Ontario Cancer Treatment and Research Foundation, headed initially by Gordon E. Richards (with his radium tube).

HMP (Provenance unknown).

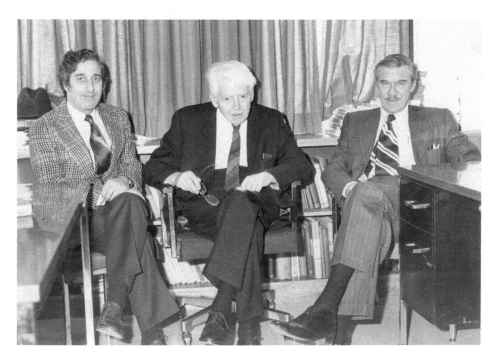

30. Psychiatry: Three Successive Department Heads, 1970s

Aldwyn B. Stokes, 1947–67, (centre) was recruited from the prestigious Maudsley Hospital in the United Kingdom; during his long tenure he promoted research and played a capital role in the creation of the Clarke Institute of Psychiatry, opened in 1966. His successor, Robin C.A. Hunter, 1967–73, (right) was the first psychoanalyst to lead the department, yet one of his first appointments was an eminent neuroscientist. Fredrick H. Lowy, 1974–80, (left) continued the eclectic approach of his predecessors while expanding its research base. In 1980 Lowy became dean of the faculty and proved to be one of its greatest post-war leaders.

HMP, donated by Dr. Frederick Lowy.

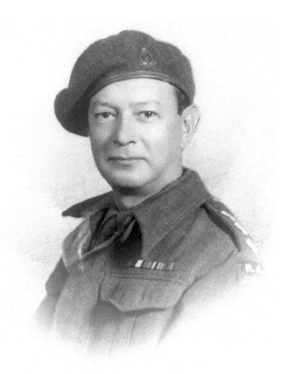

31. Physiologist Jacob Markowitz, Experimental Surgeon and War Hero, 1945

Markowitz proposed the first mammalian heart transplants (on dogs) and was part of a team that conducted the first series in the early 1930s. His surgical expertise was tested during his service with the British Army in World War II as he saved hundreds of lives in a Japanese internment camp.

Captain Jacob Markowitz in battle dress upon return to England, 1945; UTA B2004–0021/001P (01), Digital image 2004-72-1MS.

Mindful of the need to improve infant nutrition, from the mid-1920s Tisdall and Drake were devising infant and maternal foods, such as "a modified powder milk, vitone, recommended for nursing mothers."[38] Around 1930 they created two new infant nutrition products: a healthy new biscuit, Sunwheat, fortified with vitamins and minerals; and the other a substance that would dominate infant feeding for decades to come and become a code word for simplistic ideas. "Pablum," derived from *pabulum* in Latin, meaning "food," was a combination of the vitamins and minerals that growing children needed plus a ground, pre-cooked mixture of starches. It was sold by the drugmaker Mead Johnson in the United States, and, like Sunwheat, royalties from its sales supported the research at the hospital for the next twenty-five years.[39]

Tisdall, Drake, and Brown announced the introduction of Pablum in 1930 in the *American Journal of Diseases of Children*: "The cereal mixture has been used almost exclusively for the past three months in the Hospital for Sick Children, an institution with over 300 beds. It has been found to be just as palatable as any of the finely milled cereals at present so widely used. It should prove to be a valuable addition to the average dietary, because it contains in appreciable amounts so many elements that are known to be essential to normal nutrition."[40]

Tisdall went on to write *The Home Care of the Infant and Child* and, with Alan Brown, the textbook *Common Procedures in the Practice of Paediatrics*. His expertise, however, was not confined to pediatrics: "Within a relatively short period," his colleagues Brown, Drake, and Ebbs reported in a 1949 eulogy, "Dr. Tisdall won an international reputation for his research in human nutrition." A leader of numerous national and international organizations, he "helped to improve the food standards for families on relief" and during the Second World War "originated the prisoner-of-war parcels sent overseas by the Red Cross" and "raised the dietary standards of the R.C.A.F."[41]

Of import equal to Pablum was John Robert Ross's discovery at the Nutrition Research Labs in 1933, together with Alan Brown, that children were contracting lead poisoning from the shiny lead-based paint on their toys and cribs. In 1935 Ross and Brown wrote, "Twenty-three cases of lead poisoning were treated at the Hospital for Sick Children in the past two years. It would thus appear that lead, rather than strychnine or illuminating gas as was previously thought, is probably the most common single cause of poisoning in children. Of these 23 cases, 10 had cerebral symptoms on admission and 5 of these died," while another "resulted in a cerebral sclerosis with mental retardation." They went on to describe the symptoms of "latent" and "late" lead poisoning in young children, noting that these "are somewhat different from those found in the adult. Abdominal cramps, wrist drop [from peripheral nerve damage] and blue lines on the gums occur very rarely in children."[42] The same year, Ross and Colin Lucas of the Department of Medical Research proposed a widely used test for detecting minute amounts of lead in urine.[43] The Ontario government banned lead-based paint in 1936 from use in toys and children's furniture.

Ross was one of the Canadian pioneers of allergy studies. Born in Toronto in 1901, he finished medicine at U of T in 1926 and trained in the field of allergy in Boston and New York. In 1932 Ross founded the allergy division of HSC. He was also the founder of the Canadian Society for the Study of Allergy.[44]

The oxygen tent was first introduced in England in 1920.[45] But in 1929 researchers at HSC modified it for the relief of children whose respiration was severely compromised. (This is the forerunner of the hyperbaric chamber.)[46] Brown said in 1934, "The continued use of the oxygen tent, which was first used [sic] in this Department through the co-operation with the Department of Physiology, and the use of the Drinker Apparatus has resulted in the saving of many lives."[47] The Drinker "iron lung," originated at Harvard in 1928, saw extensive use during the 1937 polio epidemic, discussed below[48])

The late 1930s saw the introduction of the sulfa drugs in the Department of Paediatrics, as in other departments of the faculty. The results in children were as stunning as those in adults. Brown said of sulfanilamide, "The value of this chemical has been strikingly shown in this department in the treatment of streptococcic meningitis, which formerly was fatal in one hundred per cent of the cases, while at the present time fifty to sixty per cent of the patients are recovering. Excellent results have also been obtained in the treatment of erysipelas and streptococcic infections of the throat." They had also tried it in pneumococcal infections. Now recoveries occurred in two out of five cases "in which over the previous ten years the mortality had been one hundred per cent."[49]

During August and September 1937 a huge polio epidemic swept the city and province. Early in the outbreak, the Ontario government financed a controlled field trial to test the effectiveness of a popular zinc sulphate nasal spray as a prophylactic measure. The study involved 5,000 Toronto children with "an observed control group of equivalent size" and was administered by HSC and the university School of Hygiene under the direction of Robert Defries, acting director of the school and Connaught Labs.[50] The results, reported in November in the *Canadian Journal of Public Health*,[51] "clearly demonstrated that the spray was ineffective as a polio preventive."[52] According to Canadian polio historian Christopher Rutty, this early field trial was nevertheless significant for "its relatively high standards of professionalism, methodology, and administrative and public co-operation," the latter "reinforced by the close physical proximity between the provincial health department, the Hospital for Sick Children, and the University of Toronto's School of Hygiene and Connaught Laboratories" and the close professional and academic links among them.[53] The advantages of what was taking form as the Toronto academic health sciences complex were already beginning to have an impact on research.

One of the most alarming effects of the 1937 epidemic was the large number of cases involving respiratory paralysis, which prior to the invention of the iron lung usually resulted in death. The first iron lung in Canada was an early Drinker model acquired by HSC in 1930, and it was still the only one in the country as of August 1937, as first one child and then a second requiring it was admitted. In response to this emergency, HSC staff under the leadership of Superintendent Joseph H.W. Bower hastily constructed on 26 August a makeshift machine from "an experimental respirator for premature infants" attached to "wooden box" and by the next day had completed plans to build additional metal respirators.[54] In all, twenty-seven iron lungs were manufactured at HSC during the epidemic. Most were used there or at the neighbouring Toronto General Hospital, but a number were shipped to other hospitals, including the original wooden lung, which was flown to Denver by the *Toronto Star* to treat a patient there. "The dramatic story of the 'Herculean efforts' at HSC to manufacture iron lungs drew intense press attention" in both the local newspapers and farther afield.[55]

The surgical staff of the hospital developed "a type of splint which could be easily applied and which would prevent, to a large degree, the deformations which so quickly follow the acute stage of the disease [polio]."[56] Orthopedic frames and splints were manufactured at the Ontario government's expense at HSC as well as Hamilton General and London's Victoria Hospitals and distributed throughout the province. These were the first standardized devices available in North America and could be shipped within "minutes" as opposed to the days or weeks required for custom-built splints. "By late November ... nearly 2,000 splints and frames had been provided free by the Ontario government." They quickly became known as the "Toronto splints" and until the early 1940s were the standard throughout North America, with the (US) National Foundation for Infantile Paralysis stockpiling as many as 150,000 in New York City in 1939.[57] The devices were praised by American doctors at a January 1940 meeting on the "Fight Infantile Paralysis Campaign" chaired by Eleanor Roosevelt at the White House.[58]

As the number of polio cases grew, the province took over the old Grace Hospital in Toronto and on 29 September it became the 150-bed Ontario Orthopaedic Hospital, dedicated exclusively to pediatric polio patients and staffed by HSC physicians and surgeons under the direction of Alan Brown and surgeon-in-chief David E. Robertson.[59] These tremendous achievements in the face of a terrible disease did not go unrecognized: HSC was on its way to world fame.

As a result of the efforts of Alan Brown and other leading Canadian pediatricians, the Royal College of Physicians and Surgeons of Canada (RCPS(C))recognized pediatrics as a separate medical specialty in 1939. The first qualifying examination in the new discipline, however, was not held until 1946, probably because of the war.[60]

In 1951 the Hospital for Sick Children moved from the old quarters on College Street to a new building on University Avenue – where it remains today, though much expanded. The initial facility consisted of 632 beds, which was expanded in 1964 to 810 beds with the construction of the Gerrard and Elm Street extensions.[61] At a special two-day conference in October 1951, all the old residents in pediatrics were welcomed to the new hospital, and a painting of Alan Brown was presented to him "at a great reunion dinner."[62] As the new hospital was opening, its scientists were making a significant contribution to research on the polio and Coxsackie viruses, in clinical studies under Nelles Silverthorne and lab work directed by Andrew J. Rhodes, who had just joined the hospital to take charge of the virus laboratory, in cooperation with Connaught Medical Research Labs.[63] Simultaneously, work supported by the US National Foundation for Infantile Paralysis, the polio research charity, was going forward on the testing of gamma globulin with poliomyelitis antibody with a view to developing a serum that might give protection against polio[64] (for further details see the discussion in chapter 5).

When Brown retired in 1952, he left a massive scientific legacy, converting the Hospital for Sick Children into what a 1960 obituary in the *New York Times* called "one of the world's leading child treatment and research centers."[65] He also left a legacy to Canadian pediatrics. Brown said in 1949, "During the last thirty years the Hospital for Sick Children has trained approximately 73 per cent of the paediatricians in Canada. This, I think, is somewhat of a record for any institution in performing this type of service."[66] His eulogists concurred with this assessment; in fact, the *New York Times* credited him with "the training of 90 per cent of the pediatricians trained in Canada." On announcing his death in 1960, the *Canadian Medical Association Journal* cited his tenure as "the Golden Age of pediatric training in this country," and an accompanying "Appreciation" stated, "His influence on paediatric teaching and practice was astonishing, and few individuals have influenced the health of the nation as he did."[67]

## Lawrence Chute

In 1952 A. Lawrence Chute succeeded Brown as chief physician at the children's hospital. In a nod to the Royal College's recognition of the specialty, Chute at once changed his hospital title from "physician-in-chief" to "paediatrician-in-chief," remaining, as Brown had been, professor of pediatrics; therewith a new era began.

Lawrie Chute was born in 1909 in India into a missionary family, his father Jesse a Baptist minister and his mother Pearl Smith Chute an 1895 graduate of the Ontario Women's Medical College; she was a medical missionary in Akidu, India.[68] Lawrie was, however, educated in Canada, earning a BA at Victoria College in the University of Toronto in 1931, a master's degree in physiology in 1932, and an MD in 1935. As a medical student his main interests were said to have been rugby and the annual class musical, Daffydil, although he was the class silver medalist. After interning at the General and HSC, he took a PhD at London University in 1939, then returned to Canada as an assistant in the Banting and Best Department of Medical Research and a staff member at HSC. During the war he was injured in North Africa in an accident, convalesced in England, then did research on wound shock, proceeding in 1945 to Deaconess Hospital in Boston to study diabetes under Elliott Joslin.[69] In 1947 he returned to the Banting Institute and in 1949 rejoined the Hospital for Sick Children as assistant director of the research laboratories, with a strong research interest in childhood obesity.

On his watch, Chute had to cope with the funding changes that were convulsing medicine in the province, with the education of increasing hordes of medical students, and with space demands that led to the opening of a new wing of the hospital on Gerrard Street in 1964.

How was one to accommodate the medical students who needed some pediatric exposure in order to do family medicine but didn't want to specialize? This was a chronic problem at HSC. In 1957 Chute said that the student desperately needed some final-year clinical experience in the outpatient department at HSC because "[i]t is here that he must learn the technique of history taking and the management of both parent and child." Yet the third-year exposure to pediatrics was an insufficient clinical experience for this work. Far from being a monopolist, Chute was in favour of setting up children's wards staffed by members of the Department of Paediatrics in all the teaching hospitals.[70] In 1962 the question of masses of rotating interns (140 in number) at HSC again surfaced: it was, said Chute, a disadvantage of the "concentration of children's services in one large institution."[71]

In the late 1950s a government hospitalization plan was just being introduced that would pay the hospital costs of all patients, abolishing the large public wards that had previously been hallowed sites of teaching and making all patients, essentially, "private." At the time, this threatened to cause problems across the board in academic medicine and certainly in pediatrics. Chute noted in 1958 "the very large percentage (65–70 per cent) of semi-public patients on our public wards. While much use is made of these patients for teaching, it is not a satisfactory answer for the markedly diminished number of [public] patients who are directly under the supervision and control of the teaching group ... This situation will become even worse with the advent of the Government Hospitalization Plan."[72] In January 1959 the Hospital Insurance Plan was introduced and the question of "control" of the teaching beds immediately surfaced.[73] Previously, the private patients had been exempt from teaching. Now there were so many that they really should be integrated "into a clinic type of organization with group rather than private control."[74] In fact, all would become "private" patients, in that the government paid for their care.

The opening of the Gerrard Street wing in July 1964 offered a solution to the public/private issue. "The major step [will be] our re-organization for teaching, namely the formation of a clinic to include all patients of the teaching staff both private and public." This would not only ensure an "adequate volume of patients for clinical teaching" but would also "promote increased participation through discussion at all levels between staff man and resident and among the general paediatrician, the specialist, and the research worker."[75] (The new wing had extensive lab facilities as well as beds.) On 1 July 1964, "Paediatric Consultants" was established, after a three-year study by the accounting firm Clarkson Gordon, to deal with the advent of universal medical insurance and the disappearance of the "public," or indigent, patient, "formerly the source of teaching material."[76]

In 1966 Lawrie Chute resigned as chief of pediatrics at HSC to become dean. Harry Bain succeeded him.

### Harry Bain

Harry Bain was a person of the North. Born in 1921 in Cache Bay, Ontario, the son of a lumberman, he attended North Bay Collegiate Institute and then U of T on a scholarship, graduating in medicine in 1944. His future, he told the yearbook, was "to settle down near Hudson Bay."[77] Fate, however, took a hand. After service in the war, he trained in pediatrics at HSC and the Children's Hospital of Winnipeg. His heart beat northwards. In 1969 he created the Sioux Lookout Project, to provide medical care to native Canadians (a project to which the federal government responded with alacrity[78]). And after his retirement in 1986 he returned to North Bay, where he died in 2001 at age eighty. After his passing, his wife Barbara said, "He was a Cache boy until the day he died. He loved the bush, he loved fishing."[79]

Yet the great vortex to the south drew him for his career, and after Winnipeg he joined the Department of Paediatrics at the Children's Hospital in Toronto, where he became pediatrician-in-chief in 1966. During his term the Foundation of the Hospital for Sick Children was established in 1973.

Overcrowding on the wards with med students persisted under Bain, making it difficult to create subspecialty services (which would be totally over the heads of the teeming students). Residents in the new Department of Family and Community Medicine had started turning up at HSC and the decision was made in the early 1970s to ship them out to three peripheral community hospitals for their training in pediatrics: Mississauga, Toronto East General, and Scarborough General Hospitals. (Clerks weren't sent out to the periphery because there were no residents in pediatrics to supervise them.) Bain felt ambivalent about this expedient: a third of the practice of these family physicians would be pediatric, and it was imperative that they have at least four months of training under qualified pediatricians. The ultimate result of this overcrowding was a decline in the quality of education: on Bain's watch U of T students lost their countrywide first place in pediatric questions in the national licensing exams (LMCCs).[80]

In these years, the Department of Paediatrics underwent a great expansion, growing from twenty to more than sixty "geographic" (offices at the hospital) full-time appointments, "so that," as medical reporter Charlotte Gray put it, "a complete tertiary pediatric facility was developed."[81] The subspecialties mushroomed as well. In 1972 a nurse-practitioner training program was begun.[82]

The expansion did not, however, include a perinatal program of the kind being set up at Women's College and Mount Sinai. This long remained a sore point: the inability to provide comprehensive care of infants in the last few months of pregnancy and the first few of life. Neonatology was strong at HSC but perinatology was not (see also obstetrics and gynecology, chapter 19). In 1974 the hospital lamented, "The lack of an obstetrical unit at HSC precludes the possibility of developing a complete perinatal program."[83]

But science forged ahead. During Bain's term, in 1972 Aser Rothstein, one of the great leadership figures in the history of the hospital, became director of the Research Institute of HSC (see pp. 276–278). Allan Okey, who later became chair of pharmacology after working at the institute, said that the institute's main thrust was not children but science: "It was an institute set up to say, 'What are some of the important scientific issues?' If they have something to do with pediatrics and children that's a bonus, but I think first and foremost they wanted excellence in the research, and tried to get the very best investigators." HSC and the other Research Institutes had a powerful magnetic influence on researchers elsewhere in Canada. Toronto was known, Okey said, as "'the black hole', because typically the resources here were sufficient to lure good investigators."[84]

### David Carver

In December 1976 David Carver was appointed chair of pediatrics and pediatrician-in-chief at HSC. Born in Boston in 1930, Carver graduated from Harvard College with a bachelor's degree in 1951 and with an MD from Duke in 1955. Pediatric microbiology and immunology were his specialty fields, and he had an international reputation as a pediatric virologist. He had joined the staffs of the Albert Einstein College of Medicine and Johns Hopkins School of Medicine before accepting the chairmanship of the Toronto department. Therewith, after decades of faculty leaders recruited in Great Britain, one of the first American chiefs arrived on campus.

Under Carver, the Department of Paediatrics underwent some dramatic changes. New divisions, such as pharmacology and nutrition, were created; others, such as neurology, were expanded; new chiefs were appointed, more full-time staff were taken on. Whereas the department previously had almost no Medical Research Council of Canada scholars, by 1983 it had six. Teaching was restructured; clerks and family practice residents were confined to general wards and outpatient clinics, while specialty wards were reserved for pediatric residents in their later years. As one reviewer commented, "The historical separation between the university and the Hospital for Sick Children seems to be disappearing as a result of Professor Carver's belief in the importance of integrating the activities of the hospital and the university more closely."[85]

During Carver's tenure, HSC and the University of Toronto also adopted a new approach to academic leadership. "To enhance the process of renewal and a continuous infusion of new ideas," chiefs were granted five-year term appointments, renewable only once, in contrast to the unlimited appointments in the United Kingdom and United States.[86]

### Robert Haslam

As a result of this change in policy, Robert Haslam took the baton in 1986 from Carver as pediatrician-in-chief of the hospital and chair of the university department. Haslam was a native of Saskatoon, his father the chair of physics at the University of Saskatchewan. "During my youth," he said in a 2005 autobiography, "my father was never quite reconciled to my wish to become a physician … because, in his mind, medicine was not a science like physics but, rather, an art."[87] A 1960 graduate of the University of Saskatchewan medical school, he trained in pediatrics and child neurology at Johns Hopkins and the University of Kentucky, then spent five years as director of the John F. Kennedy Institute (now known as the Kennedy-Krieger Institute) in Baltimore. In 1975 Haslam returned to Canada as head of the fledgling Department of Pediatrics at the University of Calgary and chief of pediatrics at the Alberta Children's Hospital.

From the get-go, Haslam had a significant management problem to confront: medical graduates of the U of T had simply not been selecting residency programs at the hospital for further training. During Haslam's tenure, the attractiveness of training at the Hospital for Sick Children greatly improved. An external reviewer said in 1991 that the percent of applicants from U of T "had increased from none to few per year over the preceding many years, to 32 (13%) in the past year. This very significant improvement from what must be regarded as a very unsatisfactory circumstance to a laudable one, was achieved, in Dr. Haslam's judgment, by the attention that Dr [Rayfel] Schneider and Dr [Alan] Goldbloom had made to the improvement of the undergraduate and graduate teaching programs."[88]

Yet many students required exposure to pediatrics. And it is interesting that, even at this late date – after the hospital had bent itself in two trying to accommodate all the medical students, clerks, interns, and family practice residents seeking exposure – the training problem had not been solved. In January 1990, Haslam told the faculty "Self-Study" group, organizing for the next of the endless site visits and assessments, that the clerkship in pediatrics was much too short. "More time is needed to give proper exposure to the full range of illnesses experienced by children. Four weeks represents the shortest clerkship in North America; the average is six to seven weeks. Students' performance on the MCCQE [Medical Council of Canada Qualifying Examination] has not been good (below the national average). The Chair [Haslam] believes this is largely because students at the University of Toronto do not take Paediatrics very seriously."[89]

Haslam met the decrease in the number of resident slots imposed by the ministry in these years by creating a salaried Clinical Assistant Program. A highlight of Haslam's tenure was the successful negotiation with the Ministry of Health in 1991 of a practice plan – a means of funding education and research through the billings of the pediatric group. Paediatrics was thus the first department in the faculty to accomplish this: "Indeed, our Paediatric agreement was the first major agreement of its kind in Ontario."[90]

The grand highlight of the Haslam years was moving into the hospital's new 817,000-square-foot patient care centre in January 1993. "It's overwhelming," he said in a *Globe and Mail* article. "It's as though we've all been marching towards Jerusalem, and now finally, our long pilgrimage is at an end."[91] Given the overcrowded and outmoded conditions in the University Avenue hospital, this was no exaggeration. "By the late 1970s it was clear to everyone that a new hospital was badly needed," another piece in the *Globe* explained. "The physical space – mainly four-bed and two-bed rooms set along endless, windowless corridors – was inadequate and depressing ... In addition, many of the patient rooms were too small to hold all the necessary medical and nursing equipment." Anxious parents of seriously ill children were reduced to "camping out on cots or chairs." In contrast to this dismal scene, the new eight-story wing – "constructed around a glass-topped Atrium" featuring fountains, "full-size trees," and an overhead moving sculpture of "larger-than-life pigs and cows on a trapeze" – provided individual patient suites with daybeds for parents, and "several large playrooms ... strategically located across from the nursing stations to allow staff to monitor activity."[92] Eight weeks later the first patients moved into the Atrium.

The Atrium was significant not just as a swell new accommodation but because it marked the implanting of a genuine research culture at the hospital. Numerous though scientific achievements had been at HSC, they had occurred almost as by-products of providing first-class care. HSC surgeon-in-chief John Wedge said in June 1996, "A substantial effort has been made over the past year to integrate research and teaching with clinical programs in the hospital. Traditionally, research at the hospital has been viewed as a separate initiative rather than an endeavour that should pervade the entire hospital culture." They have poorly funded teaching and research training. But a leaf has turned, "and a new capital campaign has embarked on raising funds for thematic areas of research which parallel clinical programs. Previous capital campaigns have been almost exclusively focused on 'bricks and mortar' but the current one is seeking funding for endowed chairs, research programs identified as specific themes and a research training centre to support the development of future researchers." Those in the hospital Department of Surgery anticipate "major benefits in enhancing our support for surgical scientists."[93] This was a tardive note, one that the faculty as a whole had long since struck.

## Hugh O'Brodovich

Hugh O'Brodovich, appointed chair and pediatrician-in-chief in 1996, came from within HSC itself, although an international search had been undertaken (on 30 July 1995 the *New York Times* ran an advertisement headed "Health Care Excellence" and seeking "an accomplished professional" with "administrative experience, exceptional clinical skills and leadership abilities, and a strong background in research"[94]). Like Haslam, O'Brodovich hailed from Western Canada. Born in Saskatoon, he completed his medical degree and specialty training in pediatrics and pediatric respiratory medicine at the University of Manitoba, followed by a three-year research fellowship in pediatric pulmonology at Columbia University in New York. He returned to Canada in 1981 as an assistant (later associate) professor of pediatrics at McMaster University in Hamilton and staff pulmonologist at its Medical Centre before being recruited to U of T and HSC in 1986. In 1990 he was promoted to a full professorship[95] and four years later succeeded Henry Levison as chief of the Division of Respiratory Medicine at the hospital.

O'Brodovich added a new dimension to the department's research program with his expertise in the cellular and molecular mechanisms of lung disease. In cooperation with members of the Division of Neonatology, he helped establish a Medical Research Council Group in Lung Development and in 1990 became head of the respiratory research division of the Research Institute.[96] The same year his group reported in the *Journal of Applied Physiology* that administering the sodium transport inhibitor amiloride to newborn guinea pigs before their first breath resulted in respiratory distress, hypoxia, and failure to clear their fetal lung liquid.[97] This finding was important for indicating that the neonatal respiratory distress syndrome was initiated not only by surfactant deficiency but also impaired fluid clearance from the lung's airspaces.[98]

An external review in 2000 found that, under O'Brodovich, the department "continues to be the pre-eminent academic pediatric program in Canada. Its academic productivity in terms of [peer reviewed] publications is at a leadership level internationally ... HSC continues to be an incubator for academic pediatric leaders globally."[99] This statement proved prophetic. In 2006 O'Brodovich left HSC and in January 2008 he became physician in chief at the Lucile Packard Children's Hospital and chair of pediatrics at Stanford.[100]

## The Subspecialties of the Department of Paediatrics

The many subspecialties of a huge department such as pediatrics cannot be covered comprehensively without turning the book into an encyclopedia. Nonetheless, some of the stories need telling. In the background was the transformation of pediatrics itself from a primary-care specialty to a discipline heavily peopled with subspecialists. A committee noted in 1974, "The role of the paediatricians in

Canada has not yet been clarified. 25 years ago almost all did a large proportion of primary care. Now one-third do exclusively primary care, one-third consulting ... and one-third mixed." So training had "to be geared to the production of three types – primary care, general consulting, sub-specialty."[101]

In 1969 the Independent Planning Committee indicated the size of the problem: "There are 18 general services in Paediatrics, including an out-patient department and emergency ... the Department has, in addition, 19 specialty services (cardiology, neurology etc)." In addition, "[i]n 1966 the ratio of full-time to part-time clinicians was 1:3. Today, the ratio approaches 1:2 and may rise to 1:1. This change in ratio reflects the accelerating increase in the development of sub-specialties and the increasing emphasis in the Department on research."[102]

Another large shift in subspecialty operations occurred in 1980, as the practice of letting general pediatricians admit their patients to subspecialty areas, such as cardiology or neurology, and caring for them there, came to an end. Henceforth, said the Self-Study of 1983, only "staff physicians who have been certified by the appropriate division chiefs as having subspecialty expertise in their area" would supply care. "This means that the individuals are full time physicians who are specifically working in the divisions under consideration. This change has recognized the reality of physicians being truly in charge and also eliminated problems for both house staff and parents in understanding who to deal with."[103] The rise of the subspecialties occurred, therefore, in a dynamic environment where such concepts as "general" community pediatrician and "primary care" were being squeezed out by the relentless drive towards specialized research knowledge that has been seen on almost every page of this book.

## Division of Neonatology

In the early years of the Hospital for Sick Children, admission was restricted to "[c]hildren ... from two to fourteen years of age," although younger infants could be brought to the out-patient department "for medical advice."[104] This rule was not always followed: the 1906 annual report explained that babies under two years old were admitted for surgery and that numerous other exceptions had been made to the age rule "as a number of urgent and deserving cases have come to us that could not be turned away." At this point, with the opening of a separate nurses' residence, additional space was available and "a reasonable number of ... little tots" were now to be accommodated in a new ward.[105]

Two years later, in 1908, the hospital reported, "The rapid improvement made by the patients of this age indicates that the [infants'] department has proved eminently beneficial."[106] Nevertheless, infant mortality rates remained high, with 45 percent of deaths between 1875 and 1908 occurring among patients "under one year of age."[107]

A true neonatal service began at HSC with two important advances. The first specialized neonatal ward at the hospital opened in 1915 with individual glass

cubicles "to allow isolation and to minimize cross-infection"[108] for the nurtur-
ance of the newborn. It was said to have been modelled on the newborn babies' wards at the Pasteur Hospital in Paris. According to the 1915 annual report,
which featured a photograph of the "cubicle floor," the new ward was unique in
Canada and represented the state of the art "with running water, hot and cold."
The facility was evidently needed, given that the youngest infant admitted the
previous year had been "only 10 minutes old," and the hospital was by now caring for "premature babies," one of whom weighed only "2 lbs. 5 oz at birth, but
had since doubled in weight."[109]

Exsanguination transfusion, as seen in chapter 4, is the progressive replacement of small amounts of the child's blood with donor blood. Lawrence Bruce
Robertson returned from transfusing soldiers during the First World War to
begin transfusing infants at HSC after the war and set up one of the first transfusion services in North America, which between October 1922 and September
1923 performed over 120 exsanguination transfusions on infants and children in
the hospital, "usually for septicemia, gastroenteritis, or severe burns"[110] (many
of these under the influence of a later discredited theory that "toxins" of various
kinds, infiltrated the blood from the colon or an infected tooth, causing systemic
disease). That is the background of the first published pediatric transfusion.

In 1925 Alfred P. Hart, a U of T medical graduate in 1911, introduced exsanguination ("exchange") transfusion to treat severe neonatal jaundice. "It was my
fortune," Hart wrote, "to be called by Dr. Murray of Parkdale, to see ... [a] baby
born on December 18, 1924." Hart, thirty-six at the time, was on the pediatric
staff at HSC. The infant seemed healthy, but, "as the father informed me, they
had had six boys born previously all apparently as healthy and strong at birth
as this baby. They all, however, had developed jaundice within the first twenty-
four hours, and the condition had become progressively worse until death occurred in from three to eleven days." Dr Hart diagnosed icterus gravis (severe
jaundice) of the newborn and decided to wait and see how things transpired.
"On the second day, the father stated that he could see jaundice beginning to
appear on the tip of the nose but as it was evening and only artificial light could
be used I could not see it myself." The next day, however, the baby was "distinctly jaundiced," although the liver was of normal size. On the third day the
child was much worse, the liver palpable at the margin of the rib cage, and the
stool and urine full of bile.

Going over the literature, Hart could "not find many suggestions for the treatment of these cases." One authority suggested "small doses of calomel [mercu-
rous chloride] for the infant." Hart feared that some toxin was circulating in the
body destroying the liver cells. "I felt that if something drastic was not done
at once the child was certainly going to die." He decided to refer the child to a
colleague for an "exsanguination transfusion," which his late colleague Bruce
Robertson had recently described, "in the hope of removing a sufficient amount
of toxin to prevent the progress of the disease." John L. MacDonald at HSC

removed 300 cc of blood from the anterior fontanelle, "at the same time transfusing 335 cc. of blood into the internal saphenous vein at the left ankle." The
doctors also administered a small amount of glucose. "The donor was a healthy
male not belonging to the family."

The results? "By the following morning the jaundice was much less intense."
It had entirely vanished by the fourth day. At five and a half months the child
had experienced "no return of the jaundice since and is gaining and developing as any normal baby." This is a remarkable story and, possibly, aside from
Robertson's own contribution in 1921on erethroblastosis fetalis, represents the
first contribution of the Hospital for Sick Children to the international scientific
literature.[111] Hart's technique was adopted worldwide for the treatment of what
was later identified as Rh negative factor, and this achievement was acknowledged in his 1954 obituary in the *New York Times*.[112]

The main figure in the history of neonatology at the children's hospital is Paul
R. Swyer. Born in London in 1921, Swyer earned a bachelor's degree at Cambridge in 1940 and a medical degree in 1943. He interned at Middlesex Hospital
in 1947–8, then trained at the Brompton Hospital for Diseases of the Chest and
at the Hospital for Sick Children at Great Ormond Street in London in the late
1940s and early 1950s. In 1953, while at Warwick Hospital, he and G.C.W. James
described "hyperlucent lung syndrome" – or lessened unilateral attenuation of
X-rays as they pass through the lung, meaning reduced blood flow in connection with overdistended alveoli (air sacs) – that may follow a severe infection
and that became eponymously known as the "Swyer-James syndrome."[113] In
1953 he came to the Hospital for Sick Children in Toronto as a fellow in cardiology. The neonatal intensive care unit was founded in 1962, and Swyer served
from 1967 until his retirement in 1986 as chief of the Division of Neonatology.
In 1964 Swyer and his fellow Maria Delivora-Papadopoulos conducted one of
the first North American trials of intermittent positive pressure ventilation for
the neonatal respiratory distress syndrome, in this case, hyaline membrane disease.[114] In 1970 Swyer and colleagues introduced intermittent negative pressure
artificial respiration as a way of aiding pulmonary blood flow and preventing
lung deflation.[115]

During Swyer's tenure, neonatal mortality in Toronto dropped abruptly.
Even though the neonatal unit at HSC was often way over its fifty-bed capacity, in 1971, "[t]he latest figures for neonatal mortality for Metro Toronto [1969]
showed that at 12.1 deaths per 1000 live births, the neonatal mortality was the
lowest ever recorded," down from twenty "since the intensive care unit in the
Neonatal Division came into being."[116] In 1975 Swyer published the first textbook on neonatal intensive care.[117] He is considered one of the international pioneers of the discipline.

Following Swyer's retirement in 1986, Barry Smith and Martin Post were recruited from Harvard University to bring in research expertise in the cell and
molecular biology of the lung, Smith as head of the Division of Neonatology

and Post as head of neonatal research. Their research focus was further enhanced with the recruitment of clinician-scientist Keith Tanswell from the University of Western Ontario in 1989. Between 1988 and 1993 Smith headed up a
multi-investigator Medical Research Council Program Grant in Lung Development, which was continued under Tanswell's leadership as a Canadian Institutes of Health Research (CIHR) Group Grant until 2009. Smith left HSC in 1996
to become dean of health sciences at Queen's University in Kingston, Ontario,
and was succeeded by Tanswell. Sadly, Smith's tenure there was brief because
he was diagnosed with ALS in 1998 and died in June 2001 – but not before contributing a personal account of his experiences to *Living Lessons*, a monograph
on humane palliative care.[118]

Keith Tanswell became head of neonatology following Smith's departure.
Like Paul Swyer, he was of English origin, born in Dorset in 1946 and educated
in the United Kingdom, obtaining his MB and BS from St Mary's Hospital Medical School of London University in 1969. He first came to Canada as a senior
resident in pediatrics at Queen's in 1975–6, then went on to do a fellowship in
neonatology, followed by research training at Queen's and at Duke University.
From 1979 to 1982 he was a staff neonatologist at Kingston General Hospital and
an assistant professor of pediatrics at Queen's, and from July 1982 until his recruitment to HSC he held a series of positions at Western and St Joseph's Health
Centre in London, rising to a full professorship in pediatrics and deputy director of the Lawson Research Institute at St Joseph's. Tanswell built upon the
research focus begun by Barry Smith, recruiting additional clinician-scientists
and investigating regulation of lung development and injury, oxygen toxicity,
and free-radical biology. In 1996 he became the inaugural holder of the University of Toronto Chair in Neonatal Medicine endowed in by the hospital's Wom-
en's Auxiliary.[119] By 2000 the division was represented at three sites, including
Sunnybrook Hospital and Women's College Hospital, and included eleven full-
time neonatologists.[120]

### Division of Cardiology

John D. Keith founded the Division of Cardiology at HSC when he arrived at
the hospital in 1938 and for decades remained the central figure. He was among
the many distinguished clinicians who came to Toronto from the prairies. Born
in Winnipeg in 1908, he reached Toronto at age four. Graduating in medicine in
1932 – during which time he was the captain of the football team – he interned
in the pediatric department of the Strong Memorial Hospital in Rochester, New
York, then spent five years of postgraduate study at the Children's Hospital
in Birmingham, England, under Sir Leonard Parsons, with a research interest
in rheumatic fever. In 1938 he accepted a post at HSC to found a cardiac department and clinic and three years later wrote a classic article on prognosis in
rheumatic heart disease.[121] As his eulogist, cardiologist Vera Rose, said in 1989,

"At that time heart disease in children was mainly diagnosed as rheumatic in origin and little was known about congenital heart disease."[122] After the war he returned to HSC, just as cardiac surgery was exploding. It now became, as Keith later put it, "extremely important to decide what specific lesion was present."[123] Therefore, a kind of renaissance in cardiology occurred. Keith was first in Canada to undertake cardiac catheterization in children and first in North America to do angiocardiography in this population.[124] When in 1947 he persuaded the chief of surgery at the hospital that a cardiac surgeon was needed, William Mustard, recently recruited to HSC as a general and orthopedic surgeon, was sent to Johns Hopkins for a month to study with pioneer heart surgeon Alfred Blalock.[125] The first cardiac operation at HSC was performed later the same year. Thus began a close partnership between cardiology and heart surgery which has continued to the present and has played a major role in the hospital's decades-long pre-eminence in cardiac care.

Keith compiled a large database on congenital cardiac defects and drew on it in a number of contributions. After the war, he created the section at the Ontario Medical Association on cardiology; in 1952 this turned into the Ontario Heart Foundation, which subsidized much of the work of the division. In 1958 Keith, together with Richard D. Rowe and Peter Vlad, later a cardiologist at the State University of New York at Buffalo, edited what was to become one of the classic texts of pediatric cardiology, *Heart Disease in Infancy and Childhood*.[126]

Summing up Keith's influence, Rose said, "Under his direction in the division of cardiology more than 100 fellows were trained and many now practice as division chiefs in pediatric cardiology in all parts of the world."[127] Similar observations would be made in tributes to his two successors, Richard Rowe, who headed the division between 1973 and 1986, and Robert M. Freedom, chief from 1986 to 2000. In a 1988 obituary of Rowe, Freedom spoke movingly of his "human legacy. His trainees populate the globe ... Those individuals fortunate enough to have been trained by Dick Rowe could not help but be touched by the humanism and compassion of the man."[128] And in a biography published just before Freedom's own death in 2005, two of his colleagues emphasized that Freedom's "most significant and longest lasting contribution has been made in the very large number of fellows that have had the opportunity to work with him at the Hospital for Sick Children. They have come from every corner of the globe, and are a living tribute to his care for children, dedication, and kind heart."[129]

By the time Keith retired in 1973, HSC was already of sufficient stature in pediatric cardiology to attract Richard Rowe back from Johns Hopkins, where he had risen to the position of Harriet Lane Professor of Pediatrics and director of the Helen B. Taussig Children's Cardiac Center. Rowe had a particular interest in newborns with heart conditions, and under his leadership the Toronto team pioneered the use of "left heart and retrograde cardiac catheterizations in the neonate and young infant."[130] As with each of the division's chiefs, he was a prolific author, enjoyed a close relationship with the Division of Cardiovascular Surgery, and made significant advances in the field, as well as progressively expanding its clinical and research activities. Rowe stepped down as chief in 1986 but remained active in the division until his death in January 1988. His passing occurred six weeks before his planned retirement.[131]

HSC's world-class reputation in cardiology continued and assumed a higher international profile as Bob Freedom took charge of the division between 1986 and his official retirement at the end of 2001 (following a year's sabbatical during which he began to write and edit his eighth and final textbook, *The Natural and Modified History of Congenital Heart Disease*[132]).

In his inaugural vignette in the Department of Paediatrics' Annual Report for 2000–1, newly appointed Chief Andrew Redington described the Division of Cardiology as "one of the largest and most successful in the world." The pediatric cardiology training program "is the largest in Canada and one of the largest and most sought after in North America … Its fellows have populated cardiology groups throughout the world, many going on to become leaders of our specialty."[133]

### Division of Endocrinology

Among the oldest divisions of the Department of Paediatrics was endocrinology, which dated back to Gladys Boyd's insulin clinic in 1923. According to historian Michael Bliss, insulin was slow to be introduced to the hospital because Alan Brown had taken a dislike to Banting when he was a resident there. In November 1922, Banting and Boyd together resurrected a comatose eleven-year-old girl, Elsie Needham, "after many hours of deep unconsciousness."[134] (By January she was back in school.) Boyd herself was just four years out of medical school (where she had been director of the Undergraduate Medical Women's Council) and twenty-eight at the time she saw Elsie. Endocrinology at HSC really began with her, though she did not subsequently join the academic staff. Teaching in the subject apparently commenced with Chute's return to HSC and its research laboratories in 1949, after the war and his several years of research. At the hospital Chute conducted landmark clinical studies on the use of animal growth hormone in treating pituitary deficiency and the long-term complications of juvenile diabetes; in addition he was instrumental in establishing the Canadian Diabetes Association. The diabetes program continues to be a focal point of the division's activities.[135]

In the 1954–5 session the hospital founded a metabolic ward "for the study of various metabolic disorders under controlled conditions," directed by Andrew Sass-Kortsak.[136] Born in Hungary in 1916, he had completed his medical degree at the University of Budapest in 1940, going on to train with the renowned physiologist Fritz Verzar at the University of Basel, Switzerland. While there, his research attracted the attention of HSC physicians, and he was invited to join its staff in 1949. The ward, technically part of the hospital's new Research Institute, was a self-contained service, and its function under Sass-Kortsak and Chute was mainly endocrinological. (Sass-Kortsak went on to make important contributions at the institute, particularly in the investigation and treatment of Wilson's disease, a metabolic liver condition. A position as research professor was created for him in the Department of Paediatrics in 1966 and he became head of the Research Institute in 1981.[137])

In 1970 an endocrinology division was formally established under John D. Bailey. In the late 1960s, however, Bailey and his group were conducting the only research in "Endocrinology" reported by the hospital, and an endocrine section must already have existed in some form.[138] Following its establishment the division quickly became known for pioneering pediatric endocrine research and clinical studies. Of particular importance was the creation in the mid-1970s of a newborn screening program for congenital thyroid deficiency.[139]

### Division of Hematology (after 1981 Hematology/Oncology)

Pediatric medicine's first footprints in hematology were at the "Rh" laboratory at Winnipeg (named for rhesus monkeys, whose blood was found to contain the Rh factor in 1940) and at the Montreal Children's Hospital just after the Second World War. Bernard Laski, who trained in New York after graduating from U of T in 1939 (in the heyday of Toronto's medical anti-Semitism), is said to have introduced hematology to the Department of Pathology of the children's hospital in Toronto in the late 1940s while simultaneously involved in private practice. Pediatric hematologist Alvin Zipursky writes of the HSC scene in those days, when 300 exchange transfusions for hemolytic disease of the newborn were being conducted annually, "The technique in those early years was very crude, performed, according to one source, 'by letting blood drip into the saphenous vein and out of a slit radial artery into a bowl.'"[140]

In 1962 John Darte, one of Canada's first pediatric oncologists, left the Princess Margaret Hospital to found the division of hematology at HSC (see p. 265). After Peter McClure succeeded Darte as head of hematology in 1968, "an active, sophisticated clinical and laboratory service was developed."[141] The emphasis in the 1970s was on hemophilia, treated on an outpatient basis. "Haemophiliac patients may now lead an essentially normal life," said Chute in 1972, with patients and their parents administering their own injections.[142] The hematology division established an outpatient treatment facility in the 1971–2 session for blood transfusions, platelet transfusions, chemotherapy, and other procedures. By this time 90 percent of their hemophiliacs were being treated as outpatients.[143]

In the 1970s and 1980s the stunning advances in bone marrow transplantation in leukemia – and later in stem cell transplantation – added important new tools to the armamentarium in pediatric hematology and oncology. In 1972 HSC began a bone marrow transplantation program and, as an HSC executive pointed out, "the hospital soon became known as a leading centre for this procedure."[144] In 1980 pediatric oncology moved from the Princess Margaret Hospital to HSC.

Hematology and oncology were combined in 1981, when Zipursky (a 1953 medical graduate of the University of Manitoba) came from McMaster University to succeed McClure. In 2002 the bone marrow transplantation program at HSC was the designated centre for pediatric stem cell transplantation in Ontario and undertook seventy transplants during the session.[145]

### Division of Infectious Diseases

The scientific study of infectious diseases at HSC goes back to 1899, when William Goldie, who had graduated in medicine three years previously, thereupon training in the Department of Pathology and Bacteriology, was appointed physician-in-charge of infectious diseases at HSC. He retired from the position in 1911, while retaining an academic appointment in the Department of Medicine.[146]

The infectious diseases story resumes with George McNaughton, who grew up in Toronto and finished his medical studies in 1931. He trained in pediatrics at HSC and held teaching and resident positions at Presbyterian Hospital, part of Columbia University, in New York and at Cook County Hospital in Chicago. In 1935 he joined the Hospital for Sick Children, serving as registrar from 1936 to 1946. Of McNaughton it was said somewhat movingly at the time of his death in 1967, "His own little world was the infectious disease wards of the Hospital for Sick Children, and the falling mortality records of this department during his tenure of office are an everlasting testimony of his skill, his knowledge, and his efficiency. The kindness of his heart seemed to radiate to his little patients."[147]

In the following year, the 1968–9 session, Crawford Anglin, a 1943 graduate, took over the "extremely heavy service and teaching commitment" of the infection service.[148] His tenure saw a big decline in meningitis mortality, from 10–15 percent to 2.9 percent in 1971. "This has been accomplished by a team effort, the team consisting of doctors, nurses, bacteriologists, neurologists, and others," Anglin reported. The division was now studying meningitis "in tiny babies during the first month of life … The mortality in this group is still distressingly high (greater than 50 per cent) and one of the objectives for the 1970s is to rectify this situation."[149]

Like many early staff members, including some division chiefs, Anglin held a part-time position. In 1979 Ronald Gold was recruited from the United States as "the first full-time head of the Division of Infectious Diseases at the Hospital for Sick Children."[150] In 1997 the infectious diseases ward was eliminated, but the division continues to exist.

### Division of Nephrology

The Division of Nephrology blossomed when C. Phillips Rance, a 1942 U of T medical graduate, agreed to head it; together with Robert Jeffs and William Harvey, in the 1966–7 session he established a renal dialysis unit.[151] They were soon following about thirty patients in different stages of chronic renal failure: eight were on chronic dialysis; kidney transplantation had begun in the late 1960s and by May 1969 four patients had had renal transplants using cadaveric kidneys.[152] In 1971 Gerald S. Arbus returned from postgraduate training in Boston and New York to take charge of the rapidly expanding dialysis and transplant service.[153] Under Arbus's direction the unit changed from peritoneal dialysis to hemodialysis, "and our effort is in the direction of returning these children to as normal a life as possible."[154] The years ahead saw "an enormous upsurge of activity within the dialysis field," which along with renal transplantation was the core mission of the nephrology division.[155]

## Division of Neurology

George F. Boyer was the first neurologist at the Hospital for Sick Children. Stemming from Kincardine, Ontario, he graduated from high school in 1903, from medicine at U of T in 1907; he was said to be possessed of "a bright, sunny disposition, and … endowed with intense energy."[156] After training at Cleveland Lakeside Hospital and in London, England, he was originally appointed to the Toronto General Hospital, then to HSC as a consultant (not a staff physician) in 1912. In 1932 he organized an epilepsy "subdivision."[157] It was in all likelihood Boyer who established in Toronto the value of electroencephalographic studies "in children presenting behaviour problems or suffering from convulsive disorders … in distinguishing between convulsions and functional attacks." He also confirmed that the drug Dilantin (phenytoin) controlled grand mal attacks but not petit mal.[158]

In 1949 W. Wray Barraclough succeeded Boyer as consultant neurologist. Barraclough, a 1916 U of T graduate, had trained in Toronto; at Johns Hopkins University; at the National Hospital, Queen Square in London; and at London Hospital. He was a member of the Royal College of Physicians, London. In 1952 he stepped aside for William A. Hawke, a Toronto MD from 1930, who also was MRCP and who covered both neurology and psychiatry, eventually founding the Department of Psychiatry at HSC in 1968.

Neurology was granted full divisional status at HSC in the 1966–7 session, with John Stobo Prichard its full-time head. Prichard is a major figure in the history of Canadian neurology, and it was he who established training in pediatric neurology in this country. Prichard and Richardson later organized a training program in adult neurology. Prichard was one of the few Welshmen on the faculty, in contrast to the many Scots. Born in Barry, Wales, in 1914, he earned a BA at Cambridge in 1935 and a medical degree in 1938. After five years in the war, he trained in neurology at Queen Square, Hammersmith Hospital, and Massachusetts General Hospital, then immigrated to Canada in 1950 to organize the electroencephalographic lab at HSC at about the same time that John Scott was doing so at the General.

Prichard's students may be found all over the world. His eulogist and former pupil J. Alexander Lowden said in 1987, "Wherever he travelled with his wife Joan, they visited old friends and were warmly welcomed." At HSC

Prichard undertook a number of initiatives. He began combined neurolog-ical-neurosurgical rounds, he organized a dedicated ward for neurological patients, and he "encouraged the establishment of an active research pro-gram in neurosciences." He took a strong interest in developmental disabili-ties, helping organize the Surrey Place Centre, and after he retired from the chiefship of the Division of Neurology in 1977, he established the Child De-velopment Clinic (later the Child Development Centre, which in 2005 moved to Bloorview) and a research program in learning disabilities. Lowden, who ended up in Montreal, said, "On a personal note, I have Stobo to thank for encouraging me to enter a career in science when I was a half-trained paedia-trician. When my family and I returned to Toronto after completing a PhD, Stobo was there to ask us to dinner, to support my efforts in setting up a lab, to encourage me in those first nervous steps of a new investigator on his own."[159] Among Prichard's three children was Robert, a later president of the University of Toronto.

As a sign of the times, it was an American, William J. Logan, who followed the Welshman Prichard as the next head of the neurology division at HSC in 1978. Logan finished medical studies at the University of Chicago in 1963, then trained in pediatrics at the Johns Hopkins Hospital and the Cincinnati Chil-dren's Hospital, in neurology at Stanford and Johns Hopkins. He spent several years at the National Institutes of Health in Bethesda, thereupon proceeding to the University of Virginia School of Medicine, where he established a labora-tory for neurotransmitter neurochemistry, as director of pediatric neurology.

It was on Logan's watch that in 1993 Gabrielle deVeber introduced the epi-demiologic study of pediatric stroke to HSC. A 1984 medical graduate of Mc-Master University, deVeber created at HSC the Canadian Pediatric Ischemic Stroke Registry, which brought together data from all sixteen Canadian chil-dren's hospitals, creating by 2005 a population base of data on incidence, risk factors, and treatment on over 1,300 children. In 1995 she initiated a two-centre outcome study for children with focal, non-progressive cerebral disorders, in-cluding stroke, and developed an outcome measure – the Pediatric Stroke Out-come Measure – that subsequently was widely adopted internationally. These data permitted the assessment of several risk factors, including coagulation dis-orders, chicken pox, and cardiac surgery.[160]

In 1996 O. Carter Snead III, the head of the division at this writing, took of-fice, continuing the tradition of appointing highly visible US investigators. In 2005 neurology and neurosurgery merged into a single Clinical Neurosciences Unit.[161]

### Paediatrics Was Not the Only Department at HSC

In a big, complex hospital there are many departments. Each has its own story. But this history of the faculty shall tarry only at a couple of special interests and conclude with the Research Institute. For the Department of Psychiatry at HSC see chapter 14.

*Department of Radiology*

One of the gemstones of the Hospital for Sick Children was the Department of Radiology, which began in 1919 with the appointment of Albert H. ("Bert") Rolph. Previously, imaging at the hospital had been conducted under the guidance of radiographers. Rolph was born in 1880 to a prominent Rosedale family. He took first a degree in arts – indeed developing later in life such widespread artistic interests that he became viewed by his colleagues as something of a dilettante. He graduated in medicine at U of T in 1906, interned at HSC, then took several professional degrees in England. During the war, he cut his teeth on radiology at the Canadian base camps in England and France, then, at the behest of HSC board member Sir Edmund Osler, returned to Canada to be hired as a radiologist in 1919. The following year the T. Eaton Company donated the hospital's new radiological equipment and again in 1940 newer equipment, in this technologically fast-changing field. By 1950, for reasons unknown, the Eaton family had given radiology at HSC almost half a million dollars.

In 1936 Rolph propelled radiology at HSC into the public eye by trucking a cumbersome army field X-ray device up to Callandar, Ontario, where he had dinner with Allan Dafoe, the physician of the Dionne quintuplets, and the following day took X-rays of the famous quints. Rolph, alas, rather lost control of the department amidst his many artistic interests, and by the time John Munn joined the service in 1946 as an assistant radiologist, the doctors were taking the radiographs home or piling them under patients' beds.[162] In 1947 Munn would turn radiology at HSC into a university department.

Munn was born in 1913 in Ripley, Ontario, and graduated in medicine from the University of Western Ontario in 1938. After training in radiology at the Toronto General Hospital between 1941 and 1943, he served overseas with the Royal Canadian Army Medical Corps, returning after the end of hostilities to direct the radiology service of the Discharge Centre at Exhibition Grounds in Toronto, then hopped over to HSC where in June 1946 he became assistant radiologist under Rolph. Because he was quite green about the pediatric side, he trained in Boston and New York at children's hospitals, then returned in January 1947 to lead pediatric radiology at HSC. In the 1948–9 session Munn brought radiology at the hospital into the university system.[163]

At HSC under Munn, science ruled. Right off the bat, he ended the practice Rolph had introduced of irradiating supposedly enlarged thymus glands. Writes the historian of radiology in Toronto, "Once Munn demonstrated to the staff that the thymus normally changed size and shape in the course of respiration, they agreed that the practice should be stopped."[164]

Meanwhile, cardiologist John Keith had been working on cardiac catheterization, and in 1948 Munn and Keith developed a four-frames-per-second angiography camera to see if infants with cyanotic heart disease were operable. Munn helped ignite interest at HSC in fibrocystic disease of the pancreas, establishing that it could be diagnosed radiographically without passing a tube down the child's esophagus to see if the gastric juices were diagnostic of the illness. Munn later said, "You'd hear on rounds that you couldn't do this, couldn't do that. I used to step over the boundaries and set them back." Munn and John Darte joined in the fight against the X-ray machines that once existed in shoe stores to check the fit. From 1964 on, he figured among the first radiologists to determine the diagnostic signs of child abuse.[165] By the time Munn stepped down in 1967 the radiology service at HSC consisted of four members, one of whom was Bernard Reilly.

The Reilly era began in October 1967 as Barney Reilly became head of radiology. Reilly was a Scotsman who earned a Glasgow MB degree in 1949. In 1950 a Saskatchewan anti-tuberculosis organization brought him to Canada, and after training in Boston as Munn had done, he finally wound up as a pediatric radiologist in Saskatoon in 1959. In 1961 he came to the North York General Hospital as a general radiologist, then moved in 1967 to HSC back into the pediatric side.

Reilly expanded the radiology department from four members to thirteen, investing in loads of new equipment for the new wing of the hospital that would be finished in 1971. And he opened up pediatric neuroradiology, engaging Evert Kruyff as the first specialist in 1961 (who, like his counterpart Karel terBrugge at the Western, was a Dutchman).[166] Yet the stellar figure in the history of neuroradiology at HSC – and the founder of the field in general – was Derek Harwood-Nash.

It was Harwood-Nash who helped Barney Reilly build the hospital department while at the same time pioneering the radiologic investigation of the child's brain and nervous system. Born in Bulawayo in what was then Rhodesia, Harwood-Nash was educated at the University of Cape Town and graduated with an MB in 1960 at the same time as his close friend Alan Hudson. They interned in surgery together, and both entered a fellowship program in neurosurgery at HSC under Bruce Hendrick. Harwood-Nash then became interested in radiology and trained under George Wortzman at the Toronto General Hospital, receiving his diploma in medical radiology in 1966. In 1968 he became director of neuroradiology at the hospital. Harwood-Nash wrote his first high-impact article in 1971 on the significance – or lack thereof – of skull fractures "without clinical abnormalities of the sensorium or the central nervous system" in children. Conducted with Hendrick and Hudson, the research found that such fractures were "of little significance."[167] In 1976 Harwood-Nash and Charles Fitz published their classic monograph *Neuroradiology in Infants and Children*, which, as eulogist Michael Huckman put it, had the result of "giving birth to the specialty of pediatric neuroradiology and making Toronto its capital … 'Sick Kids' soon became the Mecca to which men and women from all over the world flocked to be trained in his section."[168] In the years 1978 to 1988 he succeeded Reilly as chief radiologist of the hospital. A faculty report in 1983 called neuroradiology at HSC "the crown jewel of the department. The group has a well recognized international reputation for clinical and academic work."[169]

The advent of computed tomography and magnetic resonance imaging caused a revolution in pediatric radiology: "Do you want to see the scan first, or the patient?" as Robin Humphreys posed the dilemma.

> This question, a prelude to the consultation on a new patient, echoes repeatedly through hospital corridors every where. It wasn't always like this. In the 'BC era' (Before CAT scanning), a respected former university chairman of pediatrics would utter, 'Don't do something! Stand there and observe the child.' Indeed that was about all one could do. Consider the options for the small patient with symptoms of 9 months duration that suggested the possibility of a brain tumour ... The child would be subject to a primitive xray procedure that consisted of injecting air into the brain ventricles (air pneumoencephalography). After a while, the air would percolate through the ventricles and maybe cap the front edge of a tumour ... An operation would be planned for which the surgeon often felt at a disadvantage. What were the actual dimensions of the tumour and into what critical structures had it insinuated itself?

These injected air–type examinations that some characterized as "barbaric" gave way, Humphreys said, in the mid-1970s to CT scanning. "Neurosurgeons were liberated. Pathological processes could be confirmed, as could the detail of their anatomical relationships to adjacent brain structures ... At last the surgeon possessed an imaging tool that could provide one with an intelligent list of diagnostic possibilities and, in the event an operation would be required, the roadmap for surgical approaches." A decade later magnetic resonance imaging (MRI) followed, an even greater revolution because now individual brain structures could be outlined. "The printed MRI pictures resemble the black and white photographs of the brain that are found in the traditional atlases of anatomy, with which all medical students are familiar. The many additional manipulations of the MRI sequences have provided by now [2002] greater confidence than ever before, with respect to the precise diagnosis of the disease condition in the nervous system." This was, said Humphreys, especially true of the spinal cord.

From imaging it was just a hop, skip, and jump to "image guided therapy," about which Humphreys also waxed eloquent. In May 2002 HSC's Image Guided Therapy Suite opened. Humphreys said, "Instead of traditional, invasive surgery, surgeons, radiologists, physicians and anaesthetists work together using needles, catheters, wires and probes inserted through small incisions, in combination with imaging equipment and tiny cameras, to examine and treat patients." He gave the example of a child with "a fluid collection around the brain." The CT scanner in the unit weighed 1.3 metric tons and moved on floor rails. "The C-Arm, which weighs 1.4 metric tons, moves on ceiling rails over the examining table."[170] The effect of this technological progress on the diagnosis and treatment of disease has been incalculable. If one had to range beyond the introduction of antibiotics and the improvements in surgery that have made a difference in children's health, the imaging revolution would be high on the list.

*Department of Surgery*

Surgery always arouses alarm in patients and loved ones. But when children are the patients, the alarm is special. The surgeons at HSC have always had a special kind of status.

In 1898 Clarence L. Starr was appointed as a junior surgeon at HSC, with bone tuberculosis his specialty. When in 1913 the post of surgeon-in-chief was created, Starr, as the first incumbent, reorganized the service with one chief and a subordinate staff; all staff surgeons had university appointments.[171] As seen earlier, in 1921 William Gallie succeeded Starr. When in 1929 Gallie moved over to the General as professor of surgery, David Edwin ("Eddie") Robertson took his place at HSC.

Robertson was a distinctive figure. Born in 1883 in Milton, Ontario, at age six he came to Toronto; he was educated at Harbord Collegiate and then the Faculty of Medicine at U of T, graduating in 1907. (Known to his fellow medical students as "Scotch," he occupied "positions of honor and trust in the Hockey and Football Clubs."[172]) After postgraduate study in England and Germany, he returned to Toronto to accept a surgical appointment in 1912 at the Hospital for Sick Children. After the war he found himself "carrying the responsibility of the surgical service almost single-handed."

In 1929, Robertson succeeded Gallie as surgeon-in-chief at HSC, "which position he occupied with great distinction until his death [in 1944]." At HSC he led a campaign against appendicitis, reducing the death rate from 15 percent in 1922 to 0.1 percent at the time of his death. In surgical innovation, in 1932 he performed the first lung lobectomy at the children's hospital and in November 1940 did the first ligation at the hospital for patent ductus arteriosus. The late 1930s, of course, saw the revolutionary introduction of the sulfa drugs, and in the fall of 1939 Robertson began treating osteomyelitis (infection of the bone) with them, "in this manner changing entirely the clinical picture of this disease."[173] In 1936 Robertson captured the nation's attention, entombed in the Moose River mine collapse, as he was saved in a dramatic rescue after ten days in the rubble.[174]

With Robertson's death in 1944, Arthur Baker LeMesurier became chief of surgery at the children's hospital. Thus another storied figure in the history of surgery in Toronto comes into view.

LeMesurier was born in Darjeeling, India, attended the University of Toronto Church School and Upper Canada College, and graduated from the U of T Faculty of Medicine in 1910. During his studies he is said to have "played in every University tennis tournament, and with the University cricket team."[175] After training as a resident in surgery at HSC and in New York – and after five years of military medical service during World War I – he joined the surgical staff of the children's hospital in 1920, remaining there until his retirement in 1950. He was surgeon-in-chief from 1944 to 1950. LeMesurier was known for a number of scientific contributions, including a traction technique for fractured femurs that he developed during the war and which is known as LeMesurier Traction. He is known as well for the studies that he and Gallie undertook on free grafted fibrous tissues, such as fascia and tendon (called "living sutures"), and a long-term follow-up study of an amputation technique used during the war called the Symes amputation, in which LeMesurier determined that this technique – above the heads of the metatarsal bones – was superior to others. He said that "[n]ot one had to be re-amputated and that their ends are causing less trouble than any other stump." He also originated a technique for the repair of cleft lip that became known worldwide as the LeMesurier Technique, introducing a new era in the treatment of cleft lip patients.[176]

In 1950 Robert M. Wansbrough succeeded LeMesurier as surgeon-in-chief at HSC. "Tim" Wansbrough was born on a farm near Grand Valley in 1900. He matriculated in 1918 and graduated in medicine in 1924. He then trained in surgery at HSC under Gallie, joining the Department of Surgery in 1928. Said his eulogist in 1956, "His appointment coincided with the depletion of the attending staff at his hospital ... For many years this threw a great volume of work on the shoulders of the newest member of the staff," leaving little time for research. He was again in uniform during World War II, and after his return worked even harder than before, "leaving him with no time for more leisurely academic pursuits, even had he wished these." After becoming professor and chief of surgery in 1951, "he suffered from an attack of cardiac infarction. Undaunted by this he did not spare his energy, and died on duty [1956] with an extension of the same lesion."[177]

In 1956 Alfred W. Farmer replaced Wansbrough as head of surgery at HSC. Farmer is a crucial figure in the history of the department because he originated the divisional system that was then widely copied. He grew up in St Catharines, Ontario, and studied medicine at U of T, where he also excelled in sports, graduating in 1927. He trained in surgery in Toronto, followed by a year of plastic surgery in England, from which he returned in 1931 to join the surgical staff at HSC. Just after becoming chief of surgery, Farmer set up the five (later six) specialty divisions in surgery: neurosurgery, under William Keith; plastics, under William Lindsay; cardiovascular, under William Mustard; orthopedics, under Robert Salter; and general, under Stuart Thomson; the division of urology was formed later, under Robert D. Jeffs.[178] As Fred Kergin, head of the campus Department of Surgery, said, "This has resulted in better patient care, in greatly enhanced productivity in clinical and basic research and in the provision of a unique opportunity for training in the various specialties in paediatric surgery."[179]

In 1966 Farmer stepped down as chief of surgery, succeeded by Robert B. Salter, whose personal activities as professor and chair of surgery are described in chapter 7. During Salter's tenure subspecialization galloped forward. Highly specialized and complex procedures started to become normal. At HSC in September 1966 the first set of conjoined twins at the hospital were separated; in January 1969 the first kidney transplant at HSC was conducted.[180] Robin Humphreys comments of the Salter years, "By this time, the pediatric identity was weaving its way through the various subspecialties of surgery. Formerly, a 'pediatric surgeon' was a general surgeon who ... was very experienced and comfortable operating upon various organ systems in the child's body. Now, the individual surgical disciplines were becoming subspecialized, and full-time surgeons with extra training in their respective pediatric surgical specialty were joining the staffs of children's hospitals."[181] (Salter's more than 300 former postgraduate students honoured him by forming the Salter Society, an organization that meets regularly.)

In 1976 Robert Filler came up from Boston to become HSC's next surgeon-in-chief. Filler, a pediatric general surgeon who had graduated in 1956 from Washington University in St Louis, helped the hospital score a large humanitarian – and public relations – triumph in 1979 by rescuing a seven-month old Brooklyn baby named Herbie Quinones, Jr., whose parents were too poor to afford US health care, from a condition in which he could not swallow food without cutting off the flow of air to his lungs (tracheomalacia), leaving him, as the *Toronto Star* put it, "in what nurses at the Brooklyn Hospital called 'dying spells.'" Alerted to the child's need, the *Toronto Star* newspaper brought Herbie to Toronto, and after the successful operation Metropolitan Toronto chairman Paul Godfrey organized the "Herbie Fund" to bring children from all over the world to Toronto for life-altering or life-saving surgeries. By 2009, when Herbie himself celebrated the thirtieth anniversary of his operation, the Herbie Fund had brought more than 600 children from 88 countries to the children's hospital in Toronto for operations that literally gave them their lives. Filler, a member of the Division of General Surgery who had been hired from Boston in 1976, had readily sprung in – and for free.[182]

In December 1994 Filler passed the baton to John H. Wedge, a pediatric orthopedic surgeon, as surgeon-in-chief at the hospital. And in January 2005 Wedge gave way to James Wright, previously program head of population health sciences at the Hospital for Sick Children's Research Institute. The tenures of these latter individuals are too recent for historical evaluation.

I have avoided use of the term "Sick Kids" in this discussion, even though that today is the hospital's official name. This is doubtless just stuffiness on my part. Yet it is of interest that the phrase "Sick Kids" is actually a coinage of hospital public relations and has only been adopted officially in recent years.[183] Among clinicians of the faculty, the hospital was always referred to as "the Children's Hospital," or else "HSC." This is just a footnote about the triumph of public relations over medical tradition.

### HSC Research Institute

In a broad sense, the Research Institute of HSC goes back to a small chemistry laboratory that Duncan Graham authorized in 1918. Named the Nutritional Laboratory in 1929, its tasks, as seen, included the development of Pablum cereal and Sunwheat biscuits.[184]

In a narrower sense, the institute as such dated to the early 1950s. In the background was a polio epidemic. The work of Rhodes's team at HSC on the polio vaccine aroused international attention as the disease seemed to spread rapidly, chilling parental hearts. In September 1952 Chute, who had just become chief physician at HSC, described Rhodes's work. "In poliomyelitis we still have a potent enemy capable of warping the body and spirit of our youngsters, but there is a gleam of hope on the dark horizon," he said. "Laboratory workers have recently found a method for growing the virus of poliomyelitis in a variety of living tissue cultures. Formerly this disease could only be kept going in living monkeys or in some cases in mice. This made its study difficult. Now the virus can be grown in a test tube." Chute said that Andrew Rhodes, director of the hospital's virus laboratory, "is engaged in the study today of polio and his work has provoked ... widespread interest."[185]

In December 1953, HSC announced that it was founding a Research Institute, with microbiologist Rhodes, previously at the Connaught Laboratories, at its head. As the *Globe and Mail* explained, "Rhodes has been a key figure in several major research developments, one of them the production of a polio vaccine as a result of collaboration between the hospital, the laboratories and the National Foundation for Infantile Paralysis, New York." Since July 1953, Rhodes had been in charge of the hospital's various unrelated research programs. "Until now," hospital officials said, "there had been no way of co-ordinating research." "The institute would take over direction of all present research, would take administrative burdens off research workers' shoulders." A research committee would guide the institute, composed of Rhodes, Lawrie Chute, chief of the Department of Paediatrics, and Robert Wansbrough, chief of the Department of Surgery. The funding apparently would come from some of the revenues that Frederick Tisdall and Theodore Drake had collected in royalties from Pablum for their pediatric research foundation, and it was clear that the hospital would like to see big research stemming from such a long-term commitment happen again.[186] "We hope to be able to develop several research teams to investigate a number of problems," Rhodes told the *Toronto Daily Star*. "One of the difficulties in the past has been that the lack of a continuing program has discouraged young research workers, and many have left after only one or two years. With more funds available, more continuity can be given and better facilities provided."[187]

Building on this base of research in virology, the Research Institute steadily added other components. Sometime after he took office in 1956 Farmer created "a very active division of surgical research in the Research Institute."[188] In the fall of 1956, "a radioisotope laboratory with animal facilities became available for use."[189]

When Rhodes stepped down in 1956 to become director of the School of Hygiene, Robert Rolf Struthers took his place two years later. Sixty-five at the time, Struthers was formerly professor of pediatrics at McGill University and associate director of the Rockefeller Foundation's Division of Medical Education and Public Health.

In the 1961–2 session W. Stanley Hartroft, a 1941 medical graduate of the University of Alberta and PhD scholar, became director of the Research Institute. Hartroft had been a member of the Department of Physiology until the early 1950s, when he progressed to Washington University in St Louis. Now he was returning to Toronto as director of the Research Institute at HSC with a part-time appointment in the Department of Physiology.[190]

In the early 1960s, the hospital began aligning its research stars into the institute on a full-time basis, in particular Andrew Sass-Kortsak, who was studying copper storage in Wilson's disease; Donald Fraser, who was looking at calcium metabolism in children; Paul Swyer, who was working on cardiac problems in neonates; and Robert Ehrlich, who was researching growth hormone. Several other workers, including cardiologist John Keith, had part-time appointments.[191]

The grant money flowed freely and private contributions picked up. These were years of great expansion in the Research Institute, which by the mid-1960s had formal sections on allergy, cardiology, endocrinology, genetics, hematology, metabolic disease, neonatology, neurology, and virology. Some of the sections, such as neurology, had only one investigator (Prichard); others, such as metabolic disease, had several.[192] By 1970 the institute had thirty full-time scientists plus twenty-five part-timers whose full-time work lay in patient care.[193] In 1973 the Hospital for Sick Children Foundation was established, which greatly increased the funding of the Research Institute, turning it into a scientific power centre.

In 1972 a capital event in the life of the Research Institute took place: Aser Rothstein, an immense scientific figure, became director. Born in Vancouver in 1918, he attended high school there. He went to college at the University of British Columbia and the University of California at Berkeley. In 1943, he received a PhD in biology from the University of Rochester. Rothstein spent most of his career in scientific research at US government agencies: he assisted at the Atomic Energy Project to develop a nuclear weapon in 1943–5 and spent the ensuing decades at federal science laboratories working on such issues as the toxicity of uranium, which led Rothstein, still in government service, to membrane biology (the few students of this area called themselves "the Transport Workers Union").[194] He finished his US government career as co-director of the Atomic Energy Project from 1965 to 1972.

Rothstein had one of those outsized personalities that people talk about decades afterwards. Allan Okey, later chair of pharmacology, recalled Rothstein from his own days at the Research Institute: "Aser was a person of great integrity and somebody with a lot of wisdom and quiet leadership, because he wasn't a bombastic kind of a person, but someone who was a 'get on with it' kind of guy, who did what a lot of the younger scientists always hope that their superiors will do, that is to simply say, 'How can I create an environment where good things can happen?' I saw that as the way things worked at Sick Kids."[195]

Accepting the directorship of the Research Institute at HSC meant returning to Canada. What drew Rothstein back to his country of birth? "It was the idea of establishing an Institute with the whole spectrum – from very basic to very applied research – that has intrigued me, because that gives the most immediate knowledge transfer from what we know about biological systems to using it in practical diagnosis and treatment."[196]

In April 1972, Rothstein sent a memo to senior staff on how the research foci of the Research Institute need to be sharpened, along the lines of interdisciplinarity, expectations of progress, and impact: "[We] should choose research areas on the basis that we can make a special contribution because of our unique facilities or unique collection of talent. We should not choose an area of research unless we can develop an outstanding effort that will contribute effectively to our service to the community."[197] It is interesting that he did not say research that would raise the institutional profile but rather research that would benefit the community.

On campus and off, the consensus grew in the 1970s that the Research Institute was acquiring visibility. As Bain told the long-range planners in November 1974, "The consensus was that it has had a great impact and has achieved international recognition … It represents an outstanding example of basic research applied to the clinical situation."[198]

Under Rothstein, certain operating rules were worked out. All research done in the hospital occurred "in the domain of the Research Institute," as Rothstein told the faculty's Science Policy committee in December 1976. The institute paid the salary of any staffer who spent at least 50 percent of his or her time in research. Also, all members of the institute had academic appointments at the university, though the institute was independent of the university bureaucracy and its director reported directly to the HSC trustees.[199]

When Rothstein retired from directing the institute in 1986, it had grown to over 500 full-time employees, ranking as one of the top two such centres in the world.[200] Lou Siminovitch, who had been instrumental in recruiting Rothstein, later told university president David Naylor that "[Rothstein] transformed a very modest research program at the Hospital for Sick Children to one of international excellence [and] provided a model and standard of quality for all future hospital-based institutes."[201]

Splendid though the evolution of the Research Institute had been, several observers decried the separation of the institute from the hospital's clinical departments. By 1991 James Friesen, director of the institute, was said to receive almost no input from the huge Department of Paediatrics, a discussion that might have been useful in identifying research problems and marshalling resources. "As the Research Institute now exists," wrote one external reviewer in 1991, "it might as well be wholly separate from the Hospital corporately and geographically." There was, effectively, a disjunction "between the clinical and research endeavors of the Hospital."[202]

The further story will be pursued in chapter 28.

### Coda: The Bloorview Children's Hospital and the Hugh MacMillan Rehabilitation Centre

In 1899 the same group of women who had founded the Hospital for Sick Children met again to discuss an institution devoted to the care of children with chronic illnesses and physical disabilities. From this came the Home for Incurable Children, with its fifteen beds, located first on Toronto's Avenue Road, then at a bigger site on Bloor Street East permitting (by the 1950s) fifty beds. By this time a number of physicians from HSC were cross-appointed to what became called in 1959 Bloorview Hospital, Home and School. (Four years later, in 1963, it was rechristened Bloorview Children's Hospital.) Bloorview also became a training site for occupational and physical therapists from the faculty.

Bloorview vaulted from a chronic care facility to a research centre. In 1967 a visiting physician from Massachusetts General Hospital wrote to Fred Dewar, surgeon-in-chief at the General, about the Orthotics and Prosthetics Research Laboratories at Bloorview: "This group of laboratories has already become known internationally for its work on electrically stimulated prostheses for children. There is an unusually good scholarly and research environment here, as well as superb clinical facilities. And I was happy to note that there were several engineering students assigned to this unit doing their theses." Disappointingly, he encountered no trainees in orthopedics.[203]

HSC and Bloorview signed a memorandum of agreement in 1983 to weave Bloorview's population of disabled infants and children into the postgraduate program and the treatment team concepts of HSC and to give HSC residents some exposure to neurorehabilitation. Yet a review two years later found it discouraging that little research was being conducted at Bloorview.[204]

In February 2002 Bloorview became fully affiliated with the U of T, with Golda Milo-Manson of the Department of Paediatrics as chief of medical staff.[205]

All the staff would shortly have appointments in the campus Department of Paediatrics, making Bloorview the largest subspecialty training centre for developmental pediatrics in Canada.[206]

Meanwhile, in 1957 another facility, the Ontario Crippled Children's Centre, was established on Rumsey Road. In the 1969–70 session a one-month rotation was implemented there to "provide specialized instruction in rehabilitation medicine."[207] This facility was also involved in pioneering electrically powered prostheses for children. In 1971 William F. Sauter of the centre designed the first child-sized electric hand for an eight-year-old. This device, produced and marketed by the Variety Village children's charitable organization as the VV 105 hand, resulted in the development of progressively smaller myoelectric hands for children as young as eighteen months.[208] These prostheses were only of benefit to young patients with below-elbow amputations, so in 1983 Sauter's group devised an electric elbow and hand assembly light enough to be used by a three-year-old.[209]

In 1985 the facility was renamed the Hugh MacMillan Medical Centre, in honour of a physician who ran its hospital section in the early 1960s despite severe disabilities from polio. In 1990 the name was changed to Hugh MacMillan Rehabilitation Centre.

In 1996 the Hugh MacMillan Rehabilitation Centre merged with Bloorview Children's Hospital to become the Bloorview MacMillan Children's Centre. Subsequent changes in structure and title will not be followed here.

Many consider the Hospital for Sick Children to be Toronto's most glittering medical ornament. No other Toronto hospital has such worldwide recognition, and scientifically the researchers and clinicians at what is now universally called "Sick Kids" lead their respective international packs. That this institution emerged from a handful of women activists in the late nineteenth century intent upon saving children, and found its scientific furtherance in a handful of Ontario plowboys straight from the farm, is only a bit short of miraculous. I promised at the beginning of this book to abstain from superlatives, yet here they are called for.

# 11   Research

This brings me to a brief discussion of what constitutes a great medical school. It is, of course, one that will produce graduates who will give the best possible service to our sick ... It means, too, that it is staffed by first-class teachers, men and women who can help their students to learn and teach them to think for themselves. It also means that it has among its staff, men and women who are capable of conducting effective research and for whom there is sufficient financial support to enable them to carry on such studies. Once a school has achieved that position it has a right to the adjective great."[1]

William Gallie, 1957

Gallie was right and wrong. He was right that Toronto had absorbed the English emphasis on clinical excellence and close relations between teachers and students in medical education. He was, however, engaging in wishful thinking in the belief that, before the Second World War, Toronto occupied a prominent position among the world's research universities. It didn't. The English tradition was a double-edged sword. As President Claude Bissell reflected in his memoirs, "The tone at Toronto was formed by teachers who had graduated from English universities, and England had always been skeptical of any attempt to pursue scholarship in an institutional system. There the important point was to give a good first degree, and then leave scholarship to follow its own natural evolution." Bissell said that Toronto displayed "the typical colonial attitude: if one really wanted to pursue formal graduate studies, one went to a leading American or European university; the resources in Canada for advanced work were slim." Insulin had been a vast anomaly. Up to the 1960s, most departments of the faculty were not animated by the spirit of discovery, although here and there spectacular successes had occurred. Bissell said that in the 1950s the faculty was "strongly oriented towards practice and might well have expressed surprise if it had been suggested that this was not its whole duty."[2]

A bit of framing: not just in Toronto but in North America as a whole the primacy of research rushed forward in academic life. As Stanley Joel Reiser, at the time director of the history of medicine program at Harvard Medical School, noted in 1978, "At most university hospitals and medical schools during [the 1950s], research had become the keystone of the medical arch."[3] Toronto was thus part and parcel of the surge in the New World to pick up the scientific baton that had slackened in the hands of the war-torn Old World. The new language of science was no longer German and its main fortresses no longer Berlin and Heidelberg, but Bethesda and Southern California. And Canadians aspired to do more than just pad along behind.

An interest in science is not the same thing as a devotion to research. From the very beginning, the Faculty of Medicine was keyed into the importance of science – microscopes, departments of physiology, visiting lectures by William Osler: all was in place to distance medical Toronto from the bleeding and purging of yore. Yet mere commitment to science is not research. And until around 1905 almost nothing was said about contributing to the great international Niagara of research, as opposed merely to producing scientifically literate physicians for the population of Ontario.

This deficiency started to be noted. In a memorandum to a provincial commission on the University of Toronto in 1905, Alexander Primrose, secretary of the faculty, referred "to the absolute necessity of providing for research work. If one were to enquire into the growth of the larger universities on this continent and in Great Britain it is quite obvious that an important and essential feature of the development of progressive institutions has been … the provision of research laboratories … if this country is to keep abreast of the advances made in scientific Medicine elsewhere."[4]

Primrose and his colleagues tended to see Britain as the model. Primrose, after all, had been educated in Edinburgh. Yet the continent of Europe, especially Germany, provided a more apt model than the United Kingdom. Dean Charles K. Clarke, who had visited the great research centres of Germany, such as Emil Kraepelin's university psychiatric hospital in Munich, said in 1914, "If the schools of Germany in Berlin or Heidelberg or Munich are regarded throughout the world as being in the front rank," it was because "much of the work has been done which makes the medicine taught to-day more helpful and more hopeful that than which was taught thirty years ago." What might Canadians learn from this? "The proper outlet for an enquiring mind is the critical training of systematic experimentation. No one can be expected to go far in medicine … who gets no ideas of his own from his studies, who has not the opportunity to put his ideas to the test, and who is not trained in the balancing of evidence obtained by scientific experiment. Medical Research is just this."[5] Clarke's field was psychiatry. But in internal medicine, surgery, and other fields as well, the heavy hitters were in German-speaking Europe. Yet for cultural reasons Toronto did face more towards London and Edinburgh than Berlin and Vienna.

A big part of the research story is funding, and some funds to subsidize this work were present. In 1912 a Medical Research Fund was created through "gifts from citizens."[6] As well, in 1915 the generosity of Colonel Gooderham made possible the erection of the Connaught Antitoxin Laboratories (see pp. 59–60). In 1915–16 the federal government established at the university a special fund of $15,000 to investigate the "problems connected with the functional re-education of returned soldiers." From 1920 onwards, the federal government earmarked for the university $60,000 a year for "scientific research," and the province set aside $10,000 a year to support the research of Banting and Best. In the summer of 1925 private funds endowed the Banting Research Foundation with $600,000. Thus, in 1926 President Falconer said, "A survey of the past six years of the life of the university indicates that the greatest development has lain in the movement for research, especially in the scientific departments."[7]

This theme of rather gentlemanly part-time research coupled with sputters of funding persisted through the interwar years. In 1937 Dean Gallie expressed delight that interdisciplinary research seemed to be occurring in the faculty. Examples included the collaboration between physiology and surgery on heparin and the study "of the nature of nerve impulses and muscle contraction conducted by Drs. Solandt, Smith and Botterell of the Departments of Physiology, Anatomy and Surgery." There was also the collaboration between Guy Frederic Marrian of biochemistry and Melville C. Watson of the Department of Gynaecology and Obstetrics on "the female endocrines." The Department of Medical Research had played a role "in aiding all other departments, and particularly the clinical, in the research problems which present themselves from time to time." Gallie also mentioned collaboration in teaching, as in "the neuropathological laboratory under Prof Linell, Dr Hyland and Dr K.G. McKenzie."[8]

After the Second World War, the pace quickened. In 1947 President Sidney Smith noted, "On all sides ... there is a growing interest in medical research. Appointments and promotions should be made with this objective in mind." Dean Joseph MacFarlane added, "The tremendous advances in medical knowledge in the past two decades have resulted in correspondingly increased obligations on the part of medical schools everywhere ... The medical school of today is no longer a school solely for the training of undergraduates, although that is its most important function. In order to maintain teaching at a high standard, all its teachers must be interested in the broad field of research and graduate training."[9] This is the first definitive acknowledgment that a primary function of a medical faculty is research, alongside the education of family physicians.

It is probably MacFarlane who gets the credit for bumping up the faculty's originally close to nonexistent interest in research. Behind the research boom that began in the post-war years were many circumstances: veterans returning from the war eager to make scientific contributions after facing death for six years; freshly available government funds, including from the newly founded

National Institutes of Health in the United States; the curiosity-inspiring land-side of new and effective pharmaceuticals such as penicillin. But the research wave at the faculty was also dean-driven. A series of deans, of whom Joseph MacFarlane was the first, were lashing the research whip, converting a comfortable gentleman's club of the pre-war years into a research-driven faculty.

Making possible all this new research was a large step-up in funding in the early 1950s. After years of stringency, MacFarlane could hardly believe his eyes: "There are considerable funds available from sources outside the University – the National Research Council, the Defence Research Board, the federal health grants, the Canadian Life Insurance Officers Association … The Kellogg Foundation has for two years supported travelling fellowships for advanced graduate students in special fields. Four of our younger staff appointees were elected as Nuffield scholars." The list went on and on.[10]

President Sidney Smith was not slow to act on these insights. In February 1947 he asked MacFarlane to convene a committee on research in the Faculty of Medicine and to provide an overview of funds available. MacFarlane convoked the barons of the faculty on 20 February in the Faculty Room of the Dean's Office – a group that included William Gallie, Alan Brown, Arthur Ham, Ray Farquharson, and Charles Best, among others – to consider getting research up and running. In March, MacFarlane crunched some numbers to see what kinds of funds were available for research. The results were pathetic: Across the faculty, the percentage of the department budgets expended on research usually hovered between 10 and 30 percent. In the Department of Medicine it was 45 percent but the amount allocated was only $5,800 for 1946–7. Obstetrics and gynecology and physiology had zero; pathological chemistry had allocated "none for current year."[11] It was a faculty that spent little on research and had even less space for it. At the university where insulin had been discovered, by 1947 serious research had basically come to a halt.

## What To Do?

The quintessential researcher is not the family doctor but the clinician-scientist. After the Second World War, the awareness started to dawn that medical researchers needed systematic training in the basic sciences. This was the beginning of the clinician-scientist. The story goes back to 1946, when the faculty met to decide what plans should be made for postgraduate study. They devised a "[p]roposal regarding the establishment of a graduate school in the Faculty of Medicine, University of Toronto." This would enroll postgraduates taking the course for the Master of Surgery degree, the four diploma programs (Public Health, Industrial Hygiene, Psychiatry, and Radiology), and students wishing to pass the various certifying exams of the United States and the United Kingdom. Nothing came of this. But it was the first thought that medical training might involve advanced graduate study.[12]

In 1949 James Dauphinee in the Department of Pathological Chemistry noted that the residents were too busy to spend more than a year doing research. "It is not possible for them to accomplish much in the way of investigation during this time. They just begin to know their way about the laboratory when the time comes for them to stop and go elsewhere, and the work which they have begun so well may remain unfinished. Steps are, therefore, being taken to encourage a number of the Fellows to work in the Department for two years or more and if possible to proceed towards a graduate degree."[13] This then in embryo was the clinician-scientist program that Bernie Langer was to propose in surgery and Eliot Phillipson, much later, in medicine. By June 1951 three MDs had earned the faculty's basic research degree, the bachelor of science (medicine), one of them from the Department of Pharmacology.[14]

By the late 1950s the very environment of Toronto itself had started to change in a way favourable to recruiting researchers. People might find it attractive to come here. The city was changing from Presbyterian grey to an ethnic robe of many colours. Bissell said, "A genuine city was beginning to emerge with some sense of style and a growing pride and confidence in itself." Toronto was becoming "a place of alluring variation," in contrast with Ottawa, "a pleasant but dowdy town." (Bissell had been president of Carleton University in Ottawa.)[15]

A generation gap began to emerge between the old hands, who saw themselves mainly as clinicians and teachers, and the new guard, who viewed their mission as research. And so the old hands began to feel a bit disconcerted. In 1962 Dean Hamilton and John Oille, the latter a truly old hand (he had graduated with his MB from Toronto in 1903), in a brief to the Royal Commission on Health Services, noted uneasily that "the large and increasing volume of funds available from granting agencies for research work is to a degree down-grading teaching and weakening administration." Although research was important, they allowed, "the answer is … to augment support for teaching and administration."[16] Talk about being on the wrong side of history!

Against this enrooted resistance to research as a primary mission, the increasingly research-oriented university moved forward. In 1959 the Faculty Council deliberated which of two degrees might be preferable: a PhD in medicine or a doctor of clinical science.[17] Of course freshly minted MDs were free to enroll in PhD programs. Yet as was pointed out in the discussion, "[a]fter a long medical course the individual must spend a minimum of three years to take a PhD and a further three or four years to become clinically qualified." A few Stakhanovites such as Jack Laidlaw had done just this. Yet most shrank from endless years without income. "It would seem desirable that there should be some way in which these two types of training might be integrated into a more concentrated course."[18] Nowhere in Canada had this been previously organized.

After this meeting, MacFarlane and Lawrie Chute had a talk with the dean of the School of Graduate Studies (SGS), who thought "that the PhD degree was too confining and rigid to fit the requirements of the proposed programme." The SGS dean urged them to bring in a research doctoral degree in the Faculty of Medicine.[19]

It was thus a small step forward that in 1960–1 the doctor of clinical science degree was introduced, available to doctors of medicine "who look forward to a career in medical research and who would wish to maintain comparable academic status with their colleagues who have proceeded to higher qualifications in the Royal College of Physicians and Surgeons."[20]

So in the early 1960s the faculty began a heavy swing on the pivot from teaching to research. Evidence of the old faculty's attachment to teaching were the world-beating textbooks that came out of anatomy, pathology, physiology, histology, and pharmacology. "In those days," reflected Colin Bayliss in 1988, a member of both the Departments of Surgery and Physiology, "teaching was the major activity of this Faculty. About twenty years ago, the feeling developed that there should be more breadth to our academic pursuit, and that is when research became the major endeavour ... During the '60s and '70s funding was relatively easy, so a lot of people went into research in a big way. Over the years, teaching became more of a second class activity, although at one time it was first class."[21]

By the early 1960s an unfamiliar obstacle posed itself: the problem in the faculty regarding research was not really money but space in which to conduct research. The dean said in 1962, "The total spent on research in the past academic year exceeds, by a small margin, the budget of the Faculty ... The most pressing need today is for space ... nearly every department lacks adequate research space ... The assurance of a new building on the corner of Elizabeth and College Streets to house basic science and investigative laboratories to complement existing space in the Banting Institute does not answer the immediate problem."[22]

In 1964 a special committee of the university's Board of Governors chaired by Dean Hamilton reported on the needs of the medical school, signalling "the need to increase full-time staff in both basic science and clinical science, and to provide adequate space of research and teaching." Toronto was becoming so uncompetitive that foreign medical schools were hiring away our staff.[23] On the subject of inadequacy, Dean Hamilton pointed out how understaffed the faculty was: "In both basic and clinical sciences there are 94 persons paid a full-time salary. 59 of these are paid in whole, or in part by grants from outside agencies." They teach not only 600 medical students but students in rehabilitation medicine, dentistry, pharmacy, and so forth. "An average for an American school teaching medical students alone is 130 for a class of 100. There should really be at least an additional 100 full-time teachers supported by the University." He continued, "The public should be made aware that there is a definite crisis in relation to teaching and research in the medical schools."[24]

*From the British to the American Model*

In these years the cultural orientation of the faculty began to swing from the United Kingdom to the United States. By the late 1950s, those medical graduates of Toronto who opted to leave the country voted overwhelmingly to remain in North America and not migrate to England. In 1957, of 5,700 living graduates of the faculty, 1,077 – or 19 percent – gave their address in the United States, 133 in the British Isles (and 42 "foreign").[25] Thus, Dean Hamilton's remarks in the previous section were accepted as self-understood, and nobody at the Faculty Council asked indignantly about the teacher/student ratio at the Middlesex Hospital in London. At that same meeting, Bill Bigelow volunteered that "if the school is to be a top-ranking one it is necessary to accept American standards of excellence and this involved more University funds and more full-time staff ... If this whole situation were presented to the Board of Governors in a way that business men understand, he felt sure that the Board would support the Faculty."[26] American standards of excellence: this was a definitive turning of the page.

Individual researchers were quite sensitive to the difference between the English and the American models. Canadian tradition lay with the former; the future, much though it hurt to say it, with the latter. Bigelow told colleagues in 1965, "In the clinical departments ... research has only become part of the activity and responsibility of a staff member in recent years. In Canadian medical schools we have tended to follow the older British system of appointing members of the staff ... who are outstanding clinicians, teachers and administrators. It is only in recent years that new clinical appointments have been made to young men with strong orientation to research. This is an important trend and one that must be encouraged, as it keeps us in line with the American standards of excellence and allows communication with that country and membership in their senior societies."[27]

This reorientation started to appear in various circles, some of them faculty members of British origin who could see the handwriting on the wall. In 1964 psychiatrist Daniel Cappon, a member of the team restructuring the faculty, wrote Dean Hamilton, "To my mind we are moving ... towards a natural line of cleavage between: (a) traditional clinical Medicine, related to teaching and secondarily to research (along the service-centred British lines). And (b) academic Medicine, in which research is primary and teaching secondary ... (the more modern U.S. model)." Cappon, who was British, said he inclined more towards the former but conceded that the "advanced centres" had probably already reached the latter.[28]

Amidst all the goodwill about pressing forward on the American model, in the mid-1960s there was a prise de conscience about how inadequate the previous status of research had been. Following a critical assessment of the administration of Canadian medical schools by the Association of American Medical

Colleges in 1963, in March 1964 the Faculty Council formed a committee to consider the organization of the university's Faculty of Medicine. Called the Committee on Structure and Organization of the Faculty, it was chaired by Bill Bigelow and reported in November 1965 rather devastatingly about the status of research in the faculty. "It was quite remarkable," the committee found, "that there was no organization at Faculty level and no Standing Committee on Research," despite the fact, as Dean Hamilton observed, that "the funds for the prosecution of research now exceed the University budget allocated to the Faculty of Medicine." Furthermore, "The present budget of the Faculty is grossly inadequate to maintain present standards indefinitely, let alone to permit the development necessary to keep up with today's demands." The recommended changes in the report "cannot be implemented without a considerable increase in expenditure on the central administration of the Faculty." The committee strongly endorsed the report from the Board of Governors' special committee on hospital renovations and on the need for a Medical Sciences Building.[29]

The Structure Committee report of 1965 was thus crucial in the slow pivot in Toronto medicine from the British model to the American. The British privileged teaching, as did older members of the faculty, many of them of Scottish origin in particular, who were keen on attentive teaching of the medical students. The American medical schools privileged research, and Toronto at least was henceforth bent upon following that model.

Until the mid-1960s the faculty had been so haphazard about the systematic organization of research that it had no research committee. Then in 1965 President Bissell organized the formation of a Research Board; mounting a research committee became virtually mandatory for the Faculty of Medicine. There was an important role for the hospitals in implementing this new research model: providing space. The special committee of the Board of Governors had recognized this and the Faculty Council did as well: "The individual teaching hospitals must provide research space." And the new Research Committee of the faculty would ginger them along.[30] Thus, in the mid-1960s there came together a confluence of trends favouring research: the shift from the English to the American model, a new emphasis on research within the university as a whole, and the elevation of the clinician-scientist to academic ideal.

This confluence began to shift the whole pattern of care. In 1966 Dean Hamilton said that the "clinical scientist" will make care in teaching hospitals superior to that in community hospitals. "The clinician who is attracted to the teaching hospitals is one with an inquiring mind that continually seeks and probes to find out what is causing disease. He wants and demands facilities to do research and the time to do it." A hospital without laboratories cannot retain "its top flight clinical scientists. They move to the hospital that will encourage and support investigation and the kind of medical care that results from it for there is no doubt that the quality of medical care is directly related to research." Community physicians find such academic utterances a breathtaking expression of arrogance. Yet this was the worldview of the 1960s, in which research had just been discovered like a precious jewel lying in the gravel.

With the conflation of good academic research and good patient care, care shifted from the family doctor to the community hospital, and complex cases from the community hospitals to the academic centres. Hamilton continued, "The pattern of medical practice and care in the community is changing, with the general hospital providing more and more care of the kind formerly given by the general practitioner, this being imposed upon the specialized referral hospital." This change also concerned family medicine: there would have to be expanded outpatient and emergency departments. "Ambulatory care departments or centres must be created to give treatment for 24 hours per day, staffed preferably by practitioners primarily concerned with family practice. Such centres will become of major importance in teaching medical undergraduates."[31] The implications of the faculty's new research orientation were thus considerable.

Let me set these events in a North American context: the exploding demand for physicians, the soaring research budgets – especially funds flowing from the coffers of the National Institutes of Health in Bethesda, Maryland – and the increasing insistence on multidisciplinarity among university departments and among health science faculties. Embodying this virtual euphoria about medical education, health care, and research was Lowell Coggeshall's 1965 report to the Association of American Medical Colleges, a report that was widely attended to in Toronto and on other Canadian campuses. Coggeshall had headed a blue-ribbon committee, and in his report he said, "The enormous expansion of medical education, research, and service, especially in the past two decades, has resulted in greater changes than have occurred during any other period in medical history." In addition to beefing up medical education, the report called for "reduc[ing] barriers between instruction and research."[32] Research would enter the classroom; medical students and trainees would enter the lab. It was not just that research would benefit humankind; it would benefit the training of physicians. The Coggeshall report thus gave a crucial, and ironical, push in the pivot of Canadian medical faculties – which in the British tradition had always been great in medical education! – from British-style education to American-style research.

There was also a local context. Toronto's career as a poor country cousin poking along behind McGill was about to come to an end with a huge new infusion of funds.

### Space and Money

It took a great deal to get the provincial government to sit up and listen to the Faculty of Medicine. But attention sharpened in 1963 when Dean Hamilton wrote President Bissell that, in Bissell's words, "the faculty, generally believed to share with McGill, primacy in the country, was actually slipping badly into a secondary position ... The main causes of decline were the continuing reliance on part-time teachers, the split between the clinical and the basic sciences, and the lack of facilities for research."[33]

Falling behind McGill for a lack of space! This was especially painful given that the faculty was unable to take advantage of the new government funds becoming available for research because there was no space for the new labs.[34] In 1966 the federal government established a Health Resources Fund to support capital expenditures for educational purposes in health care; 50 percent would be contributed by the province and 50 percent by the federal government.[35] At the same time the province established the Senior Co-ordinating Committee, chaired by the deputy minister of health (following its dissolution in 1972, its responsibilities were assumed by the Health Science Education Committee). "The Senior Co-ordinating Committee was responsible for making recommendations to the Minister of Health and the Minister of University Affairs on the capital programmes required to develop educational and research arrangements for health disciplines."[36] The provincial Hospital Services Commission would dole out the cash as universities and hospitals asked for it.

Dean Chute told the department chairmen in October 1967 that the Ontario government was going to start funding grant applications "relating to the problems of health within this Province." He laid out the application procedures. The forms could be obtained from the Health Grants Section, Research and Planning Branch, of the Department of Health.[37] The chairs must have been delirious. Nothing like this had ever happened before! As usual, Wightman agonized about the new funds, saying shortly after Chute had opened the cornucopia, "We seem to be standing on the verge of a new era. We are all waiting to see how it will be defined. It is evident that we are being offered support from government which may entail some loss of freedom. On the other hand we may find that an opportunity is being offered to us which we have never had before ... It is to be hoped that a solution can be found before we are all suffocated by the output of these Xerox machines on campus."[38]

The amounts of money available seemed overpowering. In September 1974 Dean Holmes told the Faculty Council that the provincial Health Resources Development Fund had made $100 million available "for the health sciences Complex in Toronto. Of this sum, $90 million is ... for hospital development, $10 million for on-campus development, to include any health science Faculty."[39] The province started making teaching and research funds available to fuel full-time practices as the Ontario Health Insurance Plan arrived. One could earn a living in a specialty because, as pathologist Kenneth Pritzker explained, "it was open-ended. All you had to do was get your patients, and everything would be paid for, and the supply exceeded the demand."[40]

In 1976 a provincial committee chaired by Howard Petch (president of the University of Victoria in British Columbia and formerly academic vice president of the University of Waterloo) reported on requirements in the province for health research, concluding that the province should provide "adequate capital facilities," facilities for innovative new research, the avoidance of duplication of facilities, and resources to support research in the teaching hospitals and their teaching programs. As for Toronto, large amounts of research space were recommended for all the teaching hospitals. The committee reached the pregnant conclusion that "[c]ash flow problems should not be permitted to inhibit the sensible planning of research facilities."[41] (For more on funding issues, see chapter 12.)

### Institute of Medical Science

A huge bound forward was the foundation of the Institute of Medical Science (IMS) in 1968 – the official date, although it was up and running the previous year.

In the 1960s, concerns about the medical school's relatively poor research record converged with worries about the faculty being not sufficiently part of the university but rather a professional facility for physicians. Bissell wanted medicine to be a "unifying discipline, part science, part human calculus, part mystery," and he looked for ways to rope the faculty more securely into campus life. Simultaneously, the Department of Medicine wanted to introduce graduate degrees issued by the School of Graduate Studies for aspiring clinician-scientists who were starting to animate the research side of things by studying in the basic science departments. Bissell and graduate dean Ernest Sirluck discussed how to "unite clinical experience and knowledge with the pure sciences" and to that end proposed, with the Department of Medicine, a Centre for Medical Sciences.[42]

In March 1964 Jack Laidlaw told Dean Hamilton that a number of clinical departments were "keenly interested" in having various faculty members supervise MA, MSc, or PhD research. They wanted to implement this via the School of Graduate Studies, rather than via the "Doctor of Clinical Sciences," which was controlled by the faculty and seen as a kind of Mickey Mouse affair. But SGS "might question whether at the present time there is a satisfactory atmosphere (eg 'band of graduate scholars') and whether there are enough satisfactory supervisors." Also, "[i]t might be worth stressing that during the past two decades there has been an increasing tendency in clinical departments to study fundamental biological processes, both physiological and pathological, not only in the human being but in animals and isolated tissues as well."[43] Laidlaw, who was to become a major player in the story, thus helped initiate it.

Planning for such an entity advanced with remarkable speed. Wightman evidently broached the idea to Associate Dean Edward A. Sellers, and at a meeting of the senior committee of the faculty in September 1966, Sellers "reported on the proposal to establish in the graduate school an interdepartmental organization which would form a graduate department representing the interests of the clinical departments and which might be known as an 'Institute of Medical Science.' He [Sellers] had acted as chairman of an organizing committee which had discussed the proposal with the heads of departments. The procedure was left to a committee composed of himself, Profs. Laidlaw, [Donald] Fraser, [Andrew] Sass-Kortsak, and [Abraham] Rapoport." Jack Laidlaw then succeeded Sellers as chair of the organizing committee; the thought was that he might also be chair of the proposed graduate department.[44]

About this time Bun McCulloch was becomingly increasingly unhappy with the opportunities to train more investigators in clinical research at the Ontario Cancer Institute. He found the basic science departments of the faculty unresponsive and, given that he knew Laidlaw well – the two had lived in the same student residence at the University of London while Laidlaw was earning a PhD there in 1948–9 – "it was a natural evolution," said McCulloch, "that Laidlaw began to include [me] in his discussions. Laidlaw's group determined to establish a route by which medical graduates could take MSc or PhD programs with the rigour that such programs required."[45]

Wightman, clearly pleased at this coup for the Department of Medicine, noted in the spring of 1967 growing interest in "integrative" science: organ research "which may carry us vertically into the basic sciences, and bring them into closer relationship with us. The way for this has been prepared to some extent by the degree to which investigative activity has been fostered in clinical departments ... and the growing interest of basic science departments in things which have a clinical relationship." This is nurtured "by the present movement to establish a clinical arm in the School of Graduate Studies – multidisciplinary, but of special interest to the Department of Medicine." By January 1967 Laidlaw was calling the new institute "the "graduate department of Human Biology."[46] By the summer of 1967 SGS had accepted the "new Clinical Sciences Institute. This will enable clinical divisions of the school to enroll graduate students directly, and hopefully will greatly increase our supply of clinical scientists for the educational institutions so urgently needed by our own expanding school."[47]

At this point, the proposed institute was clearly conceived as the research arm of the Department of Medicine, despite Wightman's hospitable declaration that "our departments" would be welcome to use the new "Division of Clinical Science."[48] All staff were cross-appointed from other departments. The institute, however, offered core seminars of its own and was not just a collaborative program.

Laidlaw and McCulloch placed a premium on critical feedback. Laidlaw described the seminars that McCulloch and Till held at OCI: "You'd listen to them criticize the presentation and you would think that the speaker had killed their mother. And so Bun was great. The two of us were a great pair and we set up something novel that had high standards." Up to then, residents with an interest in research "might go to a physician that they thought highly of, and in a very informal way they would get some training and they might or might not write it up. It was just a mishmash. We felt that we needed some discipline in this."[49]

"Quality was an important thing," Laidlaw said in an interview.
"And being part of the School of Graduate Studies was a guarantee of quality?"
"Yes, exactly."

In the summer of 1967 the Institute of Medical Science opened its doors under Jack Laidlaw, in association with the core band of researchers on the executive committee from the Department of Medicine: Sass-Kortsak, Fraser, Rapoport, and Robert Volpé. (These would later be joined by other such research stars as George Steiner from medicine and physiology and Harvey Stancer from psychiatry.) In September 1968 the Ontario Council on Graduate Studies approved its degree programs (MSc, PhD). The IMS therewith became the graduate department for twelve of the fourteen clinical departments. (Clinical biochemistry and pathology had their own graduate departments.)

In 1969 Bun McCulloch became the graduate secretary. The IMS was to serve as the graduate arm of the clinical departments, he said. "Historically, prior to the founding of the Institute, clinical departments had no direct access to graduate students, and individuals wishing to prepare for careers as clinical investigators undertook this through a basic science department, and upon completion of training were qualified in a discipline rather than as clinical investigators."[50] So the real purpose of the institute was to produce clinical investigators trained in the basic sciences. In contrast to the graduates of other departments, IMS students were experts in clinical investigation rather than in a given discipline. The institute would serve as an umbrella for research" in the clinical departments of the faculty, as the phrase went.

What was the problem with the previous system? McCulloch said, "Dr Laidlaw and his colleagues were concerned that no formal mechanism existed for training in medical research as opposed to professional education ... The informal approach ('apprenticeship system') did not result in any recognition of a successful completion of a programme because of the lack of assessment procedures ... IMS was founded in order to provide structured graduate programmes leading to recognized degrees, MSc and PhD."[51] Or, as Laidlaw put it, the purpose of the institute was "to provide an interdisciplinary research experience in the area of human biology."[52] The IMS was similar to the Department of Experimental Medicine at McGill, though the latter lacked the centralized structure.

By 1975 IMS had widened its staff somewhat, including not only thirty-two members cross-appointed from medicine, but eleven from pediatrics, nine from surgery, and smaller contingents from other departments.[53] (Two-thirds were from clinical departments, one-third from basic science departments.) Yet all appointments at this point were from the faculty, with the exception of a few from the School of Hygiene, which was abolished in 1975, its staff joining the Faculty of Medicine. In 1975 Laidlaw decamped for McMaster University. Mc-Culloch succeeded him in that same year as director before becoming, in 1979, the associate dean in the School of Graduate Studies. At that point, the founding period of IMS was concluded.

By 1983 John Leyerle, dean of the SGS, called IMS "probably the strongest graduate program in the life sciences at the University of Toronto."[54] In that year Aubie Angel, an endocrinologist (MD from Manitoba in 1959), who had arrived in Toronto in the early 1970s along with the rest of the McGill cohort that included Charlie Hollenberg and Mel Silverman, became director of IMS.

Over time, the interest of medical graduates in linking basic research to clinical research seemed to diminish and that of nonphysicians increased. Originally conceived for medical graduates, IMS opened its doors increasingly to PhDs interested in clinical research, though Laidlaw wished to restrict these to the truly "outstanding."[55] By 1981, of the institute's forty-seven graduate students, two-thirds were medical graduates, one-third were PhD candidates with bachelor of science degrees. (By then, it had 112 graduate faculty drawn from 15 departments within the School of Medicine.)[56] Such was the upsurge in enrolment that the leaders of the institute asked rhetorically, "Is the clinician-scientist really vanishing?" as was widely feared in the United States. In Toronto the answer was no.[57]

In 1991 surgeon Ori Rotstein became associate director of IMS, his job being to bring the Department of Surgery into the graduate training program. "I was the liaison between surgery and the IMS in clinician-scientist training," he later said in an interview. The Department of Surgery had previously been developing its own surgeon-scientists independently, and now they were to come on board the IMS.[58]

## MD/PhD and Clinical Investigator Programs

An important step in qualifying physicians as scientific investigators was the MD/PhD Program, created in 1981 under the leadership of Mel Silverman.[59] It was the first such program in Canada and remained the leading one. The enrollees in the program were expected to complete both MD and PhD degrees within seven to eight years and were fully funded. Silverman, said Ori Rotstein, "was like a dog with a bone. He'd push and push and push and push, and now the program's established and now I think they're doing extremely well."[60]

Over time, the MD/PhD graduates shifted from appointments in basic science departments to clinical departments, to firm up clinically oriented teaching and research within those departments. They thus started to supplement the PhD scientists in the clinic who had been translating fundamental scientific findings into the clinical context and vice versa. "Much of that role now has been transferred to clinician-scientists appointed to clinical departments," found a report in 1988. In that year roughly half of the applicants to the program were graduate students intent upon becoming clinician-scientists.[61]

In 1996–7 the Royal College Clinician Investigator Program was established in the faculty and by 2000 included over eighty MD trainees in full-time graduate studies. Said the faculty's plan for 2000–4, "Many of these trainees will complete their initial research training in the Faculty of Medicine obtaining either a MSc or PhD degree and then train outside of U of T, usually in a prestigious center in the USA or Europe and return to Canada as highly skilled researchers." Said the 2000–4 plan of this and the IMS program, "The graduates of these programs are the future academic and research leaders in Medicine across Canada. Over the past ten years, between 80 to 90% of these graduates have been recruited into academic research positions in Canada" (and approximately 50 to 60 percent of them would be at the U of T).[62]

### Kick Back

In 1972 the Long-Range Planning Committee of the Faculty Council struck a "Science Policy Sub-committee" – numbering among its members Bun McCulloch, George Connell, Eliot Phillipson, and Lou Siminovitch – which truly found itself tapping about in the dark. Nobody knew how much research was going on at the hospitals or in the Medical Sciences Building, and the subcommittee was a bit disoriented about how to proceed. They thought that perhaps the various hospitals and institutes might establish "research committees." Indeed, the Science Policy Sub-Committee should "make every effort to help them in their activities." Site visits might be useful too, just to find out what was going on. It was the first time anybody on the faculty had given any thought to how one might try to get broad-based research moving.[63]

In January 1972 the Science Policy Sub-Committee began visiting the teaching hospitals to learn what research was going on. Existing research was being done, as Lou Siminovitch pointed out, mainly by PhDs "because qualified medical researchers are not available, and they won't become available because there is no security in a funded grant position." Groups should be formed across hospitals, he said, on the basis of specific research problems, such as calcium metabolism and cardiovascular immunology. Should all hospitals not share alike? No, said Siminovitch. "He felt that to reach levels of excellence in certain areas it might be necessary for the 'rich to get richer' and that a democratic allocation of funds was not always best."[64]

What the members of the subcommittee (which became in December 1973 the Science Policy Committee) found in their hospital visits was not encouraging. Most of the teaching hospitals did not have research directors. The sums dedicated to hospital-based research were paltry, and some of the teaching hospitals, such as the Wellesley, were willing to make no concessions to research at all in terms of protected time.

By May 1974 the committee had worked out a document on "Research Planning in the Faculty of Medicine," but in a preliminary circulation it encountered huge hostility, especially from members of the basic science departments. The committee decided not to submit it to the Faculty Council, where it would certainly be voted down. Why was there such hostility to research planning? the members asked. Some reasons: "Fear that a bureaucratic structure will take control ... Feeling that there is already too much bureaucracy and red tape interfering with research. That planning is a departmental function, and should not be taken over by a Faculty-wide committee." There had been some planning in the clinical departments, "for example, the Departments of Surgery, Medicine and Pathology organized and planned an endeavour that was funded to the amount of $1M by the Heart Foundation."[65] The alienation that was to demarcate the basic science departments from the rest of the faculty had already begun.

It is interesting that the Science Policy Committee – as well as its sister the Long-Range Planning Committee – never really accomplished much. Both were agents of the Faculty Council. The reason, as Dean Holmes rather embarrassedly explained to the Science Policy Committee at its final meeting in April 1979, was that in the "democratization of the governance of the Faculty in the late 60's and early 70's, during which period the Science Policy Committee was created," there was a "dichotomy between the legislative and executive functions of the Faculty ... A review of the [Science Policy] committee's activities shows that for the most part attempts to develop its own initiatives have been thwarted." The same was true, the dean said, of the Long-Range Planning Committee. But now the dean intended to get serious about promoting research in the faculty, and he needed a committee capable of executive action. In November 1978 Holmes proposed the formation of a Faculty Research Committee.[66] He envisioned a small advisory committee of six department chairs as a research committee, chaired by Aser Rothstein, head of the Research Institute at HSC. It was the executive of the faculty that was now going to gin up research.[67]

In this lackluster research picture of the 1970s and early 1980s there were, however, several bright lights. One was the Department of Medicine under Charles Hollenberg, who had become Eaton Professor of Medicine and head of the department in 1970. Hollenberg had driven forward the divisional system within medicine, each subspecialty present in a hospital division and the hospital divisions yoked together like pistons in the university division. He said in 1978 that in chest disease this had worked. "By comparison, efforts to co-ordinate research in Cardiology have been less successful. A strong division exists at the Toronto General Hospital, for example, but this has tended to overshadow programmes at other hospitals." He continued, "It is undesirable to have a concentration of strength in one hospital only." (Siminovitch, an elitist, had exactly the opposite view.) Again, one realizes the importance of a single dynamic figure such as Charles Hollenberg in pushing forward the research mission of a big department with hundreds of members such as medicine. Once Hollenberg linked the divisional structure to the accomplishment of research, the big locomotives in medicine started to move out of the yard.[68]

But outside of medicine and surgery, research in the other departments lay fallow. In November 1977, the Long-Range planners delivered a searing indictment of research at the faculty as then practiced. One bears in mind that large amounts of public funding had become available. Yet the explanations the Long-Range planners conceived were more cultural than financial. Yes, the faculty did encourage research to some extent, "partly for its own sake" and partly "to create scholarly, scientific physicians." (There was at this point no talk of Toronto joining the handful of elite research universities.) But above and beyond producing doctors who had a nodding familiarity with research findings and questions, the culture of research in the medical faculty was paltry. Disciplinary boundaries "tend to hinder modern research endeavours where multidisciplinary and trans-sector and -departmental endeavours are desirable." Also, "[t]he overall economic climate of the Faculty, the University and the country as a whole tends to be inimical to sustained research endeavours." The space for labs was inadequate, especially in the teaching hospitals, and the hospitals themselves, under financial pressure, saw research and teaching as competing with patient care. But, said the long-range planners, these two functions can't be separated. "Clinical faculty and hospital administration must recognize that exemplary clinical care cannot exist in an environment that lacks a good research program – one nourishes the other." Clinical faculty themselves had little impetus to do research, when research "carries with it a financial penalty which is, in many instances, intolerable to the individuals concerned." The planners concluded that currently, "[c]linical research activity is insufficient; multidisciplinary research [is] only rudimentary"; and "the effective interaction between the three sectors, in furtherance of the Faculty's scientific objectives, is inadequate."[69] In sum, the balance of five years of work by this committee, a core band of dedicated scientists, was that Toronto had not yet got its research act together.

The definitive pivot of the faculty towards research occurred in the deanship of Fred Lowy, who took office in July 1980. Lowy had his work cut out for him. He later said, "I felt the big challenge was to continue ... moving the direction of this medical school from its historically provincial orientation to more ambitious national and international objectives." They had become a "national leader." "Yet our internal organization and recruiting patterns were not really geared to the new direction." Of Canada's sixteen medical schools, he said, only four "have the capacity to become excellent as judged by international standards. And those few have the responsibility to carry Canada's colours internationally. The University of Toronto stands foremost in that regard and our responsibility is the greatest." Furthering medical research at the University of Toronto was, in other words, a national mission.[70]

In cold print, this institutional chest-beating, originally intended for internal consumption, makes the faculty seem arrogant and self-absorbed. Yet it is striking that since the 1920s the medical faculty of the University of Toronto has had a sense of national mission. These larger ambitions sparked departmental insecurities. At a meeting in December 1982, the basic science chairs expressed alarm at the growth of the hospital research facilities as competitors for funding. Lowy tried to put events into a larger frame. Hospital research, he said, "is not new ... What is new is the increase in both basic science and clinical research in recent years, and more recently the decision by several of the large general hospitals to make a substantial commitment of resources for research purposes. While agreeing that in the past there was no coordination of research ... across institutions, he regarded the current situation as an opportunity for the University to take an active leadership role in this area, and it was his opinion that Hospital Board Chairmen would be receptive to this approach." Initial steps, Lowy said, were already underway.

The university delivered a one-two punch on research. One was Lowy becoming dean of medicine in 1980. Two was George Connell, a former head of biochemistry, becoming president of the university in 1984. Connell was like a bulldog on making medicine at U of T a great research faculty. It caused consternation in September 1987 when he appeared at a meeting of the Education Committee, expressing rather austere thoughts: "The Faculty have to be dedicated and committed to the ideal," he said, "be willing to experience some pain and discomfort to achieve this idea of a research university. In his opinion, neither of these conditions exist at present at U of T."[71]

Meanwhile, a crisis was brewing. In June 1985 the basic science chairs learned that the faculty's success rate in grant capture had dropped beneath the national average: "[The faculty] does not do as well on a per capita basis as a number of other medical schools, ranking about fourth or fifth. Also, we have not been doing well in Medical Research Council committee membership." G. Harvey Anderson, associate dean for research, pointed out that from a slate of 30 names submitted the previous year "only one was selected."[72]

In the background of these unhappy local events, an international revolution was taking place in molecular biology. Lowy wanted to make sure the U of T Faculty of Medicine kept abreast, which at that point was not at all a sure thing. In the fall of 1985 he told the faculty, "We cannot shrink from participating in today's biological revolution." He quoted George Keyworth, a scientific adviser to President Reagan: "Biological sciences stand on the brink of understanding that I can only liken to the brink that Einstein saw for physics in 1905." Lowy said, "The pace of discovery nowadays is bewildering ... It is now a truism that the biomedical research of today determines medical practice tomorrow." Recently, Lap-Chee Tsui and Manuel Buchwald at HSC had discovered the chromosome containing the gene for cystic fibrosis. And Tak Mak in medical biophysics had "isolated the gene which codes for the T-lymphocyte receptor, the fundamental recognition unit of the immune system." Yet Lowy was unhappy with the current state of research at U of T: "Our research grants per full time faculty member are not the highest in Canada; our investigators' papers are not in the very leading international journals ... as often as we would like."[73] There had never been such decanal pressure on the faculty to keep up.

### The Hospital Research Institutes

Lowy's dream of a first-class research faculty was to be realized, but it happened as a result of circumstances quite outside the faculty's control: the rise of the hospital Research Institutes.

Every teaching hospital came to have its own research institute. The Hospital for Sick Children was the first, established in 1953, followed by the Toronto Western Hospital in 1958, Mount Sinai Hospital in 1975, the Toronto General Hospital in 1985, Sunnybrook in 1989, and St Michael's in 1994.

These were well-financed operations that quickly came to overshadow research done at the medical school, although the hospitals were part of the academic health science complex, and all the staff simultaneously held university appointments. Arthur Slutsky, vice president of research at St Michael's Hospital and a veteran scientist, said in an interview, "My guess is that research grants and funding of research in, let's say, 1975, was 10 percent in the hospitals, 90 percent in the university medical school." Today, by contrast, "80 percent of research is done in the teaching hospitals, and 20 percent in the university medical school."[74]

Compared to the faculty's basic science departments, the Research Institutes had the disadvantage of offering five-year renewable contracts rather than tenure. But they had the advantage of less teaching, although Research Institute scientists still craved graduate students. They also made fundraising easier. Slutsky noted, "Because the Research Institutes were smaller, probably there was a little more access to foundation money from donors. If you're at the University, with 30,000 faculty or whatever, if you want donations, where do you go? It's huge. Here, it's a relatively small place, you know the president of the foundation, and it's just probably a little bit easier to get foundation money." Slutsky added, "If you come into hospital and I save your life, you'll probably want to donate. You'll probably feel pretty good about it, that's a pretty good donation. So it's probably easier for hospitals to get funds from donors."[75]

In the early 1980s the question of hospital Research Institutes started to glimmer on the faculty's radar. In 1982 Lowy said hospital research "is not new ... What is new is the increase in both basic science and clinical research in recent years, and more recently the decision by several of the large general hospitals to make a substantial commitment of resources for research purposes [the

Research Institutes]. While agreeing that in the past there was no coordination of research ... across institutions, [Lowy] regarded the current situation as an opportunity for the University to take an active leadership role in this area."[76]

The campus basic science chairs asked themselves what to do about hospital research in the basic sciences: Should the university cross-appoint all the hospital investigators in the new hospital-based research units? A subcommittee of Donald W. Clarke, Keith Moore, Harold Atwood, and Jim Friesen looked into it.[77] The subcommittee decided that the faculty basic science chairs should be involved in the appointments process and the selection of candidates. Immunologist Brian Underdown, associate dean of basic science, was to carry the ball in discussions with the hospitals.[78]

The clinical chairs were equally uneasy, but Underdown assured them in February 1983 that "all research space whether located on campus or in the teaching hospitals would be regarded as 'University space.'" There was, after all, a Hospital University Research Coordinating Committee (HURCC) to ensure that things didn't go too badly off track. Yet the clinical chairs were not satisfied: "To date clinical departments have not been involved in the planning of the research thrusts of the hospital research institutes."[79]

Uneasiness grew. In October 1983 at the Faculty Council, members feared that hospital financial advantages would draw away the graduate students into milieus "where the ... quality of supervision has been less than optimal for their needs. There is a fundamental difference in philosophy between a hospital Research Institute with its mandate to do research, and a basic science department whose mandate extends beyond scientific productivity to scholarship with its didactic role and with relationships to other departments in carrying out its research and teaching." Moreover, the basic scientists would be dispersed among the hospitals, "often resulting in relative isolation, and a serious weakening of the home department." And how about teaching, with which the basic science departments felt swamped? The members of the Research Institutes would do little. How about "role models" for the graduate students? In hospitals "the provision of care must take priority over the acquisition of knowledge for its own sake."[80]

Aser Rothstein, head of the Research Institute at the children's hospital, attended the meeting and tried to soothe the agitated spirits. Research Institutes were the wave of the future, he said. "It is clear why it is happening – hospitals still have the ability to mobilize resources whereas universities have difficulty; hospitals recognize that research is good for the hospitals, not just for the university, in enhancing the hospital's image and role." A possible disadvantage: "Hospital scientists may have more time for research, but must 'publish or perish.'"[81]

Associate Dean Clarke also tried to assure the ruffled basic scientists: the partnership has "a simple quid pro quo, i.e. the hospitals wish to develop research – this increases their image, and allows them to recruit personnel of high caliber. To develop research, hospitals require the availability of graduate students and University appointments. In return the University acquires the opportunity to develop new programmes in new space which would not otherwise be available."[82]

The whole exchange makes clear how threatening faculty scientists and clinicians found these great hospital Research Institutes that were shooting up a couple of hundred yards away on University Avenue.

Feelings deepened. In the spring of 1985, Dan Osmond, a professor in the physiology department, saw a "mind-boggling feast and famine juxtaposition of proliferating multi-million dollar research institutes and nearby University Departments undergoing painful budgetary squeezes that threaten essential teaching functions ... and decrease the time available for research." He said they were capable of denaturing the university's mission: "Like the proverbial camel with its nose in the nomad's tent, the Institutes will find themselves mostly outside when it suits them, but with the option to creep as far inside as their clout and well-timed political wriggles will carry them. In the end, of course, the tent takes on the shape of the camel." He also feared the teaching-burdened campus professors were at a disadvantage compared to the Research Institute scientists in competing for research funds and graduate students. "The University Departments will expend their energies in nurturing students through the demanding undergraduate and early graduate years, only to have them snatched away in their prime. There could be a 'brain drain' from the University to Institute for the wrong reasons." Osmond concluded, "Creating an overcrowded, viciously competing scientific scene in Toronto that turns scientists against each other, and turns off students that come to us, will weaken rather than strengthen us."[83]

Once again Rothstein was on the scene, a one-person fire brigade. To this onslaught of resentment he responded, "It is like trying to tell Alberta, which is expanding rapidly now, that they can't expand because Toronto already has the money and we don't want to share, even though they may be putting up better competition for the funds." He added that there were certain kinds of research, such as on patients, that could be done only in hospitals. He made a second point about what would be called in very short order "translational research": making progress in basic science relevant to the clinic: "In the hospitals, where you have a lot of basic research people working side by side, waiting for the same elevator, in the same coffee shops, with people who are faced with bedside problems, it is amazing how much conversation goes on that ends up in a very rapid knowledge transfer."[84]

In the years ahead, the Rothstein approach triumphed and the grudging suspiciousness of the campus departments was forgotten. In 1987 Acting Dean Harvey Anderson pointed out that half of all Connaught Awards – a campus-based award program – had gone to hospital-based scientists. The faculty scrambled even more to support cross-appointments. Indeed, Anderson suggested that the lagging and underfunded basic science departments might hook themselves to the Research Institute stars. On the subject of "how to foster the development of basic science research, particularly in the Medical Sciences Building," Anderson said, "efforts should be made to take advantage of the growth in the hospital sector through the potential offered by cross-appointments."[85]

By the new century, the Research Institutes had virtually taken over the training of graduate students: two-thirds of those in the faculty's basic science departments were supervised by scientists in the hospital Research Institutes –so much so that the hospital institutes needed to appoint research training directors.[86] (On the faculty's rebound into molecular research in the new millennium, especially in the Terrence Donnelly Centre for Cellular and Biomolecular Research, see chapter 28.)

What had made Toronto such a successful academic centre? In a 2009 interview, Don Cowan said it was the hospital Research Institutes. Once upon a time, the Medical Sciences Building was important, he said. "The interesting thing is that the real power not only of clinical but other kinds of research are the hospital institutes. The power has drifted away from the University." The institutes are "vastly better funded." Cowan noted, "Now the University continues to be important because the university controls the granting of degrees, controls academic rank, and teaching appointments ... But [the Research Institutes] are one of the things that's made the University of Toronto a really research-intensive medical school."[87]

# 12 An Academic Health Sciences Complex

Communication within the Faculty of Medicine has always been difficult ... Not only does physical separation of the members of the department militate against a cohesive unit, the hospital in which the individual works is a separate and distinct entity where, in my opinion, the cohesive forces of the individual discipline are greatly modified by the daily contact and necessary inter-relationships with all other clinical disciplines. The hospital is just as much an institution as the University and conflicts between these institutions will continue until a time is reached [with] more harmony than exists now.[1]

John Hamilton, Vice President, Health Sciences, 1969

The relationship among faculty, hospitals, and provincial government, as it evolved in the late 1960s, is daunting in its complexity and will not be rehearsed here – any more than is necessary to understand the outcome (and why this book is about much more than a single Faculty of Medicine). What came out of the negotiations was something called an Academic Health Sciences Complex (AHSC), an organic association among faculty and teaching hospitals. There is nothing quite like Toronto's health sciences complex elsewhere, and it explains a good deal of the distinctiveness of the Toronto story.

One should gain some distance up front: this book is really about two institutions, the Faculty of Medicine and the teaching hospitals of the University of Toronto. Their stories are inseparable and intertwined. It was members of the faculty who made clinical discoveries that redounded to the advantage of the citizens of Ontario and of humankind. It was the hospitals that provided the frame. (And it was the practice plans, which constitute a kind of third player, that supported teaching in the hospitals.) All players were nestled together in an "academic health sciences complex," meaning the arrangements that a medical faculty and its teaching hospitals work out, for better or worse, among themselves. There are two models: "operational aggregation," in which, as in some

American centres, the hospitals and university are governed under the same roof, and "operational disaggregation," in which university and hospitals are governed separately. Toronto corresponded to the latter.[2] In Toronto, the "tripod" of care, education, and research of the AHSC was distributed among the players rather than concentrated under a "single owner" that controlled medical school and hospitals alike.[3]

The U of T is distinctive in two ways. Unlike some other Canadian provinces, Ontario does not have comprehensive regional health authorities, so the Toronto health science complex was never integrated into a larger governing body but followed its own dynamic. Second, the Faculty of Medicine at Toronto was forced to coexist with a number of large teaching hospitals without controlling them. This compelled compromises, some of which have benefited health care and research, such as the hospital Research Institutes, some of which have not, such as the parochialism of the individual hospitals that the university was at pains to rein in. Thus in the larger picture, Toronto has taken a distinctive course.

But the motor driving this story forward was science, not administrative exigencies. And science swelled with a great lionhearted roar. As Dean John Hamilton said, "Originally teaching hospitals had no affiliation with universities. Medicine was mainly an art in which science played a small part. As science came to play a larger and larger part, the provision of the necessary scientific personnel and laboratories by the hospital was impossible and association with a university became a necessity. Today [1962] no one would think of establishing a medical school apart from a university."[4] The story is thus kind of win-win: scientific advances steadily increased the power of physicians to investigate patients and relieve their complaints. The hospital boards realized they could better offer quality care with academic medicine. And the patients benefited from hospitals in firm alliance with a university faculty because physicians were now able to influence the course of disease, something virtually unheard of in the therapeutic powerlessness that constituted most of medicine's 2,000-year history.

### "The Big House"

From the get-go there were three teaching hospitals: the Toronto General Hospital, St Michael's Hospital, and the Toronto Western Hospital. Yet early in the story, the action was at the General, the "Big House."

At the beginning, organized bedside instruction at the General did not exist. William Gallie remembered the years around 1900: "There was no attempt at staff organization or even at segregation of patients, except that the surgical, obstetrical and medical patients were kept in separate wards. The contact of students with patients was solely on the occasion of clinical lectures or at the bedside during group clinics. There was no such thing as clinical clerkship or as sharing in the investigation or in the diagnosis and treatment of the patients. It certainly was bad."[5]

The narrative arc of the story is the faculty's increasing demands for control over the General. As medical historian James Connor explains, "[The faculty] wanted all patients placed under the charge of university clinical staff ... They hoped that a university advisory committee could be struck to guide intern staff and admit hospital patients." In 1904 the Toronto General Hospital board acceded to the formation of such a committee, and over the next two years the doctors' committee let the hospital know their needs.[6]

The basic problem was that the faculty required a university hospital for teaching purposes but was unable to pay for one. In the Toronto General Hospital Act of May 1906, it was stipulated, "The trustees shall allow any medical student of the University of Toronto to visit the wards of the hospital and attend them for the purpose of receiving instruction from the members of the Faculty of Medicine of the University of Toronto," upon the payment of a fee.[7] TGH therewith became the teaching hospital of the U of T. As Dean Charles K. Clarke said in 1908, "The ideal situation for the University would be to have a University Hospital under full control of the University, but this seems to have been impossible unless the University or the Government on its behalf had been willing to assume the total expense of the hospital. In return for the $300,000 paid by the Government in 1906–07 the University possesses by statute the right to have its students instructed clinically by its professors in the hospital, and the University is represented on the Board of Trustees by four members, but the Trustees as a whole reserve for themselves the right ... to appoint the staff."[8]

A reorganization took place in 1908 that created the Departments of Medicine, Surgery, Obstetrics, Gynaecology, and Ophthalmology; otology, rhinology, and laryngology were combined. Medicine and surgery were divided into three services each. Connor explains, "Doctors appointed to the General's visiting staff could not serve on the staff of any other general hospital." This reorganization caused a realization among physicians "that the medical community had split into 'haves' and 'have nots.' Specialist practitioners who held formal appointments at the University of Toronto as well as the Toronto General Hospital had become a super-elite within the fraternity. Those who held hospital appointments in the city's other hospitals occupied a lower rung; those who did not hold any hospital privileges ... ran the risk of being pushed to the margins of the profession." Connor argues that this formalized relationship bound hospitals and university together as never previously. "In the past the clinical education of doctors had been at the discretion of the hospital. In 1908, the Toronto General became, in all but name, a university hospital, in which medical education was another of its integral obligations." When Abraham Flexner visited Toronto, preparing for his famous report released in 1910, the reorganization impressed him.[9]

University president Robert Falconer was keen to move the university and the Faculty of Medicine into the league of major research institutions. To this end, he pleaded for closer faculty-hospital relations. In 1911 the Toronto General Hospital Act was amended to stipulate that the hospital board should make new appointments only after recommendation by a joint hospital-university committee, made up of four members from the hospital and four from the university. Flavelle and Byron Walker, chairman of the university Board of Governors, inked an accord which established the Joint Hospital Relations Committee. In addition to the provincial stipend, the university also began to pay the hospital $25 a year for the hospital privileges of each student.[10] In 1911–12 Charles K. Clarke, who had been dean of the faculty, also became superintendent of the hospital, "cementing" what the president of the university called in 1912 "the close connection between the hospital and the university."[11]

The Joint Hospital Relations Committee endured for years – until another university act in 1971 – and ensured that all medical staff at the hospital would have university appointments; many indeed were chairs of their campus departments. What continually threatened to destabilize this tranquil relationship was the onrush of science.

There was a new milestone in 1928, when the university signed an indenture agreeing to "provide space and facilities for both basic and applied research to the staff members of the Toronto General Hospital." These facilities were at first situated in the Banting Institute, later at other campus facilities.[12]

*Early Clashes*

This loose framework provided splendid opportunities for clashes. There was a basic tension between the hospitals' reluctance to allow students to take on responsible work, such as history-taking and doing physical exams, and the faculty's desire for them to learn through hands-on practical experience. Should the final-year students help out in surgical procedures? The hospital said no, the faculty pushed. FitzGerald said in 1935, "Unless the student is made a part of the hospital organization, the same as an interne, he never ... takes a serious interest in practical, clinical work. The result is that he graduates with a wealth of laboratory and text-book knowledge but very little real clinical knowledge such as he acquires with great speed if he is fortunate enough later to be appointed to an internship." FitzGerald wanted the sixth-year students made into non-residential junior interns.[13]

And how about the new medical graduates who wanted to continue as "internes" in surgery? Were they to be selected by the Department of Surgery or the hospital? A solution was worked out in 1947, initially apropos the veterans hospitals such as Sunnybrook, then applied to all the teaching hospitals. MacFarlane said, "I have talked this matter over with the Professor of Surgery and it is hoped that after the first of July we will receive most of our new internes from a joint selected board with representatives from all the teaching hospitals. We would seek people who had had at least the [surgery] rotation and preferably their senior year." Janes, professor of surgery, said, "So far as surgery is concerned the program is already underway and they have agreed that they will refer applications to a Joint Committee of the committees of the teaching hospitals. The group will be considered as a whole."[14]

There were few further changes in hospital-faculty relations until the advent of hospital insurance in 1958–9 really upset the apple cart. If all patients were now "private," and thus off-limits for teaching as the previous private patients had been, where would the teaching patients come from? As MacFarlane said in 1959, "The advent of hospital insurance in Ontario has been viewed with … some concern by those responsible for the maintenance of undergraduate teaching and of resident training." The Hospital Insurance Commission had held two further meetings during the year, he said, with representatives of the medical schools and teaching hospitals. The commission was ill-disposed to get involved in the question of what constituted an adequate teaching unit and preferred to leave it to the hospitals and the medical faculties to work things out. The Toronto faculty had a committee under neurosurgeon Harry Botterell that was to consider faculty-hospital arrangements.[15] So as far as the province was concerned, university and hospitals would just have to make their own deal.

But it was not just the problem of teaching beds. The problem of research conducted in hospitals became acute in the early 1960s. In the 1963–4 session, the Board of Governors of the university struck a special committee on medical education chaired by John Hamilton that reported in May 1964. The special committee decided to centralize basic science research on campus and simultaneously to decentralize clinical research by supporting, in the major teaching hospitals, "the creation of research facilities, both experimental and clinical." Given that the big teaching hospitals were all developing parallel teaching and research programs, the board felt that it made sense to create a "campus-based complex of basic science and joint research space [in] an attempt to meet the problem of interdisciplinary research which is considered to be the greatest development to which medical science can look forward."[16] What was opaquely called the "Health Sciences Complex," intimately linking hospitals and university, was about to take form, part of the push coming from the university side.

## The Health Sciences Complex

This story goes back to the early 1960s, just after John Hamilton became dean. The provincial government asked the university to consider enlarging the medical class to 250 students per year, and the faculty agreed to this if facilities were to be made available. The Medical Sciences Building came out of this bargain. At the same time, the number of patients in the veterans hospitals was falling off, and the suggestion arose that Sunnybrook might become a teaching hospital. Government largesse loomed. In 1966 the federal Health Resources Development Fund was established, making it possible for the hospitals to expand and to employ greatly increased numbers of staff on a full-time basis. Capital expenditures for education purposes in the health field soared.[17] Thus a surprising governmental open-fistedness created expansive thoughts.

In 1964 the University Teaching Hospitals Association (UTHA) was founded. It was basically an association of hospitals. As obstetrician William Paul later recounted the story, "UTHA began as a 'club' of trustees of affiliated teaching hospitals to discuss common problems." The member hospitals retained their independence. The association consisted of the board chairs of the seven affiliated general hospitals, plus the four specialty hospitals (HSC, etc.), plus five members from the university, including Paul himself, and the president and vice-provost for health sciences. Thus the UTHA board was dominated by lay figures, given that nonphysicians headed all the hospital boards. The UTHA had a management committee made up of administrators of all the member hospitals and a medical advisory board.

A second pathway to the Academic Health Sciences Complex was struck in July 1964 when John B. Neilson, a specialist in preventive medicine at the University of Western Ontario and chairman of the Ontario Hospital Services Commission (OHSC), toured the province's medical schools. As he wrote to the provincial minister of health Mathew Dymond (who also was a physician, graduating from Queen's in 1941), "Concern was expressed in most schools about the possible adverse effect on the availability of teaching patients if and when a so-called 'Medicare' plan develops in the Province. The consensus of opinion was that the most efficacious way to meet the situation was by the development and designation of 'clinical teaching units' in the teaching hospitals. The Complex would thus evolve about these teaching units."[18]

In October 1964 John Robarts, premier of Ontario, announced that the province intended to "upgrade teaching facilities in the health sciences" (see also chapter 25). A plethora of briefs from the interested parties arrived at the Ministry of Health. In January 1966 the government established a Senior Co-ordinating Committee, under the chairmanship of the deputy minister of health, Kenneth Clayton Charron, a medical graduate of U of T (1934) – who originated from Kirkland Lake and was previously director of Health Service, Department of National Health and Welfare, in Ottawa – "to co-ordinate planning of health services and education." The committee was to make recommendations to the various ministries and then to see that the appropriate department of the Ontario Hospital Services Commission implemented them.[19] By September 1968 the U of T Faculty of Medicine had completed its brief and forwarded it to the Senior Co-ordinating Committee.

The idea for such a complex seems to have germinated within the provincial government at the same time as within the university's Board of Governors.

Initially, the provincial government used the term "centre" rather than "complex." In July 1965, Dr Bernard L.P. Brosseau, a provincial health official, told Neilson that health care today is based on the idea of cooperation among the health sciences professions. "The Health Sciences Centre is the organization that can accomplish this by providing joint educational facilities and integrating the teaching of those subjects that are a common requirement. The Health Sciences Centre concept was developed to meet the requirement for joint training that will make possible the team approach in the field of health ... It is generally agreed that the faculty of medicine should act as the co-ordinating agency for the Health Sciences complex and that the centre should be an integral part of a university." Brosseau continued, "It is recommended that the Health Sciences centre approach be considered in Ontario for the teaching of the health sciences ... Whenever possible a university teaching hospital must be physically part of the centre." Further, "[a]dequate research facilities must be provided for all members of the teaching staff. This will require that a research laboratory be proved for each full-time member."[20] Thus the province saw the faculty at the core of a health complex embracing all the teaching hospitals. This was a much more integrated, organic vision than the previous joint committee had possessed.

Under the aegis of this concept of "complex," floating in the air in the mid-1960s, small steps began proceeding. At a December 1966 meeting of the faculty's senior committee, Dean Chute commented "on the importance of all applications for research going through the heads of departments, even those administered by the hospitals ... He will bring this to the attention of the hospital administrators also."[21]

On 12 August 1966 the chairmen and the administrators of the Toronto teaching hospitals met, agreeing to form an Advisory Co-ordinating Committee. Lawrie Chute, dean of medicine at U of T, was chair, and the heads of the other teaching hospitals – including the New Mount Sinai Hospital, which now started to be drawn into faculty events – were also present. Chute said afterwards of the meeting, "There was agreement that Toronto should develop as a major centre, rather than each hospital going its own way. However, the suggested combination of hospitals [into teaching 'hospital schools'] was a new idea and did not receive immediate approval. It had been agreed that there should be a University Hospital Joint Board with the senior administrators meeting monthly, and the full Board including the Chairmen of the Hospital Boards, meeting twice yearly to resolve the more serious problems."[22]

It was at this August meeting that the hospitals and the faculty bought into the premise that "[t]he Medical Education Program of the University of Toronto will, in future, be based in a central basic science complex on the campus and on several semi-autonomous Affiliated Institutions composed of groups of Teaching Hospitals and other Health Institutions all of which have separate ownership." A central coordinating committee would be required. "As there is as yet no legislative authority for a Medical Centre, the successful operation of the proposed committee or board … will be based on agreements made in good faith by the constituent members." Such a board will provide a "direct channel of communications" to the university and to the Boards of Trustees of the various hospitals. "The Provincial Government, and in particular the Ontario Hospital Services Commission, are vitally interested in this development because of the potential capital and operating costs involved."[23]

The wheels ground rather slowly. It was only at a meeting of the Senior Co-ordinating Committee in August 1969 under Charron that "[t]he recommendation to develop a new institution was made on the advice of the Ontario Council of Health, after a review of the manpower situation in Ontario." It was noted, "The universities in the province are being asked to develop a programme over a ten year period … It is then proposed to co-ordinate the programmes of the various universities into a provincial plan, which will be reviewed and up-dated annually."[24] The province was thus very much the midwife of the academic health science complexes that came into being at all the Ontario medical schools.

In the background of these events was the huge increase in government spending on health care that had taken place since the Second World War. This was touched on in the previous chapter. The Ontario Hospital Services Plan went into effect in January 1959, enrolling over 90 percent of the province's population for monthly premiums of $2.10 for a single person and $4.20 for a family. The Ontario Hospital Services Commission was conceived to implement the plan. As a result of this provincial largesse, the number of hospital beds per 1,000 of the population increased in Ontario from 4.1 in 1947 to 6.0 in 1965, then plateaued. Not only did the hospitals increase in size, but the personnel in the hospitals soared too, from 165 per 100 beds in 1953 to 186 in the mid-1970s. The number of patient days in hospital and the number of physicians registered in Ontario (from 4,200 in 1941 to 14,500 in 1975!): both increased.[25]

In addition, in 1969 the province started participating in a federal shared-cost health insurance program. "In 1972 a new Ontario Health Insurance Act merged the hospitalization and medical care insurance plans into a single government-operated health insurance plan for the province." The average annual real rate of growth increased every year by about 10 percent.[26]

It was too much. Alarmed, the province began to pull back in the late 1960s from this health-care machine that was gobbling an ever greater percent of the gross provincial product. "By the mid-1970s," writes economic historian K.G. Rea, "the Ontario government was redirecting its efforts with respect to the provision of health care services … seeking to cut back the system."[27]

Thus, the atmosphere of happy self-congratulation of the budget boom years came to an end. There would have to be cost savings, and cooperation between the university and the teaching hospitals was necessary to achieve them. The university and the hospitals would have to be cheese-paring about hospital organization and curriculum planning. Dean Chute said in 1969 that never before had the university worked with the hospitals at this micro-level, and though the experience produced much fury among the clinicians – "the Heads of Departments meet[ing] weekly, and on occasion twice a week, for an average of four or five hours per session" – there arose from it an intimacy between hospitals and medical faculty that had not previously existed.[28] The coordinating committee was responsible for telling the government the capital needs of the Health Sciences Complex in the coming years. Further documents communicated figures that, in the stringency of the late 1960s, struck the government as astronomical.

As the faculty and the hospitals wrestled with these budget issues, the Ministry of Health steamed. In December 1967, a ministry memo charged, "There is a lack of co-ordinated planning within each University programme, however, in Toronto this deficiency is much more acute and manifesting itself in a series of demands for capital programmes which surely go far beyond the bounds of realistic requirement and the availability of capital support. Expansion programmes for teaching hospitals are being planned by the individual institutions, without the accord of the University. The proposals for the Toronto General, Toronto Western are typical of this."[29] A week later the ministry fumed that the teaching hospitals in the Toronto area had forwarded expansion plans totaling a third of a billion dollars. They noted "[f]actors bearing upon the unsatisfactory state of planning ... The framework for a total Health Care Delivery system has not yet been fully devised." The ministry said, "Hospitals are submitting proposals independently of Universities." The general conclusion was this: the Health Science Centres must run a much tighter ship.[30]

In fact, at the provincial level, coordination was awful. In October 1967 the Ontario Hospital Services Commmission (OHSC) met with the main provincial teaching hospitals. One hospital gripe concerned "the lack of communication between the university medical schools and the hospitals." Appointments were made "without consultation with the hospital administrators. The hospitals objected to the fundamental principle that it was acting in the capacity of a paying agency for another body. In many cases the hospital's first notification was a letter from the Commission stating that the Commission had approved the appointments as submitted by the dean of the medical school. The hospitals were then expected to provide office space and include the salaries in their budgets."[31]

But the Ministry of Health was at pains not to cut costs at the expense of research. By the late 1960s the need for research had been sufficiently internalized that it required no further justification. In July 1968 Charron told Dymond, "There are several factors which need to be considered and kept in perspective with regard to health sciences development at the University of Toronto." One of those factors was research: "Arrangements for financing of the health sciences should take into account the service and research component (particularly clinical investigation) as features which are unique to the health sciences and beyond the university orbit."[32]

In 1968 the university's Board of Governors became involved, setting up a Medical Survey Committee (the "Borden Committee") that met in the summer "to integrate all health services within the university and especially to examine the hospital-university relationships." Dean Chute appointed five members of the faculty to meet with this committee, and in September these five forwarded to the board's committee a big needs document.[33]

At an early December 1968 meeting, the Faculty Council heard the views of its own review committee, which had been constituted to examine plans for the faculty made by the Board of Governors' Borden Committee. In this December meeting the Faculty Council put forward again the idea "that there be a common planning group to plan together with representation from each hospital and the Faculty. The [hospital] boards of trustees and the [university] Board of Governors did not appreciate the necessity of this. This proposal had been put forward twice in the last two years, to plan together, eg duplication inadequacies etc. In this way neither hospitals nor university would be the boss but there would be a middle group."[34]

Meanwhile, the ministry was cutting budgets and reducing training slots. In November, H.S. Martin, chair of the OHSC, asked U of T to resubmit a lesser budget. At a meeting of the Faculty Council on 11 December 1968 a ministerial decision to cut the number of teaching beds was announced. How to proceed? "Subsequent discussion pointed to the need for co-ordinated planning, although the Dean [Chute] stated that all previous attempt to achieve this on a University-Hospital basis had failed." The Faculty Council continued, "During the meeting the need for a planning group to coordinate the needs and aspirations of the teaching hospitals and the University became increasingly apparent."[35] Thereupon, the faculty constituted an Independent Planning Committee (IPC) to draft the resubmission. The IPC consisted of the board chairs of the teaching hospitals plus the top faculty executives. At the end of 1968 the IPC drew up a document specifying the conditions that must be met for becoming a teaching hospital, a clinical department, an affiliated hospital, and so forth.[36]

On 1 October 1969 the Independent Planning Committee submitted its report, recommending "the immediate formation of a formal association or system of the Health Science Faculties of the University and the presently affiliated hospitals and institutes."[37] The preparation of the IPC report was a real bonding exercise. The faculty chairs and other executives were "to establish the closest possible liaison with intra-hospital planning committees in each teaching hospital." There were numerous references to "the University-teaching hospital complex."[38]

The Independent Planning Committee aimed at the creation of a Health Science Resource Centre: "The very existence of this Committee ... evidences the imperative need for a permanent and formal organization whereby the affairs of that [faculty-hospital] partnership in education may be more efficiently conducted ... The unwillingness or inability of the Faculty of Medicine and the teaching hospitals to collaborate in the period 1965–68 in the formulation of planning programmes for medical education (even in the face of emergent circumstances) led to the formation of this Committee – which the Faculty Council saw as an ad hoc committee which would disband itself when its functions had been fulfilled." To the contrary, they needed a permanent "structure." If they didn't act there would be legislation. "The teaching hospitals and the Faculty of Medicine are, in a sense, but one institution – a school for the instruction of undergraduate and post-graduate medical students in the interests and for the welfare of the people of Ontario." It is thus interesting, after decades of inertia, to see the faculty and the hospitals forced into bed with one another by the Ministry of Health in a funding crisis – and in the process of becoming intimate, just to extend this perhaps unfortunate metaphor – to acquire an easy and cooperative working relationship that had never previously existed.

Under the ministry lash, therefore, the faculty and the teaching hospitals declared willingness to drag themselves into a more permanent union: "The Committee accordingly recommends the immediate formation of a formal association ... of the Health Science Faculties of the University of Toronto and the presently affiliated teaching hospitals ... to provide an organized means whereby the planning ... of the University teaching complex may be co-ordinated in the interests of assuring more efficient operation and the elimination of duplicate ... facilities."[39]

Dean Hamilton played an interesting and hitherto unknown role in these negotiations. According to an OHSC interoffice memo headed "Toronto Health Sciences Complex," of 15 June 1971, a week previously, two ministry officials had met with Dean Hamilton "to discuss the downtown Toronto hospital situation:" "Dr Hamilton agreed that the OHSC should commission the role study [which hospital does what] for the downtown Toronto hospitals." Further, "Dr Hamilton agrees with reducing teaching beds, more than enough now and we could even accept St Michael's Hospital moving 'outside Toronto.'... In general we all agreed that the University should, can and will adapt itself to service requirements of the community.... Only minimal research space is required in addition to what is now provided. The only space that will be needed is the small amount required to support the beds in clinical investigation units." Hamilton was equally accommodating on other points that would have outraged his colleagues had they known of his acquiescence: "Sufficient classroom space is already available if it were properly scheduled." "Dr Hamilton supports the elimination of duplication of highly specialized facilities." Part of the Hospital for Sick Children might be given to the School of Dentistry (!), and finally, "Dr Hamilton would support a move to remove some of the independence of the hospitals as well as the University in order to develop and implement a more rational use of facilities."[40] Hamilton had, essentially, given the ministry cover for the drastic organizational changes and budget cuts that lay ahead. In fairness to him and to Dean Chute, both men were very much under fire from a faculty upset about massive changes at the last minute, and Hamilton, at least, may have thought timely concessions to the ministry the swiftest way of putting the kerfuffle behind.

There is no doubt that an attached ministerial budget memo headed "Toronto Health Sciences Complex" was brutal: a number of hospitals have already received construction funds. "No additional funds will be available to these institutions within this decade." The hospital bed capacities must all be reduced: the TGH would lose 160 of its 1,100 beds, Sunnybrook 86 of its 600, SMH 294 of its 600, and so forth. Facilities for postgraduate training were to be capped at four times those for undergraduates. "Only minimal research space will be provided in addition to that currently available in the Medical Sciences Building," the memo noted. Hospitals were encouraged to share auditoriums and classrooms, and there would be no "sixth medical school" for the province within this decade.[41] In fact, there was none for more than three decades: The Northern Ontario School of Medicine, hosted jointly by Lakehead University in Thunder Bay and Laurentian University in Sudbury, admitted its first students in September 2005.[42]

Thus, the new relationship between teaching hospitals and faculty was to resemble "federalism." In March 1967, in response to a query from the Toronto General Hospital, Chute gave his view of the relationship between university and the hospitals: "The medical school should be visualized as a type of federalism made up of ten components, rather than as four or five autonomous units. Some of the larger centres will be complete units, but it is unlikely that the smaller ones will be."[43] The Health Sciences Complex represented a huge step forward in hospital-faculty cooperation. It was cooperation wrested from unwilling hospital boards and a hesitant faculty by a provincial government intent upon cost-saving and alarmed at its own earlier generosity. Yet in terms of science and patient care, it was an undoubted step forward.

### The Academic Health Sciences Complex Takes Wing

The negotiations to establish an Academic Health Sciences Complex will not be followed here in detail. Yet two points of interest emerged. One, participants became increasingly interested in putting resources into primary care, rather than the expensive specialties. At a September meeting in 1969 some participants wondered "whether the production of family practitioners is being neglected. It was suggested this should be given careful consideration when discussing priorities."[44] This was an important spur to founding the Department of Family and Community Medicine.

Second, the university's claim to manage hospital resources was becoming ever more evident. At the same September meeting "Dr Hamilton reported that some time ago the University began taking an inventory of all space available for teaching purposes for the Health Sciences. It is proposed to treat this as one block of space to be allocated as practically as possible for the implementation of all Health Science programmes. This is not easy but progress is being made."[45] Not easy indeed; the faculty claim to control great blocks of hospital square footage was breathtaking.

By the end of September 1969, Charron gave Dean Chute two months to develop a "master plan" for the Health Sciences Centre.

The hospitals had to respond. In March 1970 James Douglas Wallace, an Albertan who had joined the General in 1966 and soon became medical director, then executive director, told the Board of Trustees that it have no choice but to join the coming Academic Health Sciences Centre. He said that in February he had attended a conference organized by the Senior Coordinating Committee on cooperation among the provincial university Health Science Centres, the teaching hospitals, and other educational entities. "It was made abundantly clear that our future development is dependent upon co-operation with the University of Toronto, the CAAT Colleges [Colleges of Applied Arts and Technologies] and other Teaching Hospitals in the area." A provincial proposal was also distributed "to develop an organized Health Sciences Complex in Toronto as a result of the report submitted by the Independent Planning Committee. Toronto General Hospital can no longer exist in isolation as a major teaching and research centre. Such a formalized relationship will result in some loss of autonomy. However, as Government is now responsible for practically all of the financing for hospital, medical and educational services, it is doubtful, at this time, how much autonomy we really have." Wallace urged the trustees to "support any plans ... in the development of a major health sciences complex ... In my opinion, it is no longer logical or possible for one component of a complex to develop, or perhaps survive, in isolation in the health field."[46] What Wallace, a veteran clinician and hospital loyalist, recommended was, in essence, abject surrender of the hospital's former independence.

What inducements could there be for the hospitals to thus abandon their autonomy to a Health Sciences Complex? Two months later, in May 1970, it became clear, as Wallace reported to the trustees, "The Senior Co-ordinating Committee of the Province will not approve individual plans for financing through the Health Resources Development Fund until such organizational plans have been finalized."[47] So no more money until they sign on.

Another way of getting the hospitals on board was to make their chief physicians into "professors." In medicine, Wightman said that to coordinate hospital teaching programs, "the physician-in-chief at each hospital has been given the rank of Professor and asked to assume responsibility for the teaching assignments in his own hospital."[48] (Unlike in the Faculty of Arts, in medicine, the title "professor" is highly valued and represents a source of prestige over other "doctors.") This began making the hospitals partners in postgraduate training, which reached its fullest expression, as was seen, in the 1990s in the Research Institutes, when the number of graduate students in the hospitals outnumbered those in the basic science departments (see p. 301).

In this manner the Academic Health Sciences Centre began in Toronto; this was not the first in Canada, for Alberta had established the initial such centre, followed by a second at McMaster University. But with the giant Faculty of Medicine and its many teaching hospitals, Toronto's was certainly the most imposing.

It became "Health Sciences." The plural of *Science* was soon accepted, and in Toronto the Health Sciences Centre held the faculty and the teaching hospitals together in an organic connection, not a mechanical union. Phillipson later likened the Academic Health Sciences Centre in Toronto to "a balanced environmental ecosystem, involving the University, teaching hospitals, research institutes, and faculty members. Like all ecosystems, challenges affecting one component of the system quickly exert a ripple effect on all elements, highlighting the need for a collective response if the balance in the system is to be maintained."[49] The mechanics of creating health science complexes for each set of medical schools and teaching hospitals in the province were complex but basically involved the Ontario council of deans and the council of hospital administrators sitting down across from each other at the table and drawing up contracts ("meaningful written agreements") that "should prevent many of the misunderstandings that have arisen in the past," as Wallace told the TGH trustees.[50]

Was the faculty happy with the new Academic Health Sciences Complex? Highly suspicious was the first reaction. All the planning of the late 1960s had just made everybody miserable. In 1970 Dean Chute said, "Undoubtedly the most pressing problem facing the Faculty of Medicine ... is to redefine its relationship with its associated teaching hospitals." He said that current agreements were totally inadequate for the new era of government insurance programs and formula-financing for the universities. The hospital trustees, on their side, depended on the university for the approval of new capital budgets. And the university Board of Governors were looking at large new budgets unrelated to traditional concepts of academic activities. Said Chute, "There is, to my mind, a very great danger that the educational programme and needs of the Medical School will be dictated by the professional demands of hospitals rather than by the University ... The University and the hospitals which serve its educational needs must work in much close relation to one another than has been the case in the past."[51]

*Role Study*

The province wanted badly to know how hospital services overlapped and what programs could be cut. In October 1971 the Senior Co-ordinating Committee proposed a "role study" for the Toronto Health Sciences Complex, wanting to learn "the role of each hospital in relation to other hospitals as well as to the community. Facilities will be shared to the greatest extent possible in order to ensure that public money has been wisely spent." OHSC wanted "emphasis on family physicians," including "[m]ethods of delivering health care other than on an in-patient basis, especially ambulatory services, including family practice units and home care programs."[52] (One hears the drums on behalf of family medicine beating ever more loudly. See chapter 24.) The consultants Kates, Peat, Marwick & Co. would undertake the study.

Within the Health Sciences Complex, the hospitals began planning cooperatively, something unheard of previously. The Role Study of 1972 called for various hospital groups to form "clinical complexes." Following this report, "the four hospitals located near Queen's Park and University Avenue decided to form a coordinating committee, now called 'The Queen's Park Hospitals.'"[53] In April 1972 John Hamilton, vice president of health sciences, suggested to Dean Chute that a "Tri-Hospital Complex Coordinating Committee" be created for the three general hospitals in the "College Street–University area" (Mount Sinai, the General, Women's College); he said that HSC would send an observer; "co-ordination of services" was the objective, the Ministry of Health was not involved. "In achieving these general objectives, it is understood that each general hospital shall retain its individuality and integrity through maintenance of its own Board of Trustees and separate management." It was not proposed that "the Complex Co-ordinating Committee establish a permanent secretariat," but it must have a budget.[54]

The reactions to this committee's recommendations of August 1972 showed that force majeure would be required to get the hospitals to coordinate services. Walter Hannah, chair of the subcommittee on obstetrics and gynecology, said that "even though the Role Study recommended that one of the three obstetrics units in the complex be phased out, the subcommittee felt that all three were needed. "In general terms ... no general hospital is complete without the basic four departments, Medicine, Surgery, OB/GYN and Family Practice." All were busy and had 85 percent occupancy, "which for obstetrics is considered to approach a maximally acceptable occupancy rate." Also, teaching would suffer. As for gynecology, it can't exist in isolation without obstetrics. But maybe there could be a single neonatal ICU, with divisions in each of the three obstetrics departments.[55] A similar subcommittee on "emergency services" reached an identical conclusion: nothing could be sacrificed. All three hospitals would continue to have emergency departments, even though they were only a stone's throw apart. Indeed, the General kicked back with particular fury at the suggestion that it lose its emergency and trauma service, even if Mount Sinai was organizing a splendid new one.[56] Stronger medicine was needed.

In 1973 the UTHA set up a planning committee to determine the disposition of the $100 million from the provincial Health Resources Development Fund for the health sciences complex in Toronto ($90 million for hospitals, $10 million for campus). The committee, chaired by John Law, was composed of the chairmen of the boards of the General, the Western, St Michael's, and Sunnybrook. This committee in turn set up a "working party" consisting of the executive directors of the four hospitals and the dean of medicine. "The plans of the four hospitals concerned have been reviewed, a site visit to each institution has taken place, and a retreat has been arranged to co-ordinate this information."[57] This committee was now in a position to make actual decisions about who got how much money.

From within the faculty, requests for consolidation were acceded to grumpily, if at all. In January 1973 Hollenberg said that the Departments of Medicine in the three "trihospitals" would set up a "coordinating committee" that will try to determine what services can be coordinated.[58] Fred Fallis in family medicine stonewalled: there was no hope of integrating the three hospital family medicine departments "because the respective hospitals depend upon these units as a source of referred patients. Any integration of personnel and function would therefore disrupt admitting patterns and referrals."[59]

In 1973 the faculty formed its own Planning Strategy Committee with all the deanery in attendance, in addition to faculty barons W. Robert Harris, chair of the Long-Range Planning and Assessment Committee; Lou Siminovitch, chair of the sub-committee on science policy; and Charles Hollenberg and Donald Wilson, the important clinical chairmen.[60] In November 1977 the dean appointed William Paul, former chair of obstetrics and gynecology, as the inaugural associate dean of institutional affairs, "in recognition of the growing involvement of the medical school with the network of teaching hospitals and community hospitals, the UTHA, and in recognition of the fact that moves appear to be underway for the development of a District Health Council for Toronto."[61]

In retrospect, these efforts at more or less voluntary centralization were almost doomed to fail. Hamilton saw this clearly: when told that the Committee of Clinical Chairmen at their March 1973 meeting had expressed reservations about the ability of Women's College and Mount Sinai to cooperate in medical education and research, Hamilton, now vice provost, said how dismayed he was "that the clinical chairmen seem to be repudiating responsibility of acting in concert ... [This] ... strengthens my belief that the Queen's Park Hospitals integration will never progress."[62] They would have to be compelled. This was indeed the route the province would take in a decade's time: mergers would have to be mandated. Yet in the meantime, the network of ties between faculty and hospitals was becoming ever thicker.

## Getting Some Teeth into Things

Hospital autonomy is often regarded in a negative way in the Faculty.[63]

Louis Siminovitch, 1973

The actual control the faculty had over the hospitals was rather minimal at ground zero. There were research policies, but governance was separate.

By the mid-1970s faculty policies towards research in the teaching hospitals had been worked out. The rule at the University of Toronto, as articulated in

Howard Petch's 1976 report on health research in Ontario, was, "At least one in ten full-time equivalent staff of a hospital should be engaged in laboratory research. In addition, space should be provided for two-thirds of the remaining staff for research with patients or fundamental research." Moreover, under faculty leadership there was already a health-complex-wide effort to develop unique research initiatives at each institution, such as the rheumatic disease research unit at the Wellesley Hospital, clinical immunology and neurosciences at the Western, and cardiovascular at the General. One limitation on the application of faculty policy across the board, said Petch, was that some of the independent facilities such as the Princess Margaret Hospital and the Addiction Research Foundation were provincial institutions, and such influence as the faculty had been able to achieve "appears to be the result of individual leadership and initiative, rather than organizational arrangements."[64]

Building an Academic Health Sciences Centre involved a series of bilateral agreements between the faculty and each of the teaching hospitals, establishing for that institution a hospital-university Joint Relations Committee. The agreement with St Michael's Hospital, for example, was concluded in July 1979 and made provision for a separate committee to administer that particular nexus.[65]

To give all hospitals a greater voice at the Ministry of Health, in 1979 the University Teaching Hospitals Association (UTHA) disbanded in favour of the Hospital Council of Metro Toronto (HCMT). It was formed to deal with the newly established District Health Council for Toronto, a provincial body, to enable all the hospitals of Toronto to speak with one voice and was intended to build links, having a planning committee involving both hospital and university representatives, and a university-hospital relations committee. This latter committee would have a subcommittee known as the "Dean's Committee," with deans, hospital executive directors, and so forth.[66] Yet this did not further links among the teaching hospitals, and faculty–teaching-hospital relations stayed at the level of bilateral agreements between the university and each hospital. Moreover, the relations between the dean and the hospital executives were described as "sporadic."[67]

In June 1981 the president and chairs of the hospital boards held a big meeting at Simcoe Hall, the university's administrative centre, and resolved to build links on research and other matters of common interest. They agreed on "[t]he establishment of a committee under Faculty leadership, with representatives from each hospital, to examine the issue of the Health Sciences complex as a whole … The Board Chairmen gave an undertaking not to unilaterally establish new initiatives affected the rest of the complex without prior discussion."[68]

Accordingly, in 1982 a Hospital University Research Coordinating Committee (HURCC) was established, chaired by Brian Underdown, associate dean of research. This committee brought together the hospital research directors. (Also, in November 1983, the Faculty Council approved hospital participation in the faculty's restructured research committee.[69])

How else might the hospitals be brought into line with faculty policy? Make the tenure of the hospital department chiefs subject to the same five-year renewable limitation as the university department and division heads. These efforts began in April 1981, as Dean Lowy mentioned to the university clinical chairs that he had this in mind. At this meeting, "Dr Hollenberg recommended that the review process should incorporate the principle that it is a joint University/hospital process in which the University and the hospital are equal partners."[70] All parties assented to this by February 1982.[71]

Thus occurred the slow knitting together of hospital and faculty. Both sides surrendered autonomy. In the early 1980s hiring decisions in the faculty ceased to be entirely departmental but were shared with the hospitals. In 1984 Dean Lowy told Alan Hudson, then chair of the university Division of Neurosurgery,

"Until the last two years decisions regarding the allocation of university teaching and research programs in hospitals were entirely departmental ... This is no longer the case now – we are engaged in a more explicit partnership with the teaching hospitals and there has been acceptance, by all the Boards of the Fully Affiliated Hospitals and the University, of the need for all parties to consult before reaching major decision that affect other institutions ... We believe that this Health Science Complex can best develop through differentiation of function and mutual support. The Faculty alone does not have the resources to do this. We are now expecting hospitals to contribute major resources (space, equipment, salaries) to support research activities that were once considered university responsibilities. Hospitals have also agreed with the need for central mechanisms for allocation of new major facilities and programs (e.g. Trauma Units, Open Heart Cardiovascular Units, MRI Units, Lithotripsy Units) ... In effect, agreeing to those things, Hospital Boards have agreed to limit their autonomy to some degree, in the interests of developing a better Health Science Centre."

Lowy pointed out that some kind of adjudication system was necessary for conflict resolution, and in September 1983 he proposed such a system of review committees, which was accepted by all the teaching hospitals.[72] Thus, in the space of a few brief years – and under the leadership of a dynamic dean, Fred Lowy, who took office in 1980 – the integration of faculty and teaching hospitals had progressed remarkably.

Lowy kept striving for a more formal body, however, to advance this linking, rather than just the latticework of review committees surrounding appointments and similar structures for cooperation that were developing at the micro level. Lowy organized a "President's Council" to bring together hospital executives and faculty brass. By February 1982 it had met once "and approved in principle the concept that the University and the teaching hospitals should plan as one unit the development and shrinkage of the system [apropos cutbacks], rather than all institutions proceeding independently."[73] This was pretty vague.

Later in 1982 Lowy therefore organized the Task Force on Faculty-Hospital Relations, chaired by Joseph T. Marotta, chief of neurology at the Wellesley and one of the faculty barons. In May Marotta reported what he had learned. Various structures for faculty-hospital contact were already in place, including the following: (a) The Dean's Committee, chaired by the associate dean of clinical and institutional affairs and including university representatives plus the CEOs of the eleven affiliated teaching hospitals. This was an offshoot of the University-Hospital Relations Committee under the aegis of the Hospital Council of Metro Toronto, with objectives similar to those of the old University Teaching Hospitals Association. It offered a forum for discussion but had little role in decision-making. (b) The Committee of Clinical Chairmen, which Marotta called "a good forum for communication and discussion but it is not particularly effective in decision making and long range planning." And (c) The University-Hospital Relations Committee – a committee also under the aegis of HCMT, with members drawn from hospital trustees and administrators, clinicians, and university representatives. "There is considerable redundancy between its role and that of the Dean's Committee. It is more effective in terms of communication than decision making."

The Marotta task force concluded in May 1982 that there was no good forum for decision-making. "The major weakness of the organizational structure appears to lie in the relationship between the CEOs and the Clinical Chairmen."[74] So the big disconnect in the system lay between the senior administration of the hospitals and the university chairs of the divisions and departments.

On the basis of that task force, in December 1982 Lowy recommended to the President's Council the creation of a University of Toronto Health Sciences Complex Management Advisory Committee, which included university officials and the executive directors or presidents of the then eleven fully affiliated teaching hospitals.[75] This was more like it. This was a body that could have some bite but soon gave way to another entity with more power.

*Hospital Mergers*

The next hurdle in university-hospital relations was the hospital mergers of the late 1980s, especially the merger of the Toronto General Hospital and the Toronto Western Hospital in 1986. In January 1986 the university had two committees in place to track the merger: (1) a committee composed of chief executive officers under Hollenberg; and (2) a clinical planning committee under Marotta.[76] Edward M. Sellers had the responsibility for merging the two systems of undergraduate medical education, where the hospital coordinators threatened to clash with the faculty administration. As he explained in April 1986, the hospitals had "responsibilities for providing an environment for education"; university departments had a "responsibility for the conduct, quality and implementation of their educational programs." Sellers wanted more hospital "resources" for medical education, pointing out "that while each hospital has two coordinators with responsibility for undergraduate education [meaning hospital and campus coordinators], they have no formal relationship to one another."[77]

There were also governance implications in the merger. In April 1986 Lowy said that "up to now the University Governing Council has not formally recognized the interdependence of the hospitals and the Faculty of Medicine, and there is no formal mechanism whereby the hospitals and the Governing Council interact. The report takes the position that Governing Council should adopt a formal posture vis-à-vis the teaching hospitals." What might that formal posture be? Lowy said the faculty executives with most knowledge of hospital affairs were the university department chairs. He told a meeting of the university clinical chairmen that W. Vickery Stoughton, president of TGH, "has given assurance that he is prepared to accept the pivotal role of departmental chairmen in this process." This, therefore, was the seminal event in knitting hospitals and faculty together: a formal hospital role for the university departmental chairs as delegates of the Board of Governors of the university.[78]

In June 1986 the Joint Faculty/University Hospital Planning Committee (JPC) came into being, consisting of Lowy as chair; Joseph Marotta, who was associate dean of clinical and institutional affairs; Bernard Langer, chair of surgery; Walter Hannah, professor of obstetrics and gynecology; Stoughton of TGH; Sister Christine Gaudet, CEO of St Michael's Hospital; and D. Martin, president of HSC.[79] The dean had his own Strategic Planning Committee.

Together, these two bodies would guide hospital mergers. Several were on the horizon: Sunnybrook was to be merged with either Women's College or the Wellesley; the Princess Margaret Hospital would soon move to hospital row on University Avenue and was ripe for a takeover. Sunnybrook in particular offered the faculty an alternative vision from being a single entity clustered about Queen's Park to a faculty with, as Lowy put it, "[t]wo academic foci whereby the University would develop the Bayview site jointly with constituent institutions, and over time create there a true academic focus with a strong basic science component and the appropriate infra-structure." There was great enthusiasm for this latter model, Sunnybrook integrated into the Health Sciences Complex to become "a major teaching hospital."[80]

The 1990s saw a further wave of hospital mergers, including Sunnybrook with Women's College Hospital, the Clarke Institute of Psychiatry with the Addiction Research Foundation and the Queen Street Mental Health Centre (chapter 14), and Princess Margaret Hospital with The Toronto Hospital (chapter 13). This decade also witnessed the formation of the Toronto Rehabilitation Institute (chapter 23).

Following the merger that blended the General and the Western together into The Toronto Hospital in 1986, there were three major liaison organizations to bring faculty and teaching hospitals together: (1) the old President's Council, now called the Hospital-University Board (HUB), chaired by the vice provost of health sciences and including chairs of the hospital boards; (2) the Faculty of Medicine's Teaching Hospitals Advisory Committee, chaired by the dean and including all the hospital CEOs (this had been previously known as the Health Sciences Complex Management Advisory Committee, but it had not been effective and was restructured); (3) the Hospital University Research Coordinating Committee (HURCC), established in 1982 and chaired by the vice provost of health sciences and research directors from all teaching hospitals.[81]

This considerable institutional carapace sounded complex but in fact could be boiled down to a simple formula. As Stoughton, now president and CEO of The Toronto Hospital, said in 1990, "The hospital's priority is patient care, the University's is teaching. This tension, coupled with an increased tertiary care role, can lead to conflicts with respect to education ... The issue is not really one of conflict, then, because teaching and research enhance patient care."[82]

Yet this rather anodyne formulation concealed the real conflicts of interest that persisted between hospitals and universities. A case in point: in 1990 a group of fundraisers at The Toronto Hospital wanted to find the money for a chair in neurosurgery for the hospital. This sounded like a good idea, right? Not at all. Bernie Langer, head of surgery, immediately blew the alarm whistle to Dean Dirks: "The creation of a Toronto Hospital 'Chair' ... will pre-empt any possibility of developing a University Chair in Neurosurgery. This will inhibit the development of a University Division of Neurosurgery, and it will also make it very difficult to appoint the University Chairman of Neurosurgery in any other hospital but The Toronto Hospital." He said that if it were possible for hospitals to buy university chairs in this manner – meaning the university head would always be situated at that hospital – "I am sure that many of them could find the two million dollars necessary to have a Chairman in that hospital in perpetuity."[83] In fact, in the 1991–2 session, the Dan family donated a chair in neurosurgery to the university, not to the hospital.[84]

To better partner hospitals and university, in January 1992 the Toronto Academic Health Science Council (TAHSC) was created, including a mixture of hospital and campus executives. Its purpose was to link the locomotives together. An accreditation team noted in May 1992 "the critical interdependency of the Faculty and the hospitals ... the hospitals are absolutely dependent on the medical school for faculty appointments and graduate and postgraduate programs. The TAHSC concedes the Faculty's strong centralized focus and control of teaching." The team said this would avoid a re-enactment of the teaching hospitals differentiating themselves as medical schools, as had happened in London, England, with Guys, Barts, and other hospitals. "The unity of purpose evidenced by the TAHSC is in contrast with the lack of coordination between hospitals at the time of the previous visit [1990]."[85] In 2004 this body became the Toronto Academic Health Science Network (TAHSN).

One more integrative body might be mentioned, among the welter that grew up in later years. In September 2001 the Hospital/University Education

Committee (HUEC) was created, following the recommendation of the Urowitz/ Whiteside Task Force on Medical Education to, among other things, recruit clinical teachers for teaching the undergraduate medical education curriculum.[86]

The tug of war between faculty and teaching hospitals turned into an embrace, in the midst of which the medical faculty found themselves. As Eliot Phillipson put it in 2002, "It would be an understatement, to say the least, to describe the relationship between the University of Toronto and its clinical faculty as one of complexity and ambiguity. Consider, for example, that clinical faculty members hold appointments in the University and are accountable to it for their academic performance." Yet they receive neither compensation from the university nor tenure. They are accountable to the hospital, "whose corporate structure and governance are independent of their university." And they "derive their income from neither the University nor the hospital, but rather from self-employment earnings (ie clinical practice) that flows through independent practice plans."[87] Phillipson nonetheless professed astonishment that the system worked so well.

To ensure that it continued to work well, in 2005 the University Governing Council established the Clinical Faculty Policy that made possible full-time university appointments for physicians in the ten fully affiliated hospitals and part-time and adjunct university appointments for physicians engaged in teaching medical students and postgraduate medical trainees in community-affiliated hospitals. The affiliation agreement between the hospitals and the university required that all full-time physicians in the hospitals be simultaneously appointed to the university and be promoted up the academic ladder in an identical manner. The Clinical Faculty Policy ensured the integration of clinical care with education and research and was a capstone to a century's development.

In retrospect, as the Health Sciences Complex twisted and bucked in the fire hose of change, it created a constant and ongoing need for new structures to encase it. The story of these structures possesses a certain drama because it shows how institutions that, at the beginning, stood separate and alone became fused into a powerful organism for treating patients effectively, training physicians to be state of the art, and fostering world-class research.

# 13  Cancer Care

What once characterized the Toronto approach to cancer was the separation of the surgical treatment of cancer from medical and radiotherapeutic approaches. Cancer surgery took place in the big teaching hospitals. Chemotherapy and radiotherapy were centred in the Ontario Cancer Institute and the attached Princess Margaret Hospital. This separation was overcome only in 1995 with the move of the Ontario Cancer Institute from Sherbourne Street to join the row of hospitals on University Avenue.

In the Faculty of Medicine, until 1991 radiotherapy (radiation oncology) and diagnostic radiology were united in the same unit, the Department of Radiology. It is here that the story begins. The early radiologists were also radiotherapists, and almost from the beginning, Gordon Richards, the professor of radiology, pressed for establishment of a treatment unit. In May 1931 the "Cody Commission" was convened by the provincial government, chaired by Canon Henry John Cody, chair of the university's Board of Governors, who would shortly become president of the university itself. As Donald Cowan explains in his study of cancer care in Ontario, in February 1932 the Cody Commission "recommended the establishment of radiation treatment centres in the three cities with medical schools (Kingston, London and Toronto) ... These became known as Ontario Institutes of Radiotherapy" (OIR). The OIR in Toronto was opened in 1934 under the headship of Gordon Richards in the remodelled Dunlap Building on University Avenue,[1] which therewith became the seat of the Department of Radiology. The institute specialized in radium and X-ray treatments, a matter in which the university was "deeply interested."[2] The availability of these new therapies hit a deep nerve with the public, and in 1943 a government act incorporated the Ontario Cancer Treatment and Research Foundation (OCTRF) to take responsibility for cancer control, of which Richards became the managing director in the 1944–5 session.[3]

Thus cancer care arrived on the faculty's plate. In the 1946–7 session, the faculty established a general research committee, a subcommittee of which included university departments interested in cancer; the subcommittee had "under its review and guidance the whole field of cancer research."[4] When the Wellesley Hospital amalgamated with TGH in 1948, Richards and the chair of the TGH trustees met with the Minister of Health to discuss the possibility of making the Wellesley Division of the Toronto General Hospital "an institute/hospital for the treatment of cancer." The TGH trustees wanted the future cancer hospital to be part of TGH, which would have meant expanding the Ontario Institute for Radiotherapy.[5] But OCTRF resisted this. Neither won, and in 1951 Premier Leslie Frost announced that the new cancer hospital would have an independent board yet be headed by the chair of the TGH trustees, Norman Urquhart. In 1952 the cancer institute was incorporated in an act of the provincial legislature. The institute's board included members from the OCTRF, the U of T, and the major teaching hospitals. They had to establish buildings for treatment and research on cancer. In 1957 the act was broadened to include the operation of a provincial hospital, which meant that the Ontario Cancer Institute would include research facilities plus a clinic, to be situated next to the Wellesley Division of the TGH. In 1958 the clinic portion became "Princess Margaret Hospital."[6]

### Ontario Cancer Institute – Princess Margaret Hospital

The advantage that Princess Margaret had in those days [was] the clinicians working almost cheek to jowl with the basic scientists. It didn't happen anywhere else in the city.[7]

Donald Cowan, 2009, referring to the 1970s

A building on Sherbourne Street for the Ontario Cancer Institute was commenced in 1954, and by late 1957 researchers had already begun to occupy their space. The hospital, with its eighty-seven beds – ten in a children's ward – accepted the first patient on 1 May 1958.

The founding director of OCI was Clifford Ash, a radiotherapist born in Edmonton, Alberta, in 1909 and medical graduate of the University of Toronto in 1934. After interning at Toronto Western Hospital, Ash spent several years with the Indian Medical Service, where he was officer-in-charge of the military hospitals in Bangalore, Madras, and Cannamore. Back in Toronto in 1938, Ash joined Richards at TGH as a radiation therapist and in 1952 became professor of therapeutic radiology within the Department of Radiology as well as director of the new Ontario Cancer Institute. At the time of his death in 1981 he was praised for attracting "outstanding staff" to the new institute.[8] Indeed, the men and women he attracted were world-class.

The eight-story building included four stories for patient care and three for research on cancer and on radiation (the eighth story was the basement, which housed much of the radiation equipment and workshops). The Ontario Cancer Institute with attached clinical centre was thus simultaneously one of eight provincial treatment centres sponsored by OCTRF, just as the OIR had been. But the Princess Margaret Hospital (PMH) as its successor was also one of the teaching hospitals of the U of T.[9] (PMH did, however, receive some of its operating budget and capital directly from the Ministry of Health.) The Princess Margaret Hospital only admitted patients whose cancers were potentially responsive to radiotherapy. Chemotherapy might be used as an ancillary treatment; there was no cancer surgery, which would be divided between TGH and the other teaching and community hospitals. The radiotherapists at PMH were positive in outlook and forward-leaning in approach. Bernard Cummings, later head of radiation oncology, comments, "From the beginning the radiation oncologists showed a willingness to challenge traditional concepts of the utility of radiation. In this they were helped by the coincidence in the opening of the hospital with the availability of the much more effective modality, Cobalt-60 radiation."[10]

As OCI was being organized in 1956, Harold Johns agreed to lead research in physics. Johns therewith "created," as James Till put it, "almost single-handedly, the field of Medical Physics in Canada, and then developed one of the most outstanding medical physics programs in the world."[11] The purpose of clinical physics included calibrating the therapy machines, measuring the dose of radiation delivered at various tissue depths, and developing new ways of delivering radiation treatment. Johns's most important achievements lay in "devising isotope-based techniques (cobalt and cesium) for delivering energetic radiation doses." He came up with "these high-energy beams [that] could reach deep tumours without damaging the skin," as McCulloch put it. Johns would drive to the nuclear reactor at Chalk River to fetch radioactive cobalt in a lead-lined pot in the back of a truck," his son-in-law Clive Greenstock said.

Johns initiated his work in Saskatoon. By placing radioactive cobalt in a lead container with a single pinhole, he allowed a radiation beam far stronger than previously available X-rays to be focused on deep-seated malignant tumours. This became what *Maclean's* magazine called in 1952 the "cobalt bomb."[12] The Cobalt-60 machine, "mounted in casing that was attached to a movable fitting in the ceiling of a therapy room," was called "the stripper" and was used among other purposes in preparing patients for bone marrow transplantation.[13] A Canadian 37-cent stamp issued in 1988 depicted Johns and celebrated his discovery of cobalt-60 radiation therapy.

In the history of the Faculty of Medicine Johns emerges as a major figure in bridging basic science and treatment. His parents were missionaries, and Johns's father decided to come to a new university opened in Chengdu, West China, in 1910 to teach mathematics. That is where Johns was born five years later. He earned a BA at McMaster University in 1936 and a PhD in physics from the University of Toronto in 1939. Until 1956 he lectured in physics at the Universities of Alberta and Saskatchewan, publishing *The Physics of Radiology* in

1953, a standard text for years. In 1956 he was called to the Ontario Cancer Institute as head of the physics division (an institute department). In 1962 he succeeded Ham as the head of the Department of Medical Biophysics (a university department). "We used to have a session at Princess Margaret for the trainees," said Bernard Cummings, later head of radiation oncology, who came to PMH in 1974. "It was called the hot seat. Harold would pluck somebody out of the audience, sit him down in a chair in front, and grill him – and that could be very, very uncomfortable. You had to understand the basics with Harold. He was a tremendous teacher, very effective, and very well liked."[14]

Lou Siminovitch, a colleague of Johns's at OCI in medical biophysics, has left a portrait of Johns as a researcher intensely interested in biology while being a physicist. "Fortunately, although Harold Johns and I differed enormously in our personalities (and our abilities to play squash, curl or water-ski), we got along well ... I learned a great deal from Harold, who had tremendous leadership skills. In addition, he possessed considerable scientific flair and expertise, and it is my conception that he was the source of the great strength in [radiotherapy] that one now finds in Canada." And then Siminovitch came to the core of things. "Harold Johns was a true academic. He loved science." He recalled, "I spent countless hours trying to educate Harold Johns about biology. Harold had a phenomenal curiosity and really wanted to know. But I believe that he found it difficult to absorb the uncertainties of biology, as compared to the realities of physics."[15] Johns, being "a great believer in physical, almost violent activity," as Ernest McCulloch put it, periodically organized scientific retreats at his cottage where, amidst the waterskiing and cooking, he urged the department's graduate students to acquire scientific competence both in physics and biology.[16]

Ernest McCulloch himself emerges as one of the seminal figures in the history of Canadian science for his co-discovery, with Harold Johns's student Jim Till, of stem cells (see chapter 5). McCulloch was twelve years younger than Johns, born in 1926 in Toronto, where he attended Upper Canada College. He earned a medical degree from the University of Toronto in 1948, editing the U of T medical journal. After training at the General, he passed his fellowship in medicine from the Royal College in 1954. He was a research fellow under Wightman at the General until joining the Department of Medical Biophysics at OCI in 1958. He then spent the years from 1968 to 1988 in various capacities, including director, at the Institute of Medical Science on campus while remaining involved with research at OCI. It might be remarked that, apart from stem cells, McCulloch's "major work has been concentrated on normal and malignant blood formation," as a 2011 obituary issued by the University Health Network put it. "With his colleague Dr James Till, he devised the first functional assay (the spleen colony assay) for primitive blood cell precursors (pluripotent stem cells of CFU-S) ... The discovery of the spleen colony assay for stems cells and its exploitation were major stimuli for the development of the field of experimental haematology."[17]

After Arthur Ham agreed in 1956 to head research in biology, he and Harold Johns brought on board a first-class team: Johns's students Gordon Whitmore and Jim Till joined in 1956, researching at the Connaught Labs until the new building was completed in 1957. John R. ("Jack") Cunningham came in 1958 and began the work in treatment planning systems for which he would later become known. Interestingly, Johns's students tended to migrate from physics to biology. Cummings remembered them as "a very strong group of physicists ... If British Columbia had recruited them from Saskatoon, British Columbia would have developed in the way that the OCI did. It was a question of where that group went."[18]

Siminovitch came to OCI because he had been a National Cancer Institute of Canada fellow, reporting to Ham. Ham got to like him and recruited him for OCI. Siminovitch arrived carrying in his satchel the research issue of somatic cell biology. He had never worked with cancer. Siminovitch insisted that biochemist and microbiologist Rose Sheinin come on board, as well as bacteriophage specialist Clarence Fuerst and immunochemist Bernhard ("Hardi") Cinader.[19] Ham also recruited Allan Howatson and Arthur Axelrad from the Department of Anatomy, and of course McCulloch from the Department of Medicine at TGH.

The OCI researchers wanted an academic connection, but there was a big problem: the basic science departments in the Faculty of Medicine refused to appoint them.[20] Also, physics at OCI had been refused by the campus Department of Physics. This stiff-arming meant the OCI scientists would be unable to have graduate students unless they founded their own department – which is what happened. Ham convinced the faculty to accept the new Department of Medical Biophysics and very shortly it was a big success. For Siminovitch, the environment recalled the intensity of Paris, where he had been a postdoc at the Pasteur Institute in the late 1940s (see pp. 686–687). "We did all sorts of original things," he said, "that had never been done at the university. For example, we all went to a lake up north, to Harold Johns' cottage, for a few days. We did all our own cooking, we lived in the cottage, and people just talked about things that they hoped to do. Then we had these meetings all the time that brought people together. Having to form this department against the university, that brought us together." At that point McCulloch wasn't even a scientist; he was a hematologist. "Till knew no biology, and McCulloch knew no physics. We all grew up together. My independent science career started there, McCulloch's science career started there, Whitmore's science career. We all were starting together, we were new and starting together, and nobody bothered us."[21]

When the Department of Medical Biophysics opened in 1958, it had two divisions: biology, headed by Ham, and physics, headed by Johns.[22] They saw themselves as stars. McCulloch said, "The formation of the Department of Medical

Biophysics fostered a research climate characterized by a firm intention to make a contribution to cancer research at a world level." This was not a big compliment to the faculty: "The negative attitude of the university insured that the scientific staff saw their allegiance to the Ontario Cancer Institute rather than the university disciplinary departments."[23]

From the very beginning, the work of Ham, Johns, and Siminovitch made the research labs of the OCI "unique international centres of cancer research," as McCulloch said.[24] In 1959 McCulloch, Siminovitch, Axelrad, and Ham reported isolating a tumour virus similar to the one that NIH researchers had found in leukemic mouse tissue and identified as a polyomavirus,[25] a genus of viruses capable of inducing tumours in experimental animals and, in some cases, humans; one branch of the polyomavirus was known as SV 40. SV 40 opened up "gene splicing," and the polyoma tumour viruses were hot subjects.

In the 1960s, the Till-McCulloch group attracted a series of productive students. In 1965 Alan Ming-ta Wu, fresh from taking an MD degree in Taiwan, entered the graduate program in medical biophysics. McCulloch later said of his student's untimely death at age 42, "[Wu] was first to show the extensive differentiation capacity of the pluripotential hemopoietic stem cell. This he did through a demonstration of functional heterogeneity among the clonal progeny of CFU-S through chromosome marker and cytochemical studies. As part of this work he was able to produce a mouse with a hemopoietic system that was entirely derived from a single cell." In 1968 Wu completed research for his dissertation and accepted a post at the University of Wisconsin, later at the National Institutes of Health in Bethesda. There, "he gave the first unequivocal evidence that cells of the lymphoid and of the myeloid lines of differentiation belonged to the same clone, a concept that is now universally accepted." When Wu returned to the University of Toronto in 1976, sadly just five years before his death of a brain tumour, he had developed "a unique system for long-term culture of the progenitors of human T lymphocytes." A scientist of great self-discipline, he was said to drive himself just as hard in marathon running as in the lab, and in the five years before he died he completed ten of them.[26]

In addition to the research wing of OCI, the clinical wing, called the Princess Margaret Hospital, had several major figures, including radiotherapist Clifford Ash as chief physician; Harold Warwick as medical oncologist; and radiation oncologists Vera Peters, John Darte, Walter D. ("Bill") Rider, and James ("John") Simpson.

With Siminovitch's departure in 1969 to found the Department of Medical Cell Biology in the new campus Medical Sciences Building, Jim Till became head of the Division of Biological Research. In 1971 Gordon Whitmore replaced Harold Johns (who obeyed a faculty ten-year retirement rule) as chair of the Department of Medical Biophysics. Johns remained head of the OCI's Division of Physics until his retirement in 1980. In 1975 John Darte – who had left in 1968 for Memorial University – replaced Ash on his retirement as director of OCI.[27]

## Toronto Sunnybrook Regional Cancer Centre

In 1972 the Ontario Cancer Treatment and Research Foundation (OCTRF) decided to establish a cancer treatment centre at Sunnybrook Hospital, the North Toronto Cancer Clinic, to serve the growing northern tier of Metropolitan Toronto.[28] A decade later, in 1982, the Toronto Bayview (later Sunnybrook) Regional Cancer Centre opened, under Richard "Derek" Jenkin, a pediatric radiation oncologist, one of the first in Canada. Following Jenkin's move from PMH, the pediatric radiation treatment program was also relocated to the Sunnybrook centre. The program returned to PMH after that hospital relocated close by the Hospital for Sick Children. In the 1993–4 session, the Sunnybrook Oncology Program and the Toronto Bayview Regional Cancer Centre Oncology Program merged, and Ken Shumak was appointed CEO of the centre and director of oncology at Sunnybrook. The program merger offered surgeons "better access to cancer centre resources."[29] Carol Sawka of the Department of Medicine succeeded Shumak in 1999. And in 2002 Shun Wong, who relocated his practice and research laboratory from the Princess Margaret Hospital, was appointed head of the Department of Radiation Oncology at Sunnybrook and head of the Radiation Therapy Program. The cancer centre at Sunnybrook was important for the history of cancer treatment, but it was also important for the history of Sunnybrook. Said Don Cowan, who became chief physician at Sunnybrook in 1974, "The thing that really helped Sunnybrook finally break out was the fact that the Cancer Centre went there." [30] With the help of the Reichmann family, they built a research institute that represented, said Cowan, "a turning point in the recognition of Sunnybrook as a bona fide academic centre."[31] In January 2004 all the regional cancer centres integrated, or merged, with their host hospitals.

## Medical Oncology at PMH

Medical oncology, the treatment of cancer with drugs, at OCI went back to the late 1950s. It was O. Harold Warwick, Canada's pioneer medical oncologist, who established the medical service in 1957–8. Brought up in New Brunswick, he graduated with an MD from McGill in 1940 as gold medalist. He had heard about the new drugs for treating cancer and went to Britain to find out more about them, training at the Chester Beatty Institute in London and becoming a member of the Royal College of Physicians in 1947. After a short period at McGill and the Royal Victoria Hospital in Montreal, he came to Toronto in 1948 as executive director of the Canadian Cancer Society and the newly formed National Cancer Institute of Canada. He worked half-time as a clinician at TGH, caring for cancer patients, researching, and teaching. In 1955, at the behest of radiology head Clifford Ash, Warwick joined the Department of Radiology at the General as a consultant in medical oncology. In 1959 he was the first worker in North America to give the early vinca alkaloids to patients.[32] Don Cowan later said of Warwick, "He was Canada's first medical oncologist, although the term wasn't coined until many years later. He had done work at Edinburgh on nitrogen mustard in the immediate post-war years,[33] and later at Princess Margaret, Cowan says, "he did the first major study in the world on vinblastine." Warwick and Edmund Yendt in the Department of Medicine "did some major work on hypercalcemia in cancer ... So I say that Harold was a bona fide medical oncologist because he cared for cancer patients, taught – he was my first bedside teacher in medical school – and did research; he was not just a drug pusher."[34]

Warwick left OCI in 1960 to become dean of medicine at the University of Western Ontario. After a brief interregnum with Donald M. ("Mac") Whitelaw as chief of medicine (who clashed with Ash), in 1965 the Princess Margaret Hospital recruited Daniel Bergsagel from MD Anderson Hospital in Houston to be chief of medicine. Born in Outlook, Saskatchewan, in 1925, Bergsagel had graduated in medicine at the University of Manitoba in 1949, taken a DPhil at Oxford, and gone to the United States as a staff physician in medical oncology at MD Anderson from 1955 to 1965. "For the first time," said McCulloch, "the OCI Department of Medicine would be led by a doctor specially trained in the medical aspects of cancer care." Bergsagel had ambitions for Toronto and tried, for example, to recruit Emil Freireich, who would shortly move to MD Anderson to become head of medical oncology. Bergsagel was a key figure in transforming OCI into a major international cancer centre.[35]

Under Bergsagel's guidance, in 1973 Princess Margaret Hospital introduced a two-year course in medical oncology for trainees who had first completed their Royal College Fellowship in internal medicine. This was the first such organized program in Canada and a real feather in Bergsagel's cap. There were medical oncologists in Canada before this program but most trained, at least partially, out of the country. The little program was, however, almost stifled by a shortage of training slots. The country was crying out for medical oncologists, yet annually PMH could accept only three applicants. In addition, by 1979 the North Toronto Cancer Clinic was about to open at Sunnybrook and would demand at least one trainee. Each of the Toronto teaching hospitals as well had opened medical oncology units. "We will need more trainees," wrote Bergsagel in 1979, "to take advantage of the training opportunities in these hospitals."[36]

In 1990 Ian Tannock replaced Bergsagel as head of the Department of Medicine at PMH. Tannock, a medical graduate of the University of Pennsylvania in 1974, established in 1996 that a prednisone combo gave palliation to some patients with symptomatic hormone-resistant prostate cancer who had been unresponsive to prednisone alone.[37] He is also remembered for a scorching indictment of routine screening for prostate cancer using Prostate-Specific Antigen (PSA). How did we cure symptomless prostate cancer? he asked in 2002 in the *Lancet*, tongue in cheek. We cured it by making all the patients symptomatic with fear after discovering their PSA was positive. "No longer do patients arrive for yearly check-ups enjoying their lives in blissful ignorance of their cancer.

Now they arrive monthly, flustered and anxious, some of them with graphs or computer printouts in hand." They no longer have symptomless prostate cancer but symptomatic prostate cancer; the actual reduction in mortality from the test had been minimal.[38]

It was not only members of the Department of Medicine at PMH who administered chemotherapy but until well into the 1980s members of the Department of Radiation Oncology as well. Cummings clarifies, "Many radiation oncologists had trained in the UK as 'clinical oncologists,' a specialty in which trainees learn to use both radiation and chemotherapy (this situation continues in UK and in some Scandinavian countries, generally in parallel with the specialty of medical oncology). Prior to and during my time at PMH (since 1972), much of the chemotherapy and hormone therapy for breast, prostate and colorectal cancer was provided by radiation oncologists, who gradually withdrew from this practice in the 1980s as more medical oncologists were recruited, and as more Canadian-trained radiation oncologists joined the staff since the latter are not trained to give chemotherapy."[39]

Darte died of a heart attack in December 1975 only six months into his tenure, and Raymond S. Bush became director of OCI the following year. Ash had earlier seen OCI as mainly a radiotherapy institute, but Bush had a broader vision of comprehensive cancer care.[40] Ray Bush was born in Toronto in 1930 but grew up in London, England, earning a bachelor's degree in science in 1951 from the University of London. He then worked as a physicist. Back in Canada, he graduated in medicine in 1961 from Toronto, completed a radiation oncology residency at the Princess Margaret Hospital, and joined the staff of PMH in 1966. In 1977 Bush led a team, including later chair Mary Gospodarowicz, that achieved virtually complete cures (85 percent) in localized non-Hodgkin's lymphomas.[41] After serving as director of OCI, he returned in 1988 to the academic practice of radiation oncology. He died two years later of lung cancer. (Incredibly, many of the radiation oncologists in these early years were smokers, including Bill Rider, who died of vascular disease, and John Simpson, who died of lung cancer. Vera Peters was also a heavy cigarette smoker and almost certainly died of lung cancer, not breast cancer as some sources indicate. In the early 1970s, the special staff lunch area in the PMH cafeteria was said to be just "solid smoke.")

Under Darte and Bush, OCI began to broaden its mission, expanding cancer care to several treatment modes and no longer just radiation. Vera Peters, for example, led a trial in 1985 that established that older patients with more extensive lymphomas might be offered either combination chemo and radiation therapy or chemotherapy alone, sparing them the side effects of radiation.[42]

Under Bush, OCI started taking students with medical backgrounds from the Institute of Medical Science as researchers. To be sure, the chemotherapy program was a huge success, but by 1982 Bergsagel's medical oncology unit was being worn down with service demands. The province had refused to fund chemotherapy programs at some of the peripheral general hospitals, and the patients were all streaming to Princess Margaret. Some represented a special burden. Bergsagel said in 1982, "The staff are interested in lymphoma patients and attract a large number of them. Treatment is so difficult to start for these patients that it is not always feasible to have the family doctors assisting with their care. This group of patients responds well initially, but when relapse occurs after primary treatment, they are never well again. The group takes up 40% of the medical beds. At this point it is difficult to turn these patients away after they have been followed here for 5 years."[43] So medical oncology was overrun.

Where to get fresh staff recruits? The problem of getting undergraduates interested in medical oncology was becoming acute in those years. The students received virtually no teaching in the undergraduate program and thus had no basis for choosing it as a field. "Very few undergraduates come here," the medical oncologists at PMH agreed. "The staff would be anxious and willing to participate in undergraduate teaching in oncology because they feel that if a high caliber student is to be attracted to oncology, he must be exposed to it early in his training."[44] So there was a recruitment bottleneck, not that the service ever had trouble finding trainees from across Canada, yet the leadership wanted top-drawer candidates interested in research.

### PMH Moves to University Avenue

The university clinical departments and the hospital departments at Princess Margaret remained for a long time two solitudes. For a review in 1982, Gerard Burrow, university head of medicine, came over to Sherbourne Street for a meeting. At the meeting, research at OCI was discussed and Burrow learned that the four new members of medical oncology "are all doing basic research." Burrow became interested and said, "It is a problem he faces at the University. He had not realized that the whole hospital here is involved in research, whereas in other teaching hospitals their only concerns are patients and teaching."[45] It was an interesting comment on the differential penetration of the research spirit in the early 1980s.

In 1985 a provincial role study recommended redevelopment of the OCI/PMH, "and," says Cowan, "in 1986 the Minister of Health approved funding for redevelopment."[46] There was to be a new OCI and after much agonizing, a University Avenue site was decided upon, just north of the Mount Sinai Hospital and across from the TGH.[47]

The faculty was heavily involved in these decisions. In 1987 a committee was struck to "Study the Impact of the Relocation of the Princess Margaret Hospital"; it had a number of subcommittees, one of which was Don Cowan's Oncology Co-ordinating Council.[48] It would supply faculty input to the repositioning of cancer care.

With the move to the west side of University Avenue in 1995, services began to merge between TGH (now part of The Toronto Hospital) and the Princess Margaret Hospital. To be sure, Mount Sinai gained the thoracic oncology program led by Bob Ginsberg and the sarcoma program –which acquired the status of a world leader – directed initially by Fred Langer and then by Bob Bell. Most of the other cancer action, however, involved the General. In the 1989–90 session, "a Comprehensive Cancer Care Centre is being planned that will involve collaboration between the Princess Margaret Hospital and the University Avenue area hospitals." The OCI/PMH had now approved a Department of Surgical Oncology, created in 1994.[49] In June 1996 the new comprehensive care program announced the heads of its clinical services: radiation oncology: Bernie Cummings (Department of Radiation Oncology); medical oncology: Armand Keating (Department of Medicine); and surgical oncology: Bob Bell (Department of Surgery).[50]

In 1988 Bush resigned as director of OCI after a long period of tension surrounding the need to expand the Sherbourne Street quarters but lack of funds for doing so. Don Carlow became director, changing his title to "president and CEO."[51] In 1991 an administrative reorganization occurred involving the creation of vice presidents of research and oncology and a number of new divisions, the details of which would range too far afield from the Faculty of Medicine.

But in these changes, medical oncology loomed ever more in importance. Said a 1991 report, "The rapid acquisition of knowledge pertaining to the therapeutic application of cytotoxic drugs through the late 60's and 70's resulted in the emergence of the discipline of medical oncology. The initial role of internists appointed to PMH changed from that of 'physician responsible for the medical management of patients receiving irradiation' to one of cancer specialist [in] the therapeutic use of cytotoxic drugs."[52]

Epidemiology became increasingly significant. The National Cancer Institute of Canada had an Epidemiology Unit at the University of Toronto, and as early as 1981 a group of epidemiologists led by Anthony B. Miller developed a protocol for breast screening for cancer.[53] In the 1990s, one of the new divisions of the OCI was epidemiology and biostatistics. And a research team headed by Norman Boyd, in the Department of Medicine, discovered in 1995 that "mammographic densities are an indicator of increased risk of breast cancer" and that the quantitative classification of densities might serve as a risk metric.[54] The discovery was of importance in determining the frequency of breast screening.

In 1993 radiation oncologist Simon Sutcliffe replaced Carlow as CEO and would stay in the saddle until the merger with the Toronto General (or "the Toronto Hospital," as the joint General-Western administrative construct was called). The move to the new quarters on University Avenue in 1995 was nigh, and, unbeknownst to OCI, the end of its independence was also approaching. In July 1994 Sutcliffe was appointed head of the TTH Cancer Program, serving as a link between the two institutions that left their boards intact. In November

1994, the boards of OCI/PMH and The Toronto Hospital passed resolutions to form a Joint Oncology Program. Alan Hudson (TTH president and CEO) was chair of the management committee, and Simon Sutcliffe (OCI/PMH president and CEO) was program director. The management committee would report to a joint board steering committee, chaired by the dean of medicine.[55] In February 1996, after a clash of will with Alan Hudson, Sutcliffe resigned.[56] In the summer of 1996 the Health Services Restructuring Commission completed an initial report on "restructuring the Metropolitan Hospitals," proposing among other initiatives "the transformation of the OCI/PMH to the Princess Margaret Comprehensive Cancer Centre," a clunky term that never caught on with the staff and which the board itself eventually rejected. Further recommendations involved merging much of the clinical care at TGH, the Mount Sinai Hospital, and the Princess Margaret Hospital at its new site.[57]

In September 1996, Donna Stewart in the Department of Psychiatry was appointed chief of women's health for the PMH/TTH Joint Oncology Program.[58] Stewart was a major figure in women's health care in addition to being an international authority on psychosomatic illness.

In December 1997 the merger of the Toronto Hospital and the OCI/PMH was finalized to form what became called in 1999 the "University Health Network," driven by Alan Hudson and Peter Crossgrove, chair of the Board of Trustees of the Toronto Hospital.[59]

Peter Crossgrove's role in all this was central. Don Cowan says,

> He was chair of three different boards during the merger process. At the beginning he was chair of the TTH board and very much in favour of Alan Hudson's vision of the merger with PMH. In 1995, shortly after he gave up the TTH chair, he accepted the government's invitation to become chair of the OCI/PMH board, continuing to support the merger. He did acquire 'a few more merger scars' (he had been deeply involved with the TGH/TWH merger in 1986), but under his leadership the PMH board and most of the staff came 'on board.' In the Spring of 1997, just weeks before the OCI/PMH board voted in favour of the merger, Crossgrove moved on again to become chair of the newly formed Cancer Care Ontario (from OCTRF). Anthony Fell took over the OCI/PMH board.[60]

As Don Cowan, one of the faculty's main utility hitters over forty years, reflected, "Thus in 1997, the OCI/PMH, which had developed from the old Institute of Radiotherapy in the TGH, had returned home. This circle had closed."[61]

Cancer care in Toronto finally became rationalized. In the 1998–9 session, the University Health Network announced that its branch, the Princess Margaret Hospital, has "welcomed all oncology programs from across the Network into our modern facility." They had twenty surgical oncologists and fifteen medical oncologists, in addition to some twenty-five radiation oncologists. For the first time, surgical and medical care of cancer in Toronto were united.[62] In 2003 a collaborative agreement was signed between Cancer Care Ontario (CCO) and the University Health Network, rationalizing cancer care.[63] In January 2004, as mentioned earlier, the integration of the cancer centres into the host hospitals took place. This meant that CCO no longer ran the centres and was not responsible for hands-on patient care, which devolved to the hospitals. Instead, CCO became a planning organization and major adviser to the Ontario Ministry of Health (by this time "Long-Term Care" had been added to the title of the Ministry of Health) on cancer issues, stressing quality and setting standards and evidence-based guidelines.[64]

### Department of Surgery

Not only was there no surgery [at PMH], but there was no Department of Surgery. There was no surgeon sitting at the table of decision-making, with the head of medicine, the head of radiation oncology, the head of research.[65]

Donald Cowan, speaking of the 1970s

Surgeons have always operated for cancer. All general surgeons were cancer surgeons. "There were few real surgical oncologists," said Cowan, "few people trained as surgical oncologists, as they are now."[66] At the Toronto General Hospital, the gynecological surgeons specialized in pelvis (Peter Vernon, an ob-gyn doctor, was a trained gynecological oncologist); the head and neck surgeons had those cancers (David Briant, an ENT surgeon, had trained in cancer); the orthopedic surgeons operated on the osteosarcomas; and the general surgeons did everything else, including breast and gut.

The first involvement of the Department of Surgery of the University of Toronto in an oncology program occurred in the 1934–5 session, when surgical representatives affiliated themselves with the aforementioned Institute of Radiology. Harold Wookey, Robert Harris, and Robert Janes were among the surgeons who, as Gallie said in 1935, "have had an excellent opportunity to observe the effect of radium and X-ray in the treatment of malignancy and to form an opinion as to when radiotherapy can be expected to be of value. The plan of organization which provides that decisions on treatment shall be made by the expert in radiology and by the clinical specialist seems to me [Gallie] to have overcome the difficulties that have so often wrecked similar experiments."[67]

There events stood for the next half century, as the Department of Surgery had no further interdisciplinary ventures. Before the 1990s the great bulk of cancer surgery was undertaken in community hospitals, not academic centres, and often, because of the high mortality, referred to as "salvage work." Many surgeons, it must be said, found something off-putting about the radiation oncologists at Princess Margaret. (The reverse was also true.) Bill Rider, a skilled and innovative radiation oncologist, had a rough edge or two, said Cowan.[68]

To be sure, clinicians at the Princess Margaret could refer their patients to surgeons at the Wellesley Hospital if the patient had originally come from there. Yet, said Cowan, "If the Wellesley had recruited surgical oncologists and put their research efforts in that direction (they preferred immunology, rheumatology and some excellent endocrinology, such as Bob Volpé), they could have been one of the outstanding cancer centres in North America. The cultures of the two institutions were different. Wellesley had a lot of private practices and, yes, some of the 'carriage trade.' The two were different – different cultures – and each found it difficult to reach out to the other. They didn't have an Alan Hudson and Peter Crossgrove (and probably the resources) to make it happen."[69]

In the 1989–90 session the Department of Surgery organized a surgical oncology program, with Hartley Stern appointed director and chairman of the Oncology Planning Committee. Several divisions – particularly the Divisions of Neurosurgery, General Surgery, Thoracic Surgery, Orthopaedic Surgery, and Urology – were said to be "in the process of organizing oncology programs and recruiting clinical-scientists."[70] It is thus at this surprisingly late date that a real surgical oncology program begins, and just in time for the "planned move of [OCI] to University Avenue."[71]

Sunnybrook Hospital hosted the Toronto Bayview Regional Cancer Centre, and in 1992–3 Ralph Gilbert was appointed head of surgical oncology there; Denny DePetrillo started the surgical oncology program at PMH in 1990, and in 1993 this program joined the global budget of the Department of Surgery. (On DePetrillo's leadership of the Division of Gynaecologic Oncology in the Department of Obstetrics and Gynaecology, see chapter 21.) Hartley Stern said of the cancer surgery program, "This has been a significant advancement for surgical oncology." He continued in his 1993 report, "Planning at both ambulatory cancer centres [Sunnybrook and PMH] and within the University program has become increasingly multidisciplinary and site group directed." (Site group means the affected organ.) Bearing this in mind, the Department of Surgery now changed the structure of its oncology committee. "The new University Committee is now composed of representatives from all surgical disciplines including our Department, Otolaryngology and Obstetrics and Gynecology."[72]

In the 1993–4 session, a Division of Surgical Oncology was created in the Department of Surgery as a joint venture between Princess Margaret and the Toronto Hospital, with Robert Bell as the acting chair, replacing Stern, who had just decided to move to Ottawa.[73] The University Avenue hospitals were setting out to develop a comprehensive cancer care program. "This joint venture has paralleled the development of closer ties between Sunnybrook and OCTRF which also offers surgeons better access to cancer centre resources." Bell, in the surgery annual report, noted that all divisions of the Department of Surgery had expertise in cancer surgery – in neurosurgery, for example, Mark Bernstein and Paul Muller becoming expert in the management of astrocytomas, a common type of tumour in the central nervous system composed of astrocytes.[74]

The science pedal was pushed in the 1994–5 session when Bernard Langer took charge briefly of the Surgical Oncology Program at the Toronto Hospital. Langer's focus was no longer just coordinating clinical care but bringing basic science to bear in malignant disease. As part of this effort, a group of surgeons organized Toronto's first surgical oncology laboratory in the Samuel Lunenfeld Research Institute of Mount Sinai Hospital.[75] As Martin McKneally later observed, with Langer's entry on the scene, cancer surgery in Metro Toronto began to shift from the community hospitals to the big teaching hospitals with surgical oncology programs. "It was only when Bernie Langer and Alan Hudson started exerting their surgical leverage that complex cancer surgery stopped in hospitals underpowered to deal with its complications and high mortality."[76]

As seen, consolidation of The Toronto Hospital and the Princess Margaret Hospital resulted in a comprehensive program of cancer care, the Comprehensive Cancer Care Centre, and in 1995–6 the surgical wing of this centre became directed by Bob Bell, who was henceforth head of surgical services in the Joint Oncology Program. DePetrillo accepted a post at Cancer Care Ontario as coordinator in surgical oncology for the province.[77]

In 1998 the Royal College accepted a General Surgery Surgical Oncology Fellowship at U of T, in a program jointly administered by Sunnybrook and The Toronto Hospital together with Princess Margaret Hospital. In July the first two fellows began their tenure. Ralph Gilbert at the Sunnybrook cancer centre was said to be one of the spark plugs of the program. The Department of Surgery announced, "The presence of a critical mass of postgraduate surgical oncology trainees has allowed the initiation of a core curriculum in surgical oncology which will begin in September 1998 ... Professor Wedge [chair of the department] encouraged the development of the core curriculum by allowing the Surgical Oncology Committee to merge with surgical oncologists from gynecology, otolaryngology and ophthalmology to form an umbrella committee for the fellowship programs." This represented an important advance. "In the past, Canadian surgeons planning to pursue a career in oncology generally left Canada for fellowship training under the auspices of the Society of Surgical Oncology [a US organization]. The University of Toronto General Surgical Oncology Fellowship has been designed to meet the criteria of the Society of Surgical Oncology Fellowship."[78]

With an academic superstructure in place, surgical oncology took off in Toronto. In January 1999, twenty-two surgical oncologists moved into the Princess Margaret Hospital "to carry on practice in a multi-disciplinary cancer care centre. This is a significant change for surgical practice in Toronto."[79] (These surgeons conducted their outpatient clinics in PMH, and some had office space. Yet all major surgery continued to be performed in TGH or Mount Sinai because PMH did not have the operating rooms or inpatient space needed for this additional load.) In 2001 Jonathan Irish, an otolaryngologist, became head of surgical services at PMH.[80] McKneally said that under the leadership of Irish at

PMH, with the support of Bob Bell, surgical oncology blossomed as a discipline, "bringing to an end an era of unidisciplinary management dominated by radiation therapy."[81]

## The Division of Hematology/Oncology of the Department of Medicine

Cancer care came to medicine much later than to surgery, and by the nature of its biochemical complexity cancer care was dispersed throughout the medical specialties and the basic medical sciences. It would rob too much of this material of context to detach it from its master narratives and concentrate it all in this chapter. But here the adult Division of Hematology and Oncology of the Department of Medicine will be discussed, as well as the numerous interdisciplinary and collaborative programs drawing internists together with other specialists. The story of pediatric oncology finds its home in the section on hematology/oncology in the Department of Paediatrics of the Hospital for Sick Children.

The concept of a division of hematology existed in embryo as early as 1956, mentioned in a Department of Medicine report under "Haematology" that touched on Ernest McCulloch's work "in maintaining growth of leukaemic leukocytes in tissue culture."[82] McCulloch would shortly continue this work at the Ontario Cancer Institute (see p. 339).

Kager Wightman originated interest in hematology at the General, although he was not formally the founder of the division. Cowan remembers, "Hematology and oncology were great interests of his. He had an influence in guiding many trainees toward careers in that direction. When I was a student and a postgraduate trainee, he treated large numbers of patients with leukemia and lymphoma, patients with solid tumours and of course benign blood disorders. It was Kager who guided me into the area. I know that Bun [Ernest] McCulloch had a great regard for Kager."[83] Wightman was a member of the international, the American, and the Canadian societies of hematology. When in 1966 the "Wightman Club" was being founded by Kager's students, there was a question of its "heraldic crest." McCulloch suggested that the crest include a microscope "to indicate the Professor's interest in haematology."[84]

In 1958 John Crookston, who had earned a Toronto MD degree in 1947 and a subsequent PhD at Cambridge, was appointed head of the Division of Hematology and Blood Transfusion, in the Department of Laboratories of the Toronto General Hospital.[85] In 1960 he took over the clinical fellowship program in hematology at the General from Wightman, who had become the professor of medicine, and this marks the birth of the division in the Department of Medicine.[86] Nell Farquharson said in an interview that before Crookston's appointment, "hematology was done by my father ... They made their own slides, they didn't have an official area. On each ward there was an area for making blood films." Among the veterans of these early days were Irving Rother, a 1943 U of

T graduate who had matriculated at Riverdale Collegiate in Toronto (and who starred at basketball in med school), and Don Cowan, a 1956 Toronto graduate who had trained in medicine and was interested in the blood cancers. Farquharson remembers "Don jumping up and down, getting slides showing the X chromosome … Chromosomes were part of hematology." She continued, "Slowly hematology went from being all just hematologists. It started to split off, so there was someone in charge of the blood bank, someone in charge of coagulation, some clinical people."

Nell Farquharson went down to the United States to study; when she returned in the mid-1960s, "[t]hey weren't even calling themselves hematologists, they were calling themselves oncologists, they even dropped the term." It was Kager Wightman who steered the division towards oncology. "He was the first person at the General, anyway, and maybe in Canada, to bring along the idea of giving more than one drug to a patient. Everyone thought he was going to kill people. We were handing out tablets of melphelan [a derivative of nitrogen mustard] or myleran [an alkylating neoplastic agent], you know, single drugs, and he got the idea that probably it would be better to give several drugs, attacking cells in a different manner." Farquharson herself was the first clinician in Toronto to administer Adriamycin (doxorubicin). She got it from NIH "and supplied it for the city." Later in life when she developed breast cancer, she was treated with Adriamycin and said to herself, "That's my drug!"

Did Toronto become an important trial centre for cancer drugs? Not really, Farquharson said. There were no trial nurses and she couldn't get the clinicians to cooperate and "get these doctors in different hospitals to make out their forms … So I just decided I was sick of it, I'd just be an Indian, I don't want to be a chief in charge of these drugs."[87]

When Bernie Langer returned from his visit to various US clinics in 1963, he brought with him – in addition to an interest in liver transplantation – a detailed knowledge of the use of drugs in the treatment of cancer. This had been the original rationale for the trip. Langer said in an interview, "The field of chemotherapy in the management of cancer was in its infancy … Up until that time, surgeons managed all cancer, radiation therapists managed cancer that surgery couldn't look after, but the physicians really had very little role in it, and the idea that physicians might take an increasing role … led Fred Kergin [head of surgery] to believe that we should have some surgeons trained to know something about chemotherapy." That was Langer's job. He was "to go and visit the centres where chemotherapy was being developed. Nobody here knew anything about that." So Langer visited a surgical cancer centre in Madison, Wisconsin; Roswell Park in Buffalo; MD Anderson Hospital in Houston; and Memorial Sloane-Kettering Hospital in New York. He brought back an expertise in "regional perfusion" with chemotherapeutic drugs.

Given that Langer was among the few members of the faculty who understood anything of chemotherapy, he gravitated towards the likeminded: Don

Cowan in the Division of Hematology and Harold Warwick, the other medical oncologist in town.

Cowan, a classmate of Langer's, was among the few members of the faculty to have grown up on a farm in Newfoundland in the days before it joined Confederation – though he did attend high school in Brantford. He had wanted to study scientific farming at Guelph and return to Newfoundland, but fate intervened in the form of a job in a medical records department, and he decided to "take a whack" at medicine, graduating from U of T, as mentioned earlier, in 1956.[88] He had trained in pathology at Columbia-Presbyterian Hospital in New York, took clinical training with Kager Wightman at the General and at the Princess Margaret Hospital, and fellowed in hematology-oncology in London, England. In the mid-1960s he was in the Department of Medicine at TGH. A third member of this little oncology group was obstetrician-gynecologist C. Peter Vernon, who was cross-appointed to the Princess Margaret Hospital. Vernon, who had graduated in medicine from Toronto in 1954 and done the grand tour in the United States and Europe, was a specialist in the surgical treatment of gynecological cancer. He is considered by some the first real cancer surgeon in Toronto.

Langer said, "We set up a clinic where we would all attend together. It was Don Cowan, Peter Vernon, and myself. We saw one another's patients, and when one was away on holiday, we would manage their patients." Langer agreed that this "was the first beachhead of oncology at the General Hospital." (Similar multidisciplinary clinics already existed at PMH.)[89]

In 1970 Cowan became city-wide coordinator of the postgraduate training program in clinical hematology. He didn't exactly leap at the opportunity, but one day he was in his lab at Princess Margaret and got a phone call from Charlie Hollenberg. "He said he wanted me to coordinate hematology for the city. That was about the last thing I wanted to do, get involved in any kind of administrative stuff." But Cowan had not yet met Hollenberg, who had only just arrived, and thought he should go over and see him. "I can't remember exactly what happened, but I remember standing out on College Street sort of dazed, having agreed to do what he wanted me to. In fact, I can remember him fixing me with his steely blue eyes. 'Don,' he said, 'those of us in academic medicine have a responsibility to do these things.'"[90] In 1974 Cowan ceded the helm and went up to Sunnybrook to become chief physician.

By the mid-1970s, the Ontario Cancer Institute had pulled together a good deal of the interest in oncology, and the hematology division of the Department of Medicine was giving itself more over to hematology as such, for example, the role of platelets in coagulation. The focus was clinical research rather than basic science.[91] Toronto General Hospital was becoming, as Hollenberg said in 1973, "a major referral center for patients with coagulation defects and indeed, most of the postgraduate education in this particular aspect of hematology occurs at this institution."[92] Oncology as such was said, at least in this division, to be "inadequately developed."[93]

So in hematology there was a shift away from cancer. The members of the division were cross-appointed to the Department of Laboratory Hematology at the General and constituted an integrated service, with emphases on sickle-cell disease and thalassemia, often getting referrals from the hematology clinic at the Hospital for Sick Children after the patients had reached adult age (a clinic that Bill Francombe had founded in 1986 and ran for many years). One bears in mind that there were once few such patients as most did not survive to adulthood. Yet the link to cancer research was preserved: the division ran clinics for leukemia and lymphoma.[94] And in 1986 Michael Baker, head of oncology at TGH, was appointed chief of hematology, thus insuring the integration of hematology, oncology, and the hematology laboratories.[95]

In 1970 bone marrow transplantation began at OCI for patients with acute leukemia.[96] The investigators, led by Ernest McCulloch, had first to solve the problem of separating the stem cells from the cells causing graft-versus-host disease (GVH), a frequent complication of bone marrow transplantation involving a reaction caused by incompatible donor cells in the tissues of the host. They achieved this through "velocity sedimentation." "The apparatus has been suitably scaled up and tested, and clinical experiments to test this hypothesis are currently under way at our institution," they reported in April 1972.[97]

Later in 1972 was issued the first report on "bone marrow transplantation in patients with acute leukaemia" from the internists and radiation oncologists at OCI. Cowan, part of the team, remembers the excitement: "Rick Miller and Bob Phillips had developed a cell separation technique" to retain the stem cells. "We had a meeting every Monday noon," said Cowan. "We were ready to do the transplant. Bob got up and left the meeting and said, 'okay, continue, it's in your guys' hands now, you're the clinicians.'" Cowan remembers running down the hall after him: "Bob, you're the expert, you've got to be part of this team." And he was.[98]

The patients were prepared for the transplant with high doses of cyclophosphamide, an anti-cancer agent of the nitrogen mustard group, and whole-body irradiation. They thereupon received bone marrow grafts from a sibling with an identical immune constitution. The lymphocytes were also removed to prevent graft-versus-host disease. The results of such drastic procedures were not auspicious and the authors concluded, "While the separation procedure [of lymphocytes] appears a promising method for reducing the severity of GVH in bone marrow transplants, one must seriously question the usefulness of bone marrow transplantation in the treatment of acute leukemia."[99]

Yet these were early days in the therapy of a desperate illness. The investigators learned from their mistakes and resolved to press on. After the first failure they gathered together and said (in an internal memo), "Our intention is to build on this experience; we anticipate not only that we can improve our methods of marrow transplantation but also that we will learn more about acute leukemia ... Just as our previous work has involved laboratory experimentation and the translation of the results into clinical practice, we intend to approach the solution of our problems by fundamental research and by clinical study."[100] It would be hard to find more impressive evidence of reasoning back and forth between basic science and clinical medicine – to the ultimate benefit of leukemia patients worldwide.

In 1986–7 TGH and the university established the U of T Autologous Bone Marrow Transplant Service, a national resource for patients with leukemia and malignant lymphoma. It was headed by Armand Keating, an Ottawa graduate in 1976, who had just arrived in Toronto.[101] By 1991–2 this was called the Autologous Bone Marrow Transplantation Program; still led by Keating, it was said to be "a last resort for patients with leukemia, lymphoma or Hodgkin's disease." The hospital explained, drawing upon Joseph Brandwein (who in 1990 moved to St Michael's), "An autologous transplant involves 'harvesting' a patient's own bone marrow while he or she is in remission. The patient is then given chemotherapy or radiation treatment to destroy all remaining cancerous cells, and reinfused with the harvested marrow which regenerates itself."[102] This new program, in addition to the application of the new chemotherapies, meant that by the late 1980s the combined hematology divisions of TGH and TWH – now merged – made hematology at the Toronto Hospital the "leading referral centre in the country for leukaemia treatment."[103]

In the history of pediatric oncology in Canada, John Darte occupies a special role. Born in 1920 in Welland, Ontario, he earned a bachelor's degree in biological and medical sciences at U of T (St Michael's College) in 1942, then, after starring in rugby, graduated in medicine in 1944. He trained as a pediatrician at the Hospital for Sick Children, then in hematology and radiotherapy, becoming, as William Meakin said in an obituary, "the first multidisciplinary pediatric oncologist in Canada, if not in North America."[104] Following several further years of training in the United Kingdom, including the Christie Hospital of the Holt Radium Institute in Manchester, he returned to Toronto in 1957 as a pediatrician at HSC and a radiotherapist at the Princess Margaret Hospital, where he founded the pediatric unit. McCulloch recalls Darte as "a remarkable man; huge in stature, he was gentle in manner." Sometime between 1957 and 1962 he conducted with the help of McCulloch "three marrow transplants as a treatment for leukemia," said McCulloch. "These were certainly the first human transplants in Canada and may have been the first in the world. One temporary remission was obtained."[105] (This overlooks the role of E. Donnall Thomas in Cooperstown, New York, in 1956 – winner of a Nobel Prize in 1990 for this achievement. Yet the Darte-McCulloch bone marrow transplant was certainly a significant moment despite their failure to write it up!)

In 1962 Darte founded the hematology division of HSC. Between 1968 and 1975 he served as founding chair of the Department of Pediatrics at Memorial University in St John's, Newfoundland, returning then to Toronto to become the second director of the Ontario Cancer Institute and the Princess Margaret Hospital until his untimely death in December 1975 shortly thereafter.

### Coordinating Medical Oncology

There was a long history of unhappiness in the faculty about the fragmentation of oncology: radiotherapeutic approaches were substantially hived off at OCI, but well into the 1970s there was some radiation treatment provided on machines in Sunnybrook, Toronto General, Toronto Western, and St Michael's Hospitals by radiation oncologists who visited from PMH and conducted some clinics in those hospitals. Surgery was offered in the teaching hospitals, and medical oncology was spotted about here and there. In the mid-1970s Robert Harris, head of the Long-Range Planning and Assessment Committee, said, "The Committee recognized that there was a deficiency in the emphasis on Oncology in some of the ... teaching hospitals. In addition, the Committee was made aware of a lack of co-ordination of all programmes in Oncology, and the anomalous location of the Therapeutic Radiology programme in the Department of Radiology in dissociation from other Oncology programmes."[106]

This separation was a burr under the saddle of the teaching hospitals. Kathleen Pritchard, head of medical oncology at Women's College, told the recently constituted Task Force on Oncology in 1985, "At present, the majority of the radiation and medical oncology community of the University of Toronto are isolated in the Princess Margaret Hospital and the Toronto-Bayview Clinic ... Unfortunately, the communication between the Princess Margaret Hospital and, as far as I can tell, the Bayview Clinic, and the surgical community is extremely poor. There is little common ground between these groups: there is a large degree of antagonism which has existed for many years and I think that this is reflected in a singular lack of co-operation in the areas of teaching, patient care and research between these groups."[107] (In fairness, there were numerous clinics at Sunnybrook and PMH where surgical consultants participated with the oncology staff, but collaboration in some areas was indeed limited.[108])

The third arm of cancer care was medical approaches. To nurture this arm, in 1973–4 a joint postgraduate program in medical oncology was established, as seen earlier, and based at PMH, directed jointly by Daniel Bergsagel and John Simpson.[109] Cowan noted, "For several years the trainees in both medical oncology (Bergsagel) and radiation oncology (Simpson) did a common first year during which they trained in both disciplines and then went one way or the other. This plan ultimately fell apart, and although trainees often rotated back and forth it was not as formal."[110]

Surgical and medical approaches allied with each other at the General. In June 1978 the Goldie Rotman Oncology Unit opened at the Toronto General Hospital. The Rotman family had donated a sum of money in memory of their mother for a multidisciplinary ambulatory unit with six examination rooms, a radiotherapy room, and offices. The Rotmans also contributed towards the purchase of a Whole Body Scanner.[111] The oncology unit was a joint project of the hospital Departments of Medicine and Surgery and had initially a somewhat uneasy relationship with the Princess Margaret Hospital.[112] Michael Baker, simultaneously deputy director of the Division of Hematology and head of the Oncology Group, was director of the Rotman Oncology Unit.[113]

By the 1984–5 session, the four hospitals in the University Avenue area – the Hospital for Sick Children, the Mount Sinai, the General, and Women's College – had initiated a coordinated program for cancer treatment and research, with combined weekly oncology rounds and coordinated meetings. This became the "University Avenue Oncology Group." The TGH annual report said, "Regional clinics for the University area will be operated for leukaemia at TGH, sarcoma at Mount Sinai and skin cancers at Women's College." In addition, "[t]he research programme will be consolidated in the Max Bell Research Centre and the Charlie Conacher Research Wing." A whole group of new investigators was coming in. By this time, at the Rotman Oncology Unit in the Mulock Larkin Wing at TGH there were twenty-four clinics in operation, with over 20,000 patient visits a year.[114] By 1985–6 the General Hospital had become the centre for the Lung Cancer Study Group.[115]

Dean Lowy, meanwhile, had established in 1984 an oncology task force to tie the various threads together. The background was this: in 1983 the District Health Council of Metro Toronto issued a report on oncology services in Metropolitan Toronto, recommending that the faculty of medicine integrate cancer treatment within all the hospitals and the province's cancer care centres. Then an external review of the Department of Radiology in 1984 recommended that radiation oncology be established as a separate department. A "role study" of OCI/OCTRF conducted by consultants also recommended some kind of coordinating body for oncology. So Dean Lowy established a task force on oncology in July 1984 that was to consider a possible Oncology Coordinating Council and detaching radiation oncology from the Department of Radiology. The task force was chaired by Burnett Thall, a member of the U of T Governing Council and a trustee of the Ontario Cancer Institute, as well as senior vice president and director of the *Toronto Star*. The task force alone was a real accomplishment. As Kathleen Pritchard told Thall in February 1985, "In the seven years I have been employed as an oncologist in the University of Toronto, this is the first time that I have received correspondence from the 'University' as a member of the 'oncology group.' I regard this correspondence alone, as a forward step."[116] Seventeen oncologists joined the task force, which between August 1984 and March 1985 had ten meetings.[117]

The task force recommended in 1985 the formation of a university Oncology Coordinating Council (established the following year under Donald Cowan). The task force also recommended the establishment of a Department of Radiation Oncology. Maybe there should be a Department of Clinical Oncology? The faculty shied back from this, just as they had shied back from a Department of Neuroscience. At a meeting of the clinical chairs in October 1985, "[i]n the discussion the issue of an all-encompassing Department of Clinical Oncology was raised. It was pointed out that this had been examined by the Task Force but was rejected as too disruptive to the other departments concerned."[118]

Cowan reached out with his Oncology Coordinating Council (OCC) to all the major players in the far-flung cancer scene, and they were numerous. He liaised with the Ontario Cancer Institute, the Toronto Bayview Clinic, the OCTRF, the Department of Medicine Oncology Committee, the oncology coordinator, "the committee looking at radiotherapy in the downtown area, and the OCI/OCTRF Senior Planning Committee." Cowan's council would have about twenty members, in addition to representatives from education and research (by 1987 TGH had added an Oncology Research Laboratory).[119] At a meeting of the clinical chairs in June 1986, Cowan "noted that his style was consultative, co-ordinated, and on occasion, coercive, and he hoped to be able to provide leadership in Oncology. He regarded the departmental structure as integral to the University."[120] Cowan left the OCC in 1989 and in that year the Oncology Interdepartmental Division was created, headed in 1990 by Gerry Goldenberg (of the University of Manitoba) as assistant dean of oncology.[121]

Out of Cowan's OCC came the concept of a "Division of Preventive Oncology" that Hollenberg, now president of OCTRF, floated as early as 1992.[122] But the division "never really took off," as Bernard Cummings, later head of radiation oncology, agreed with an interviewer's question. "I think because those of us who were involved couldn't see what it added to what we were already doing."[123] By 2000 the division was being "wound down."[124] Instead, training in medical and radiation oncology in the teaching hospitals became organized by informal consultation among directors of education. (There has to be some coordination to meet the requirements of the Royal College.) Cummings said, "[The residents'] program directors get together and say, 'I've got three trainees, and we'll need three months for each of them,' and our education director would sort out when they should come, and negotiate."[125]

On the model of the United Kingdom, cancer care at Princess Margaret for gynecology and lymphoma had always been coordinated with "tumour boards," where representatives from the different disciplines discuss the care of each new patient. In other tumour sites at PMH and at Sunnybrook, the system had been somewhat more informal, organized for all cancers by "site groups,"[126] meaning that representatives of the different cancers, say gastrointestinal, met once a week, including the medical oncologists, radiation oncologists, pathologists, imagers, and surgeon oncologists. "Then within that will be subgroups," said Cummings, "with, say, a specific interest in esophagus cancer, and they'll get together and design treatment programs and research programs for patients with an esophagus cancer." The site group would have a head, rotated amongst

the disciplines. More formal tumour boards are currently replacing these informal structures at the request of Cancer Care Ontario.[127]

### Department of Radiation Oncology

Since the days of Gordon Richards, the Toronto tradition of radiology had been
to allow imaging and therapy to develop separately within the department. Radiotherapy, later called radiation oncology, had never been a formal division of
the department, and it was, as Bernard Cummings put it, "managed with benign neglect by the imagers."[128]

Indeed one of the big radiology stars of the past was a radiotherapist: Vera
Peters. Born in 1911 and raised in Thistletown, Ontario, Peters graduated in
medicine from the University of Toronto in 1934, where she played basketball
and hockey and was the president of her sixth-year class. In 1936 Gordon Richards, the head of radiology, perhaps recognizing her extraordinary scientific energy and personal drive, persuaded her to embark on a personal apprenticeship
under his guidance. In the course of her career Peters made several scientific
discoveries and was probably the first female physician of the faculty to have
achieved real international distinction.

Peters's signal contribution occurred early in her career: on the basis of cases
treated under Richards's direction between 1924 and 1942 at the Ontario Institute of Radiotherapy, she demonstrated in 1950 that Hodgkin's disease, a disease uniformly looked upon as fatal, could be treated radiotherapeutically, with
a five-year survival rate of 51 percent and a ten-year rate of 35 percent. She determined the importance of early diagnosis and treatment and that the affected
lymph nodes required "intensive irradiation."[129] In essence, she was the first to
show that early-stage Hodgkin's could be cured. This 1950 paper, and the 1958
follow-up, changed fundamentally the treatment of lymph cancer.[130]

Peters's fame in breast cancer rests on her approach with conservative surgery – lumpectomy or breast-conserving surgery – followed by radiation. Her
retrospectively controlled, case-matched study compared radical mastectomy,
physically deforming and psychologically devastating to many, to lumpectomy
(also called wedge resection) plus post-operative radiation. There turned out to
be no statistical difference in local recurrence or survival. Hence radical mastectomy was unnecessary. Peters's was the first controlled study making this
important point. In concluding, she turned fiercely against the proponents of
radical mastectomy: "No woman in true clinical stage I breast cancer should
fall victim to the mental anguish or physical morbidity of radical ways. Our social conscience should dictate our professional conscience. Those who would
seek help from us do so in bewilderment ... We who should epitomize hu-
manitarianism all too frequently turn it aside in an effort to pursue outmoded
ways ... Prophylactic radiation and prophylactic mastectomy could, with few

exceptions be eliminated in early breast cancer. This study shows what I have long known to be true: that radical methods are not in the best interest of the patients."[131]

Peters's later work did fundamentally change thinking about breast malignancy. She came to understand that breast cancer is a systemic disease and that local lymphatic spread may not be as important as spread in the systemic blood system, bypassing the lymph nodes. These were immense contributions. She became known as the great advocate of conservation in the treatment of breast cancer. In 2010 she was named to the Canadian Medical Hall of Fame.

Peters was also something of a role model for this early generation of female physicians. She had a "very successful marriage [and] pulled off this whole business of mother and physician," said Don Cowan in an interview. And she also stuck to her guns when she knew she was right. A senior female radiation oncologist, Sarah Donaldson, at Stanford University told Cowan, "There were very few female oncologists and the faculty in radiation oncology was predominantly male with uniform leadership by men. Some of these men were dominant and dictatorial. Donaldson remembers that Vera could stand up to the strongest of these men, in small groups or international meetings and hold her own and win the debates. She was willing to stand up to such individuals as virtually no one else, male or female, could." Donaldson concluded, "[I]f Vera Peters can do it so can I."[132]

So the radiation oncologists were a lively lot. Yet they were trapped in the departmental structure of the faculty together with the diagnosticians – with whom they had nothing in common save once having shared a technology. Thus, for years the radiation oncologists had contemplated breaking free yet collided with decanal resistance to adding yet another department.

The first chief of radiation oncology was Clifford Ash, a student of Richards, who in 1950 became inaugural director of OCI as well.

Ash was succeeded on retirement in 1975 by Bill Rider, who grew up in Darlington, England, but finished medical studies in Edinburgh in 1945. He trained in the Edinburgh Royal Infirmary, then in 1956 was persuaded by Ash to join OCI. After Darte was appointed director of OCI, he asked Rider to serve as director of radiation oncology "over a handshake at the Westbury Hotel." Rider's conception of the job was "to massage the 'Brownian Movement' in the right direction, not to direct by fiat."[133]

Even before coming to Toronto, Rider was well known for a 1955 paper on multiple myeloma, the first in the literature on combination chemotherapy.[134] Rider strongly favoured efforts to preserve organs if possible. This meant irradiating tumours first and reserving surgery for failure.[135] Rider and Douglas Bryce – head of otolaryngology, who in 1955 became the departmental representative to the old Ontario Institute of Radiotherapy – contributed to that tradition by insisting that patients with laryngeal cancers be seen jointly by a radiation oncologist and an otolaryngologist. Not all laryngeal cancers required "the universal loss of the larynx."[136] As Cummings said, "They were both committed to laryngeal preservation. So we were treating with radiation much more advanced larynx cancers than they were in many parts of the world, where it was assumed that any thing other than a very early cancer required a laryngectomy"[137] (on Bryce see pp. 492–93). Cummings later affirmed the robustness of what some called the "Toronto approach" to radiotherapy: "There's one overriding theme in Toronto, and that has been what I'd call organ conservation. There's been a conscious attempt to preserve normal anatomy and function, as opposed to saying that certain tumors should always be excised, and then we'll irradiate that area and try to make sure they don't come back."[138] This approach applied, for example, to retinoblastoma in children or, as seen, to the preservation of the larynx and the conservative management of breast cancer. Cummings himself implemented the conservation approach in anal cancer.[139]

When the Ontario Cancer Institute opened in 1958, Bill Rider was part of the radiotherapy team from the beginning. "We opened with five physicians and twice as many talented researchers," he later said, "in a milieu of excitement about the future." Clifford Ash, the first director of OCI, gave them their head, emphasizing "service to the patient directly, and indirectly through education and research." Rider continued, speaking in 1982, "In a quarter century we have progressed from a 'nothing outfit' to the 'leading edge' such that many outsiders have referred to us as the 'Mecca.'"[140]

Each cancer centre in Ontario was responsible for training radiation therapists, and in 1960 radiation oncology took on this responsibility for training in Toronto and for some other locations. This prevailed until the consolidation of training programs at the Michener Institute and at Hamilton in 1999.

The teaching of radiation oncology to medical students originated not with the radiation oncologists in the Department of Radiology but with the physicists in the Department of Medical Biophysics at OCI on Sherbourne Street. In 1960 the faculty sought the participation of medical biophysics in a curriculum review; Arthur Ham, head of the department, said that if the department were to contemplate "the teaching of radiation medicine and radiation biology ... the thought should be introduced that there should be a course in radiation medicine in Medicine ... We have to provide a good outline of what we think medical students should know about radiation and its effects and ... what years of the medical course these subjects should be taught."[141] (Disappointingly, when a quarter of a century later the dean of medicine did get around to including oncology in the undergraduate curriculum, no one from the Department of Medical Biophysics was included.[142])

Yet stirrings about a separate university Department of Radiation Oncology started to become loud much later, at the time of a review of the hospital Department of Radiation Oncology at Princess Margaret in 1982. Rider, chief of the hospital department, said he was quite keen on separating from the university Department of Radiology. "During Dr Ash's time there was talk about a separate

Department of Radiation Oncology, but he did not want it." Rider noted that the University of Western Ontario, Queen's, and McGill all had separate departments.[143] At the review Joe Marotta asked radiation oncologist Andrew Harwood "if he had any feeling of belonging to the Department of Radiology at the University. Dr Harwood said he had no personal feeling of belonging, and in fact could not see the relationship between radiation oncology and diagnostic radiology."[144]

On Rider's retirement in 1985, William Duncan, the head of radiation oncology in Edinburgh, briefly became the new head. Bernard Cummings, with his insider's seat, offers the following positive account: "Duncan strongly supported the independence of radiation oncology as a specialty, but the suggestion of a standing apart by radiation oncologists was a position wholly foreign to Duncan's approach to clinical care and research. He strongly encouraged multidisciplinary clinical care. After Duncan completed a 5 year term at PMH, he was not offered reappointment, but was recruited back to Edinburgh where he again became Professor and Chair."[145]

In 1991 Bernard Cummings himself became head of radiation oncology. It would be Cummings, along with Derek Jenkin and Don Cowan, who steered the group to department status.

There came for the radiation oncologists a surprised realization that radiation oncology was absent in the undergraduate curriculum, and this realization helped lead as well to the founding of a department. With the advent of the "block curriculum" in the 1980s the subject was simply whisked away. Simpson said it had once been the case that "every clinical clerk came to PMH for a one week rotation. This was cut out in spite of pleas from the staff and the high ratings given the rotation by the clerks. On several occasions attempts have been made to persuade the curriculum committee to reinstate the rotation. The University of Toronto is the only university in Canada which does not provide any regular exposure to clinical oncology."[146] Cummings said, "I think most undergraduates' notion of what oncology involves is based on their experience on surgical floors. They see the patient who has the diagnosis, has the initial surgery, and after that relatively little exposure to what else goes on with those patients."[147]

In the early 1980s, therefore, radiation oncology was dead keen to strike out on its own. The ice actually started to break up in 1984 with an external review of the Department of Radiology that said "radiation oncology played no part in the residency program or undergraduate training program of the Department of Radiology" and that it was "archaic" to keep the two together. "Radiation oncology should be made a full medical school department."[148]

Then there was the backlog. Cummings said what really had propelled the province to fund a separate department "was the waiting list problem, where we weren't able to treat all the patients at Princess Margaret Hospital or at Sunnybrook. There was a lot of bad publicity for everybody concerned, and the government was anxious to be able to show that it was doing something for cancer ... because we were mammothly short of radiation oncologists, physicists, and radiation therapists."

It was also helpful that in 1983 the District Health Council of Metro Toronto recommended that the university "initiate the integration of oncology services among the teaching hospitals, the Provincial cancer treatment centres and other hospitals."[149]

Thus it came to pass that in July 1984 Dean Lowy commissioned the aforementioned task force under Burnett Thall to consider "the desirability of establishing a separate Department of Radiation Oncology and/or a Department of Oncology." In May 1985, this task force recommended accordingly.[150]

A "Provincial Role Study of Cancer Services in Ontario" in 1985, commissioned by the OCI/OCTRF, recommended the creation of a department of radiation oncology "to lessen medical ignorance about the treatment of cancer with radiation."[151]

Said a faculty committee in 1991, "In summary, since 1983 there have been 8 independent reports formulated by expert reviewers all recommending the establishment of a Department of Radiation Oncology." By 1995 there would be fifty radiation oncologists at the PMH and Toronto Bayview Regional Cancer Centre (TBRCC) at Sunnybrook. "A departmental structure with clear academic identity is the organizational structure strongly preferred."[152]

In 1990 Minister of Health Elinor Caplan told Dean Dirks that the province would fund a Department of Radiation Oncology, and by January 1991 the faculty learned that the Ministry of Health had allocated $444,000 a year to support it.[153] That same month saw a "Draft Proposal to Establish a Department of Radiation Oncology."[154] Later in 1991 the Governing Council approved the new department and Bernard Cummings became its first chair.

Cummings, a New Zealander, graduated from the University of Otago School of Medicine in Dunedin, New Zealand, in 1967 and, after training in clinical oncology for two years in a hospital in Christchurch, spent a year as a resident in radiation oncology at PMH, where Bill Rider had agreed to take him on. Rider then agreed that Cummings pass a further year, in 1973–4, at the Royal Marsden Hospital in London, England. And in 1974 Cummings returned to join the Department of Radiology in Toronto as a lecturer and rose through the academic ranks.

Why didn't he return to New Zealand instead? "Here," he said in an interview, "there were very stimulating people to work with, like Ray Bush and then on the laboratory side, people like Gordon Whitmore ... There were just a far larger number of patients, a far greater variety, and an opportunity to do things that I didn't think I'd get elsewhere." He was not surprised on arrival to find that over half of the radiation oncologists in Canada were British-trained, and certainly more than half at Princess Margaret had emigrated from the United Kingdom.[155]

Cummings saw radiation oncology as a field ripe for research and wanted to make sure that Toronto followed the international pattern of recruiting residents receptive to research training. Currently in the United States it is said that about half the recruits in radiation oncology have a PhD or other research qualification. The proportion is lower in Toronto, but about a quarter of the trainees or junior staff have formal research training. "It's recognized," said Cummings, "that radiation oncology offers tremendous opportunities for research, because for people who have both a physics and a biology interest it offers a merging of the developing computing and engineering skills on one side, and the biology on the other." Of course the same was true in diagnostic radiology, yet in radiation oncology they had patients of their own, "and many people want to have patients on an ongoing basis."[156] In the Department of Radiation Oncology, residents were given up to a year to spend in research. Combining the two hospital departments of radiation oncology at PMH and Sunnybrook into a single university department created one of the largest academic departments of radiation oncology in the world. In 2010, the combined radiation oncology faculty of sixty-one included seventeen clinician scientists, with numerous others involved in education and clinical research.[157]

On Cummings's watch a university-based program for training radiation therapists was approved by the Governing Council in 1998, and inaugurated the following year, to augment the technical competence certificate that such therapists got from the Michener Institute. (Previously this had been in the hands of each of the major radiation treatment centres.) The program was established "to respond to the requirement that radiation technologists have a baccalaureate degree as an entry requirement to practice."[158] Under the direction of Pamela Catton and Mary Gospodarowicz, the program later developed a master's degree and even a PhD track.

### Should There Be a Department of Oncology at the University of Toronto?

Why not just have a Department of Oncology, rather than limiting it to radiotherapy? This, according to Cummings, had been the original vision of many in the late 1980s. The story is an interesting example of how academic politics shapes public health policy. Cummings said that the pathologists had been "adamantly opposed, they did not want to have primary appointments in Oncology and a secondary appointment in the Department of Pathology." (James Phillips in pathology said, "It would be impossible to separate oncology pathology from the rest of pathology."[159]) Also, said Cummings, most of the medical oncologists, urged on by Hollenberg, preferred to stay in the Department of Medicine. So the brief of the organizing committee had just drifted from oncology in general to radiation oncology.

There was also opposition to a Department of Oncology at the decanal level. In his response to the external review of the Department of Radiation Oncology in 2000, Dean Naylor put the kibosh on the entire idea: "I agree that many years hence it is possible that we would organize more of the faculty along disease-specific lines rather than by discipline; but at present I can see absolutely no rationale for organizing a department of Oncology. Indeed we have just disbanded the IDDO" (the Interdepartmental Division of Oncology – Goldenberg stepped down officially as director in 2001). Naylor defended the decision as part of the need to further rationalize and simplify the faculty's structure by not creating new departments with "some of the tangled lines of accountability and authority that currently exist ... Specifically, any interdepartmental thrust in oncology would have to be organized under multiple departments, be accountable to a council of departmental chairs, and be catalyzed by major external funding. Otherwise, there is no reason why such a structure cannot be created by the involved individuals or departments on a less formal programmatic basis."[160]

So why might a formal Department of Oncology be needed at all? What is a department good for, in other words? Why not simply let the radiation oncologists continue under the imagers' regimen of benign neglect? Because, said Cummings, research is at stake. "While [belonging to the Department of Radiology] worked well at the social and local administrative level, [the radiation oncology group] was not realizing its potential. It was not as powerful a potential force as a structured department. There was really no push to do academic work. People did it if they wanted to." In the past, said Cummings, the only people who had a track record of academic research were Vera Peters, Ray Bush, Derek Jenkin, and Bill Rider. But then a new cohort of radiation oncologists came on line from about 1974, "and there was a recognition that the medical records at Princess Margaret Hospital were a goldmine ... It was mainly by retrospective studies initially, and then we moved from retrospective chart analysis to prospective clinical trials."[161]

Isn't this interesting? That such an apparently trivial matter as whether a group of clinicians constitute a "department" can have such far-reaching consequences for the public health and patient welfare? Out of the Department of Radiation Oncology came innovations in the administration of radiotherapy that were of great benefit in the treatment of patients with cancer and touched the lives of millions.

# 14    Neuroscience and Psychiatry

The University of Toronto had tremendous but scattered strength in neuroscience. Basic, clinical, behavioural: all have their stories, but it took forever for these great resources to come together.

## Psychiatry

Psychiatry in Toronto did not have a promising beginning. Psychiatric patients were kept in underground cells of the Old York Gaol on King Street until a new jail was built.[1] Said Mr J.H. Tuke, brother of the noted English psychiatrist Daniel Hack Tuke, who visited the facility in September 1845, "It is one of the most painful and distressing places I ever visited. The house has a terribly dark aspect within and without and was intended for a prison. There were, perhaps, 70 patients, upon whose faces misery, starvation and suffering were indelibly impressed. The doctor pursues the exploded system of constantly cupping, bleeding, blistering and purging his patients ... The foreheads and necks of the patients were nearly all scarred with the marks of former cupping, or were bandaged from the effects of more recent ones ... Everyone look emaciated and wretched."[2] This was psychiatry in the pre-scientific era. The Provincial Lunatic Asylum opened in 1850.

### Asylum Psychiatry

In 1853 Joseph Workman, an Irish immigrant who had graduated in medicine from McGill University in 1835 and lectured on obstetrics and materia medica at John Rolph's Toronto School of Medicine, took over direction of the new Provincial Lunatic Asylum (as it was called before 1871, after which it became the Asylum for the Insane, Toronto). Workman, retaining his clinical faculty status as emeritus professor of obstetrics, regarded formal training of future alienists (asylum psychiatrists) as a crucial necessity. He established three part-time residential positions for medical students as clinical assistants or externs who earned a modest stipend while living and working on-site at the asylum. Among these aides was the young Charles K. Clarke, later professor of psychiatry.[3]

Following the retirement of Workman, in 1875 Daniel Clark became superintendent. Clark, from southwestern Ontario's Port Dover area, was a Toronto School of Medicine graduate, a US Civil War surgeon veteran, and member of the provincial medical council.

Formal academic instruction in psychiatry in Toronto dates from the course of lectures that Clark initiated at the asylum in 1882 for medical students at the Trinity Medical School and the Toronto School of Medicine.[4] In 1887 at the reopening of the faculty, Clark accepted a university appointment as "extra-mural professor of mental diseases," in essence establishing a precursor to the psychiatry department of the university.

Clark earned a footnote in Canadian history by testifying in 1885 at the trial of Louis Riel – leader of a First Nations resistance movement –that Riel was insane. In 1891 Clark became president of the Association of Medical Superintendents of American Institutions for the Insane, the forerunner of the American Psychiatric Association.[5] His lectures were supported by printed class notes, published in 1895 as *Mental Diseases* – evidently "the first psychiatric textbook for senior medical students produced in Canada."[6]

When Clark stepped down as extra-mural professor of medical psychology in 1903, John C. Mitchell replaced him for the short period 1903–6; Mitchell was appointed superintendent of the Provincial Hospital for Epileptics in Woodstock in 1904, then in 1905 superintendent of the Brockville Hospital for the Insane. In 1900 Nelson H. Beemer also became an extra-mural professor of medical psychology. Beemer, a medical graduate of the Victoria University medical department in 1874, was superintendent of the Mimico asylum (a suburb of Toronto) and retained the extra-mural post until his death in the 1934–5 session.[7] Neither man has left much of a trace (although Mitchell was president of the Ontario Medical Association in 1903–4), and their memory is overwhelmed by that of their successor: Charles Kirk Clarke, superintendent of the Toronto Asylum, founding professor of psychiatry in 1907, superintendent of the Toronto General Hospital, and dean of the faculty.

Clarke was born in 1857 in Elora, a village in Upper Canada, of a notable family: his father was the former Speaker of the Ontario Legislature. Charles qualified in medicine at the Toronto Medical School in 1878, having begun his career in psychiatry as a clinical assistant (as noted earlier) under Joseph Workman at the Toronto Hospital for the Insane. From 1881 to 1905 he was assistant superintendent, then superintendent, of the Rockwood Hospital for the Insane at Kingston and simultaneously professor of psychiatry at Queen's University. Behind his promotion as superintendent at Rockwood there is a story: as psychiatric historian Cyril Greenland tells it, Clarke became repelled by the political intrigues then prevailing in provincial institutions and resolved to leave government service, when "on the morning of August 13, 1885, while he and William Metcalf, medical superintendent, were making their ward rounds, a patient, Patrick Maloney, stabbed Metcalf in the abdomen, inflicting fatal wounds. Following Metcalf's death, Clarke reluctantly withdrew his resignation and was appointed medical superintendent at Kingston. He accepted this appointment, he said, 'in order to protect several hundred defenceless creatures from a political hireling who might be pitchforked into the position.'"

Clarke continued, "I love psychiatry, but hate politics: I felt that much could be accomplished if the politicians could be fought off with any degree of success."[8]

In 1905 Clarke returned to the Toronto Hospital for the Insane, replacing Daniel Clark, who resigned at the age of seventy. Two years later he became full professor of psychiatry at the university and, in 1908, dean of the Faculty of Medicine, a post in which he continued until 1920. In 1911, while still dean, he became superintendent of the Toronto General Hospital.

Clarke was not able to avoid politics in Toronto. In 1907 the provincial government sent him as part of a commission to Europe to look at models for modern psychiatric services, which Toronto much needed. He returned thoughtful about institutions he had visited, such as Emil Kraepelin's university psychiatric hospital in Munich. Clarke wrote in 1908, "[Germany] today has left all other countries behind in psychiatric studies ... Her Psychiatric Hospitals have placed psychiatry on a high plane." This, he concluded, was what was needed in Toronto. The government had given him hope of building such a hospital within the near future. "The laboratories will be thoroughly equipped for the purposes of pathological investigation," he rhapsodized, "studies of the body-fluids, bacteriology, physiology and psychology; and the research side of the work will be of just as much importance as the purely medical." Just as in Munich, they would have in Toronto a university department of psychiatry with a psychiatric hospital (Clarke used the German term "clinic") of its own.[9] This hospital, adumbrated in 1908, opened its doors in 1925 as the Toronto Psychiatric Hospital. (A makeshift reception hospital was briefly organized in the old private patients' pavilion at the former site of the Toronto General Hospital on Gerrard Street from 1913 to 1920.[10])

But the First World War intervened, and for today's reader it is interesting that Clarke anticipated in 1916 the concept of post-traumatic stress disorder, acquired in combat and treatable in special facilities. As the casualties were invalided home, the psychological carnage was appalling. "New conditions have arisen since the use of high explosives and the mental strain during action seems to be of the most severe character," Clarke wrote, "with the result that we encounter numerous cases of mental stress requiring special treatment." How were these men to be cared for? In nursing homes? Clarke found such facilities "unsuitable in every sense of the word – patients do badly and conditions are not favourable for their recovery." In asylums, "they become, in all probability, one of a herd rather than individuals to whom special treatment must be given ... It is wrong to let these men bear the stigma of being certified inmates of a hospital for the insane." Clarke proposed the establishment of a special hospital for the trauma victims of combat. "This hospital should be equipped with the most modern scientific, hydro-therapeutic, and electric apparatus demanded in the care of such patients ... [and] should not be too great a distance from some large public hospital where necessary apparatus and laboratories are to be found, to carry on the scientific investigations which are absolutely necessary." He added, "It is only fair and just that the provisions asked for should be made, as these men who suffer from mental and nervous troubles ought to be pitied and assisted just as much as those who have had physical disability."[11] (Thanks to Clarke's foresight, Canada did care more appropriately for its psychologically wounded veterans than other countries.)

Clarke, it must be said, was not an entirely benign figure in the history of Canadian psychiatry. In 1914 he opened a Social Service Clinic at the General where young women in some kind of sexual trouble might easily be diagnosed as "mentally-retarded" and sent away to provincial institutions. Alarmed at the growing influx of "mental defectives" among immigrants, after the First World War he pleaded for such "eugenic" measures – meaning improving the human race by selective breeding – as the segregation of those with "hereditary mental disability" in special asylums.[12] In encouraging such measures, he very much breathed the spirit of the times.

In 1907, the year in which Clarke was appointed professor, another significant event occurred in the history of Canadian psychiatry: Clarence Hincks graduated with an MB from the University of Toronto. Hincks stemmed from St Marys, Ontario, his father a Methodist cleric, his mother a former schoolteacher who adored Hincks and coached him in his studies. Medical degree in hand, he did not train in psychiatry but rather drifted around a bit, working for example as the district medical inspector for schools in West Toronto, when in 1913 he saw an advertisement for the Fourth International Congress of School Hygiene, to be held in August in Buffalo. In hopes of finding someone to help him understand his pupils' woes, physical and otherwise, he attended and heard of a test of intelligence that had been developed by Théodore Simon and Alfred Binet in Paris. "To Clare's knowledge," writes historian Charles Roland, "they had not yet been used at all in Canada." Hincks returned to Toronto full of enthusiasm for determining how intelligent his students were. He was, of course, among the many who stumbled into the minefield of "intelligence" and its testing, and the Simon-Binet test later became accused of imposing social metrics of intellectual excellence instead of scientific.

Charles Clarke thus asked Hincks to help with an outpatient "Feeble-Mindedness Clinic" that was being organized in 1914 for the Toronto General Hospital.

Hincks became enthralled with the blooming concept of "mental hygiene" – measures one might take, including "eugenic," to keep the population mentally healthy. After a visit in 1917 to the New York offices of the National Committee for Mental Hygiene, Hincks returned to Canada to co-found (with Clarke) in Ottawa in 1918 the Canadian National Committee for Mental Hygiene, an organization that later became the Canadian Mental Health Association.[13] The organization, very much a presence on the psychiatric scene today, has no intrinsic connection to the University of Toronto and the narrative will not be pursued here, except to point out that in the 1920s and 1930s the "mental hygiene" disciplines were often animated by the same concerns about immigration and the feared degeneration of the native white stock that motivated much social psychiatry in those days. Clarke, who in 1918 became medical director of the committee, gave the inaugural keynote speech. An editorial in the *Canadian Medical Association Journal* summing up Clarke's work noted, "Tests of mental deficiency have amply revealed to how great an extent a proper application of the study of psychiatry is required in our state." Further, "[t]he interest of intelligent men and women must be directed to the conservation of the mental health of the race by developing the qualities of foresight and judgement."[14] Today, people accept the concept of "mental health" as on the whole positive, forgetting that it was born in the sewer of eugenic thinking that flowed through much late-nineteenth- and early-twentieth-century psychiatry.

*University Psychiatry*

As stated, in 1907 Clarke became professor of psychiatry. In 1920 a faculty committee headed by Alexander Primrose had been struck to advise on the distribution of a grant from the Rockefeller Foundation. This committee noted "the recent remarkable development of this [Psychiatry] Department and the wide spread interest taken in it by the community at large." Psychiatry must therefore be imbedded in the university curriculum. The committee members also "advocate the erection of a psychopathic Hospital of at least 85 beds in or near the grounds of the Toronto General Hospital to provide clinical facilities for teaching and research." The new psychopathic hospital should include "adequate laboratories for research in metabolism and pathology and psychology."[15] Voices had been loud in Toronto for many years on behalf of the creation of such a hospital, and before the war, as noted, a commission had travelled to Germany to see if Emil Kraepelin's university psychiatric hospital in Munich might provide a model for such a hospital.[16] Here, the Faculty Council came out four-square for such a facility. The following week they emphasized even more emphatically that "there is an urgent demand for recent graduates to become trained as psychiatrists for many positions which are open to them, and these can only be met at present by these men being forced to go the United States ... for the necessary training."[17]

An added stimulus to the timely construction of such a hospital was the Rockefeller Foundation's stipulation that the hospital actually be built before the $1 million grant envisioned for the faculty was paid out.[18]

As the new psychiatric "Reception Hospital" opened in 1925, Clarence B. Farrar succeeded Clarke as chair of psychiatry, one of the first Americans to accept a major faculty appointment after the long string of Englishmen and Scotsmen. Farrar was remarkable if only for his longevity in office: He retired in 1947 and was for over thirty years (from 1931 to 1965) editor of the *American Journal of Psychiatry*. Farrar was born in 1874 in Cattaraugus, New York, an upstate village where his father was an insurance broker. He graduated with an arts degree from Harvard in 1896 and earned a medical degree at Johns Hopkins University in 1900. He then worked for two years as an assistant physician at the Sheppard Pratt Hospital, a private psychiatric facility on the outskirts of Baltimore. An event that shaped Farrar's life greatly, turning him towards biological psychiatry, was the two years from 1902 to 1904 that he spent in Heidelberg in the lab of Franz Nissl (who is remembered for a stain for nervous tissue named after him). Farrar then returned to a staff job at the Pratt from 1904 to 1913; he worked for three years, from 1913 to 1916, at the New Jersey Hospital for the Insane at Trenton, then ruled by an eccentric figure, Henry Cotton (who believed that the highway to mental health lay in removing such sources of "focal infection" as infected teeth and colons).

World War I brought Farrar to Canada. Keen to serve the cause, in 1916 he enlisted in the Canadian army (the United States, of course, entered the conflict only in 1917), and, because Canada lacked psychiatrists for dealing with the mentally wounded men then being invalided home, Farrar was transferred to Ottawa for service with the military hospitals commission. In 1923 he left government service to become superintendent of a private psychiatric hospital in Guelph, Ontario, called the Homewood Sanitarium. Clarke met the dynamic young Farrar through their mutual colleague (and future dean) John Gerald FitzGerald and was impressed by him; with Clarke's death in January 1924, in 1925 Farrar became his successor.[19]

Farrar's twenty-two-year reign as professor of psychiatry and director of the Toronto Psychiatric Hospital (TPH) saw the rise of a solid academic program. The 1931–2 session witnessed the founding of a three-month course in psychiatric nursing for nurses from the general hospitals.[20] In the 1932–3 session, the department hooked up with School of Graduate Studies "for work leading to the Ph.D."[21]

One of the earliest holders of the PhD in psychiatry was Ruth MacLachlan Franks, a medical graduate of U of T in 1926, who earned her PhD in 1936 with a thesis on depression in women. She was said to be "the first doctor to be granted a Philosophy Degree in Psychiatry by a Canadian university." Franks trained in psychiatry at TPH and thereupon was psychiatrist to the Women's College Hospital from 1926 on. She worked as an assistant psychiatrist at the

Zurich University Psychiatric Hospital at Burghölzli in 1930–1 and was later involved in occupational therapy.[22]

In 1935 a one-year diploma program (DPsych) was established to train psychiatrists, mainly those who worked in the provincial mental hospital system ("Ontario Hospitals").[23] (At the same time "CB" Farrar, as he was known, led efforts to create a provincial Board of Psychiatric Examiners to vet all applicants for posts in the provincial hospital service.[24]) The first six DPsych diplomas were handed out in the fall of 1936.[25]

*The Farrar Years*

In psychiatric therapeutics, a page was turned in the late 1930s with the introduction into psychiatry of the new "physical therapies." First came insulin coma, or injections of insulin to induce a series of hypoglycemic shocks, used for the first time in Canada in Nova Scotia in March 1937 and at the Ontario Hospital, New Toronto, two months later, as a new "insulin unit" opened under Norman Easton.[26] By 1940–1 the Toronto Psychiatric Hospital as well had acquired an insulin unit under Burdett McNeel. In collaboration with the Department of Medical Research, the study of the biochemistry of schizophrenia began, using the electroencephalograph (EEG) and lab tests among other means of investigation. Much of this research was ultimately given up, perhaps prematurely, as electroconvulsive therapy came to replace insulin coma. But the work is interesting as an example of a profoundly biological approach to psychiatry.[27]

All of this new investigation prompted a more formal organization of psychiatric research. In the 1938–9 session, a research unit was organized at the Toronto Psychiatric Hospital, funded by a grant from the Rockefeller Foundation and given jointly to the Department of Psychiatry and the Department of Medical Research. It was under the aegis of this grant that much collaborative research of a biological nature was shared in the next decade by the Departments of Psychiatry and Medical Research. For the purpose of research, a twenty-bed ward was set aside on the third floor of the hospital, with clinical staff provided by the Department of Health "and with laboratories for biochemistry and EEG equipped and staffed by the Department of Medical Research," it was said in 1939. "Initial studies now under way will compare the effects of various types of pharmacologic shock." The workers were deemed to be especially interested in schizophrenia.[28]

Thus it was that an interdisciplinary team from the Banting and Best Department of Medical Research (BBDMR) and the Department of Psychiatry began the second of the new physical therapies: Metrazol convulsive therapy, or use of a chemical agent to induce therapeutic convulsions. (Metrazol was a brand name for pentylenetrazole.) Metrazol convulsive therapy was introduced internationally in 1935, in Toronto in 1939, but it does not seem to have been widely practiced here, although McNeel led a team at the Toronto Psychiatric Hospital that studied it.[29] Gordon R. Hall in the BBDMR headed a group "engaged on the problem of the physiological significance of metrazol and insulin shock therapy in the treatment of schizophrenics," in conjunction with the Departments of Psychiatry and Public Health and the Committee on Mental Hygiene. Hall also looked at electrical patterns in the brain during shock "as recorded from the exposed area striata [sic] of the cortex" with the BBDMR's recently constructed EEG machine, evidently studied in animals. The Metrazol research continued under Hall's direction at the Department of Medical Research and was supported by a grant from the Scottish Rite Masons and the Rockefeller Foundation until the Second World War, when the treatment went out of style. The 1942 report of Norman Easton and Joseph Sommers, staffers at the Toronto Psychiatric Hospital, on the 23 percent risk of vertebral fractures in Metrazol convulsions, helped mark the end of interest in chemically induced therapeutic seizures.[30]

The third, and the safest and most effective, new physical treatment was electroconvulsive therapy (ECT), or use of electricity to induce convulsions. This was administered in Toronto for the first time in 1941, apparently at the research unit of the Toronto Psychiatric Hospital, under the supervision of a recent diploma-holder in psychiatry, Lorne Proctor, who received his MD in 1938. Proctor, who was apparently cross-appointed between the outpatient psychiatric department of the Toronto Western Hospital and the Toronto Psychiatric Hospital, said that by 1944 ECT had been administered at these institutions (and at the Ontario Hospital New Toronto) to 400 patients, procuring a recovery rate in depression of around 80 percent[31] – a result typical of the success of convulsive therapy in mood disorders. Clearly, the Department of Psychiatry was on board for biological approaches to mental illness from the earliest days.

The department's rather extensive dalliance with lobotomy began in the 1941–2 session, in collaboration with neurosurgeon Ken McKenzie (see pp. 78–79). Farrar said in 1942, "Improvement in a group of involutional melancholics [midlife depression] and a group of catatonic schizophrenics following bilateral frontal leucotomies has been observed."[32] Abe Miller continued this work in psychiatry, in collaboration with McKenzie. In 1949 "Dr G[rant] C Beacock and Dr A[braham] Miller have continued an investigation into the clinical criteria associated with good prognosis in a group of patients submitted to prefrontal leucotomy."[33] Elsewhere, interest in lobotomy vanished in the early 1950s with the introduction of chlorpromazine and the other antipsychotic drugs. Yet Miller soldiered on and in 1967 published a follow-up study of 150 patients lobotomized between 1948 and 1952. The results, he said, were rather encouraging. Although virtually all had a "personality defect," 67 percent "improved sufficiently to live out of hospital." Miller believed there was a continuing role for prefrontal lobotomy in "selected cases of intractable mental disorder."[34] The conclusion is rather startling, as by 1967 lobotomy had been swept from psychiatry by psychopharmacologic agents.

In the 1920s, Sigmund Freud's psychoanalysis started to make headway in Toronto, though not necessarily in the Department of Psychiatry. Freud's acolyte and biographer, the London psychiatrist Ernest Jones, had spent 1908–13 in Toronto as a neuropathologist at the Toronto asylum, though he actually did little to kindle enthusiasm for analytic doctrine. In the graduating class of 1924, the yearbook teased Muriel Fetterly that she was "specializing in psychoanalysis, hockey, long histories and blushing."[35] (She proceeded on to the Department of Hygiene of Cornell University in Ithaca, New York, an authority on calcium metabolism.) The first flicker of interest in psychoanalysis in the department occurred in the 1951–2 session, as Edward J. Rosen and Daniel Cappon were said to "continue to pursue their research in the field of psycho-dynamics."[36] The uptake of psychoanalysis in Toronto seems to have been slower than in comparable American cities, and Montreal was the big entrepôt for psychoanalysis in Canada.

Meanwhile, interest in biological psychiatry continued apace. In the 1939–40 session, John Dewan, a University of Western Ontario graduate (1932) who had earned a PhD in biochemistry at Cambridge University, returned to Toronto to begin research. In 1946 Dewan would become the director of the newly modernized outpatient department.

*Stokes*

Research received a great boost in 1947 when Aldwyn B. Stokes of the Maudsley Hospital in London, England, replaced Farrar as professor of psychiatry. Recruiting Stokes as chair of the department was a bit of a coup for the university because Stokes was situated right in the royal road in British psychiatry that led to knighthoods and prestigious chairs. Born in 1906 in Newport, England, he read physiology at Oxford at Jesus College (obtaining his Greyhound colours for rugby and his Authentic colours for cricket). He studied medicine at King's College Hospital Medical School in London, graduating in 1931. He was a house officer in medicine at King's College Hospital from 1932 to 1934, thereupon training in psychiatry at the Maudsley Hospital as an assistant medical officer, then medical officer, from 1935 to 1939. In the late 1930s, on a Rockefeller Travelling Fellowship, he studied periodic catatonia with Rolf Gjessing at the Dikemark Mental Hospital in Norway. He served as deputy superintendent then superintendent of the Mill Hill branch during the war – the Maudsley was evacuated – and returned to the Maudsley as superintendent.

Apparently seeing his way to a professorship in London blocked by Aubrey Lewis, in 1947 Stokes accepted the chair at the University of Toronto. He simultaneously became director of the Toronto Psychiatric Hospital, which post he resigned in 1961 "to devote all his efforts to the development of the university department" until his retirement in 1971, as his eulogist Fred Lowy, then chair of the department (later dean), said at the time of Stokes's death in 1978. Lowy pointed out that Stokes had played a capital role in "the marshalling of forces and resources which resulted in the construction of the Clarke Institute" in 1966.[37]

Although Stokes was eclectic in the inclusion of social and community psychiatry and psychotherapy programs, his basic orientation was biological. "Psychiatry is concerned with a breakdown in living," he wrote in 1951. "The breakdown is biological and issues from genetic, physical, psychological, or social causes. The pattern of causation effects secondary consequences which penetrate the human biological system even to the molecular physical level."[38] Though the meaning of this is not completely clear, it is apparent that Stokes did not direct his considerable energy towards converting the Department of Psychiatry into a psychotherapy institute. He began his tenure by recruiting Rolf Gjessing, whom he knew from the catatonia research, to come from Oslo to Toronto to set up a metabolic clinic and laboratory at TPH. Dewan later described the atmosphere at the hospital: "It was a real live place. You felt things were happening. Reaching out. They weren't accepting everything simply because it was in front [an apparent reference to psychoanalysis]. When Dr. Gjessing came it was a great morale booster."[39] Metabolic research on catatonia became the battle flag under which brain investigation advanced. After Gjessing left, his collaborator Allan Gornall in the Department of Pathological Chemistry carried this research forward.

In 1952 Stokes recruited John Lovett-Doust, whose specialty was physiological psychiatry, from the Maudsley to head the research laboratory. At the Institute of Psychiatry at the Maudsley, Doust had worked on the production of "experimental psychoses" with LSD.[40] (David J. Lewis at St Michael's Hospital among others continued this work in the late 1950s, at the cutting edge of the new discipline of psychopharmacology: using psychotomimetics, or drugs causing psychosis, to produce clinical states thought comparable to schizophrenia.) In 1959 the laboratory gained a small research unit of six beds, and a whole row of biological studies progressed. In 1958 John Dewan and William Spaulding in the Department of Medicine, who in 1947–8 had been physician to TPH, published *The Organic Psychoses: A Guide to Diagnosis*. In the foreword, Stokes slammed the field's neglect of the biological to the advantage of psychoanalysis: "It is astonishing, particularly when cellular and chemical pathology are in rapid advance, that the field of the organic psychoses has been relatively neglected in practice."[41]

Under Stokes, in 1947–8 a children's clinic was organized at HSC, the beginning of pediatric psychiatry in Toronto. It became included in the training program of the Department of Psychiatry. Yet the future of child psychiatry lay in cooperation with the Department of Pediatrics at the Thistletown Hospital, the county branch in West York of the Hospital for Sick Children, which in 1959–60 joined the two-year training program with TPH.[42] In July 1968 the establishment of a separate Department of Psychiatry at HSC took place with the appointment of Quentin Rae-Grant as professor of child psychiatry and psychiatrist-in-chief of the hospital. At the same time John Fotheringham became medical director of the Mental Retardation Centre (in the former quarters of TPH at Surrey Place), and the new Hincks Treatment Centre (for adolescents) opened under Angus

M. Hood.[43] The Clarke Institute of Psychiatry, the successor of the Toronto Psychiatric Hospital, would later add its own child and adolescent unit. Child psychiatry was thus well established in Toronto by the late 1960s.

TPH was an Ontario Hospital, and its administration lay in the hands of the provincial government. In 1947–8 Stokes set up an "academic council" for the Department of Psychiatry as advisory to the university "to promote the educational development of psychiatry within the general medical framework."[44]

At the beginning of his tenure, Stokes also moved forward on postgraduate education, adding to the department in 1946 a full four-year training program after internship that would lead to the fellowship of the Royal College (unlike the one-year diploma program or the PhD program). It was open to any medical applicant and not just to members of the Ontario Hospital Service. Liaison to general-hospital psychiatry would be vouchsafed through Sunnybrook Hospital and the Hospital for Sick Children. (The General had as yet no psychiatry department.) The Department of Medicine founded a psychiatric unit at the Wellesley Hospital in 1949 that was also included in the program – see farther on. Postgraduate trainees who were not members of the Ontario Hospital Service would receive a subsistence payment.[45] In September 1948 the provincial government gave a large mental health grant to the Department of Psychiatry that funded training fellowships, increasing the number of postgraduate trainees from five in 1946 to eighteen in 1949. (Of seven candidates in 1948, five obtained the diploma, two the specialist certification of the Royal College.[46]) Loath though the provincial government was to surrender control of TPH, it acceded to "the principle that men entering the postgraduate course are completely under the aegis of the University."[47]

By the 1952–3 session, graduate training had been expanded to include the psychiatry division of the Toronto Western Hospital and the Brookside Clinic Hospital (for alcohol addiction). "Altogether there are now nine centres of instruction within the University framework of medical education," said Stokes.[48] In 1956–7 the Ontario Hospital at Queen Street, the main Toronto mental hospital, was brought into the training program. In 1964–5 the diploma program was lengthened to three years.

Stokes was eclectic rather than wholly biological in orientation, for, coming from the Maudsley, he endorsed the principle that the psychiatrist should have broad training in the community. In addition to the teaching hospitals, he developed associations with the Family Court and other organizations "to broaden the field of experience for psychiatrists in training."[49] He wished to see psychiatry influence nursing education and sought a liaison to the School of Nursing: "It is becoming increasingly apparent that to effectively influence illness she needs not only a technical skill on the organ level of disease but also a penetration into the emotional difficulties of the patient." There was a role in psychiatry for occupational therapy, not just handicrafts but "weaning from the hospital to the vocational responsibilities of community living." Morton Teicher, the hospital's first chief of social work, was greatly expanding psychiatry's reach into the lives of patients and their families. Cyril Greenland, with an MSc in social work (and PhD in the 1980s), later continued this trend. And under John Seeley, during whose association with the department a major study of mental health in the Toronto district of Forest Hill was completed,[50] the staff sociologists emphasized "social interaction in a community."

Social psychiatry was to be emphasized in the teaching program "so that preventive work with the community agencies, with the schools in the field of vocational rehabilitation, and on such problems as alcoholism, epilepsy, and chronic illness is not disregarded."[51] Stokes reached out to Delbert Wollin in neuroradiology and Eric Linell in neuropathology. Stokes and Manville W. Sloane in pathology (who also had a PhD in neuroanatomy) studied "the pathology of the thalamus."[52] Stokes has often been sent up because of a rather orotund speaking and writing style, but he opened up the Department of Psychiatry from the cramped confines of TPH to the world.

Relief from the lack of space at TPH was at hand. In the 1952–3 session, the Ministry of Health agreed to "the establishment of a new Psychiatric Institute,"[53] which, however, would not open its doors for another thirteen years.

As is known, the research agenda of the department until the mid-1950s was overwhelmingly biological. Yet the psychoanalytic note became increasingly insistent, a matter of interest because in those years, south of the border, psychoanalysis had virtually taken over psychiatry. In his 1954 report Stokes said that the department was adding a complement: "The holders of these posts will give an increased emphasis to the developmental aspect of psychiatry including the psychoanalytical."[54] It was Daniel Cappon who in particular picked up the torch of psychoanalysis, in the 1954–5 year initiating a formal program: "The point of departure in a very complicated area of inquiry is dream content and structure in patients suffering from physical disease."[55] Alan Parkin was the chief figure, a Toronto graduate who had trained in psychoanalysis in London, returned to Toronto in 1954, and two years later created the Toronto Analytic Study Circle. Parkin attempted to establish a training program in the department but was not initially successful. (Daniel Cappon led the "section on psychodynamics.") Parkin did, however, increasingly influence his colleagues, and his work started to be noticed in departmental publications in the early 1960s.[56]

The delays in building the new psychiatric hospital became infuriating. In 1958 Dean MacFarlane grumbled that psychiatry desperately needed a new building: "In a field where costs of medical care are greater than for any other illness, a field which in the past has lagged far behind other branches of Medicine in research and enquiry, but in which there are successively brighter lights burning in a previously darkened horizon … it is disappointing to report that our central physical facilities … are primitive and outmoded. The delay in plans to correct this situation is difficult to understand."[57] Finally, in the 1959–60 session the province authorized building the new psychiatric hospital.[58]

The biological wing within the department was further reinforced with the arrival of Harvey Stancer at TPH. Stancer, born in Toronto in 1926, had earned a PhD in pathological chemistry at Toronto in 1953 and an MD in 1955. He then began a vast Cook's tour that took him from McLean Hospital in Belmont, Massachusetts, to the Maudsley, to the Psychiatric Institute at Columbia University. After his Royal College certification as a psychiatrist in 1962, he became the head of neurochemistry at TPH until 1966, then, with the move to the Clarke Institute of Psychiatry, chief of the clinical investigation unit and head of neurochemistry until 1976. He was the professor of psychiatric research from 1974 until 1981 and head of the affective disorders unit from the late 1970s to the early 1980s. Vice chair of the department until 1985, he retired in 1991, a figure of such magnitude on the biological horizon that the department's later annual Research Day was named after him.

On the clinical investigation unit, Michael S. Ross and Harvey Moldofsky proposed in 1977 the use of pimozide as an alternative to haloperidol, another antipsychotic laden with side effects, in the treatment of Gilles de la Tourette's syndrome.[59] In 1993 Moldofsky, the founder of sleep studies in Toronto, became director of the Centre for Sleep and Chronobiology, which had just been established the previous year.

Psychiatry was trying hard to join the medical mainstream after so many years at the margins. In December 1965, Stokes asked Dean Hamilton for space for psychiatry in the new Medical Sciences Building: "Even a small representation within the pre-medical Science Division of the Medical Complex would be important as a present representation of what many of us think must be of greater moment in the future when Departments of Medical Sciences in the Faculty of Medicine will be a usual arrangement."[60] Nothing came of this.

Events rushed ahead. On 18 May 1966, the Clarke Institute of Psychiatry opened, a few blocks west on College Street from TPH. The clinicians formed a medical partnership "for the collection and distribution of medical fees in a teaching institution."[61] Six months later, in December 1966, Stokes stepped down. A new era began.

When the Clarke opened in 1966, it was as an independent institute with a board of its own, not as a provincial hospital in thrall to the Ministry of Health. Edward Turner, at the time professor of forensic psychiatry and head of the Metropolitan Toronto Forensic Service, said later that this autonomy was the key to the Clarke's success. "Dr [Mathew] Dymond, then Minister of Health, was an enlightened man who saw the merits of having an institute responsible to a board of trustees and not directly to the government. And I believe over the years his wisdom has been proven. It [the board] has kept us at arm's length from government directives and with moderately generous funding, the Clarke has been able to develop imaginative programs."[62]

*Psychoanalysis and Competing Views*

Six months after Stokes's departure, the department held its first seminar on psychoanalysis, "Projective Object Relations."[63] This coincided nicely with

Robin C.A. Hunter's appointment as the chair of psychiatry and director of the Clarke Institute. Hunter, a psychoanalyst, was born in Jamaica in 1919 and graduated from Calabar High School there in 1938. He came to Canada in 1940 and enlisted in the Royal Canadian Air Force. Shot down over occupied Europe, he spent four years as a prisoner of war. Returning to Canada, he began medical studies at McGill and earned an MD in 1950. After completing in 1953 training at the Allan Memorial Institute, which was the Department of Psychiatry of McGill University, Hunter served as a "registrar," or resident, at the Maudsley until 1955, then returned on staff at McGill. In 1964 he became head of psychiatry at Queen's University, then accepted the chair of the department at Toronto in 1967. Hunter was a graduate of the Canadian Institute of Psychoanalysis, the first analyst to lead the department.

Yet among Hunter's first appointments were not other analysts but, in 1967, an internationally known scientist in brain research: Oleh Hornykiewicz of the University of Vienna, known for showing in the early 1960s that a lack of dopamine characterizes Parkinson's disease and that L-dopa treatment relieves its symptoms.[64] (There was a kerfuffle in 2001 when Hornykiewicz was passed over for a Nobel Prize in this area.) Born in Sykhiw in Poland (now Ukraine), Hornykiewicz earned an MD from the University of Vienna in 1951 and ended up as chair of the Institute of Biochemical Pharmacology there. In connection with the Departments of Psychiatry and Pharmacology in Toronto, Hornykiewicz set up his own brain research laboratory and for many years spent long annual stretches in Toronto, serving as a world-class resource.

Having to serve two masters – the faculty and the ministry – psychiatry in these years was torn between science and service obligations. Psychiatry had one foot in such research facilities as the Clarke Institute, which had few patients and was not well adapted for teaching. The other foot was in traditional clinical settings such as the Ontario Hospitals, where service responsibilities were overwhelming. Neither was a resource of the University of Toronto nor an ideal setting for training. Under those circumstances, as a report pointed out in 1969, the opening of hospital psychiatry departments was long overdue.[65]

*The Story of the Hospital Departments of Psychiatry: Beginnings at TGH*

The advantages of the neuropathic wards in the Toronto General Hospital quickly attained recognition, and for this the profession must always be deeply indebted to the enthusiasm and the activities of Dr. Campbell Meyers.[66]

Lewellys F. Barker, 1927

The tale of psychiatry in these years cannot be told in a straightforward manner because most people, clinicians included, had a horror of "insanity" – something seen by psychiatrists in asylums. Anything less than full-bore psychosis was brought to neurologists, where it was treated as "nervous disease." So the heads of medicine all held psychiatry at arm's length and encouraged "neurology" in its stead. In those days, neurologists often offered a large dollop of psychotherapy to psychoneurotic patients in addition to treating organic brain diseases that for the most part were incurable.

This is therefore a story with two tracks. The first track – the asylum – began earlier. The second track is the psychiatric story in the general hospitals.

In May 1906 D. Campbell Meyers established the "nervous wards," also called "neurological wards," at TGH. These were, according to Meyers in 1911, "the first in Canada."[67] Meyers said, "These wards were advocated and established for the treatment of ... all Functional Neuroses ... these wards were not established for the treatment of the insane." Immediately, one sees psychotic illness being triaged from neurology and "nervousness."

Meyers had hoped that a separate ward for "acute insanity" might also be founded at the General, but this turned out to be impossible. In any event, the twelve-bed "Nervous Wards" were a great success, and by 1907 "the establishment in Toronto of a distinct and separate Psychopathic Hospital and Clinic" was anticipated – which, alas, did not occur until 1925. Meyers said, "The results have demonstrated clearly that the development of the acute insanities may be prevented in a very large proportion of cases, when treatment is commenced sufficiently early."[68]

Yet the Nervous Wards were haunted by apparently "nervous" patients who on admission turned out to be fully psychotic and made everyone else even more nervous. In 1908, therefore, Clarke (superintendent of the Toronto Asylum and shortly to be superintendent of the General as well) was brought on board to help out with the "insane" patients.[69] It is of interest that English psychiatrist Ernest Jones, the acolyte of Sigmund Freud mentioned previously, spent the years before the First World War in Toronto as a pathologist at the Toronto Asylum and from 1909 as an assistant psychiatrist in the Nervous Wards.[70]

The Nervous Wards came to an unhappy end in 1911 as Clarke, now superintendent of the hospital, abolished the service on the grounds that psychotic patients were wandering about unsupervised: "The institution is not equipped to deal with these people satisfactorily or with safety to patients and nurses."[71] That was the end of inpatient psychiatry at the General for the next half century.

TGH also had an outpatient psychiatric service. As Clarke told the story, "In 1909 when Superintendent of the Toronto Hospital for the Insane, I felt that something should be done to establish an Outdoor Clinic for psychiatric cases. It was only too evident that patients would be reluctant to seek help in a hospital for the insane." So TGH superintendent John Nelson Elliott Brown approved of the plan and secured the trustees' permission for "placing at our disposal a room in what was known as the Ward Clinic, a little house on the corner of Chestnut and Christopher Streets in the east end. These details are given as it was the first Clinic of the kind to be established in Canada. Dr Ernest Jones, the well known psychiatrist, who was at that time Associate Professor of Psychiatry, and also serving as Pathologist at the Toronto Hospital for the Insane, was assigned to the duty." Then with the building of the new TGH on College Street, "the Clinic house" disappeared.[72]

TGH had established in December 1911 a Social Service Department under a registered nurse, Norah Holman, apparently an American.[73] Dr Helen Mac-Murchy provided the medical leadership and for two years chaired the Ladies' Committee, which financed a social worker to do follow-ups.[74] It was under the aegis of this department that in April 1914 the newly formed juvenile court clinic opened its doors, aided by Miss E. De V. Clarke, a social service nurse. The purpose of such a clinic? C.K. Clarke said, "I had always felt that the greatest work of any Social Service Department was that of discovering defectives in a community and providing proper care and treatment for them." (Clarke refers here to having "defectives" admitted to institutions for mental retardation.) The university Department of Psychology became involved, administering IQ tests. The big problem here, Clarke said, was "dealing with the many delinquents of the moron class – children who are not only out of place in industrial schools for normals, but a menace where the population is of the mixed variety as far as mentality is concerned." The new clinic was kept very busy protecting the community from such cases. (It is unsurprising, given these views, that Clarke seems also to have been anti-Semitic, asserting that children of Jewish immi-grants belonged to "a very neurotic race" who should be closely watched for mental deficiency and "the weaklings weeded out remorselessly."[75])

Thus, by 1914 TGH had an Out-Patient Department Clinic for Feeble-Minded, staffed by Clarke, Clarence M. Hincks, who is seen as the founder of child psy-chiatry in Canada, and Oswald C. Withrow, a 1902 medical graduate of the university who stemmed from Oxford County.[76] In 1915 the feeble-minded de-partment was transformed into a "Psychiatric Clinic" under Hincks, the pri-mary mission of which seems to have remained "the mentally abnormal of the city." Hincks gushed, "Dr C.K. Clarke is, of course the mainspring of the or-ganization, and is the last court of appeal in all difficult cases." Whereas in 1912 the mentally ill had been such a menace that they couldn't be permitted to roam the hospital (and their "Nervous" service abolished), in 1915 Hincks said, "The wisdom of inaugurating a Psychiatric Clinic at the Toronto General Hos-pital has now been well proven."[77] Hincks became increasingly emphatic on the subject of mental retardation. "Toronto is roused at last," he said in 1916. "The terrible menace of the feeble-minded has shocked the community." The Psychi-atric Clinic had discovered how many of them were criminal, and immigrants too! Happily, the Psychological Laboratory of the University of Toronto and the Medical Social Service were both recruited to expose these evils.[78]

Meanwhile, Jane Grant had supplanted Holman as the head of the Social Ser-vice Department; she gratefully acknowledged in 1916 the work of the clinic: "It is to this centre that all branches of hospital social service or general social ser-vice must look for its salvation. Eliminate the feeble-minded and insane from our communities and all social work would be a joy." By early 1919 the clinic had examined almost 5,400 cases, from "high grade imbeciles" on down to "moron" and below. "This in itself indicates the magnitude of the problem in one locality and incidentally proves that the most pessimistic of the prophets in Ontario have far underestimated the number of defectives in the Province." Of the "defectives," only 55 percent had been born in Canada. "This points most clearly to the fact that immigration ... must be far more carefully supervised than has been the case in the past."[79]

In 1926 the Psychiatric Clinic was transferred to the newly founded Toronto Psychiatric Hospital;[80] one understands now why the prospect of reviving a psychiatric clinic at the Toronto General Hospital in the 1960s was received with something less than enthusiasm.

Until the mid-1940s, psychiatry and neurology at the General were one. The further neurology story appears later. The psychiatry story continues here.

*The Psychiatry Story Continues, but at the Wellesley Hospital*

There had been a neurology, or neuropsychiatric, service at the General under Goldwin Howland. After Howland's retirement, in 1949 Ray Farquharson eliminated the service at the Toronto General Hospital itself and created a psychiatric unit at General's Wellesley division, directed by Herbert Hyland and including J. Clifford Richardson and J. Allan Walters. From the outset, the new unit was available to the Department of Psychiatry for postgraduate training, although, as a division of the Department of Medicine, it was not otherwise connected to psychiatry. Stokes, however, was said to give the unit his "active support."[81]

The new unit was soon involved in undergraduate education as well, given that, as Farquharson put it, "The Department has always been aware of the importance of instructing medical students in the understanding of patients' emotional difficulties, which are part of all illnesses." Allan Walters lectured to upper-year students "on clinical methods of psychological examination."[82]

The rise of psychiatry in the Toronto teaching hospitals thus revolves around these three figures: Herbert Hyland, Allan Walters, and Ric Richardson. (One bears in mind that none of this story is related to the Department of Psychiatry after 1925 at the Toronto Psychiatric Hospital and quite uninvolved in the general hospitals.)

Hyland was born in Toronto in 1900 and graduated with an MD in 1926. His interest in psychiatry was said to have been touched off by a summer internship at the Ontario Psychiatric Hospital in Whitby. Hyland spent the late 1920s in further training abroad, particularly at the National Hospital for the Paralyzed and Epileptic (as this famous neurological hospital was then called) in Queen Square in London, where he acquired the "London Membership." (He was in fact a Fellow of the Royal College of Physicians.) According to Max Findlay, it was neurosurgeon Ken McKenzie who revived interest at TGH in neurology, causing Hyland to be appointed in 1930 to the Department of Medicine as a junior demonstrator.[83]

Hyland was an early player in what was conceived around 1931 as a neuroscience program, when Eric Linell became professor of neuropathology. Linell at the Banting Institute was to "coordinate" the work of McKenzie in neurosurgery, Jason Hannah in neuropathology at the Toronto Psychiatric Hospital, and Hyland in the Department of Medicine at the General. Dean FitzGerald said, "This step has been planned for some time and results of great theoretical interest and practical importance should emerge therefrom."[84] The program came to nothing, but Hyland became interested in the study of migraine and epilepsy with the new technique of electroencephalography, or examination of the electrical patterns of the brain.[85]

In the polio epidemic that swept Toronto and the province in the fall of 1937, it was often necessary to put the patients into mechanical respirators, or "iron lungs," which, as Duncan Graham put it, speaking of the work of his colleagues, "prolonged immobilization of the spine and ribs definitely imped[ing] the recovery of the paralysed muscles."[86] Hyland and colleagues made a considerable discovery: that the paralysis of the muscles of respiration in the iron lungs could be lessened with physiotherapy. The team wrote in 1938, "Active movement is probably the most important single factor in the program of physical treatment, calling into play and exercising the entire neuro-muscular unit. Muscle training was commenced as soon as the slightest sign of voluntary contraction could be seen in the muscle."[87]

During the war, Hyland's interests became more expressly psychiatric. In 1942 he and Richardson, from their base at No. 1 Neurological Hospital in England, published an article on "psychoneurosis" among the troops, finding that it constituted "over half the total number of cases." Four-fifths of the patients had "evidence of nervous instability prior to enlistment."[88] In 1949–50 Hyland succeeded Robert G. Armour as head of neurology and as head of the medical service on Ward G of TGH.[89]

Walters, a leading "neuropsychiatrist," which meant training in psychiatry and neurology, was born in Napanee, Ontario, in 1906; he earned a medical degree from the University of Toronto in 1933. He worked for two years at the Ontario Hospital, Whitby, then, after interning at the General, spent several years in England at, among other institutions, the Maudsley and the National Hospital at Queen Square. He was delighted to return to Toronto in 1940 when Graham asked him to cover the neurology service while Hyland and Richardson were off to war. Walters is known in the international literature for his description of a kind of hysteria known as "regional pain syndrome," which he first published in 1959 in the *Journal of the Canadian Psychiatric Association* (and in 1961 in *Brain*).[90] He was "admittedly lacking an immersion in Freudian psychology,"[91] as his eulogists put it somewhat mildly, for psychoanalysis was all the rage after the war, and Walters adhered to a biological concept of psychiatry.

"Ric" Richardson had a similar somatic perspective on psychiatry. Born in 1909 in Owen Sound, J. Clifford Richardson's interest in the brain was strengthened as an undergraduate in medicine by an elective with Eric Linell. After graduating in medicine in 1932, he served a year as autopsy fellow at the Banting Institute under Oskar Klotz, where he decided to specialize in neurology. In the mid-1930s he spent several years at Queen Square, passing his membership examination for the Royal College of Physicians in 1937. Back in Toronto, Richardson and Hyland published a widely cited paper on cerebral ("berry") aneurysms in 1941, based on 118 cases of spontaneous subarachnoid hemorrhage seen at the Toronto General Hospital between 1928 and 1938.[92] (The finding drew the attention of the Toronto neurosurgeons, in particular William Lougheed, who joined the neurosurgery division in 1956 and pioneered operations for, in Cosbie's words, this "far from hopeless condition.")[93] During the war Richardson and Hyland collaborated on a study of psychoneurosis in the military. They were among the early clinicians using electroshock, although they did not introduce it to Toronto.[94] It is thus interesting that Richardson, as many neurologists of his generation, moved at the borderline between neurology and psychiatry. In 1946 Richardson got his fellowship in neurology, and he and Hyland joined Armour on the neurology service on Ward G until it was divided among other public wards in 1948. Thus he and Hyland moved to the Wellesley in 1949, and that hospital came under the suzerainty of the General.

Richardson and Hyland, says historian-neurologist John Wherrett, "were anxious to develop training in neurology"; in 1944 they began to take fellows for a year, many of whom went on for further work at Queen Square.[95]

Richardson made several important scientific contributions, including work in 1951 with Mary Tom in neuropathology on benign islet cell tumours and cerebral hypoglycemia, in which they were first to describe lower motor neuron changes secondary to severe hypoglycemia. "The name 'hypoglycaemic amyotrophy' might be suggested as a suitable one," they said, to describe such "extensive lesions of the lower motor neurons with consequent muscle atrophy."[96] The term caught on. Yet in these years Richardson's interests were veering in the direction of neuropsychiatry, and in 1952 he described "epileptic attacks with predominant psychic symptoms" and the usefulness of the electroencephalogram in differentiating them from "neuroses."[97]

Just as a footnote on the history of electroencephalography in Toronto, the service had begun in 1938, then was discontinued during the war for lack of personnel. After the war, Richardson insisted that it be restored. John Scott was chosen for the post, having trained at the Montreal Neurological Institute and Queen Square in physiology and in clinical encephalography. When in August 1949 Scott returned, he was appointed to re-establish the EEG department, with a post in both physiology and medicine.[98] This represented what Findlay calls "a unique Clinical Neurophysiology Service" for the divisions of neurosurgery and neurology.[99]

In 1959 Richardson, Roger Chambers, and Peter Heywood described the severe brain damage that might accompany an interruption of the cerebral oxygen supply, concluding, "Many of these tragic cases of severe cerebral anoxia and hypoglycemia can be prevented by ... measures such as careful attention to adequate airway in unconscious patients," findings that had a significant impact on emergency medicine.[100] The scientific high point of Richardson's career occurred in 1963 as he, together with Professor Jerzy Olszewski and John Steele, a Toronto neurology resident, described a disease involving dementia (that may resemble an agitated depression), plus defects of ocular gaze and axial dsytonia together with damage in subcortical structures. They labelled the new disease "Progressive Supranuclear Palsy," or PSP.[101]

The psychiatric unit at the Wellesley represented, as psychiatrist Robert Pos put it, "the first major inroad of psychiatry into the teaching general hospitals" and was part of a growing integration of psychiatry into mainstream medicine.[102] Meanwhile, "Psychological Medicine" had snuck back into TGH, in association with the Division of Neurology. The Dean's Report for 1956–7 mentioned "Neurology and Psychological Medicine" as part of the Department of Medicine at the General. But there were no psychiatrists associated with it, only neurologists such as Hyland and Richardson and some internists.[103]

In 1960 the Wellesley became an independent hospital again. It could no longer serve as the neuropsychiatric outpost of the General. The time had come to return psychiatry to the Toronto General Hospital.

*Division of Psychiatry in the Department of Medicine at TGH*

There were essentially two separate departments of psychiatry until 1967: one was based at the Toronto Psychiatric Hospital under the leadership of the professor of psychiatry; the other was based in the Department of Medicine at the Toronto General Hospital and its filial the Wellesley Hospital. Until 1967, the professor of psychiatry had no control over this second track in the General Hospital. The animus against psychiatry in the Department of Medicine at the General had been very deep. In 1951 Stokes said, "The problems of nervous and mental disorder constitute a vast area of study, the development of which is certain to be slow. To many, working in the well-tilled lands of organ medicine, the territory is a rejected wasteland, depreciated for its barren returns."[104]

It was under the aegis of the Wellesley Hospital neurologists, or "neuropsychiatrists," that psychiatry began its return to the General Hospital. In 1960 Richardson left the neuropsychiatric unit at the Wellesley to succeed Hyland as head of neurology at the General.

Simultaneously, Allan Walters left the neuropsychiatric unit at the Wellesley in 1960 to head a separate psychiatric service at the General. Cosbie calls him the "unofficial head of psychiatry at the General Hospital."[105] Wightman, chair of medicine, accepted rather reluctantly that the times were trending towards psychiatry in general hospitals. In 1962 he said, "A Psychiatric Unit at the To-ronto General Hospital seems imminent, after long discussion. The develop-ment of psychiatric units in general hospitals is a matter which seems to find universal support in theory, but presents certain difficulties in practice in a local setting. It is still the feeling of the members of the Department of Medicine that a close liaison between the psychiatrists and the internists in the hospital is a matter of great importance."[106]

By 1960 a psychiatric division had been created at the General as part of the Department of Medicine; interns started rotating between psychiatry at the General and TPH and the Ontario Hospital on Queen Street.[107]

Things started to come together. In 1962 Robert Pos joined Walters, and Stokes, who wished to coordinate psychiatric services among all the teaching hospitals, was said to be strongly behind Pos and Walter's ambitions to establish an auton-omous department of psychiatry.[108] Stokes had organized a General Hospitals Committee in 1963 to liaise between the university department and the hospital departments. In 1966 Walters resigned as chief of the psychiatric service and in 1968 was replaced by Pos, a real firebrand.

Pos came from the Netherlands, where he was born in 1927 in Amsterdam and educated there in medicine, graduating with an MD in 1951. He interned in Amsterdam in 1951–4, came to Canada, and interned at the Toronto General Hospital in 1954–5. He earned a DPsych diploma in 1958, then stayed in Toronto until late in his career (earning, however, a PhD at the University of Utrecht in 1963). From 1958 to 1962 he was a staff psychiatrist at the Ontario Hospital on Queen Street, then joined the psychiatry service at the General, where in 1968 he became psychiatrist-in-chief.

Events were moving in the direction of independence for general hospital psychiatry. At a December 1966 meeting of the Joint Hospitals Committee, the body that coordinated faculty and hospital policies, it was said, "At present, in the general hospitals, psychiatry is considered as a sub-department of Medi-cine. It is now suggested that for optimum development in this area psychiatry should have departmental status ... with the Head of the Department a member of the Medical Advisory Board of the Hospital. It was requested that the admin-istrators inform their hospitals of this new University policy."[109]

*Department of Psychiatry, TGH*

The crucial event in achieving autonomy is authority over one's budget, and in the 1966–7 session the budget for hospital psychiatry was transferred from the Department of Medicine to the Department of Psychiatry.[110] Wightman saw here loss and decline, as he said in 1968: "With the advent of a new Profes-sor of Psychiatry, a valued limb of the Department of Medicine in the teaching hospitals has been amputated and autonomous Departments of Psychiatry are being set up in the hospitals. While this is consonant with the modern trend towards specialization, one regrets the loss of integration which it entails. The same forces are acting to produce a separation of Neurology, Cardiology, and all the rest."[111]

Each of the new Departments of Psychiatry now had a psychiatrist-in-chief. At the General it was, of course, Pos; at Sunnybrook, Wilfred E. Boothroyd; at the New Mount Sinai, Stanley E. Greben; at the Wellesley, R. Ian Hector; at Women's College, Lois M. Plumb; at the Western, Alan J. Preston; and at St Michael's, William J. Stauble. Their theoretical orientations ran from Pos's interest in physiological psychiatry to Greben's in psychoanalysis. It scarcely meant the dominance of psychoanalysis, yet it was a foot in the door.

At the General, it was decided in 1968 to renovate the Burnside building, previously dedicated to obstetrics, "for the purpose of providing 60 psychiatric beds."[112] The space was needed because in 1967 a new provincial Mental Health Act mandated all general hospitals to "provide in-patient care, ambulant patient services, emergency care, day care, and community consultation."[113] In the 1970–1 session an acute psychiatric service was organized at the General.[114]

This was the beginning of a great expansion in hospital psychiatry. By the mid-1980s, under TGH psychiatry chief Paul Garfinkel, there was a mood and nutritional disorders team run by Sidney Kennedy, an acute care team under Robert Buckingham, a general psychiatric unit under David Goldbloom, a self-harm program under Jon Ennis, and a behavioural medicine and anxiety-disorder unit under Richard Swinson. The outpatient division had grown fiercely: the eating disorders program, established in the 1984–5 session, was seeing 300 new patients a year, and the department had added an outpatient clinic for Alzheimer's patients under Harry Karlinsky.[115]

Other hospital psychiatry departments developed more specialized interests, such as psychogeriatrics and adolescent psychiatry at Sunnybrook; psychoanalysis at the Mount Sinai Hospital (in 1984 Stan Greben at Mount Sinai was appointed first professor of psychotherapy[116]); psychophysiology at Toronto Western Hospital; and group therapy at St Michael's Hospital. Indeed, so disparate were some of these interests that the Self-Study of 1983 tattled, "Many [psychiatry] staff were recruited when funding was free and their interests vary enormously, not always in concert with the academic goals of the department. This is particularly true of certain teaching hospitals."[117]

*Psychiatry at the Clarke Institute*

Spread out over two adult mental hospitals and a number of general hospitals, psychiatry at the University of Toronto was a big deal. In 2005, with 686 primary appointments, psychiatry was one of the largest departments in the faculty. The department pulled itself into the academic top drawer in several ways. This began under Robin Hunter.

In 1969–70 Hunter organized a research committee, with G. Peter Brawley as chair. By 1971 some ninety-nine projects were underway.[118] Given that the teaching hospital departments were now all part of the university department, this required a bit of digestion. As well, all the teaching hospitals were said to be "redirecting" their efforts "into community involvement and care."[119]

In the faculty as a whole, "diploma program" usually meant the opposite of "research degree." The Department of Psychiatry now proposed to make research part of the diploma program. In November 1973 psychiatrist Henry B. Kedward told the Faculty Council's Committee on Postgraduate Medical Education, "[We now] provide the basis for a new Diploma with a research emphasis which, it is hoped, will be appropriate to contemporary circumstances." They wanted to encourage scholarship by the residents, which the Royal College exam did not do. "Without this stimulus and aim it is unlikely that many residents will strive for excellence and make special efforts in scholarly enterprises and without the institutional support of a Diploma the few who do pursue scholarly endeavours will be disadvantaged."[120] The department proposed a formal dissertation program.

In 1973 Hunter stepped down to become associate dean of clinical sciences, and in July 1974 Frederick H. Lowy became chair of psychiatry and director of the Clarke Institute. Lowy had been trained as a psychoanalyst yet had an eclectic view of the psychiatric mission, and in his stewardship of psychiatry and later role in the faculty as dean, which he assumed in 1980, he proved himself one of the greatest leaders of the faculty in the post-war period.

Fred Lowy was born in Grosspetersdorf, Austria, in 1933 and fled the Holocaust aboard a ship named the *Serpa Pinto* to Canada; Lowy was, as a journalist noted, "among the few hundred Jews Canada accepted during the Nazi advance across Europe."[121] Lowy earned an arts degree from McGill in 1955 and an MD in 1959. He took his medical training at the Royal Victoria Hospital in Montreal and his psychiatric training at the Cincinnati General Hospital, long a fortress of psychoanalytic thought, from 1962 to 1965. He returned to Montreal as a demonstrator in the Department of Psychiatry at McGill; there from 1965 to 1970 he completed his analytic apprenticeship at the Canadian Institute of Psychoanalysis. In 1971 Lowy was called to the Ottawa Civic Hospital, an important psychiatric hospital, as psychiatrist-in-chief and, as stated, came to Toronto in 1974 as professor of psychiatry and director of the Clarke Institute. In Toronto, he was very much a new broom.

Lowy tried to deepen the involvement of psychiatry in undergraduate education and told the long-range planners in December 1974, "Psychiatric experience is gained only over a long period of time and therefore block teaching is not entirely appropriate to Psychiatry ... 70 to 80% of patients have emotional problems, many of which could be treated by family physicians rather than requiring a psychiatrist." He continued, "Many family practitioners received their training in psychiatry in settings not appropriate to the type of problems they are likely to encounter in daily practice."[122]

Just as Lowy's deanship would be characterized by a drive towards research, so was his chairmanship. After taking office in 1974, Lowy appointed Harvey Stancer to a chair as research professor; under Lowy, Stancer served as research coordinator for the department, presiding over a two-story research building next to the twelve-story tower, funding coming heavily from the Ontario Mental Health Foundation.[123] Lowy was entirely sympathetic to the biological side of the discipline and in February 1978 promoted Donald V. Coscina, a PhD psychologist (who later departed for Wayne State University), "to Head of the new section of Biopsychology Research ... The goal of this interdisciplinary section is to design and perform experiments with animals which promote further understanding of behavioural and biological factors in human mental illnesses."[124]

Forensic psychiatry was another Lowy initiative. In May 1977 the Metropolitan Toronto Forensic Service was inaugurated as the result of an Ontario Government Order-in Council. Located at the Queen Street Mental Health Centre (formerly the Ontario Hospital, Toronto) and operated by the Clarke Institute, "METFORS" employed R. Edward Turner as psychiatrist-in-charge, professor of forensic psychiatry, and director. The Forensic Psychiatry Division of the Clarke consisted of, as one source put it, "the forensic service of the Clarke Institute, the family court clinic of the Clarke Institute and the forensic service at QSMHC. This constitutes what is probably the largest integrated university teaching service in forensic psychiatry in North America." A rapid assessment unit to help the courts, it comprised twenty-three beds to assess and treat thirty- to sixty-day referrals.[125]

In 1980 Vivian Rakoff succeeded Lowy as chair of psychiatry, and if there were to be a prize for the most engaging, reflective, and articulate speaker and writer among the faculty leadership in those years, Rakoff would win it hands down, for his wit and off-hand wisdom are recalled with great fondness. He was not an analyst. Born in Cape Town, South Africa, in 1928, Rakoff earned two arts degrees – the MA in 1949 – at the University of Cape Town. He came to London in 1950–1 as a psychologist at the Tavistock Clinic, receiving an MB from the University of London in 1957. He interned in London, then trained in psychiatry back home again at the Grote Schuur Hospital from 1958 to 1961. Coming to Canada in 1961, he apprenticed at McGill until 1963, then at the Jewish General Hospital, passing from associate director of research from 1963 to 1967 to professor of psychiatry in 1968. In 1974 he accepted a position as professor of psychiatric education in the Department of Psychiatry at Toronto, was psychiatrist-in-chief at Sunnybrook from 1978 to 1980, then became professor, chair of the Department of Psychiatry, and director of the Clarke Institute in 1980. Rakoff published widely on a range of topics from the experiences of concentration camp inmates to adolescent psychiatry. Yet his name may be best remembered for the positron emission tomography (PET) centre named after him – opened in 1992 under Sylvain Houle – for which Rakoff ardently lobbied the provincial government and which helped raise Toronto's profile significantly in the world of biological research.

During Rakoff's tenure, the tension that had been simmering between psychotherapeutic and social approaches on the one hand and neurobiological on the other came to the surface. In 1985 external examiners expressed concern about an evident underdevelopment of biological approaches to brain and mind. Rakoff responded defensively, "My personal feeling is that we have, as a Department, bridged the gap between neuropsyche and neurosoma. However, I feel a small but nagging concern, that in our enthusiastic entry into the neurobiological side of our discipline, we may forget our equally important commitment to psychosocial issues."[126] The neuropsyche had become well nigh extinct in many American departments of psychiatry. Rakoff struggled to keep it alive in Toronto.

In 1990 Paul Garfinkel succeeded Rakoff as professor of psychiatry. It is an interesting comment on the distance between the general-hospital and asylum branches of Toronto psychiatry that he was the only psychiatrist-in-chief at the General ever to have ascended to the university chair. Garfinkel was an international expert on eating disorders and an eminently scholarly figure. During his tenure, several organizational changes took place. In March 1997 the Health Services Restructuring Commission of Ontario, established in 1996, recommended merging into a single corporation the Addiction Research Foundation, the Clarke Institute of Psychiatry, the Queen Street Mental Health Centre, and the Donwood Institute (for the treatment of addiction disorders founded by R. Gordon Bell –"the man who first brought Antabuse to Canada" – in 1967[127]). In November 1997 Garfinkel became president and CEO of the new corporation which, the following year, was named the Centre for Addiction and Mental Health (CAMH).

On Garfinkel's watch, the department began to profile itself in research on psychopharmacology, especially the work of Shitij Kapur and Gary Remington, acolytes of pharmacologist Phil Seeman (see pp. 441–442), on the dopamine and serotonin systems in schizophrenia.[128] Together with Robert Zipursky and PET scan specialist Sylvain Houle, they established in 1996 that low doses of the antipsychotic drug haloperidol might be quite adequate to treat a psychotic episode, because at low doses the D2 receptor (dopamine receptor), apparently important in the therapeutic response, was almost completely occupied with molecules of the drug.[129]

Donald Wasylenki succeeded Garfinkel as chair of the department in 2000. Wasylenki, who earned his MD from the University of Saskatchewan in 1971 and trained at Toronto (also receiving a master's degree and psychoanalytic training), was a leading research specialist in community psychiatry and the organization of mental health services. During Wasylenki's tenure, the department grew greatly, sprawling by 2009 across eight fully affiliated teaching hospitals. Its residency program was the largest in North America. It had seventeen endowed chairs and two endowed professorships. In 2003 Wasylenki established a clinical-scientist training program on the model of those in medicine and surgery, and by 2009 twenty-seven residents were pursuing PhDs. External assessors praised "the consolidation of the neuroscience program," which included "the fields of combined genetic and neuroimaging, pharmacogenetics, epigenetics, and animal models of schizophrenia" – this in contrast to the heyday of psychoanalysis in the 1970s.

An external review in 1999 found the Department of Psychiatry at the top of its game. Seven percent of medical students at U of T went into psychiatry, compared to the North American average of around five. The postgraduate program was said to be "the largest on the continent." The reviewers were somewhat dismayed that the department "is not quite as prominent internationally as one would expect from its size." Yet the silver lining was that "[t]his reflects a process of transition, in which a department that had been primarily clinical is being converted into a research centre." Paul Garfinkel, the chair at the time, was rather stung at the accusation that the department lacked international prominence and pointed to "the huge amount of funding that comes to the Department from international peer-reviewed sources ... and the many spectacular people we have recruited and developed over the decade and their prominence in the international arena."[130]

Indeed, in the next years the department leapt ahead in research. An external review in 2004 said, "The research effort in the Department of Psychiatry ... has been outstanding," and "[t]he department is now amongst the top few productive departments in the Faculty of Medicine." The Clinician Scientist Training Program was seen as the crown jewel of the research effort, "one of the outstanding initiatives of the current Chair's [Wasylenki's] tenure, and should go a long way to ensure the development of a cadre of young, academic psychiatrists to be the next and future leaders of academic psychiatry in Canada."[131]

*Ontario Hospital, Queen Street*

The Toronto asylum was the birthplace of psychiatry at the faculty. Yet the founding of TPH essentially short-circuited the asylum from academic psychiatry. The slow reintegration of this historic asylum into the life of the faculty began in the 1951–2 session, as a new academic unit was authorized at the Ontario Hospital, Queen Street, "which will be accorded university status as a teaching mental hospital." Eric Linell, the founder of neuropathology in Toronto, began making periodic visits to the unit.[132]

Late in the 1950s, life at Queen Street began to take on the spirit of the times. In the spring of 1959, Donald J. McCulloch was, according to Robert Pos, "conducting his own unique experiment in psychiatric ambulatory care with Farrell

Toombs," who was a professor of human relations at the university.[133] McCulloch graduated in medicine from U of T in 1948, earned a diploma in psychiatry, and came to run the Community Mental Health clinic at the hospital, which then had the address 999 Queen Street West. This was the beginning of community psychiatry in Toronto, with an alternative flavour.

In the 1967–8 session, the Ontario Hospital, Toronto, changed its name to the Queen Street Mental Health Centre.[134] Simultaneously the asylum experienced a complete reorganization, as active treatment was separated from the "infirmary-nursing-domiciliary programs," and treatment teams moved out to various areas of the city of Toronto.[135] With the founding of CAMH, "Queen Street" became seamlessly reintegrated into academic psychiatry, and the old buildings, with part of the much-admired historic brick walls still about them, thus completed a century and a half of evolution from one of the most regressive aspects of psychiatric care in Toronto to among the most progressive.

### Department of Psychiatry at the Hospital for Sick Children

In January 1937 a clinic "for the mental care and adjustment of problems during childhood" opened at the children's hospital, its complement drawn from the full-time staff of the Department of Paediatrics.[136] Under Stokes in the 1948–9 session, this clinic became incorporated into the postgraduate training program of the university Department of Psychiatry. Said Stokes in 1949, "This extension of training facilities will allow a focusing on the problems of functional illness in children."[137] In the 1950s William A. Hawke, a U of T medical graduate of 1930, headed the "neurology and psychiatry" service of the Department of Paediatrics (he was also director of developmental pediatrics from 1968 to 1972), with a special interest in "childhood schizophrenia." In the 1967–8 session a formal Department of Psychiatry was established at HSC under Hawke, who then stepped down in September 1968 as Quentin Rae-Grant became psychiatrist-in-chief and professor of child psychiatry.[138]

Born in Aberdeen in 1929 and a medical graduate of that university in 1951, Rae-Grant had trained first in surgery at Aberdeen, then in psychiatry at the Maudsley, receiving his diploma in 1958. He served as the director of child psychiatry at the Jewish Hospital in St Louis, was on staff at Johns Hopkins University, had several research posts including chief of the social psychiatry section at the National Institute of Mental Health in Bethesda, Maryland, before coming to Toronto. Previously, the Division of Psychological Medicine of the Department of Paediatrics had been headed by William Hawke; at the time that Rae-Grant came to Toronto as inaugural departmental head, there were two other full-time psychiatrists in the department and several part-time, who already had a child psychiatry training program in place with three residents at child settings across Metro Toronto.

With ample funding available, Rae-Grant built the department to nine full-time psychiatrists by 1985 and numerous part-time appointees. He organized a consultation service to the child abuse and sexual abuse programs. Seven regional centres were affiliated with the university department, including twenty-one residents. The diploma program in child psychiatry, initiated in 1972, involved a dissertation, and residents were taught by the head of their dissertation committee to do research, presenting their results at an annual Child Psychiatry Day. Rae-Grant encouraged active research programs in all the centres and with "very substantial outside grant support." As a result, individuals from around the world began coming to Toronto for training in the Child Psychiatry Diploma Program. In a review of North American programs in child psychiatry in the early 1980s, Toronto ranked second. In 1977 Paul Steinhauer and Rae-Grant produced a popular text, *Psychological Problems of the Child and His Family*, published in Toronto by Macmillan. It was brought out in 1983 as *Psychological Problems of the Child in the Family* in a greatly expanded and revised edition by Basic Books.[139] Steinhauer later became director of postgraduate training in child psychiatry. He was a collaborator in composing the Family Assessment Measure (FAM) – which became widely used internationally. He later initiated the Sparrow Lake Alliance and Voices for Children.[140]

In the 1971–2 session a Mental Health Clinic at HSC "blossom[ed] into full operation. This clinic, a part of the General Medical Clinic, provides immediate access to psychiatric assistance by Dr. Saul Levine from the Department of Psychiatry. It allows us to assess severe behaviour disorders and identify specific psychoses at their onset," said Rae-Grant.[141]

In 1976 an Adolescent Unit was opened, under great admissions pressure with the closure of a comparable unit at Queen Street. Klaus Minde led the department's efforts in infant psychiatry and William Wehrspann in the treatment of sexually abused children. Rae-Grant himself was to become a national leader in psychiatry and president of the Canadian Psychiatric Association in 1982–3.[142] In 1987 he accepted the chair of child psychiatry at the University of Western Ontario.

### Alcohol and Drug Addiction Foundation/Addiction Research Foundation

The Alcoholism Research Foundation (ARF) was established in 1949 by a provincial act to do research on treatment and rehabilitation in alcoholism. H. David Archibald, a social worker with a degree in alcoholism studies from Yale, was hired by the Liquor Control Board of Ontario as the foundation's first executive director. Given that a tenth of the total provincial health budget was expended on the effects of alcoholism, this was not an unwarranted deployment of resources. The first facility, Brookside Hospital, was opened in 1951. Three years later, ARF organized in-house research. In 1961 the foundation expanded its mission to include drugs, becoming the Alcoholism and Drug Addiction Research Foundation, then shortened to Addiction Research Foundation.

Reg Smart, a scientist, recalled an international meeting organized by ARF in those early days. "It was exciting to think just everybody who knew anything about the alcohol studies field was in this one room. Of course, a few years later with the development of the ARF and with the development of the institutes in the United States and other countries, you would need a very, very big room to have all of the experts. Now, probably, there's no room in the world that would contain them all."[143]

The ARF was not a part of the university, yet Archibald wanted a strong connection to it. (He also wanted to distance the foundation from Alcoholics Anonymous, or AA.) The foundation's medical staff were cross-appointed through the Department of Medicine and held faculty appointments; the university had the right to approve all clinical staff. For example, in the session 1964–5 John L. Silversides at the Toronto Western Hospital, a neurologist in the Department of Medicine, became chief physician.[144]

It would take the narrative too far afield to review the history of this important agency. But in 1971 an eighty-bed Clinical Institute to combine care and research was established at ARF; this was the clinical research division of the foundation and was considered a teaching hospital of the Faculty of Medicine. Many clinical staff held cross-appointments between the Research Division of the ARF and the Clinical Institute.[145] The foundation also had a long-term contractual agreement with the Department of Pharmacology to finance the research of the ARF scientists interested in basic research in alcoholism and drug topics. In 1974 four full-time pharmacologists, plus technicians and graduate students, were seconded to ARF, their salaries paid by the foundation. Indeed, much of the pharmacology research budget stemmed from the foundation.[146] With the Department of Psychiatry – within shouting distance of the ARF after the opening of the Clarke Institute at the corner of College Street and Spadina Avenue – there had typically been little interaction. In 1998, however, ARF was merged into the Centre for Addiction and Mental Health.

## Neurology

The complexity of the central and peripheral nervous systems and the incredible array of diseases that can affect them results in Neurology being divided into more subspecialty fields than probably any other branch of medicine.[147]

Anthony Lang, 2006

Unlike many other centres, neurology in Toronto was a division of the Department of Medicine and neither a department of its own, nor – unlike in German-speaking Europe where neurology began – a part of psychiatry. The classic German term was "nerve doctor" (*Nervenarzt*), meaning combined expertise in nervous system and behavioural disorders. In Canada, neurology belonged traditionally to internal medicine and not to psychiatry. Yet without a doubt, in Toronto as everywhere else, neurologists saw plenty of patients whose problems were psychiatric rather than organic but who did not wish the stigma of being diagnosed as "mentally ill."

The story of academic neurology in Toronto goes back to 1892, when neurologist Donald Campbell Meyers was appointed to the newly founded St Michael's Hospital. Meyers, who graduated from Trinity Medical College in 1888 and became a licentiate of the Royal College of Physicians of London the following year, opened his own private sanatorium on Simcoe Street in 1894 (which in 1897 moved north to Heath Street, then on the outskirts of the city, and became "Dr Meyers' Neurological Hospital"). In 1905 he was still also serving as "Neurologist to St Michael's Hospital."

In 1906, as seen, Meyers persuaded the province to establish the twelve-bed "Nervous Wards " at TGH.[148] (In a reflection of how entwined were the early roots of psychiatry and neurology, the Department of Psychiatry at the Toronto General Hospital was named "The Campbell Meyers Department" at its beginning in 1967.) The wards were closed in 1911 as TGH moved to a new location. Evidently unhappy with this closure, in 1911 an anonymous individual offered an "entirely unsolicited" grant of $2,500 towards the founding of a "Neurological Pavilion" in the new TGH buildings then going up on College Street.[149] In 1914 this pavilion became a neurological clinic with Goldwin Howland at its helm.[150]

By 1920 this clinic had turned into the "sub-department of Neurology" in the Department of Medicine. Said a later account, "Since 1919 [Goldwin Howland] has been in charge of teaching in Neurology and Psychological Medicine."[151] A 1920 document from the Department of Medicine referred to "the proposed Sub-department of Neurology," where "50 percent of their [time will be devoted] to teaching and hospital work, 50 percent to research."[152]

Howland was born in Toronto in 1875 into a prominent family whose ancestors included Sir William P. Howland, a father of Confederation, and William H. Howland, a mayor of Toronto (who, it is said, helped the city through his reform efforts to acquire the name "Toronto the Good"). "Goldie" Howland graduated in medicine in 1900, having spent the summer of his second year as a medical officer at the Brockville Asylum for the Insane. He trained in neurology in London, acquiring membership in the Royal College of Surgeons in 1905 among other English qualifications; he also studied in Berlin. One biographer calls him "the first consulting neurologist in Canada."[153] He co-described, along with Walter Campbell and Ernest Maltby, "dysinsulinism" from an islet cell tumour in 1929, a tumour that Roscoe Graham successfully resected (see p. 119).

A major neurological appointment at the General was, as has been seen, Herbert Hylton Hyland, who joined the Department of Medicine in 1930. He, Richardson, and Walters formed the nucleus of neuropsychiatry at the Wellesley

Hospital discussed earlier. In the late 1930s they and others congregated in an informal organization called the "Thirteen Club" to discuss common interests in the "neurological sciences."[154] Yet neurology remained weak. In 1945 McKenzie said, "More team work is necessary in some hospitals before really strong departments worthy of attracting post-graduate students, can be developed. I believe that neurology is one example – at the moment in the U. of T. there is little or no team work in this important subject."[155]

After the war, Richardson and Hyland worked under Robert Armour, whose own appointment went back to 1919 in Howland's neurology clinic.[156] They were in Ward G, the neurology section of the Department of Medicine, until Farquharson, who wished to discourage the medical subspecialties, divided that ward in 1948 among the public wards at the Toronto General Hospital.[157] Shortly thereafter, Richardson and Hyland went over to the Wellesley Hospital to found in 1949 the new neuropsychiatry service. In the same year Hyland succeeded Armour as head of neurology at the university and as senior physician in charge of neurology and psychiatry at the Toronto General Hospital.

At the General, with the opening of the new Centre Block (later the Urquhart Wing) in 1958, neurology obtained a teaching service of its own. After 1960 Richardson built a formidable training program for neurologists, which was now considered entirely separate from psychiatry (the last reference to the unit for "Neurology and Psychological Medicine" occurs in 1956–7).[158] His colleague John Wherrett said at the time of Richardson's death in 1986, "As much as any individual, 'Ric' Richardson influenced training of neurologists in Canada … He took a very personal role in the instruction of trainees in the clinical discipline of neurology." Wherrett recalled, "On Monday evenings throughout the fall, trainees joined Dr. Richardson and his wife in the living room of their charming house perched on the side of a Toronto ravine [on Avondale Road in Rosedale] for 'fireside seminars,' presented by the trainees and followed by refreshments. These popular occasions gave the trainees and the Richardsons an opportunity to get to know each other well, and established a tradition since maintained." "The culmination of his efforts," said Wherrett, "was the establishment of the Chair in Neurology [1982], for which he was the first incumbent."[159]

Richardson intended to retire in 1975, and as this time approached Hollenberg, head of medicine, said that it was urgent "to recruit a replacement for Dr. J.C. Richardson as Director of the Division of Neurology, Toronto General Hospital. This appointment is probably one of the most important of its kind in the country and a good deal of care will have to be taken."[160]

In 1975 John Wherrett succeeded Richardson as director of the university Division of Neurology. Wherrett, a Queen's graduate in 1955, had in 1963 established the first neurochemistry lab at the General, with particular interest in the genetics of the lipid storage diseases. In the 1984–5 session, he was succeeded by John G. Humphrey.

The Division of Neurology booked a number of important scientific contributions. Anthony E.T. Lang specialized in movement disorders and cast new light upon the "Parkinson Puzzle." Lang, who in 2000 occupied the Jack Clark Chair at the U of T's Centre for Research in Neurodegenerative Disease, completed a medical degree at the University of Toronto in 1975, then trained in neurology at Toronto and in movement disorders at Kings College Hospital and the Institute of Psychiatry in London. After his return to Toronto in 1982, he originated the movement disorders clinic at the Toronto Western Hospital, which became the largest such clinic in Canada and of worldwide importance. In 1997 a team led by Lang and neurosurgeon Andres Lozano proposed pallidotomy in the management of advanced Parkinson's disease ("significantly reduces levodopa-induced dyskinesias and off-period disability").[161] Lang in general was associated with the view that efforts to restore dopamine were insufficient to arrest the progression of the disease and that a "multisystem" approach should guide the therapeutics.[162]

Peter Carlen was a major figure in the understanding of the basic neurobiology of brain disease. Born in Edmonton in 1943, Carlen earned an MD at the University of Toronto in 1967, then trained in medicine at the Montreal General Hospital and in neurology at the Toronto General Hospital. He fellowed at the neurobiological unit of Hebrew University in Jerusalem between 1972 and 1974. Returning to Toronto, he headed the neurology program at the Addiction Research Foundation and served as staff neurologist at the Toronto Western Hospital. In 1989 he became director of the Playfair Neuroscience Unit at the Western. Among Carlen's achievements was the discovery in 1978 of the reversibility of brain damage from alcoholism with abstinence;[163] the 1999 discovery that intracellular calcium regulation is altered and raised in aging neurons;[164] and the discovery in 2002 that a form of mental retardation known as "fragile X" is related to a decrease in expression of the glutamate receptor subunit GluR1 glutamate.[165]

James A. Sharpe had an important international reputation in neuro-ophthalmology and was director of the Neuro-opthalmology and Neuro-otology Centre at the University Health Network. Born in Brantford, Ontario, Sharpe finished medical studies at the University of Western Ontario in 1966, began his training in medicine at McGill and the Royal Victoria Hospital in Montreal, then between 1968 and 1972 completed a residency in neurology, neuropathology, and ophthalmology at U of T. After fellowing in neuro-ophthalmology at St Michael's, the Bascom Palmer Eye Institute at the University of Miami, the University of California in San Francisco, and Queen Square at the University of London, Sharpe became head of the Division of Neurology at Toronto Western Hospital in 1986, then of the University Health Network. Sharpe was known for his work in disruptions of the smooth-pursuit mechanism of the eye and the mechanism of nystagmus,[166] and he took a leadership role in numerous neurological societies and journals at the national and international level. He was probably the leading Canadian neuro-ophthalmologist.

The Division of Neurology wanted to break free of the Department of Medicine, just as the cardiologists and other divisions were straining to do. In 1973 "responsibility for appointments and coordination of academic programmes in neurology at the teaching hospitals [was] delegated by the Chairman of the Department of Medicine to the Professor of Neurology."[167] This meant de facto independence. Then there were mergers, forced by financial pressure of the kind that other departments were experiencing as well. In the 1984–5 session, the academic activities of the neurology divisions of the General Hospital, HSC, and the Mount Sinai all became "integrated ... in an attempt to maximize the resources of the three institutions."[168]

During these years neurology was pulled in two directions: one by those such as Wherrett who wanted to see it established as a separate department and one by those in the Department of Medicine and the Dean's Office who wanted instead to see a campus neuroscience program arise of which neurology would be the clinical arm.

In March 1987, a dean's committee chaired by Bill Tatton proposed formation of a Department of Neurology. Charged with developing neuroscience at U of T, the committee was "to determine how best to bring the rapid explosion of fundamental neuroscience research into the clinical sector in a more effective way. The committee examined various options and concluded that the best approach was the creation of a Department of Neurology with ... a strong scientific component." The back-and-forth after this time-bomb landed on the table was interesting: Gerard Burrow, head of medicine, was opposed, wanting neurology to remain a division of the Department of Medicine. Bernie Langer in principle objected "to the breaking up of departments into smaller segments." He gave the example of neurosurgery, which had autonomy yet remained in the Department of Surgery. He didn't think "that providing departmental status for Neurology [was] ... the right approach toward achieving the goal." Yet he agreed with Burrow that they needed "to move at an early stage to a programme in Clinical Neuroscience."[169]

The neurologists themselves formed a committee under Jim Sharpe to consider the issue. Dean Lowy was sympathetic to their idea of constituting a separate department, and the clinical chairs' committee voted in May 1987 to approve "the establishment of a Department of Clinical Neurological Sciences."[170] In 1988 a spokesperson for The Toronto Hospital said, "During the past year, the Faculty announced its intention to establish a Department of Neurology. Final arrangements have not yet been completed." "The University of Toronto," it noted, "is possibly the only medical centre of stature in the world that does not have a Department of Neurology or Neurosciences. The new Department is planned initially at The Toronto Hospital."[171] Yet it didn't happen. When Sharpe became division director of neurology at The Toronto Hospital in 1989, he told

Dean Dirks that the neurologists wanted to be a department of their own, not a division within a Department of Neuroscience.[172] Dirks stonewalled the neurology department idea on the grounds that "we should first solve the financial problems of the Neurosciences before we embark on the whole academic process."[173] The new department was stillborn, and the division of neurology has remained to this writing part of the Department of Medicine.

The story is part and parcel of the failure of the neurosciences to make institutional headway at the University of Toronto. Indeed, there is a rather poignant note from Associate Dean Joe Marotta to Dirks in June 1990, lamenting that since 1981 "the superb neuroscience department" that once was hoped for "has consisted of fits and starts, hope, lack of hope, anger, joy, academic justification, status quo ... but no finalization." Marotta concluded his letter, "As I leave the office, I am deeply saddened by my inability to make progress in this area."[174]

## Neurosurgery

Neurosurgery, of course, is a division of the Department of Surgery. But its history fits better here. This story left off in 1958 in chapter 5, with the opening of the new neurosurgical unit at TGH and the jubilation attending the rise of a successful young field. The narrative thread here is the coalescing of the various "neuro" specialties into a clinical neuroscience unit, though it would take a long time before it was called that.

When Harry Botterell returned to the General after the war, his first task, according to neurosurgeon Max Findlay, was to "convince McKenzie of the need for a neuroradiologist." McKenzie had hitherto been reading his own films and thought that quite adequate. The epicentre of Canadian neuroradiology in those days was the Montreal Neurological Institute (MNI) at McGill, and a series of its graduates found their way to Toronto. Douglas C. Eaglesham was the first, appointed in 1945 and said to have "raised the whole standard of neuroradiological diagnosis at the Toronto General Hospital." Delbert Wollin, another MNI graduate, succeeded Eaglesham in 1948, and when Wollin left TGH for a post in Calgary in 1959, George Wortzman, another MNI trainee, filled his shoes.[175]

Wollin recalled the neurosurgical operating room ("D-OR"): "Harry [Botterell] would sit there with a cup of coffee while his residents were operating. God help them if they did not tell him if they got into trouble. But he did not interfere with them, and Dr McKenzie didn't either. It was quite a contrast from my own training [at the MNI] where it sometimes seemed that the neurosurgery residents could come and go but never turn a bone flap. At the General Hospital the residents were given the responsibility, with very careful supervision, of treating brain tumors, herniated discs and all this sort of stuff."[176]

On 8 November 1958, the new Neurosurgical Unit was dedicated at TGH. In the ceremony, Kergin "paid tribute to the major part that Robert Janes had played in establishing the department within the General Hospital and the disciplines which had contributed to its progress: Eric Linell and Mary Tom had established neuropathology; Douglas Eaglesham and Delbert Wollin had organized neurological radio-diagnosis; and John Scott brought with him from England electroencephalography. But, said Kergin, it was the close liaison with the neurologists Herbert Hyland, JC Richardson and Allan Walters, that had contributed since the pre-war era to the clinical and research study of the patients and which had established the value of having this surgical division embodied in the General Hospital."[177]

William Lougheed offered one source of continuity from the old unit to the new. In the 1960s he pioneered the use of the microscope during brain surgery, reporting in 1969 a series of forty patients with ruptured aneurysms "repaired with the operating diploscope."[178] As Findlay and Robin Humphreys judged these achievements, "Bill was a world pioneer in hypothermic brain protection from cerebral circulation arrest and he became one of the world's first, and certainly Canada's first neurosurgeon, to bring the microscope into the operating theatre. Microneurosurgery was born."[179]

In 1971 Lougheed made history by performing a venous bypass graft of an occluded internal carotid artery, in a patient whose internal carotid artery on the other side was also almost completely occluded. (The internal carotid arteries supply blood to the front part of the brain.) He took a leg vein (a piece of the saphenous vein) to construct the anastomosis. The success of the operation emboldened the neurosurgeons: "We would now be prepared to do an endarterectomy [an excision of the plaque-thickened wrapping of an artery] on ... the intracranial carotid artery since this is not difficult and allows a satisfactory anastomosis to be completed. This operation is a long and tedious one."[180] (An anastomosis is joining two blood vessels.) In the early 1970s, says Findlay, Lougheed started to run out of energy. Yet it was as late as 1989 that he performed his last operation. In 1990 neurosurgery was transferred to the Toronto Western Hospital.

In 1963 Tom Morley became head of the Toronto General Hospital Division of Neurosurgery – the flagship division – and would lead his colleagues for the next fifteen years, until 1979. He also headed the university division. Born in Manchester, Morley studied medicine at Oxford, graduating with an MB in 1943. He trained in neurosurgery at Manchester with Sir Geoffrey Jefferson and emigrated to Toronto in 1952, qualifying for his Canadian Royal College Fellowship in 1953 (he already was a fellow of the Royal College of Surgeons in England). He consulted at Sunnybrook between 1954 and 1960 when it was still a veterans hospital, then joined the neurosurgery division at the General. Under his chairmanship at the hospital, some fifty neurosurgeons finished their training.

In 1979 Alan Hudson assumed leadership of the university division, introducing the surgery department's surgical-scientist program to the division. In the

1982–3 session, Ron Tasker succeeded Morley as hospital division head. Tasker, born in 1927, had grown up in Toronto, finishing his medical degree in 1952 and training both in neurosurgery and in physiology in the Banting and Best Department of Medical Research. He was a McLaughlin travelling fellow at the Massachusetts General Hospital and the University of Wisconsin in 1959–60, joining the staff at the General in 1961, where he was a Markle Scholar. Griff Pearson called Tasker's stereotactic surgery program "almost unique" in Canada and "one of the major units in North America."[181] (Stereotactic surgery uses a system of three-dimensional coordinates to locate the exact site in the brain to be operated on.) Among other achievements, Tasker is known for co-authoring, with Philip L. Gildenberg, the *Textbook of Stereotactic and Functional Neurosurgery* (1998).

Under the leadership of Tasker and Hudson, neurosurgery participated in the explosive growth that swept imaging and other modes of investigation in the 1980s. In the 1982–3 session a neurosurgical intensive care unit opened at the General; available in the division were CT-guided stereotactic neurosurgery that obviated the need for ventriculography, the previous painful technique that involved injecting air into the central nervous system (CNS), then turning the patient upside down so that it could circulate through the ventricles; there came as well intraoperative ultrasound, the use of evoked potentials during operations to guide the treatment of CNS lesions, and "a program for cerebrovascular embolization procedures in otherwise intractable lesions."[182] (The ventricles in the brain contain the cerebrospinal fluid.)

With the appointment of Chris Wallace in 1988–9 at the Toronto Western Hospital, a Cerebrovascular Research Laboratory came into being, that, together with the neuroradiologists and radiotherapists, anchored the University of Toronto Brain Vascular Malformation Study Group.[183]

In 1988 the two neurosurgery divisions at TWH and TGH merged; Charles Tator succeeded Alan Hudson as head of the university Division of Neurosurgery. In the 1990–1 session he became the Leslie Dan Professor of Neurosurgery and the head of the hospital division as well as of the university division. The Toronto Western site was chosen for several reasons. As Tator later said, "A basic and clinical neuroscience research unit, which already contained three major neurosurgical laboratories, was located at Toronto Western. Another factor was that a major new neuroradiological facility containing clinical and research magnetic resonance units and new neuroangiography suites had been constructed there." The TGH trauma unit was transferred to TWH.[184]

Tator, born in 1936, had grown up in Toronto and earned a medical degree from the U of T in 1961 and a PhD in neuropathology in 1965. He was co-director of the Playfair Neuroscience Unit and had a lively research interest in spinal injuries, a Toronto tradition going back to Albin Jousse at the Christie Street Hospital.

In the 1995–6 session, under Tator's direction, interhospital subspecialty committees in spinal neurosurgery and peripheral nerve surgery were established.

Michael Fehlings headed the spinal committee, which envisioned multicentre trials of decompression for acute cord injury.

Fehlings became one of the key neuroscience players in the new century. A U of T medical graduate in 1983, he trained in surgery at Queen's University from 1983 to 1984, then in neurosurgery at U of T from 1984 to 1990. He earned a PhD from the Institute of Medical Science in 1989 under the supervision of Charles Tator with a thesis on calcium channel blockade and direct current electrical stimulation in promoting recovery from experimental spinal injuries. In 1990 he became a Fellow of the Royal College. In 1988 he had joined the spinal injury research lab of the Playfair Neuroscience Unit, then fellowed from 1991 to 1992 in the neurosurgery research lab of the New York University Medical Center. In 1992 he came on staff in the Department of Surgery and as a staff neuroscientist at Playfair. He became the holder of the Robert O. Lawson Chair in Neural Repair and Regeneration at the Western in 1999 and simultaneously research director of the Division of Neurosurgery.

As a result of this spinal research, mortality in spinal cord injury was reduced from 40 percent in the early 1980s to approximately 5 percent by 2008. (One bears in mind, of course, that mortality in such injuries was being reduced in most developed countries in these years. Still, it was an achievement.) In the fall of 2008 a University of Toronto Spinal Program was founded, under the co-leadership of Fehlings of the Division of Neurosurgery and Albert Yee of the Division of Orthopedic Surgery.[185]

When in 1999 William Hutchison, together with a team that included neurosurgeons Ron Tasker and Andres Lozano and physiologist Jonathan Dostrovsky, discovered the first cortical pain neurons in the cingulate cortex, it ended up on the front page of the *Globe and Mail* as well as in *Nature Neuroscience*.[186] Hutchison embodied perfectly the rewards of appointing basic scientists in the Department of Surgery. He did an MSc in pharmacology with Harold Kalant, then a PhD in Canberra, Australia, in a lab founded by Sir John Eccles, Nobel Prize winner in 1963 for his work in neurophysiology. After further study in Germany, Hutchison returned to Toronto in 1992 to work with Jonathan Dostrovsky on the neurophysiology of pain in animal models. He also scrubbed in with Ron Tasker in thalamic surgery. "This discovery," said Val Cabral, research program coordinator of the Department of Surgery, "involved the development of basic research describing the alterations in basal ganglia neurophysiology with Parkinson's disease, dystonia and other movement disorders."[187]

In 1996 at the Toronto Western Hospital, neurosurgeon Mark Bernstein, a 1976 graduate of the University of Ottawa, performed the first outpatient awake craniotomy in the world (inpatient awake craniotomy in Canada having been pioneered by Wilder Penfield at McGill in the 1920s), beginning a series that would include forty-six outpatient awake craniotomies by 2000. Bernstein concluded, "The procedure may be psychologically less traumatic to patients than standard craniotomy for brain tumour."[188]

The neurosurgery division became a powerhouse in the Department of Surgery. In July 1999 James Rutka at the Hospital for Sick Children was appointed chair of the division.[189] Under Rutka, the division became "one of the strongest programs in North America." It received annual grants in the order of $5 to 8 million. Its huge volumes of over 7,000 operations per year were more than double those of its US competitors. The division had seven chairs and Rutka would add several more.[190]

### Division of Neurosurgery, HSC

The neurosurgical advances which have emanated from Sick Kids have reached nearly every neurosurgeon who has operated upon a child.[191]

Richard Ellenbogen, 2007

By the late 1950s, pediatric neurosurgery was beginning to take on a distinct identity in such centres as London, Paris, Boston, Chicago, and Toronto, which had free-standing children's hospitals with dedicated pediatric neurosurgeons. "But then," writes Robin Humphreys, "it was not uncommon for surgeons operating upon children also to carry a part-time adult practice. Nonetheless, the momentum was underway."[192] Readers earlier saw the "Three H's," students of McKenzie and Botterell, come on stage. In 1952 E. Bruce Hendrick, having completed the Gallie Course in surgery, began training in pediatric neurosurgery at the Children's Hospital in Boston. When he returned in 1954, "with his youthful vigor and military brush cut" (as Humphreys said), he became Canada's first full-time pediatric neurosurgeon. He was joined in 1964 by Harold Hoffman, then in 1970 by Robin Humphreys.

Amidst the clatter of china in the coffee room at HSC in the 1960s and 1970s, a whole neuroscience program came together around the germinal point of neurosurgery. The three H's slowly took retirement and gave way to the "two Jims," Jim Rutka and Jim Drake. James Drake joined the division in 1988; at the hospital's Research Institute he opened the hydrocephalus research laboratory, the first such laboratory in the hospital's history. Drake called attention to the "frustrating dichotomy between technological advancements and clinical outcomes [that makes] hydrocephalus one of the most understated and complex disorders that neurosurgeons treat."[193]

James Rutka arrived in 1990, in the vanguard of the Surgical Scientist Program, and opened the second research lab. Rutka attended York Mills Collegiate (high school) in Toronto and majored in chemical engineering at Princeton. He studied medicine at Queen's University, graduating in 1981, then trained in neurosurgery at U of T under Alan Hudson. Funded by the Medical Research Council of Canada, he earned a PhD in tumour biology at the University of California at San Francisco. Back in Toronto in 1990, Rutka and Drake alternated clinical duties and research stints in the lab, each spending two weeks first in the one, then the other – a system that has proven so successful that it has also been adopted by neurosurgeons Ab Guha and Andreas Lozano and by Mike Tymianski and Chris Wallace.[194]

Rutka's major research interest was brain tumours. Humphreys said that Rutka "combines the investigational aspects of tumour biology with therapeutic programs designed for brain tumour control."[195] In the 1997–8 session, together with Mark Bernstein and Ab Guha, Rutka established a brain tumour centre on the third floor of the McMaster research building of the Hospital for Sick Children, for which Sonia and Arthur Labatt donated $5 million, a joint effort at HSC, the Toronto Hospital, and U of T; Rutka was the first director and Mark Bernstein and Ab Guha associate directors. They were to have 3,000 square feet of lab space at HSC in addition to Guha's lab. (There was also a Gerry and Nancy Pencer Brain Centre at TTH, which Mark Bernstein helped develop.)[196] In 2002 Rutka and others identified the gene responsible for medulloblastoma, the commonest brain cancer in children. His team found that a subset of children with medulloblastomas had mutations in a gene called SUFU, a tumour-suppressor gene that had recently been identified. SUFU suppression predisposed children to medulloblastomas by modifying the "sonic hedgehog" (SHH) signalling pathway (the sonic hedgehog gene series, also discovered at the Research Institute of HSC, plays a big role in embryonic development).[197]

The neuro specialties began to coalesce at HSC, a development which highlights the ability of the hospitals to lead the way in interdisciplinary convergence. In the mid-1960s the Department of Anaesthesia developed a neurosurgical subspecialist in Robert Creighton. John Relton became the neuroanesthetist for spinal surgery. The neuroradiologist Derek Harwood-Nash has been previously mentioned. Margaret Norman had launched the neuropathology program, succeeded by Laurence Becker. John Stobo Prichard drove the Division of Neurology forward; it was immediately adjacent to the neurosurgical Ward 5G. William Logan succeeded him, continuing the epilepsy program. Humphreys recalls the "rollicking and productive sessions" on combined neurology and neurosurgery rounds at 8:00 in the morning on Fridays.[198] In 1986 the epilepsy monitoring unit was established, initially as a two-bed unit, later growing to four private rooms. It served mainly the monitoring of children with intractable seizures, in order to map out the functional cortex with the aid of various neuroimaging studies. (Most of the children do not have focal lesions.) According to Hiroshi Otsubo, director of the Neurophysiology Laboratory at HSC, the program was transformed with the introduction in 1997 of intracranial invasive video electroencephalogram monitoring.[199]

Neurosurgery at the children's hospital was among the most successful divisions in the faculty. The faculty Self-Study of 1983 noted, "a continuing stream of Americans at the Hospital for Sick Children, which is the only place in the continent where they can obtain their experience in paediatric work."[200] As

Robin Humphreys prepared to replace Harold Hoffman as hospital division head in 1996, an external reviewer described the division "as the best in pediatric neurosurgery in the world and the standard to which all others aspire."[201]

As Humphreys himself approached retirement, he looked back on the rush of life in a busy department: "In the last 5 years, HSC neurosurgeons have performed 3,473 surgical operations which lasted 9,501 hours."[202] In June 2003 he stepped down.[203] In 2005 neurology and neurosurgery merged into a single Clinical Neurosciences Unit.[204]

### Neurosciences: Playfair

Addressed earlier was the rather improvised program in neurosciences that Eric Linell tried, unsuccessfully, to pull together in the early 1930s. Again in the 1951–2 session, Linell aspired to "close co-operation with Dr D[elbert] Wollin in the field of Neuro-Radiology. He attends our weekly conferences with the physicians, surgeons, and psychiatrists. Dr Linell and members of his staff go to weekly neuro-radiological conferences at the Psychiatric Hospital. It is a great pleasure to be closely associated with this important development of Radiology."[205] This sounds like a neuroscience program avant la lettre. But it did not turn into a formal collaboration.

Neuroscience reached its first firm footing in the faculty in 1978 with the establishment of the Playfair Neuroscience Unit at the Toronto Western Hospital. The story is this: Helen Scott Playfair, the wife of Stuart Playfair, who owned the Tampax Corporation, died in 1959 of Parkinson's disease. In 1960 Mr Playfair donated 6,000 shares of the Tampax Corporation to the University of Toronto, worth about $1 million at the time, $40,000 of which were to be used to "to equip a laboratory under the supervision of the Division of Neurosurgery to investigate problems of Parkinson's Disease."[206] Early in 1961 a committee was struck to administer the Playfair Memorial Fund; it agreed that a "neurological laboratory," administered by electrophysiologist John Scott, should be supported. A second laboratory of neurosurgeons Ronald Tasker and Stanley Schatz in the Banting Institute was also to be supported. The Playfair Committee met and agreed that only interest was to be spent.[207]

What followed was a textbook example of how ill-suited academic committees are to move important projects forward. By December 1961 plans had changed: the committee would fund a neurochemical laboratory, to be directed by Wherrett at TGH once he returned from completing his PhD.[208] (This laboratory was established in 1963.) But even better: plans were afoot for a new Clinical Research Building at the northwest corner of College and Elizabeth Streets. The Research Laboratories of the Neurological Sciences Group might be situated there.[209] (These laboratories were never built, and the Standardized Patient Program is the latest in a series of faculty centres to occupy the 88 College Street site, a former church.) By 1964 Playfair funds were supporting Tasker's lab at the

Banting Institute, the electron microscopy room, Calvin Ezrin's endocrine lab in the Banting Institute, and Wherrett's lab on the eleventh floor of TGH, in addition to the electromyography equipment. By 1965 the Tampax stock was worth over $2 million and the fund was generating $40,000 revenue a year, supporting the work of Ric Richardson, Ron Tasker, Neill Rewcastle, John Wherrett, and John Scott.[210] (The impression must not arise that these were not worthy projects, merely not the kind of monument that the Playfair family had in mind.)

In October 1965 Richardson and neurosurgeon Tom Morley were asked to take the lead in pressing Dean Hamilton for "the establishment of an Institute of Neurological Sciences within the University."[211] But the following year Associate Dean Edward A. Sellers has another idea: a neurology centre was needed to coordinate research and graduate teaching. In March 1967 Richardson met with Mr Playfair at his home on Rosedale Road to tell him of these rather dispersed results. The following month committee members considered "a clinical-neurosciences committee to obtain temporary space and facilities for neurological research."[212] In July 1968 Mr Playfair died.

Eight years had now passed since the bequest. On 16 January 1969 the Neurosurgical IHCC (the neurosurgical division) met at the Faculty Club. On the agenda was a "University Neurosciences Institute or Department." The minutes noted, "The Meeting was not particularly in favour of such a development, because it could not see in what it would benefit from the re-organization; it might very well in fact, be worse off."[213] In subsequent bureaucratic demarches, the neurosurgeons made clear that the establishment of a "Department of Neurosciences" was not "palatable" to them. In April 1969 the Playfair committee decided to petition for 10,000 square feet of dedicated lab space somewhere for "core neurosciences." Further complex bureaucratic manoeuvring took place. In December 1969 Ernest Sirluck, dean of the School of Graduate Studies, explained to a working party of the Playfair Committee that a "Neurological Institute" would be in the SGS, not the Faculty of Medicine.[214]

In November 1970 the Playfair Committee was informed that there would be a one- to two-year delay because Sirluck was retiring. By June 1972 the Playfair stock was worth around $6 million. Yet despite the hotness of the stock, many of the players were still lukewarm. In September 1972 Richardson told President Evans, "The submission for such a Neuroscience Institute has been received rather coolly by the pertinent faculty and graduate school committees."[215] There was a meeting with the Playfair family, who were apparently upset. Evans asked Hollenberg to take the situation in hand. By the fall of 1972 Hollenberg was chairing the Presidential Advisory Committee on the Playfair Fund. Now we know there would be action. Hollenberg was a real leader, and what was lacking in this sad story of the development of the neurosciences at the University of Toronto was leadership.

Hollenberg coaxed from the faculty's Sub-committee on Science Policy the decision that a future Neurosciences Physical Facility was to be situated in a hospital, not in the Medical Sciences Building.[216] By January 1973 grand plans were laid out: they would use the Clinical Center at the National Institutes of Health in Bethesda as a model, "a central team of 15–20 major investigators," and so forth.[217] By June 1973 Dean Chute had considered the possible sites and, following the energetic urging of neurologist William (Bill) McIlroy, recommended the Toronto Western Hospital. And this is what came to pass: in November 1978 the Playfair unit was opened at the Western under William Tatton. In achieving this result, Hollenberg had apparently rubbed so many people the wrong way that he was not included on the search committee for director of the institute. Associate Dean Jan Steiner advised Dean Holmes, tongue in cheek, "It was suggested that you might perhaps speak to Dr. Hollenberg and break the news to him gently."[218]

Because so much capital had been dribbled away over the years, only $3 million remained in the endowment, the revenue of which was not sufficient to fund a unit as originally conceived.[219] Yet the Western was offering two floors of the research building they were constructing and would supply animal facilities and support services. Playfair money sufficed to support five scientists, and a few others were financed separately. The Playfair family decided to terminate its support as of June 1985 and the university shouldered the burden of funding the unit. The Playfair unit made important contributions to campus neuroscience, but it did not bring the investigators together. Ron Tasker, for example, had the standing offer of a lab at Playfair but preferred to move his lab from the General to the Medical Sciences Building. F. Griffith Pearson, professor of surgery, said, "The geographic location represents a major obstacle."[220]

Although Playfair had a somewhat circuitous origin and was not the equivalent of a department or institute, it nonetheless played a considerable role in the Toronto neuroscience story. Ross Fleming comments, "Establishing the Playfair laboratories at Toronto Western Hospital, where 'bench' to 'bedside' research could occur, allowing surgeon-scientists to quickly and efficiently move from operating room to laboratory and back, had a powerful catalytic effect in gradually transforming TWH into a major neuroscience centre, attracting such leaders as Carlen, Tator, the powerful neuro-radiology team [Gordon Potts, Karel terBrugge], and ultimately becoming the site to which the entire TGH neurosurgical program moved where the University Health Network has become one of the world's outstanding neurosurgical programs." Thus, Fleming offers some perspective from a clinician-scientist who, as he says, "watched the Toronto neurosurgical science from the front row for 63 years."[221]

### Neurosciences: A Second Track

Playfair had not solved the university's neuroscience problem, the dimensions of which emerged around 1990 with a glossy 154-page catalogue entitled "Research Activities in the Neurosciences" that stated, "There are approximately

170 neuroscientists in the Faculty of Medicine."[222] This figure, moreover, excluded all those outside the faculty.

The stumbling about Playfair touched off a discussion of neuroscience in the university community. In February 1966 Dean Hamilton had approved the concept of a neurological sciences institute in the Toronto General Hospital.

In 1973 an Institute of Neurosciences was approved but not funded.[223] The rest of the neuroscience community began to grumble about all the money going into bricks and mortar at Playfair. Wherrett complained to Dean Holmes, "Under the present plan only a small part of the Neurosciences community ... could be supported ... We believe that it would be unwise to dissipate much of the Fund's capital ... in building ... We recommend that a substantial fraction of the disposable monies be available by competitive application for all neuroscientists in the University and not limited to members of the proposed Playfair Laboratory Unit."[224]

Discontent arose within the Dean's Office as well. In 1982 Donald W. Clarke, physiologist and associate dean of basic sciences, observed of the neurosciences, "There is ... concern that this is an area which has not reached the level of development which might be expected, given the resources and personnel available within the University and the teaching hospitals." Dean Lowy agreed, "This is an example of an interdisciplinary area which is not well coordinated at present due in part to the strong departmental structure which is the tradition at this University."[225] Lowy struck a committee on the neurosciences and a long period of bureaucratic shuffling ensued that will not be reported here.

Bill Tatton emerged as the major player in the campus neuroscience scene. In the summer of 1983 he became associate dean of neurosciences; he was already vice president of research at the Western and professor of physiology. He and Gordon Potts, the star neuroradiologist and chair of the Department of Radiology, began consulting on acquiring a magnetic resonance imager.[226]

Time passed. A neurodegenerative centre emerged on the horizon in 1987, partly financed by Mark Tanz, that would open in 1990 (see later for more details). Playfair was up and running. In April 1987 Lowy felt it time to try for a "Department of Clinical Neuroscience."[227] Yet nothing happened.

John Dirks became dean in July 1987 and decided to have another kick at the neuroscience can. In September 1990 he said, "Because of our long tradition of neuroscience discoveries and because we have one of the strongest and largest neuroscience communities in North America, I have proposed the establishment of an Institute of Neurosciences that will bring together eminent neuroscientists ... Our concept is to develop the Tanz Neurosciences Building as the nucleus for the Institute."[228] In December 1990 he struck a Neurosciences Executive Committee "to discuss the present status of neurosciences."[229] There was already a Collaborative Graduate Program in Neurosciences (called "PIN"), founded in 1985 and initially coordinated by John Yeomans. Could something more substantial not be organized about the nucleus at the Tanz? In May 1991 this executive committee proposed an institute of neurosciences, noting "the barriers that have precluded the development of an Institute, over the past 20 years." An institute had been proposed in 1973 but was never realized owing to money problems. "At the present time, the rationale for constituting an Institute is very strong."[230] But it must not have been strong enough, because at a neuroscience meeting in January 1992 there were "strong objections" from unnamed quarters to such an institute and the idea was dropped.[231] There things rested. Anticlimactically, in the faculty's plan for 2000–4, a "neurosciences network" was rather feebly put forward.[232]

In the meantime, in 1995 at the Western Division of the Toronto Hospital a Neurosciences Centre for the training of residents in neurosurgery and neurology was established. The Playfair Neuroscience Unit at the Western was the research arm of this centre. With a grant from the Krembil Foundation that permitted a great expansion of its programs, this became the core of the Krembil Neuroscience Centre. Thus Playfair was the basic science arm of neurosciences, Krembil the clinical arm with Fehlings as the director.

### Centre for Research in Neurodegenerative Diseases

In 1984 the faculty suspended its rather half-hearted search for donors for an endowed chair in the neurosciences on the grounds that it was conflicting with the university's larger fundraising campaign. They had only raised $65,000 for such a chair. Yet from the ruins of this failed effort emerged a proposal from the Department of Physiology for a neurodegenerative disease program.[233]

By June 1985 the Neuroscience Planning Committee, led by Bill Tatton in physiology, drafted a proposal for a "Canadian Research Centre for Neurodegenerative Diseases." Things began to look more promising in September 1986, when Mark M. Tanz, a Toronto business figure whose mother had died of Alzheimer's disease, made an offer to donate a number of millions of dollars for the development of a Neurodegenerative Disease Centre in the Botany Building when it was vacated in 1988. About ten investigators, some cross-appointed from various departments, would form the core of the centre, which was seen as augmenting the faculty strength in the basic sciences.[234]

By May 1987 the funding was finally nailed down: Tanz was donating $4 million, in return for which the centre would be named after him. Other sources such as the Alzheimer's Society were contributing an additional $5 million. Donald Crapper-McLachlan, who graduated in medicine in Toronto in 1957 and was cross-appointed between the Division of Neurology at the Toronto Western Hospital and the Department of Physiology – studying environmental and genetic factors in neuron death in degenerative brain disease – would be the interim director while a big search was launched for director.[235]

In June 1990 the Neurodegenerative Disease Centre in the Tanz Neuroscience Building officially opened as a partnership among the university, the

Alzheimer's Association, and a number of private donors, notably Mr Tanz and his friends, who contributed $13 million. After four years' tenure, Crapper-McLachlan turned over the interim directorship of the centre to Peter Carlen, also in the neurology division of the Toronto Western Hospital. And in May 1995 Peter St. George-Hyslop, the noted investigator of degenerative diseases, and also on staff at the Western, took over the directorship on a regular basis.

Important science came from the Centre for Research in Neurodegenerative Diseases. In 2002, St. George-Hyslop himself was the principal investigator in a trial on the possibility of an Alzheimer vaccine. In mice, the use of amyloid-beta peptide was effective in reducing Alzheimer-like neuropathology and spatial memory impairments. Yet a trial of this agent in humans was discontinued because "a few patients developed significant meningoencephalitis cellular inflammatory reactions."[236] As well, St. George-Hyslop and colleagues in 2006 identified cyclohexanehexol inhibitors of amyloid-beta aggregation as affecting amyloid in Alzheimer's. "These therapeutic effects ... support the idea that the accumulation of A-beta oligomers has a central role in the pathogenesis of Alzheimer disease."[237] Research on blocking the synthesis of amyloid became an important international research strategy.

It is a comfort of sorts that from the wreckage of the larger neurosciences project at the University of Toronto, at least this little gem of a centre, named in 2010 the Tanz Centre for Research in Neurodegenerative Diseases, was saved.

There is one more chapter in the neuroscience story and that is told later. It is interesting that when acknowledged leaders such as Charlie Hollenberg reached their strong arms into these pots, events moved forward. When academic committees, with their need for consensus among squabbling constituencies, tried to advance the ball, nothing happened. Hollenberg never presented himself as a titan, a Canadian version of Robert Moses, the titan builder of the Port Authority of New York. But he was a real leader, and often that is what is needed.

### Baycrest Hospital and the Rotman Research Institute: An Efflorescence of Neuroscience

In 1918 the Jewish community of Toronto founded Baycrest Hospital to care for the needs of elderly family members. For decades, the hospital had no connection to the Faculty of Medicine. In gerontology – which was the hospital's raison d'être – undergraduate contact in the 1970s was limited to "the occasional student to ... take an elective in geriatrics through Baycrest." As for postgraduates, junior interns from Mount Sinai might serve a one-month rotation at the Baycrest Hospital.[238] And that was it.

Mindful of the general increase in academic research, in 1983 the Board of Directors of the hospital revised the mission statement to include "research and education in aging." This expression of interest in research was to reach an extraordinary flowering.

In 1988 Baycrest opened discussions with the University of Toronto about a possible affiliation. This was in preparation for launching the following year, in 1989, a formal program of research: the Rotman Research Institute in Cognitive Neuroscience under Donald Stuss as director.

Stuss, a psychologist, had earned a PhD in 1976 from the University of Ottawa, fellowed in neuropsychology in Boston, then came on staff in 1978 in neurology and in psychology at the University of Ottawa; he also directed the Department of Psychology at the Ottawa General Hospital. In 1989, as stated, he came to Toronto to launch the Rotman Institute and in 1991 became vice president of research for Baycrest, as well as director of the Rotman Research Institute (RRI). Stuss, considered one of the world's foremost neuropsychologists, wrote with D. Frank Benson in 1986 a seminal study, *The Frontal Lobes*; in his 1992 work on frontal dysfunction after traumatic brain injury, Stuss found that disturbance of executive "frontal" abilities is very common in closed head injury. The article cast a spotlight on disruptions of executive function in traumatic brain injury.[239] In 2000 he used the Wisconsin Card Sorting Test to localize different processes in the frontal lobes.[240]

Stuss's tenure at RRI was a whirlwind. He organized in 1992 a clinical research unit. Stuss established a research partnership with the Centre for Addiction and Mental Health on the downtown campus. A major coup was his recruitment of Endel Tulving, a former chair of psychology in the Faculty of Arts and Science, as inaugural holder of the Anne and Max Tanenbaum Chair in Cognitive Neuroscience. Tulving is remembered for his hypothesis in 1972 that episodic memory differs from other kinds of memory.[241] In 2005 Tulving received a Canada Gairdner International Award for revolutionizing the field of memory research.[242]

The RRI drew together a high-powered battery of academic talent intent upon investigations ranging from behavioural neurology to cognitive rehabilitation to neuropharmacology. There was now a rush of new foundations. In 1995 the hospital established a Clinical Epidemiology and Evaluation Unit to study health issues in older adults. In 1996 the Kunin-Lunenfeld Applied Research Unit (KLARU) was organized, separately from the RRI, with the goal of conducting translational research; it merged the clinical research unit and the clinical epidemiology unit and opened two years later with its first director, David L. Streiner.

In 1996 Baycrest became a fully affiliated teaching hospital with U of T. At the same time, a series of research chairs and centres were established: the Max and Gianna Glassman Chair in Neuropsychology; another Anne and Max Tanenbaum Chair in Cognitive Neuroscience; the Sandra A. Rotman Chair in Neuropsychiatry in 1999 with Helen Mayberg as the incumbent (who therewith came from the University of Texas at San Antonio to Toronto, where she was to pioneer the study of deep-brain stimulation for treatment-resistant depression[243]); and a centre endowed by Ben and Hilda Katz in gerontological social work. There were other foundations as well, too numerous to list. Such an outpouring of community support for scholarly endeavour is unique in the history of medicine in Toronto and represents an extraordinary vote of confidence in the ability of academic enterprise to make lives better.

Baycrest joined various international networks for the study of frontal temporal dementia, cognitive rehabilitation, and functional imaging. The downtown hospitals, Sunnybrook, and several other Ontario universities became networked together with Baycrest in 2001 in the Behavioural Research and Imaging Network (BRAIN), led by Randy McIntosh at the Rotman Research Institute. Together with Sunnybrook and the Ottawa Health Research Institute, Baycrest organized in 2003 a Centre for Stroke Recovery, as the province provided matching funds for research into post-stroke interventions. The following year a number of smaller clinics at Baycrest for the study of mood, memory, and stroke were amalgamated into the Brain Health Centre Clinics. A Centre for Integrated Molecular Brain Imaging, part of an international network funded by the Lundbeck Foundation, was established in 2005 using PET and MRI technology for the study of addictive and mood disorders.[244]

The story thus has a provisional happy end, led by this remarkable research complex in North Toronto that for most of its half-century history had been a home for the elderly.

**Envoi**

Neuroscience is one of Toronto's biggest stories. And even though all of its bits did not coalesce into a single administrative unit, Ross Fleming emphasizes, "What Toronto has 'works,' and works extraordinarily well. Each component seems to thrive under its own relative autonomy, usually within its parent department, but with strong collaboration between various components." The frustrated researchers and administrators, said Fleming, never found the "Holy Grail" of a single neuroscience department.[245] But what they did was not to be sneezed at.

# 15  Anatomy

They were giant people, those people.[1]

Fred Dewar, 1930s

Until recently, anatomy had always been considered the queen of the medical sciences. Its teaching once formed the fundamental core of basic medical education, and it went without saying that all medical students would dissect a cadaver and memorize the origins and insertions of the muscles, the osteology of the bones, and the course of the major blood vessels and nerves. Acquiring all this information served more ritualistic than practical functions, yet it was part of the ritual of becoming a doctor, in Toronto as well as elsewhere.

The teaching of anatomy in Toronto goes back to the earliest days of medical education in the 1820s. When the faculty was refounded in 1887, an anatomy department sprang back to life as well, chaired by James Henry Richardson as the first professor of anatomy. Richardson, born in 1823 in Presqu'Isle, Upper Canada, attended the first course of lectures of the medical faculty of King's College (as the U of T was then called); he then decamped for England, where, as Ross G. Mackenzie – who has written a history of the Department of Anatomy – explains, Richardson studied at Guy's Hospital for three years and obtained in 1847 the Diploma of the Royal College of Surgeons, England. He returned to Toronto to teach anatomy until the medical school of the university was abolished in 1853 and thereafter became professor of anatomy in the Toronto School of Medicine. Richardson also practiced surgery at the Toronto General Hospital. Interestingly, at the time of the visit of the Prince of Wales to Canada in 1860, Richardson proposed "that all native Canadians joining the procession … should wear the Maple Leaf as an emblem of the land of their birth."[2] This gesture was said to have created the maple leaf as Canada's national symbol.

The course in anatomy was very thorough then and students dissected the whole body twice. "Medical students in those days probably knew their anatomy much better than they do now," wrote John Oille in 1964, looking back on a fifty-year career in medicine that began with his graduation in 1903. (By contrast, physical examination was taught almost not at all, and Oille had to learn percussion from the country doctor in Sparta, Ontario, with whom he worked after finishing his studies.[3])

From 1896 to 1907 Alexander Primrose, who was met in an earlier chapter, headed the Department of Anatomy. Then in 1907 James Playfair McMurrich took the baton. Born in 1859, McMurrich was educated at Upper Canada College and awarded a bachelor's degree from the University of Toronto. McMurrich was not a physician; he took a PhD from Johns Hopkins in 1885 in biological studies, held various posts in the United States, then from 1894 to 1906 was professor of anatomy at the University of Michigan. From 1922 until 1930 McMurrich was inaugural dean of the School of Graduate Studies and stepped down at the same time from both the anatomy post and the deanship. While at Michigan, in 1902 – in what was to become a tradition of textbook writing for the faculty – McMurrich authored a manual of human embryology called *The Development of the Human Body*.[4] A seventh edition appeared in 1923. It was during McMurrich's tenure that the anatomy department moved from the Biology Building to the newly built Anatomy Building, opened in 1923 and now called "the McMurrich Building." "Anatomy with him," said his eulogist, "was set on a high scientific plane, far above that of a mere adjunct of surgery."[5]

Playfair McMurrich inspired gentle parodies such as this, composed by med "stude" William S. Stanbury, 3T0 (class of 1930) of Exeter, Ontario – who ended up practicing in Leeds, England – for *Epistaxis* the opening night of Daffydil in 1928 (following the First Lords Song in Gilbert and Sullivan's "HMS Pinafore"): "When I was a stude I served my term / With Jimmy Watt of the McMurrich firm. I studied bones and knew them well, / For I picked up the stakes whenever they fell. / I threw those bones so successfullee, / That now I'm a member of the Facultee."[6] (James C. Watt was a professor of anatomy.)

Gilbert and Sullivan notwithstanding, innovation came quickly in anatomy. In the late 1920s Malcolm J. Wilson, a 1916 U of T graduate, introduced X-ray demonstrations. The staff also began offering "demonstrations of surface anatomy, in which the men students alternate in acting as subjects while models are engaged for the women students."[7] A committee struck in 1920 to consider the allocation of the large Rockefeller grant among departments was "strongly of the opinion" that histology and embryology, currently in the Department of Biology, should be transferred to anatomy.[8] The foundation was willing to donate half a million dollars towards the construction of an Anatomical Institute, so their opinion had some weight, and the institute opened, as stated, in 1923.

On the subject of textbooks, in 1930 the author of one of the faculty's biggest international hits took the helm of the anatomy department: John Charles Boileau Grant. Grant is celebrated in the history of the faculty as one of the trilogy of textbook writers who, aside from insulin, gave the faculty its international claim to fame before the 1950s – the other two being William Boyd on pathology and Charles Best on physiology. Grant was born at Loanhead near Edinburgh in 1886, his father a Presbyterian minister. His mother, a Boileau, was a direct descendant of Etienne Boileau, a thirteenth-century mayor of Paris.[9] Grant finished medical studies at the University of Edinburgh in 1908, a classmate of his lifelong friend Boyd, then worked for two years as a demonstrator in anatomy at the University of Durham in Newcastle-on-Tyne.

After a distinguished war record as a medical officer, marked, as his biographer P.V. Tobias puts it, "by conspicuous gallantry and devotion to duty while under attack," Grant followed his friend William Boyd to Canada in 1919 to take up the professorship of anatomy at the University of Manitoba. He was lured to Toronto in 1930 and set as his first task the creation of a museum of anatomy, with the specimens in characteristic four-sided jars, "set on revolving bases, hence, each specimen had four surfaces to present, each was specially illustrated and labeled. These the student, seated and with text-book or notes beside him, could study in comfort." (Advantageous though the current "problem-based" medical curriculum may be, it is dispiriting to think that today's students no longer have the grasp of anatomy that this method conferred.)

Grant was kind to his students. Dewar recalled his "funny squeaky voice, and it somehow reminded you of a mouse every now and again. He had a wonderful sense of humour and when the day's work was done, you were up at his house. You always got a good drink too, and his wife was charming." He was pathologist Boyd's brother-in-law. "Between the two of them they certainly made the basic science portion of our medical school just tremendous. They were giant people, those people."[10]

Grant became known in Toronto for a dramatic lecturing style that involved, as all the great anatomy professors prided themselves, on being able to draw the intricate organs of the body on the blackboard in living colour ambidextrously, both hands moving in sync at once. Barney Berris remembered Grant's lectures: "His style was very formal and he always wore his academic robe when he taught. He walked back and forth in front of the room with short steps and would stop only when he wished to draw something on the blackboard. He made the structural science of anatomy come to life. He related the sites of the body organs to function ... which is why his book was titled Method of Anatomy."

Indeed, *Method of Anatomy*, published in 1937, was Grant's first book. By 1991 it had gone through eleven editions. His *Handbook for Dissectors* appeared in 1940, known more simply as *Grant's Dissector*. In 1943 his third great book appeared,

*Atlas of Anatomy*, which by 1991 was in its ninth edition.[11] Even though *Gray's Anatomy*, first published in 1858 from St George's Hospital in London, dominates televised images of anatomy, it was *Grant's Anatomy* that conveyed anatomical knowledge to generations of medical students across the globe.

Recruiting Grant was a coup. In 1931 Dean Primrose celebrated the past achievements of the famous anatomist, including his undergraduate teaching. It is characteristic of that generation that nothing was said of his publications but much made of Grant's military record as "medical officer in the Grenadier Guards and later with the Black Watch, winning the military cross with bar."[12] These clinicians and scientists were still under the influence of their military experiences in the First World War, and it would, alas, all come again in the Second World War as once again the members of the faculty trooped off to arms. Military service was a far more powerful bonding experience than science.

One more thing about Grant: "[He] began the department tradition, which continues to this day, of having demonstrators wear blue-collared lab coats so they could be easily identified in the dissecting laboratory."[13] (The demonstrators themselves were mainly surgical trainees about to sit the primary exam of the Royal College.[14])

"The 'Grant Days' can only be described as exciting and stimulating," writes anatomist Ross Mackenzie, who remembered them well. "It was during his period that the Department of Anatomy was repeatedly voted by the graduating class as the best department during their undergraduate course." Grant lectured three times a week, always on the area of the body under dissection in the laboratory. "The students were required to spend approximately twelve hours each week dissecting in the gross anatomy laboratory where they were under the supervision of an adequate number of demonstrators."[15] (It was during the Grant Days in the 1942–3 session that a histology lab technician named Harry Whittaker, a kind man beloved of several generations of medical students, was appointed.[16])

At the end of the Second World War, Grant was especially pleased that the faculty had begun considering plans for postgraduate courses. He wrote in 1945, "There is greater satisfaction in offering anatomical facilities to graduates who have decided upon definite careers and who are certainly going to make use of the anatomical knowledge they acquire than to undergraduates with indefinite ideas of the future."[17]

With the appointment of Arthur W. Ham in 1932, Grant established a Division of Histology in the department. Ham was one of the great scientific figures of the faculty, in addition to being an international tennis star. He was born in 1902 in Brantford, Ontario, and educated at Brantford Collegiate Institute; he graduated with an MB from U of T in 1926. Ham thereupon worked for two years in the Department of Pathology under Oskar Klotz. Yet, as he later said, he showed "more preference for a racquet than a probe and became Ontario's tennis singles champion, playing between 1926 and 1928 internationally on Canada's Davis Cup teams."[18]

It was, however, Klotz who sparked Ham's lifelong interest in bone metabolism. From 1929 to 1931 Ham trained in cytology under Edmund V. Cowdry at Washington University School of Medicine in St Louis, then worked as Cowdry's assistant before returning to Toronto to accept an appointment in 1932 in the Department of Anatomy. "To his subject he brings enthusiasm and activity," said Dean FitzGerald, welcoming Ham to the faculty.[19] Ham's first paper in 1930 was a pioneering effort that described the role of "osteogenic cells" in the repair of fractures, a process in which, Ham said, adult bone cells played no role.[20] The paper represented, as one of his eulogists put it, "the major thrust of his research: to seek to understand mechanisms of bone repair and bone biology."[21] In 1950 he published the first edition of his great histology textbook, which became known as *Ham's Histology*, in the same way as other such eponymous Toronto textbooks as *Grant's Anatomy* and *Boyd's Pathology*. The textbook reached, under editor David Cormack, its ninth edition in 1989. The textbook was, it must be said, something of a nightmare for medical students though a scientific triumph: It contained over seventy pages on bone metabolism.[22] In 1957 Ham joined the Ontario Cancer Institute, and his further career will be chronicled there. After his first wife, Dorothy Ross, died in 1976, he acquired a certain celebrity by marrying in 1981 *Toronto Star* society columnist Lotta Dempsey Fisher.

Ham changed the teaching of histology, which has the potential of being a very dry subject. In 1941 Grant said, "The outlook of Histology, now in charge of Dr A.W. Ham, has changed considerably during the last decade, the tendency now being to study as living things the materials which comprise the human body and to consider them physiologically as well as anatomically ... Although the study of the living cell, as in tissue cultures, has had an effect in bringing about this change, the rise of endocrinology has had a still greater influence ... Anyone privileged to see the profound and sudden changes that certain hormones can produce in the architecture of the tissues can scarcely refrain from regarding (and teaching) Histology as the study of living material."[23] Ham's former students recalled his lively style. Said Barney Berris, "His teaching was notable for his infectious enthusiasm and obvious interest in his subject. Many of our teachers ... spent little time discussing medical research. However, Dr. Ham referred to medical research often in his course, describing how important it was in expanding the frontiers of medicine and how exciting it was to be involved in research."[24]

Ham brought a high note of science to the Department of Anatomy. In 1952 he led a small team studying, in rats, liver tumours that had been induced to grow in the medium of the yolk sacs of chick embryos. The team succeeded in maintaining three of these tumours in serial cultivation for two and a half years.[25] In particular, Ham sparked research on carcinogenesis and leukemia, supported by the Foster Bequest Fund of the university and the National Cancer Institute, that he would shortly take with him over to the Ontario Cancer Institute in the late 1950s.[26] Arthur Axelrad collaborated in this research and in 1966 succeeded Ham as professor of histology, thus giving up his post at OCI in the Department of Medical Biophysics.

In 1956 John W.A. Duckworth succeeded Grant as chair of anatomy. Like Grant, Duckworth was a Scotsman and graduated in medicine from the University of Edinburgh in 1936. After interning at the Royal Infirmary, he joined the Department of Anatomy at Edinburgh. He served in the Royal Navy during the war, then returned to the anatomy staff at Edinburgh, where he remained until becoming a member of the department in Toronto in 1952. Four years later he became head.

Duckworth resigned in January 1965 and the question of transition arose. Who would be the next professor of anatomy? Rather uncharacteristically (for someone who had no interest in administration), Ham put himself forward for reasons that are quite interesting and cast light on the later abolition of departmental status for anatomy and its conversion into a division of the Department of Surgery. In early 1965 Ham was at the Ontario Cancer Institute, though still a professor of histology. He wrote Dean Hamilton that no one in the department was really suitable as chair and that he, Ham, would accept an interim appointment. "My role over the next couple of years would be that of trying to ... create more of a research atmosphere and make the Department more productive this way and make it increasingly attractive for further staff. I think because of my age and also because I think they all like me and think I could help them in research I would get their co-operation."[27] This became the Achilles heel of the Department of Anatomy, their failure to restart a research program after Ham took the cancer research with him to OCI.

It was not Ham who became the next professor of anatomy – though he did serve as interim chair for a year – but James S. Thompson, who assumed the chair in 1966. Jim Thompson became one of the barons of the faculty. He was born in 1919 in Saskatoon, Saskatchewan, into an academically distinguished family; his father was an internationally known biologist who became president of the University of Saskatchewan. Thompson enrolled in medicine at the University of Toronto, graduating in 1945. He worked for two years at the Banting Institute before joining the anatomy department of the University of Western Ontario in 1948. From 1950 to 1963 he was a member of the anatomy department of the University of Alberta, coming then to Toronto, where he chaired the Department of Anatomy from 1966 to 1976. Because of his leadership skills, he frequently served in important posts in the faculty, for example, as the speaker of the Faculty Council for nine years, as his eulogist and fellow anatomist Keith Moore points out, "the first person to hold this prestigious position." His research interest was genetics, and in 1966 he and his wife Margaret ("Peggy") Thompson, professor of medical genetics, published *Genetics in Medicine*, another of the U of T textbooks that enjoyed international success and translation into several languages. Thompson was greatly beloved by his students (including the present author). "[H]is door was always open," as Moore says. "Dr Thompson knew most students by name and repeated this feat each year."[28]

In the 1967–8 session, the department was separated into two divisions – gross anatomy, embryology, and neuroanatomy versus histology.[29] It was apropos this separation that Jim Thompson made a fatal mistake. At a meeting of the long-range planners in February 1974, Thompson said, "Anatomy is essentially a teaching department and until 1966 there were few PhD's granted and relatively little research conducted. Since 1966 there has been an increase in research particularly in the Histology Division."[30] In 1975 Thompson told Dean Holmes, concerning the separation of the department into two divisions, "The original division of the department into Histology and Gross Anatomy included the assumption that members of the Division of Histology would be expected to carry the major portion of the research load in the Department and that the members of the Gross Anatomy Division would be required to carry the major portion of the teaching load."[31] Essentially, this reduced the anatomists to service providers alongside the histologists, who were to profile themselves as scientists. And in a faculty navigating at flank speed towards research, this was a heading towards demotion. As the long-range planners noted in a 1976 report of the Department of Anatomy, "Insufficient research. Very urgent."[32]

Over the years to come, the anatomy division would end up with a huge teaching burden. This was the difficult situation that Keith Moore inherited in 1976 when he agreed to leave the University of Manitoba and head the Department of Anatomy in Toronto. In negotiations with Associate Dean Jan Steiner, Moore asked that the staff be beefed up, "to strengthen the research and graduate programs of the Department of Anatomy." Steiner replied that the request was, alas, impossible but hoped that Moore would come anyway.[33] Moore did indeed accept the appointment and during his tenure wrote a large textbook, *Clinically Oriented Anatomy* (1980), that enjoyed great international success.[34]

The crucial turn came in October 1984 as an external review of the department found its research activities inadequate and the division between anatomy and histology "polarizing." In 1985 the histology division was abolished.[35] Patricia Stewart, a basic scientist, was appointed graduate coordinator, and she attempted to wrench the department in the direction of cell biology.[36]

In 1985 Martin J. Hollenberg, Charles's brother, became professor and chair of the Department of Anatomy, succeeding Moore, who ascended to associate dean of basic sciences. Hollenberg had earned his medical degree at the University of Manitoba and a PhD in anatomy at Wayne State University, and he previously had served as dean of medicine at the University of Western Ontario. On his watch, in 1990 the department was renamed the Department of Anatomy and Cell Biology. There were further changes in leadership. But it was too late.

In March 1997 Dean Arnie Aberman created an Anatomy and Cell Biology Task Force to reorganize the department.[37] In October the task force recommended dissolving the Department of Anatomy and Cell Biology, merging gross anatomy with the Department of Surgery, and merging the cell biology component with the Department of Medical Biophysics.[38]

In 2002 the cell biology unit was closed and the Department of Anatomy became a division of the Department of Surgery. The Governing Council shuttered the master of science and doctor of philosophy programs in the department the following year.[39] And that was the end of the Department of Anatomy.

Yet the scientific and teaching record of this small but vibrant academic division was considerable. Anatomist Ian Taylor, a very personable Scotsman, received in 2008 the Harry Whittaker Memorial Teaching Award. And division head Michael Wiley was selected for the W.T. Aikins Award for developing innovative instruction materials. Cindi Morshead, who as a graduate student in the Department of Anatomy made the discovery of adult neural stem cells under the direction of Derek van der Kooy,[40] returned to join the division's tenure stream in 2003; at her lab in the Donnelly Centre for Cellular and Biomolecular Research she did leading-edge investigation of stem cells and their precursors.[41]

In 1972 British anatomist David Sinclair, head of the department in the University of Aberdeen, wrote unwittingly a fitting epitaph for the Department of Anatomy in Toronto: "British anatomists are nowadays assured that all that is needed in the medical curriculum is a thorough knowledge of sociology and molecular biology, with perhaps a dash of psychology thrown in, and that 'ambulance man's anatomy' is more than adequate as a preparation for clinical practice in the wards. At the same time postgraduate knowledge of the subject is assessed by amateurish (and occasionally puerile) 'true or false' questions. It is therefore refreshing [to learn] that some surgeons at least, are interested in gross anatomy, and may occasionally make use of it."[42] The man's bitterness is palpable at the fate of anatomy, once the queen of the medical sciences.

# 16 Physiology/Banting and Best/Biochemistry/ Pharmacology/Nutrition

There was a time when all these subjects blended together, subsumed before the First World War under the general heading "Physiology." Today, in historical irony, the boundaries among them are disappearing once again as a molecular revolution prompts the generalization that all basic sciences are essentially studying the same thing: what happens inside the cell. As this is written, we are not quite yet ready for such a general statement because in basic sciences such as physiology the systems approach still counts. One thinks of neurophysiologist Jonathan Dostrovsky's collaboration with Andres Lozano in surgery and Helen Mayberg in psychiatry[1] on deep brain stimulation to relieve treatment-resistant depression,[2] work that owes little to research at the molecular level. Yet today the basic sciences are recovering the unity that physiology lent them before the Great War, and in the story of putting medicine in Toronto on a scientific basis, this cast is full of characters.

## The Department of Physiology

A recurrent theme ... was the emerging importance of physiology as a medical science that should be crucial in integrating new molecular knowledge into realistic models of human bodily function.[3]

External review, Department of Physiology, 1999

In the 1880s there were only two notable sites in North America for the teaching of physiology: Johns Hopkins University under H. Newell Martin and Harvard under Henry P. Bowditch, both notable names in the history of medicine. Toronto became a third site beginning in 1885 when Archibald B. Macallum, a student of Martin's, began introducing medical students to "the modernized type of physiology," by which he meant science based on first-hand experimentation.

Born in 1858 in Belmont, Ontario, Macallum earned a BA from the University in Toronto in 1880 and was awarded the medal in natural science. He was the first formidable scientific figure in the Faculty of Medicine.

Macallum had a great mentor, the zoologist Ramsay Wright, who served first as professor of natural history at University College, Toronto, in 1874, then as professor of biology from 1887 to 1912, and was one of the great guiding scientific spirits of the university in the late nineteenth century. (Wright's chair was called ""Biology and Physiology" from 1887 until 1892, when it became simply "Biology," but it is unclear if Wright actually lectured in physiology.)

Macallum was a student of Wright's (see chapter 3) and became a lecturer in biology in 1883. With the opening of the faculty in 1887, physiology was established by the provincial legislature as a university chair, and Macallum continued teaching a course in physiology to the medical students that he had begun in 1885, patterned, as he said, "after that in Cambridge under Sir Michael Foster." (Macallum was at this point quite a junior figure, as it was only in 1888 that he earned a PhD from Hopkins and a medical degree from Toronto in 1889.) In 1892 Macallum became the professor of physiology, a post that he held until 1908.[4] Based in the Biology Building, Macallum's Physiological Laboratory was modelled after Michael Foster's group at Cambridge; in 1897 he established a PhD program, the first PhD program in Canada according to Sandra McRae. (The first graduate was Frederick Hughes Scott in 1900, who then completed an MB at Toronto in 1904 and went on to make a name for himself in neuroscience in England and as professor of physiology at the University of Minnesota.)[5] Out of the Macallum school came a series of further physiologists, such as Maud Menten and James B. Collip, who occupied prominent posts in other US and Canadian universities.[6] After the completion of the new Medical Building in 1903, Physiology moved from the Biology Building (where it was part of the Faculty of Arts) to share space with the Faculty of Medicine.

Harold Atwood and Mladen Vranic, who have written the official history of the Department of Physiology, assign to Macallum a capital role in the development of the University of Toronto: "He fought hard and completely succeeded in transforming the University of Toronto's Medical School into one of the leading schools in North America. He also was largely responsible for a fundamental change in the view of the University as primarily a teaching institution," and left as a legacy the "establishment of research." He supervised the first student to receive a PhD from the University of Toronto (and also appointed the first woman lecturer in the university, Clara Benson, of the Faculty of Household Science). His Royal Society obituary stated, "Macallum's monument is the Medical School of Toronto."[7] Physiology played a capital role in training medical students to think scientifically, and McRae, who has studied the development of physiology at Toronto in detail, remarks, "Laboratory work in physiology, histology, and microscopy became the key courses used in modernizing the medical curriculum, reveal[ing] the essential role that laboratory teaching and research played as a bridge between biology and medicine at the University of Toronto."[8]

Biochemistry was somewhat slower to develop, as it evolved from a specialty called "Physiological Chemistry," "a designation," Macallum said, "contested in the early 'eighties' by physiologists who held that the subject covered should be regarded as belonging to Physiology and by chemists who maintained that it was but Organic Chemistry." In Toronto, biochemistry began to be taught in 1884 to undergraduates in arts and in medicine but, Macallum said, "it was only in 1888 that it began to rank with physiology in the extent of the instruction involved." In 1908 Macallum's chair in physiology was split; Macallum became the professor of physiological chemistry, and Thomas Gregor Brodie was summoned from England to be the professor of physiology.[9]

Brodie, an Englishman who had qualified for membership in the Royal College of Surgeons in 1890, had worked previously as a lecturer at St Thomas's Hospital Medical School in London, progressed to director of the research laboratories of the two Royal Colleges, then taught physiology at the Royal Veterinary College. According to Atwood and Vranic, "He was considered one of the leading experimental physiologists of the English-speaking world."[10] Three years after his arrival in Toronto, in 1911 he received the distinction of Croonian Lecturer of the Royal Society. During his tenure in the Toronto chair, "[h]e determined to make Toronto a great School of Physiology," as his eulogist said at the time of his death during the war in 1916, and suggested that physiology in Toronto was indeed world-class.[11]

After Brodie's death, Winifred Cullis, lecturer in physiology at the London School of Medicine for Women and co-investigator with Brodie, replaced him as professor of physiology for the 1917–18 term.[12] (She was one of the first female lecturers in the Faculty of Medicine, if not the first, and the first woman to hold a professorial chair in a medical school in England.[13])

In 1918 the Scotsman John James Rickard Macleod became professor of physiology. Macleod's life and the "great events" of his tenure, namely the discovery of insulin in the Department of Physiology of the University of Toronto, are discussed in chapter 4, pp. 49–56. Still, it is interesting to dwell for a moment on the huge amount of research on insulin going on in the Department of Physiology by 1923. Walter Campbell later described the significance of this advance along a broad front: "I am well aware that there were others who could have done it [insulin research], but the fact is that our group covered adequately all phases of insulin use and published it before any one else … It may be regarded as initiating clinical investigation along many lines both in Toronto and elsewhere in North America."[14]

With Macleod's return to Scotland in 1929, Charles Best became head of the department at age thirty. Best was already world-famous because of the insulin discovery. He further anchored his own scientific reputation and that of the Department of Physiology in 1937 with his textbook, co-written with Norman

B. Taylor, *The Physiological Basis of Medical Practice*.[15] Vranic says of the textbook, "When I studied medicine in Zagreb, the Best and Taylor book was considered to be the best source of information for a student in medicine. This book put the medical school in Toronto on the international map with respect to the teaching of physiology."[16]

Research on insulin and carbohydrate metabolism ran like a red thread through the history of the Department of Physiology after the 1920s. This interest intensified after Best became head of the department. Reginald Haist worked on the insulin content of the pancreas and on the particular cells (beta cells) that controlled the production and secretion of insulin. Many members of the department investigated different drugs for the treatment of diabetes, including the sulfonylureas as oral agents. The work of Vranic and Gerald Wrenshall in studying the responsiveness of various tissues to insulin is discussed farther on. Finally, Otakar and Anna Sirek investigated vascular changes in diabetes, especially the effects of growth hormone on blood sugar and amino acids.[17] Insulin and carbohydrate metabolism thus provided over the years a scientific backbone for the department.

But it was not just insulin. The Second World War shaped the work of the department as well. Among its members serving overseas was Jacob Markowitz, and this is a story that combines science with personal heroism. Markowitz, born in Toronto in 1901, graduated in medicine from U of T in 1923 and earned a PhD in physiology in 1926. After serving on the staff of the experimental medicine department of the University of Minnesota until 1930, he joined the Department of Physiology at Georgetown University as a professor until 1932, then returned to Toronto as a research associate. In 1937 he wrote his pioneering *Textbook of Experimental Surgery*,[18] which reached a fifth edition by 1964.

While at Georgetown, Markowitz proposed the first mammalian heart transplants and in 1933 became part of the team that conducted them, although the animals failed to survive more than a few days.[19] Markowitz described heart transplants in dogs as a routine procedure: "The exercise of transplanting the heart is a good one. The surgeon gains insight into the surgical anatomy of this organ and incidentally learns much about vascular anastomosis … A surgeon who can successfully transplant the heart may be reasonably sure that he is adept in the technic of vascular anastomosis."[20] This was pioneering work. Mladen Vranic comments, "Markowitz and [Aaron] Rappaport were considered the world's best experimental surgeons with respect to dog surgery."[21] (On Rappaport see farther on.)

Markowitz was a remarkable figure, adept not only at transplanting hearts but in organizing transfusion services. When the war broke out, he signed up with the British Army and served at Singapore, which fell in February 1942 to the advancing Japanese force. Later in the session, the dean told the faculty, "Word has … been received that Dr. Jacob Markowitz is a prisoner of war."[22] Markowitz's experiences in a Japanese internment camp were truly horrible, but he acquitted himself nobly and attended to the medical care of hundreds of sick and wounded comrades. "We had a large number of men," he later said, "who had to have their legs amputated because they were going crazy with pain from tropical ulcers, or were suffering from severe infections of their shin bone … By means of novocaine, which we were able to purchase in the 'black market,' our doctors in one camp alone did a most charitable work removing legs from 115 people, of whom over half were alive at the end of the war." Markowitz organized a transfusion service, keeping the donors' blood from coagulating by whipping it with a stick. (He had described this technique in cardiac transplantation his 1937 book.) For his "development of simple techniques for jungle surgery and his ingenious methods of improvisation that saved hundreds of lives," as the citation read, he received in 1946 one of the highest British military honours: the Order of the British Empire.[23] Markowitz returned to the Department of Physiology after the war.

Upon Banting's death in 1941, Best became head of the Banting and Best Department of Medical Research (BBDMR) as well. As John T. Murphy, later chair of the Department of Physiology, said in 1979, "During [Best's] ensuing stewardship of these two departments, and fueled by the gradual appearance of substantial financial endowments as a result of the discovery [of insulin], BBDMR began to act in many ways as a research arm of the Department of Physiology." This relationship received "physical embodiment" when both moved into the new Best Institute in 1955.[24] In the years from 1941 to 1965, when Best was head of both departments, the work of both tended to blend together. Under Best, the Department of Physiology considered itself something of a separate entity, "not closely associated with the Faculty of Medicine," as President Claude Bissell later pointed out. Best "developed his own institute where he pursued his researches in an intimate atmosphere, apart from the rest of Medicine: he was wary of the faculty and fearful of bureaucratic interference. He had a feeling that his faculty was not really concerned with fundamental research, and that it gave little heed to the recognition that came in regular waves to him from universities and learned societies all over the world."[25]

Charles Best embodied both BBDMR and the Department of Physiology. By 1947 he had long been world-famous, was constantly feted abroad, and had a great sense of his importance and that of his department. At that point – long before the Weston gift – President Sidney Smith had begun raising money "towards the cost of the new building to accommodate the extension of Dr. Best's work," spurred by a fear of losing Best to a competing campus. Best had had an "Institute of Physiology" in view for some time and had been active in fundraising, lining up substantial grants from the Eli Lilly Company and various private donors.[26] By the 1948–9 session, architects' plans were available "for a new building on College Street beside the Banting Institute. This will be known as the Charles H. Best building and will house the Department of Physiology," Dean MacFarlane said.[27] The move took place in June 1954.

Best was concerned about the future of BBDMR and was greatly relieved when these concerns were resolved in 1960 through the generosity of Canadian business magnate Garfield Weston. According to Best's wife Margaret, the gift was made during a social visit on 1 April 1960: "Garfield and Charley sat on one side of the room and talked while we (the ladies) sat on the other side but near to them and talked. Garfield had intimated to Charley that he wanted to do something to help his research. Pretty soon Garfield got up and came across and said 'Margaret, I have just given Charley a million dollars.' … He wanted everything done just as Charley wants it. Charley had contemplated for some little time setting up something to endow the Banting and Best Department and then along came this generous and thrilling gift."[28] That October President Bissell "announced the formation of the Charles H. Best Foundation and the presentation of the Weston cheque for one million dollars."[29] The endowment was set up outside the U of T to be "used specifically and solely by the Banting and Best Department." This arrangement was approved by President Bissell and some members of the faculty, but not at all by Dean MacFarlane, who complained about it to other department heads and in at least one case claimed that "there was already too much medical research."[30] According to Vranic, the interest from this foundation "is still used to support research in the Banting and Best department."[31]

Although Best's legacy was enormous, one piece of it was toxic: his reluctance to collaborate with the clinical departments. Vranic recalled, "During the era of Best the word was, you have to be wary of the Greeks even if they bring presents. So at the time when I came to Toronto [1963] this was applied to the clinical departments. In other words, don't trust the clinical departments. Best felt that we have to be isolated from the clinical departments." This seems to have been, moreover, the attitude of the basic science departments in general, not just of physiology.

Vranic spent years trying to overturn this doctrine through interactions with the Department of Medicine, collaborating with John Challis, his successor as head of physiology, in obstetrics, and together with John MacDonald collaborating with neurology and neurosurgery. Vranic said, "Once you show something in dogs, everyone says, 'that's very nice.' But then the moment you start to do experiments in humans and you can confirm it, the clinicians say, 'ah ha.'"[32]

In 1965 Reginald E. Haist succeeded Best as the chair of physiology, leading the department away from Best's focus upon diabetes. New staff came on board in the areas of cardiovascular, renal, gastrointestinal, and neurophysiology. Physiology and BBDMR began to drift apart again, and with the move of the Department of Physiology from the Best Institute into the new Medical Sciences Building in 1969, the administrative separation received geographic embodiment. In 1967 BBDMR was recognized in the faculty as an independent department, although it did not receive graduate department status.

Haist himself had graduated in medicine in 1936 and finished a PhD in the Department of Physiology in 1940. His own scientific work focused on diabetes, especially the beta cells of the islets of Langerhans. On campus, however, he is better remembered for chairing an advisory committee in 1964 at the behest of President Claude Bissell to look at procedures for academic appointments. The "Haist Rules" tightened up a number of university practices in the area of promotion and tenure. (After retirement in 1975, he embarked upon a successful career as an artist, and his last exhibition, held at the Arts and Letters Club – a genteel gathering place for artistically inclined academics – in May 1987, was said to be "one of the most successful of the various exhibitions held by that club.")[33]

The study of diabetes was growing thin. Under the lash of Lou Siminovitch, cell physiology was rushing into prominence, and that was not a strength of the department. When the long-range planners asked Haist in 1974 about "the lack of emphasis on Cell Physiology," Haist explained "that in the past this branch of Physiology separated off to be included in the Department of Biology … As a subject it has been taken over largely by the Zoology Department. There is no input by the Physiology staff into the Cell Physiology taught by the Department of Zoology."[34]

In 1975 John T. Murphy became chair of the department. An American born in 1938 in Yonkers, New York, with an MD from Columbia in 1963 and a PhD in neurology and neurosurgery from McGill in 1968, Murphy had lectured in physiology at McGill and at one of the campuses of the State University of New York before coming to the Department of Physiology at Toronto in 1970. His research fields were electrophysiology, electromyography, and brain mechanisms in the control of voluntary movement. Research grants received by members of the department doubled after 1975. Said the dean in comments for the external review of the Department of Physiology, "The recent development of the Playfair Neurosciences Unit of the Toronto Western Hospital under Dr W.M. Tatton has been a major advance in neurosciences generally and neurophysiology in particular."[35]

Vranic comments on the Murphy years, "What was initiated during that time, and further developed during the next decade, was to divide research topics in the department into the following platforms: Brain Research and Integrated Neurophysiology (B.R.A.I.N.) Platform (48 members), Cardiovascular Platform (25 members), Endocrine and Diabetes Platform (22 members), and Reproduction and Development Platform (19 members)." Vranic adds, somewhat parenthetically but the comment is worth noting, "The large number of people included in the platforms reflects that our department now has 120 professors, and that the platforms now include academics that are not appointed, or cross-appointed in physiology. In my opinion, presently our department is one of the strongest in the Faculty of Medicine, and has an important international impact. It also reflects a very close relationship between basic and clinical academics."[36]

In 1980 Murphy stepped down because he wanted to train further in neurology, and in July 1981 Harold Atwood became chair of the department. Atwood, son of U of T zoologist Carl Atwood and brother of novelist Margaret Atwood, was born in Montreal in 1937 and educated at the University of Toronto with a BA in 1959 and at Glasgow University with a PhD in 1963; he taught at the University of Oregon from 1962 to 1964 and the California Institute of Technology in 1964–5, joining in 1965 the Department of Zoology of the University of Toronto. Atwood was known for his research on synaptic differentiation and long-term changes in synaptic efficacy.[37] He was a somewhat unconventional choice for chair of physiology. As he himself later explained, "He [Atwood] had no formal connection with traditional Departments of Physiology, and his most significant research was on invertebrate organisms. 'You are the first invertebrate to impress the 'mammals,' wrote a colleague on hearing of the appointment." Yet Atwood's scientific focus was not so much invertebrates as synaptic transmission and neuromuscular physiology, and he fit right into a department which, in those years, was preoccupied with the rapidly rising hospital Research Institutes and the demands of their new members for cross-appointments in the basic science departments of the faculty including physiology.

In scientific terms, among the achievements of the department during Atwood's tenure was Harald Sonnenberg's co-discovery of atrial natriuretic factor (ANF), a precursor of the hormone that regulates renal and cardiovascular homeostasis, for which he received a Gairdner Award in 1986. This breakthrough happened as follows: in 1980, Sonnenberg was part of a team led by Adolfo de Bold, a professor of pathology at the Queen's University, which discovered the peptide hormone ANF. De Bold had determined that granules in the cells of the atrium regulated water and electrolyte balance, but he needed a bioassay for diuretic substances. So he phoned Sonnenberg, who "was searching for a natriuretic hormone," said de Bold, "and had a rat bioassay for that purpose." Sonnenberg invited de Bold to give a seminar in Toronto, and de Bold sent him some atrial extracts. Weeks later, "to my unbelieving ears, Harald phoned me to say that the injection of atrial extracts produced a diuresis and natriuresis that was immediate and incredibly strong." This was ANF. Astonishingly, the prestigious *Journal of Clinical Investigation* rejected their findings, and so the researchers submitted the paper to *Life Sciences*, "where it was quickly accepted and published in 1981."[38] The paper went on to become a "Citation Classic" (highly cited) as defined by the Institute for Scientific Information.[39] (Vranic comments, "The idea of an undetected natriuretic hormone was originated by Jim Pierce, who also collaborated closely with Sonnenberg. Unfortunately, Pierce died in a car accident before it was discovered that this new hormone is located in the heart."[40])

Sonnenberg graduated from the University of Alberta, then earned a PhD in 1964 from the Free University of Berlin. In 1967 he became a member of the Department of Physiology and gained international renown by perfecting a technique involving the microcatheterization of the medullary collecting duct of the kidney to demonstrate his theory that this duct controlled the reabsorption of sodium. Shortly thereafter he became involved with de Bold's research.

From 1991 to 1995 Mladen Vranic (pronounced "VRAN-itch") was chair of the department; like many other chairs, he was a student of Best's. Vranic was born in Zagreb in 1930. The story is this: in 1941 Croatia was ruled with the help of the Germans by fascists called Ustashe. Because of his Jewish origin, Vranic and his family escaped to Dalmatia, which was partly under occupation and partly annexed by Italy. The Vranics spent one year in an Italian concentration camp, which was, as he described it, "very humane." Yet big peril lurked: "The danger was that the Germans were desperate to have the Italians deliver the inmates to a German camp. This became particularly dangerous when Italy collapsed in 1943. My family was saved by a Yugoslav partisan boat, which also carried wounded partisans. They finally arrived in Southern Italy, which was already under allied occupation." After the war, Vranic returned to Zagreb to earn a medical degree in 1955, writing a dissertation in the area of diabetes, and a doctorate of science in 1962. At a conference in Geneva in 1962, he began making inquiries about working with Best in Toronto, and with the help of the Sireks and Göttingen endocrinology professor Werner Creutzfeldt (son of Hans-Gerhardt Creutzfeldt, discoverer of mad cow disease), the application caught Best's eye. Vranic came to Toronto a year later as a postdoctoral fellow and joined the department two years later. He told a journalist, "'I came here in 1963 and expected to stay for two years. But 46 years later, I am still here,' says the professor of medicine and physiology, who has green eyes, bushy eyebrows and a slow, deliberate manner of speaking."[41]

After his arrival in 1963, Vranic worked with Wrenshall and Geza Hetenyi, a Hungarian émigré scholar with an MD in 1947 from the University of Budapest and a PhD from Toronto in 1960; they were investigating tracers for the measurement of glucose turnover to help clinicians avoid "deadly errors." Vranic began publishing on the subject in the early 1970s.[42] He found that the hormone glucagon is produced in the stomach as well as in the pancreas.[43] "The discovery helped differentiate the roles of insulin and glucagon in the control of blood sugar in diabetes." In 1980 there was a huge finding: obese people are "resistant to the effect of insulin on glucose metabolism."[44] But it turned out, as George Steiner and Vranic also showed in 1980, that fat people did not have a monopoly on insulin resistance: it could also occur in lean people with high triglycerides. This was the first application of the tracer method to human beings.[45]

Vranic's main contribution using tracer methods was identifying the relationship among exercise, stress, and the management and prevention of type 2 diabetes. Under the sponsorship of the Kroc family, the owners of McDonald's restaurants, Vranic organized in the late 1970s a big meeting at the Kroc family's ranch in California that "gave a boost to the whole field."[46]

David MacLennan, a colleague and friend, summarized Vranic's research contributions as follows:

Vranic was a leading figure in diabetes research for over five decades, making major contributions in at least five areas. He pioneered the quantification of factors involved in diabetes pathogenesis, developing precise methods to dissect the effects of diabetes on the liver and the periphery, and participated in the first clinical studies on insulin resistance and hypertriglyceridemia. He showed that hepatic glucose cycling increases markedly in diabetes and that glucose cycling in the liver is an early marker of diabetes, making it a potential target for pharmaceutical intervention. He pioneered new concepts of the role of exercise in diabetes, leading to precise methods for controlling insulin, allowing type 1 diabetics to participate in the Olympics and clinicians to recommend exercise and healthy eating habits to prevent type 2 diabetes. His discovery of extrapancreatic glucagon changed prevailing views that each hormone is synthesized only in a specific gland. Finally, he showed that hypoglycemia is a major problem in insulin treatment of Type 1 diabetes and went on to develop methods for amelioration of hypoglycemia in insulin-treated diabetics.

He continued, "The importance of Vranic's achievements has been recognized nationally and internationally by his election to Fellowship in the Royal Society of Canada, the Canadian Academy of Health Sciences and the Canadian Medical Hall of Fame. He was awarded an honorary MD from the Karolinska Institute, Stockholm and he is a Member of the Order of Ontario and an Officer of the Order of Canada."[47]

In 1995 Vranic was obliged to step down because university policies then in force mandated retirement at 65. John R.G. Challis, previously professor of physiology and of gynecology and obstetrics at the University of Western Ontario, became chair. In Toronto, Challis led studies of the hypothalamic-pituitary-adrenal axis in pregnancy, finding, for example that elevated corticotropin-releasing hormone was a marker of preterm labour.[48] Born in Cambridge, England, in 1946, Challis earned a doctorate in science from the University of Nottingham in 1967 and a PhD in physiology from Cambridge in 1971. After research posts at the University of California at San Diego, Harvard, and Oxford, he came to McGill in 1976, then to the University of Western Ontario in 1978, where he became cross-appointed in 1981 as a professor of obstetrics and gynecology and a professor of physiology, with a research interest in the endocrinology of pregnancy. (At Toronto, he was also vice president of research between 2001 and 2007.)

Challis wanted to "further modernize the traditional physiological mode," as Atwood and Vranic explain in their history. He reached out to colleagues in the Research Institutes with cross-appointments and initiated collaborations with the clinical departments, especially obstetrics and gynecology. The faculty complement of the department grew from 75 to about 100.[49] In 2008 Challis left Toronto to take up a post as president and CEO of the Michael Smith Foundation for Health Research.

In 2001 John F. MacDonald succeeded Challis as chair. MacDonald, trained in physiology and neuroscience at the University of British Columbia and other institutions, was originally appointed at U of T in the Department of Pharmacology, then moved to the Department of Physiology in 1990 to become a founding member of the Medical Research Council Group in Nerve Cells and Synapses (which Harold Atwood established, stepping down from his chair six months early to lead it). The MRC Group exemplified interdepartmental and interfaculty cooperation (medicine and pharmacy). MacDonald and neurosurgeon Michael Tymianski collaborated in research on the early treatment of stroke, based on the idea that inhibiting a certain enzyme activated in a stroke will turn off the switch that causes apoptosis, or programmed cell death.[50] During his tenure, the department obtained eleven Canada Research Chairs as well as the prestigious Michael Smith Chair in Neurosciences and Mental Health (whose holder Min Zhuo in 2006 identified the location in the brain of the pain mechanism[51]).

MacDonald's tenure is also remembered because he increased the department's enthusiasm for collaboration with the Research Institutes. Previously, colleagues had been fearful that the institutes were going to steal their graduate students. Under MacDonald, as Vranic put it, "the environment for graduate students in our department is more collegial." Owing to government grants, physiology grew to be as well equipped as the institutes, and increasingly people were recruited on cross-appointments, part paid by physiology, part by the institutes. "And we share students. For us right now the institutes are extremely important," said Vranic.

An external review in 2006 found that "the Department of Physiology grew because it embarked on what has proven to be a very successful strategy of forming collaborative relationships." And then something very Canadian was noted: "It became clear to us that the successes enjoyed by the Department were needlessly down-played because of a perceived wish to not take undue credit." [52]

## Banting and Best Department of Medical Research (BBDMR)

I've been around when there has been pressure to earn one's keep in terms of tuition units based on the number of bodies you teach. When that happens, there's this emphasis on teaching which can only be met at the expense of the research side. So having one department in the Faculty that's dedicated to a research mission reminds the University of its mandate for research. It points out to the University that it is not all about teaching, that the acquisition of knowledge is as important as the dissemination of knowledge.[53]

Bernard Schimmer in 2009

In the jubilation over the discovery of insulin, in May 1923 the province passed the Banting and Best Medical Research Act, providing an annual grant to the Board of Governors for the establishment of the Banting and Best Research Fund. This led to the creation of the Banting and Best Chair of Medical Research, of which Banting himself was the first holder and therewith the first research professor in Canada. In addition to support from the provincial grant came the Insulin Fund of the Connaught Laboratories, as well as private donations.[54]

In 1928 the university signed an indenture agreeing to "provide space and facilities for both basic and applied research to the staff members of the Toronto General Hospital." These facilities, to be called the Banting Institute, were situated across College Street from the hospital and connected to it by a tunnel.[55]

In 1930 the university established the Banting and Best Department of Medical Research with Banting as its chair. For the next decade, he directed research in the BBDMR laboratories, which were located on the fifth floor of the institute that bore his name. Until 1967 the BBDMR was outside the Faculty of Medicine and reported directly to the president.

On 16 September 1930, the Banting Institute was opened. Lord Moynihan of Leeds, president of the Royal College of Surgeons of England, gave the formal address. The historic connections with British medicine were overpowering: "Lord Moynihan unveiled a portrait of Lord Lister ... presented by the late Dr. F. LeM. Grasett and Dr. H. [sic] St. George Baldwin, both of whom were house surgeons with Lister." (Frederick LeMaitre Grasett and Edmund St. George Baldwin had already assumed places of British honour at a celebration of "Lister Day" in 1927;[56] they were cousins and both were Edinburgh-trained surgeons in the 1870s who had emigrated.) At Baldwin's death in 1931, Dean FitzGerald noted that he had been among the earliest to "assist in the dissemination of the gospel of asepsis."[57] Beneath the portrait in the library was "embedded in the wall ... a brick with a suitable inscription stating that it was removed from Lister's Ward in the Old Glasgow Royal Infirmary, now demolished." As an illustration of the former Anglophilia of Toronto medicine this is exquisite, but the wind would soon blow from the south. At the time of its opening, the Banting Institute housed the laboratories of the BBDMR and the Departments of Pathology and Bacteriology (then a single department), and Pathological Chemistry, as well as the clinical Departments of Medicine, Surgery, Obstetrics and Gynaecology, Ophthalmology, and Otolaryngology.[58]

In 1936 Banting brought Bruno Mendel to the department from Holland, where Mendel, a German Jew, was seeking refuge from the Nazis. A protégé of the great biochemist Otto Warburg, Mendel was interested in the cholinesterases, important for those aspects of the nerve impulse that are transmitted by acetylcholine. Cholinesterase consists of "true" and "pseudo," and it was Mendel and his lab in 1943 that sorted the classification out.[59] Mendel remained in the department as head of the Subdepartment of Cellular Physiology until returning to Holland in 1950.[60]

A second scientific triumph of the young BBDMR was Wilbur Franks's rubber antigravity flying suit, which helped the Allies achieve air superiority during the Second War. Franks, a fifth-generation Canadian born in Weston, Ontario, in 1901, earned his MD in 1928 and joined Fred Banting at the institute. Franks initially did research on Metrazol therapy in schizophrenia with fellowships from the Hartford Retreat, a private US psychiatric hospital. But in the later 1930s Banting anticipated the outbreak of hostilities in Europe and began discussions with experts from the Armed Services of what the institute might be able to contribute. David H. MacLennan, Franks's eulogist, tells the story from here: the air force called Banting's attention to "the particular problems of black-out from high G forces." Franks, too, was familiar with the problem of centrifugal force. His research on carcinogenesis at the institute used a centrifuge, in which "[t]he test-tubes kept breaking, resulting in a dangerous mess. One day he found that test-tubes floated in water were protected against centrifugal force. He came to the conclusion that the same principle might be used to protect a human being. On September 14, 1939, four days after the invasion of Poland, he ran his first experiments by accelerating mice encased in a protective layer of fluid." The philanthropist Harry MacLean gave Banting and Franks $5,000 and Franks started making a rubber antigravity suit. "Within a few months they had a man-sized version of the one that mice had worn."

At Camp Borden the investigators tested the suit in a Fleet biplane, with Franks "protected by the suit and the pilot unprotected. Later, at the time of Dunkirk, a Spitfire and pilot were made available temporarily to Dr. Franks in Canada and forces in excess of 8 G's were achieved with the pilot remaining conscious. The suit was perfected into an operational model and was introduced into the Air Force in 1942, providing Allied pilots with superiority in the air."

As part of this research Franks also built a human centrifuge, and MacLennan reminds readers that NASA adopted the device at the beginning of the American space program. "If you saw the film 'The Right Stuff', you will recognize that the astronauts trained in a centrifuge derived from Franks' design."[61]

### After Banting's Death

On 22 February 1941 Fred Banting perished in an airplane accident, and Best became the chairman of BBDMR, simultaneously serving until 1965 as chairman of the Department of Physiology. Vranic recalls seeing Best at a meeting in these years, "a tall, strong, and vigorous man who during the discussion, raced enthusiastically from one part of the room to another, sharing the microphone with all who wished to engage in the discussion."[62]

Important work was conducted at BBDMR. There was a diabetes team consisting of Gerald A. Wrenshall, a PhD scientist with a background in physics (who himself had diabetes, sought out Best, then took another PhD in physiology); Walter S. Hartroft, an MD with a doctoral degree in pathology; and Best himself. In 1954 they established experimentally, as well as in human subjects, that there were two types of diabetes: one involving "profound loss of beta cells and of the extractable insulin of the pancreas within relatively short times after the onset of the diabetes"; the other, seen in humans with mature-onset diabetes, "where pancreatic insulin and beta cell granulation are much more abundant and show little tendency to change with duration of the diabetes."[63] These were later called type 1 and type 2 diabetes.[64] As Vranic sums up the significance of the paper, "The surprise was that Type II diabetic patients had insulin in their pancreas. Accordingly Type II diabetes has to be due in part to insulin resistance."[65]

BBDMR did not conduct only diabetes research. In 1958 Aaron Rappaport defined the basic unit of liver function as the acinus, which, Vranic said, "revolutionized our view of hepatic physiology and pathology."[66] Rappaport had one of the more colourful personal histories in the faculty and illustrates perfectly the tremendous enrichment that immigrants from Europe brought after the war to Toronto. Born in 1904 in a small town in Austria, Rappaport graduated in medicine from the German University in Prague in 1929. He trained in surgery in Berlin from 1929 to 1933, then, with the Nazi rise to power, fled to the Cochin Hospital in Paris. From 1935 to 1941 he was head surgeon in the Jewish Community Hospital in a small town in Romania; from 1942 to 1948 he joined the surgical staff of the Hospital Love-of-Men in Bucharest. In 1948 he came to Toronto as a research associate in the Department of Medical Research, where he earned a PhD in 1952 and wrote several important articles on experimental liver ischemia.[67] He joined the Liver Research Unit in the Department of Medicine at Sunnybrook Hospital in 1978. Such was the recognition of his work on the architecture of the liver that the basic constituent of liver structure is sometimes referred to as "the acinus of Rappaport."

After 1965, Charles Best became inactive as director of BBDMR because of his gathering illness. Donald Clarke from the Department of Physiology served as acting chair until the appointment in 1968 of Irving Fritz. Fritz, who had no historical ties to the Department of Physiology, had by this time shed his original strong interest in diabetes (he had trained with diabetologists at the University of Chicago). He now changed the research focus to metabolic control and signal transduction (what happens from the time a hormone binds on the cell surface to its ultimate effects on metabolism). He was fascinated by the role of carnitine in the utilization of fat for energy production and discovered the carnitine-acyl transferases in the inner membrane of the mitochondria. In the words of his eulogist David MacLennan, who succeeded Fritz as the chair of BBDMR, Fritz "was a pioneer in the area of regulatory aspects of substrate translocation across mitochondrial membranes."[68] (Fritz received a Gairdner Award for this work in 1980.)

In the 1960s the weather vane of faculty appointments started to shift from Scots to Americans, and Fritz was one of the earliest. He was born in Rocky Mount, North Carolina, and earned a dental degree at the Medical College of Virginia in 1948, then a PhD in physiology at the University of Chicago in 1951, followed by postdoctoral work in Copenhagen, where he discovered the role of carnitine in fatty acid oxidation by mitochondria. After a research year in 1955–6 at the Michael Reese Hospital in Chicago, he accepted a post in physiology at the University of Michigan and progressed to Toronto in 1968.[69]

Fritz's tenure began a period of renewal. David MacLennan later said in an interview, "Irving Fritz was hired to bolster research. Best had hired a lot of young people, starting in 1941, who were coming to the end of their appointments. As an incoming Chair, Fritz was able to hire a new cadre of young people, starting in the late 1960s."[70]

Fritz had no interest in asking BBDMR members to teach, a point that rankled with the colleagues in physiology, who did plenty of teaching. He told MacLennan, "I'm going to protect your teaching, and in turn I expect you to be excellent in research. I respect excellence."

MacLennan said, "To me this was like a clarion call. 'If you want excellence, I'll give you excellence.'" And he did so in a long career that produced 330 papers that have been cited more than 20,000 times.

With Fritz's arrival, the faculty decided to separate the Department of Physiology and BBDMR. Bernard Schimmer said, "Reginald Haist was appointed chair of Physiology, and Irv Fritz was appointed chair of Banting and Best. The Physiology Department moved to the Medical Science Building, Banting and Best stayed here [in the Best building], and expanded during Fritz's time to occupy the building. It was at the same time that the University changed the status of Banting and Best. The Department had originally reported directly to the President, and around this time, the Department was made part of the Faculty of Medicine, and the endowments of the Department came under control of the Faculty of Medicine."[71]

Historically, the Banting and Best Department of Medical Research was divided into various "sections," including the section Eric Baer founded in the late 1940s on "synthetic chemistry." Baer, born in Berlin in 1901and trained in chemistry, taught in Berlin and Basel until his migration to Canada in 1937; he was among the (very few) Central European academics of Jewish origin hired in the Nazi years at the University of Toronto.[72] Baer was an international leader in the synthesis of phospholipids, where he, in the words of Irving Fritz, "established the optical and absolute configuration of naturally occurring glycerides and phospholipids." This is important because studying the role of phospholipids in cells membranes and blood clotting would not be possible without the "availability of pure compounds prepared and characterized by Dr. Baer and his colleagues." Fritz said that Baer's death in 1975 "marks the passing of an era of classical organic synthetic chemistry which began with Emil Fischer,"[73] one of the founders of organic chemistry in Germany before the First World War.

Efforts of the Banting and Best Department of Medical Research to acquire its own graduate program were unsuccessful. It hadn't mattered so much under Best because then the distinction between the Department of Physiology and the Department of Medical Research had made little difference. In 1961 Best tried to get the School of Graduate Studies to establish an independent graduate program. They wouldn't but as a consolation offered to rename the physiology graduate program "the Graduate Department of Physiology and Banting and Best Research." Best accepted this, although it was "in fact antagonistic to the spirit of his proposal to separate BBDMR from Physiology in the Graduate School."[74]

After Best, the wall between the two departments grew even higher. In 1970 Fritz tried to "have a separate BBDMR Graduate Program in Metabolic Control in the School of Graduate Studies," but the Senate rejected this, "primarily because of the difficulties envisaged in having a new graduate program accepted at a Provincial level at a time when general financial support was diminishing." Then in 1972 BBDMR tried to persuade graduate dean Ernest Sirluck at SGS "to initiate an umbrella graduate program within several basic science departments concerned with the education of cellular and molecular biologists." But with the exception of Siminovitch's Department of Cell Biology, none of the basic science departments was interested. Bernard Schimmer confirmed this in an interview: "When Fritz came in, one of the things he wanted to do was establish a graduate program, and he, together with the faculty, developed a very forward-looking graduate program. But it was turned down, largely due to opposition by the other basic science departments."[75]

Both Fritz and Dean Holmes were uneasy about the quality of research being done in the department. In April 1974 Fritz told the long-range planners "that while at least 2 members of the department are doing work of very high quality, he considered that there should be several more doing work of equally high caliber."[76] Fritz said that if cross-appointing could be increased, "as [the colleagues'] research propensity declines, they could move unilaterally into their cross-appointed department and still carry out a very useful teaching function." Dean Holmes commented, "There is a desire to increase the quality of research done within the department."[77] The long-range planners were looking towards phasing BBDMR out.[78]

To increase research, Fritz encouraged collegiality. MacLennan later said, "He brought a lot of excellent people together, with different interests, and they were in a small building, a confined space. They had nothing to do but research … With the different interests, people would bring in new technologies." He gave the later example of Bernie Schimmer coming in with cell culture (in 1969), and suddenly "everybody was using cell culture." MacLennan continued, "By having this cross-fertilization among people with different ideas and different technologies, this was the ideal place to move things forward."[79]

Joining the faculty had thus been something of a two-edged sword for BBDMR. On the one hand, they did have increased opportunities for reaching out to others in interdisciplinary research. On the other, their teaching-free status was resented by other basic science departments, who saw themselves swamped with teaching obligations, none more so than anatomy. In 1975 Jim Thompson, professor of anatomy, suggested to Holmes, "The question of whether the teaching should be done by the BBDMR raises the question of whether this is basically to bring the members of that Department into the teaching or to improve the teaching currently given to the medical students." If the former, then maybe BBDMR members could "act as demonstrators in the Histology program."[80] Members of the department were horrified at this and similar suggestions.[81]

By the end of Fritz's tenure as chair of BBDMR in 1978, relations between the physiology department and BBDMR had been badly strained, the major issues being teaching, including their joint listing in the graduate school, and research endowments. David MacLennan recalls the efforts to deal with these problems. "A Basic Science Faculty retreat was called in which the agenda soon dissolved into an airing of grievances against the BBDMR by John Murphy, Chair of Physiology, and Rose Sheinin, Chair of Microbiology. As acting Chair of BBDMR, I bore the brunt of the charges against the BBDMR and the threat of dissolving the BBDMR and incorporating its members and its resources into other departments. Fortunately, Keith Dorrington, Chair of Biochemistry and the Associate Dean for Basic Sciences, held a higher opinion of the value of maintaining a research department within the Faculty of Medicine, especially one with its tradition of research excellence."

MacLennan continued: "I initiated discussions with Dorrington and the BBDMR faculty, which quickly led to the implementation of a series of obvious steps, which have since benefited both the BBDMR and its cognate Departments. The joint listing of Physiology and the BBDMR in the graduate school was terminated. Each BBDMR faculty member was then cross-appointed into a Department which already had a graduate program and proceeded to teach at both graduate and undergraduate levels. The payoff to the BBDMR (in addition to diminished hostility) was a sudden and exceptionally valuable increase in the graduate student population in the Best Institute; the payoff to the cognate basic science departments was an equally sudden influx of new teachers (6 in Biochemistry; 3 in Physiology, 1 in Medical Genetics, 1 in Pharmacology, 1 in Microbiology and so forth), which lowered the teaching burdens of staff in these departments."

Canadian Tire was involved in the department as well. MacLennan noted, "One of the BBDMR endowed funds is the Billes Estate, the inheritance of about 7% of the Canadian Tire shares held by the Canadian Tire co-founder, J. W. Billes. Because the income from these shares was consistently low, all of the inheritors won the right to sell them and reinvest at a higher return. Alerted to this sale and the probability of a 5-fold increase in the yearly return from the Estate, I again initiated discussions with the BBDMR Faculty and then went to Dean Fred Lowy with a proposal to share the income from the Billes Estate with the Dean's office in return for a guaranteed BBDMR complement of 14 faculty. In addition, we proposed that the Billes bequest be recognized in the form of the creation of the J.W. Billes Chair of Medical Research in the BBDMR," of which MacLennan became in 1987 the inaugural holder.[82]

On the basis of the bang-up job MacLennan had done as acting chair between 1978 and 1980, he was confirmed in 1980 as the chair of BBDMR, a position he held until 1990. Born in Swan River, Manitoba, in 1937, MacLennan earned a PhD in biology from Purdue University in 1963, then after six years at the University of Wisconsin, where his postdoctoral fellowship was quickly converted into a research assistant professorship, he accepted a post in 1969 in the BBDMR. His first research accomplishment was in 1970 purifying the sarcoplasmic reticulum calcium pump, one of the basic motors of ion transport in cellular metabolism.[83] Through his cloning in 1990 of the DNA encoding the partner of the calcium pump in regulation of muscle contraction and relaxation, the calcium release channel, he was able to identify the genetic basis for malignant hyperthermia in both humans and pigs and to patent a test for porcine malignant hyperthermia, which has generated millions of dollars through the University of Toronto Innovations Foundation.[84]

On MacLennan's watch, the sails began to fill again. Research flourished as molecular biology became a widely used tool, and the future of BBDMR was no longer under a cloud. The question of teaching was resolved as members of the department agreed to accept a commitment of around one-fifth of their time.[85]

Between 1990 and 1995 Cecil C. Yip chaired BBDMR. Born in Hong Kong in 1937, Yip was educated in Canada, receiving a bachelor's degree from McMaster University in 1959 and a PhD from Rockefeller University in 1963. Charles Best brought him back to Canada in 1964 to join the BBDMR. Yip is known for having discovered the insulin receptor in 1978[86] and, with Peter Ottensmeyer in medical biophysics, for having described in 1999 the three-dimensional structure of that receptor.[87] On campus, Yip was vice-dean of research from 1993 to 2002; his major achievement was his role in the establishment of the Terrence Donnelly Centre for Cellular and Biomolecular Research (CCBR), of which he became inaugural co-director in 2002.

In April 1996 the department began a second uptick in fortune as James D. Friesen was appointed chair. Friesen had just stepped down from heading research at HSC when the call came from Arnie Aberman: "Are you interested in being Chair of BBDMR?" Friesen said he would come over and talk to the search committee and as part of the negotiations asked for $1 million for new positions. "It sounded like a lot of money to me but it probably wasn't."[88] Given that times had changed from a decade earlier, Aberman agreed to the money, and the Friesen years saw many new hires as well as an influx of research funds.

Jim Friesen was born in Rosthern, Saskatchewan, in 1935 and, after earning a BA at the University of Saskatchewan in 1956, came to Toronto for a PhD in medical biophysics in 1962. After appointments at the Institute of Microbiology in Copenhagen, the National Cancer Institute of Canada, Kansas State University, and York University, he arrived at the University of Toronto as chair of the Department of Medical Genetics in 1981. In scientific terms, Friesen in 1976 became the first Canadian scientist to clone a gene (see p. 426), and in 1984 he and Danish colleagues identified a ribosomal mechanism in which the protein component, which is the final product of the ribosome, "comes back and sits on the beginning, or just upstream of the gene, and stops it from being translated."[89] As a means of feedback control, "[i]t's a very elegant method in a very primitive organism."[90] Friesen said that they preceded Masayasu Nomura in the discovery.

Thus, as Fritz had done three decades earlier, Friesen revitalized the BBDMR. In 2002, external reviewers described him as "energizing and transforming the Department." He "spearheaded" a faculty and university application for $53 million for the construction of a new research building that would eventually house the Centre for Cellular and Biomedical Research. The BBDMR ranks, said the reviewers, "in the upper tier of research departments in Canada, and has a strong international presence." As a research department with minimal teaching obligations, but whose members have tenure, the department had a singular kind of intellectual mobility: "BBDMR is uniquely positioned among departments to rapidly respond to emerging scientific trends, because it need not maintain a teaching program in a fixed subject area. It is therefore free to assemble highly interactive multidisciplinary teams." The reviewers pointed to the department's new focus on genomics and proteomics. All of the department's graduate students were registered in other "home" departments. Yet they seemed to consider the Department of Medical Research their home: "They greatly value the multidisciplinary nature of BBDMR, exposure to varied experimental systems and methodological approaches, the interactive and collaborative environment, and the closely-knit social interactions between students."[91]

Friesen gave a new unity to the department's research. In 2000 he wrote, "The BBDMR is at the centre of one of the most exciting eras in biomedical sciences. The research objective of the Department is 'to study cellular processes at the molecular level.'" The department, he said, would give special emphasis to "gene expression and signal transduction" using the methods of functional genomics and proteomics. The new centre that he and Yip had organized, Friesen said, would be crucial in achieving this goal.[92]

In 2001 David MacLennan reflected on the future of BBDMR. He celebrated Friesen's chairmanship partly for Friesen's "insight into the qualities in young scientists that make them leaders. His appointments of Aled Edwards, Ben Blencowe, Charlie Boone, Tim Hughes and Andrew Emili bring new directions … in proteomics and genomics to our Department … Thus our young staff are among the best funded in the Faculty and are certainly among the most enthusiastic and productive." (On these young scientists see chapter 28.) MacLennan said that Jim Friesen and Cecil Yip had recognized that the new science would require "unprecedented sums of funding for research" and lots of space and that the two investigators had been the leading force behind the new CCBR. According to MacLennan it was Friesen and Lou Siminovitch who had recognized the need for enormous new funding in this path-breaking research and had suggested that the province "support genomics research through the Ontario Genome Initiative, now expanded to the Ontario Genome Institute"[93] (see p. 691).

## Department of Biochemistry

Archibald Byron Macallum was introduced in an earlier chapter. In 1885 he began lecturing in physiology to the medical students and arts undergraduates. But how about biochemistry itself, an outgrowth of physiology? Although different sources give different dates, most consider that the Department of Biochemistry was founded in 1908, when Archibald Macallum switched from the chair of physiological chemistry to the chair of biochemistry.[94]

These early physiologists and biochemists were not insignificant figures. By the turn of the century, Macallum was already a physiologist of international stature, a Fellow of the Royal Society in 1906. In 1906 William Osler is said to have urged his appointment to the presidency of the university. Yet at the time, Macallum's conversion to biochemistry was in full swing and it is unlikely he would have abandoned his active lab for such a post. From the foundation of the *Journal of Biological Chemistry* in 1905 onwards, Macallum was involved in fledgling biochemistry organizations. Says his biographer J.M. Neelin, "Again he used these forums to promulgate his scientific opinions and policies. These events could only strengthen his conviction that biochemistry was the new wave from which his university must not be omitted." Macallum advocated splitting the physiology department in 1908 into physiology and biochemistry departments.[95] In the judgment of emeritus biochemistry professor and historian Marian Packham, "Macallum's most notable contribution to the U of T was the establishment of research and scholarship as essential functions of the university." Formerly, it had been "primarily a teaching institution, involved in the preservation and dissemination of knowledge, but not with its advancement. He was instrumental in the establishment of the Ph.D. degree [achieved in 1897] that he saw as a research degree requiring a thesis."[96] In 1915 Macallum chaired a PhD advisory Board of Graduate Studies that led to founding of the School of Graduate Studies in 1922.

Macallum was thus one of the main champions of scientific medicine in Toronto. "The University of Toronto had a well-established and even distinguished research tradition in physiology long before anyone had even heard of insulin," says Sandra McRae, an academic historian who has studied the department. McRae sees Macallum, despite his abiding interest in marine invertebrates, as exerting "a profound influence on the growth of scientific medicine at Toronto, not least through his support for and exemplification of the research ideal."[97] Said one biographer, "It is generally acknowledged that the international reputation of the medical school of the University of Toronto owes much to his untiring diligence and unfaltering resolution."[98]

As seen, when the physiology chair was split in 1908, Macallum became professor of biochemistry. When he stepped down from the chair of the department in 1917 to head the wartime Advisory Council on Scientific Research, Brailsford Robertson succeeded him the following year – for one year – to return his native Australia in 1919.

In 1919, Andrew Hunter settled into the chair. Hunter, a Scotsman born in Edinburgh in 1876, had taken a medical degree there in 1901, taught in Edinburgh, then studied in Berlin and Heidelberg for the next four years as a Carnegie Research Fellow. He came to Cornell University in 1908, worked for the US Public Health Service in 1914–15 as biochemist in charge of the pellagra investigation, then progressed to Toronto in 1915 as professor of pathological chemistry. In 1929 Hunter returned to Scotland as chair of physiological chemistry at the University of Glasgow. (He then came back to Toronto in 1935 as professor of pathological chemistry.) Hunter was a distinguished scientific figure and author of the classical study *Creatine and Creatinine* in 1928.[99]

Under Hunter, the department moved in 1921 from the Faculty of Arts to the Faculty of Medicine. In 1924 Hunter began the practice of weekly seminars in the department that have continued to the present. Said E. Gordon Young, historian of Canadian biochemistry, "Andrew Hunter was an elegant, meticulous experimentalist, a devoted scientist, and an able teacher. He dressed fastidiously and spoke slowly and deliberately, with careful diction. Many students declared 'Andy's' courses the most lucid lectures in the whole Faculty of Medicine." Yet his "seemingly cold personality," possibly only "Scottish reticence ... inspired admiration rather than affection in his students," in Young's view.[100]

In 1929 Hardolph Wasteneys, another scholar of British origin, took the baton from Hunter. Born in Richmond, England, in 1881, the eldest son of Sir William Wasteneys, Hardolph grew up in Australia, working as a government biologist. He went to California around 1909 to learn about water purification, then found himself at the Rockefeller Institute in New York in the laboratory of Jacques Loeb, working on cellular oxidation.[101] Loeb thought so highly of Wasteneys that he said to him, "Why don't you work towards a PhD?" Thus Wasteneys earned a PhD from Columbia University in 1916 without a previous undergraduate degree. Jack Laidlaw said Wasteneys was "[o]ne of the most remarkable human beings in the whole Faculty of Medicine. He was an extraordinary humanist. And the underdog, he was looking to help the underdog every hour of his life."[102] Wasteneys is indeed recalled for his commitment to the University Settlement during the Great Depression, helping the destitute with various relief programs.

In 1918 Wasteneys came to Toronto as associate professor of biochemistry and, as stated, succeeded Hunter as chair in 1929. He remained chair for over twenty years, retiring in 1951, and thus truly shaped the modern department. Scientifically, Wasteneys is remembered for the work he did with colleague Henry Borsook (who later moved to the California Institute of Technology) on methods for the fractional analysis of "incomplete protein hydrolysates," especially in a 1930 article.[103] He appointed a succession of highly productive new scholars, including Herbert Kay, Guy Marrian, Leslie Young, Gordon Butler, and, in 1939, Jeanne Manery Fisher, the first female professor in the department.

Born in Chesley, Ontario, in 1908, Jeanne Manery earned her BA in physiology at the U of T in 1932, her PhD in 1935 (marrying zoology professor Kenneth Fisher in 1938). After a postdoctoral fellowship at Harvard from 1936 to 1937, she joined the Department of Physiology at the University of Rochester, then returned to Toronto in 1940 as a demonstrator in the Department of Biochemistry, where she remained for the rest of her career (appointed only in 1948 as "part-time" assistant professor, "full-time" in 1953; these distinguished female investigators faced discrimination and hurdles in terms of opportunities and career advancement, an important issue even today). At Toronto, Manery Fisher became a mentor of many women scientists. Although internationally known for her work in electrolyte metabolism and active transport through plasma membranes, she shared the same status as other female staffers. As Marian Packham remembers, "Even in the 1940s, keys to the Medical Building were not issued to women staff members ... because it was not 'seemly' for them to work in the evenings unchaperoned!"[104]

In 1951 Arthur M. Wynne became head of the Department of Biochemistry, remaining in office until 1960. Therewith one of the major figures in the history of biochemistry in Toronto treads upon the stage. Born in Brigden, Ontario, in 1891, Wynne obtained a BA in biochemistry from Queen's University in 1913, an MA the following year, then went to work with Herbert B. Speakman – who brought with him from England bacterial cultures for the industrial production of acetone – at British Acetone Ltd, housed at the Gooderham & Worts distillery in Toronto. Acetone was then being used in the manufacture of munitions. After the war this group moved to the University of Toronto and was established in 1919 as the Department of Zymology (later known as enzymology), with Speakman as head. In 1925 Wynne earned a PhD in zymology. At the time of the merger with biochemistry in 1929, Wynne received the rank of assistant professor. Old-timers remember these years as a time of crushing teaching loads, as biochemistry offered instruction to students of faculties across the university. Yet Wynne supervised twenty-one PhD candidates, and his eulogist said in the 1971–2 session that "[h]e must be given a large share of the credit for the flourishing state of his field in Canada today."[105]

Starting in 1960, Charles S. Hanes led the department for five years. Toronto-born in 1903, he joined the staff in 1951 from Cambridge, where he had earned a PhD and "where," says Packham, "he had been involved in developing the technique of paper chromatography in connection with research on phosphorylase." Further, "Dr Hanes initiated the procedure of appointing the Departmental chairman for a five-year term (renewable once) thus taking the chairmanship away from being 'a life sentence,' as he termed it." Hanes retired having had the satisfaction (or not) of seeing members of his department appear for the first time on television, as three of his colleagues in 1963 presented a program for the CBC *Live and Learn* series on the nature of biochemistry.[106] Hanes, who became professor emeritus in 1965, was among the last representatives of the Oxbridge school of lone scholars in little labs. He had a horror of "big science." Said his eulogists, "In his view science in the universities was best pursued by small groups comprising a professor, a technician, two or three graduate students and the occasional postdoctoral fellow."[107] This eminently British view would shortly be overturned by a very much rival American concept.

In 1965 George Connell became professor of biochemistry and head, overseeing a major expansion of the department. Connell was one of the main leadership figures in the history at mid-century of the faculty. Born in Saskatoon, Saskatchewan, in 1930, Connell received a BA from the University of Toronto in 1951 and, as one of Hanes's first graduate students, a PhD in biochemistry four years later. He took a postdoctoral fellowship at the School of Medicine of New York University in 1956–7, then joined the biochemistry department of the University of Toronto. During his five-year term as chair, in 1972 he became associate dean of basic science; in 1974 he became vice president of research and planning and in 1977 accepted the presidency of the University of Western Ontario. He returned to Toronto in 1984 as president of the University of Toronto.

Connell was an important scientific figure. In 1962 he and Gordon H. Dixon in the Department of Biochemistry – together with subsequent Nobel Prize winner Oliver Smithies, then at Connaught (later at the University of Wisconsin's Department of Medical Genetics) – determined that there were three common genetic types of haptoglobin, a serum protein that binds with hemoglobin. The three had been colleagues in Toronto for years, working also with geneticist Norma Ford Walker at the Hospital for Sick Children (whom Smithies refers to as "my first real, albeit informal teacher of genetics").[108] Smithies's previous work made this haptoglobin discovery possible: a conversation in 1954 with Andrew Sass-Kortsak at the children's hospital firmed up Smithies's thinking about starch gel electrophoresis.[109] Connell, Dixon, and Smithies used this technique and reported the results of their haptoglobin research in 1962.[110]

On Connell's watch, biochemistry became among the first departments to leave the old Medical Building and, in July 1968, take up quarters in the new Medical Sciences Building, joined there later in the year by other colleagues who had inhabited the old Knox College building on Spadina Crescent. It was also Connell who initiated collaboration with the hospital Research Institutes, just then beginning to rise. In 1965 Connell gave a status-only appointment at the Research Institute of the Hospital for Sick Children to Bibudhendra (Amu) Sarkar, who in 1993 discovered the copper-histidine treatment for Menkes disease, a fatal neurodegenerative disease of genetic origin[111] – the first of many such appointments.

In 1970 George Ronald Williams continued the tradition of British heads of biochemistry. Born in Liverpool in 1928, he earned a PhD from the University of Liverpool in biochemistry in 1951, fellowing in 1952 in the Banting and Best Department of Medical Research. While on leave in 1956 at the Johnson Foundation of the University of Pennsylvania, Williams helped elucidate, with Britton Chance, the sequence and function of the respiratory enzymes in oxidative phosphorylation.[112] After Williams returned to the BBDMR, he moved over to biochemistry in 1961 and to the chairmanship in 1970 (and the principalship of Scarborough College in 1984). "In his first year as chairman," says Packham, "the Department reached an all-time high enrolment of 66 graduate students,"[113] which has only been surpassed in recent years.

Packham generously praised her colleagues while muting the importance of her own work. In 1968 she co-authored with J. Fraser Mustard one of the most important pieces of basic science research to emerge from the faculty in these years: the conclusion arising from their previous work that such nonsteroidal anti-inflammatory agents as aspirin inhibited the aggregation of platelets on blood-vessel walls: "The administration of ASA to rabbits (in doses which inhibited collagen-induced platelet aggregation) impaired hemostasis, prolonged platelet survival, and diminished the amount of deposit formed in an extracorporeal shunt."[114] By implication, the daily consumption of aspirin might forestall heart attacks. Packham was born in Toronto in 1927 and earned a PhD in biochemistry at U of T in 1954. In 1963 she acquired a research appointment at the Ontario Veterinary College in Guelph, where she had a radioisotope lab. It was at Guelph that much of the experimental laboratory work on the platelet project was done; then in 1965 she joined Mustard's group at the Blood and Vascular Disease Research Unit at U of T, and the following year, when Mustard went to McMaster, she joined the Department of Biochemistry at the University of Toronto as a lecturer. In 1967 she presented at a meeting their finding that such nonsteroidal agents as phenylbutazone and aspirin inhibited platelet aggregation in response to various aggregating agents. On the Mustard team (and later his biographer), she was responsible for much of the writing.[115]

James Fraser Mustard himself was not a member of the Department of Biochemistry.[116] Yet given the importance of his work with biochemist Marian Packham, herself one of the department's outstanding scientific figures, it seems appropriate to discuss his involvement with the University of Toronto here. In Toronto he had appointments in medicine from 1957 to 1963 and in pathology in the early 1960s, giving lectures during that time. Among the most distinguished scientists in post-war Canada, Mustard was born in Toronto in 1927, graduated with an MD from Toronto in 1953, and earned a PhD from Cambridge University in 1956 for research on platelets, then a highly neglected subject. Mustard had little interest in clinical medicine but a keen taste for laboratory research, and in 1958 he became a research fellow based at Sunnybrook of the Canadian Heart Foundation. In 1960 he and several other investigators, including two physiologists at the Ontario Veterinary College in Guelph, found that in pigs microthrombi composed of platelets form on the normal walls of pig aortas and that in some models "the pattern of deposits corresponds to ... the lesions in the early stages of swine atherosclerosis."[117] Thus platelet aggregation might lead to atherosclerosis (and, by implication, to strokes and heart attacks).

In 1963, together with Robert L. MacMillan, Hugh Smythe, and Kenneth Brown, Mustard established the Blood and Vascular Disease Research Unit at 86 Queen's Park (currently the site of the McLaughlin Planetarium). Of this small but important lab, hematologist Jack Hirsh (a 2000 Gairdner Award winner) later said, "All the places where I did basic science research were excellent (London Postgraduate Hospital, Washington University at St Louis and Toronto), but I'd say my time with Dr Mustard at the University of Toronto was the most productive. And that influenced me in coming back to Canada [to McMaster University]."[118] In 1966 Mustard left Toronto to chair the Department of Pathology at McMaster, where he and others were helping John Evans establish the new Faculty of Medicine. Mustard later became the president of the Canadian Institute of Advanced Research and was a senior figure on the national and international horizon. Another group of researchers scooped Packham and Mustard in print on the first report of the aspirin-platelet finding, but in 1970 they published a comprehensive overview of platelet research including the aspirin finding.[119] In 1977 Keith J. Dorrington, a molecular immunologist who had come to the campus in 1970 from Cambridge University, took over from Williams as chair for a total of six years while simultaneously serving as vice-provost of health sciences. Marian Packham succeeded him as acting chair in 1983, and in 1984 Harry Schachter became head.

Schachter, a world-famous glycobiologist, was born in Vienna in 1933 and educated at the University of Toronto. He earned a bachelor's degree in 1955, a medical degree in 1959, and a PhD in biochemistry in 1964, after which he immediately joined the department. In 1976 he transferred his lab to the Research Institute of the Hospital for Sick Children, where he studied inborn disorders involving the glycosylation of proteins.[120] Schachter accelerated the opening of the department to the new currents in biochemistry. At Schachter's initiative, in 1990 the department increased its commitment to a kind of biochemistry known as "structural biology." He and Jeremy Carver initiated the Protein Engineering Network Centre of Excellence, called PENCE. Needing a crystallographer for structural work, in 1991, after an extensive search, they appointed Emil Pai from Heidelberg, who had performed pioneering work in the field. Pai's recruitment served as the nucleus for the recruitment of other structural biologists to Toronto, many associated with biochemistry.

Yet, according to Packham, these were years of some discouragement in the department with low staff morale. There were few new appointments. Moreover, "[d]uring the fall of 1990, the very existence of the Department of Biochemistry was threatened because of the problems created by falling budgets."

At heated meetings the Basic Science Assembly of the faculty discussed "the restructuring suggestions of the Dean's Advisory Committee that would have merged eight [basic science] departments into five along interdisciplinary and programmatic lines," in a BIG department (biochemistry, immunology, genetics). This plan was, however, never adopted.[121]

Then came the era of change with Peter Lewis and Reinhart Reithmeier. In the history of the department in the late twentieth century, the tenure of Peter Lewis is regarded as a turning point. Lewis served as chair between 1991 and 2001, a decade that Packham sees as "revitalizing" the department.[122] Following a bachelor's degree from the University of Calgary, Lewis earned a PhD in biochemistry at Cornell University in 1972. Then, after a stint at Portsmouth Polytechnic and the University of California at Davis, in 1974 he joined the Department of Biochemistry in Toronto, where he later (in 1998) directed the Program in Proteomics and Bioinformatics. In 2002 he became vice-dean of research and international relations in the faculty (in 2010 associate vice president of research).

Lewis recognized the importance of big interdisciplinary initiatives. The era of the single investigator was over. Large cross-departmental teams were funded by the university's Academic Priorities Fund, which was set up by the provost in 1994 to keep the university competitive in a time of budgetary restraint. The fund was intended to break down the boundaries between departments (at least two had to be involved), and under Lewis large research groups started to come together. In 1992 the department formed a new protein structure group, also involving scientists at the Hospital for Sick Children and Princess Margaret Hospital. An external review in 1995 marked the new program in structural biology as "outstanding." Indeed, protein structure became one of the department's core strengths. In 1998 Lewis became director of the new multidisciplinary Program in Proteomics and Bioinformatics that he had helped found, which a 2001 review found to have "world-class stature." In biochemistry, molecular biology, bioinformatics, and structural biology were clearly the wave of the future. "The common denominators," as Lewis pointed out, "are questions about the molecular mechanisms of life."[123]

Biochemistry continued to embrace the growing strength of the hospital Research Institutes. Lewis said, "The collaboration makes both of us stronger." The Canada Research Chairs and the Canada Foundation for Innovation catalyzed this development, creating the resources to "recruit and retain top people," as Reinhart Reithmeier put it.[124] By 2010 the department had recruited twenty people over the previous ten years. "Peter Lewis inculcated that culture of collaboration," Reithmeier said. Hospital and faculty meshed smoothly in biochemistry: nuclear magnetic resonance (NMR) machines owned by the children's hospital were located on campus in the Medical Sciences Building, creating a state-of-the-art research and training facility headed by Lewis Kay, an internationally renowned biochemist and NMR spectroscopist. HSC scientists ranked among the department's top teachers. The hospital faculty were treated in the department as "one of the family," not as second-class citizens.

The campus-based and the hospital-based faculty pursued numerous collaborative projects and were able to procure resources that neither would have on their own.

Packham said of the trajectory of the Department of Biochemistry over the past hundred years, "With close to 60 faculty members, Biochemistry is a research powerhouse publishing over 1,000 papers in the last five years (as of September 2010). Its graduate enrolment continues to grow and attracts top graduate students from across Canada and around the world ... Throughout its over 100-year history, Biochemistry has met many challenges and continues to thrive as the fundamental molecular life science."[125]

## Department of Pharmacology

The Department of Pharmacology at the University of Toronto was one of the first such departments in North America. In the early days, pharmacology was taught together with therapeutics and was usually called "materia medica." As James K.W. ("Ken") Ferguson, a later department head, explained, the term *pharmacology* was recognized at the time as "an experimental science for the investigation of the actions of drugs," practiced in only a few centres in Great Britain and Europe. It was obvious, Ferguson continued, that James Thorburn, the first professor, "had no intention or expectation of starting a department of experimental pharmacology in the near future. There was no money and no space for it" in the fledgling unit. Thorburn's use of the term seems to have been influenced instead by the leaders of the field in Edinburgh, in particular Thomas L. Brunton's *Textbook of Pharmacology, Therapeutics and Materia Medica* (1886 and subsequent editions), which "was first on the reading list for his students."[126]

Thorburn was born in Queenston, Ontario, in 1830, his father a long-time member of the Upper Canada Assembly. He took his medical training at the Toronto School of Medicine, proceeding on to a postgraduate MD in Edinburgh.[127] By the time he became professor of pharmacology and therapeutics in 1887 he was fifty-seven years old and "had been practicing medicine in Toronto for 32 years."[128] In addition to several other prestigious appointments, he was medical director of the North American Life Insurance Company from 1881 to 1904 and taught medical jurisprudence and later materia medica and therapeutics at the Toronto School of Medicine until it was taken over by the faculty in 1887. Thorburn retired from the university as professor emeritus in 1890 but remained active in medicine until his death in 1905, publishing a total of three editions of the *Manual of Life Insurance Examinations* and becoming president of the Canadian Medical Association (1895) and the Ontario Medical Council (1897).

### MacCallum and Successors

Thorburn was followed in the pharmacology chair by James Metcalfe MacCallum. An 1886 medical graduate of Toronto's Victoria University, he spent two years studying ophthalmology in London before returning to a varied practice in Toronto. "Specialty practice in the little city of 140,000 was not easily established so soon after graduation," Ferguson explained,[129] as well as being a relative rarity during this period. In addition to practicing both ophthalmology and otolaryngology, MacCallum "assisted the professor of gynecology" (Uzziel Ogden) and in 1890 accepted an appointment as lecturer in the Department of Pharmacology and Therapeutics, becoming the professor the following year.[130]

"The connection between ophthalmology and pharmacology seems a little tenuous," Ferguson remarked, "but there was some. Cocaine had been introduced as a local anaesthetic only a few years earlier and was under active investigation" in both disciplines, as were "many of the drugs with actions on the autonomic nervous system with ... interesting effects on the eye."[131] During his tenure the title of the professorship was changed to "Materia Medica and Therapeutics," evidently in accordance with the designations used by the provincial College of Physicians and Surgeons; "Perhaps Dr. MacCallum felt that teaching a course called pharmacology was a little pretentious."[132] MacCallum eventually returned to his original specialty, becoming an associate in ophthalmology in 1903 and leaving the department in 1907 to undertake additional training in ophthalmology in London and Germany before returning to the staff of the Department of Ophthalmology.[133] (His subsequent career there is detailed in chapter 19.)

The real history of pharmacology in Toronto begins with Velyien Ewart Henderson, who in 1908 published a pharmacology textbook, one of the earliest examples of the classic genre of "Faculty" textbooks that Boyd and Grant made famous.[134] In 1909 the university funded a post in pharmacology as Henderson became "associate professor of pharmacy and pharmacology."[135] Henderson, who became one of the beloved senior figures in the history of the faculty, was born in Coburg in 1877 and grew up in Toronto; he attended Upper Canada College, matriculating in 1895 and "leaving College with the proud title of 'Head Boy.'" He studied science in the undergraduate program at U of T, did famously, and when he graduated in 1899, entered directly into the second year of medicine; he received his medical degree in 1902. "Vel" was widely known as an athlete, in addition to being intellectually brilliant, and figured on the McGill/Toronto Varsity team that met the Oxford/Cambridge team at some point during these years.[136] He worked from 1902 to 1903 as a demonstrator in the Department of Physiology at the University of Pennsylvania, returning to Toronto in 1904 as a lecturer in pharmacy and pharmacology, where he ascended to the professorship in 1912. It was after his service in the Great War that he began the scientific career that made him, as one eulogist put it, "Canada's foremost pharmacologist." With W. Easson Brown in 1923 he introduced ethylene as an anesthetic gas. Attempting to improve on this, in 1929 fellow pharmacologist George Herbert William Lucas and Henderson introduced cyclopropane, establishing its efficacy in preclinical trials.[137] Cyclopropane was a great scientific accomplishment and it became adopted around the world.

Lucas, born in Parkhill, Ontario, in 1894, received a PhD from U of T in physical chemistry in 1923. He was associated with Banting for the next three years, then in 1926 joined the Department of Pharmacology. In 1928 Lucas, in the words of his eulogist, "encountered cyclopropane as a chemical oddity, proposed its pharmacologic investigations, and then found with Dr Henderson its ability to smoothly anaesthetize animals." Banting submitted to investigation as a volunteer. Lucas achieved international recognition for the discovery as, "for many years, cyclopropane was a most widely used general anaesthetic throughout the world." His interest in toxicology brought him, at the request of the Ontario Jockey Club in 1934, to investigate the doping of racehorses. "He then served for many years as analyst for racing commissions in Ontario, Quebec and Manitoba and became president of the international 'Association of Official Racing Chemists.'"[138]

Allied to pharmacology in the early days was the discipline of therapeutics (later therapeutics was closer to medicine; see chapter 8 for details). In 1908 Robert Dawson Rudolf occupied the chair of therapeutics. Rudolf was born in Pictou, Nova Scotia, but moved with his parents to England at the age of five. He finished medicine at the University of Edinburgh in 1889, studied in Berlin and Paris, and then trained as resident physician to the Royal Infirmary and the Hospital for Sick Children in Edinburgh. "From 1891 to 1896 he was medical officer to indigo planters at Behar, India," said his eulogist, yet continued his research and graduated with an MD from Edinburgh (he was certified as a Member of the Royal College of Physicians of London in 1902). He began his career at Toronto as demonstrator in anatomy, then in 1897 became a demonstrator in medicine, in 1903 an associate professor of medicine, and in 1908 professor of therapeutics. In 1910 he became a Fellow of the Royal College of Physicians, a higher grade than member, and was said to be "the first physician practicing in Canada to receive this distinction."[139] At the time of his retirement in 1934, his textbook, *The Medical Treatment of Disease*, first published in 1921, was in its fourth edition.[140] Popular with the medical students, Rudolf won this accolade in *Epistaxis* in 1921: "R is for Rudolf, who dabbles with drugs; / His prescriptions they say, will make hair grow on jugs. / He laments of the dangers that man undergoes / And teaches the treatment for frost-bitten toes. / Whenever you meet him he's always a smile; / He's one of the few that makes living worthwhile."[141]

Under Henderson, the discipline of pharmacology marched into the 1920s as the Department of Pharmacy and Pharmacology. As the Department of Hygiene and Preventive Medicine moved to the newly constructed School of Hygiene, pharmacology gained new lab space by taking their old quarters in the Medical Building.[142] Henderson launched the beginnings of a Canadian "formulary," or list of approved drugs, in the 1930–1 session.[143] He completed it in 1945 just before he died, and in 1946 the Canadian Medical Association brought out a revised version as the *Physicians' Formulary*,[144] adopted by the Department of Veterans Affairs as its official formulary.[145]

After Henderson's sudden death from a coronary in August 1945,[146] James Kenneth Wallace Ferguson headed the department. Ken Ferguson was born in Tamsui, Formosa, in 1907, when the island still belonged to Japan. He received a bachelor's degree from U of T in 1928 and an MD in 1932, then trained in physiology as a National Research Council Fellow at Cambridge University. After further work at the University of Western Ontario and Ohio State University, in 1938 he returned to Toronto to join the Department of Pharmacology. Following wartime service in the Royal Canadian Air Force (RCAF), he became chair of pharmacology in 1945 and took over responsibility for keeping the *Physicians' Formulary* up to date. In 1955 he became the director of the Connaught Laboratories. Among his scientific achievements, Ferguson discovered in 1941 the oxytocin hormonal reflex in childbirth (the "Ferguson reflex"[147]).

On Ferguson's watch, the Faculty Council approved the discontinuation of Latin in the writing of prescriptions, as well as the conversion from apothecary and avoirdupois weights and measures to the metric system. "Breaking with a long tradition," Ferguson said, "the decision was hard to make, but necessary, since the consistent use of Latin in prescribing has become well-nigh impossible in recent years."[148]

*Werner Kalow*

In the post-war years, one of the central figures in the department was Werner Kalow, a scientist of great international distinction. Born in Cottbus, Germany, in 1917, Kalow studied medicine at the University of Königsberg (now Kaliningrad), graduating in 1941 in time to serve on a German merchant ship – a blockade runner – and to be captured and interned as a prisoner of war in Arizona, where he was the camp doctor. In 1947 he started studying pharmacology at the Free University in West Berlin. Yet he was influenced not so much by his own professors as by such British pharmacologists as John Gaddum and their work on dose-response curves, a matter of complete disinterest in Berlin at the time. Between 1949 and 1951 he trained in pharmacology at the University of Pennsylvania under Carl Schmidt, who had co-discovered the sympathetic stimulant ephedrine. In 1951 Ken Ferguson, chair of the Department of Pharmacology of the University of Toronto, had a chat with Kalow about Toronto, a university familiar to Kalow because biochemist Bruno Mendel had discovered the enzyme pseudocholinesterase there in 1943. (As stated earlier, Mendel joined the BBDMR in 1936 and ultimately became head of the Subdepartment of Cellular Physiology, remaining until he returned to his home in Holland in 1950[149] – so Kalow would have just missed him.) Ferguson was thus able to persuade Kalow to abandon his job prospects at Penn and come to Toronto, where he stayed for the remainder of his career.[150]

Early on at Toronto, using the spectrophotometer, to which Mendel didn't have access, in 1956 Kalow found a genetic variant of pseudocholinesterase (now butyryl-cholinesterase), which controlled the brief half-life of the muscle relaxant succinylcholine, often used during general anesthesia.[151] This turned out to have an ethnic distribution. Studying medical students at Toronto, he and colleagues found an ethnic variation in the metabolism of the barbiturate drug amobarbital: Chinese students had greater urine concentrations than non-Chinese students. "We had found a new interethnic difference in drug metabolism," he later said.[152]

In 1962 Kalow laid the basis of the field of pharmacogenetics, or genetically modified drug response, with his pioneering book, *Pharmacogenetics: Heredity and the Response to Drugs*. He found, for example, hereditary modifications of a cholinesterase in the metabolism of succinylcholine. A patient with an atypical cholinesterase would remain apneic much longer after administration of the agent than a normal patient, and this was under genetic control.[153]

There were further genetic discoveries. In his 1962 book, Kalow had explored the genetics of spiking fevers and muscle rigidity during anesthesia. He and anesthetist Beverley Britt coined the term "malignant hyperthermia" in a 1968 article that found "familial involvement" in a subset of patients with hyperrigidity and hyperthermia under anesthesia.[154] In 1970 Kalow and colleagues in the Departments of Pharmacology and Anaesthesia found that malignant hyperthermia with rigidity of muscles under general anesthesia was a different disease from malignant hyperthermia without rigidity. "Our findings indicate," they said, "that malignant hyperthermia with rigidity is caused by an inborn metabolic error in skeletal muscles which renders the muscle susceptible to disturbances of intracellular calcium distribution."[155] This was a finding of great interest and moreover confirmed Kalow's hypotheses about pharmacogenetics: inborn errors of metabolism are genetic, and here such an error modified drug response, in this case to the anesthetic halothane. (David MacLennan at the BBDMR went on to identify in 1992 the molecular basis of the disorder, so it is an interesting Toronto story.[156])

When Ferguson departed to become director of Connaught Labs in 1955, Harry Cullumbine briefly replaced him, then resigned in 1957–8 to go to Philadelphia "for personal reasons."[157] In July 1958 Edward A. Sellers became head of pharmacology.

Sellers, who later in life figured among the barons of the faculty, was born in Winnipeg in 1916. He attended Ridley College, a private prep school in St Catharines, Ontario, then returned to the University of Manitoba to earn his MD in 1939, winning on graduation the gold medal as the student with the highest standing in the class. After military service during the war, he finished a PhD in physiology at the University of Toronto under Charles Best in 1946. He was appointed to the Department of Pharmacology, which he then left for physiology and the Department of Medical Research, returning to pharmacology as chair in 1958. (In 1965 he was appointed associate dean of basic science, receiving responsibility for establishing the basic sciences in the new Medical Sciences Building that opened in 1969.)

On Sellers's watch, Harold Kalant, another international heavyweight, became a member of the department. Kalant hailed from Toronto, born in 1923, studied at Bloor Collegiate Institute, and graduated with an MD from the university in 1945, where he won, according to *Torontonensis*, "innumerable scholarships."[158] He trained in pathological chemistry, earning a PhD in 1955, after which he worked in the Canadian defence industry before joining the Department of Pharmacology in 1959. Kalant became well known in the area of chemical dependency, and typical of his great output was a review article he wrote in 2001 on the pharmacology of "ecstasy," an amphetamine of street abuse.[159] He became a lead scientist at the Addiction Research Foundation.

When in 1965–6 Sellers left to become associate dean, Kalow succeeded him as department chair. There is a long tradition of departments of pharmacology being interlaced with the pharmaceutical industry, and Toronto's was no exception. Just before becoming head, Kalow was on leave at the Boehringer company in Ingelheim, Germany, and contemplated taking a post there until Edward A. Sellers, on a European trip, convinced him to return to Toronto; after Kalow was back, W.G. Bruce Casselman resigned to become medical director of Geigy Canada.[160] There were many such contacts. A financial boon for the department? Not really. Allan Okey said of the 1990s, when he was chair, "Virtually no money ever flowed there directly from the pharmaceutical companies."[161]

By the 1970s the department would, in Kalow's estimate, "rank equally with Harvard and McGill."[162] Kalow himself acted as a magnet for the recruitment of such international stars as Stephen Spielberg at HSC in adverse drug reactions and Jack Uetrecht on drug hypersensitivity. (Similarly Phil Seeman later acted as a magnet for such bright young talents in psychopharmacology as Hubert Van Tol and Hyman Niznik – who did his PhD thesis with Seeman.)

Yet several observers commented that even though pharmacology was strong in basic research and addiction work (getting almost $1 million a year in research funds from the ARF), clinical pharmacology was a serious deficiency.

It was therefore an important step forward when in the late 1970s divisions of clinical pharmacology were founded at HSC following a donation from the Reichmann family and at Sunnybrook. The Division of Clinical Pharmacology and Toxicology at HSC was established in 1978 as part of the Department of Paediatrics; the Division of Clinical Pharmacology was established around the same time at Sunnybrook as part of the Department of Medicine by Martin Myers, who was then succeeded by Frans Leenen and Edward M. Sellers as division directors. (In 2000 Sellers and Rachel F. Tyndale discovered that inhibiting a certain liver enzyme [CYP2A6] with the drug methoxsalen reduced smoking in a laboratory setting. The finding suggested a novel way of curbing tobacco dependence.[163])

As for other scientific achievements among the clinical pharmacologists, Neal Shear was among the first, as colleague Shinya Ito put it, "to define and characterize the in vitro phenotype of patients with drug hypersensitivity."[164] Notable programs included Gideon Koren's work at HSC on "Motherisk," meaning reproductive toxicology: in 1999 Koren and co-workers in the Division of Clinical Pharmacology and at the children's hospital found that exposure to organic solvents increased substantially the risk of major fetal malformations. The finding, published in the *Journal of the American Medical Association*, came as a bombshell and was widely reported.[165] Okey said of Motherisk, "It's a resource for people all around the world to get the most objective advice you can about the risk to the offspring when the mom's exposed in pregnancy."

### Philip Seeman

In 1977 Philip Seeman, another international star, succeeded Kalow as chair of the department. In 1974 he discovered the existence of a receptor for dopamine in the brain that seemed associated with the illness schizophrenia. Indeed, over his career in the Department of Pharmacology of U of T, he made a number of important discoveries.[166] Born in Winnipeg in 1934, Seeman graduated in medicine from McGill in 1960. An American classmate of his recommended interning at Harper Hospital in Detroit. "But the internship there made me realize that my best efforts at curing the sick were limited. I never seemed to cure anybody – the patients kept coming back, their high blood pressure still high or their asthma still severe … That's when I decided to go into medical research to do something which might have some long-term and wide impact."

Seeman visited his wife Mary Szwarc-Seeman, a research fellow at Manhattan State Hospital and later a distinguished scientist in her own right, in New York. "The sight was overwhelming. Here were two thousand patients [at Manhattan State] who had schizophrenia or psychosis. The scene was unforgettable. I had no idea that schizophrenia was so common, 1% of the world, and that it started so early in life. Anyway, Mary said, 'Why don't you work on schizophrenia?' and then she said, like a wife says to a husband, 'Why don't you do something useful?'" In 1966 Seeman earned a PhD at Rockefeller University in life sciences, after which he came to the Department of Pharmacology of the University of Toronto.

"As a first step, I decided to see how antipsychotic drugs worked by looking for 'the antipsychotic receptor,' if there was such a thing. And if I could find that spot, then I would see if anything was wrong with the schizophrenic brain. They all said I was wasting my time, because nobody believed that a 'thinking disorder' as complicated as schizophrenia could be corrected or localized to a specific receptor for the wide variety of antipsychotic drugs." Seeman's research contributed to making the 1970s and 1980s the "era of neuroreceptors" in the history of psychiatry.

Finally, Seeman continued, he discovered an "antipsychotic receptor" in the brain in 1974, "here at this wonderful university, and named it the 'antipsychotic dopamine receptor.'"[167] It was christened the "D2 receptor." Seeman's discovery caused great excitement. Around this time other investigators were making similar discoveries. In 1993, thanks to the intervention of Vivian Rakoff, chair of psychiatry, the Ontario government donated funds that let the Clarke Institute of Psychiatry buy a brain imaging unit for positron emission tomography (PET) scanning. This was thrilling for Seeman: "So we can now see these receptors in people, and when these receptors are overactive, one gets hallucinations and delusions. And when two-thirds of a patient's dopamine receptors are occupied in the brain by the medicine, then the hallucinations and delusions are usually gone. So, the art of psychiatry is becoming the science of psychiatry."

In 1993 Seeman, together with pharmacology colleagues Hong-Chang Guan and Hubert H.M. Van Tol, made another important discovery: that dopamine D4 receptors were elevated in schizophrenia.[168] This opened the way to a search for D4 receptor blockers as a possible treatment.

Seeman will also be remembered for having begun in 1975 a small pharmacology textbook, *Principles of Medical Pharmacology*, published by the department, that Harold Kalant and colleagues in the fourth edition in 1985 grew into a major international textbook; at this writing it is in the seventh edition.[169]

### Allan Okey

In 1989 Allan Okey took over as chair. Okey was born in La Crosse, Wisconsin, and earned his undergraduate degree at a local college, followed by a pharmacology PhD from Southern Illinois University in 1969. His Canadian career began (two years before the degree was awarded) in 1967 at the University of Windsor in the biology department. In 1980 he joined the Division of Clinical Pharmacology at the Research Institute of the Hospital for Sick Children; he was cross-appointed to the campus Department of Pharmacology, initially on a status-only basis. Only when Okey was asked to be chair of pharmacology in 1989 did he join the department full-time.

In his research, Okey developed methods which led to the first demonstration that the aryl hydrocarbon (AH) receptor is not peculiar to laboratory animals but exists also in human tissues and cells. Although the AH receptor initially was of interest because of its role in regulating drug-metabolizing enzymes and in mediating toxic effects of environmental chemicals, this receptor subsequently has been shown to underlie fundamental biological processes such as cell proliferation and differentiation.[170]

"We were in the time when the resources were dramatically shrinking," said Okey of the early 1990s. The department shriveled during his tenure from fourteen tenure-stream positions to six, and its teaching strength was maintained only by cross-appointments and status-only staff. Okey encouraged collaborations among the basic pharmacologists on campus and the clinical pharmacologists in the hospitals. "It used to be two solitudes," he said. "But we saw value in having our students receive training that included an understanding of what clinical pharmacology is like, that pharmacology and therapeutics aren't all molecular biology and biochemistry." Despite the severe contraction in its complement of tenure-stream staff, the department fulfilled not only its role in medical education but also administered two separate BSc programs that were in great demand from arts and science students – one in pharmacology, the other in toxicology. Moreover, the graduate program in pharmacology became the largest such program in North America with over 120 MSc and PhD students at its peak. Okey later said, "I would like to think that my recruitment of key cross-appointed and status-only staff, including the clinical pharmacologists, made it possible for the Department to do well educationally during the lean years."[171]

For years at the university there had been interest, as zoologist Donald Chant, vice president and provost (and anti-pollution activist), put it, "in bringing some focal point to the diverse toxicological activities going on here." The Department of Pharmacology would have been a logical place for such a program, and it was felt that a joint program with the University of Guelph made sense, given the latter's interest in veterinary medicine and agriculture; around 1979 a working party was established to study the feasibility of establishing a joint centre. In April 1980 both universities approved a preliminary proposal and organized a steering committee under Chant. The province was to be petitioned for the substantial sum required for such a centre, which envisioned hiring thirty-five professional staff for the University of Toronto alone. Unfortunately, the project sat idle and ultimately was dropped in its full amplitude because of funding cutbacks.[172] Then in the new century the toxicology project was revived as an integral part of the Department of Pharmacology, and in November 2007 the department's name was changed to the Department of Pharmacology and Toxicology.[173]

## Department of Nutritional Sciences

The department is certainly one of the few nutrition departments in a faculty of medicine in North America and among a handful of nutrition programs worldwide that are based in medical schools and that are highly successful.[174]

External review, 2002

The study of nutrition as a medical science in Toronto went back to the origins of the School of Hygiene and the opening of its new building in 1927, when Earle W. McHenry was appointed to undertake "glandular studies" with Charles Best. McHenry, born in Streetsville, Ontario, in 1899, had at the time a master's degree and counted as an "assistant" in the hygiene school until he completed his PhD in biochemistry in 1929. McHenry earned his place in history by preparing in 1928 a soluble liver extract for oral use in the treatment of pernicious anemia[175] – a disease of great interest to Farquharson and Graham in the Department of Medicine. The highly purified intramuscular liver extract that McHenry perfected in 1931 was used by the two clinicians and resulted in their 1933 article on the new treatment (see p. 183).

In 1941 McHenry became head of the new Subdepartment of Nutrition in the School,[176] and in 1946 he was appointed professor of nutrition and head of the Department of Public Health Nutrition. At the time of his death in 1961, McHenry had a large international reputation that included a textbook, *Basic Nutrition*. In 1956 nutrition was organized at the school into a little two-person department, and McHenry's student George Beaton (PhD in 1955) succeeded him in the chair.

At the time of the dissolution of the School of Hygiene in 1975, therefore, nutrition research and teaching had a long and distinguished history in Toronto. Just before the dissolution, in 1974 a task force recommended that a new Department of Nutrition and Food Science be created in the Faculty of Medicine – quite appropriately, in terms of the enormous contributions that McHenry and others had made to medicine. Nutrition was therefore one of the four new departments in the faculty in 1975; it joined as a basic science.[177]

Beaton stayed on as chair and was obliged by the Governing Council in 1975 to include in his department the nutrition component of the Faculty of Food Sciences – Nutrition, Dietetics, and Food Chemistry. The Faculty of Food Sciences was being dissolved and the other components turfed to arts and sciences. Said a report by nutritionist Henry Berry, "This has created formidable and unenviable problems for the Chairman of the Department [of Nutrition], namely, staff from previously separate departments who are at conflict and disproportionately tenured, and a divided location at opposite ends of the Campus."[178] The rather anemic little nutrition department now had twelve full-time staff – divided between the FitzGerald Building on College Street and the Lillian Massey Building on Bloor Street West – one PhD candidate, and little in research grants. Beaton complained that he hadn't been able to get authorization for anything and that the whole situation seemed paralyzed.[179] But the long-range planners, to whom Beaton had been making these laments, saw the glass as half full rather than half empty and made to Dean Holmes a positive recommendation: "We are impressed that this Faculty has in its various divisions the potential to make the University of Toronto a world leader in Nutrition, and that its Department of Nutrition and Food Science will play a key role in this development."[180]

The bright light in the new department was G. Harvey Anderson, who in 1976 organized a nutrition course for the medical students, said to be the first such "free standing" course given to medical undergraduates in North America.[181] Anderson is the star of this story, from 1981 to 1991 chair of the department and in 1992 acting dean of the Faculty of Medicine. Anderson was the pre-eminent scientific figure in studies of nutrition in the faculty after the old Department of Nutrition, inherited from the School of Hygiene in 1975, was broken up and replaced with the Department of Nutrition and Food Science.

Born in Provost, Alberta, in 1941, Anderson received his first two degrees at the University of Alberta, then took a PhD in nutrition science from the University of Illinois in 1969. After a research fellowship at the Massachusetts Institute of Technology in 1969–70, he joined the University of Toronto, receiving a professorship in the department in 1978. Leadership in this department, somewhat in turmoil after joining the faculty, fell on his shoulders.

As he assumed the chair in 1981, Anderson had a large deadweight problem to confront. The Self-Study of 1983 said that the "major weakness" of the department "is the existence of a relatively large number of non-productive staff members. Dr Anderson identified at least four appointees who are unable or unwilling to do research at levels approaching the usual standards of competence, much less creativity. Dr Anderson rhetorically asked how he could restructure a department with limited resources if one-third of his allotted FTE [full-time equivalents] were non-productive, with tenure?" Yet Anderson was hopeful of a future "based on an aggressive drive to obtain outside support for programs to which he feels deeply committed." The Self-Study continued, "If successful, it could serve an extraordinarily important role in bridging [nutrition and the basic sciences] and in facilitating interchanges among basic and clinical scientists interested in all aspects of metabolism and metabolic regulation."[182] This analysis turned out to be quite prescient.

By the time that Anderson stepped down from the chair in 1992 to become acting dean, he had recruited several promising figures, often in collaboration with St Michael's Hospital. In 1980, just before he assumed the chair, he had been influential in hiring British scientist David Jenkins to the department. Jenkins, who originated the concept "glycemic index," was cross-appointed to St Michael's Hospital, and his work is discussed in the context of that hospital (p. 630). Vladimir Vuksan, who had a research interest in ginseng, had joined the department in 1986 and St Michael's in 1990, becoming associate director of the hospital's Risk Factor Modification Centre. Internist Lawrence Leiter in the Department of Medicine at St Michael's frequently collaborated with such Department of Nutrition workers as Jenkins, Mi-Kyung Sung, and John L. Sievenpiper.[183] Sung herself and A. Venketeshwer Rao were prominent in efforts to identify a treatment role for soybean saponins in colon cancer.[184] Nutrition was a department that came alive, after so much travail, under the healing hand of Harvey Anderson.

In 1992 Heather Maclean became chair, succeeded in turn by Michael Archer in 1998. In 2007 the department acquired a degree program for the professional nutrition stream, the MSc in community health, public health nutrition, to produce hospital dietitians. And the department had an academic graduate program in the MSc/PhD nutritional sciences stream. In a review in 2002, the external assessors praised "[t]he wisdom of the University of Toronto in retaining the department as a separate entity with the broad mission of basic, clinical and community science aspects of nutrition," a wisdom borne out "by the extraordinary progress and success of the department over the past 5–7 years." They called nutrition a "'signature program' for the university." Responding to the review, Dean Naylor pointed out "the extraordinary turnaround from a few years ago, when there was debate as to whether the Department would even continue to exist!"[185] Indeed, it did seem like a good call.

# 17 Medical Biophysics/Biomedical Engineering/ Immunology

The institutions in this chapter are all Johnny-come-latelies. But they show the dynamism of change in medicine. Age-old disciplines such as anatomy wither and become appendages of other departments. New institutions are thrown off by the remorseless process of change and rise up, such as the marriage of physics and medicine, the marriage of engineering and medicine, or the science of the immune system. By the next time someone takes a crack at writing a history of the Faculty of Medicine these departments too, in their turn, will seem antiquated and hoary – in exactly the same way that an anatomy museum does today with its pickled specimens in their glass jars – and other disciplines that lie as yet aborning will rule the roost.

## Department of Medical Biophysics

Medical Biophysics is ... a Department unlike all the others. It has no significant budget for faculty, it has no jurisdiction over space, and it does not make primary appointments. In essence, the Department functions as a program of graduate studies for students who are enrolled in one of its component entities.[1]

External review, 1996

The Department of Medical Biophysics was founded in the Faculty of Medicine on 1 July 1958. It owed its existence to a decision in 1955 by Dean Andrew Gordon of the School of Graduate Studies that, as Harold Johns put it, "all graduate training must be carried on at the University campus." At the Ontario Cancer Institute, scientific work was jointly conducted by Arthur Ham at the Division of Biological Research and Harold Johns at the Division of Physics. Yet because the institute was off campus over on Sherbourne Street, it appeared that the students of those OCI staff who did not have faculty appointments would not qualify for enrolment. Ham was a member of the anatomy department and

Johns of the physics department, so for their personal students there would be no problem (although the students would have to work on campus). Yet many other members of the OCI physics division in particular did not have faculty appointments and, unless something were done, they would be unable to supervise students. The head of the Department of Physics, W.H. Watson, was frankly hostile: doctors and researchers were like cheese and chalk, he argued: "The research man would not be allowed to practice."[2]

To solve this problem, senior executives – including M. Wallace McCutcheon, head of the OCI Board of Governors; John MacFarlane, dean of medicine; Clifford Ash, director of OCI; Ham; and Johns – put their heads together and decided, Johns said, "to create a university department comprising both the Divisions of Biological Research and of Physics, which would in effect make the Ontario Cancer Institute part of the University of Toronto as far as graduate training was concerned." The head of this new department would be the head either of biological research or of physics research. The department would be situated in the Faculty of Medicine.

What was the new department to be called? There were various proposals such as "Biophysics," "Radiobiology," and so forth. But Ham insisted strongly that the department have a name "with the broadest implication – Biophysics," and given that it was to be situated in the Faculty of Medicine, he accepted the qualifier "Medical Biophysics." Initially there were problems with prerequisites: biology students would need a whole raft of physics courses to qualify, and vice versa, but once the SGS realized that the new department was attracting first-class students, the office became more indulgent about formal prerequisites, "so that today the student's course load is tailored to the type of research problem he is attacking."

The new department attracted students from a wide variety of backgrounds, including, in 1970, eight students with medical degrees among the forty-one graduate students in the PhD program. Johns, speaking of himself in the third person, said, "Dr Johns' main concern was to establish the Biophysics Department as an outstanding research group, and to insist on productive and original research from each student, before the PhD was granted. In this, he was eminently successful, and graduates from the department were in demand in many of the world's leading cancer research centres."[3]

In theory, Ham chaired the new department from 1958 to 1961. Yet preoccupied by his histology textbook, he quickly lost interest in the drudgery of academic administration, and Lou Siminovitch became the de facto head of the department. Siminovitch said that Ham "was nearly always occupied pecking away with two fingers on his old typewriter. So … I began to take on many of the administrative duties, such as equipment purchases … and even responsibility for some recruitment. Very early, therefore, Dr Ham asked me to take on the role of head of the Division of Biological Research." Johns concurred, and Siminovitch ended up running the department.[4] (Siminovitch was not really a cracker-jack administrator. In an interview, Jim Friesen laughed at the notion. "Nobody will ever categorize Lou as an administrator. He is as far from an administrator as it is possible to be."[5])

So what was Siminovitch's contribution? "He was a builder rather than an administrator," said Jim Till. "He played a fundamental role in building several of the most outstanding research environments in Canada, at the Ontario Cancer Institute (1956–69), the Hospital for Sick Children Research Institute (1970–85), and the Samuel Lunenfeld Institute at Mount Sinai Hospital in Toronto (1983–94)."[6] At the University of Toronto, he was a builder of the Departments of Medical Biophysics and Medical Genetics.

Friesen said of the years after Siminovitch's research on the polyoma virus and stem cells, "He got so-called somatic cell genetics going. You take a human cell, or a mouse cell, and put various selective pressures on it, and you'd get various kinds of mutants that are interesting. People said, 'It's impossible, it can't be done because they're diploid [having two sets of chromosomes] and you'll never get recessive mutations and most mutations are recessive. It won't work.' Well, it did work, because there's all kinds of shedding of duplicate chromosomes that goes on in cultured cells."[7] Out of somatic cell research came stem cells, for example.

Stem cells were the big science story to come out of the department in those years, recounted in chapter 5. That story was the result of a collaboration between McCulloch and Till. Shortly before their team work began, McCulloch had played a pivotal role in a separate collaborative program, one that was based on studies of a tumour virus that McCulloch had recovered from a mouse mammary tumour and cultivated serially in cell cultures. Axelrad, Ham, Allan Howatson, and Siminovitch were all involved in this research, as the virus induced a variety of tumours in newborn Swiss mice and hamsters. Kidney tumours, for example, developed so quickly that the animals often died within two weeks. The researchers became known as the "polyoma group," for a tumour virus that could induce a variety of cancers.[8] By the early 1960s research in the department had grown to grand dimensions, with eight postdoctoral students, thirty-two graduate students, and investigation going on in four main areas: cell and radiation biology; studies on virus and tumours; immunology and immunochemistry; and clinical and isotope radiation physics.[9]

In 1968 it was decided to shift the group interested in cell biology to the Medical Sciences Building. Originally they were to remain part of the Department of Medical Biophysics, but, under Lou Siminovitch's leadership the following year, they constituted themselves as a separate undergraduate department. The graduate students remained with the Department of Medical Biophysics. Johns said, "This arrangement will enable Cell Biology to have access to students from Physics and Chemistry backgrounds, who are being attracted in increasing numbers to the Department of Medical Biophysics."[10] (On the evolution of the Department of Medical Cell Biology, see pp. 689–693.)

In 1971 Gordon Whitmore succeeded Johns as head of the Department of Medical Biophysics. Born in Saskatoon, Saskatchewan, in 1931, Whitmore attended the University of Saskatchewan for his first two degrees, receiving an MA in 1954, and was a student of Johns before proceeding along with Till to Yale for his PhD in biophysics in 1957. Johns brought him and Till to Toronto in 1956, a year before they were awarded their degrees, as physicists in the just-opened OCI. McCulloch said that Whitmore was "at the forefront of the international radiation biology research community";[11] and Whitmore collaborated with Mortimer Elkind on a major reference book, *The Radiobiology of Cultured Mammalian Cells* (1967).[12] By now, there were also groups in medical biophysics at TGH and HSC.[13]

The department's record at "grant capture" stood out in the university, which on the whole had not done badly at this activity. Orthopedic surgeon W. Robert Harris, head of the Long-Range Planning and Assessment Committee, commented in 1975, "Dr Whitmore says he cannot remember the last time a grant application was refused. This 100% success rate is the best we have heard of, followed closely by BBDMR, which I recall had an 86% success rate."[14]

The Department of Medical Biophysics was a rather curious amalgam for the university, given that, with the exception of some physics research, its central focus was a single disease, cancer, and that the department was, as R. Mark Henkelman pointed out in 1986, "essentially contained within medical research institutes such as the Ontario Cancer Institute, the Ludwig Institute and the Radiological Research Laboratories. Thus, for many staff members, their academic appointments are secondary to their primary appointments within the research institutes." The university provided almost none of the budget, yet the university mattered greatly as a source of graduate students.[15]

In 1976 Robert Allan Phillips succeeded Whitmore as head of the department. Phillips was born in St Louis, Missouri, in 1937 and took a PhD in molecular biology at Washington University in St Louis in 1965. A leader in cell immunology, he had his office at the Hospital for Sick Children and was the first departmental chair situated outside of OCI. The situation was as follows, Phillips explained in 1986: "The department of Medical Biophysics was created at the OCI. However, as the number of cross appointed faculty has increased, mainly in genetics, the size of the faculty has increased to the point where there are more than half of the faculty outside of the OCI and more than two thirds of the graduate students are in laboratories outside the OCI." So in 1981 Phillips formally split the graduate programs, making Friesen responsible for the genetics program and R. Mark Henkelman for the medical physics program, and Phillips himself headed the cell biology program.[16] The genetics program had a strong affiliation with the Hospital for Sick Children and became involved in the study of the genetic diseases of children.

The dissociation between the main OCI site and the chair's new office prompted a general review in the faculty, which concluded that an additional graduate department might be created "more suited to the areas of strength and philosophies of the major groups of Medical Biophysics outside the OCI."[17]

In 1986 the faculty decided to split the Department of Medical Biophysics into two units. The unit of cell biology and medical physics would continue to be situated at OCI on Sherbourne Street as the Department of Medical Biophysics. A new graduate Department of Medical Genetics would be created, to be run by the existing undergraduate Department of Medical Genetics, which Jim Friesen had headed since 1981.[18] Of the department remaining at Sherbourne Street, the medical physics program had eleven full-time members in 1986, the cell biology program twenty-six.

In 1987 Frank Peter Ottensmeyer, born in Essen, Germany, in 1939 and educated at the University of Toronto (with a PhD in biophysics in 1967), took the baton from Phillips, returning the Department of Medical Biophysics to its home at OCI. (Ottensmeyer may be remembered for his despairing opinion in 1990 that graduate MDs were too old to be trained as research scientists: "He felt ... the age of this cohort on average, about 32 years old was typically too late to begin a productive research career."[19])

In the late 1980s the Department of Medical Biophysics acquired Sunnybrook as a second site in addition to OCI. In 1996 the 110 graduate students of the department were distributed at these two sites among three divisions. The first was the Cell and Molecular Biology Program, which was the largest. Most of its members were at OCI, though five were at Sunnybrook. One of the segments of this division was the Amgen Institute, headed by Tak Mak. Second came the Medical Physics Program, its largest component in medical imaging at Sunnybrook, with five members. The most recent division was the Molecular and Structural Biology Program, centred at OCI.[20]

Immunology had always been close to medical biophysics, and in the fall of 1992 Richard Miller, previously chair of immunology until 1990, was appointed chair of medical biophysics.[21] In 2002 James Lepock, chair of physics at the University of Waterloo, succeeded him.[22]

Medical biophysics had its origins, as has been seen, in a cancer research institute and retained this character, as external reviewers put it in 2006, of "differ[ing] from any other Department in being almost entirely an academic home for scientists at several of the major Research Institutes in Toronto." The great majority of medical biophysics staff were at OCI/PMH and Sunnybrook, yet significant contingents found themselves as well at the Hospital for Sick Children, the Toronto General Hospital Research Institute, the Samuel Lunenfeld Research Institute at Sinai, and the Rotman Research Institute at Baycrest. "The Research Institute culture of Medical Biophysics," the reviewers pointed out, "presents both significant advantages and also major challenges." Among the advantages were the excellent support for students and faculty and the close links to clinical programs that facilitated translational research. Among the disadvantages was that the Department of Medical Biophysics had little control over hiring or research direction and that its staff often identified more with the hospital Research Institute than the university department. Yet there was one unshakable core concept that had been present from the beginning: "Research is the heart of the student's program in Medical Biophysics."[23]

### Institute of Biomaterials and Biomedical Engineering

Biomedical engineering is a hybrid, the offspring of two dynamic man-centered science-based professions, Medicine and Engineering ... well-established disciplines [that] have been cross-fertilizing each other with the discreet exuberance of elderly professors who have just discovered that intercourse can be enjoyable as well as productive.

Edward Llewellyn-Thomas, 1973

Toronto had a distinguished history of applying engineering solutions to medical problems, as the work of Bill Bigelow and Gordon Murray showed. In late 1961 Arthur Porter, then head of industrial engineering, and James Ham, head of electrical engineering, had a conversation about moving the university into a new branch of engineering: biomedical. The Institute of Bio-Medical Electronics was founded in 1962, with Norman Moody, the former head of electrical engineering at the University of Saskatchewan, as its first director. At Saskatoon, Moody had developed an analogue computer for the rapid analysis of indicator dilution curves. "Can one doubt," Moody said, "that the marriage of the two disciplines of medicine and engineering, will produce people with a much deeper insight into the mysteries of nature and nature's living machines than can be obtained by separate studies in these fields?"[24] It was a joint venture of the Faculty of Applied Science and Engineering through its Department of Electrical Engineering.

The following year, 1963, Edward R. ("Tommy") Llewellyn-Thomas, a McGill medical graduate in 1955 and medical research associate at the Ontario Hospital in New Toronto, joined the new institute. In addition to his medical research, Llewellyn-Thomas was known for his science fiction novels (written under the pseudonym Edward Llewellyn). He also had a background in engineering, having studied it at London University and served with the Royal Engineers during World War II. As Bill Francombe later said, "While in medical school Tommy was employed as an Electrical Engineer at the Montreal Neurological Institute, where he worked with some of the giants of neurological science such as [Herbert] Jasper and [Wilder] Penfield, at that time engaged in their pioneering work on mapping the electrical activity of the brain." After graduation, he practiced family medicine for several years "on a small island in the Bay of Fundy, often travelling in a fishing boat to other islands to visit patients." Then he moved to Toronto to join the Defence Research Medical Laboratory and studied aspects of aerospace medicine, especially psychopharmacology in space. He joined the Department of Pharmacology as a part-time lecturer in 1959, full-time in 1964, when he also became a professor in the Department of Electrical Engineering. In 1974 he was appointed associate dean of undergraduate affairs, which he occupied until the time of his death in June 1984.[25]

Founding the institute created an auspicious bridge between the university and industry. The institute opened its doors with the aid of a gift from the Johnson Wax Company "for the support of a laboratory in Medical Electronics." It was to be fostered jointly by the Faculty of Applied Science and Engineering and the Faculty of Medicine and chaired by Moody. Dean Hamilton said at the time, "It is anticipated that the collaboration between the two faculties will have very far reaching results in many fields of medicine and biology."[26] The following year Hamilton called the institute "the first official marriage of engineering and medicine in Canada."[27] It was anticipated that, with Llewellyn-Thomas's appointment, graduate students qualified in medicine would be attracted to this new field. This actually never happened, yet early on, members of the institute made a number of important contributions to medicine, such as Llewellyn-Thomas's special camera that followed the movements of the eye, featured in 1969 on the cover of *Scientific American*.[28] Although students joined the institute from their home departments, faculty usually had salary support from their department of primary appointment.

By the late 1960s the Institute of Bio-Medical Electronics was established in renovated quarters in what is now known as the Rosebrugh Building, with six scientists and fourteen cross-appointed staff. In a collaborative graduate program, most of the eleven PhD students had co-supervisors: one from the Faculty of Applied Science and Engineering, the other from the Faculty of Medicine.[29] By 1970 Moody was able to claim, "During the seven years of its existence the Institute has developed into the leading centre for research and education in medical engineering in Canada and is rapidly establishing a world-wide reputation."[30]

Research contributions began to flow. For example, the 1968 PhD thesis of Michael Albisser[31] (supervised by Llewellyn-Thomas and Bernard Leibel of the Banting and Best Institute) studied glucose regulation and proposed a computer controlled closed-loop artificial pancreas. It was in 1974 that Albisser and colleagues reported the first use of an extracorporeal system to maintain glycemia in the normal range during consumption of meals.[32] In the 1966 President's Report[33] Norman Moody stated, "Our research on gamma ray cameras has resulted in a clinical instrument now in use at the Sick Children's Hospital." This is perhaps the first report from the institute of a practical diagnostic imaging system. It is of interest to note that Michael Joy, who worked on the development of this type of camera for his PhD, became an institute faculty member and was the first to report and test a new MRI imaging modality, called current density imaging.[34]

In 1973 the institute's name was changed for a second time from Institute of Biomedical Electronics and Engineering to the Institute of Biomedical Engineering.[35] The change was needed to reflect the broadening involvement of the institute in departments other than electrical engineering. Perhaps it made things sound slightly less techy because the institute was starting to take fire for its remoteness from medicine. One faculty report in the mid-1970s said, "Present problems: No built-in liaison between hospitals and University biomedical engineers. Very urgent." Also, "Not enough students with medical background entering field."[36] In the President's Report of June 1972 Moody reported, "The Institute presents a decade of progress with some pride. From an original staff of two, and a graduate student population of a single person, it now has ten academics, 2 research associates, a supporting staff of 7 and 40 graduates."[37]

From 1974 to 1983 Richard Cobbold, an expert on the physics and engineering of medical ultrasound, was the director, succeeded in 1983 by surgeon Walter Zingg, who had been associate director. Cobbold in collaboration with Wayne Johnston (surgery), for example, had led a team that reported in 1982 a technique for quantifying disturbed blood flow in carotid artery disease using Doppler ultrasound.[38] During Cobbold's term Morris (Mickey) Milner was appointed adjunct associate professor. Milner was formerly responsible for the biomedical engineering program at McMaster University before joining the Ontario Crippled Children's Centre as director of rehabilitation engineering. His appointment served to greatly strengthen the biomechanics program as well as ensuring very close collaboration between the two organizations, especially in relation to graduate student supervision and the delivery of courses.

Zingg was a biomaterials researcher with a medical background. Swiss-born with an MD in 1950 from the University of Zurich and an MSc in 1952 from the University of Manitoba, he had come from Manitoba to the Hospital for Sick Children in 1964 and to the institute in 1972. Previously, he had collaborated closely with Albisser and Leibel: his collaboration at the institute with Michael Sefton, for example, ranged from cardiovascular materials to insulin pumps. Biomaterials historian John Brash comments, "Walter's contributions were mainly in the development of animal models for evaluation of materials and devices. The A-V shunt dog model for blood compatibility testing, for example, has generated much valuable information"[39] (see also p. 227 for his work with Bernard Zinman).

In 1976 Cobbold and Zingg offered the long-range planners a vision of their mission: training biomedical engineers and scientists through the School of Graduate Studies. To be sure, medical students were at something of a disadvantage "because they don't have all the mathematics and physics necessary to cope with Biomedical Engineering." But they were trying to get them up to speed. Another colleague added that the students, largely from engineering, were said to be "of extremely high calibre and bring with them personal support from external granting agencies which is an enviable situation." There were to be three kinds of graduates: the clinical biomedical engineer (MHSc), the industrial biomedical engineer, and the biomedical engineer (PhD).[40]

When Zingg took over as director in 1983, he resolved to align the institute more with the Faculty of Medicine. Few physicians, he said, enrolled in its programs, and those who did tended to enter the field of anesthesia.[41] In 1984 the Clinical Engineering Program was introduced under Alfred Dolan, offering a master's of health science (MHSc) degree. It had been approved in 1975 but put on ice because of budgetary problems. In 1985 Zingg introduced a visual sciences laboratory and in 1986 a medical acoustics lab, with support of the industrial liaison program of the Natural Sciences and Engineering Research Council. In a 1987 assessment of the institute's course, Zingg wanted to build to the institute's strong suit: "We are the only Institute that can 'build the bridge' between Medicine and the Physical Sciences and Engineering."[42] Around the same time Paul Wang developed a sustained-release insulin implant.[43] These implants, which are widely used in veterinary medicine and for diabetes research, are made by a small but successful commercial company (LinShin Canada) founded by Paul Wang.

Two years later, in 1989 Zingg stepped down and Hans Kunov, an engineer with a specialty in acoustics and hearing, became director. During Kunov's tenure, the institute introduced into the Faculty of Applied Science and Engineering undergraduate curriculum for the 1993–4 year a biomedical option for the third and fourth years of the Engineering Science Program. This represented the first formal undergraduate biomedical engineering program that the institute was responsible for delivering. Meanwhile, in an unrelated development, in 1986 the Centre for Biomaterials was established primarily by Dennis Smith, Walter Zingg, Michael Sefton, and Robert Pilliar as a joint project of the Faculties of Dentistry, Medicine, and Engineering and aided by financing from the provincial Ontario Centre for Materials Research.

In 1998 the Centre for Biomaterials (in the Mining Building), the Tissue Engineering Group, and the Institute of Biomedical Engineering (in the Rosebrugh Building) merged to form the Institute of Biomaterials and Biomedical Engineering (IBBME), an interfaculty institute that reported to the deans of applied science and engineering, medicine, and dentistry.[44] In 1999 tissue engineer Michael Sefton replaced Kunov as director. Sefton was involved in developing artificial "organoids" to substitute for human organs in transplants.[45] This represented a movement towards a more direct involvement in medicine, one reinforced by the arrival in Toronto in 1995 of Molly Shoichet and several others. This led to a strong interest in stem cell engineering, molecular imaging, and nanotechnology, all reflected in the hiring of a cluster of Canada Research Chairs in the 1990s and the early twenty-first century.

The 1998 merger that created IBBME was most timely because, according to external reviewers in 1999, it presented "a unique opportunity for the University of Toronto to develop world leading research activity in this area."[46] In 2001, with the financial support of the Whitaker Foundation, the IBBME organized a new Graduate Program in Biomedical Engineering under the direction of Michael Sefton, permitting it for the first time to register graduate students directly without needing a home department.

## Department of Immunology

Immunology has a very long history, both in general and at the University of Toronto. In general a burst of research from 1890 to the First World War established the existence of such concepts as antibodies and blood groups. At the University of Toronto, an "optional class in Immunology" was initiated for the medical students in the 1922–3 session.[47] Yet such basic immunological concepts as "the immune system" emerged only in the 1960s, its molecular basis in the 1990s. And so the real history of immunology is actually quite brief. Yet investigators at the University of Toronto made some important contributions.

In the 1960s immunology, driven by the discovery of radioimmunoassay, started to take off as a discipline. (This is an assay method for determining the presence of substances, often small proteins, by gauging the relationship between their radiolabelled and radiounlabelled portions.) The hospitals pressured the faculty to develop an immunology program. In 1967, under the leadership of executive director John Law, the Medical Advisory Committee of the children's hospital struck a Committee on Immunology. The committee saw immunology as a department of the hospital and a division of the Research Institute, led by a senior scientist with a university appointment, "probably in the Department of Cellular Biology."[48]

In August 1968 Law told Dean Chute that the hospital needed to start a program but that it would be difficult to attract a first-class figure "unless departmental status in the University is available." Moreover, "[t]here is danger that a number of hospitals will attempt, as we have, to start a separate, independent department that will duplicate space, budget and compete for staff unless a total, co-ordinated plan is developed by the University." Therefore, the faculty had to act: "Immunology will develop in Toronto one way or another. The choice from a University standpoint is not whether there will be Immunology ..., but whether it will be fragmented, duplicated or co-ordinated by the University."[49] In Toronto, the impetus to develop the field thus began with a hospital administrator.

In 1972 the Institute of Immunology was founded within the Department of Biochemistry as a PhD program of the School of Graduate Studies with offices in the Medical Sciences Building. According to biochemistry historian Marian Packham, Keith Dorrington and Robert H. Painter were important in its genesis. Dorrington, a biochemical pharmacologist from Sheffield, had joined the Department of Biochemistry in 1970 and organized a large work group in molecular immunology. Biochemist Robert H. Painter as well was cross-appointed to the new institute.[50]

Director of the institute was Bernhard Cinader.[51] "Hardi" Cinader, a short, balding man with a white chin-beard, was born in Austria, trained in London, and moved from England to Canada in 1958 as head of the immunochemistry subdivision of the Ontario Cancer Institute. With his appointment as head, he served as the founder of the Institute of Immunology and directed it for ten years. As Dean Naylor pointed out on the occasion of Cinader's death in March 2001, "He was the driving force behind the establishment of the Canadian Society for Immunology in 1966" and was its inaugural president. In 1969 he became the founding president of the International Union of Immunology Societies.[52]

Yet there was a long gap between establishing an institute and building a department. Institutes could be evanescent things; in Toronto departments, for the most part, had the solidity of steel – and cost deans considerable sums in administration. Cinader's proposal in November 1972 to establish a Department of Immunology met with grumbling. "Of particular concern were ... the budgetary implications in setting up another new department, and the question of whether a plan for the establishment of a department which initially would have only 1.5 members, would gain the approval of the University Administration."[53] Also, the existing Institute of Immunology had not yet been approved by the School of Graduate Studies or the Minister of Colleges and Universities, so raising the ante to a department was said to be premature.[54]

Interest in immunology quickened. The institute sought to shift from the SGS to the Faculty of Medicine, as Cinader held out the promise of being able to identify immunologically individuals who are responsive, for genetic reasons, to specific treatments. At the HSC a Division of Immunology was established in 1971–2. The institute, with its cross-appointed staff, had in 1974 an initial intake of thirteen graduate students, but Cinader saw the potential as much greater.[55] Cinader also wanted in the hospitals a core group of research immunologists "with a primary commitment to research who could act as consultants but not be required to treat patients." He aspired for immunology to have the same tight focus that Siminovitch had been able to achieve on mammalian somatic cells.[56]

Yet despite Cinader's enthusiasm, the Institute of Immunology was not really coming together. In November 1980 Dean Lowy convoked an ad hoc committee on the subject, peopled with such faculty heavyweights as Hollenberg and Rose Sheinin, to see what could be done. Lowy said, "Despite the presence of at least 30 individuals of world stature in Immunology, the profile in Immunology within the Faculty is low, its efforts poorly coordinated and the number of students relatively small." Maybe it should be a department because "[i]n general departments have more strength than institutes insofar as they have a formal structure and power."[57] Four months later, in February 1981, this committee recommended the creation of a Department of Immunology.[58] It would have ten full-time staff.[59]

In July 1984 the Department of Immunology was founded, with Richard G. Miller as chairman. "This marks the first time in fifteen years that a new department has been established in the Faculty," said a news bulletin.[60] Rick Miller, who hailed from St Catharines, Ontario, was born in 1938 and educated at the University of Alberta with a master's degree in science in 1961 and a PhD in physics and biology at the California Institute of Technology in 1966. Thereupon Jim Till had recruited him as a postdoc to the Ontario Cancer Institute. McCulloch referred to him as a "leader in cell immunology."[61]

The new department was organized on the hub-and-spoke principle, the department's central hub being at the Medical Sciences Building, the spokes at the hospitals: the Ontario Cancer Institute, the Hospital for Sick Children, the Toronto Western Hospital, and Mount Sinai. An external review in 1989 found research at the Medical Sciences Building in molecular immunology thriving, with "international stature." But research in clinical immunology in the hospitals was underdeveloped, and the Departments of Medicine, Surgery, and Paediatrics needed to develop their own units with a distinctive clinical focus on immunodeficiency and inappropriate immune responses.[62]

This discussion leaves the impression that all the faculty's immunology resources were concentrated in the department. The opposite was true. Simultaneously, the Departments of Medicine and Surgery were organizing a huge transplantation effort, with immunology the basic science undergirding. By the 1983–4 session there were forty-six principal investigators in the immunology/transplantation program, with fifty-five graduate students and a total research funding of over $6 million. Of these forty-six, only twenty-three were on the university campus. All, of course, had departmental affiliations, but only seven were with the Department of Immunology. (Eight were affiliated with pediatrics.)[63]

It is thus unsurprising that, when Michael Julius – based at the Wellesley Hospital (and later the vice president of research at Sunnybrook) – became chair in July 1993, a burning issue was the "us" (campus) versus "them" (Research Institute) syndrome because the institutes were picking off the best candidates with higher salaries. "All that changed," said Julius, "with the appointment of Arnold Aberman as Dean of the Faculty. In addition to being a superb facilitator, he insured that Faculty resources are devoted to the best science ... Thus, we were in a position to provide competitive start up packages." Recruitment for the "node" (the suite of offices and labs for the department) in the Medical Sciences Building picked up. Julius was also helped by the "strong liaison" the department maintained with the firm Pasteur-Mérieux-Connaught (PMC), the French-based successor of the Connaught Laboratories, whose vice president of research, Michael Klein, was a member of the department. PMC contributed $15 million, distributed over ten years, "to those Canadian applicants whose research efforts are conceptually aligned with PMC's mandate, specifically, vaccine development."[64]

Yet, just as other basic science departments successfully resolved the "us versus them" syndrome by embracing the institutes, so did immunology. By the new century, immunology under the chair, Michael Ratcliffe, had become sufficiently interwoven with clinical medicine that 85 percent of the members of the department were based in the hospital Research Institutes. An external review in 2006 concluded that, in the units at the Medical Sciences Building and Sunnybrook, "the Department is pre-eminent in Canada in the field of basic immunology." Given sufficient attention to translational research, "[i]t can aspire to being one of the best Departments of Immunology in North America."[65]

# 18 Laboratory Medicine (Pathology/Microbiology/ Pathological Chemistry)

At the heart of basic science is the chemistry of disease. Pathological chemistry as it was once called – or in its modern garb clinical biochemistry – brings biochemistry to the bedside. At the University of Toronto, chemistry, microbiology, and pathology converged in the 1990s in the Department of Laboratory Medicine and Pathobiology, "pathobiology" being a neologism so recherché that Toronto has the only such department in the world. How these events unfolded illustrates this volume's theme of leadership lashing the horses ever faster towards research.

## Pathology

The study of pathology and bacteriology at the University of Toronto went back to 1892, when John Caven, scion of a distinguished Ontario family, was named professor of pathology. Born in St Mary's, Ontario, in 1861, he was also pathologist to Toronto General Hospital. Caven's father was the Reverend Dr William Caven, principal of Knox College, and his younger brother William P. Caven a well-known physician and member of the Department of Medicine. In 1896 the post became the chair of pathology and bacteriology.[1]

When Caven became ill in 1900, John J. Mackenzie assumed the chair. Mackenzie sprang from the same Scottish roots as so many of his colleagues. Even though he himself was born in 1865 in St Thomas, Upper Canada, "many in his family attained eminence as leaders in Institutions of learning both in Scotland and elsewhere," as his eulogist at the time of his death in 1922 noted. Among these distinguished forebears were Principal Rainy, "a leader of the Church in Scotland," and "Professor Kennedy of New College, Edinburgh," who graduated in 1886 from the natural science department of the University of Toronto, much "under the spell" of Ramsay Wright. On Macallum's advice, Mackenzie went to Europe and studied anatomy at Leipzig under Wilhelm His (discoverer of the "bundle of His") and physiology under Professor Karl-Friedrich-Wilhelm Ludwig; Mackenzie also worked in Berlin in the laboratories of Emil du Bois Raymond and of Robert Koch, the virtual founder of the science of bacteriology. With this kind of sterling international preparation, Mackenzie returned to Toronto in 1887 as a fellow in biology under Wright. For the next decade he worked as bacteriologist for the provincial Board of Health – the second such post in Canada following one in Quebec – simultaneously lecturing in the subject at the Royal College of Dental Surgeons. As a public-health scientist, he expedited the introduction of diphtheria antitoxin and in 1895 imported a supply from the Institut Pasteur in Paris. In 1896 he became instructor in bacteriology at the University of Toronto and earned the MB degree in 1899. With the evident precondition out of the way that he be a "doctor" in addition to scientist, in 1900 he succeeded John Caven as chair of pathology and bacteriology in the Faculty of Medicine. As Ramsay Wright said at the time of his appointment, "Mackenzie possesses a very extensive knowledge of the literature of modern Pathology, facilitated by his mastery of French and German, a weapon equally useful to the teacher and to the investigator."[2]

In the 1911–12 session the department moved to a new building in the Toronto General Hospital complex, the Pathological Building.[3] Immediately a problem of space presented itself that would dog the department for decades:[4] They simply did not have enough room for both service work and science. In the 1930–1 session the department moved to the Banting Building, where the same problem recurred as the department developed a formal relationship with the new provincial Pathology Laboratory under former faculty member Joseph E. Bates.[5]

Mackenzie died prematurely in 1922 of an infection acquired during the war – while leading the laboratory section of No. 4 Canadian General Hospital at Salonica – and Oskar Klotz took the chair. A native of Preston, Ontario, Klotz grew up in Ottawa (where he starred on Ottawa's War Canoe that took the national championship in 1898). In medical school at Toronto he was "one of the best-liked men in the year" (class of 1902) and further delighted his classmates by planning the menus for the annual feast that the Dinner Committee staged for the class.[6] From 1905 to 1910 he was appointed to the pathology department of McGill University and the Royal Victoria Hospital. In 1910 he became professor of pathology and bacteriology at the University of Pittsburgh; the years 1921–3 he spent "on a special mission for the Rockefeller Foundation in South America." His appointment at U of T began in July 1923.[7]

Klotz was among the earliest investigators of lung cancer, at a time when few had any idea it was caused by cigarette smoking. It had once been an unusual disease. "Of late there has been an increasing interest in malignant neoplasms of the lung," he wrote, ominously, in 1927, "and the presence of cancer is found to be far from rare." On the basis of his own experience in Pittsburgh and Toronto, he said, "It is evident that primary malignant disease of the lung is much more frequently encountered during recent years than in the past." He had no clue what might be causing it, perhaps increased dust in the air. "Some attribute the increased incidence to cigarette smoking, but we have no direct evidence in support of this view."[8] (Norman Delarue in the Department of Surgery came closer to getting it right; see p. 164.)

Towards the end of Klotz's tenure, Thomas Henry Belt emerged as a significant figure in pathology. In 1934, in research based on extensive autopsies, Belt called attention to the high frequency of pulmonary embolism, found in about 10 percent of adult autopsies. He gave something of a "natural history" of the phenomenon: "Pulmonary embolism, in the majority of instances, is not a single but a recurrent event, with small emboli as forerunners and larger ones as a climax."[9] He called attention to "circulatory embarrassment" as the cause: gathering "cardiac incompetence slows the venous circulation and increases the likelihood of thromboses in the leg and pelvic veins."[10] Belt was born in Ancaster, Ontario, in 1902, "a son of the manse," where his father was an Anglican clergyman. He entered the University of Toronto in 1922 for medical studies, was the class president of the third year, the editor of *Epistaxis* in the fourth, and chairman of Daffydil in the fifth, and graduated with an MD with honours in 1928.[11] After finishing his studies, he trained in pathology under Klotz, then spent a year in Germany under Karl Aschoff in Göttingen and Bernhard Fischer-Wasels in Frankfurt. Thus equipped, he returned to Toronto in 1931 and rejoined the Department of Pathology, becoming pathologist to the Toronto Hospital for Consumptives and coroner's pathologist for the City of Toronto. In 1937 he left Toronto for a post at the Postgraduate Medical School in London. His eulogists ascribed to him "a vigorous personality, humorous and tolerant, a good teacher and a critical observer," although his last years were clouded by illness and an early death in 1945.[12]

### William Boyd

In 1937 William Boyd, professor of pathology at the University of Manitoba, took the chair of pathology in Toronto. Boyd was one of the faculty's international stars, and generations of medical students worldwide learned pathology from his fluently written textbooks. Born in 1885 at Portsoy, a fishing village in Scotland, Boyd earned a medical degree from the University of Edinburgh in 1908. He served as medical officer and pathologist at several British mental hospitals and then was stationed in France with a field ambulance at the outbreak of hostilities. A university friend, Alexander Gibson, had gone to Winnipeg and urged Boyd to come out to Canada. (Gibson similarly recruited John C.B. Grant for the chair of anatomy.) In 1915 he was "requisitioned" from the front to Canada – Canadian medics needed to learn pathology – and he ended up in Alberta for twenty-two years. Following John Grant, he came to Toronto in 1937 for a further fourteen years – succeeding Klotz – going then finally to Vancouver for another three at the University of British Columbia. It was in Winnipeg that in 1920, as a pathologist as the Winnipeg General Hospital, he wrote a widely noted account of the epidemic of encephalitis lethargica, a worldwide plague that had surged from 1917 to around 1926, in that city.[13] In 1925 in Winnipeg he wrote his *Surgical Pathology*, followed by *The Pathology of Internal Diseases* in 1931 and in 1932 his *Textbook of Pathology* (the last edition of which, the ninth, appeared in 1990[14]).

Boyd was an engaging writer, though he did not necessarily warm to the task and noted in his "commonplace book," or literary diary, "Some five years ago I spent a month in bed in an Edmonton hospital, and as I had nothing to do, in a weak moment I conceived the idea of writing a book. At first it was great fun planning the lines along which it would develop, and so on, but it was far greater fun finishing the blamed thing off, and shoving it in the mail. You come home tired in the evening, and find the beastly thing lying on your desk with some knotty problem awaiting solution ... there was only one person hated the thing more than I did and that was my wife."[15]

All of Boyd's textbooks were "phenomenally successful," as his biographer H. John Barrie put it, but it was his *Textbook of Pathology* that made his great reputation. "It is easy to make the fatal mistake," Boyd wrote, "of regarding pathology as being concerned merely with states, particularly the state at the moment of death. But disease is not a state; it is rather a process ever changing in its manifestations, a process which may end in recovery or in death, which may be acute and fulminating in its manifestations, or which may represent the slow ageing of the tissues brought about by the sharp tooth of time."[16]

Said Barrie, "His books did not display unusual expertise of the author in any one field, but they had a readability which reflected his own obvious joy in reading, his mastery of the arresting phrase, simile or anecdote to enliven his subjects and his ability to place the facts of pathology in their clinical setting." Said one colleague to a young lecturer, "It doesn't matter what book you recommend to the undergraduates, they will all read Boyd."[17]

In the classroom Boyd practiced question-and-answer in teaching. Barney Berris remembers, "Dr Boyd was a superb teacher. He walked into the lecture theatre with slow, deliberate steps ... He spoke slowly and his speaking style was like his writing, simple and colourful, with a poetic lilt." He had a bit of a lisp. "In his first lecture he asked ... 'Is Bewis heah?'" Berris, startled, put up his hand, and Boyd said,

"Bewis, today we are going to discuss rheumatic ('weumatic') fever. What do you know about rheumatic fever?"

"Nothing, sir."

"Good," Boyd said. "Today, I'm going to tell you something about rheumatic fever and then you and the others are going to try and figure out what the pathology and clinical manifestations of rheumatic fever might be."

Boyd went on to ask questions, and the students answered as best they could, "and the discussion went back and forth." Berris said, "This was my first experience with this kind of interactive teaching. It went on all year and kept us spellbound."[18]

Boyd rearranged the collection of pathological specimens in the "museum" to give an overview of the progression of disease rather than just illustrating gross pathology. And he instituted with the Department of Medicine "clinical-pathological" weekly conferences for medical graduates, later known as "CPCs" and today a familiar part of hospital routine in matching clinical diagnoses premortem (often wrong) to pathological diagnoses postmortem (inevitably, and embarrassingly, correct).[19]

Boyd saw pathology as the royal road to medical knowledge. "There is only one way to become a pathologist, and that is to work for some years in a department of pathology," said Boyd.[20] (He urged the students to think first in terms of the patients' symptoms and not their underlying organs.) "It is disturbed function rather than disordered structure which is responsible for the symptoms of the patient. To give a name to some lesion, and to make it fit into some accepted scheme of classification, is a very limited concept of pathology ... The person of central, indeed commanding interest, is the sick man, woman or child, and it is the undergraduate, when he begins to practice medicine, who is going to relieve the sick person's suffering by virtue of knowledge supplied by the scientist ... A world of disordered function lies revealed in any lesion, if we only have the eye to see it."[21]

Boyd's great contribution to pathology lay thus not at the level of characterizing disease but in urging his colleagues to ask the question why. Much later, after the venerable Department of Pathology had merged into the Department of Laboratory Medicine in the 1990s, the chair of the merged department, Avrum Gotlieb, looked back on Boyd as a model for all the members. "William Boyd understood the noble role that the field of pathology played in the grand scheme of medical practice and he did his best to inform the medical profession about pathology." Gotlieb quoted Boyd's *Pathology for the Physician*, the eighth edition: "The purpose of pathology is not merely to learn a set of facts about things, but to study the causes of things, and why things happen."[22]

When Boyd died in 1979 at age ninety-four, his colleague Emmanuel Farber said, "Without a doubt he had more influence on the teaching of Pathology than any other Canadian, or for that matter any other medical teacher in the Western World."[23]

### Bacteriology as a Division of Pathology

In the history of therapeutics, the bacteriology division of the Department of Pathology has a footnote. Penicillin for medical use was begun in England in 1939.

The Second World War saw a dramatic effort to mass-produce enough to make it available to military physicians. In Canada, this task fell partly to the Department of Pathology and Bacteriology, where, over in the old Knox College Building on Spadina Crescent (as the "Spadina Division" of the Connaught Labs), they were cultivating penicillin full-blast.

The antimicrobial story goes back to the late 1930s, when Philip Harvey Greey, a U of T graduate in 1928 and member of the Division of Bacteriology, was helping to introduce, first, the sulfa drugs and then penicillin. As part of Duncan Graham's interest in sulfapyridine ("Dagenan"), Greey and colleagues compared sulfapyridine with other agents in experimental work on the pneumococcus, finding it superior.[24]

In the fall of 1941 Greey began work on the production of penicillin, enlisting help from investigators in the Department of Medical Research. Greey described the problems: "A shortage of facilities for the sterilization of large volumes of culture fluid was encountered. The Toronto General Hospital generously made its large autoclaves available … Each evening the night duty nurses sterilized the culture media that were planted with the mould the next morning." Towards the end of 1942 a pilot plant was established in the Banting Institute, financed by the National Research Council, and early in 1943 the first batches of penicillin for clinical use started to flow. The Connaught Laboratories began to ramp up production, as indeed did a number of commercial firms, almost all of it meant for the armed forces. Ray Farquharson chaired a Joint Services Penicillin Committee, situated at the Christie Street Military Hospital in Toronto, to supervise training and distribution, and Greey, on behalf of the National Research Council, adjudicated clinical requests for the precious substance. Greey recalled the "penicillin girls" at the Banting Institute: "For nearly a year through their efforts, enough penicillin was made in the small pilot plant to satisfy the Canadian needs for those urgent civilian cases … Some 300 patients were treated, and in many cases recovery was attributed solely to penicillin."[25] By 1945, said Dean Gallie, "[o]ver 300 patients were treated with the penicillin prepared in this department in collaboration with the biochemical group of the Banting and Best Department of Medical Research."[26]

The bacteriology division of the pathology department got its start in the 1933–4 session when Greey, who had joined the department a year after getting his medical degree and had been lecturing in bacteriology since 1930, was placed in charge of "the diagnostic clinic in Bacteriology."[27] By the 1939–40 session a Division of Bacteriology existed in the department, with William L. Holman, a McGill graduate of 1907 who had come to Toronto with Klotz in 1924, as its head. In 1946 Greey succeeded Holman as professor of bacteriology and associate director of the Department of Pathology.[28]

In the 1950–1 session the Department of Bacteriology became independent from the Department of Pathology. Much later, the faculty attempted to re-merge bacteriology, now called microbiology, with pathology and thus end its independence. Chair Leslie Spence commented on the prospect of rejoining pathology and microbiology in a proposed Department of Laboratory Medicine, "In 1952 we were emancipated and we have no desire to return to a state of servitude."[29] However, let's not get ahead of the story.

### John Hamilton

In the summer of 1951 John Hamilton succeeded Boyd as chair of pathology. Hamilton served as dean from 1961 to 1966, and his life is discussed more fully in chapter 29. Suffice it to say that he was originally a Toronto graduate and student of Klotz's, that he was forty when he took over pathology, and that he had been hired away from Queen's. Internationally, the old method of teaching pathology by organ system had gone out of style, replaced by experimental pathology and teaching students "the dynamic nature of pathological processes," as Hamilton put it after returning from a teaching seminar at French Lick Resort in Indiana. He felt the techniques of the department he had inherited from Boyd a bit pokey.[30]

It was on Hamilton's watch that in 1959 one of the more arresting figures in the history of the department came on board, Jan Steiner. Steiner, an émigré from the Holocaust, was born in a village in Moravia in 1916. He studied medicine at the Charles University in Prague, fled, and thereupon served in the French Army and the Czech regiment of the British Army until 1941. He completed an MB degree at Liverpool in 1943, then took postgraduate study at Oxford, earning an MD. After some years in general practice in Lincolnshire, England, he migrated to Canada and took up an assistantship in pathology at the Sinai in 1955. Four years later, in 1959, after apparently clashing with Harold Pritzker, he went over to the university Department of Pathology at the Banting Institute and rose through the ranks until lured away by the Chicago College of Osteopathic Medicine in 1977 and the University of Chicago in 1980. Informal chats with Steiner at the Banting Institute inspired a number of Toronto scientists and clinicians; here, and as associate dean, he epitomized the spirit of scientific curiosity and fast-lane investigation. Kenneth Pritzker said, "Steiner was another one of these charismatic, psychothymic characters. With great enthusiasm he brought in experimental pathologists from all over the place from the United States to give a lecture here and there. It was really an outstanding exercise."[31]

In 1961 Alexander Charles Ritchie succeeded Hamilton as head of pathology. Ritchie, a New Zealander, was born in Auckland in 1921 and finished medical studies there in 1944. He progressed to a DPhil in pathology at Oxford in 1950, then emigrated to Canada to spend the years 1954–61 at McGill. When he came to Toronto at age 40 to head the pathology department, he was also pathologist-in-chief at the General.

Under Ritchie, pathology's chronic space crisis grew worse. The autopsy fa-cilities at the Banting Institute were said to be "far inferior to the facilities found in most small hospitals."[32] The department ditched the pathology museum that had existed since the turn of the century and that Boyd had so proudly rede-signed, but space was still scarce.[33] Ritchie began using the term "grotesque" to describe the autopsy service.[34] In 1969 the Independent Planning Committee found that "the present facilities of the Department are inadequate from a clini-cal standpoint and are totally inadequate for teaching and research. One clinical teacher ... stated that the existing facilities in Pathology in all hospitals, for both clinical teaching and research, 'range from atrocious to bad.'"[35]

Yet there were some triumphs. In 1968 in the hospital Department of Pathol-ogy at TGH, Alexander G. Bell, a researcher in the Department of Genetics at the children's hospital, organized a cytogenetics laboratory and also provided genetic counseling – this around the same time that a similar lab was being organized at HSC (see pp. 693–694).[36] In 1968 Malcolm Silver, a PhD in pathology and soon to be departmental chair, delighted cardiac surgeon Bill Bigelow so much with his study of the pathology of heart valves that Bigelow had previ-ously implanted, including "some of the early, unsterilized, homograft valves that were placed in the descending thoracic aorta as much as five and six years ago," that Bigelow wanted Silver to do all the cardiovascular pathology work sent to him: "This pathological information is completely unique."[37] Ritchie set up in 1967–8 in the Medical Sciences Building a Division of General and Experi-mental Pathology, with Henry Zoltan Movat its first head; Movat, of Romanian origin, took his MD from Innsbruck, Austria (in 1948), and a PhD from Queens, joining the Toronto department in 1957.[38]

Yet the spirit in pathology in those days was not peppy. One mid-1970s report identified it as "[a] 'depressed' department. Very urgent [need for action]."[39]

### Emmanuel Farber

In 1975 Emmanuel ("Manny") Farber became chair of pathology. Farber was Jewish, born in Toronto, and subject to the anti-Semitic bigotry of the day. Here is surgeon Bernie Langer on the subject: "Manny Farber ... was silver medalist in Medicine [in 1942], and couldn't get an internship at the Toronto General. So he went to Hamilton and did his internship, then he went to Pittsburgh and trained in pathology and then became head of their Research Institute, and even-tually, when I was Chairman [of surgery], he was recruited back here as Chief of Pathology at the Toronto General Hospital, and Chairman of the Department ... It says a lot about the change that took place during the span of his career. He couldn't get a job as an intern, he came back as Chair of the Department."[40]

At Pittsburgh, Farber became well known for his research on the pathogen-esis of cancer, especially in the liver. In an interview, Kenneth Pritzker, chief of pathology at Mount Sinai, added, "Farber was a very well-known experimental pathologist. So he was really at the top of his game, and in his late 50s, he came to Toronto. He was an enthusiastic guy, with a lot of American attitude – because he had lived for the most part in the United States." He said, "What I remember most about him was his enthusiasm, his unbridled enthusiasm." Pritzker once went to him with a problem. Farber asked, "Why do you think they call it research, kid? You look again."[41]

Farber's energy and dynamism were said to have caused a "renaissance" in the department. Pritzker continued, "The whole idea was that they wanted professors and chairs who were investigators. This was certainly the vision for Pathology, and in those days there was access to special money if you could get a real star." Farber hired several people as investigators, Pritzker said, "and he had a sort of mini-industry that was the core of the research component. Then he was successful in stimulating research at each of the teaching hospitals."

On Farber's watch, said the Self-Study of 1983, "The main academic goal of the department has become the study of disease at a cellular level. In the past, the department has had an 'honest journeyman' image. A major effort is now being made to create an area of academic excellence." Among the seventy-three staffers, those whom Farber identified as "old-fashioned" had started to leave, whereas residents and young researchers were keen to join the newly research-oriented department.[42]

At the time of Farber's retirement in 1985, the mood in the pathology department had swung about completely. An external review in 1984 said, "The Department enjoys an excellent national and international reputation as a research and training center in experimental pathology. This reputation is based primarily on Dr Farber's eminence as an experimental oncologist." The current research funding of the "graduate department" of almost $3 million was called "a remarkable achievement." Farber was little involved in "service pathology." "The revolutions of the past decade in molecular biology, neurobiology, immunogenetics and oncology have already influenced the recruitment efforts of other academic departments." There was evidently a sharp split between "the practicing clinical pathologist" and "the pathologist confined to laboratory medicine." "The triple threat pathologist [RST triad – research, service, teaching] is a dying species."[43]

### After Farber

In 1985 Malcolm Silver, returning from the University of Western Ontario where he had spent the previous five years as head of pathology, succeeded Farber. He inherited a department with only five tenured positions, but thirty-eight full-time and seventy-nine part-time and volunteer staff, plus thirty-eight residents, seven postdocs, and twelve graduate students – a compliment to Farber in their number and variety yet a sad comment on the faculty's inability to make more tenured appointments. A 1990 review said of pathology in Toronto, "This research activity makes Toronto one of the largest and best funded University Departments of Pathology in Canada and the Department would also rank well above average in North America."[44]

Merger was in the air. Dean Aberman was keen to cut costs and the molecular revolution was erasing departmental boundaries. In January 1987, Silver proposed to Dean Lowy a merger of the Departments of Pathology, Clinical Biochemistry, and Medical Microbiology into a single "Department of Pathology and Laboratory Medicine." "This may seem like a naked grab for power by the Department of Pathology," he said, "but the logic of amalgamation in the future is inescapable." He explained that other universities were doing it and that "collaborative research can be encouraged."[45] This evoked an enraged response from the chairs of the other departments involved.

Nonetheless, in June 1994 Andrew Baines (the chair of the Department of Clinical Biochemistry), Silver, and Aberman held discussions about a possible merger between clinical biochemistry and pathology. A committee chaired by Peter Pinkerton, who was appointed in both departments, was convened in November 1994 to study the matter, recommending in January 1995 that such a merger also include the microbiologists.[46] By November 1995 Silver's second term as chair was ending. To facilitate the merger, it was agreed that the same person would be appointed chair of pathology and chair of clinical biochemistry.[47] The following month, that person turned out to be cardiovascular pathologist Avrum Gotlieb.

The dynamic Gotlieb was one of the stars of the faculty. Born in Montreal in 1946, he was entirely educated at McGill, receiving an MD in 1971. He was board-certified in pathology in the United States in 1976. A staff pathologist at St Michael's Hospital in 1978 and at The Toronto Hospital in 1980, he became in 1983 director of the Vascular Research Laboratory of the Department of Pathology, based at the General. In 1983 he and Silver published *Cardiovascular Pathology*, in its third edition at this writing. It would be Gotlieb who led the Department of Pathology, and the microbiologists and the clinical biochemists, into the Department of Laboratory Medicine in 1997.

## Department of Pathology: Division of Neuropathology

It was at Ken McKenzie's instigation that Oskar Klotz created a Division of Neuropathology in 1931, with Eric Linell at its head.[48] Born in Ashton-on-Ribble in England in 1891, Linell was educated at boarding school, then began medical studies at the University of Manchester, receiving the bachelor of medicine in 1914. After service in the navy, he returned to Manchester for the MD degree, which was conferred in 1920. He turned to anatomy and was appointed in 1923 to the University of Toronto, where neurosurgeon Ken McKenzie kindled his interest in neuropathology. Neurosurgeon Tom Morley, who eulogized him at the Faculty Council at the time of his death in 1983, said, "Like McKenzie, Linell entered a specialty that had not existed before in Canada and full-time neu-ropathologists were rarer in the world even than neurosurgeons." In the absence of a mentor, Linell proved a splendid autodidact and in 1931 transferred from anatomy to the Department of Pathology, where Oskar Klotz asked him to establish a Division of Neuropathology. Mary Tom accompanied him from anatomy. "Linell and Tom, with their postgraduate students in clinical neurology and neuropathology, produced a steady flow of articles with a strong bias towards the solution of clinical problems." He was something of a picture in eccentricity, from his standard slice of pie and glass of milk at Lawrence's Lunch, "a slit in the façade of stores and offices at College and Bay which have now disappeared," to the "half a dozen loaded pipes ranged and ready to go in front of him on the formalin-sodden cutting board [and] the enormous brown tea pot that needed his two hands to lift and pour." He was, Morley thought, "the last man in Toronto to wear a bowler hat to work."[49]

In the Division of Neuropathology, Mary Isabel Tom was the microscopist. Born in Goderich, Ontario, in 1896, she studied theology for four years at Trinity College, then decided to join the medical school, where she played hockey. She graduated in medicine from U of T in 1922, next to such luminaries as Ray Farquharson and Joe MacFarlane, and chose as her motto, "All life, all fire, Never rests, never tires."[50] Neuropathology often collaborated with the neurology division of the Department of Medicine in various researches and she was a frequent publisher, as for example when she first-authored a paper with Clifford Richardson in 1951 on hypoglycemia in an islet cell tumour that had caused unusual changes in the spinal cord.[51] (The islet cells produce insulin, and a tumour that hyper-produced insulin would cause low blood sugar.) She shouldered the bulk of examining the tissue that came over to the Banting Institute from the hospitals.

It is interesting that as early as 1931–2 the discussion of neuroscience on campus was raised. In that session FitzGerald and Graham asked Linell to become a coordinator for neuroscience on campus. Clearly, neuropathology was seen at the centre of the neuroscience web[52] (see p. 371). In 1937–8 Ric Richardson, just finishing a long stretch of postgraduate work in neurology, was appointed as a fellow in neuropathology. He had just joined the Department of Medicine and would, collaborating with Mary Tom, "devote special attention to the study of diseases of the nervous system."[53]

Further integrating the neurosciences, in 1951–2 Linell began making periodic visits to the Ontario Hospital, an asylum on Queen Street. As well, in the 1951–2 session, Linell began working closely with neuroradiologist Delbert Wollin, who had finished medical studies in 1939. Wollin attended the weekly conferences in pathology with "physicians, surgeons, and psychiatrists." And "Linell and members of his staff go to weekly neuro-radiological conferences at the Psychiatric Hospital. It is a great pleasure," said Hamilton, "to be closely associated with this important development of Radiology."[54]

In 1957 Linell stepped down in retirement from, as Hamilton said, "[t]he only centre in Canada devoted exclusively to the examination and study of the pathology of the Central Nervous System[;] it has served in this school to correlate the efforts of neurologists, psychiatrists, neurosurgeons, anatomists and others in further knowledge in this important area."[55]

In 1959 Jerzy Olszewski became professor of neuropathology. Born in Poland in 1913 on an estate near Wilno managed by his father, Olszewski finished his medical studies at Wilno in 1937 and started training there in neurology, only to be interrupted by the war. He resumed in 1944 at the University of Freiburg, working with the great neuropathologist Oskar Vogt, then in nearby Neustadt in the Black Forest (earlier in Berlin); Olszewski received a second MD degree from the University of Freiburg in 1947, thereupon immigrating to Canada, where he arrived at the Montreal Neurological Institute in 1948, and took a PhD at McGill in neuroanatomy in 1951; at McGill he continued the work he had begun with Vogt on the cytoarchitecture of the cerebral cortex. He taught neuroanatomy and neuropathology at McGill until leaving for a post at the University of Saskatchewan in 1956, where his interests veered ever more towards neuropathology. He was called to the chair in Toronto in 1959. His career in Toronto was alas short-lived as he died in 1964. His eulogist said, "Dr Olszewski became one of the best known and most respected neuropathologists in the world."[56]

In his brief tenure, Olszewski worked hard to build up the research side of the division, expanding postgraduate training and bringing students from all over the world. John G. Humphrey organized a special lab for muscle diseases, and Calvin Ezrin opened up the study in Toronto of the hormones of the anterior pituitary gland. There were generous private donors to the program. A long-awaited electron microscope was finally up and running.[57]

Linell, Mary Tom, and Olszewski left to neuropathology at the university a brilliant legacy. The further story may be followed in chapter 14 on the neurosciences.

## Microbiology

Many of the major advances in basic medical science in recent years have come from those interested in microbiological concepts and methods. This is because it has been realized that the experimental material in microbiology lends itself readily to biological investigations at the molecular level.[58]

Louis Siminovitch, 1966

To reprise, in the 1950–1 session bacteriology became an independent department, with Philip Greey the head.[59] Penicillin and the other antibiotics had scarcely been introduced than resistance to them was growing, and Greey, in this small department, undertook studies of the increasing resistance of the microorganism staph aureus: "Perhaps these findings indicate that the end of the antibiotic era in the treatment of staphylococcal infections in hospitals is near at hand."[60]

Yet the world of science was moving beyond studies of antibiotics. Siminovitch disliked even the name "Bacteriology." He wrote pharmacologist Harold Kalant in January 1965 that many Departments of Bacteriology had changed their name to Departments of Microbiology and "teach all aspects of virology, certain aspects of mammalian cell culture *in vitro*, and degrees of genetics and biochemistry of microorganisms." Microbiology, he said, deserved a place in the coming Medical Sciences Building. For such a department "a minimum size group would be about 8–9 senior investigators, which should include members competent in bacteriology, virology, animal cell culture, and possibly electron microscopy."[61]

In the 1967–8 session Arthur E. Franklin took over as acting chair from Greey, who retired.[62] Franklin, who was born in 1921 in Saskatchewan, had a background in biochemistry, with a PhD from McGill in 1951. He had been a research associate at Connaught, then was a microbiologist at the Banting Institute from 1955 until he began his new job. With his interest in virology and strong basic science background, he corresponded to the requirements Siminovitch had set out. Yet the problems of the little department were deep.

In 1969 the Independent Planning Committee concluded dismissively, "The Department of Bacteriology is said to be the weakest Department in the Faculty of Medicine." Its numbers were insufficient for service needs, and "research in Bacteriology ... has not kept up to modern demands." Only at the Hospital for Sick Children could serious research be said to occur.[63]

Readers will be struck that, so often when the problems of a department seem demoralizing, a dynamic academic leader is brought in who rights the ship and sets it on a proper course. And this happened in what was still being called "Bacteriology" with the appointment of Norman A. Hinton in 1970.[64] Hinton, a native of Kapuskasing, Ontario, was born in 1926 and earned an MD at Queen's in 1951. This was followed by graduate training in bacteriology. In 1955 he joined the staff at Queen's where he became chair of the Department of Microbiology, serving simultaneously as bacteriologist at the Kingston General Hospital. Hinton had turned the Toronto appointment down already once, as did a number of other distinguished microbiologists, when first offered the headship of what Edward A. Sellers, head of the bacteriology search committee, referred to as a "neglected" department. "There was agreement that ... medical microbiology in the Faculty and affiliated hospitals was in a sad, or even precarious, state," Sellers told Dean Hamilton in June 1969. When Hamilton refused to pump funds into the department, Sellers resigned as chair of the search committee.[65] Hinton then subsequently accepted, having apparently secured a playable hand from the dean.

Under Hinton, bacteriology roared back to life, with seven full-time posts, a pumped-up research budget, a new unit at Sunnybrook, new labs at several of the teaching hospitals, an interhospital infection control group that met monthly with attendance of over a hundred, and cross-appointments to the Department of Microbiology in the School of Hygiene.[66] The concept was that the department would consist of the hospital departments of microbiology without a big campus presence (but only three hospitals had such departments: the General, HSC, and, as mentioned, Sunnybrook).[67] Hinton changed the name from the Department of Bacteriology to the Department of Medical Microbiology.

And this brings us to a big problem that Hinton faced. In a separate narrative, the School of Hygiene had its own Department of Microbiology, founded in 1933. It also had a separate Department of Parasitology. This was clearly an anomalous situation: to have two departments of microbiology on the same campus, one department called the Department of Microbiology attached to a School of Hygiene, the other a rump called the Department of Medical Microbiology attached to a medical faculty.[68]

When Hinton came to Toronto from Queen's, he is said to have "asked for the Chairmanship of a single unified Department of Medical Microbiology ... This was apparently not possible to accomplish," said Robert Harris, chair of the Long-Range Planning and Assessment Committee, "so instead he was made Chairman of two departments: one in Medicine, the other in the School of Hygiene. This proved to be an impossible arrangement so Dr. Hinton withdrew from the School of Hygiene." Now, in 1974, the School of Hygiene was being dissolved, and something had to be done with their Department of Microbiology. At this point, Hinton again demanded one department and space in the hospitals to accommodate its members.[69] He told the long-range planners that the department at the School of Hygiene "has become segregated from service, patient care, residency training – loss of contact with applied Microbiology." He wanted one Department of Microbiology "with both basic science and clinical responsibility."[70] For a second time, Hinton's request was refused because of the political difficulty in merging these two unwilling entities with different pasts and personnel. Hinton stayed on as the chair of the faculty's Department of Medical Microbiology.

In 1975 the dynamic Rose Sheinin became head of the Department of Microbiology and the Department of Parasitology, both inherited from the School of Hygiene and now merged into a single department. Sheinin herself, born in Toronto in 1930, had been educated at U of T, finishing with a PhD in biochemistry in 1956. She fellowed at Cambridge and the National Institute for Medical Research in London in the mid-1950s, then in 1958 accepted a research associate fellowship in the Division of Biological Research of the Ontario Cancer Institute, where she remained until 1967. Appointed to the Department of Medical Biophysics in 1967, she accepted the professorship of microbiology-parasitology, as stated, in 1975.

The faculty now had two microbiology departments: Medical Microbiology (the successor of the Department of Bacteriology), under Hinton, and the

Department of Microbiology and Parasitology (inherited from the School of Hygiene), under Sheinin.

Faculty pressure on the two departments to merge was strong. But the former School of Hygiene people were resistant: Almost all had tenure; many had ceased to be scientifically productive and did not wish the bother of a merger. Without new blood, the Department of Microbiology-Parasitology, said Sheinin, would not survive.[71]

Things did not go well with microbiology-parasitology after 1975. It was, Sheinin allowed five years later, a scientific catastrophe: "The former Department of Microbiology had been allowed to fall into a state of mediocrity, particularly at the level of research, with minimal expectations for the future." In the interval, she had made a number of positive changes. Yet she told Dean Holmes in January 1980, "Unless steps are taken *immediately* to avert it, the possibility exists that the Department of Microbiology and Parasitology will wither and die within the next two to four years."[72]

The pressure from the faculty was like a blowtorch. By June 1981, the staff at microbiology-parasitology in the FitzGerald Building (the old School of Hygiene headquarters) had come around under duress: they were prepared to support a merger (Lowy told the Faculty Council a couple of weeks later that they were in fact digging in their heels[73]). But the staff of Hinton's Department of Medical Microbiology had voted twenty-two to thirteen against a merger,[74] possibly because the hospital members of this department did not have tenure, were scientifically productive, and resented being chained to a dead weight. Although some of the medical microbiology staff were cross-appointed to the microbiologist-parasitologists in the FitzGerald Building, none of the latter were cross-appointed to the former. (Such mergers at the University of British Columbia and McGill, it was said, had also recently failed.[75])

To make a long story short, in 1983 medical microbiology and microbiology-parasitology merged to constitute the Department of Microbiology, under Leslie Spence,[76] who had just succeeded Hinton as chair of medical microbiology. Born in St Vincent, West Indies, in 1922, Spence was British-educated at Bristol University for his MB in 1950, then a University of London diploma in tropical medicine and hygiene in 1951. He worked until 1962 as a medical officer for the government of Trinidad, then directed the country's virus laboratory and taught virology at the University of the West Indies until 1968, when he came to McGill to teach microbiology. In 1972 he joined the Department of Medical Microbiology in Toronto, which he chaired a decade later, becoming simultaneously microbiologist-in-chief at the Toronto General Hospital.[77]

Yet the merged department did not manage to surmount the problems that had dragged the old one down. A devastating external review in 1984 said, "This department suffers from a neglect so serious its viability as an academic unit is threatened."[78] The FitzGerald microbiologist-parasitologists, said Ken Pritzker in an interview, were very unhappy at the changes. At the hospital level the microbiologists were really infectious disease people who had been "co-opted." But at the faculty level, "What they always had in microbiology was a group of basic scientists, but that was the group that was left over from the School of Hygiene." To get them to go along, Pritzker continued, "there was a carrot, and the carrot was that the University came up with a large number of new positions. And every one of those positions went to a campus-based person. That proved to be a true carrot and a reality, because over that decade there was tremendous growth of the research capacity" and much more interaction with the other basic science departments. "There were many common programs."[79]

Spence retired in 1988, succeeded by John Penner in 1989 as acting chair, becoming officially appointed as chair in 1992. In this situation of drift, in 1994 the faculty formed a task force to consider what to do about the Department of Microbiology, and in 1996 the Faculty Council voted to terminate it.[80] The Department of Microbiology thus came to an end.

### Department of Pathological Chemistry

Emphasis continues to be placed on the importance to the physician, when studying a patient, of understanding as thoroughly as possible the disturbances in biochemistry and physiology to be found in association with the metabolic and other diseases, how they have been brought about, how they themselves may produce important signs and symptoms, how they may be recognized, and how they may best be treated.[81]

James A. Dauphinee, Head of the Department of Pathological Chemistry, 1958

The Department of Biochemistry, a basic science department housed in the Medical Sciences Building, is considered elsewhere in this volume. Clinical biochemistry, or pathological chemistry as it was once called, is more at home in the hospitals, for clinical biochemistry means tests and the like. Indeed, a Clinical Pathological Laboratory was established at the General in 1906.[82] Much later, clinical biochemistry, like microbiology and pathology, would also be folded into the new Department of Laboratory Medicine in the mid-1990s, but here are a few words about its long and distinguished history.

Who needed pathological chemistry? Did biochemistry and the Department of Medicine not cover all the bases? Here is Walter Campbell on the significance of this subject: "Prior to 1915 medicine in Toronto developed almost exclusively along clinical lines ... The founding of a chair in Pathological Chemistry was a recognition of a need for a fuller understanding of disease in terms of an alteration of the normal physiological chemistry of the body." Campbell, writing in the 1960s, mentioned his own paper on mercuric chloride nephrosis, or damage to the kidney from a toxin, as "the first to unify the two departments in this field."[83] Also a "series of papers by Hunter and Campbell on creatine were groping towards this understanding, a small beginning perhaps, but foreshadowing the changes which, both here and elsewhere have changed clinical medicine profoundly."[84] Pathological chemistry arose from the concept that the clinician needed to understand in biochemical terms what was happening in the body, whether in nephrosis, a degenerative disease of the renal tubules that spills protein into the urine, or high creatine phosphokinase in the lab report, meaning the patient has recently had a heart attack.

These eminently practical questions began to be asked in 1909, when John B. Leathes came to Toronto as the first professor of pathological chemistry. He returned to London in 1914 to take a chair in physiology at Sheffield.

Born in London in 1864, Leathes stemmed from a distinguished clerical and medical family, one of his mother's ancestors a physician to Henry VIII. He enjoyed a classical education, in an era when that meant being able to speak Latin, and once delivered a speech in Latin on the occasion of the visit of the English prime minister, Mr Gladstone, to his school, Winchester. Gladstone is said to have replied in English. Destined for the clergy, Leathes rebelled and headed towards medicine, obtaining the MB in 1893 and the fellowship in the Royal College of Surgeons the following year. With his poor eyesight he evidently made a terrible surgeon and detoured instead in the direction of physiology, working with Ernest Henry Starling at Guy's Hospital on the action of veratrine. He then spent four years training in physiology on the Continent, notably with the famous Oswald Schmiedeberg in Strassburg (then a German city). Back in England in 1899, he served for the next decade on staff in physiology at St Thomas's Hospital Medical School. As the new chair in pathological chemistry was established in Toronto in 1909, Leathes was appointed professor. In 1912 at a building adjacent to the General Hospital he established new laboratories for graduate students, as well as a biochemical laboratory in the medical wards of the General and a second laboratory at St Michael's Hospital, with a colleague from his department in charge of each laboratory. Notes his biographer Rudolph Peters, "This shows how alive Leathes was even at this early time to the value of the clinical biochemist." In 1914 he left Toronto, accepting the post of professor of physiology at Sheffield. Peters said of Leathes's general approach to clinical biochemistry that he was mindful of "the importance of breaking down the barrier between preclinical and clinical studies so that the modes of thought in the laboratory could be brought into clinical medicine ... In this way, where possible, disease became explained as a diversion from the normal."[85]

In 1915 Andrew Hunter, a Scotsman, followed Leathes in succession to the chair as the beginning of a long though varied association with the University of Toronto: Hunter held the chair of pathological chemistry from 1915 to 1920, held the chair of biochemistry from 1920 to 1929, and, after heading the Department of Physiological Chemistry in Glasgow, was again the professor of pathological chemistry in Toronto from 1935 to 1945.[86] Hunter's life is considered in chapter 16, but here it might be reminded that he was thirty-nine when he took the chair in Toronto and had received a thorough scientific preparation in

Berlin, Heidelberg, and his native Edinburgh. As he arrived in Toronto, he was a leading figure in the discipline.

When Hunter transferred to biochemistry in 1920, Victor John Harding, an Englishman, became the professor of pathological chemistry the following year. Born at Bury in Lancashire in 1885, Harding studied chemistry at the University of Manchester, graduating with a bachelor's degree in 1906 and a doctoral degree in 1912. After three years at Owen's College in Manchester in research, around 1915 he was appointed demonstrator in chemistry at McGill University. In 1920 he accepted a post at the U of T as professor of pathological chemistry and remained head of the department until his death in 1934. In research, he was distinguished for a series of papers on the toxemias of pregnancy begun while at McGill, concluding that "the primary aetiological factor in the nausea and vomiting of pregnancy is lack of glycogen in the maternal liver."[87] As his eulogist puts it, he "established the now wide spread use of glucose therapy in Hyperemesis Gravidarum ... Doctor Harding's researches in pregnancy metabolism have ... had a very tangible influence in rationalizing therapy; of this, the obstetrical text books of to-day bear abundant testimony."[88]

Then in 1935 Hunter returned. "In submitting this first of what may be called my 'Second Series' of Reports from the Department of Pathological Chemistry," he said, "I cannot help commenting upon the great expansion which the department has undergone since I last reported upon it in 1920. Physically, of course, the department, to which I have returned, is an entirely new one, occupying premises more commodious and, in many ways, more convenient than those with which I was familiar in the old Pathology Building." In 1920 there were one professor and a lecturer plus a couple of part-time staff, "and the head of the department operated his own typewriter." By 1935–6, said Hunter, the teaching staff had grown to four full-time members. "This doubling of the staff has been accompanied ... by an increase in [the department's] contribution to medical and scientific research," the number of those "actively engaged in research" rising from two in 1919–20 to eight in 1935–6. Instruction in the department, he said, had changed little since the days of Leathes.[89]

Hunter, a classroom veteran, was mindful of the inherent difficulty of teaching basic science to medical students: "The position of Pathological Chemistry as a fourth-year subject [second clinical year] has this disadvantage, that the student engages upon it before he has had any experience of clinical medicine and before, therefore, he can appreciate its value or obtain practice in its application. From this point of view it might be better to postpone the subject to the fifth year; but to that course there would be a still more serious drawback, for it would create a gap of one year during which the student would be taught no chemistry whatever, and during which he would be apt to forget those biochemical facts and principles which are the foundation and necessary precursors of his work in this Department."[90] The comment is no less apposite today, when in problem-based learning educators struggle to get students to understand the rationale of what they are doing before they see patients and not to forget it until after their exams.

It was only with the arrival of James Dauphinee to replace Hunter as chair of pathological chemistry in 1947 that the department became led by a Canadian, indeed by one of the very few British Columbians to make it eastward in medicine in those years. Dauphinee was born in New Westminster, British Columbia, in 1903 and, after a master's degree at the University of British Columbia in 1923, earned a PhD in biochemistry at the University of Toronto in 1929, an MD in 1930. Thereupon he was a Mickle Fellow, which he spent in 1930–1 at St Bartholomew's Hospital in London; he then interned in Toronto and joined the Department of Medicine in 1933–4, where he served as a demonstrator until 1941; he was in the Royal Canadian Army Medical Corps during the war (in Belgium, attending a diphtheria epidemic among the troops). He returned to Toronto to the Department of Medicine, taking the professorship of pathological chemistry in 1947.

Dauphinee, "a reticent man," contributed greatly to putting the Department of Medicine on a scientific basis through his biochemical contributions. In the 1947–8 session, the faculty formed a general committee to investigate "certain radio-active therapeutic agents shortly to be available from the Chalk River project and supplied through the National Research Council." Research with "tracer substances" was already underway in the Department of Medicine.[91] In 1949, together with physicist William Paul, he established the first isotope lab at the Toronto General Hospital. In 1950 at the General he established a steroid assay laboratory with Allan Gornall. At Sunnybrook he set up a Clinical Investigation Unit in 1951, which he ran until 1966.[92] Dauphinee is a historic figure who, according to his colleague and eulogist Andrew Baines, introduced "the first controlled clinical studies done in Toronto." Baines said, "He introduced to the Toronto General Hospital many analytical techniques and discoveries we now take for granted including: flame photometry, filter paper electrophoresis, enzyme assays and ceruloplasmin."[93]

This steroid laboratory had actually been in the works for several years, and it was Gornall, not Dauphinee, who was the chief player. In the 1948–9 session, Gornall had taken leave from the Department of Pathological Chemistry on a Nuffield Fellowship and was working with Guy F. Marrian, the professor of biochemistry in Edinburgh, who had joined the Toronto biochemistry department during the war years. Once Gornall returned from Edinburgh, it was intended that he guide the work of the steroid lab. "This laboratory," said Dauphinee, "will be devoted to the study … of fundamental and clinical problems in the realm of endocrinology and it is hoped that it will serve a very useful purpose, not only as a research laboratory, but also as a source of stimulus and information for all those who are interested in the endocrine field."[94] The steroid laboratory opened up in Toronto the study of the endocrine system and invited widespread collaboration among medicine and psychiatry, among other fields, on such matters as the role of the adrenal cortex in periodic catatonia.[95]

The Radioactive Isotopes Lab, which William Paul ran, also sparked a wide gamut of research, as members across the faculty used such resources as radioactive phosphorus to study various conditions. (This William Paul, born in Toronto in 1918, is not to be confused with the William Paul in obstetrics and gynecology, who was also a faculty leader.) Paul the biophysicist, who was among the founders of the disciplines in Toronto, took a PhD in pharmacology in 1948, fellowed in Cambridge in 1948–9, then from 1949 to 1953 joined the pharmacology department. From 1953 to 1983 he was a member of the Department of Pathological (Clinical) Chemistry. In 1950 James Ferguson, the professor of pharmacology, said apropos Paul, "It seems timely to remark that biophysicists are increasingly important members of any progressive faculty of medicine. Some thought must be given to the problem of providing permanent places in our organization for persons with this special training."[96] Indeed, the Department of Medical Biophysics was just dawning, though Paul stayed with the biochemists. In the 1952–3 session, the Atkinson Foundation supported equipping the new labs of "biophysics" as a sub-department of pathological chemistry, under Paul's direction.[97]

During his tenure, Dauphinee soon adumbrated a scheme that Bernie Langer would later bring to fruition in the Department of Surgery as the clinical scholars program. The problem, he said in 1949, was that they want residents to gain some scientific training, but the current time isn't adequate. "For the most part, these Fellowship Candidates find it impossible to remain in the study of basic science more than the required year … It is not possible for them to accomplish much in the way of investigation during this time. They just begin to know their way about the laboratory when the time comes for them to stop." Dauphinee said that steps were being taken to permit them to work at least two years "and if possible to proceed towards a graduate degree."[98]

In the 1965–6 session, Allan Gornall took the baton from Dauphinee as professor of pathological chemistry. His tenure would see the emergence of the hospital departments of clinical chemistry as the main balustrades of the university department. Gornall, an Easterner, was born in River Hebert, Nova Scotia, in 1914. He gained a bachelor's degree from Mount Allison University in 1936 and a PhD in pathological chemistry from the University of Toronto in 1941. After wartime service in the navy, he joined the department in 1946 as a lecturer and rose through the ranks. In 1949 Gornall and colleagues authored a much-quoted article on a simple procedure for determining the total protein, albumin, and globulins in serum that became a "Citation Classic".[99]

Immediately upon taking office, Gornall ensured that all the hospital heads of clinical chemistry were cross-appointed to the university department, making it clear that he attached much importance to this "liaison."[100] "We have suggested that in the future the University Department of Pathological Chemistry should be made up of Departments of Clinical Biochemistry established in each of the teaching hospitals of the Toronto Medical Centre."[101] He continued, "The

Department will aim to create a first-class centre of biochemistry in a clinical setting, with approximately equal numbers of basic scientists and medically qualified biochemists on its staff." To this end they established in 1967–8 a Diploma Course in clinical chemistry, the first in Canada.[102] The plan was to shift the research centre of gravity away from the Banting Institute and into the hospitals, each of which would have its biochemist-in-chief and an academic as well as a service section.[103] A Departmental Council organized in 1970–1 had equal elected representation from the Banting division and from the hospital divisions.[104]

Just as clinical biochemistry continued to gallop forward in the hospitals, it galloped out of the undergraduate curriculum, to Gornall's dismay. The new "block" curriculum that came in during these years did not have space for all subjects, and radiotherapy (see ch. 11) and clinical biochemistry were among those chopped. In 1970 "[t]he staff of this department has felt rather keenly the expropriation of its responsibility for providing a course in clinical biochemistry to medical students."[105]

## Department of Clinical Biochemistry

In 1971–2 the name was changed from "Pathological Chemistry" to "Department of Clinical Biochemistry." The change was perhaps an ill omen because it marked the beginning of the Long-Range Planning barons' efforts to abolish the department entirely and make it a division within the Department of Biochemistry. As George Williams, chair of biochemistry, pointed out in 1974 somewhat invidiously, "Recruitment and publications of the [pathological chemistry] department suggest that it is not producing a programme in clinical Biochemistry but essentially another Biochemistry department with fundamental research in Biochemistry."[106]

Dean Holmes set up a review committee in May 1975 headed by psychiatrist Robin Hunter that determined radical changes in clinical biochemistry were necessary: essentially to shift the centre of gravity to the hospitals and at the same time to make them research-oriented. There were really two parts of the department at the time: the Banting-based academics and the teaching-hospital-based service groups. "This dichotomy is unfortunately characterized by very different professional and academic life-styles … Gornall was retiring, and his successor must be hospital-based, the Chief Clinical Chemist at the 'hub' teaching hospital."[107]

The action followed the script. In July 1977 David Goldberg followed Gornall in succession. He had been biochemist-in-chief at the children's hospital for the previous two years. Born in Glasgow, Goldberg had earned his PhD there in 1965 and MD in 1974; he had been recruited to HSC from the University of Sheffield. On Goldberg's watch the department essentially functioned as two units, as the 1983 Self-Study observed, "one small central academic-oriented unit and a larger service-oriented hospital unit with separate funding and, by and large, separate objectives." The central core at Banting and HSC were said to have "real areas of strength."[108]

By the end of Goldberg's second term in 1987, talk of major change was circulating: clinical biochemistry should be folded into a larger Department of Laboratory Medicine. In February 1987 Goldberg fired off a furious letter to Lowy protesting such a merger. Possible mergers were being dealt right and left. Goldberg told Lowy, "It may amuse [you] to learn that in developing our recently submitted Long Range Plan for the Department of Clinical Biochemistry, we agonized on whether or not we should make a bid to take over the Department of Pathology, but ultimately concluded that the prize was not worth the effort."[109]

In 1988 Andrew Baines became the last chair of the Department of Clinical Biochemistry. He was also to serve in 1994 as vice-dean of education. Baines, born (1934) and raised in Toronto, graduated with an MD from the University of Toronto in 1959 and earned a PhD in pathological chemistry in 1965. He joined the department in 1968 and, having a humanistic streak, served as principal of one of the university's colleges, New College, beginning in 1974. In 1984 he became biochemist-in-chief at the Toronto Hospital and department chair in 1988.

Baines presided over the end of the department. In the previous pages I have already noted a meeting that Baines, Silver in pathology, and Aberman held in June 1994 about a possible merger of the two departments. In November 1994, the Pinkerton committee was formed,[110] and in January 1995 the committee recommended that three departments – clinical biochemistry, pathology, and microbiology – be brought together in a new department.[111] And that was that.

## Towards a Department of Laboratory Medicine and Pathobiology (Formerly Department of Clinical Biochemistry, Department of Microbiology, Department of Pathology)

Many students are identifying pathology and laboratory medicine as an intellectually satisfying way of practicing clinical medicine. They enjoy being at the crossroads of basic science and clinical medicine and being able to move from bench to bedside and back.[112]

Avrum Gotlieb, Chair, Department of Laboratory Medicine and Pathobiology, 2001

In January 1995, as seen, Peter Pinkerton's committee recommended that the current Departments of Clinical Biochemistry and Pathology, together with the medical microbiologists, be brought together in a new department. A committee chaired by Bernard Langer of the Department of Surgery was then struck "to develop a detailed merger proposal." They reported in June 1995. Members of all three units voted for merger.

On 1 January 1996, Avrum Gotlieb was appointed acting chair of both the Department of Clinical Biochemistry and the Department of Pathology; shortly after his appointment he chaired a Steering Committee to implement the merger, reporting on 20 September 1996. The three departments then voted again yes. So now the whole plan was sent to Faculty Council for approval. (Just as a footnote: when in March 1996 the Faculty Council approved a motion terminating the Department of Microbiology, it created a new department for teaching medical undergraduates called the Department of Medical Genetics and Microbiology.[113] This new department was, however, outside the purview of the Department of Laboratory Medicine and was in 2007 folded into the Department of Molecular Genetics.)

In January 1997 the Faculty Council voted to have just a single graduate and a single undergraduate department for pathology, clinical biochemistry, and microbiology in the new Department of Laboratory Medicine and Pathobiology.[114] In July 1997, Gotlieb became acting chair of the new department.[115] He said later, "The original merger of the university departments in 1997 was carried out for academic reasons and not for financial ones. LMP achieved the intended goals of the merger which were that faculty in laboratory medicine and pathobiology integrate their education and research expertise to create a large thriving department."[116] In January 1998, the division heads were announced: Division of Clinical Biochemistry (Eleftherios Diamandis), Division of Medical Microbiology (Don Low), and Division of Pathology (Wedad Hanna).[117]

On the intellectual origins of the new department, Kenneth Pritzker said in an interview that there were two motives for merging the three departments into one. The first was economical, the driver here being Arnie Aberman. The second was intellectual: "In the lab world, some of us recognized that there were so many overlaps between the various lab departments that if you were going to develop things that were new, you had to merge them … We were all very isolated, and the folks weren't even talking to each other during their training, and then they would be placed in departments. When I became chief [of pathology] at Mount Sinai, there were probably 32, 36 chiefs or something like that, of very small departments, scattered around. Now there are six." What should the new department be called? Pritzker did a study of what other such departments were called. "You couldn't use the word 'Pathology.' I felt strongly that the department should have a name that was similar to other departments in the world. Well, I lost that battle because they called it 'Laboratory Medicine and Pathobiology.' We're the only department of pathobiology in the world."[118]

By 2001, the centre of gravity of laboratory medicine in Ontario was clearly Toronto: over 50 percent of the laboratory physicians in the province were employed at the Academic Health Sciences Complex and practiced academic laboratory medicine, as Gotlieb pointed out in 2001.[119] Indeed, historically the Department of Pathology at U of T had "trained many of Canada's specialists and current leaders in laboratory medicine," as external reviewers commented in 2001. "The Department has an immense base of professional and material resources." They found the department to be "an outstanding department of pathology when viewed in comparison to other departments in Canada and throughout North America." But there was a warning note: "The tendency to lose departmental cohesiveness as clinical and investigative faculties polarize, is a continuing challenge, one seen in all pathology departments aspiring to engage in research." Gotlieb wanted to add – as did every department in the faculty – investigators with both clinical training in pathology and research training. But they were scarce in the marketplace and, again as in so many other departments, he had set out to train his own. "This is clearly one of Dr. Gotlieb's most cherished personal goals," said the reviewers, striking a poignant note.[120]

Gotlieb had reason to be proud. In 2004 he said he had "the largest department of its kind in Canada and one of the largest worldwide. Laboratory Medicine and Pathobiology has over 200 faculty, over 60 residents and clinical fellows, 150 graduate students ... and as the second most successful clinical research department in the Faculty of Medicine, brings in over $23 million per year in research and awards."[121]

In Pritzker's opinion, "the consolidation of the departments gave the Department of Laboratory Medicine a huge critical mass. It's one of the top ten pathology departments in the world."[122]

# 19  Ophthalmology and Otolaryngology

## Department of Ophthalmology

On the importance of ophthalmology, from a 1974 planning document: "In any year 16% of the people have an ophthalmic examination. This is a personal contact, one charged with emotion for the patient, this is the daily hour-in and hour-out life of the staffman. At least 1500 of these contacts are made each day by the members of the Department. They present personal problems, personal tragedy, preventative medicine, economic productivity, and at all times need for the expertise offered. This relationship is going to grow because in the increasingly complex environment, the industrial environment of productive people, the economic value of vision, and anxiety which is related to vision, is going to increase."[1]

Department of Ophthalmology, 1974

Ophthalmology began in Toronto in 1850 as S.J. Stratford opened the Toronto Eye and Ear Infirmary, which then vanished in 1863 "when Dr. Stratford left for other parts," as the official history of the Department of Ophthalmology puts it.[2] "Two years later, in 1865, Dr. Abner Roseburgh re-established the clinical facility and was shortly joined by his brother-in-law, Dr. R[ichard] A[ndrews] Reeve." Reeve had just graduated from medicine at Queen's. In 1872 he was appointed to the Toronto General Hospital, the institution's first specialist of any kind.[3] (Ophthalmology and otology were combined at this time. Only in 1905 did the General establish a Department of Otology and Laryngology separate from ophthalmology.) In 1887, with the refoundation of the faculty, Reeve became Toronto's first professor of ophthalmology.

In 1914 James M. MacCallum succeeded Reeve. Born in 1863 in the hamlet of Eglinton north of Toronto, MacCallum graduated from the medical department of Victoria University in Toronto in 1886, then sought postgraduate training at Moorfields Hospital in London. Back in Toronto in 1888, he set himself up as an oculist and ophthalmologist and ranked among "the city's foremost specialists."[4] He entered the faculty in 1892, following Thorburn as professor of therapeutics, and thereupon in 1903 joined the Department of Ophthalmology and Otology, ascending to the chair in 1914.[5] According to the departmental history, MacCallum "was a remarkable man in that he had a gruff exterior, but underneath he had a heart of gold ... He will be especially remembered for his interest in the work of budding artists ... and even financed a group of those young Canadians who later became renowned as Canada's famed Group of Seven."

In 1920 the Faculty Council passed a motion for the hospital department to become a teaching department, given the "wonderful opportunities to develop along scientific lines." (Ear, nose, and throat was also included in motion.)[6] A faculty committee headed by Alexander Primrose proceeded to recommend for ophthalmology and otolaryngology the same unitary structure that was seen applied in earlier chapters to medicine and surgery: a single powerful head of a single service, with the difference that the head would serve only half-time rather than full-time as in the big departments. "A staff, under the direction and control of the Head, will be constituted to meet the requirements of the Department."[7] This, then, marked the beginning of the powerful departmental system so characteristic of the Faculty of Medicine of the University of Toronto.

Indeed, a series of powerful heads then followed. In 1929 William Herbert Lowry succeeded MacCallum in the chair of "Ophthalmology and Otology." Born in 1880, Lowry studied medicine at Trinity, graduating in 1901 – two years before the medical faculty of Trinity University merged with the University of Toronto. He was "one of the first surgeons in Canada to become interested in the treatment of detached retinae, and was proficient in the surgical repair of this condition which heretofore had rarely responded to treatment." A whole cohort of young ophthalmologists grew up under his wing.

In 1924 the department began receiving specimens of diseased eyes for examination in its laboratory; by the early 1930s, under the guidance of research fellow Alexander E. MacDonald, this had expanded to almost a hundred per year from all over Ontario, and the department routinely conducted pathological examinations for the provincial laboratory as well.[8]

Somewhere in the force field between poignancy and exasperation lay MacDonald's other research work. One problem suffered among the young men invalided back from the front in the war was the presence of "intraocular steel foreign bodies." MacDonald was trying to "cut down the size of the magnet [needed to extract them] without sacrificing the force required ... He hopes that funds may be made available so that this work may be carried out to a satisfactory completion. He thinks that a grant of $50 would be sufficient for this purpose."[9] How maddening to think that the faculty's circumstances in the Depression were so straitened that a $50 grant for these wounded young veterans with bits of metal in their eyes should have been problematic!

In the 1930s A. Lloyd Morgan began the experimental transplanting of corneas in rabbits. "If the technique can be perfected," said Lowry in 1935, "a lot of persons, who are now nearly blind from corneal scars, will be helped considerably." This had worked, he said, in England and on the Continent. The U of T may do a human eye within a year.[10] Three years later, Morgan's transplant technique had succeeded and the first human received a cornea in Toronto in the 1937–8 session.[11]

Lowry's successor, Walter W. Wright, took office in 1941. The following year he organized the ophthalmology training program for postgraduates, combining facilities at the General and the Hospital for Sick Children. In the 1941–2 session, they took on a single trainee.[12] Gallie later said of this fledgling program, "Until ten years ago there had never been an eye specialist trained in Canada. When one of our graduates wished to go into this specialty he had to go for a number of years to England or the United States. But ten years ago, the University decided to support this department as it had already supported Medicine and Surgery. A young, highly qualified professor was appointed on a part time basis, who proceeded to organize a programme of postgraduate internships and study somewhat similar to that of the great clinical departments, and soon we had here in Toronto a school for ophthalmologists."[13]

In 1946 Alfred J. Elliot, a 1937 U of T graduate, became chair. Simultaneously ophthalmologist-in-chief at the Toronto General Hospital, he had "sufficient salary to enable him to devote a large part of his time to academic duties."[14] Among those duties was growing the postgraduate program, which by the late 1940s had been extended from two to three years. Elliot also began to link the different hospital teaching programs together. "A satisfactory system of rotating the internes through the four teaching hospitals was developed in order to utilize as much as possible the clinical material available at each hospital."[15] Elliot himself was said to be "the first to bring under the aegis of the University the Departments of Ophthalmology in the other hospitals of the city."[16] In 1947–8, the department began planning for an eye institute, which, among its various achievements, would rank highest of all in the public mind.[17]

And indeed, the most visible legacy to the Canadian public of the Department of Ophthalmology was the Eye Bank, which grew out of a conversation in May 1950 between Col. Edwin Albert Baker – cofounder of the Canadian National Institute for the Blind (CNIB) who had been blinded in both eyes during World War I – and Elliot. In exchange for a $500 donation from the CNIB, the department established the eye bank at the Banting Institute. In 1955 Hugh Ormsby, the eye bank's first medical director, and Oscar B. Richardson, director of the eye pathology laboratory, secured funding from the federal health department for research in corneal transplantation.[18] Under the leadership of Ormsby, in 1956 the Department of Ophthalmology, giving preference to the now aging veterans who had been blinded by mustard gas in World War I, began undertaking corneal transplants. (Baker had to go to Ottawa and plead

for the retention of their veterans' pensions for these men who could now see.[19])
In this 1955–6 session, "Mrs. R. MacKneson has organized an eye bank for the
procurement of eyes suitable for transplantation and the distribution of such
eyes to surgeons who wish to perform corneal transplantation operations."[20]
Ormsby and Prasanta Basu – who at that point still had an appointment at a
clinic in India – described in 1959 a technique for the long-term storage of corneal grafts that made possible the concept of an eye "bank." The storage, moreover, reduced the antigenicity of the grafts.[21] With its links to CNIB, the Eye
Bank became a prized national resource.

In 1961 J. Clement McCulloch, who completed medical studies at the U of T
in 1939 and was ophthalmologist-in-chief at the Western, succeeded Elliot as
professor of ophthalmology. Under McCulloch, research blossomed in the department and grants flowed in.[22] 1967–8, the department brought in a diploma
in ophthalmic science.

The Eye Bank had now become a major project in the department, processing more than 500 eyes a year, which the bank then sent to hospitals across the
province for service in transplantation.[23] Said McCulloch in 1969, "Not only are
more eyes being received but, with improved surgery techniques, the indications for corneal transplants have expanded and the number of transplanta-
tions being done is increasing. In addition, the Eye Bank has been performing a
larger function in assisting eye banks in neighbouring districts." The Eye Bank
also supplies "vitreous for vitreous transplantation and is now developing a
technique using cobalt sterilized fascia lata for repair of ptosis and other plastic procedures about the eyes and lips."[24] By 1971, over 5,000 eyes had been donated, of which more than 2,600 were used for corneal transplantation. Over
50,000 people had signed donor cards pledging their eyes. In this joint program
with the CNIB, now directed by George A. Thompson, the Eye Bank lab under
Basu was also supplying sclera and vitreous, offering suture material from cadaveric fascia lata to ophthalmic plastic surgeons in Canada and the United
States.[25] Research in the department had now shifted to the laboratories at 1 Spadina Crescent, and the only research being done in hospitals was that involving
patients.[26]

Talk of an eye institute surfaced repeatedly. Yet things were not so simple.
When Ronald Pinkerton, head of ophthalmology at Queen's University, visited
the department in 1979, he called attention to the pitfalls of such an institute.
"This poses conflict with the referral pattern in the six separate institutions and
their autonomy, and if more widely oriented to serve the entire province has potentials for conflict with the other four medical schools in the province."[27] The
comment is interesting for its unabashed self-interest.

The research drum beat ever more loudly, but the ophthalmic community
was split on the subject, and it was a split not untypical of many specialties.
On the one hand, there was a core of researchers doing scientific work, one of
whom, Michael Shea at the Banting Institute, wanted an ophthalmic institute.

On the other, there was a large group of community ophthalmologists, creating a "wide gap between earnings of private practitioners and academic staff" and making recruitment to the academic department difficult.[28]

In 1982 Clive B. Mortimer, a Cambridge MB of 1954 (and later MD) who had been on staff at the General for twenty-five years, was appointed chair. On Mortimer's watch, the department adopted a group-practice plan. As well, ophthalmology was becoming an increasingly technology-driven field, and in 1983 the department purchased a "YAG" laser for capsulotomies and iridotomies, located at the General for use by all hospital departments. ("YAG" stands for the type of crystal used in "photodisruptive lasers.") Mortimer said that the ministry had funded it "on the understanding that no hospital would undertake to purchase a machine for at least one year."[29] As he explained on another occasion, "It seemed ridiculous that we should have five YAG lasers in Toronto, one at each teaching hospital, when in fact one YAG laser could do the work for all the hospitals. That was really our first effort at sharing and inter-hospital cooperation."[30] In 1987 Mortimer led the move of most of the department from the General to the Toronto Western Hospital.

At the level of science, outstanding was Brenda Gallie's work on retinoblastoma, a terrible childhood cancer.[31] Gallie, the granddaughter of William Gallie, was cross-appointed to the Hospital for Sick Children and the Ontario Cancer Institute. In 1982 she proposed a genetic origin for retinomas and retinoblastomas. In 1989 a team led by Gallie identified the genetic mutation in retinoblastoma.[32] And in 1996 she recommended a combination of standard anticancer drugs and cyclosporine, followed by laser therapy and cryotherapy.[33]

Finally, a development was achieved in 1988 devoutly wished by the department for years: the opening of an Eye Research Institute, to "bring together clinicians and basic scientists in a central investigative facility," under the leadership of William P. Callahan, chairman of the board of the Eye Research Institute of Ontario (ERIO) at the Toronto Western Hospital. Funded by a Ministry of Health grant, the institute was conceived as "a free-standing structure with University affiliation," as was the case with the Clarke Institute of Psychiatry and the Addiction Research Foundation.[34]

In 1992 Graham Trope became chair and reorganized the department. Moving along with the grand current of clinician-scientist programs then sweeping the faculty, he introduced an ophthalmic scientist program. The department's Vision Science Research Program set out to build links to the basic sciences.[35]

Recent changes in leadership in ophthalmology will not be pursued here given that it is too close to the story for objectivity. But it has a nice codicil: in April 2001, Tony Clement, the provincial minister of health, visited the Ontario Division of the Eye Bank of Canada "to mark National Organ and Tissue Donor Awareness Week and to announce that the Ministry has more than doubled the Eye Bank's base funding from just under $0.4M to $1.07M."[36] A small department had effected some big changes in people's lives.

## Department of Otolaryngology – Head and Neck Surgery

A chair in otolaryngology goes back in some form to the beginning of the faculty, as Richard A. Reeve, one of the early deans, held the chair of ophthalmology, otology, laryngology, and rhinology from 1887 to 1903. In 1903 the chair was divided among ophthalmology and otology, which Reeve continued to teach, and the chair of otolaryngology, professed by George Raymond McDonagh, who therewith became the faculty's first dedicated otolaryngologist.

McDonagh was forty-seven when he ascended to the chair of laryngology and rhinology in 1903. Born in 1856, he had graduated with an MB from the Toronto School of Medicine in 1876, studied in London and qualified as a licentiate of the Royal College of Physicians the following year, then embarked upon a career that made him "one of the foremost men in his specialty in this country," as his eulogist said at the time of his death in 1917.[37] From the beginning of the faculty's refoundation in 1887, McDonagh lectured in laryngology and rhinology.[38] Why he stepped down from the chair in 1914 is unknown, but in that year David James Gibb Wishart succeeded him as professor and head of otolaryngology.

Wishart as well had deep roots in Toronto medicine. In 1905, and quite possibly before, the Toronto General Hospital displayed on its organizational table the specialty "Rhinologists and Laryngologists," showing David James Gibb Wishart and Geoffrey Boyd.[39] In 1906 a "Nose and Throat Department" was listed.[40] The hospital's Annual Report for 1914 featured a prominent section on the "Oto-Rhino-Laryngological Department," claiming that at the General, "for the first time in Canada, with the possible exception of the Royal Victoria Hospital, Montreal, Oto-Rhino-Laryngology has come to its own. It represents the endeavour of the nose, throat and ear specialist to build up, within the too often smothering embrace of a large General Hospital, a department at once comprehensive in scope and complete in detail." And the poor previous practitioner! "He has had to take the spare corner, the untrained nurse, the for-the-moment-available house-surgeon, and the general operating room when he could get it." Happily, the specialty was also making an incursion into the undergraduate curriculum. "The fifth year medical student of to-day has begun to realize that the nose, throat and ear are factors to be reckoned with in the diagnosis of disease." The department had a dedicated suite of six rooms in the Out-Patient Building. "Each student provides his own head mirror, and by the end of his term of instruction the student who is not as familiar with the appearance of the membrana tympani or the vocal cords as he is with the language of the heart and lungs, has wantonly neglected his opportunities, and the graduate, new in cap and gown, who passes unnoted the gaping stare of the adenoid child ... has not truly risen to his course of study," said Davis James Gibb Wishart (the author of this paean).[41]

Wishart was born in Madoc, Ontario, in 1859 into the family of a clergyman. He spent several years in London earning his licentiate of the Royal College of Physicians before teaching anatomy and otolaryngology in Trinity Medical College in Toronto, where he was secretary treasurer of the Trinity faculty until the merger with the Faculty of Medicine in 1903. He also helped train female medical students in the Ontario Medical College for Women. With the amalgamation of the two faculties, he continued lecturing in otolaryngology at U of T. Wishart was an important campus figure and served as chairman of the senior committee, called the Committee on Curriculum and Examinations, for five years before his retirement in 1922. As a sign of how anglicized the faculty was in those days, as a token of gratitude at Christmas 1927 his classmates presented him with a set of Sheffield plate.[42]

Just parenthetically, it might be noted that the Department of Laryngology saw in 1912 the appointment of one of the first women as specialists in the history of Canadian medicine, Pearl Jane Sproule (see p. 548). (Married to James Manson in 1918, she took her husband's name for the rest of her career.)

Perry G. Goldsmith succeeded Wishart in 1922. Born in 1874, Goldsmith was another product of the Trinity Medical College, graduating in 1896. It was Goldsmith and his staff who introduced bronchoscopy to the Toronto General Hospital – the first American bronchoscope was constructed in 1904 – which, as Cosbie says in his history of the Toronto General Hospital, "opened the field of thoracic surgery."[43] Goldsmith steered the department increasingly towards science and said in 1936 that "the scientific publication has very greatly increased, and the attendance of the members of the department to special society meetings has surprisingly improved. I think this is the most outstanding feature of the past year's work."[44]

Goldsmith brought back from his training in the United Kingdom a typically British prejudice against specialism and preference for the generally educated physician. In 1939, at the time of his retirement, he pleaded specifically for this perspective in undergraduate education: "There is a general tendency in the best medical schools to lessen the importance of the specialists and to restrict the time devoted to them in teaching hours. There can be little argument against this viewpoint. In our undergraduate teaching [otolaryngology] we have this ever in mind, and try to arrange our instruction so as to make the student a better all-round physician rather than a poor surgical specialist."[45] This was a perspective to which such surgeons as Richard Reznick sought to return many years later. At Goldsmith's retirement, Dean Gallie said that he had brought the department "to a position of distinction among the otolaryngological teaching units of America."[46] Interestingly, Goldsmith was one of the founding members of the American Board of Otolaryngology, even though Toronto had at the time no postgraduate training program. Peter Alberti comments that "in the establishment of this organization, [Goldsmith] established the path that led Toronto to follow American rather than British training methods when a program was eventually started."[47]

There was a brief interregnum as George M. Biggs succeeded Goldsmith in the 1939–40 session, then retired a year later for reasons of health, followed in the chair in 1941 by Angus Campbell.

Campbell, who grew up in Shanty Bay, Ontario, finished his medical studies at Toronto in 1906, then, as every previous Toronto otolaryngology professor, trained in the United Kingdom. He left few footprints as chair, and his memory has almost been effaced by the giant of post-war otolaryngology: Percy Edgerton Ireland.

Ireland was appointed professor and head of the department in 1946. Hailing from Toronto, Ireland was born in 1904 and earned his medical degree in 1929, playing with the officers' training corps band during his studies. He trained in otolaryngology at Harvard. After military service during the Second World War, he applied himself to building otolaryngology at the Faculty of Medicine, as well as in the country as a whole. Said his eulogist at the time of his death in 1973, "All his academic life, he worked through the Royal College of Surgeons of Canada and the Canadian Otolaryngological Society to develop a standard of excellence in the training of post-graduate students of medicine."[48]

Of special note was Ireland's founding of a two-year postgraduate training program in otolaryngology in the 1945–6 session, which he modelled upon the training he himself had received at Harvard.[49] Soon twelve trainees were enrolled in it.[50] By the 1949–50 session, the Royal College of Surgeons had established a fellowship examination in the subject. Sniffed Ireland, "It is the proposed policy of the Department that no new appointments will be made except to those whose training is considered adequate enough for them to be placed at the fellowship level." In addition to the two-year core program, further study in basic science and for training abroad was envisaged. As well, the postgraduate program contemplated refresher training for specialists across Canada who had not had the course but wished to keep up to date.[51]

In fact, the postgraduate training program quickly evolved into a two-tier system: the basic two-year program was for "providing specialists to the non-teaching centres across Canada." The added study was for "a smaller group ... destined for teaching appointments in our own school, the University of Western Ontario, the University of British Columbia, and the University of Alberta." It is thus interesting to see which universities, in the eyes of the otolaryngologists, were and were not on the list of supposedly elite Canadian institutions.[52]

Acute mastoid infections had been the bread and butter of classical pediatric otolaryngology, making the "hard-of-hearing child" a familiar figure at the Hospital for Sick Children, where David Wishart, chief of otolaryngology, opened an elaborate clinic for testing hearing in the 1950–1 session.[53] Yet the advent of penicillin and the other miracle drugs had a truly wondrous effect on such acute infections: relieving them before they could cause hearing loss. This tells, however, only part of the story. Adult otolaryngology dealt with much more than infectious illness: hearing loss, dizziness, nasal allergies, sinusitis, foreign bodies, and non-cancerous laryngeal disease. In those days, says Alberti, "Otolaryngology existed because of a learned skill of examining the dark recesses of the upper airway and was largely a mucosal specialty."

Still, the days of mucosal specialties were numbered. There was such a falling-off in applications for residency in otolaryngology that, were it not for students from India and other countries, the specialty would have gone into a decline. ("We have this year accepted some five or six students from India," said the dean in 1953.)[54] This is comparable to the threatened decline in chest surgery caused by the advent of anti-tuberculosis treatments in these years. Unfortunately, smoking came to the rescue of both departments. The chest surgeons were saved by lung cancer, the otolaryngologists by laryngeal and other head and neck cancers. The department founded, for example, the "Lost Chord Club" to help patients who had undergone a complete removal of the larynx.[55]

And lo and behold! The advent of all the new cancers boosted recruitment to the field, so worries about securing a future generation of otolaryngologists vanished.[56]

There were technical advances in ear surgery as well. In 1934 at St Michael's Hospital Joseph A. Sullivan pioneered the treatment of an injured facial nerve by decompression or by a nerve graft.[57] In 1957 Sullivan, by now chief of the service at St Michael's, proposed modifications to the fenestration operation for deafness, a procedure that had fallen out of use because of poor results (it entails creating a new opening in the labyrinth of the ear in cases of otosclerosis). They had been refining it at SMH since 1937 and had excellent results to report: "The patient will hear as well or slightly better than he would with a hearing aid," they said.[58] In the 1960s, fenestration was surpassed by direct stapes surgery, which was simpler, quicker, and more effective. Says Peter Alberti, "It is difficult to comprehend how important the surgical treatment of deafness had become; there was a huge pool of patients with hearing loss who benefited over the next two decades," including some of Sullivan's own students at the Toronto Western Hospital.[59]

Sullivan himself was one of the more colourful personalities in the history of Toronto medicine. Born in Toronto in 1902, the youngest in "an Irish Catholic family of five children," he attended the University of Toronto Schools, then entered medicine, graduating in 1926. During his studies he was a real athlete and captained varsity hockey teams for several years, though forced to withdraw in his first year from intercollegiate football because of a broken arm.[60] In 1928 he served as the goaltender on the Canadian gold-medal ice hockey team at the Winter Olympics in St Moritz. In 1930 he began practice in otolaryngology, where he had among his patients the prime minister of Canada, John Diefenbaker. In 1957 Diefenbaker appointed him to the Canadian Senate. In 1988 he was inducted into the U of T Sports Hall of Fame, where a hockey trophy is named in his honour. At St Michael's, he organized a Hard of Hearing Clinic to which patients streamed "with difficult hearing problems from all over the world," as his obituary said. Said a friend, "He was a man who could have been a big shot but was just a plain, straight guy."[61]

Under Percy Ireland, the department took steps to gear up for research and to give the residents a more scientific grounding. In the 1958–9 session they converted their Pathological Laboratory in the Banting Institute to a Research Laboratory and wished to move it to TGH as their new "headquarters for research."[62] (Alas, there was provisionally no space so they ended up spreading the research laboratory around at different facilities, but it was the thought that counted.) Walter Johnson became their full-time director of research. In the 1959–60 session the department lengthened the residency, adding on a year for a total of three, plus a year in general surgery.[63]

Simultaneously, they reached out to the Department of Rehabilitation Medicine under Jousse in establishing a new course in audiology and speech therapy.[64] Cortical audiometry and vestibular research became a specialty of the Toronto otolaryngologists.

Sputnik, the first satellite in space that the Soviet Union launched in 1957, took a hand as well. Peter Alberti tells the story: "Space sickness was an enormous hazard for the early astronauts, and researchers within the Department in Toronto liaised with NASA and the Canadian aerospace agency to undertake much basic and applied research in dizziness and motion sickness. This funded a great deal of the department's basic and applied research through the 1960s and 70s. Toronto was known internationally for its work in dizziness."[65]

In 1966 Douglas Bryce succeeded Ireland as professor and head of the department. (Ireland became head of the department at Sunnybrook.) Bryce was born in Toronto in 1917 and earned his medical degree in 1942. After military service, he trained in otolaryngology as the program's first graduate, then came on staff at the General as chief otolaryngologist. In line with the long tenures of department heads in those days, Bryce served until 1982, and in 2008 at the time of his death Dean Whiteside noted, "Under his stewardship the Department doubled in size, turning out 6 graduates a year and formalized a post residency fellowship program. He was responsible for recruiting clinicians and scientists who created the pre-eminent Canadian Department of the day."[66]

These years were a crucial time for the field, as the antibiotics had wiped out most of its traditional case load, the infections of the ear, nose, and throat. Yet unhappily the head and neck cancers were soaring. Instead of passing these patients on to the general surgeons, who customarily operated for such cancers, the otolaryngologists began claiming the cancers for themselves, employing, however, not surgery but radiation. As Bill Rider at the Ontario Cancer Institute, who worked closely together with Bryce observed, "Doug was destined to become the leader of this evolution ... This was to be the start of an era of close cooperation between the Princess Margaret Hospital and the Department of

Otolaryngology."[67] Present department chair Patrick Gullane said in an obituary in 2008, "Dr Bryce was one of the first head and neck surgeons in otolaryngology when it was predominantly a mucosal surgical specialty." He and Bill Rider at the Princess Margaret Hospital treated laryngeal cancer "conservatively," trying radiation first before surgery (see pp. 348–349). Rider recalled they had "discovered" this conservative treatment simply because the necrosis induced by over-radiation was so appalling.[68] In a vast retrospective chart review, Bryce figured out that stepping up the radiation to "radical" with a surgical "salvage" fallback had identical results to pre-operative radiation plus surgery.[69] What therefore was the difference? The difference was that the radical radiation patients who didn't require an operation retained their speech, while those who were operated on lost it! Rider said of these findings, "It was clear that [we] could not condone the excision of the larynx in a ruthless fashion, and that laryngectomy was the last resort for survival."[70]

An international conference in Toronto that Bryce hosted in 1974 on the management of laryngeal cancer is still referred to, as Gullane points out, "as the beginning of 'The Era of Organ Preservation.'" In the pre-seat-belt era, Bryce also pioneered the techniques of laryngotracheal reconstruction.[71]

Indeed, the department under Bryce just bristled with energy. In 1967–8, they organized a program of weekly university staff rounds. The number of trainees was bumped up from seventeen to twenty-seven. At the Banting Institute, a Temporal Bone Laboratory was organized (later giving rise to the Ear Pathology Research Laboratory). And the department put together a research committee that met monthly.[72] The residents routinely now participated in research projects and were sent to courses and meetings in the United States "when their subject matter is being presented. It is felt that this is a most important part of the programme [and] … acts as a stimulus to develop interest in academic careers." Contrary to the predictions of doom a few years earlier, in the 1960s the demand for otolaryngologists was booming, and money was pouring into the department from government and industry.[73] New space for labs in the Medical Sciences Building further encouraged the research wave. In retrospect, Bryce is said to have "guided the metamorphosis of the department from the tonsil and mastoid era to the broader and more extensive field of head and neck surgery."[74] (Patrick Gullane guided the actual name change to "Department of Otolaryngology – Head & Neck Surgery" in 2004, on the grounds that "85% of our work within the UHN is head and neck surgery; head and neck oncology is performed today by otolaryngologists."[75]) This broad liaison between radio-oncologists and surgeons was unusual, as joint clinics of equals had not existed before. Alberti said, "Nonetheless it was not until the mid-1980s that surgeons in general and otolaryngologists in particular were given equal status at the Princess Margaret Hospital with the radiotherapists, and only since that happened has the modern evolution of head and neck surgery blossomed as widely as is seen today."[76]

In 1982 Peter Alberti replaced Bryce as the head of otolaryngology. Born in England in 1934, Alberti earned an MB in 1957 from Durham University in Durham, England, then a PhD in anatomy in 1963 at Washington University. He returned to Durham to train in otolaryngology and passed his English fellowship exam in 1965 (his Canadian in 1968). Alberti came to Toronto in 1967 and advanced through the ranks in the department. During Alberti's tenure, the department achieved great success. Alberti added an "Enrichment Year Program," with an emphasis on basic research to "stimulate the development of clinical scientists."[77]

Toronto's fellowship program in otolaryngology became widely renowned, fellows from other countries coming for a year or two of additional training in Toronto. Alberti gives the background: "This started with the Colombo Plan [conceived in 1950 at the Commonwealth Conference on Foreign Affairs held in Colombo, Ceylon] during the time of Percy Ireland, and I have met several of those fellows many years later in their home countries, Pakistan, China, and India, who remain grateful for their time in Toronto." Under Alberti, the program sharply expanded. "To my knowledge," said Alberti, "this program is unique; I know of no other academic department of otolaryngology with a Fellowship program anywhere near this size. It was looked at sceptically as a cynical means for foreign practitioners to establish themselves in Canada; the truth is different. An evaluation of 100 consecutive fellows in the late 1980s showed that only three remained in Canada. The international benefits of such a program cannot be overemphasized and the value to Toronto-based residents is huge."[78]

A 1987 external review found that "[t]he Department of Otolaryngology is one of the five best in North America."[79] This high ranking did not change under either of the next two chairs, Julian Nedzelski (1992–2002) and Patrick Gullane (2002–present). Although these events are too recent to merit describing in detail, Dean Whiteside's judgment in 2009 of the department under Gullane is not without interest. "Since 2002 Professor Gullane has recruited 20 academic faculty to the department, including individuals with advanced training in head and neck oncology and microvascular surgery ... as well as research investigators within each of these domains. The department also benefits from four endowed chairs and $11 million in philanthropic support." He concluded, "When asked the secret to creating a world-renowned clinical department, Professor Patrick Gullane says, 'to be successful one has to surround oneself with people that are better than you are, empower them and let them provide leadership.'"[80]

## Department of Anesthesia

We watch closely those who sleep.

Motto of the Canadian Anesthetists Society

Anesthesia appeared in the British North American colonies shortly after its introduction elsewhere. Ether was first used in St John, New Brunswick, in January 1847, only three months after it was demonstrated in Boston.[1] The use of chloroform soon followed: introduced in Edinburgh in November 1847, it was adopted by physician and pioneer anesthetist Edward Dagge Worthington of Sherbrooke, Quebec, as early as January 1848.[2] Toronto had to wait a bit longer, yet anesthesia was in use at the Toronto General Hospital prior to January 1863, when its first death from chloroform (and the second in Canada) was reported.[3]

In 1901 Samuel Johnston graduated from Trinity Medical College, and it is Johnston who is considered a leader of the second generation of anesthetists in Canada and a founder of the academic approach to anesthesia. He wrote later, "I know I was the first physician in Canada to give up general practice and go into the specialty of anaesthesia." His work marked an end to that period when "[a]lmost anyone who could hold a mask and pour on some drug was allowed to administer an anaesthetic." Surgeons John Caven and Alexander Primrose urged Johnston "to make anaesthesia a specialty and devote my entire time to it." Johnston began giving anesthetics as a house surgeon in the Toronto General Hospital on Gerrard Street in 1902–3. "As the other house-surgeons did not seem to relish the job, I gave the bulk of the anaesthetics, and made up my mind that it was possible to avoid most mishaps."

After finishing this internship, Johnston was asked to stay on at the General as an anesthetist and in 1907 began devoting himself largely to anesthesia.

He spent 1908–9 in England acquiring further training, then began teaching in Toronto: "We instructed the house-surgeons as they came on, and supervised them until they became somewhat proficient." At this point, Johnston began lecturing to the medical students, and in good order the hospital created a Department of Anesthaesia with Johnston the chief anesthetist.[4] Johnston thus worked at the Toronto General Hospital on a consultant basis from 1904 until his retirement at sixty-eight in 1936 "after many years of faithful service." As early as 1926 Johnston had eight assistants in the hospital department.[5]

Anesthesia acquired a formal existence in the faculty as a "subdepartment" of the Department of Therapeutics in the 1933–4 session as Ray Farquharson became professor of therapeutics.[6]

It is difficult to imagine today what a blessing anesthesia was to medicine and to suffering humanity. William Osler wrote in 1921, "At a stroke the curse of Eve was removed, that multiplied sorrow of sorrows, representing in all ages the very apotheosis of pain. The knife has been robbed of its terrors, and the hospitals are no longer the scenes of those appalling tragedies that made the stoutest quail. To-day we take for granted the silence of the operating-room."[7]

There were anesthetic discoveries in Toronto. In 1923 William Easson Brown administered clinically (to Fred Banting) ethylene, the anesthetic properties of which Velyien E. Henderson, professor of pharmacology, helped develop. Brown had asked, "Since a man can pass out from drinking too much liquor, why not use alcohol in its gaseous form, ethylene, as an anaesthetic?" Ethylene became a headline story in the *Globe* that year but never made it to the big time because it had an unpleasant smell and was explosive.[8]

Another discovery did succeed, however. One of the signal achievements of the faculty in the 1920s was the discovery of cyclopropane as an anesthetic by George H. Lucas and Henderson of the Department of Pharmacology (see pp. 436–437).[9] The effectiveness of cyclopropane was demonstrated in animal research; Easson Brown then administered it successfully to Henderson, but the Toronto anesthetists were not further involved in its clinical development. To the contrary, Samuel Johnston banned Brown from administering it at the General after several deaths had occurred during ether anesthesia and he was concerned about the public's confidence.[10] For this reason, cyclopropane was used clinically at the University of Wisconsin and became highly popular, introduced clinically in Canada at McGill!

In 1935 Johnston was succeeded by Harry James Shields, who guided the department until his retirement in 1952. The Department of Anaesthesia was formed in 1951. Shields was born in Toronto in 1887 and graduated with a bachelor of medicine in 1911, "while his favour with the ladies has been further enhanced by an increased expertness at dancing," as the yearbook noted.[11] In 1935 Shields organized at the Toronto General Hospital the first residency in Canada for the training of anesthetists. A generation of Canadian anesthetists were brought up in this program and affectionately referred to Shields – dancing evidently now long forgotten – as "Gramps."[12]

The first resident in anesthesia was appointed in 1936. In 1947 Shields proposed a graduate course in anesthesia of two years, "for men who have had a one year rotating internship and are desirous of proceeding to certification as specialists by the Royal College of Physicians and Surgeons." The Committee on Post-Graduate Studies of the Faculty Council approved this proposal. "Students would be registered as graduate students in the Faculty of Medicine."[13] The course, centred at Christie Street Hospital, began in July 1947 and soon had eleven residents.[14]

When Stuart Vandewater, who had just graduated in medicine from U of T five years earlier, joined the department in 1952 as a junior staffer, he was to "look after all the public ward patients." The other residents cared for the private patients of the surgeons in "P-OR," P standing for private on the ninth floor of the Private Patients Pavilion. All of the anesthetists were in individual private practices, "but the joint University/TGH appointment required them to take responsibility for the public ward patients with no fees allowed, but all could attend private patients." Around 35–40 percent of the anesthetics were given on the public wards, Vandewater recalled, and were largely administered by the residents, "about four for the whole hospital at that time, and supervised (taught?) by rotating staff." Vandewater's appointment was therefore welcomed by his senior colleagues: "a load off their hands for a year, and many long tedious, and to say the least, dangerous and challenging anaesthetics with demanding surgeons!"[15]

As noted, it was in 1951, the last year of Shields's tenure, that anesthesia became a separate department, and with Stanley Campbell who took up office in 1952 the department flourished. "Up until the present," said MacFarlane in 1952, "Anaesthesia has been a division of the Department of Therapeutics; no one seems to know just how this occurred. With the advances in this specialty and the responsibility of the school in training specialists, it seems only right that it should enjoy the same autonomy accorded to other specialties."[16] Dean MacFarlane articulated an important rationale for a separate department – linking "the advances in this specialty," meaning research, with the recommendation for an independent academic entity.

Campbell himself was born in Toronto in 1899 and entered University College from the University of Toronto Schools, just in time to leave for France as a platoon commander. He returned from war to study medicine, graduating in 1924. His yearbook entry noted, "After five years of lectures and labs, of fire ranging and fox-trotting [dancing], of clinics and class solidarity, he looks forward to consulting the innocent public."[17] The juxtaposition is poignant: with what pleasure these battle-tested veterans returned to the pleasures of student life! In 1926 Campbell joined the hospital department of anesthesia.

In 1951 the Royal College instituted a fellowship examination in anesthesia, and in the 1952–3 session in Toronto a third year was added to the postgraduate program for those wishing to take the Royal College examinations, with a year's residency at either TGH or HSC.[18] The same year a postgraduate cross-hospital anesthesia training program was established in the Toronto teaching hospitals, with rotations among the hospitals.[19] (In 1959–60 the diploma program as well was extended to three years.) By the 1957–8 session there were twenty-one residents in the postgraduate program with requests for admission coming in from all over the globe.[20] The department decided to set up its own anesthetic research laboratory under Barrie Fairlie, which opened in September 1961.[21] Fairlie later said, "We carried out a variety of mostly unremarkable studies, predominantly but not entirely of what I would now label the Consumer Report variety." They looked in particular at the performance of several mechanical ventilators and found the most popular type used in North American delivered vastly excessive concentrations of oxygen. "Thus, the patients with the sickest lungs were receiving the most toxic concentrations."[22]

The department functioned, in Fairley's account, "as a private-practice partnership known as Anaesthesia Associates." It was the associates that had hired Fairlie and that "determined department policy," not necessarily the chair of the university department. The older members of the associates were, Fairley said, not trained anesthetists but "general practitioners who gave anaesthesia in the mornings and ran an office in the afternoon."[23]

Until the 1960–1 session the head of the department did not have full professorial status. When Roderick A. Gordon succeeded Campbell in July 1961, he became simultaneously head of the Department of Anaesthesia in the faculty, with the rank of professor, and chief anesthetist at TGH, "for the first time placing this department on an equal professorial basis with other clinical departments."[24] Gordon had joined the department in 1945. From Watrous, Saskatchewan, he began preclinical studies at the University of Saskatchewan with a bachelor's degree in science, then entered medicine at U of T in 1934 and finished in 1937; he took his internship and residency at the General from 1934 to 1939 and administered anesthesia for the Plastics and Burn Unit of the Royal Canadian Army Medical Corps in Basingstoke, England, during the war.[25] (He also flirted with a brief career as a violinist before deciding to study medicine.[26]) In 1961 the department recruited its first full-time researchers, James Duffin and Beverley Britt (who established a special unit for the study of malignant hyperthermia at the General).[27] In 1976 Duffin and colleagues made safer the controls of a membrane oxygenator for cardiopulmonary bypass surgery;[28] Britt made a number of contributions to the understanding of the anesthesia complication called malignant hyperthermia and, after her article with Werner Kalow introduced the subject in 1968 (see p. 439), she edited a volume called *Malignant Hyperthermia* in 1979.[29]

In July 1964, at the instigation of the Ontario Department of Labour (which sought treatment for the "bends" in deep-tunnel workers), a hyperbaric chamber came into use at TGH under the direction of Barrie Fairley.[30] The chamber was also used to increase oxygen transport in such conditions as carbon monoxide poisoning or gas gangrene. Fairley had been instrumental in bringing in a respiratory failure unit several years previously (see p. 222). Henry Barrie Fleming Fairley was born in London, England, in 1927, graduated in medicine at the University of London in 1949, and trained in medicine and anesthesia at the London hospitals. He came to Toronto in 1955 as a clinical teacher in the Department of Anaesthesia, an early scout in the "BTA" (been to America) wave that was to hit British medicine. He wrote of the excitement of those early Toronto years, thrilled at "the opportunity to be a part of the beginning (at least at TGH) of epidural anaesthesia for obstetrics, hypothermia, extracorporeal circulation, a separate cardiovascular anaesthesia group, respiratory failure management, bronchospirometry, 'code blue' management, hyperbaric medicine, laboratory research, tutorial teaching and the medical school's system [block] teaching."[31] Fairley progressed up the academic ladder, leaving Toronto in 1969 for the University of California at San Francisco, after which Charles Bryan directed the hyperbaric chamber. (Fairley became chair of anesthesia at Stanford in 1985.) In 1965 Fairley invented "the first ventilator alarm in the world," as Bevan puts it.[32] "He designed the circuitry for a disconnect alarm and it was built by his laboratory technician Hugh Lamont," with it later becoming standard on all respirators.[33]

In 1969 John Desmond and Gordon proposed a widely adopted means of measuring blood loss during transurethral prostatic surgery, important to avoid circulatory overload because of intravasation of dilute fluid – their measurement allowed appropriate blood replacement strategies.[34] Desmond, a medical graduate of Madras University in India in 1951, was among the earliest clinician-scientists in the department. Despite this accomplishment, however, the research record of the Department of Anesthesia to this point had not been impressive. In 1969 the Independent Planning Committee concluded rather shatteringly, "Historically, the orientation of the Department of Anesthesia in the University and the teaching hospitals was entirely to service. Until very recently there have been no facilities whatsoever for teaching, research or clinical investigation."[35] After this critique, research in the department started to ramp up.[36]

In July 1977 Arthur A. Scott succeeded Gordon as chair and anesthetist-in-chief at TGH. Born in 1923, his mother died in childbirth, making him the youngest in a family of six children raised by their father, a Presbyterian minister. He was educated in the one-room schoolhouses of rural Ontario, then joined the RCAF for the war. He entered medicine, graduated in 1953, then began general practice in Sault Ste Marie, Ontario, whereupon a colleague convinced him to train in anesthesiology. Scott took his Royal College fellowship in 1968 and joined the staff of the General, where he became director of the Respiratory Care Unit. From 1977 he led the university department, where he presided over a great expansion of the postgraduate division.[37]

Scott's tenure saw the growing integration of the hospital divisions. The authors of the 1983 Self-Study said, "The last review [1977] commented about hospital isolation. Much has been done to rectify this. There are now city-wide rounds on the second Friday of each month. The chairman goes to each, and members of all hospital staff are encouraged to attend. The chairman uses one of these rounds to give an annual report of the university affairs to the department ... The chairman attends each individual hospital departmental rounds approximately quarterly." In addition, "[t]he university/hospital axis is gradually gravitating towards the university. There have been departmental think-ins and Professor Scott believes that the department is beginning to think as a university unit rather than as a series of isolated hospital units. The chairman is, at long last, perceived as head of the university department and not only as an advocate of the Toronto General Hospital."[38] This was precisely the kind of university orientation the deans wished to encourage.

Yet like many clinical departments, anesthesia retained a strong hospital identification. One of the external reviewers noted in 1992 that "the University of Toronto, unlike many other faculties of medicine, is really a confederation of the teaching hospitals in the University of Toronto system ... A similar pattern exists in the Department of Anaesthesia in that the hospital-based partnerships were strong and generally contribute to the overall strength of the Department." Another said, "At present, the hospital anaesthesia services seem to operate as an alliance or confederation of mini-departments. Their loyalty and most of their income is tied to their hospital service. The chairman's role seems to be that of a feudal king with varying allegiances and loyalties from his princes – the hospital service chiefs."[39] As has been seen, this strong hospital identification ran through many of the clinical departments, and loosening it up in the interest of university-wide training and research was a major leadership challenge.

Still, within the hospitals important innovations took place. In January 1968 Gordon established a pain clinic at TGH under Ramon Evans and partially supported by a fund endowed by Conn Smythe, owner of the Toronto Maple Leafs hockey team, "in honour of his wife." In 1976 the Ministry of Health told Gordon the province would take over the funding of the Irene Eleanor Smythe Pain Clinic, and in 1988 TGH sold a property in Caledon Township that Smythe had earlier donated, in order further to fund the clinic.[40] By the 1987–8 session it was seeing almost 600 patients a year.[41]

The tenures of the several chairs who followed Scott after 1987 will not be discussed here, including Gerald Edelist (1987–93), who was anesthetist-in-chief at Mount Sinai; Robert Byrick (1993–2003) at St Michael's, David Bevan (2003–6) at TGH, and Brian Kavanagh (2006–present) at the Hospital for Sick Children. It is notable that three of the chairs were from hospitals other than TGH. Clearly, the university department was seen as a unifying factor.

Several landmark events are worth noting, including the big push into the neurosciences that Bevan initiated.[42] In 2004 the department formally changed its name to "Anesthesia," removing the British "a" from *anaesthesia*, in line with the change initiated by the Canadian Anesthesiologists Society and the growing de-Anglicizing of Toronto medicine.[43]

An external review of the department in 2002 found anesthesia in Toronto "one of the leading departments in Canada. This is due to a decision by the Faculty, under the excellent leadership of Dr. Byrick, to institute a 'culture' that emphasizes research and teaching. The product of this effort has been a significant increase in research funding, faculty involvement in research, high quality publications, and interest on the part of young physicians to enter a career in anesthesia."[44]

How anesthesia had changed since Osler's day! For the anesthetists at the Toronto General Hospital in 1989, "Patient care is provided to one of the most challenging groups of patients seen in any hospital in North America [the Toronto Hospital]. The tertiary nature of the surgical practice, the increasing number of elderly patients and the growth of the tissue and organ transplantation services has increased the complexity of, and the demand for, anaesthesia around the clock."[45]

### Department of Radiology/Medical Imaging

The Department [at TGH] has been viewed by many as the "flagship" of radiology at the University of Toronto and a premium department in Canadian radiology.[46]

The Toronto Hospital, *Annual Report*, 1988–9

In the beginning radiotherapy – meaning treatment with radium and X-rays – and radiology, or diagnostic imaging, were closely intermingled. Within the Faculty of Medicine, they remained combined in a single unit, the Department of Radiology, until the establishment of a separate Department of Radiation Oncology in 1991.[47]

### Diagnostic and Therapeutic

Radiotherapy began in Toronto with William Henry Beaufort Aikins's radium treatments, and Aikins is considered the founder of radiotherapy in Canada. After graduating with an MB in 1881 from the Toronto School of Medicine, Aikins did a kind of grand tour of postgraduate study in Europe, stopping in London, Vienna, and Paris, returning then to Toronto to start up a general practice. Marie and Pierre Curie discovered radium in 1898, and Henri Becquerel noted its effects on living tissue in 1901, marking the takeoff of radium therapy. In 1907, Aikins returned to Paris, visiting the Laboratoire Biologique du Radium. As his biographer, radiation oncologist and historian Charles Hayter, writes, "Like other doctors of the day, he marveled at radium's ability to produce changes in tissues which could not be achieved by any other known substance and which resulted in 'cures of a very surprising character.'" In 1909 Aikins brought a small amount of radium to Toronto and opened a private radium clinic, the Radium Institute of Toronto, at 134 Bloor Street West. The clinic soon became known across the country; Hayter estimates "that Aikins treated over 3,000 patients referred from a wide area extending from Saskatchewan to Quebec." In 1916 he became the inaugural president of the American Radium Society at its meeting in Philadelphia. Although a senator of the University of Toronto, he was not a member of the Faculty of Medicine (and is not to be confused with his uncle William Thomas Aikins, the first dean of the re-established faculty).[48]

Diagnostic radiology in Toronto began on an institutional basis in 1896 at the two big teaching hospitals, the General and the Hospital for Sick Children, although ironically the first hospital in the city to acquire an X-ray device was the Grace Hospital, a homeopathic establishment, which used it in mid-February 1896 to locate a needle embedded in a woman's foot.[49] In September 1896 the HSC's board of trustees noted that "our X-Ray equipment has just been imported from Europe, and this wonderful evolution of the scientific genius of the nineteenth century is added to the mechanical apparatus at hand. It will be sure to add to the marvellous cures already effected in this hospital."[50] TGH followed suit in November, but its first X-ray apparatus was rather unsatisfactory. In 1898, for example, surgeon Alexander Primrose was obliged to enlist the help of John C. McLennan from the physics department, who had assembled "all the necessary apparatus," in order to locate a bullet in a gunshot-wound case.[51]

In 1901 HSC became the first Toronto hospital to have a formal X-ray department[52] headed by a physician, Charles Rea Dickson, rather than a radiographer. It thus became the second oldest department of pediatric radiology in the world, pre-dated only by the Boston Children's Hospital in 1899. An 1880 medical graduate of Queen's University who had picked up a second MD in New York, Dickson came to Toronto in 1889 to open at TGH an "electrotherapeutics" department (peripheral application of mild electric currents that was a forerunner of physical therapy) and in 1890 took up a similar appointment at HSC. At the 1902 meetings of the Canadian Medical Association and Ontario Medical Association, he reported on the value of the X-ray "as a therapeutic agent in many conditions"[53] and potentially "curative when properly applied in suitable cases."[54] Indications discussed covered a wide range of conditions, including "Nevus, lupus vulgaris, tubercular joints, sclerodema, subacute articular rheumatism," and "neurasthenia,"[55] but the most promising of these was the treatment of "carcinoma of the stomach, ... of the cervix uteri, and ... many inoperable cases of malignant disease."[56] In 1906 Dickson was replaced briefly by another physician, Samuel Cummings, who had graduated with an MB from Toronto in 1888 and was said to have worked with Roentgen himself, but between 1907 and the appointment of Albert Rolph in 1919 the department was again run by radiographers, a common practice during the pre–World War I era.

Meanwhile an X-ray department had been established at TGH in 1906 under the direction of physician John McMaster, who in his widow's 1930 obituary was incorrectly described as "the first physician to introduce X-ray treatment in Toronto."[57] He was nevertheless an early pioneer of the discipline, speaking authoritatively about both therapeutic and diagnostic applications before the Ontario Medical Association in 1902[58] and at the Toronto Western Hospital the following year.[59] In August 1906 he and medical superintendent John Brown went down to the manufacturers' exhibition of the meeting of the American Roentgen Ray Society in Niagara Falls and bought a much better machine. McMaster had previously served in the hospital's "electrical department," and now in 1906 diagnostic radiology at the General struck out on its own.[60] The demand during these years, however, was not overwhelming. In October 1911 superintendent Charles K. Clarke informed Joseph Flavelle, chairman of the Board of Trustees, that in the month of September "106 Radiographs were taken, 33 X-Ray treatments and 38 Electrotherapeutics were given."[61]

Yet at the General too, the department was soon left to the technologists, as in 1911 the hospital wooed radiographer Benjamin Fenner and his assistant Percy Ghent away from HSC.[62] This was quite a coup, as Fenner had worked with Roentgen in 1897 and was cited at the fiftieth anniversary of the discovery in November 1945 as "one of the great pioneers of the industry." According to the *Globe and Mail*, Fenner was "one of the first to take an X-ray photograph of the human chest, and contributed much to the development of the large fluorescent screen" [i.e., the fluoroscope].[63] Ghent went on to become a pioneer of radiography in his own right, remaining at TGH for thirty-six years until his retirement in 1946 as chief radiological technician. In a 1952 obituary he was remembered for keeping abreast of the rapidly evolving discipline through "continuous study and experimentation" and as an effective teacher of student technicians. Like many of his medical colleagues, Ghent enjoyed numerous hobbies, among them historical and nature studies ("he ever and anon sought information about the fascinating things of nature by use of the x-ray"). He also wrote a column in the *Toronto Telegram* and was the author of various historical works including a brief biography of Roentgen and items on the history of radiography.[64]

Following its relocation from Gerrard Street to the "New Hospital" in 1913, TGH had a public wing on College Street and a private building around the corner on University Avenue, each with its own X-ray service; the one in the public area also held all of the hospital's physical therapy equipment as well as an electrocardiograph. In response to this expansion, a formal Department of Radiology was established in 1917, and Gordon Richards was appointed as its chief.[65]

Gordon Earle Richards was born in 1885 in Lyn, a small town in eastern Ontario, but grew up in Newboro in the home of a grandmother. The son of a Presbyterian minister who died when he was four years old, Richards realized early that he would have to make his own way in life. After commuting to Athens, Ontario, to attend high school, he entered the Faculty of Medicine, working his way through university and serving during holidays as a ship's purser. In 1908 he finished his medical studies as gold medalist of his year. Following his graduation he worked for a time as a mining camp doctor in northern British Columbia and afterwards moved to Vancouver, where he began practicing radiology at St. Paul's Hospital following postgraduate study in New York. With the outbreak of war in 1914 he joined the Royal Army Medical Corps and served as a radiologist in the Near East during the Dardanelles Campaign and with the No. 21 General Hospital on the Isle of Lemnos and in Egypt. It is unknown why he was discharged before the end of the war or how the General decided that he should be chosen to lead its radiology service.[66]

In contrast to the many faculty figures chronicled here who distinguished themselves in sports or cultural activities during their medical studies, or developed broad interests in addition to their careers, Richards was almost exclusively focused on work and achievement, although according to a colleague he took a month's vacation each year in the Rideau Lakes to "read the books he had wanted to read all year," as well as building boats and fishing, and occasionally "allowed himself a degree of relaxation" at other times with a game of golf.[67] In his professional life, however, he was viewed as a hard-driving perfectionist and "an almost authoritarian personality of the old-school" who maintained a certain formality in the clinic and was frequently brusque with co-workers and even patients. Yet despite his intimidating demeanour, he was deeply devoted to his patients and treated them with consideration and kindness. On Christmas Day he would spend much of the day carving the turkey at the hospital and visiting former patients with holiday treats and encouraging words before going home to his own family dinner.[68]

Upon arriving at the General, Richards immediately set about creating a proper radiology service, beginning with the establishment of an outpatient department, which in 1917 alone treated more than 1,000 patients. He also organized the department into a gastrointestinal division and a "radiographic and therapeutic" division, recruiting William Howard Dickson in 1919 as a specialist in the radiology of the GI tract. As the department evolved, Dickson increasingly handled the diagnostic side while Richards focused on the therapeutic.[69] (The history of radiotherapy in Toronto under Richards and his successors is detailed in chapter 13, "Cancer Care.")

Born in Pembroke, Ontario, in 1878, William Dickson graduated in medicine from McGill in 1908 and like Richards worked for a time as a mining-camp doctor in British Columbia. Unlike most of the founding generation of Canadian radiologists, however, he undertook systematic postgraduate training in the discipline, spending two years studying gastrointestinal pathology in New York with Lewis Gregory Cole before being recruited to TGH.[70] Dickson established a strong reputation in the GI field and was "regarded as something of an oracle in his chosen line" before his premature death in 1933 of "cardiac trouble, the original onset of which occurred in February, 1932." Shortly before his death, Dickson had begun "some fruitful research on the use of thorium dioxide as a means of enlarging the diagnostic field of radiology" along with "a group of keen junior graduates."[71] The results of this investigation were published in the *Canadian Medical Association Journal* in August 1932.[72]

Radiology entered the Faculty of Medicine in a modest way following a July 1919 meeting of the clinical department heads which recommended "that Radiology be made a separate Department of the University in charge of a Lecturer and Demonstrator."[73] In November, Richards was appointed "Head of the Department of Radiology in the Department of Medicine" with the title of lecturer.[74] In December 1920, the department was formally organized, with Richards (now upgraded to "Associate in Radiology") as head and Dickson and Rolph classed as "clinicians." Richards was to lecture to the medical undergraduates, Dickson to give clinics in gastrointestinal radiology, and Albert Rolph at HSC to offer clinics in pediatric radiology. (On the evolution of radiology at the children's hospital, see chapter 10.) A house service in radiology was to be established at the General as "one of the regular rotating services."[75] Faculty budgets in the years that followed allocated token amounts to Richards and a demonstrator, though in fact most of the teaching done by members of the department was unremunerated.

The establishment of radiology as a university department, however, allowed the Faculty of Medicine to begin offering postgraduate instruction. Until the 1920s there was no formalized training in the discipline, which was dominated by "physicists, photographers ... and amateur experimenters of all types."[76] This situation began to change during the First World War, as the army itself trained many young physicians who then returned to take up hospital positions and to call for radiology training in the medical school curriculum.[77]

In December 1921, the faculty's Committee on Post-Graduate Studies recommended both a one-month "short course" and a diploma program in radiology,[78] the latter on the British model first established at Cambridge in 1920. Richards organized both programs in cooperation with John C. McLennan, the professor of physics, and they were launched in 1922, at a fee of $100 for the short course, offered three times a year at the General, and $400 for the diploma course. In 1923 the latter produced its first two graduates: Eugene Shannon, who began a thirty-year career as head of radiology at St Michael's Hospital in 1925, and Omar Hague, who became Richards's first resident before returning to his native Winnipeg.[79] The short course was abandoned by 1929, as the Faculty Council explained, "because it is not in demand. This is doubtless due ... to the fact that short courses are provided by certain medical schools and manufacturers in the United States which, though totally inadequate, attract students away from courses of thorough training which demand more time."[80]

During his long career as professor of radiology at the university and chief of the department at the General, Richards became a leading international authority and the most prominent leader of the evolving discipline in Canada. By the mid-1920s, the X-ray service at TGH was considered second only to the Mayo Clinic as the "largest and best equipped department of its kind on the continent."[81] In addition, Richards established the first professional organization of radiologists in Canada, bringing together eighteen colleagues to form the Canadian Radiological Society in 1920. This group was dissolved in 1927, becoming instead the radiology section of the Canadian Medical Association. In December 1929 Richards arranged for the Radiological Society of North America to meet in Toronto – the only time it has ever met outside the United States – a singular recognition.[82]

In January 1937 Richards founded the Canadian Association of Radiologists by inviting radiologists from all parts of the country to a meeting in Toronto.[83] By the time he died in 1949, this organization's membership included "over ninety per cent of the radiologists in Canada."[84] His death, variously attributed to "leukaemia"[85] or "aplastic anemia," was considered to be "the result of exposure to the radium used by him in the treatment of literally thousands of patients."[86]

In May 1932 Richards recruited two young radiologists, Arthur Singleton and Malcolm M.R. ("Mack") Hall, to take over the diagnostic service from the ailing William Dickson. These individuals "completed the founding generation" of radiologists at TGH. Hall was a 1928 medical graduate of the faculty who had originally planned to become a surgeon, "but gave it up after an orthopedist tapped him on the shoulder in the operating room one day and said, 'Son, you'll never be a surgeon.'" He therefore went into radiology instead, and along with Richards and Singleton looked after the department[87] until his retirement in 1965.[88]

Arthur Carman Singleton was born in the eastern Ontario village of Newboro in 1900. His parents died when he was about ten, and he went to live with his sister Lila Isabel Singleton, who in 1916 married her childhood sweetheart: Gordon Richards. Like his brother-in-law, Singleton was obliged to provide for his own education. He matriculated from Kingston Collegiate, entering the U of T medical school in 1917. He left in the spring of 1918 to enlist in a tank battalion, then resumed his medical studies following the war, graduating with an MD in 1923. At medical school his slogan was, "T'would be a shame to neglect one's education by too much study."[89] Singleton completed his training in the United States, interning at St Luke's Hospital in Minneapolis, then spending a year with Douglas Quick in radiology at New York's Memorial Hospital. He was thus a qualified radiologist in his own right when he joined Richards and William Dickson in private practice in the late 1920s and was subsequently recruited to the department.[90] During the Second World War, he served as radiologist to the No. 15 Canadian General Hospital and was awarded an MBE. After returning to Canada in 1943 on medical grounds, he became consultant radiologist to the RCAF, a position he held until his death in 1968.[91]

Singleton went on to succeed Richards in 1950 as head of the Department of Radiology at TGH and the Faculty of Medicine. Although primarily interested in clinical work (and in particular in the private practice which he continued with Mack Hall at the Medical Arts Building on Bloor Street) rather than research and publication, he made a landmark contribution to the discipline by demonstrating that X-rays could be used to identify human remains in mass disasters. In September 1949 the Great Lakes liner *Noronic* caught fire while docked in Toronto Harbour, killing 119 of her 527 passengers. A team led by Singleton and TGH technician Tommy Hurst set up three mobile X-ray units in the Horticultural Building of the Canadian National Exhibition, which was used as a temporary morgue, then attempted to match films taken postmortem with antemortem X-rays of victims supplied by the Red Cross. Within ten weeks, the team was able to identify twenty-four of the thirty-five individuals for whom films had been provided.[92] This investigation, published in 1951 in the *American Journal of Roentgenology*, became a classic,[93] as well as attracting attention in the local press.[94]

Singleton also distinguished himself as an educator, organizing Ontario's first training course for radiographers and becoming a noted national figure in training radiologists. During the 1950s "a whole generation of Canadian radiologists got their start" under his tutelage at TGH.[95] Eulogies credit him with training around a quarter of the country's practicing radiologists. In 1949 he oversaw the upgrading of the diploma course from one to two years, in combination with internship. Its name was also changed from "Diploma in Radiology" to "Diploma in Medical Radiology" "in keeping with that of the English Colleges and of the English Conjoint Board."[96] The program was further enhanced in the 1953–4 session with the arrival of radiation physicist J.C.F. MacDonald as an instructor. The dean's report commented, "It is encouraging to note the increasing number of young doctors who are becoming interested in Radiology as a specialty and who are anxious to take the diploma in Medical Radiology."[97] Training in this area was then further upgraded as Harold Johns – the main founder of medical physics in Canada and already internationally known – was recruited from Saskatchewan in 1956 to head physics research at the Ontario Cancer Institute, then in development, and was also appointed to the university's Department of Physics (see pp. 446–447). In this latter capacity he was teaching residents in the radiology department as of the 1956–7 academic year.[98]

Like his predecessor Dickson, Singleton focused on the diagnostic side of the discipline, whereas Richards and his successor Clifford Ash specialized in radiotherapy. This schism became formalized at the General in 1950 as the hospital's medical advisory board decided that the two services would be separated geographically. Diagnostic radiology would take over the Dunlap Building until the new Central Building was opened (this took place in January 1959[99]), while the therapeutic service moved to the South Block on Gerrard Street. In 1953 residents stopped alternating between the two services,[100] and its 1954 annual report began to distinguish between the "Department of Radiology – Diagnostic," headed by Singleton as radiologist-in-chief, along with Hall and four

other radiologists, and the "Department of Radiotherapy," led by Ash as ra-
diotherapist-in-chief, along with radiotherapist Vera Peters and assistant radiotherapist Owen Millar.[101]

In July 1962 Mack Hall succeeded Singleton as head of the university department and radiologist-in-chief at the General, retiring three years later. Remembered in a 1970 obituary as "a gentle humble man,"[102] he had a brief tenure that
was unremarkable, continuing Singleton's emphasis on clinical care and lack of
interest in research.[103]

### The New Broom

A new era began in July 1965, as Richard Brian Holmes succeeded Hall as professor and chair of the university department and radiologist-in-chief at TGH.
Holmes was a native of London, Ontario, who had completed his MD at the
University of Western Ontario in 1943. Born in the wake of the First World War
in 1919, he took the Armed Forces Radiology Course at the General and served
from 1944 to 1946 with the Royal Canadian Medical Army Corps. After his discharge, he followed the new post-war trend of seeking postgraduate training
in the United States instead of the United Kingdom, undertaking a residency
in radiology at the Massachusetts General Hospital in Boston between 1947 and
1950. He was then recruited to Toronto by Singleton, where he quickly became
the leader of a new generation of radiologists frustrated with the old guard's
disregard for science and research.

As a history of these events put it, "Holmes lost no time in making clear that
a new broom was sweeping."[104] In a May 1966 presentation to the TGH Interdepartmental Planning Co-ordination Committee, he called for the replacement
of a culture based on "report[ing] a certain number of examinations per day"
with "a less hectic setting ... where some creative thinking can occur."[105] Under-
staffing in the hospital department exacerbated this problem. "Service requirements in the face of the shortages mean that the university functions tend to be
compromised," he explained in the dean's annual report for 1965–6.[106] In fact
the department was expanding rapidly during these years; by 1967 it included
eight diagnostic radiologists as well as five voluntary assistants.[107] Yet staff levels remained a problem. In 1969 the Faculty Council's Independent Planning
Committee continued to echo Holmes's concerns: "Historically, Radiology has
functioned primarily in providing services to patients. The Department is not
at present adequately staffed to perform its academic function ... Research has
lagged far behind service in relation to the other clinical specialties ... What is
now needed is radiological research programmes to attack the basic problems
of Radiology."[108]

Holmes addressed this need with the creation of the Radiological Research
Laboratories, which opened in 1971 in the Medical Sciences Building under the
direction of Eric Milne, a respected chest radiologist. In the absence of funding

from the university, Holmes raised the $18,000 for Milne's salary by cutting his own honorarium as department chair to zero and persuaded the rest of the staff to reduce their annual teaching honoraria from $250 apiece to a token $50.[109] This initiative began well, quickly obtaining numerous research grants and increasing its staff from two to eleven.[110] As of 1972 the lab was thriving, with "an excellent international reputation,"[111] and was the only one in North America "with a salaried staff, not based on temporary research grants" but funded from the department's practice plan.[112] Yet its success was short-lived: Milne left the unit in 1975, and although radiologist Barry Hobbs was seconded from the TGH labs part-time, the lab's focus increasingly turned to physics.[113] This shift in emphasis continued as Harold Johns became director in 1977.[114]

In 1981 the laboratories moved to the former Cardiovascular Investigation Unit at the General and eventually disappeared from there as well, with Toronto's small contribution to basic research in radiology eventually moving to the Toronto Western and Sunnybrook Hospitals.[115]

Other changes introduced during Holmes's tenure produced more lasting success. In the educational area, he quickly took aim at the now-outdated diploma course in radiology. In 1949 this program had been lengthened to two years and, as mentioned earlier, renamed the Diploma of Medical Radiology in keeping with the British model,[116] but by the 1960s most of its applicants were "coming from the ranks of general practice and are interested in returning to community practice of radiology," he told the dean in 1966. Rather than perpetuating this service-department approach, the faculty should seek to "attract a greater number who are interested in an academic career"[117] by emphasizing Royal College fellowship as the standard for postgraduate education in radiology.

Specialist certification without examination for experienced radiologists had been introduced by the Royal College in 1942, followed by certification exams in either diagnostic or therapeutic radiology, launched four years later, and a rigorous fellowship examination, begun in 1948. The last was very demanding: neither of the candidates who attempted it the first year passed, and Brian Holmes became the first in Canada to do so in 1952. Throughout the 1950s the pressure increased to adopt a single training standard – the fellowship examination – for all specialties. This was embraced in 1962, the Royal College requiring a general internship plus four additional years of graduate training (including one year spent in a discipline outside of radiology) to qualify for the exam.

Throughout this period the Royal College had also been active in certifying hospitals for specialty training. The General Hospital, the Hospital for Sick Children, and St Michael's Hospital had all been approved for training in radiology in 1948, with the Western obtaining certification a year later. As a result of these rising standards, the hospital programs assumed a greater role in specialty training. Holmes took pride in the General's success in this area: "[A]lmost none of the radiology residents who sat College exams from 1950 to 1967 failed," a record unmatched by the other Toronto teaching hospitals. With the rise of the fellowship program in the 1960s, the diploma stream became increasingly devalued and was abolished in 1972.[118]

During Holmes's tenure a number of new training initiatives were established in the department, including a training program in mammography centred at the Western under the direction of D.V. MacFarlane and Kenneth P. Vassal[119] and a first-ever "refresher course" in radiology.[120]

The main issue in postgraduate training during the 1960s, however, was a rapidly escalating demand for more radiologists coupled with a hospital-based training system "that was almost completely uncoordinated."[121] As of the late 1940s, Toronto had five hospitals with training programs in diagnostic radiology, including Sunnybrook's, which had joined the four downtown sites as a teaching department upon its establishment in 1949.[122] By 1969, this number had swelled to eight, with the addition of the Wellesley, Mount Sinai, and Women's College Hospitals. Holmes recognized from the beginning that these disparate programs had to be integrated into a single university-wide system. In 1968 he called for a "Toronto University Hospital System" in which the university Department of Radiology would press for increased staffing in all of the hospitals, paid for from "an academic budget for radiology"[123] (of which, however, there was little sign at this point).

From the beginning of his career in Toronto, Holmes had led efforts at collaboration, beginning with the creation of the Toronto Radiological Society along with Lou Harnick, chief at the Western (see p. 625), in 1951 and continuing in the late 1950s and 1960s with informal cross-hospital teaching initiatives such as slide presentations and evening quiz sessions.[124] These efforts picked up steam during his term as chair. In 1971 he set up a small departmental office on campus, a development which he explained represented "the full recognition of the truly academic aspects of the departmental function as opposed to the hospital service function."[125] What this actually meant was the creation of an academic department separate from the dominance of TGH, which Holmes further underlined by setting up a senior advisory committee representing all the hospitals, with Doug Sanders representing the General. By 1972 he was able to tell the dean that the individual hospital programs were "evolving into a single integrated and university-operated programme, co-ordinated by one individual who is specifically charged with this task."[126] Yet this was as far as the integration initiative went during Holmes's tenure; opposition from other hospital departments and his own close friendships with their chiefs made him reluctant to interfere with their independence.[127]

In scientific terms, the main advance during the Holmes era was the rise of subspecialties in radiology at TGH, which began in neuroradiology with the recruitment of George Wortzman in 1959 (see p. 387). A medical graduate of the University of Manitoba, Wortzman had undertaken his specialty training in Montreal, then the leading centre for diagnostic radiology. By the time he completed a residency in neuroradiology with Donald McRae at the Montreal Neurological Institute in 1959, he "had probably become the best trained young neuroradiologist in Canada" and went on to have a major international career in this evolving discipline. As radiologist-in-chief during the 1960s and early 1970s, Holmes played a major role in its development, securing large appropriations for new equipment. Neuroradiology thus was the first of the radiologic subspecialties to emerge in Toronto, rising in collaboration with neurosurgery.[128]

Indeed, it was in these years that Toronto became a major centre of interventional neuroradiology. This occurred with the 1976 appointment of Karel terBrugge, a medical graduate of the University of Utrecht in 1968 (see p. 515); under terBrugge's leadership, the Toronto Western Hospital took the baton from the University of Western Ontario (where neuroradiology had flourished alongside neurosurgeon Charles Drake) as the nation's leading centre of the interventional side of radiology, combing radiographic and neurosurgical procedures in the treatment of arteriovenous malformations, aneurysms, and ischemic stroke.[129] (On Derek Harwood-Nash's work in pediatric neuroradiology, see chapter 10.)

The most dramatic example of Holmes's success in bringing cutting-edge imaging equipment to the General occurred at the end of his run as chief in 1973 as he and Wortzman persuaded the provincial Ministry of Health and the other hospital chiefs to have Toronto's first CT (computerized tomography) scanner installed at the General on the condition that all of the hospitals would have access to it. In July 1973 the hospital board agreed to cover one-third of the cost from a $100,000 bequest, with the ministry picking up the remainder. When the scanner was unveiled at a big reception in May 1974, it became the second in Ontario. (McMaster University and the Hamilton Civic Hospital had jointly acquired the first scanner in the province and the Montreal Neurological Institute the first in Canada.)[130]

The other subspecialty in which TGH surged ahead was cardiovascular radiology, Holmes's own field, though most of the actual advances in angiography were made by other members of the generation of "Young Turks" who redefined the department during the 1950s and 1960s. Douglas Sanders, who had trained in radiologic pathology, collaborated on several important papers during this period on the use of chest angiography in determining the operability of lung cancers. Edward (Ted) Lansdown and Ronald Colapinto pioneered catheterization techniques, the latter becoming director of the hospital's angiography division in 1967 and working "not just in the cardiac field but in many areas."[131] "One of three physician sons of an Italian barber whose small shop sat by the Bloor subway station for decades" (as a 2011 obituary put it),[132] Colapinto went on to become the main pioneer of interventional angiography in Toronto during the 1970s and 1980s; he developed an improved technique for doing liver biopsies via catheter with the invention of the "Colapinto needle," catheter embolization of bleeding varices (previously approachable only through abdominal surgery), and most notably through his 1981 development of the "TIPS, or Transjugular Intrahepatic Portosystemic Shunt," which reduced mortality in emergency embolizations from 75 to 25 percent.[133]

Holmes stepped down as chair of radiology in February 1972 to become associate dean of medicine, then succeeded John Hamilton as dean from 1973 to 1980. Following his departure, Doug Sanders filled in for eighteen months as acting chair, then in 1974 Ted Lansdown was brought back from Manitoba to helm the department at both the university and TGH during a challenging period at both sites. Born in Winnipeg in 1927, Lansdown graduated in medicine from the University of Manitoba in 1957 and trained in radiology at TGH and the Hospital for Sick Children before joining the staff at the General. In 1968 he returned to his native province, initially as a radiologist at the Winnipeg General Hospital and then as director of radiology at the St Boniface General Hospital.[134]

### Lansdown

The beginning of Lansdown's tenure coincided with a 1974 review undertaken for the Faculty of Medicine's Long-Range Planning and Assessment Committee (LRPAC). The report examined all areas of the department's activities, including both diagnostic and therapeutic radiology as well as the emerging discipline of nuclear medicine. A key recommendation was that the department be reconstituted as "Diagnostic Medical Imaging" (including nuclear medicine), with radiation oncology becoming an independent department.[135] This initiative was not followed up, however, Lansdown explained in 1983, "because of the perception in university circles that there were already too many departments in the Faculty of Medicine."[136]

In addition to calling for more undergraduate teaching,[137] the 1974 report focused at length on the strength of the training opportunities in the various Toronto teaching hospitals, which were "certainly not found [elsewhere] in North America." These resources included "the section of Diagnostic Radiology at the Princess Margaret Hospital with its great volume of oncology patients and consequent experience in mammography, thermography, as well as lymphography"; HSC "with its concentration of specialists and subsequent great volume of unique radiological examinations" in pediatrics; the subspecialties of neuroradiology and cardiovascular radiology; and "the unique features in bone research and radiology" centred at the Toronto Western and Wellesley hospitals.[138] The department wished to add a postgraduate (fellowship) program, but this would require "that many more staff of recognized high academic caliber be obtained."[139] Developing the department along academic lines remained a problem, however, because at an average of $102 per annum, virtually no remuneration was provided by the Faculty of Medicine.[140]

Integrating the scattered training programs proved as problematic for Lansdown as it had for Holmes, despite mounting pressure from the Royal College, the program coordinators, and the residents themselves, who were eager to have more rotations and visit sites outside their home base. Yet the event that brought matters to a head was the inadequate program at the Toronto Western Hospital under Lou Harnick, which, however popular Harnick himself was, had not kept up with developments in the field and was providing little supervision to its residents. In 1982 the residents at the Western unanimously called for it to be dropped from the training schedule. Unfortunately this was not done, and the following year "academic radiology at Toronto received a grave slap in the face" as Royal College examiner Douglas MacEwan from the University of Manitoba recommended that the entire university department be placed on probation. As a result of this crisis, a new era began in 1984 as TWH neuroradiologist Karel terBrugge was brought in as acting chief, while Lansdown, having completed the now-standard term of ten years, was set to step down as chair.

After the Royal College put the Department of Radiology on probation, Dean Frederick Lowy brought in two radiologists from other universities as advisers. Their recommendations were "that the chair of the department be made independent of the hospitals and that radiology residents rotate across all the hospital departments." As a further break with the past, and to boost its academic profile, Lowy decided to look outside for a leader for the first time in the department's history.[141]

By 1984 the university had also become involved in MRI planning, with Dean Lowy establishing a task force chaired by Joe Marotta, associate dean for clinical and institutional affairs, to establish the faculty's stance on MRI and respond to the Metropolitan Toronto District Health Council report on diagnostic imaging. In September the committee recommended that in addition to the clinical MR scanner going to the "tri-hospitals" on University Avenue, a small-bore research scanner funded by the university should go to TWH. By this time the search committee for the new chair of radiology was interviewing MR specialist Gordon Potts, who would have a clinical and research base outside of the General.[142]

*A New Era*

In January 1985 D. Gordon Potts became chair of radiology at the university and chief at the Western,[143] thereby ending the traditional association of the department chair with the chiefship at TGH. (After Ted Lansdown stepped down as radiologist-in-chief at the General at the end of June 1984, Holmes returned as acting chief for two years until the appointment of Harry J. Griffiths in July 1986.)[144]

A native of Auckland, New Zealand, Potts had graduated with an MB from the University of Otago in 1951, then trained in radiology in Auckland and in London. After spending the latter half of the 1950s doing postgraduate work in various English institutions, including training in neuroradiology at the National Hospital, Queen Square, he joined the Neurological Institute of Columbia–Presbyterian Medical Center in New York in 1960. Among his achievements there was his invention, along with Juan Taveras, of a new somersaulting chair for cerebral pneumonography.[145] The device, reported in 1964 in the *American Journal of Roentgenology*,[146] became the standard chair until CT replaced pneumonography a decade later. In 1970 Potts became professor and chief of radiology at the New York Hospital–Cornell Medical Center, remaining there until his recruitment to Toronto in 1985.

In June 1985, Potts reported on the state of the department at a meeting of the Committee of Basic Science Chairmen: "[I]n discussions with the Dean ... it was apparent that the Department was weak in biologically-oriented research and clearly MRI was the most exciting development in medical imaging at this time." With decanal support and a loan from the president, the department was able to purchase "a GE two-tesla small bore scanner" (suitable for small animal research) which as agreed was "being installed in the basement of the North Pavilion of the Toronto Western Hospital." The unit was to be directed by Claude Lemaire, and research would be carried out in three main areas: physics, radiology, and neurosciences.[147]

In 1986, as construction of the tri-hospital MRI centre moved forward, Walter Kucharczyk was chosen as its clinical director. A 1979 U of T medical graduate who had done his residency in the department, Kucharczyk had just completed a fellowship in neuroradiology at the University of California at San Francisco and was running the MR centre there.[148] On 10 February 1987, the Tri-Hospital Magnetic Resonance Centre, located in a specially prepared site on the first floor of the Mulock/Larkin Wing of TGH, was officially opened by provincial health minister Murray Elston,[149] who applauded the "co-operative effort" of the hospitals in sharing the imager.[150]

Magnetic resonance imaging reverberated throughout the department. Kibitzing from the Department of Surgery, Martin McKneally noted how important generalist training in a discipline was. "The disruptive displacement of cerebral angiographers, once the elite of radiology, by contemporary imaging techniques is a striking example."[151]

The new spirit of cooperation extended to resident training, as Potts finally succeeded in creating the university-wide system that had proven such a stumbling block to Holmes and Lansdown. As Lansdown later remarked, "One of the difficulties on my part was that I knew everyone, which was an advantage for stability"[152] – but in this case it was also a disadvantage in making change, whereas Potts as an outsider met much less resistance. During his tenure the five hospital teaching programs were rolled into a single university-centred one, in which residents would stay at their home base for the first year, then rotate freely among all the hospital departments for the remaining three. The new system was implemented by the 1987–8 academic year.

Potts then went on to organize the university department and training program along organ-system lines, deliberately rejecting the imaging-technology approach that had proven so disruptive to the angiographers. "Radiologists have to master all the modalities in their organ system, because single modalities are vulnerable to take-over by other specialties," he explained.[153] So he reorganized the department into the divisions of cardiovascular, respiratory, GI, genitourinary, musculoskeletal, and neuroradiology. These university-wide subspecialty divisions were established by 1991–2[154] and with slight variations (such as the addition of breast imaging and vascular/interventional[155]) have continued to the present day.

During this period the hospitals' services and training programs were also strengthened. In 1987–8 the department at TGH (now officially known as the Toronto General Division of The Toronto Hospital following its merger with TWH in October 1986[156]) was able to report that "[a]fter a few years of uncertainty, we hope once again to attract bright, young fellows and dedicated, interested staff to build on existing strengths."[157]

Meanwhile the Western Division became a prominent centre in the emerging subspecialty of interventional neuroradiology. The seeds for this development were sown in 1984, while Harnick was still chief, with the creation of a formal program led by Ming-Chai Chiu, then head of neuroradiology, along with Karel terBrugge and visiting Parisian expert Pierre Lasjaunias. When Potts became chief of the hospital department in 1985, it was ready to take on an expanded role in the neurointerventional field. By the time terBrugge took over as head of neuroradiology three years later, he had developed sufficient expertise to supervise new interventional programs such as the one at the Montreal Neurological Institute and to train fellows in the subspecialty. Between 1988 and 1994, he trained twelve of them at the Western. By 1993 the Interventional Neuroradiology Program was the foremost centre in Canada for this subspecialty, receiving referrals from all over the country.[158]

Potts's success in building the department and its hospital partners was applauded in a 1990 report on the department by two outside specialists in radiation oncology. Although their main concern was to press for the establishment of an official "academic Department of Radiation Oncology within the University of Toronto," they conceded that "Dr. Potts appears to have done an admirable job of leading the department for the last five years in dealing with nine different hospitals, and improving the quality of the departments of Radiology at each of the institutions."[159]

In July 1991, the university department returned to selecting a leader from within, as Walter Kucharczyk, director of the MR Centre, was chosen to succeed Gordon Potts as chair.[160] At this point he was only thirty-four years old, "an almost unprecedented age for chairing a major department."[161] The policy of separating the university chair from the head of radiology at the General remained more or less in effect, although as the departments of the General and Western "divisions" of TTH were merged in 1990, Potts briefly agreed to serve as the head of the joint department until Chia-Sing Ho, chief at the General since 1989, took on the post in August 1991.[162]

Later the same year a separate Department of Radiation Oncology headed by Bernard Cummings was finally created after protracted negotiations with support from the provincial Ministry of Health (see chapter 13, "Cancer Care").[163] From that point on, the Department of Radiology – renamed the Department of Medical Imaging in 1994 – has consisted of the various diagnostic divisions and nuclear medicine. Yet there was a certain irony in changing the department's name on the eve of the centenary of Roentgen's discovery: As Kucharczyk pointed out, radiology had once more become a therapeutic as well as diagnostic discipline with the advent of interventional techniques such as balloon angioplasty, portal-systemic stenting, and neurointerventional procedures. "Indeed, just as we wound down our responsibilities in therapeutic radiation ... we markedly increased the number of minimally invasive procedures we perform today based on accurate image guidance."[164]

In December 1995, Kucharczyk's reappointment for a second term as chair of medical imaging, effective July 1996, was announced.[165] Radiologist Edna Becker comments on Kucharczyk's success in enlisting the hospital radiology chiefs to serve on the executive committee of the university department: "The open discussions were healthy to airing concerns and to understanding what changes were required."[166]

In the late 1990s Kucharczyk and other radiologists joined with members of the Department of Medical Biophysics, neurosurgeon Mark Bernstein, and neuroanesthetist Pirjo Manninen to develop a frameless MR navigation system to provide real-time image guidance in intracranial surgery in a specially designed operating room at TWH.[167] More recently, a team of radiologists at the Toronto General Hospital Research Institute headed by David Gianfelice developed "a safe alternative treatment option" involving a new imaging modality, MRI-guided focused ultrasound, to alleviate pain in bone metastases.[168] The many technological advances that occurred in diagnostic imaging after 2000 will not be considered here. The important message is that these dynamic chiefs had forged the study of radiology into a powerful university department.

### Division/Department of Nuclear Medicine

At a February 1948 meeting of the Toronto General Hospital's Medical Advisory Board, Gordon Richards announced that radioactive isotopes would soon be available to the hospital, and a committee of the disciplines involved was created. James Dauphinee, an internist from the Department of Medicine, was involved from the outset in his capacity as professor of "pathological chemistry," as medical biochemistry was called at the time, while Richards chaired the committee, "thus ensuring that the new investigative technology remained in the hands of the department of radiology."[169]

But a year later Richards was dead, and the university and TGH agreed to set up a joint "radioactive" lab in the Banting Institute for the use of all the hospitals. Dauphinee was named director, with William Paul from the physics department coordinating the actual use of the isotopes (see chapter 7). In 1953 the radiologists were pushed farther out of the picture as "Kager" Wightman of the Department of Medicine specifically recommended that a second isotope lab planned for the new building at TGH "should not be associated with the Radiology Department." By 1955 there were thus two isotope labs in the city headed by internists.[170] The following year Robert H. Sheppard, also from the Department of Medicine, "established a laboratory at the Toronto Western Hospital for the diagnosis and therapeutic use of I-131 [iodine-131 or radio-iodine] in disorders of the thyroid gland."[171] The initial domination of the isotope labs by these medical specialists rather than radiologists made sense given that the technology was used mainly for endocrine work in the 1950s and early 1960s. Studies of radioactive iodine in thyroid disorders continued to figure prominently in the reports of the Department of Medicine, but not radiology, during these years. The term "nuclear" was also absent at this point.[172] In 1962–3, still in the Department of Medicine, the thyroid research continued, but a new area of inquiry was opened as "Dr Joan Harrison, working with a low background whole body counter in the Department of Physics under the supervision of Professor McNeill, and with the collaboration of Dr J Finlay," was "studying calcium metabolism in normal and in osteoporotic subjects, using radioactive calcium."[173] (For further discussion see chapter 7.)

Academic interest in nuclear medicine began in November 1956 as the Committee on Post-Graduate Studies recommended that a two-week course on "radioactive isotopes" be given the following June by Gordon Butler of the Department of Biochemistry, along with physicist William Paul, Marian Packham from biochemistry, and "clinicians to be suggested by Professor Farquharson and Professor Janes." Although the diagnostic radiologists were still excluded, medical physicist Harold Johns and radiotherapist Clifford Ash were involved in this initiative.[174] Mount Sinai radiologist Bernie Shapiro later remarked that until the Royal College program was set up, completion of this course was regarded as a qualification in applying for a nuclear-medicine license.[175]

The volume of isotope work continued to grow rapidly during the 1960s, and in 1964 a new Division of Nuclear Medicine was created at TGH under the direction of Donald Wood. According to hospital historian Gerald Cosbie, William Paul was ineligible for this position because he lacked the necessary "medical qualifications." Wood in contrast "had been trained in Internal Medicine by Dr Wightman and had served under him as a Fellow in the Department of Therapeutics," followed by two years of specialized training in Nuclear Medicine at the Middlesex Hospital. Upon returning to Toronto in 1964, he had taken up "appointments in the Department of Medicine at the University and in the Department of Laboratories under Dr Murray Young at the TGH."[176]

By the mid-1960s, diagnostic radiologists were beginning to enter the nuclear field. According to the dean's annual report for 1965–6, Ronald F. Colapinto was "studying the celiac angiogram in liver neoplasia, and, with Dr D[onald] E Wood and Dr EG King, Department of Laboratories, Division of Nuclear Medicine, comparing the selective arteriogram and the selective isotopic scan of liver and pancreas."[177] TGH acquired its first gamma camera (a device that permitted radioactive scans to be imaged rather than simply measured with a scintillation counter) around 1966, and in that year a lecture course on nuclear medicine given by Wood was added to the radiology training program.[178]

The nuclear medicine program at TGH grew so rapidly during the latter half of the 1960s that it required additional space, and in 1968 the trustees approved a new isotope lab for the hospital's Burnside Building. Thanks to Brian Holmes's influence, the new Division of Nuclear Medicine was established in 1970 as part of the newly created Division of Radiological Sciences. Wood was to continue as division head, but overall control of the program moved to radiology. Second in command was David Gilday, a 1966 medical graduate from McGill who had just completed a radiology residency at Winnipeg General Hospital.[179] In 1971 Holmes reported, "The [radiology] department has for many years really consisted of two divisions, Diagnostic and Therapeutic Radiology. With the addition of Nuclear Medicine to the Department of Radiological Sciences at the Toronto General Hospital and the formation of a joint division of Nuclear Medicine between that Hospital and the Hospital for Sick Children, some of the staff were transferred to the University Department of Radiology for their major faculty appointment." The creation of additional nuclear medicine departments at the Princess Margaret and Women's College Hospitals, meanwhile, brought in still "more members to the newly emerging Division of Nuclear Medicine in the University."[180]

Yet things did not go well in the division at TGH. The Burnside Building proved unsuitable, and the Royal College found the training program inadequate and threatened to disqualify it. As a result, an effort to create a university division of nuclear medicine began in February 1972 with the release of a review helmed by Roger J. Rossiter from the University of Western Ontario. The reviewers acknowledged the hospital division's strong origins. But its status was now seriously threatened by its many problems. "By far the greatest weaknesses they suffer from are woefully inadequate space, remoteness from the general activities of TGH, and an orphan-like position in the administrative structure. The equipment in many instances is obsolete. The lack of a scintillation camera exemplifies their failure to remain current with regard to equipment." In the absence of leadership from the General, the other hospitals were moving ahead independently. The report concluded that the division was "in serious danger of disintegration."[181]

On 1 June, the radiology department convened a meeting "involving those staff with a major interest in Nuclear Medicine … A university-based Division of Nuclear Medicine was discussed," as a good basis for implementing the Rossiter Report. Wood stated that the creation of such a division would facilitate undergraduate teaching and postgraduate training in the specialty. Holmes said that he would tell Charles Hollenberg, the chair of medicine, that he was setting up a senior advisory committee on "the establishment of a Division of Nuclear Medicine."[182] Following the meeting Bernard J. Shapiro, chief of radiology at New Mount Sinai Hospital, pointed out that most of the Toronto teaching hospitals already had "practitioners of nuclear medicine who currently hold appointments in the Department of Radiology." These physicians could "form the nucleus of a Division of Nuclear Medicine." Shapiro had met informally with Wood, and both agreed that establishing such a division within the Department of Radiology was the best way of managing the discipline's "academic activities."[183] On 7 June, Shapiro further advised Holmes on the reasons why a university Department of Nuclear Medicine "would be of great value."[184]

The inaugural meeting of the Nuclear Medicine Planning Group took place on 16 June 1972, with the participants agreeing "that centralization of academic activities in Nuclear Medicine would be best achieved through the University Department of Radiology" and also that radio-pharmaceuticals were "the key supply need" for the discipline.[185]

In February 1983, the Department of Radiology was described in a self-study report as having three divisions: diagnostic radiology, radiation oncology, and nuclear medicine. "There is a perceived urgent need to develop work in Nuclear Magnetic Resonance. There is no such machine in Ontario at present."[186] (The term "NMR" or nuclear magnetic resonance soon gave way to "MRI," or magnetic resonance imaging, out of fear that the term "nuclear" would alarm patients.)

The disordered state of TGH's division of nuclear medicine was rectified after Ted Lansdown became chair. Lansdown found new space and set about searching for a new division head. Following a hiatus, David Feiglin (with an MB from Melbourne in 1967) was recruited as director in March 1976.[187]

According to its annual report for 1984–5, "the major new programme" in the Department of Radiological Sciences at the General involved "Nuclear Magnetic Imaging as part of a tri-hospital initiative" along with HSC and Mount Sinai.

In a second imaging development, PET scanners were planned for both nuclear cardiology and general nuclear medicine, a development which would mark "the beginning of a new era of diagnostic Nuclear Medicine."[188] But this bold initiative was shelved, as were several previous attempts led by Lansdown and other Toronto radiologists during the 1970s and 1980s to acquire a cyclotron and PET scanner for one of the teaching hospitals.[189]

By the mid-1980s the McMaster University Medical Centre in Hamilton had built its own scanner, the first in Ontario,[190] "and the scientists in Toronto were becoming ever more anxious" about this important gap in the nuclear-medicine armamentarium. Finally, around 1986, the subject of PET scanning came up in a chance conversation between Gordon Potts and Vivian Rakoff, the chair of psychiatry. Rakoff, a general psychiatrist, had previously shown little interest in brain biology, but he now became committed to bringing a PET scanner to Toronto. He used his powerful political connections to convince the provincial government to appropriate $7.5 million for a PET Centre at the Clarke Institute of Psychiatry. The centre opened in February 1993, making a psychiatric research institute rather than a general hospital the first facility to acquire the latest in nuclear technology. Sylvain Houle, who had become head of nuclear medicine at TGH in 1983, became its director. Houle, a Quebec native with impressive credentials in biomedical engineering and nuclear medicine, retained his appointment in the Department of Radiology but took up a full-time position among the psychiatrists.[191]

As of 2010 nuclear medicine was identified as a "department" within medical imaging. Its main focus is the university residency program, a six-year rotating course which leads to dual certification in diagnostic radiology and nuclear medicine. Directed by Marc Freeman, the residency program involves "eight hospital sites within four Imaging Departments," encompassing all of the main teaching hospitals including the "paediatric centre" at HSC, each of which "is well-equipped with state-of-the-art imaging equipment" (with the notable exception of positron emission tomography, see earlier).[192]

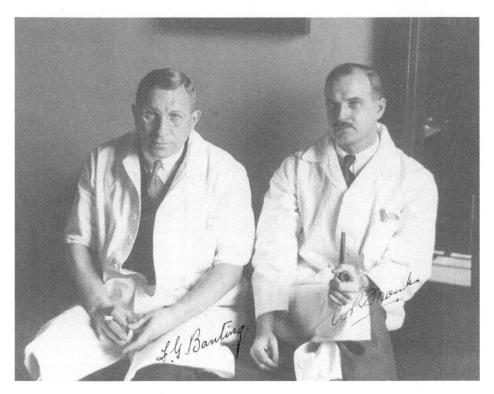

32. Banting and Best Department of Medical Research, 1930s

In the wake of the discovery of insulin, the province awarded an annual grant to the University of Toronto which resulted in the creation of Canada's first research professorship. In 1930 the Banting and Best Department of Medical Research (BBDMR) was established, with Banting as its chair. For the next decade he directed its laboratories, latterly turning his attention to military problems with his colleague Wilbur R. Franks, inventor of the first "antigravity" suit for pilots.

HMP, donated by Dr. Margaret Mason Shaw, a member of the BBDMR.

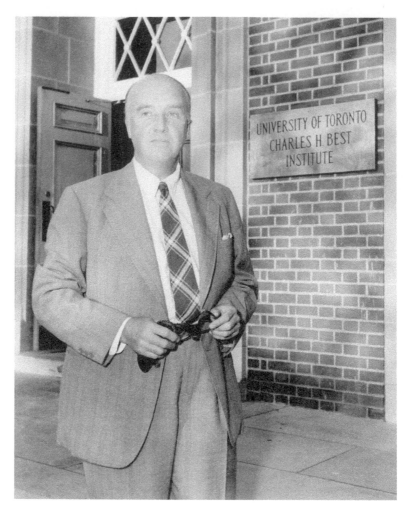

33. Charles H. Best and the Best Institute, 1954

Following Banting's death in 1941, Charles Best became head of the BBDMR as well as professor of physiology. Anxious to keep this legendary figure at the University of Toronto, President Sidney Smith helped raise the funds for a second building beside the Banting Institute to accommodate his work and that of the two departments.

HMP; Robert C. Ragsdale photography.

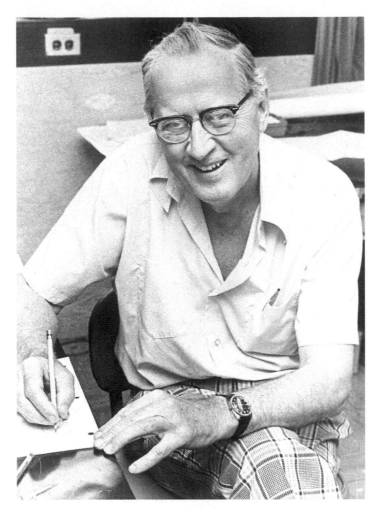

34. Harold Johns, Founder of Medical Physics in Canada

Recruited from Saskatchewan in 1956 to head the physics division of the Ontario Cancer Institute, Johns pioneered advances in radiation therapy. His major achievement was developing radioisotope techniques that could target deep tumours without damaging the skin.

Strategic Communications Department, University of Toronto.

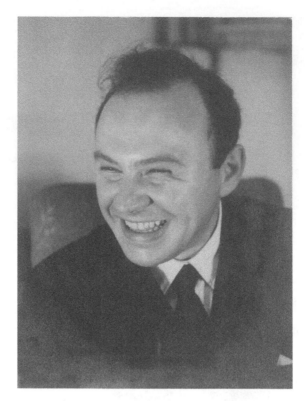

35. Immunology Pioneer Bernhard Cinader, 1960s

Austrian-born "Hardi" Cinader came to Toronto from England in 1958 as head of the immunochemistry subdivision of the Ontario Cancer Institute. In 1972 he became director of the Institute of Immunology within the Department of Biochemistry, yet the establishment of a full-fledged department did not occur until 1984. At this point in his career, Cinader has not yet adopted the "white chin beard" of his later years.

Bernhard Cinader fonds; UTA B2002-0008/001P (1).

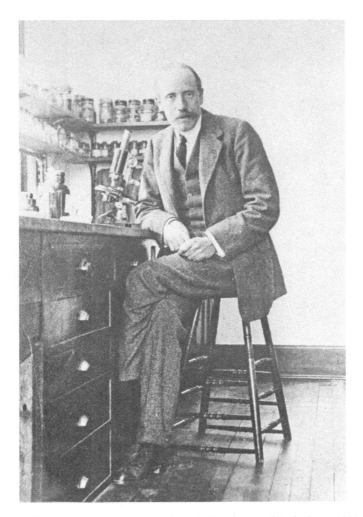

36. Laboratory Sciences: John Joseph Mackenzie, Professor of Pathology, 1900–22

The study of pathology and bacteriology in the Faculty of Medicine dated back to the 1890s. Mackenzie, the second chair, had trained extensively in Europe and was familiar with French and German scientific literature. Ramsay Wright praised his language skills as "a weapon equally useful to the teacher and to the investigator."

HMP, donated by the Medical Alumni Association, University of Toronto.

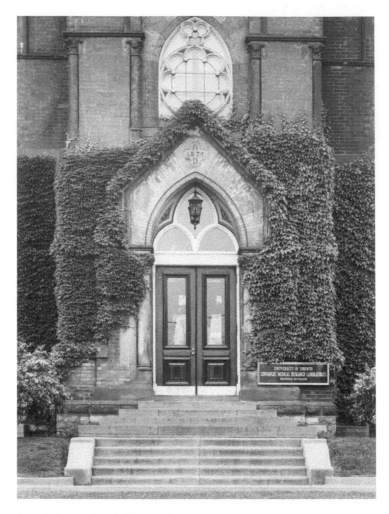

37. Laboratory Sciences: Penicillin Production

During the Second World War, the University of Toronto acquired the former Knox College building on Spadina Crescent and turned it into the "Spadina Division" of the Connaught Medical Research Laboratories. Here the bacteriology division of the Department of Pathology was involved in the mass production of penicillin and blood products for the war effort.

University of Toronto, Department of Information Services; UTA A1978-0041/029 (35).

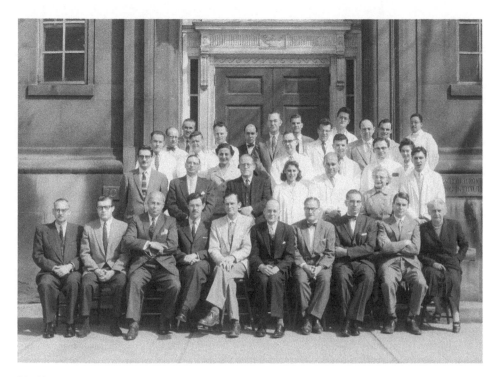

38. The Department of Pathology, 1958–9

This group assembled in front of the Banting Institute illustrates the evolution of the basic science disciplines at mid-century. Chair John D. Hamilton (fifth from the left in the front row), recruited from Queen's in 1951, modernized the department before becoming dean in 1961. Mary Tom, who pioneered neuropathology in the early 1930s, appears at the far right. The first two figures in the second row are Calvin Ezrin (an early Jewish member of the Department of Medicine) and Harold Pritzker, pathologist at the first Mount Sinai Hospital on Yorkville Avenue. Next to them is veteran microbiologist Philip Greey. In the back row, second and third from the right, are two up-and-comers: Jan Steiner, an émigré from the Holocaust who went on to become an associate dean and inspire a generation of scientists, and resident "Griff" Pearson, who later launched the lung transplantation program in Toronto.

Courtesy of Dr. Kenneth Pritzker.

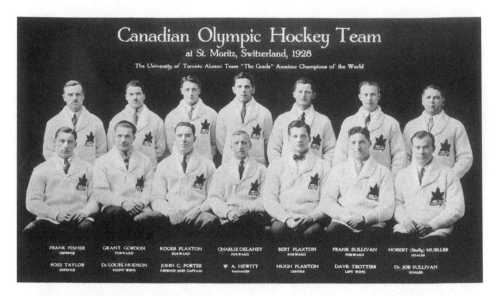

Canadian Olympic Hockey Team
at St. Moritz, Switzerland, 1928
The University of Toronto Alumni Team "The Grads" Amateur Champions of the World

| FRANK FISHER | GRANT GORDON | ROGER PLAXTON | CHARLIE DELAHEY | BERT PLAXTON | FRANK SULLIVAN | NOBERT (Stuffy) MUELLER |
| DEFENCE | FORWARD | FORWARD | FORWARD | FORWARD | FORWARD | GOALIE |
| ROSS TAYLOR | Dr LOUIS HUDSON | JOHN C. PORTER | W. A. HEWITT | HUGH PLAXTON | DAVE TROTTIER | Dr JOE SULLIVAN |
| DEFENCE | RIGHT WING | DEFENCE AND CAPTAIN | MANAGER | CENTRE | LEFT WING | GOALIE |

39. Medicine and Athletics: Joseph A. Sullivan, Olympian and Otolaryngologist

Involvement in sports is a recurring theme throughout the history of the faculty. Goalie Joe Sullivan, one of the two medical members of the 1928 Olympic Hockey Team, became a noted otolaryngologist at St Michael's Hospital, a surgical innovator, and ultimately a member of the Canadian Senate.

University of Toronto. Department of Athletics and Recreation; UTA A1979-0060/020 (30), Digital image no. 2001-77-142MS.

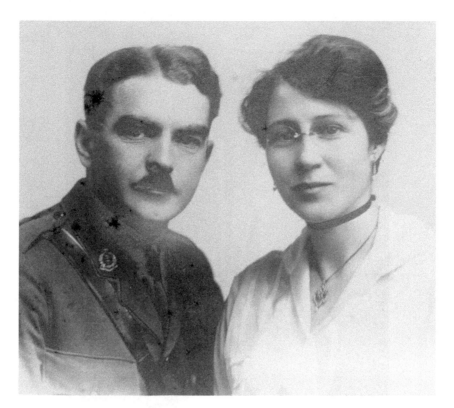

40. Gordon Earle Richards, Founding Father of Radiology in Canada

The professionalization of radiology in Toronto began in 1917 with the establishment of a formal department at TGH under the leadership of Gordon Richards, seen here with his wife Lila Singleton around the time of their marriage the previous year. Like many of his fellows, he joined the Canadian forces in 1914 and served as a captain in the Royal Army Medical Corps. It is unknown how he was recruited away to this civilian position before the end of the war.

HMP, Richards collection.

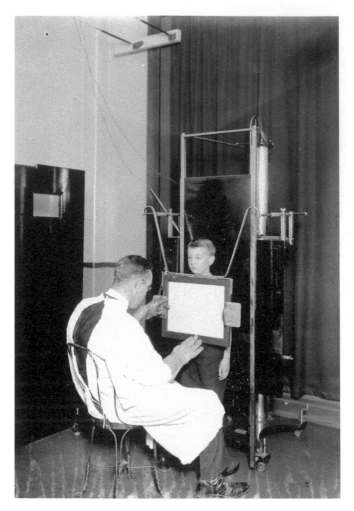

41. Diagnostic Imaging at HSC in 1917: Fluoroscopy Conducted by a Technician

A fluoroscopic chest examination done on 21 September 1917. Note the bare wires coming from the upper left. The children's hospital appointed radiologist Albert H. ("Bert") Rolph, another army veteran, in 1919.

HSC Archives.

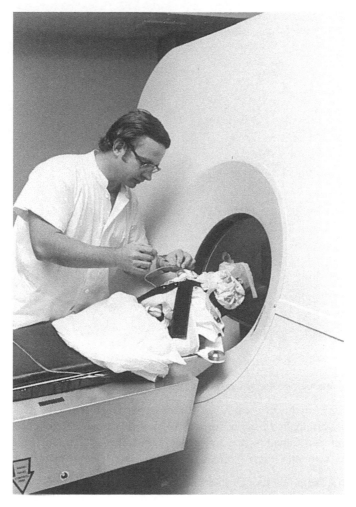

42. Diagnostic Imaging at HSC in the 1970s: CT Scan Conducted by a Neuroradiologist

Derek Harwood-Nash, who joined the staff at HSC in 1968 in charge of the new subspecialty of neuroradiology, became the world leader in the field. In 1976 he and colleague Charles Fitz published the seminal text *Neuroradiology in Infants and Children*. At the same time, neurologic investigation in children and adults alike was being revolutionized by the emergence of computed tomography, with further developments in medical imaging technologies soon to follow.

HSC Archives.

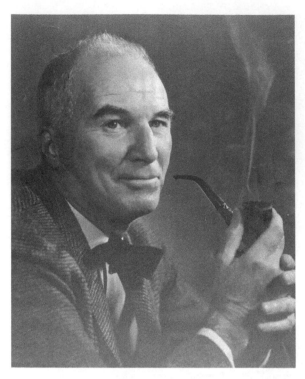

43. Obstetrics and Gynecology: Douglas E. Cannell, "The Chief," 1950–65

The leading figure in the post-war history of the department, Cannell was an unexpected choice, coming originally from the Toronto Western Hospital rather than TGH. Once in place he developed Canada's first integrated postgraduate program in obstetrics and gynecology, a "Cannell Course" comparable to the Gallie Course in surgery.

Courtesy of the Department of Obstetrics and Gynaecology.

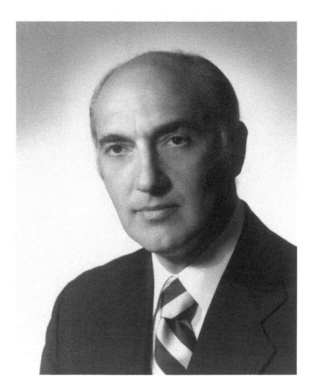

44. New Talent: Bernard Langer, Professor of Surgery, 1982–92

Medical anti-Semitism in Toronto gradually evaporated as members of the faculty became more cosmopolitan and was officially overthrown with the emergence of leaders of Jewish origin such as Charles Hollenberg as head of medicine and Bernie Langer as head of surgery at the university and TGH. Langer became one of the great builders of the faculty in the late twentieth century with the creation of the Surgical Scientist Program and the transformation of the huge Department of Surgery into a scientific powerhouse.

Dr Bernard Langer, UHN, RG 1, Department of Public Affairs and Communications fonds, TH 2.4.293.

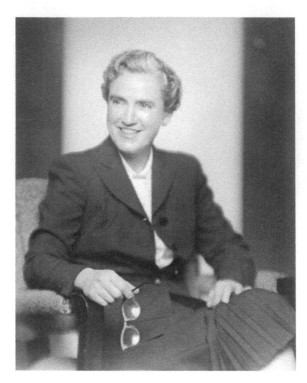

45. New Talent: Jessie Gray, Surgeon-in-Chief at Women's College Hospital, 1946–64

Jessie Catherine Gray, gold medalist in her graduating class, broke new ground for women in surgery: first woman accepted into the Gallie Course in surgery, first to become a surgical resident at TGH, and first to earn a Royal College Fellowship in surgery. During her career she racked up so many "firsts" that medical journalists named her Canada's first lady of surgery.

HMP; portrait by Ashley and Crippen photographers.

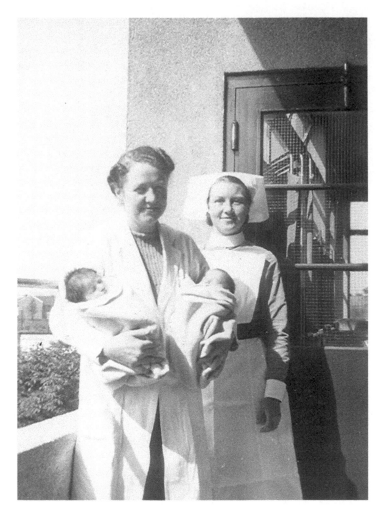

46. Geraldine Maloney, Chief of Obstetrics and Gynaecology at Women's College Hospital, 1957–66

Gerry Maloney, the first woman to achieve Royal College Fellowship status in ob-gyn, was recruited by Marion Hilliard to WCH as associate chief in charge of the educational program in 1955 to meet the university's criteria for teaching hospital status in the specialty. She succeeded Hilliard as department head two years later. Prior to this appointment she had worked at several Toronto hospitals including TGH and WCH.

Geraldine Maloney with two infants and a nurse, 1939, Miss Margaret Robins Archives of Women's College Hospital, L-03001.

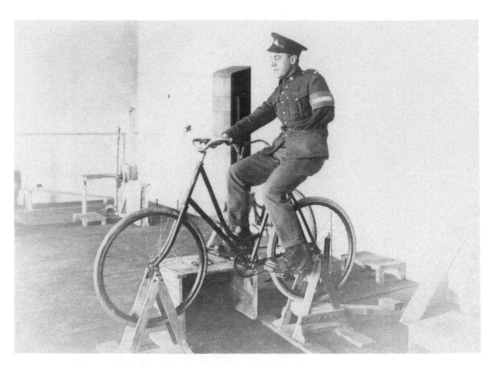

47. Rehabilitation: The Origins of Physical Therapy, 1917

In 1917 the Military Hospitals Commission established a six-month course at Hart House to train physiotherapists for the rehabilitation of injured veterans. The classes lasted until 1919 and produced 250 "Hart House Graduates."

Hart House; UTA A80-0030/002P (22).

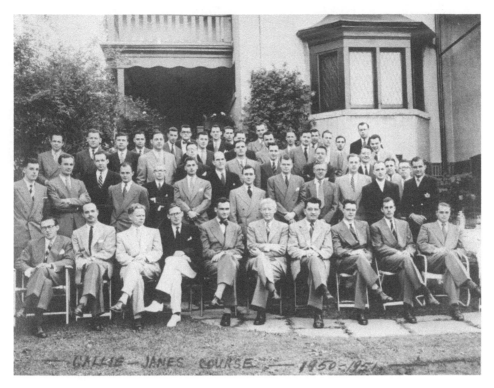

48. Robert Janes, Professor of Surgery, 1947–57, and the Post-war Boom

At the end of the Second World War, returning medical veterans inundated the Department of Surgery seeking postgraduate training. Upon becoming head of surgery Robert Janes expanded upon the pre-war Gallie Course and created a rotating residency program in the university teaching hospitals. Janes is the distinguished white-haired figure in the centre of the first row in this portrait of the Janes–Gallie class of 1950–1.

Janes Surgical Society; UTA B2000-017/001.

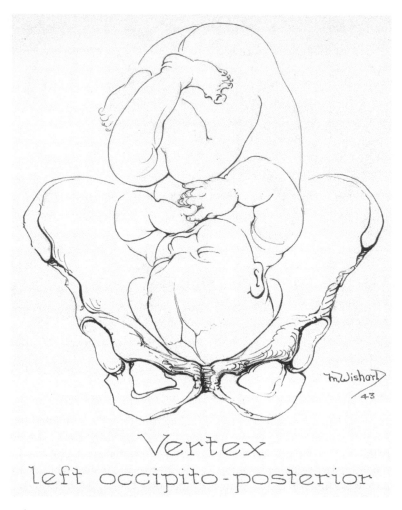

Vertex
left occipito-posterior

49. New Ideas: Art as Applied to Medicine

The creation of a new department in the Faculty of Medicine to train medical illustrators and assist other departments with medical drawings was approved in December
1945. The new unit was led by Maria T. Wishart of the faculty's "art service." Her work,
including this drawing of "relationship of child's head to pelvis," was featured in the
1946 textbook by William Scott and Herman Van Wyck, *The Essentials of Obstetrics and
Gynecology*.

University of Toronto, Art as Applied to Medicine; UTA A1997-0018/003.

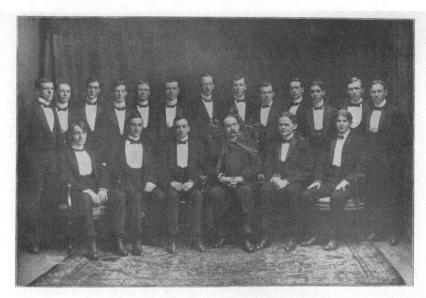

MEDICAL AT-HOME COMMITTEE. 1904-05.
UNIVERSITY OF TORONTO MEDICAL FACULTY.

*Back Row, from left to right :*
F. W. Rolph, B.A., '05.     E. A. Hodgson, Phm.B., '06.     W. Krupp. '08.     W. B. Roberts, '05.     T. Callahan, '07.     C. P. Chapin, '06.
H. M. McFadden, '07.     H. B. Wood, '07.     J. J. Garrity, '08.     H. M. McNeil, B.A., '06.     C. S. Gideon, '08.     H. E. Hammill, '08.     M. R. Graham, '06.

*Front Row, from left to right :*
H. M. Cooke, '05.     J. S. Pritchard, '05.     D. A. L. Graham, '05.     G. A. Bingham, M.B. (Tor.), M.D.C.M. (Trin.).     A. D. McCannel, Phm.B., '06.     K. C. Cairns, '05.
*Secretary.*          *President.*               *Hon. Pres.*                              *1st Vice-Pres.*          *Treasurer.*

## 50. Student Life: The Medical Society's First Annual "At-Home," 1904–5

One antidote to the rowdy behaviour of the early Meds was the organization of a formal dinner party in the British tradition of an "At-Home." Perhaps not surprisingly, this tradition was launched and presided over by "Mr. Duncan Graham, a man of gift and graces," whose formality – and exclusionary attitudes – would later dominate the Department of Medicine during his long tenure as Eaton Professor and beyond.

*Torontonensis* (1905), 191.

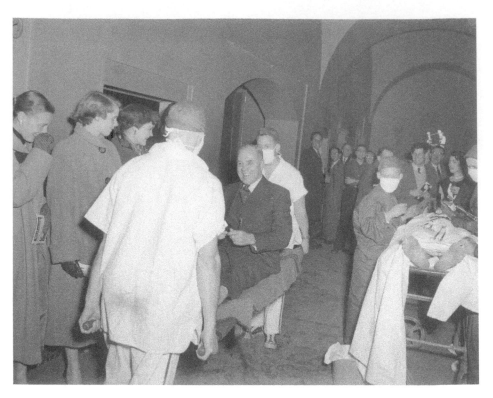

51. Student Life: Daffydil, 1953

The annual theatrical production of the medical students dated back to 1897 – with periodic suspensions for excessive vulgarity – evolving into more of a musical review in the years following the Second World War. Here Dean Farquharson gets involved in the 1953 production, being carried into the auditorium by student "stretcher bearers."

HMP (provenance unknown).

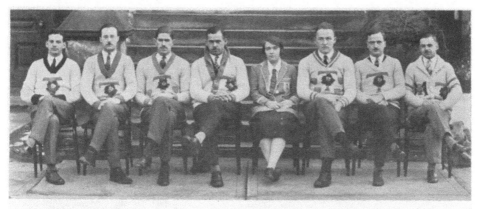

J. L. Uren,   C. W. Potter,   K. A. Fidler,   H. D. Marritt,   Miss A. M. Hilliard,   E. V. Shute,
K. C. McGibbon,   J. W. R. Webster.

## 52. Student Life: Athletics

In contrast to later generations of medical students who focused on their academic work to the exclusion of all else, participation in sports abounded during the first few decades of the twentieth century. Nor was it unusual for brilliant clinicians and scientists to have stellar athletic careers while in training. Marion Hilliard, later famed as head of obstetrics at Women's College Hospital and co-inventor of a simplified test for cervical cancer, first won varsity renown as one of the Medical "T" holders of 1927.

*Torontonensis* (1927), 72.

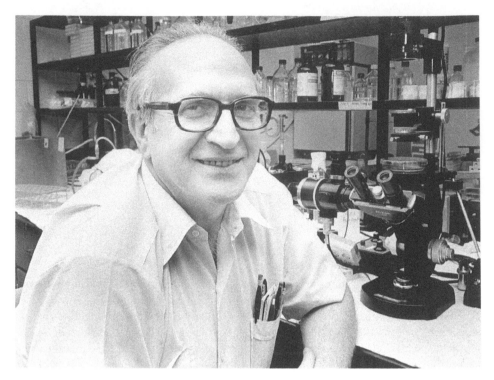

53. Molecular Medicine: Lou Siminovitch, the Builder, ca. 1965

More than any other single individual, Lou Siminovitch played a fundamental role in establishing the study of molecular biology in Toronto and the creation of several leading research institutes. At the university, he was a builder of the Departments of Medical Biophysics and Medical Genetics; and in the Toronto teaching hospitals, he was instrumental in building world-class research environments at the Ontario Cancer Institute, the Department of Molecular Genetics at HSC, and the Samuel Lunenfeld Institute at Mount Sinai Hospital.

Strategic Communications Department, University of Toronto.

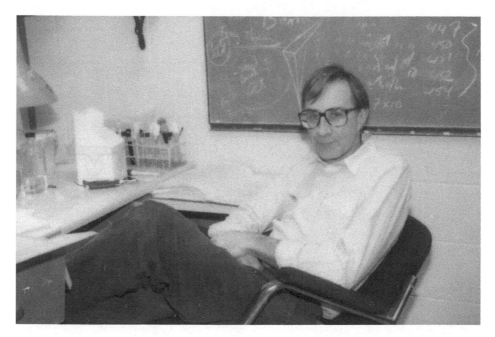

54. Molecular Medicine: Jim Friesen and the Donnelly Centre for Cellular and Biological Research (CCBR)

In November 2004, the Faculty of Medicine responded to the hospital Research Institutes with the formal opening of a magnificent interdisciplinary research facility of its own. The new centre was the brainchild of two former chairs of the Banting and Best Department of Medical Research, James D. Friesen and the late Cecil Yip. Like his mentor Siminovitch, Friesen brought together a leading team of young scientists and marshalled the tremendous resources necessary for proteomic and genomic research.

University of Toronto, Faculty of Medicine, Instructional Media Services; UTA A2007-0017 (006).

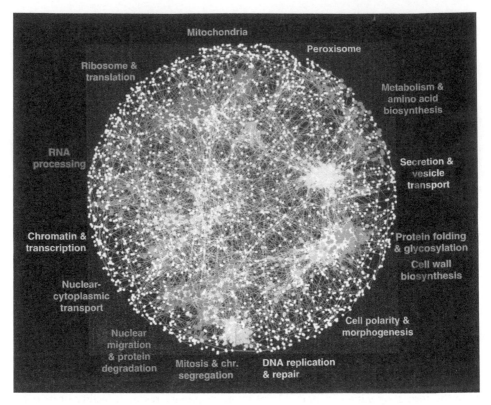

Within the figure:
Mitochondria
Peroxisome
Ribosome & translation
Metabolism & amino acid biosynthesis
RNA processing
Secretion & vesicle transport
Chromatin & transcription
Protein folding & glycosylation
Cell wall biosynthesis
Nuclear-cytoplasmic transport
Cell polarity & morphogenesis
Nuclear migration & protein degradation
Mitosis & chr. segregation
DNA replication & repair

55. Molecular Medicine: Genome Scale Genetic Interaction Mapping, 2010

In a landmark 2010 research article in *Science,* a multi-centre team led by CCBR investigators Brenda Andrews and Charlie Boone and their labs examined 5.4 million gene-gene pairs and generated genetic interaction profiles for roughly three-quarters of the genes in a budding yeast model. Genetic interaction mapping provides a functional view of the cell which can help increase understanding of complex genetic interaction networks and inherited phenotypes, including those of human disease.

Michael Costanzo, Anastasia Baryshnikova, Jeremy Bellay et al., "The Genetic Landscape of a Cell," American Association for the Advancement of Science, *Science* 327, no. 5964 (22 Jan. 2010): 425, fig. 1: "A correlation-based network connecting genes with similar genetic interaction profiles."

# 21 Obstetrics and Gynaecology

I can find no adequate reason for the choice [of obstetrics and gynaecology as a specialty] unless it be that one loves to travel by moonlight when there is no traffic; the thoroughfares are free of dust, no disturbing temptations come from open pubs ... These delights are of course compensated for by the unpleasant though flattering tendency of humanity to plan to reproduce itself under your supervision – no one else will do – during weekends desirable for a trip to the "cottage" or by the utterly puzzling facility with which nature can put full term to one of its anticipated fledglings after the first act of a delectable musical comedy.[1]

> Herman Brookfield Van Wyck, Chair of the Department of Obstetrics and Gynaecology, 1948 (written facetiously)

(NB: The history of obstetrics and gynecology at Women's College Hospital will be found under the main entry for that hospital in chapter 22.)

In earlier days, obstetrics was the keystone of medical practice. If you as a family doctor assisted the mother in her confinements, you had the family's custom for life. Accordingly, obstetrics played a fundamental role in the instruction of medical students. Gynecology in those days was more marginal, more a surgical than a medical specialty. Yet in both obstetrics and gynecology, age-old in medical time, lingered past memories of the "accoucheur" and the "women's doctor" whose specialty was hysteria and the vapours. The eighteenth-century male accoucheurs in the United Kingdom were the first physicians to rival the midwives and employed the obstetrical forceps to vanquish their female competitors. It was a tradition that had always been slightly less savory than the nobility of gaze in medicine and surgery.

As the Faculty of Medicine was being refounded in 1887, obstetrics and gynecology were separate chairs, reflecting the separation of the two disciplines at the General Hospital. The obstetrical service was housed at the Burnside

Lying-In [maternity] Hospital. Established as an independent institution in the 1850s, the Burnside had amalgamated with the General in 1877, and a new building consisting of twenty-two public and four private beds was opened in the northwest part of the Gerrard Street hospital grounds in October 1878.[2] Gynecology meanwhile began to emerge as a distinct specialty in the early 1880s with the construction of a separate "women's pavilion" with public and private wards accommodating up to forty patients.[3]

In 1887 Adam Henry Wright became professor of obstetrics.[4] As an arts student at U of T (earning a BA in 1866), he had been active in athletics and a lieutenant in the militia, seeing action in the 1866 Battle of Ridgeway against the Fenian raiders with the university company of the Queen's Own Rifles. Following a brief teaching career, he enrolled at the old Toronto School of Medicine, graduating in 1873. He practiced in Colborne, Ontario, for three years, then trained in London, Paris, and Dublin for fifteen months, taking the diploma course in 1877 that qualified him for membership in the Royal College of Surgeons of England. After returning to Toronto, Wright began what would become a large general practice. In 1878 he joined the staff of the Toronto School of Medicine and around the same time became an editor of the *Canadian Journal of Medical Science*. Between 1883 and 1886 he lectured on obstetrics at the Women's Medical College, then from the time of the reorganization of the Faculty of Medicine in 1887 until his resignation in 1912, he held the chair of obstetrics. In addition, he took an active part in university affairs, as secretary of the faculty from 1887 to 1893 and as an elected member of the university Senate from 1885. In the latter capacity he played a key role in bringing the old Trinity Medical College into the faculty in 1903.[5]

Wright also performed gynecological surgery and that in the harrowing early days just as Lister had discovered the technique of antisepsis and Lawson Tait in Birmingham was demonstrating its merit in surgery on the ovaries. Surgeon Irving H. Cameron recalled assisting in an ovariotomy, removing an ovary on which a gigantic cyst had formed. Wright had asked Aikins to assist, but he refused on the grounds that it was too dangerous: "We have had nothing but deaths in so many cases." Cameron then agreed to help out. "The operation proved to be the worst of its kind that I have ever seen, a huge cyst universally closely adherent to the anterior abdominal wall and great omentum, the liver and the stomach, whose walls had to be seared with the actual cautery to stop the bleeding." Yet thanks to Wright's skill "an uninterrupted recovery ensured. And the next four and twenty cases that we had in the General Hospital followed suit; et lux fuit! [and there was light]."[6]

As an attending physician at the Burnside Lying-In unit, Wright was involved in the introduction of aseptic procedures during deliveries in 1891 and credited this innovation with a reduction in maternal mortality. Between 1888 and 1891, before the new rules were introduced, 5 out of 519 patients had died, 3 of them from septicemia, while between 1893 and 1897 a total of 500 deliveries were performed without a single death.[7] Student activity in the unit was likewise regulated even more stringently than elsewhere in the hospital. According to a set of rules in place by 1895, "[o]nly fourth-year students could attend maternity cases and then only when accompanied by the medical superintendent or one of the other doctors on the Burnside staff; through the purchase of an $8 ticket students could be present at six births ... In keeping with the growing medical awareness that disease could be spread by bacteria through human touch, all students signed a solemn declaration that they would not visit or be present at cases of confinement ... when 'engaged in pathological operations, when recently engaged in dissecting, or when dressing putrid sores.'"[8]

Wright served as president of the American Association of Obstetricians and Gynecologists in 1890; his 1905 *Textbook of Obstetrics*,[9] based on "a large and extensive experience in this branch of Medicine,"[10] further strengthened his North American reputation. A supporter of public health reform, he was made chairman of the provincial Board of Health in January 1911, retaining this position until 1924 when the board was disbanded upon the creation of the Ontario Department of Health. At his death in 1930, Dean Primrose, who had close memories of Wright's tenure, wrote, "Many old graduates in medicine will recall the dominating yet kindly influence he exercised in the early days of the Faculty, as well as the great personal affection he had for the students whom he befriended in the most wholehearted fashion."[11]

It is difficult now to appreciate the social position of professors in the faculty such as Wright. For his retirement dinner at the York Club in 1912, present were such captains of industry as Col. Albert Gooderham, Sir William Mulock, and Sir Glenholme Falconbridge. The chair of the evening, Nelson H. Beemer, a physician in the suburb of Mimico, said that he had mentioned to a colleague a few days previously "that a dinner was to be given to Doctor Adam Wright." The friend replied, "Of course it will be held in the Arena, as that is the only place large enough to accommodate the medical friends of Doctor Wright!"[12]

One of the guests composed a poem for the occasion:

"When you and I were young, Adam,
There were no telephones;
There was no ultramicroscope;
At what went on inside.
And no X-rays for those who grope
And pry among the bones."[13]

In 1887 Uzziel Ogden was appointed professor of gynecology.[14] From 1893 to 1896 he was also the second dean of the faculty, a function that, like all deans before Joseph MacFarlane after the Second World War, he fulfilled on a part-time basis. Born in Toronto township in 1828 into a family of United Empire Loyalists, he began the study of medicine as an apprentice under a physician in Cooksville, Ontario, then entered the Toronto School of Medicine in 1845, obtaining his license four years later. After practicing for several years in Aylmer, "Canada West," he was called back to Toronto in January 1853 to begin what would become a fifty-year career in medical education. At the Toronto School of Medicine Ogden taught "materia medica and therapeutics" until 1870 and then "midwifery and diseases of women and children" until 1887.[15]

With the reopening of the U of T medical faculty in 1887, the members of the Toronto School joined the teaching staff of the new institution. Ogden continued as professor of gynecology until his retirement in 1903. As Victoria College president Nathanael Burwash put it in a 1910 obituary, "It did not fall to his lot to make a great scientific discovery." Nonetheless, Ogden was a generous promoter of new talent, offering financial as well as moral support to help "young men of promise ... rise more quickly to their deserved place on the staff."[16] He was also recognized for his promotion of scientific medical education and for staying abreast of "the newest theories, facts and methods"[17] throughout a career marked by sweeping advances.

A pioneer of medical journalism, Ogden also promoted scientific medicine through the *Canadian Journal of Medical Science*, which he founded in 1876 and edited for several years, as well as several other Toronto medical journals. His columns, advocating reforms in medical education, practice, and certification, represented the viewpoint of academically trained physicians rather than practitioners trained under the old "proprietary" system in which he had begun.

In 1903 James F.W. Ross succeeded Ogden as professor of gynecology.[18] The son of James W. Ross, who had himself been a distinguished Toronto physician and obstetrician, he completed his MB at the Toronto School of Medicine in 1878, then undertook extensive postgraduate work, including four years of study in London and on the Continent between 1879 and 1882. Following several years in general medical practice, he spent an additional year of training in gynecology and abdominal surgery in Birmingham under Lawson Tait, the leading specialist in this emerging field, and in Zurich. After returning to Toronto in 1889, he was appointed to the surgical staff of the General and soon afterwards to its newly organized Department of Gynaecology. Described by TGH historian (and ob-gyn) W.G. Cosbie as "a man of great energy and leadership," Ross was the driving force behind the establishment of the special women's pavilion in 1882 and the creation in 1908 of an outpatient clinic in a house on Chestnut Street. He was also responsible for planning the gynecological facilities at the General's new College Street site, which he did not live to see.[19]

As a pioneer of gynecology in Canada, Ross gained a continent-wide reputation for his diagnostic and surgical skill. According to a colleague, pathologist Harry B. Anderson, Ross "possessed dash and courage" as a surgeon, "with technical skill of the highest order, thoroughness with a safe conservatism." In dealing with patients, "as with all others," Anderson continued, "he was brusquely honest and straight-forward, though beneath the stern exterior he

was kindly and considerate. Neither lateness of the hour, bodily fatigue, business, nor social engagements ever prevented his promptly answering the call
for assistance, whether from rich or poor." It was thus somehow "painfully fitting" that Ross was fatally injured while answering such a call: an avid motor-
ist, he was on his way to attend a patient north of the city on 15 November 1911
when the "fore wheels" of his car "caught in a rut obscured by the recently
fallen snow" and "turned turtle into the ditch." His death two days later was
met with shock and sorrow "not only in the medical profession, but among the
public at large," and particularly by the many poor families who had been his
charity patients.[20]

With the amalgamation of the former Trinity Medical College into the faculty
in 1903, James Algernon Temple was appointed to its staff as "Professor of Operative Obstetrics and Gynaecology," a continuation of the professorship that he
had held at Trinity since 1878.[21] A medical graduate of McGill University (MD,
CM 1865; the designation "Chirurgiae Magister" (Master of Surgery) is a Mc-
Gill tradition) ,who had trained in England, Temple began a private practice in
Toronto in 1868 in association with Edward Hodder, dean and professor of obstetrics at Trinity Medical College. He quickly became one of the city's leading
physicians and following Hodder's death in 1878 succeeded him as professor of
obstetrics and gynecology at Trinity and at the Toronto General Hospital. Temple also became the last dean of the college in 1902 and in that capacity played
an important role in its amalgamation with the faculty. Although sixty years
old in 1903, he continued to serve until 1909, returning briefly in the 1911–12 session "to deliver some lectures in Gynaecology" following James Ross's sudden
death. Gynecology as a discipline was plagued in the late nineteenth century
with dangerous and meddlesome operations on women for uterine malposi-
tions and "ovarian hysteria." Like Ross, Temple's conservative approach and
"outspoken opposition to destructive pelvic operations contributed much to
the placement of a ban on unnecessary and unscientific procedures"[22] and to the
development of gynecology as a specialty.

Just as a note, Temple's combining of the two disciplines of obstetrics and
gynecology shows that the idea was not so far-fetched.[23] Yet within the faculty
they continued to operate as separate units. Gynecology and obstetrics also continued to be taught in separate parts of the Toronto General Hospital. Of gynecology it was said in the 1905 Calendar, "Small classes of students receive
instruction in diseases peculiar to women in the pavilion specially devoted to
the treatment of such patients," while instruction in obstetrics "takes place in
the Burnside Lying-in Hospital."[24]

In 1912 the Departments of Obstetrics and Gynaecology were unified, and in
November of that year the Joint Committee on University and Hospital Relations appointed Benjamin Philip Watson as the inaugural chair of the new combined department.[25] Watson was one of the faculty's first international stars.[26]
Born in a Scottish village on the Firth of Forth in 1880, he graduated in medicine

from the University of Edinburgh in 1905 at the head of his class. After interning at the Royal Infirmary of Edinburgh and the Royal Maternity Hospital, he
returned to the Royal Infirmary in the gynecologic division. In 1905 he won the
MD degree – a research degree in the United Kingdom – with a thesis on pla-
cental changes in fetal death. In 1905 he was elected Fellow of the Royal College of Surgeons of Edinburgh and began his academic career at the university,
studying gynecologic pathology for the next five years. Just before leaving for
Canada, he completed with Freeland Barbour one of the earliest textbooks of
gynecological pathology.[27]

As of 1912, the Department of Obstetrics at the General was headed by Kennedy Crawford McIlwraith.[28] An 1894 Toronto graduate who had spent a year
abroad studying obstetrics at the Rotunda Hospital in Dublin and at Queen
Charlotte's Hospital in London, McIlwraith was appointed obstetrician to St
Michael's Hospital in 1903, resigning five years later to become chief of obstetrics at the General. In 1910 he was promoted to an associate professorship in the
faculty and upon his retirement in 1933 was named professor emeritus. His colleague W.G. Cosbie later described him as "a traditional figure in the Burnside
Obstetrical Department," who had "progressed over the years from practical
midwifery to scientifically based obstetrics," and a role model for students and
trainees with "his presence at all hours of the day and night. Over a cup of coffee and a cigarette he drew from his vast experience to provide answers to their
problems at a time when manipulative obstetrics was at its zenith."[29] (Manipulative obstetrics means such procedures as podalic version that later were supplanted by caesarean delivery.)

Following James Ross's death, meanwhile, his senior assistant Frederick William Marlow became acting head of the Department of Gynaecology. In 1913 he
was named associate professor in the Faculty of Medicine and senior attending
gynecologist at the General.[30] A respected pelvic surgeon and clinical teacher in
his own right, Marlow had trained in a number of London hospitals and had
become a Fellow of the Royal College of Surgeons of England in 1903.

Upon Watson's appointment as chair of the unified department, Drs Mc-
Ilwraith and Marlow were named senior assistants in the General's obstetrical and gynecological services, respectively. Several other positions were also
"grandfathered" in this manner, but beginning in 1912, "all new appointments
recognized the combined department under Professor Watson, and his two
house surgeons alternated between Obstetrics and Gynaecology on a six-month
basis."[31] The facilities at TGH, however, remained housed separately even after
the hospital relocated to College Street in 1913. The Department of Gynaecology
was located on the third floor of the main building, while obstetrical services,
again named the Burnside Lying-In Department, were provided in a separate
building around the corner on Elizabeth Street (and in fact remained in the
old Gerrard Street facility for an additional year until the new building was
completed).[32]

Prenatal care in Toronto began during Watson's tenure with his appointment of John Gordon Gallie in 1913. According to Adam Wright's 1905 *Textbook of Obstetrics*, maternal mortality from eclampsia, or convulsions in pregnant women, was twenty-five percent; this figure dropped dramatically after Gallie, a 1910 graduate of the faculty, "applied the routine that he had learned at the New York Lying-In Hospital and the Manhattan Maternity." Regular antenatal clinics given by a social service nurse were established at the Burnside under his supervision, and although Gallie's involvement was interrupted by his wartime service, the clinic carried on, and a report on public health in Ontario showed that the maternal death rate in supervised public ward patients at the Burnside Hospital between 1910 and 1920 was less than a quarter that of the hospital's semi-private patients.[33]

With the outbreak of the war, Watson enlisted in the Canadian army, serving in the medical corps in England, Egypt, and Salonika before being recalled to Toronto in 1917 to help train young military physicians. While in Toronto, he founded the department's first laboratory of gynecologic pathology and brought his technician over from Edinburgh to help out. In 1921 Watson joined with Duncan Graham and Clarence Starr to introduce residencies in medicine, surgery, and ob-gyn respectively, with Donald M. Low becoming the first resident in the last specialty. These appointments "represented at least three years of postgraduate training, and along with the supervisory responsibility that the resident assumed came the invaluable close association with the chiefs of the department."[34]

In 1922 Watson returned to Edinburgh as the Croom Professor of Obstetrics and Gynecology, then crossed the Atlantic once again in 1926 to spend the rest of his career as the chair of obstetrics and gynecology of Columbia University.[35] He said of his Toronto sojourn, "I spent ten years there, reorganizing the department and establishing our Scottish method of teaching. The Edinburgh school has always laid great emphasis on teaching. The staff of the [Toronto General] hospital and the staff of the university looked on the teaching of students as their second most important assignment, of first importance being, of course, the care of the patients." (Nonmedical readers may not feel entirely dispirited in perusing these lines.) As he later looked back on his career, what had been the most important development in ob-gyn during his lifetime? "The extensive operations undertaken for cancer of the cervix," he answered. "These procedures could not have been thought of twenty-five years ago because the primary operative mortality would have been prohibitive. Now [1957] ... they are possible and may be revolutionary."[36] This is very much a Toronto story.

It was unusual in those years for the faculty to reach outside for a leader. When in 1922 Watson resigned, William Belfry Hendry assumed the professorship of obstetrics and gynecology. Senior members of the department alive even at this writing recall the legend of Hendry as, in ob-gyn Jim Goodwin's terms, "a great mentor."[37] A 1904 graduate of the faculty, Hendry had spent two years as a house surgeon at the General before joining the university staff as a junior demonstrator; by 1912 he was an assistant professor in the newly amalgamated Department of Obstetrics and Gynaecology. Hendry spent more than four years overseas during the First World War before returning to Toronto in 1919. Between 1922 and his retirement in 1935, Hendry – "always known affectionately as 'the Chief'" – continued to build the department.[38] Following his death in March 1939, a Faculty Council resolution stated that "he counted it his greatest achievement that he had been able to foster the careers of a large number of his younger colleagues."[39]

Perinatal care in Toronto in these years lay provisionally in the hands of the obstetricians at the General. As previously mentioned, a prenatal clinic had existed in the Burnside department since 1913, and in 1923 a Post-Natal Clinic for babies was also established there by John Gallie. Superintendent Chester J. Decker said that the six cubicles of the Post-Natal Clinic were from the outset overflowing, "as the Toronto General Hospital is at present the only hospital in the City, or even in the Province of Ontario, known to me which possesses a premature room … A large percentage of the babies cared for in the premature room are of indigent parents, and as the City does not recognize the baby, or a premature, as a patient, the Hospital bears the entire expense, which is a very heavy one."[40] By 1924 the cubicles had grown to sixteen in the "new premature room" in the Burnside. "As a direct result of this improved premature nursery service the mortality among pre-term babies has been reduced by nearly one-half," said Superintendent Decker of the year 1931.[41]

In the interwar years the department established one other specialty service, the Metabolic Ward in the Burnside Lying-In Hospital in 1923–4, under the supervision of "a specially trained nurse dietician."[42] "Here such problems as the toxaemias of pregnancy are studied by members of the staff in collaboration with the Department of Pathological Chemistry." Herman Brookfield Van Wyck, then twenty-eight and a 1915 Toronto medical graduate, was the department's liaison officer and worked with Victor John Harding, chair of the Department of Pathological Chemistry.[43] Their investigations were among the first to demonstrate "the role of salt restriction in the treatment of pre-eclamptic toxaemia."[44] Of Van Wyck the student humour paper *Epistaxis* versified in 1921, "V's for Van Wyck, just finding his place / A mighty fine fellow, he'll soon hit his pace. / Up in the Burnside he has his hands full / When things don't go right, with the forceps he'll pull."[45]

In the late 1920s John Mann joined Harding and Van Wyck's team as a fellow in pathological chemistry.[46] Of Scottish origins, Mann graduated in medicine from Queen's University as the gold medalist of the class of 1927. After completing a fellowship in pathology at Queen's and a rotating internship at the General, "he decided to specialize in obstetrics and gynaecology and was appointed senior house surgeon in this Department," joining the toxemia study the following year. His background in "pathology and biochemistry made him a valuable member of this team which made original and important observations on … the oedema of normal and toxic pregnancy."[47] Mann's greatest talent, however, lay in his "unique ability to analyse a problem and find a sound mechanical answer to it."[48] His innovations included "a completely safe and effective infant resuscitator"[49] and an improved obstetrical forceps involving "a split universal joint that permitted accurate application and guided rotation during the descent of the head through the maternal pelvis in the case of a malpresentation."[50] Mann's 1957 paper "Methods for Improving the Results of Forceps Delivery, Including an Improved Obstetric Forceps"[51] was awarded a prize by the Royal College of Obstetricians and Gynaecologists of England the following year.[52]

In the leadership of Canadian obstetrics and gynecology during this period was James Clifford Goodwin, Jim Goodwin's father. James C. Goodwin was born in 1902 in Niagara Falls, Ontario, and graduated in medicine from the University of Toronto in 1926; the yearbook acknowledged "his penchant for hard work" and high marks. He was also vice president of his graduating class.[53] He trained at Toronto, then joined the teaching staff of the Toronto General Hospital, leaving from those days several manuscript case books that show how desperate was the practice of gynecology in the days before antibiotics (introduced in the civilian population in 1945). One patient at the General in 1927 who was febrile from an infected abortion received intravenous doses of phenol, another mercurochrome.[54]

His training finished, Goodwin shared an office with Hendry in the Medical Arts Building and "built up an enormous obstetrical practice," holding staff appointments at both the General and the Wellesley. Personally, he cut a captivating figure. "Handsome, genial and outgoing, he had an easy style of speaking and was an asset to any gathering." He was one of the founding members of the Society of Obstetricians and Gynaecologists of Canada and always the dispassionate clinician: when he developed chest pain he could not determine if it was anginal in nature and decided to find out by walking up "the hill on their street on the assumption that if the pain didn't increase it wasn't of cardiac origin." The pain did not increase, yet Goodwin died of a heart attack[55] on 3 August 1953 at the age of fifty.[56]

In 1935 William Albert Scott succeeded Hendry as chair, staying in office until 1946. Scott studied medicine at U of T, graduating in 1913 as the gold medalist after earning an arts degree at McMaster University. (The U of T yearbook prognosticated incorrectly, "Bill expects to marry and start a practice in some little town out West."[57]) During his eleven-year tenure, Scott made major contributions to both obstetrics and gynecology at TGH. In addition to raising the standard of gynecologic surgery in the department, Scott organized a postgraduate training program in ob-gyn which met the requirements of the Royal College of Physicians and Surgeons and in cooperation with Gordon Richards, head of the Department of Radiology, established joint clinics at the Institute of Radiotherapy which taught interns and medical undergraduates about radiologic treatments of "malignant pelvic lesions" and also "of some benign tumours and in the control of some major disturbances of female physiology."[58]

In the tradition of Toronto medical textbooks, in 1947 Scott and Van Wyck wrote *The Essentials of Obstetrics and Gynecology*, published in Philadelphia (and without the "a" in "Gynecology," an Anglicism to which the department has clung to this day).[59] This was the first textbook from the department as a combined discipline.

In obstetrics, one of the best known research studies from the University of Toronto stemmed from James K.W. Ferguson, a member of the Department of Pharmacology, in 1941: Ferguson discovered that birth-canal reflex pathways liberate the hormone oxytocin as the cervix is dilated in labour (see p. 438).[60]

In gynecology, Toronto has an important tradition in the treatment of uterine, especially cervical, cancer. Here the central figures are gynecological surgeons Waring Gerald Cosbie and John R. McArthur. McArthur was born in Cardinal, Ontario, in 1907 and attended high school at North Toronto Collegiate. He completed medicine at the University of Toronto in 1932, trained initially at the Vancouver General Hospital, then returned to Toronto to specialize in gynecological oncology. He visited a number of centres in Europe, working in London as house-surgeon at the Soho Hospital for Women, and becoming a Member (later a Fellow) of the Royal College of Obstetricians and Gynaecologists; he returned in 1937 to the Toronto General Hospital, where, apart from his service in the Second World War, he remained. McArthur also acquired a close association with the Princess Margaret Hospital, becoming a senior consultant. "At heart though," said a biographer, "John was a dedicated Obstetrician and Gynaecologist and was revered by a huge following of devoted patients."[61]

Cosbie, born in 1894, graduated in medicine at Toronto in 1915; he was known as a brilliant surgeon. (He was also something of a historian and wrote a sturdy history of the Toronto General Hospital.[62]) His work with McArthur, and Gordon Richards in the Department of Radiology, on the radiological treatment of gynecological carcinoma dated from the late 1930s.[63] In the days before the introduction of the "Pap smear" for cervical cancer (1941), many patients who had hysterectomies for whatever reason were not simultaneously investigated for cervical cancer. This was often a fatal omission. But if a Pap smear showed a patient to have cervical cancer, how should this be managed? With a hysterectomy? On the basis of a thirty-year review of cases seen at the Ontario Institute of Radiotherapy and the Ontario Cancer Institute, Cosbie concluded that those patients often did not do well. On the basis of his experience with radiation alone,[64] Cosbie suggested, "Radiotherapy may be considered a reasonable alternative to radical operation. Radiotherapy following hysterectomy produced little benefit."[65] This finding was a milestone in shifting the treatment of uterine cancer from surgery to radiotherapy.

Herman Van Wyck's brief chairmanship from 1946 to 1950 was marked by "four years of outstanding achievement" following a distinguished career at the university and at TGH. A 1911 arts graduate of U of T's Victoria College, "he was offered a teaching career in classics" there, "and it was difficult for him not to accept." Van Wyck entered the medical school instead, however, and graduated with an MB in 1915 while serving overseas with the No. 4 (University of Toronto) Canadian General Hospital. Following his postgraduate training in ob-gyn under Watson, he spent three years as a research fellow in the Burnside's Metabolic Unit studying toxemias of pregnancy before joining the junior staff of the hospital and the Faculty of Medicine.[66]

During Van Wyck's tenure as chair, the first attempts to integrate obstetrics among the teaching hospitals in a unified service began. In the 1946–7 session he began holding joint staff meetings among the three teaching hospitals – the General, St Michael's, and the Western[67] – and a year later he reported to the dean that the staff at these hospitals have been "working in increasingly closer co-operation. Four combined staff meetings were held during the year," rotating among the teaching hospitals.[68] In the 1948–9 session, clinical conferences for fourth-year undergraduates distributed among the three teaching hospitals were introduced.[69] Van Wyck also solidified the residency program, not including internship, into "three or four years of post-graduate training – preferably one of these years being spent in one of the basic sciences."[70]

Van Wyck continued to take an active role in biochemical research when in the 1947–8 session he entered into a collaborative project with Phillip Greey in the Department of Bacteriology to study "the Rh factor problem in the Toronto area." ("Rh" stands for rhesus monkeys, in which in 1940 a blood factor problem was discovered.) By April 1948 the Rh factor had been tested in approximately 11,000 patients, in "a complete prenatal blood examination for all private obstetrical patients in the [nine] hospitals taking part."[71] This work continued for a number of years and resulted in important findings about pregnancy loss from an incompatibility between maternal and fetal blood groups that is transmitted transplacentally. (This occurs when a woman with Rh-negative blood becomes pregnant by a man with Rh-positive blood and the fetus too has Rh-positive blood.)

In 1950 the central figure in the history of obstetrics and gynecology in the post-war years assumed the chair: Douglas E. Cannell. He was something of a dark horse, coming from the Toronto Western Hospital and competing for the chair against the favoured Nelson Henderson, chief of the obstetrical service at the General. Jim Goodwin said, "This was absolutely epoch-making ... It did stir up quite a row."[72] But Cannell had been overseas in the war, always a plus with Dean MacFarlane, and in those days military service counted. Donald Nelson Henderson completed his MB in 1925 at Toronto and trained in obstetrics and gynecology there and at Johns Hopkins, becoming a noted clinician-scientist from his studies with the great American gynecologic pathologist Emil Novak. After returning to Toronto, Henderson joined the Department of Obstetrics and Gynaecology at the university and at TGH in 1930, retiring after thirty-five years' service as professor emeritus and honorary consultant in 1965. His most significant contribution to the field was a study at the Toronto Hospital for Tuberculosis, Weston, "which established the basis for non-surgical treatment of pelvic tuberculosis here and throughout the world."[73]

Douglas Cannell, known as "D.E.," was born in Gravenhurst, Ontario, in 1902, grew up in Port Carling, and attended high school at Oakwood Collegiate in Toronto, then enrolled in medicine – where he played interfaculty rugby and was as associate editor of the *University of Toronto Medical Journal* – completing his MB in 1927. He studied pathology for a year with Oskar Klotz, interned at the General, then trained in obstetrics and gynecology at the University Hospital of Case Western Reserve University in Cleveland. A eulogist later said, "His skill and gentleness in using forceps and his expertise in the delivery of breech presentations [in an era before the popularity of the caesarean delivery] reflected the excellence of that training." The eulogist concluded, "This modest, straight-forward, unassuming man with his healthy skepticism, his dry sense of humour and his infectious little chuckle, perhaps contributed as much toward the betterment of Obstetrics and Gynaecology in Canada as anyone before or since."[74]

On returning to Toronto, Cannell joined the staff of the Grace Salvation Army Hospital. At the outbreak of hostilities in 1939 he joined the Royal Canadian Army Medical Corps, serving initially with the 15th Canadian General Hospital and later as commander of the No. 2 RCAMC clearing station,[75] then was urgently called home in 1944 at the request of the university to help train medical students and residents.

In 1950 Cannell became chair of the Department of Obstetrics and Gynaecology, at the same time moving from the Western to TGH as obstetrician and gynecologist-in-chief. Cannell at once founded what became known as the "Cannell Course," comparable to the Gallie Course in surgery, "the first fully integrated University postgraduate program in obstetrics and gynaecology."[76] Central to the course was rotating for one's training among the various teaching hospitals, an innovation for which Van Wyck had already laid the groundwork. As Cannell told the dean in 1952, "The joint staff meetings of the three University hospitals have been held as usual. They have again proven their usefulness in providing an opportunity for all to become acquainted with procedures which are not common to all institutions."[77] Jim Goodwin recalled, "One thing that Cannell used to do, he'd go around – and this was something the Professor had never done – he'd attend the rounds at places like the East General Hospital, and he'd go to the St. Michael's, and he'd go to St. Joseph's, and he'd go to the Western … He brought the fold in, which was a great thing to do."[78] Cannell's position was further enhanced in 1954 as an endowment from the estate of Gordon C. Leitch, a former chairman of the Toronto Western Hospital's board, established the Leitch Chair of Obstetrics and Gynaecology as a full-time professorship.[79]

During Cannell's fifteen-year tenure, a system of full-time staff appointments was introduced at the General and extended to the other teaching hospitals, thereby improving the standard of both clinical care and "the teaching of undergraduate and postgraduate students." As the department became more academically focused, "junior members of the staff came to realize that an active interest in basic or clinical research was essential to their future careers." William Allemang undertook eighteen months' training in England on a McLaughlin Travelling Fellowship and on his return in July 1953 became supervisor of clinical investigation, the first member of the department with university support to assist the professor in academic and research initiatives.[80]

According to Jim Goodwin, "Bill Paul and Jimmy Low" were the two Cannell protégés "that started the ball rolling"[81] in terms of research. Both undertook postgraduate training abroad, becoming international authorities in the emerging field of fetal physiology. As a McLaughlin Fellow, William Morris Paul (MD from Toronto in 1947) worked at the Carnegie Institute in Baltimore with Sam Reynolds.[82] James A. Low graduated two years later, completed his residency at Duke in 1954–5, and went on to a long and illustrious career in the Department of Obstetrics and Gynaecology at Queen's University.[83] Paul was recruited as chair of obstetrics and gynecology by the University of Alberta in 1962, launching that department's "first adventure into research" by hiring Jim Goodwin and forming collaborations with the Departments of Pharmacology and Physiology, before returning to Toronto as Cannell's successor in 1965.[84] As well, in the 1961–2 session the Johnson Wax company donated funds for the establishment of a steroid laboratory in the department, and Richard Wilson, recipient of a Markle Fellowship for a year's study in Sweden, was nominated to head a new Division of Steroid Chemistry,[85] which was established in July 1963 to support endocrine investigations.[86]

A big Toronto theme has been treating cancer in as least destructive a way as possible. In 1962 gynecologic surgeon C. Peter Vernon, who had trained in Toronto, returned from an extensive apprenticeship abroad; Vernon helped develop less destructive surgical approaches to gynecologic cancer. In a 1987 eulogy, department chair Walter J. Hannah said of him, "He was a surgical innovator who was sensitive to the competing needs of surgery sufficiently radical to erase malignant disease, but sufficiently restrained to ensure a high quality of life in the surviving patient." Thus, "[h]is pioneering efforts in this area led to a more thoughtful and restrained surgical approach to gynaecologic cancer, which was a welcome departure from the surgical ruthlessness which prevailed during the early years of his professional career. For his leadership in this area, generations of women with genital tract malignancy owe him a great debt."[87]

In 1965 Cannell moved on to become executive director of the Ontario Cancer Treatment and Research Foundation, and Bill Paul became chair. The first chair to remain based at the Toronto Western Hospital rather than moving to the General, Paul proceeded to steer the department even more firmly towards research. In 1968 he said "An overall plan of research activity and distribution of research facilities in this clinical Department has been made. Our basic philosophy in this regard is that each clinical [hospital] department must have a research component in order to retain its viability." The publication list of department members started to grow.[88] (Paul went on to become associate dean of institutional affairs in the faculty from 1975 to 1980.) Yet like most of his predecessors, Paul was most fondly remembered "as a dedicated and engaging teacher to a generation of medical students and residents."[89] According to Knox Ritchie, a later department chair, his teaching was so inspiring that "students would attend the same lecture for a second time just to hear him speak."[90]

Among those mentored by both Paul and Cannell was James W. Goodwin, who followed his late father into the specialty despite an initial determination "to do anything but," until he met Bill Paul during his internship. Jim Goodwin graduated with an MD in Toronto in 1955, and after deciding he wanted to be an obstetrician after all, he nervously approached Cannell, who turned out to be "just as nice as pie" and arranged for Goodwin to broaden his clinical and scientific horizons by doing his residency at Harvard.[91] Goodwin was recruited by Paul to Alberta as a research associate and joined its Department of Obstetrics and Gynecology in 1964 after additional postgraduate training, including work in Oxford with fetal physiologist Geoffrey Dawes. On the strength of his experience in this area, Goodwin was recruited back to Toronto three years later to launch a clinical and research program in perinatology at Women's College Hospital, remaining with the faculty and serving as the inaugural director of the Perinatal Intensive Care Unit at WCH until his departure from Toronto in 1982.[92]

It was from the Amniotic Fluid Study Group at the General that in 1971 the Toronto Prenatal Genetic Diagnosis Program evolved. The General set up an antenatal genetic clinic staffed by its obstetricians and by geneticists from HSC. By 1980 the program had grown to include thirty geneticists, cytogeneticists, obstetricians, ultrasonographers, and biochemists to screen women whose fetuses might be at risk of genetic disease. Genetic amniocenteses were the main diagnostic tool, although other procedures such as fetoscopy were occasionally invoked.[93] By 1980 the program had grown to three cytogenetics laboratories: one at the General under the pathologist H. Allen Gardner, a second at HSC under Ronald Worton, and a third at Surrey Place under Joseph Berg. The number of genetic amniocenteses had increased from 6 in 1971 to over 1,000 in 1979. The service was enormously popular and the laboratories reported themselves "absolutely overwhelmed."[94]

John L. Harkins, a University of Toronto medical graduate in 1950, succeeded Bill Paul as chair of ob-gyn in 1970 and was in office until 1981. Because of the heavy service load, the research focus fostered under Cannell and Bill Paul declined significantly in these years. A 1979 review acknowledged that "the Department continues to deliver a high standard of patient care and has a good record in teaching at the graduate and undergraduate levels." Yet concerns were also being voiced "both in and outside the Department" that its "research activity has been less than optimal. This is a deficiency of many Departments of Obstetrics and Gynaecology, but the degree of productivity has been distinctly less than might be expected of a medical school of the stature of this University."[95] The department was itself aware of this problem and "has proposed appointment of a Research Director" to encourage research activity.[96]

The research deficit began to right itself when Walter J. Hannah succeeded Harkins as chair of the university Department of Obstetrics and Gynaecology in 1981. He had arrived at Women's College in July 1961 as one of the hospital's first two male staff members and in 1966 became its first male department head. He continued this legacy of "firsts" by remaining based at Women's College and continuing as chief of service there until 1986. Like his predecessors, Hannah was highly regarded for his devotion to clinical training, but he broadened the department's focus as well. According to Knox Ritchie, his successor as chair, Hannah "was the first person that turned around that very clinical culture" and achieved this in a number of ways: "[F]or instance, he started a research day in the department, where the residents presented their research." Most importantly, he began to reorganize the department across divisional rather than hospital lines and recruit staff with advanced training in the discipline's emerging subspecialties of "perinatology, oncology, reproductive biology and gynaecological urology."[97] This innovation resulted in the present subdivisions within the department.

In 1983 Hannah and seventy-nine other members of the department "made personal donations totaling $400,000 to endow the Genesis Research Foundation, a non-profit charitable organization and scientific research institution ... developed to improve the quality of health care for women through basic and clinical research." A major motive for its establishment, he later explained, was to provide a source of research funding: "Genesis is a mechanism that allows us to find the money for research that the university can't give us." By January 1992, the foundation had funded twelve projects and a further nineteen had been approved.[98]

Hannah retired at the end of June 1992 and was succeeded as chair by Knox Ritchie, who continued as chief of ob-gyn at Mount Sinai and head of the Division of Maternal-Fetal Medicine until March 2003.[99] Ritchie's tenure thus coincided with the economic downsizing and organizational upheaval of the 1990s, as health care in Toronto and throughout the province underwent extensive changes – not least in this specialty. Looking back on these events, he recalled "somebody saying that we were living in an era where there was white water most of the time ... and he never spoke a truer word."[100] Yet he believes that as a result of shrewd leadership both the department and the faculty managed to "come out of it much stronger ... you get an era of decreasing funds, and yet this Department of Obstetrics and Gynecology – and the Faculty of Medicine – have become a powerhouse during the same time. That's no coincidence."[101] In addition to playing a key role in restructuring the ob-gyn service in the University Avenue corridor, Ritchie continued to build the department on the basis of academic merit: "Now, we won't take anybody on staff unless they have done another degree, or been away, been to another fellowship somewhere."[102] He also addressed the problem of budgetary limitations by establishing a practice plan in the department, to which its members contribute 20 percent of their earnings, which "goes for academic benefit." Similar initiatives were in place in other departments, but "[w]e were one of the last holdouts against it, and that was another thing I had to do. That was probably one of the most difficult things ... But it has really enhanced the academic side of the department."[103]

One more innovation is worth noting because it became so widely used elsewhere. In January 1990, "standardized patients," professional actors coached in their obstetrical roles, started to arrive for undergraduate instruction in the gynecological exam. "This department uses a programme of 'professional patients,' ... to help students learn procedures such as pelvic examinations. At present, there are nine professional patients who go to each teaching hospital two or three times a year ... which allows students an opportunity to interact with women who can give them important feedback on their professional practices."[104]

Ritchie was succeeded in 2003 by Alan Bocking, who is chair at this writing. No attempt will be made here to evaluate his work because his tenure is too recent. It cannot be helped but observed, however, that under Bocking the department was considered by an external review to be "one of the top ten obstetrics and gynecology departments in the world."[105]

## Perinatology

Perinatal medicine at the University of Toronto has been one of the big success stories in the history of the faculty, despite a late start. Because of the Hospital for Sick Children's world-class reputation in neonatal intensive care, it was widely assumed that establishing an integrated high-risk perinatal service capable of caring for both mother and infant was unnecessary,[106] a belief that HSC helped to perpetuate. According to Knox Ritchie, they thought "that they were the only ones who could actually do it. And whenever maternity hospitals like Women's wanted to start up their own neonatal intensive care, they vehemently opposed it, and said ... the babies could come in to them, and they'd do it right."[107] Yet transporting medically fragile newborns from other sites places them at additional risk, as was acknowledged by HSC neonatologists themselves in a 1972 study.[108] The basic issue here, however, is that perinatal means care surrounding the delivery, and the Hospital for Sick Children had no obstetrical ward. Other hospitals that did were better placed to offer perinatal care.

The lack of high-risk perinatal care in Toronto was addressed during Walter Hannah's tenure as obstetrician and gynecologist-in-chief at Women's College Hospital, with the appointment in July 1967 of Jim Goodwin and John Milligan as the hospital's first perinatologists.[109] In addition to establishing a program of basic research in fetal physiology, they oversaw the construction in "the Labour-Delivery area" of "an integrated Perinatal Intensive Care Unit."[110] The new PICU began operation in the latter half of 1970 in the department's new quarters;[111] it provided, as Milligan later explained, "the first Canadian facilities geographically concentrated containing both obstetrical and paediatric modules in a totally integrated fashion."[112]

With the opening of the unit at Women's College, the value of an integrated perinatal service became apparent. "The issue soon became not whether Toronto needed a perinatal centre, but how to service all the perinatal problems in a region where more than sixty thousand births occurred every year, something that the Women's College unit couldn't possibly handle adequately." By 1978 the Ontario Ministry of Health, in cooperation with the University Teaching Hospitals Association, was calling for briefs from hospitals interested in housing a second high-risk perinatal centre.[113] Several Toronto hospitals submitted proposals, "including Sick Kids" (in an unsuccessful effort by Paul Swyer, chief of neonatology, to add an obstetrical service) and the General, which according to Ritchie submitted a weak proposal in the belief that "they would get it, hands down."[114]

As the busiest maternity service in Ontario with nearly 5,000 deliveries annually, Mount Sinai Hospital was determined to secure the ministry-approved unit. Following "a meticulously researched, painstakingly planned, and aggressively waged campaign" by Frederick R. Papsin, chief of obstetrics and gynecology and the hospital executive, the Sinai was awarded the program in January 1981.[115] Ritchie said, "Nobody thought it would go there, but the ministry ... brought somebody in from outside" to evaluate the proposals, "and they actually picked what potentially was the best thing." What probably "clinched it," he added, was that the hospital was "prepared to match the ministry money. I mean, they were prepared to go out and raise 5 million dollars to help it along."[116] (A large portion of this, some $3.4 million, was later donated by the Variety Club in support of the new facility.)[117]

The establishment of high-risk perinatology at Mount Sinai represented a quantum leap for the hospital's ob-gyn service – which in Papsin's view had been virtually ignored by the university department, despite a long tradition of outstanding clinical care and progressive approaches, including former chief Lou Harris's work on infertility and Ely Ravinsky's early experiments with fetal monitoring.[118] During construction of the new unit in the first half of the 1980s, departmental staffing was also raised to a new level. Pamela Fitzhardinge from the Hospital for Sick Children, an internationally known neonatologist, was re-cruited as chief of pediatrics in 1982.

Finding a qualified obstetrical perinatologist to head the unit, however, proved more challenging. To be sure, a fair number of Canadians (including Goodwin and Milligan at Women's College) had undertaken research fellow-ships in fetal physiology with Geoffrey Dawes at Oxford; as well, a strong pro-gram in perinatal medicine existed at the University of Western Ontario under John Patrick and Paul Harding. Yet the subspecialty was poorly developed at Toronto.[119] A 1979 review of the department found that its interaction with the pediatrics department was "limited and less than desirable," especially "in the important field of perinatology." Again, HSC's monopoly on neonatal intensive care was an inhibiting factor: "The fact that the major intensive care nursery for the teaching hospital complex is located in the Sick Children's Hospital has worked against a close interaction between obstetricians and neonatologists."[120]

Following an international search, J.W. Knox Ritchie from the Royal Victo-ria Hospital and Queen's University in Belfast, Northern Ireland, was recruited for the position. Ritchie was a 1968 medical graduate of Queen's, obtaining the three degrees – MB, BCh (Bachelor of Chirurgie [Surgery]), BAO (bachelor of applied obstetrics) – of the traditional Irish university system;[121] following a se-ries of residencies in Belfast and in what was then Rhodesia, he completed two years' training as a research officer in Oxford under the supervision of Professor Dawes. He completed his honours MD (a research degree in the United King-dom) at Queen's in 1975 with a thesis called "The Cardiovascular, Metabolic, and Endocrine Effects of Catecholamines in Fetal Sheep" and later the same year joined the staff of its Department of Midwifery & Gynaecology.[122]

Initially ambivalent about the position at Mount Sinai ("at the time I actually wasn't that interested in coming"), Ritchie was persuaded by John Patrick at Western – who "had just turned down the job" – to "come and have a look at it, and tell them where their problems are." A key factor in his decision to accept the appointment was the commitment of Gerald Turner, the hospital's execu-tive director, to "excellence" and academic leadership: "Gerry and the Board at that time decided, 'Right, the gloves are off, we're going to be competitive' ... and they were going to be as competitive as they could, in whatever area they decided to go into. I took them seriously, and I must say, they were very sup-portive, so my main aim was to make this the best possible place you could out of it."

The other deciding factor was the concentration of resources already appar-ent at the intersection of University and College: "When you looked at the geog-raphy, and the powerhouse Toronto potentially was – it wasn't yet, but it could be, if you looked at these teaching hospitals all sitting opposite each other on Ambulance Alley here. You look at Sick Kids, Toronto General, Mount Sinai. Princess Margaret wasn't there, yet, but it was Sinai that influenced them to come to that site. All of them with research institutes. And you walked up the street, and you had the basic sciences at the University just looking at you ... I don't know of any other city in the world where it has that setup ... It's unique. It makes Toronto what it is now."[123] In August 1984 he became director of obstetrical perinatology at MSH and a professor in the Department of Obstetrics and Gynaecology in the Faculty of Medicine.[124]

Soon after Ritchie's arrival, the new perinatal unit received a big boost thanks to the generosity of John Milligan at Women's College. Initially, the great majority of high-risk pregnancies were still being referred there, with Mount Sinai receiving only the "spill-over" when Women's was full. But during a lunch meeting, Milligan proposed that the two units take turns on accepting referrals, thereby allowing Mount Sinai "to take virtually half the cases" and expand its program further. This cooperation, Ritchie later explained, "wouldn't have happened in any other North American city" and was made possible only because the two directors were close colleagues working within a single university department.[125] This kind of informal collegiality has been a theme in many departments and is one of the keys to making the "matrix" work.

In 1986 the university chair of obstetrics and gynecology, Walter Hannah, gave an overview of perinatal medicine in Toronto: "As of January 1, 1986 the Perinatal Unit at the Women's College Hospital was fully operational with a 48-bed Neonatal Intensive Care Unit. The new unit at the Mount Sinai Hospital was well-established ... 30 Neonatal ICU beds. The Hospital for Sick Children maintained its 37-bed NICU. In addition to these three tertiary care hospitals, the Toronto General Hospital forms an integral part of the Perinatal Complex because of its role as an antenatal diagnosis centre and its long-standing interest and expertise in the medical and surgical complications of pregnancy." While admitting that "the costs of the programme have been substantial," Hannah said, "these must be weighed against the dramatic improvements in perinatal mortality and morbidity." Survival for preterm infants as early as twenty-five weeks' gestation was now 70 percent and for those born after twenty-eight weeks was 90 percent or higher. Moreover, "the vast majority [of survivors] showed no neurological impairment." Hannah concluded, "The perinatal programme at this University is the result of very effective collaboration of four clinical departments and four hospitals. The facilities are considerable. It will help to fill a very important need for women with high risk pregnancies ... while at the same time bringing distinction to the University as a result of the academic excellence already achieved, with even greater promise for the future."[126]

Hannah's comments were a fitting benediction for a program that had gladdened the hearts of many parents. In 1987 the Division of Neonatology of the Toronto General Hospital's Department of Obstetrics and Gynaecology, with its nine beds, received the status of a "Level II Obstetric and Neonatal Centre within the University of Toronto Perinatal Complex."[127] For a Department of Obstetrics and Gynaecology that traced its origins back to the very beginnings of the faculty in 1887, it was a nice centenary.

## 22 New Talent: Mount Sinai Hospital and Women's College Hospital

Our graduates are spread over the whole of North America and many distant lands, yet the majority were from rural Ontario until recent times. This year, of 125 students admitted to the first premedical year, 96 came from Metropolitan Toronto ... We have become a metropolitan medical school.[1]

Dean John Hamilton, 1961

Dean Hamilton prided himself that the faculty had reached out beyond the lads of the farms and small towns of Ontario to the cosmopolitan quilt that Toronto was becoming in the 1960s. And rightly so: one of the reasons for the faculty's success lay in enlarging its catchment basin from rural Ontario to a vast entrepôt with thirty-five major languages. The best and brightest from all the world were flocking to Toronto, and they and their children would teem into the Faculty of Medicine, enriching the talent pool on which academic excellence had to draw.

What a contrast with the Toronto of the 1930s! Ernest McCulloch, the cancer scientist, recalled in 1991, "I grew up in Toronto in the 1930s. I remember vividly a small mean city, a society that was frankly racist, a society that was regulated by numerous conventions with the force of law, religion that was both compulsory and repressive, parties that were formal and dull, occasional restaurants serving uniform uninteresting food and a few movie theatres. The high point of the year was the production of a Gilbert and Sullivan Opera by the employees of the T. Eaton Co!"

Then Toronto the Good began to break up. "After the war," McCulloch continued, "immigration began. The Toronto scene started to become both diversified and relaxed. Racism became unthinkable as we all met and enjoyed the new arrivals. A key immigrant group were the thousands of Hungarians, all refugees from the 1956 revolution, who emigrated to Canada, half to Toronto. Many were young professionals: physicians, scientists, engineers, and artists.

Many of those in medicine made their way to U of T, starting as fellows and associates. This was followed by a similar but smaller Czech group in 1968. Many others followed from elsewhere. They made for us great buildings, entertainment, restaurants, and, most of all, a freedom that came from membership in a multicultural community."[2]

The children of these new immigrants also went into medicine and enriched greatly the scientific Niagara of knowledge that was starting to pour from the Faculty of Medicine. Names such as Marotta, Jeejeebhoy, Mak, and Ogryzlo – unfamiliar to nonexistent before the Second World War – became stars in the faculty's pantheon. The entire world brought its new talent to Toronto, and this vast reservoir of brains, energy, and ambition turned Toronto into a research power with global reach.

Yet this is not entirely a happy story because the faculty did not reach out glad arms to all groups equally. Until the 1960s some got rather a cold shoulder, in particular, Jews and women.

### Jews

Jewish students begin showing up in the medical class in significant numbers around 1900. A number of them were born in Russia and had come to Canada as teenagers. They landed in an environment where there were virtually no Jewish physicians – Solomon Singer in 1903 was the first Jewish graduate of U of T and the city's second Jewish physician![3] They also encountered an intensely anti-Semitic environment, where local toughs shouted "Sheeny" at Jewish passers-by and pulled the beards of rabbis.[4] In 1992 Bun McCulloch, who was not Jewish, confided to his close friend and colleague Jim Till that he had just read "Mordecai Richler's little book" (evidently *The Apprenticeship of Duddy Kravitz*). "His description of growing up in Montreal parallels my own experience in Toronto in the '30s. There was clearly anti-Semitism, there was a master-race (the English) and some strange clerics (T.T. Shields was an outstanding example)."[5] Shields was a Baptist fundamentalist minister who held forth at the Jarvis Street Baptist Church. The city did not welcome these migrants from Russian and Poland with open arms.

Among the earliest Jews in academic medicine in Toronto was Leon Judah Solway, who in 1912 was in charge of the newly founded Out-Patient Sub-department in Medicine of the Toronto General Hospital, together with William Goldie. Born in Russia in 1885, Solway graduated in the university's "B and P" course in arts in 1907 and finished medicine in 1909. The university yearbook said semi-humorously that in Russia he had "suffered from Cosacky pains and a tingling sensation for the land of the free." "His frontal lobes are considerably congested and crammed up with learning."[6]

Joseph Green of the class of 2T5 (1925) – whose motto was "Came, saw and conquered" – was born in Russia in 1898, arriving in Canada in 1914 to attend high school at Jarvis Collegiate. His classmates saw him as idealistic, "to bring speedy succor to suffering humanity."[7] Noah Landis, another 2T5'er, was born in Brest-Litovsk in Russia in 1895 and known to his classmates "as a man of fine literary ability." He chose as his motto, "Dire – c'est rien, faire – c'est la chose" ("Talk is nothing, doing is what counts").[8]

These were the sons and daughters of poor Jews who had recently immigrated to Canada. They experienced a much more virulent form of anti-Semitism than did the established middle-class Jewish families in Toronto. Kenneth Pritzker, long-time head of pathology at the Mount Sinai, said, "In the 1930's, anti Semitism was most fiercely directed at the poor, the eastern European and those with limited English speaking capability. It was fueled by the depression, the rise of Nazism and the rise of socialism and communism which appealed to many of the impoverished Jewish immigrants (later, the parents of many successful U of T physicians). The assimilated Jews were a much, much smaller community and for them the anti-Semitism was 'genteel' as well as gentile. It was manifest as inability to become accepted as members of Ontario clubs such as the Granite club and of course, difficulty getting business financing from the established banks."[9]

Medical anti-Semitism in those days was raging in Toronto. Peter Carlen recalled the travails of his father, cardiologist Sidney Carlen (Katz), who graduated in medicine in 1936. Toronto General Hospital had begun accepting Jewish interns only in 1929,[10] and in 1936 Sidney Carlen was one of two. "He'd sit down at the table and everyone would get up and leave. He did a rotation at Sick Kids, got strep throat and missed a week. The chief resident wanted to deny him credit for the rotation. My father went back and stood him up against a wall and said he'd kill him." Sidney Carlen trained in internal medicine at Michael Reese Hospital in Chicago – a hospital sympathetic to Jews – and while there embarked upon a budding research career.[11]

Whatever stings these young Jewish medical students may have experienced in private did not seem to hold them back. Lillian Sher, 2T5, was president of the Medical Athletic Association and "played on the intercollegiate basketball team for four years."[12] David Eisen, who began medical studies in 1917, became inter-faculty wrestling champion in his division – featherweight – in 1920.[13] Many of the Jewish medical students buzzed with activity, and their surroundings evidently suited.

With freshly-minted MDs in hand, the road ahead was, however, a different story for the Jewish medical graduates. In the 1930s, 30–40 percent of the graduating class sought internships outside of Canada, including, one supposes, most of the Jewish students. (By 1950–1 this had shrunk to 12 percent, a sign perhaps of lessening of the anti-Semitism of the 1930s.[14])

Nor were the Jewish undergraduates always aware of bigotry (until they graduated). Barney Berris had no clue that he might be discriminated against in choosing an internship. He had grown up in Toronto in the late 1920s and 1930s and said that he heard the term "dirty Jew" only once, from a school-ground bully, whom his cousin then threw down on the ground. Yet he lived in a separate world. "There was little interaction between the Jewish and non-Jewish kids, either in the playground or walking to or from school ... My parents never said anything about who I should play with. It was simply taken for granted that all my friends would be Jewish."

After finishing medical school in 1944, Berris wanted to remain in Toronto because he was getting married. He applied both to the General and the Western, with a high standing in his graduating class: "When the appointments were announced, I discovered to my dismay that I was the only person in our class who had not been accepted or 'matched' for internship by a hospital. I couldn't understand how this could have happened and was certain it was a mistake. I went to both hospitals to which I had applied and asked to see the list of students they were prepared to accept. At first there was some resistance to my request, but when I persisted I was finally allowed to see them. I was stunned by what I saw." The long list of the General included, on the left-hand side, students near the bottom of the class. "On the right was another, very short list. It was titled 'Hebrew list' and on it were three names. The first was the name of the gold medalist in our class, and the second was another Jewish student who also had a very good record. Below the two names was the heading 'Alternate Hebrew' with my name." The Toronto Western Hospital also had a Hebrew list, with only one name on it, that of the gold medalist who had decided to go to TGH. "It was clear to me that the Toronto General Hospital had a quota of two Jewish interns and the Toronto Western Hospital had a quota of one."[15] (Berris also had a similarly unpleasant experience at McGill, so it is clear that, unhappily, the University of Toronto did not have a monopoly on Canadian medical anti-Semitism.[16])

Jack Laidlaw remembered Berris's humiliation. "Berris came and said, 'Jack, this is the story. And I know that your father is assistant registrar of the University. Can you speak to him and find out if there's anything that can be done?'" So Laidlaw did speak with his father, "and Dad looked into it and he said, 'Jack, you wouldn't believe what I found. There's a quota against Jews coming into medicine.'" Laidlaw went back to Berris and told him what his father had said.[17]

Yet Berris's encounter with anti-Semitism was not at an end. He trained at the University of Minnesota in medicine for four years. When it came time to return to Toronto, in view of his previous experiences he had no idea what reception awaited him. Yet his boss at Minnesota, Cecil J. Watson, knew Ray Farquharson, who by now was professor of medicine, succeeding the anti-Semitic Duncan Graham. Watson called Farquharson, and there was absolutely no problem at all. Watson told him, "I think everything is arranged and you will likely be appointed to the University of Toronto faculty."[18]

When Berris returned to Toronto, however, he found Farquharson backpedalling. "I would like to appoint you," he told Berris, "but it's not possible because we really don't know you." That Berris had studied medicine in Toronto was of no avail. Finally, Farquharson said, "The best I can offer you is a position as a fellow in medicine for a year and if you do well I will do my very best to have you appointed to the staff."[19]

Farquharson was true to his word, at the cost of a big drama. When in 1951 the TGH board heard of the plan of appointing a Jew, Laidlaw said, "There was substantial opposition." So Farquharson told the board that "if his recommendation did not go through, he would resign as physician-in-chief of the Toronto General Hospital."[20]

The story had a happy ending: after completing the fellowship year Berris passed his examinations leading to the fellowship degree in medicine in the Royal College of Physicians of Canada, and Farquharson asked Berris to come to his office. "I knew at once that he had good news. He was smiling and as I came through the door he extended his hand and said, 'Congratulations, we did it. You are now a member of the hospital staff with a full university appointment.'"

One of the early Jewish interns at the General was Ruth Sky, appointed in 1948, who later became a well-known Toronto family doctor. Sky overheard a nurse asking the chief of staff how the hospital chose interns for the year. He replied, according to Margaret Douglin, who interviewed Sky, "Every year we let in two Catholics, two Jews, and then all the rest." When Sky asked him for an explanation, he replied, "Well, it's always been that way."[21]

Medical anti-Semitism in Toronto was not confined to the Toronto General Hospital. When pioneering ophthalmologist Maxwell Kurt Bochner, who had just finished training in Philadelphia, returned to Toronto in 1926, he applied for privileges at the Hospital for Sick Children and was refused. As historian Lesley Marrus Barsky tells it, when a friend, Edmund Scheuer, "an affluent Toronto jeweler as well as a pillar of the assimilated Jewish community," made inquiries about the causes of this denial of privileges to Bochner, Scheuer was astonished. He wrote Bochner,

Dear Dr Bochner,
After some delay, I succeeded in getting an interview with Mr Williams [HSC administrator]. Just returning from the gentleman's office I report to you that apparently there is not a ghost of a chance of any Jewish doctor being appointed in the Staff of the Hospital.

The reason the gentleman gave to me is that all of every one of the thirty voluntary doctors on the Staff were opposed to having a Jew appointed.[22]

Until the end of the 1930s admission to the Faculty of Medicine was unrestricted in that any high school graduate with a "senior matric" was entitled to enroll. Yet the faculty became choosier after the war and implemented a quota on Jews. Bernie Langer, who graduated in medicine in 1956, said, "There was a quota. It was not an official quota, but we had a class of 150 and there were exactly 30 Jews in each class. And then I didn't know until later, but I found that there was also a quota against Catholics, which Langer put at around 20 percent. I was in a clinic group with five Catholics and five Jews, a very compatible group."[23]

Some of the documents show a prejudice against both women and Jews that is actually rather horrifying in its matter-of-factness. On 6 October 6 1944, the Committee on Admission to the First Year reported, "As in previous years your committee had to deal with a formidable array of jewish applicants, many of whom had a very good matriculation score. We have admitted 31 jews (3 being women) as compared with 32 (2 women) last year. The percentage of jews passing into the present second year is high, as the jews formed 21% of last first year, but supplied only 6% of the failures."

The report continued, "The large number of female applicants presented an equally serious problem ... This year we have had to admit 37 women, five of whom had perfect matriculation scores. That means that women plus jews constitute almost 45% of the class."[24] One is actually rather speechless in the face of this doubled-barreled prejudice and can only say that the world since then has thankfully changed.

A crack began to crease this wall of vicious anti-Semitism in 1929, when the Toronto General Hospital decided to take on one Jewish intern per year.[25] Yet Jews were not yet on staff in the big departments. As late as the mid-1940s, as representatives of the class of 1944 said, "[Jewish graduates] were confronted with Toronto's infamous 'Jewish file' which limited the number of Jews who could be given junior internships in any of Toronto's teaching hospitals to a grand total of three Jews. Worse than that, it limited to close to zero the number accepted into post-graduate training, and faculty membership was held at zero."[26]

Yet the Second World War seems to have pried open that crack into a great gap. Jewish physicians had served in the forces with distinction. Manifestly able, it seemed increasingly implausible to deny them hospital appointments. Joseph Gollom said in an interview with Margaret Douglin, "When doctors came back from their service and had been good students and had spent two or three or four years in the services and applied for appointments in the teaching hospitals, it became difficult to turn them down. Once they were in they were more than welcome because they were good students and good teachers and their scholastic standing was among the best."[27] Several observers felt that horror at the Holocaust might also have played a role. There was also a change in leadership: William Gallie, professor of surgery, and Duncan Graham, professor of medicine – both known as anti-Semitic – stepped down in 1947.

After Berris's appointment in 1951 the ice began to break up. In the 1951–2 session, Calvin Ezrin, who also was Jewish, was appointed to the rank of assistant in Wightman's Department of Therapeutics.[28] Bernie Goldman called him "the first Jewish medical person (endocrinology) hired by Farquharson ...

Cal was my first clinician in 1958."[29] (Ken Pritzker comments, "Ten years after his appointment Cal was an assistant professor even though he was one of the Faculty's few accomplished clinician scientists.") Soon after Ezrin's arrival, in 1955 Colin Woolf, a South African of Jewish origin from Cape Town, joined the Department of Medicine. From then on, the appointment of Jews ceased to be exceptional.

Bernie Langer was the first Jew appointed in the Department of Surgery of the Toronto General Hospital. (Abraham Willinsky, said Langer, was previously appointed at the Toronto Western Hospital in the Department of Surgery. Willinsky was jokingly described in the yearbook of his 1908 graduating class as "a rather well-nourished individual of decidedly Semitic appearance."[30]) As for Langer, it was Fred Kergin who, as university departmental chairman, took Langer on at the General. Langer had a tentative offer from the children's hospital. "I told [Kergin] of the offer, but that I wanted to work at the General. I think that's the first time he even thought of the possibility of me doing that. But to his great credit, he took the proposal to the rest of the staff, and after a few days he invited me to join the staff."[31]

Helen Farquharson, Ray Farquharson's daughter, who graduated in medicine in 1958, recalled in a later interview the previous anti-Semitism of the faculty: "When I started medicine [1952] – we were about the first, the vets had just left, so our class was 120, it was slightly smaller; and it took us very little time to spot that in our class group we had 10 percent girls, 10 percent Jews, and 80 percent were the rest of them. We always wondered, cause we had two Jewish girls, whether they were counted as Jews or girls."

She confirmed the Berris story. "And then my father came [in 1947 as Eaton Professor of Medicine]. He was the first one to bring a Jew on staff, Barney Berris." She noted, "My father said, 'he'd trained at Minneapolis, and he was excellent,' and I mean, he could have been a professor ... But when he brought up his name to the Board of Governors and they turned him down, my father said, 'if Dr. Berris doesn't come on staff, I'm resigning.' So that got the first Jew on staff."[32]

What broke this solid wall of anti-Semitism that existed at the General? There must have been some seminal event because whatever animus people may have harboured in their hearts, they stopped giving voice to it in public. For Bernie Goldman, the turning point was the appointment of Hollenberg as head of medicine in 1970 and Langer as head of surgery in 1982. "Bernie Langer and Charlie Hollenberg changed all that, because of their positions, because of their personalities, because of their accomplishments, and because of their fairness. That's my view."[33]

Kenneth Pritzker at Mount Sinai, who followed in his father Harold's footsteps, reflected about the nature of this extraordinary anti-Semitism in Toronto, as well as the circumstances of its ultimate disappearance: "Until the late 1960's, U of T's clinical medical Faculty was extremely inbred, i.e. graduates of U of T with only a little outside exposure. It's not widely recognized but part of the reason for the acceptance of Jews was that by the 1950's many faculty leaders had friends who had been Jewish classmates in medical school at U of T. By Harold Pritzker's time this was the case. For example my father, class of '34, was friends with John Hamilton '35, Lawrie Chute '34 (John Hamilton's successor) and many clinical teachers such as K.J.R. Wightman '36 who were in U of T Medical school contemporaneously. The friendships dated back to medical school."

Ken Pritzker continued, "By the early 1950's many of the young U of T faculty lived in North Toronto and sent their children to the same public schools. My public school class included a daughter of K.J.R. Wightman, a daughter of Rod Ross (pathologist at St. Michael's), a daughter of a pediatrician at HSC, Bob Hilliard (clinician and educator at HSC) who was Irwin Hilliard's son, a son of one the U of T ophthalmologists, and the daughter of another, as well as Fred Dewar's niece. I'm sure that none of us at that early age had any inkling how unusual this was. To some extent then, there was a community (which extended beyond medicine) of professionals, many academic, who lived together in a relatively new suburb."[34]

Thus, in private life a gathering accommodation between Jews and non-Jews occurred for younger people. But for the older generation, there was a difference between public and private. "The 'gentle' anti-Semitism was there," Berris said. "I referred many of my private patients to specialists on the Toronto General Hospital staff such as surgeons, gynecologists, ophthalmologists, and so on. But they rarely referred patients to me for medical consultation. In the thirteen years I was at the Toronto General, I had six referrals for medical consultations from the staff."[35]

Anti-Semitism very rapidly ceased to be fashionable in the faculty after the 1970s. Yet it lingered on in private as a kind of sewer gas. After Hollenberg was appointed professor of medicine in 1970, his widow Michelle ("Mimi") said in an interview, "Remarks were made to him. 'Don't we have enough Jews that are coming here?'"

> Interviewer: "People said this to his face?"
> Mimi Hollenberg: "Yeah, well, they would forget. I mean he looked like the governor of a town. So they would forget he was a Jew."
> Interviewer: "What would they say then?"
> Mimi Hollenberg: "The automatic remark was 'Oh god. I forgot.' Well you know what you forgot – you forgot that the person who is sitting with you is a Jew."[36]

### Women

The Toronto faculty's first Jewish female medical graduate was Bessie Thelma Pullan, who finished secondary school at Jarvis Street Collegiate, then entered the Ontario Medical College for Women in 1905, graduating from the Toronto medical faculty (after it merged with the women's faculty) in 1909. She married the lawyer Louis Michael Singer in 1911 and practiced as Pullan-Singer at 18 Austin Crescent. In the Jewish medical community, she became something of a point of pride, and radiologist A.I. Willinsky called attention to her in his memoirs as "the first Jewish woman doctor."[37]

In looking at the history of women in the faculty, there is really no debate about whether the glass was half full or half empty. Until the 1970s it was mostly half empty. Yet there are some points of light as early on, several distinguished women established names for themselves.

Pearl Jane Sproule is widely believed the first woman specialist in Canadian medicine. She was born on a homestead farm in Britton, Ontario, near Listowel, in 1878 and finished her MB in 1907 at U of T, where she was considered by her classmates to have "a personality endowed both by nature and inheritance with rare tact and judgement and with that most uncommon of virtues – common sense."[38] She trained in otolaryngology in Toronto, then studied in Berlin, Vienna, and London, and was admitted to the Royal College of Surgeons, England, in 1911 (as the first Canadian woman). She joined the Department of Otolaryngology at TGH in 1912, becoming chief of the service at Women's College Hospital in 1924; she finished her career there; the children's wing is named after her. Later, she married James Manson and took his name.

An early female academic in the faculty at the professorial level, if not the first, was Winifred Cullis. Thomas G. Brodie, the professor of physiology, died in 1916 during the war, and Cullis, an important English physiologist associated with him, was appointed to replace him in the Department of Physiology for the 1917–18 session.[39] A number of other high-achieving women are discussed later in the section on Women's College Hospital.

Indeed, women as academics have a brilliant and distinguished history. Yet this history is not served by the creation of myths, and the notion that Maud Menten, an important pathologist and enzymologist, somehow achieved greatness while at the University of Toronto is a myth. She was born in Port Lambton, Ontario, in 1879 and graduated with her MB from U of T in 1907, one of what were by then numerous female graduates. She gained an MD from U of T in 1911, then studied in Berlin, met Leonor Michaelis, and developed there the Michaelis-Menten equation that is considered the foundation of modern enzymology. She received a PhD from the University of Chicago in 1916 and spent the rest of her career in the Faculty of Medicine of the University of Pittsburgh. Meanwhile, the Faculty of Medicine of the University of Toronto has genuine international stars, such as the radiotherapist Vera Peters and the biochemist Marian Packham – discussed at various points in this volume – whose achievements might be better memorialized than they have been.

The great gaps in the ranks of male students and professors caused by the First World War offered an opportunity for women to come on stage, and they took advantage of it. In 1918 Dean Clarke said, "One of the striking facts ... is that women have come to us in larger numbers. In 1910 but one woman registered in the first year, and only eleven all told in attendance at that time. This session [1917–18] no less than twenty women entered the First Year, and there was a total attendance of fifty-one women. This is owing to the fact that until quite recently other institutions had closed their doors to these students."[40]

Likewise in the First World War a number of women started receiving hospital appointments faute de mieux. Thus one finds in the Department of Anaesthesia in 1915 Jennie Smillie, who finished her medical studies at U of T in 1909 (and whose name the hospital misspelled as "Smellie" – see later for more). In 1931 Mary Tom, a medical graduate of U of T in 1922, became the inaugural microscopist in the Division of Neuropathology. Over the years she was associated with several significant scientific discoveries, such as that of benign islet cell tumours of the pancreas with Ric Richardson in 1951 (see p. 372) – and yet her name has plunged almost entirely into oblivion! She is not even mentioned in the standard Who's Who of Women and Medicine in Toronto.[41]

Following the custom of the medical students' (Meds) "At-Homes," large celebratory dinners, in 1934 the Medical Women's Undergraduate Association began holding At-Homes in the afternoon, at the University Women's Club. The report to the Medical Society of the women in that year, whose honorary president was Marion Hilliard and current president Jessie Gray, closed with a steely note: "The recognition of women in our profession was not easily won by our predecessors, and we, the medical women of to-day, appreciate what they did for us and by being alert and co-operative, determine to hold fast the heritage gained for us."[42]

The medical women had by the mid-1930s become sturdy enough to enter the constitution. In the 1933–4 session, "For the first time, the women medical students were represented by their President, Miss [Marjorie] Davis, who was a voting member of the Medical Society. This will shortly be made constitutional."[43]

The number of female undergraduates in medicine in these years was not inconsiderable: in the session 1928–9, 73 of 725 medical students in all six years, or 10 percent.[44] It was an open secret to undergraduates such as Nell Farquharson in the 1950s (see earlier) that the faculty had a quota on women. Donald Cowan, who graduated in 1956, remembered, "My understanding is that the method of selection in terms of women was that they'd list them and when they got to a certain point the secretary said 'that's the end of that category' and everybody else was crossed out. The same was true for Jews."[45] Medical historian Jacalyn Duffin confirms that from late in the Second World War until the 1960s the faculty quota on female admissions was about 10 percent. And female applicants seem to have been held to a higher standard than male. (She attributes to Associate Dean Jan Steiner credit for having lifted the quota. In an interview, Steiner subsequently told Duffin how the quota system on Jews, Catholics, and women worked.)[46]

Until it was torn down in 1931, the focus of female medical undergraduate life in Toronto was Argyll House, which could accommodate about fifteen women in residence. The Medical Women's Undergraduate Associate met there, owing to the excellence of its common rooms, and the house "was most important in developing a feeling of camaraderie amongst the women in medicine." It was located near the General, and living there made "it possible for students in their senior years to readily attend their hospital duties even at night, as is the case in obstetrics," said a special committee of the Faculty Council "on living accommodation for women medical students."[47]

Handy though Argyll House was, by the early 1920s female undergraduates felt less of a need to be protected than earlier. The ample skirts of the Edwardian years had given way to the short dresses of the "flapper," and flappers there were among the female undergrads at U of T as well. Of Frances Margaret Barker, a Branksome Hall graduate in the class of 1924, it was said, "The class gasped when Marg bobbed her hair" (the bob cut is short and may include bangs). Marg also worked as a reporter for the *Varsity*, the undergraduate newspaper, and "successfully managed two election campaigns."[48]

The faculty introduced in 1919 what one would recognize as a system of mentoring for women medical students. It attempted to link them up with recent female medical graduates. Writing to Sproule-Manson, Olive G. Patterson-Cameron, and Helen Muir-Wilson as possible mentors in November of that year, a faculty administrator said, "The women medical students have been very anxious to receive the advice of some of the profession who will take an interest in their organizations and in the different girls. Your name has been suggested." Sproule-Manson and Patterson-Cameron accepted the offer but Muir-Wilson did not.[49] In 1920 Edith Hamilton Gordon, who graduated in medicine at U of T in 1915 and then obtained in 1920 the doctor of public health degree from the University of Pennsylvania (the first Canadian woman to hold such a doctorate), was appointed "medical adviser to women," a post that she held until 1939, all the while on staff at the outdoor chest clinic of Toronto Western Hospital. She organized the "Free Lances," a club that helped young women in financial need.[50]

"The girls in Medicine," to use their phrase, were seventy in number in the faculty in 1925. They called themselves "the Freshettes" and held monthly meetings at the University College Women's Union from 4:00 to 6:00 p.m., serving tea in "the cosy common-room" and listening to distinguished female speakers. "The Nabobs Tea-Party," held in "the spacious reception rooms of Argyll House," was the big event of the year. They organized for Daffydil Night and had a huge turnout for campus athletics, "competing with teams of the colleges with much larger enrolment of women. "There is amongst them … a strong esprit de corps, which is fostered and strengthened by the MWUA" (Medical Women's Undergraduate Association). Their motto was "Each for all and all for each."[51]

The Freshettes were not wimps and gave as good as they got. Here is an anonymous Freshette ("Co-Med") poetizing for *Epistaxis*, the satirical magazine that appeared annually on the eve of Daffydil:

"When I was by my mother's knee
We oft discussed what I should be.
Says I to her 'I'll be a doc.
And own a Ford, both key and lock.'
And as I ever older grew
It was the 'job' for me, I knew,
For all thought me a shining light,
My nose it was exceedingly bright.
My head it was found very long,
My feet, they too were swift and strong,
So when a youth it seemed quite plain,
The rung of fame I would attain."

[There followed several stanzas about her adventures in medical school.]

Now I begin to contemplate,
The year A.D. I'll graduate,
And after that I may survive,
If typhoid, flu and smallpox thrive."[52]

In 1953, the female medical students integrated their labs and clinics. Nell Farquharson said,

"It had been tradition that all the girls were in the same clinic group. My class looked at it and said, 'If a bunch of us have to get through three years of medicine all together, we'll hate each other.

"So we reorganized it – two of our class went up to Dean MacFarlane and asked if we could have mixed medical clinics, and he laughed and said, 'if you can get anyone to go into your clinic, you're welcome.'

"So, back we went. We had a huge common room, cause boys weren't allowed in it, and we weren't allowed in the boys' common room. We had a class list; we divided ourselves into pairs or threes, went down the class list and decided who we'd approach, so that we didn't all go up to the same chap. So one afternoon it was 'Operation Mixed Clinics.'

"We spread out through the class, and asked our respective people from our list if we could be in their clinic group. They all said 'sure,' so by the end of the day, people were coming up to us and saying, 'will you be in my clinic group?' And we'd say, 'sorry, we're taken.' It was really rather humorous."[53]

On the later discrimination against women in the Department of Medicine, Nell Farquharson said, "[The women in the department] all felt that ... they would be overlooked a bit by the men, because they worked different hours: These women had to go home, 'it's 6 o'clock, I have to go home and feed the kids,' and the chap says, 'we don't have to do that' sort of attitude ... Most of the women felt that they had had their careers slowed down because they got married and had children."[54]

Efforts to valorize the pool of female medical talent in Ontario were slow and halting, but they did exist, beginning when Ian MacDonald became dean of the Division of Postgraduate Medical Education in 1955. He is remembered in particular for the division's participation in a large effort to persuade female physicians who had interrupted their careers to return to the labour force. Begun in 1963–4 by Eva Mader MacDonald, a physician at Women's College Hospital who conducted a survey of women doctors in Canada, this effort became known as "Operation Recall." In 1967 Drs Adelaide Fleming at HSC and Ruth Kurdyak – later head of the Medical Alumni Association – circularized female physicians in Ontario about a refresher course that Ian MacDonald at the Division of Postgraduate Medical Education had got up to assist their return to practice. There was widespread interest. The Toronto course became an international model.[55]

In October 1974 the *Globe and Mail* ran an article on "discrimination in teaching hospitals." This surfaced at the meeting of the clinical chairs on 28 January 1975, who wanted to know more about it. But evidence of real discrimination against women medical students began to fade, though not to dry up, after the 1970s. When in 1981 an anonymous group of female students complained vaguely about remarks in lectures "that have been degrading to women," a furious Margaret Thompson, geneticist at the children's hospital, told Undergraduate Dean Llewellyn-Thomas, "I would like the opportunity to meet with the anonymous group of students responsible for the attached memo. I believe it is time for students to come out from behind their mask of anonymity and speak face to face with their instructors about such accusations."[56] That was the end of the story.

In 1990 in a Self-Study poll, 56 percent of female students said women were not discriminated against in medical school.[57] Demographics alone militated increasingly against discrimination. In 1992, 40 percent of the first-year class were female.[58] In 2004 women became a majority in the first-year class: 54 percent.[59]

As for women as academics, whatever shortcomings the Department of Medicine had demonstrated in treating women in the past, by the mid-1990s they had become substantially erased, at least in terms of promotion: of 176 men in the pool of junior academics eligible for promotion, by 1994–6 some 26.7 percent had been promoted; for the 51 women in the pool, the corresponding percent was 25.4. The difference was not statistically significant.[60]

## Ethnic Diversity

Toronto is now the most ethnically diverse city in the world.[61]

President Robert Birgenau, 2000

Jews and women were not the only groups subject to exclusion. In the early 1970s the number of students of Chinese origin registered as undergraduates began to increase significantly, evoking exactly the same kind of nativist reactions in the medical community as Jews had once experienced. Bette Stephenson, president of the Canadian Medical Association, once said, in a journalist's paraphrase, that "Canadian-born students are finding competition for places in medical schools tougher because of the number of foreign-born students being admitted." She had been told by medical colleagues "that about 25 per cent of the first-year medical students at the University of Toronto are of Chinese origin"; she was questioned "whether we are limiting the opportunities for Canadian students." The Chinatown Businessmen's Association in Toronto reacted furiously to this prejudicial expression, and twelve Chinese Canadian physicians, apparently in Toronto, threatened to sue the faculty if a Chinese numerus clausus, or ethnic restriction, was introduced.[62] (The term once applied to Jewish medical admissions in the United States and Europe.) None was.

The transition from a student body of Ontario farm boys to one drawn from the entire globe was accomplished in little more than a generation. By 2000, more than half of U of T students identified themselves as members of "visible minorities." Almost half were born outside of Canada; and two-thirds spoke another language at home aside from English. These changes were reflected in the student composition of the Faculty of Medicine as well as the university as a whole. Among faculty members, change was slower to come, given the lags between the beginning of one's studies and assuming a staff post. Yet the direction of change was the same as elsewhere: in the Department of Medicine, the share of new recruits who were "visible minorities" increased from 13 percent in 1993–7 to 30 percent in 1998–2000.[63]

"Toronto is one of the most culturally diverse cities in the world," said Dean Whiteside in 2009. "According to the Toronto Central Local Health Integration Network, every country of the world is reflected here. Over 160 languages are spoken and 32% of Toronto's citizens are members of visible minority groups." She added, "Most of our postgraduate MD trainees (62%) are born in Canada yet they come from a multitude of ethnic backgrounds. Just over one in three is comfortable speaking to patients in two or more languages."[64]

These are extraordinary numbers that give a clue to the success of the Faculty of Medicine of the University of Toronto. It lay partly in its richness of people. The Ontario farm boys who once ruled the faculty had actually disported themselves rather well in scientific promise. Yet that talent pool was thin, and unaided by luck – as in the insulin story – or by the chance appearance of individual genius (as in a figure such as Bill Bigelow), that talent pool would soon have been rivaled by deeper pools in other, bigger cities. What kept Toronto among the leadership in the international pack was the continual infusion of new blood from all across the globe. Women and Jews were the first new talent to mark the horizon. But then came the refugees from Eastern Europe after the war, the Hungarians and the Poles. Then came the tremendous waves of immigration from the South Asian subcontinent, from China and from Korea. And these huge and highly educated populations produced brilliant scholars and gifted clinicians, world-class scientists, and Nobel Prize candidates! Many rival centres did not have such richness to draw on, and Toronto outpaced them.

## Mount Sinai Hospital

Question to Dr Arnold Aberman, at his five-year review in 1982 as chief of medicine at Mount Sinai: "Is the Department aware of an outer limit of resources?"

   Answer from Aberman: He is not aware of where the limit exists, as history has shown that it was the excellent people who were not available – it has not been the resources that were not available.[65]

It would be difficult to find a more dramatic example of reaching out to new groups in the talent pool than the inclusion of the Jews. Although Jews had always been a strong presence in medicine in Europe since the Middle Ages, in Canada and quite specifically in Toronto, they encountered almost insurmountable barriers. One means of leaping over those barriers, other than going off to the United States for specialty training, was to found their own hospital.

   Mount Sinai Hospital began life on Yorkville Avenue in 1922 as a small twenty-bed community institution, spearheaded by a group of public-spirited women active in the then rather impoverished Jewish community peopled with recent arrivals from Eastern Europe. As the community became wealthier, their hospital migrated south in 1953 to the hospital row on University Avenue and was called the "New Mount Sinai Hospital" to distinguish it from the old. (In 1973, with the move from 550 University Avenue to a grand new building at 600 University, it was renamed simply "Mount Sinai Hospital."[66]) In 1955 the accreditation process began, as the Royal College approved a year of residency in surgery, medicine, and obstetrics and gynecology. (The hospital actually offered the residency a year before the approval. Mount Sinai's extensive involvement with obstetrics, gynecology, and perinatal care is discussed in chapter 21.)[67]

   Acceptance into the university teaching program was another matter. Berris, who replaced Mitchell Kohan in 1964 as chief of medicine at the Sinai, recalled that at the founding of the New Mount Sinai "[t]he board of directors … headed by Ben Sadowski, a forward-looking businessman and philanthropist … had great plans for the hospital. The board was determined that in time the new hospital would be accepted as a teaching hospital within the University of Toronto, a goal that seemed almost impossible in 1954 ... The board knew that if Mount Sinai could show the University that the staff doctors at Mount Sinai had training and accreditation in their specialties equal to that of the staff doctors in the existing university teaching hospitals, the University would have difficulty refusing to include Mount Sinai as a hospital for the teaching and training of students." (According to Ken Pritzker, many Jewish physicians such as Kohan, a middle-aged man, "studied and wrote the Royal College examinations; his contemporaries at TGH were given theirs."[68])

The first meeting between Dean MacFarlane and hospital administrator Sidney Liswood ended in disaster. Lesley Marrus Barsky tells the story: "As Liswood ... arrived for an appointment at the university only to be greeted by Dean MacFarlane, legs crossed atop his desk, his body language loudly proclaiming his attitude towards New Mount Sinai. 'Tell me, Mr Liswood,' asked the dean, 'where do you think Jewish medicine is heading in the next century?'"

The normally urbane Liswood was taken aback. "I don't really understand your question, Dean, but I think I do know what you're implying."

Liswood explained that the hospital would be second to none in teaching and medical care. And, says Barsky, "he turned on his heels and walked out."[69]

Under Dean Hamilton the atmosphere changed. In 1962 Mitchell Kohan succeed in getting the Departments of Medicine and Pathology at Mount Sinai accepted as fully accredited teaching departments, a year after the acceptance of Women's College Hospital in 1961.[70] When the new building of Mount Sinai opened in 1973, the hospital completed the transition from a community hospital into the first rank of the teaching hospitals.

Was there a need for a special general hospital dedicated to Jewish physicians? Yes, there was. Berris recalled the situation before the opening of Mount Sinai. Jewish physicians could admit patients to MSH if beds were available. But these doctors were denied admitting privileges at other hospitals, and they had first to refer their patients to non-Jewish physicians to get them admitted. "This was a shockingly discriminatory policy against Jewish doctors on the part of the non-Jewish medical establishment, and it lasted in Toronto from the time of the first Jewish doctors in the 1920s until the middle of the 1960s."[71]

The issue of autonomy was a sensitive one. No more than the Catholics wanted to lose St Michael's did the Jewish community wish to see Mount Sinai surrender its autonomy. In the hospital restructuring of the mid-1990s, which saw a number of institutions lose their governance, the Sinai and the Toronto Hospital did consolidate several departments: thoracic surgery, for example, moved to The Toronto Hospital, while obstetrics and gynecology came to the Sinai. In the last analysis, Mount Sinai managed to escape the fate of closure and merger of the Wellesley Hospital and Doctors Hospital because it became a major international scientific vehicle, and one could no more close it than one could close the Smithsonian or the Institut Pasteur. What follows is in no sense a history of the hospital – Lesley Marrus Barsky has already written an excellent one – but a few notes about the relationship of the Sinai and its clinicians and scientists to the Faculty of Medicine.

## Research at Mount Sinai

From the very beginning, the new hospital aspired to university rank. Pathologist Kenneth Pritzker later said in an interview, "The hospital had the ambition right from the start, right from the Yorkville days, of becoming a teaching hospital and a research hospital. They absolutely insisted that the hospital be on University Avenue and remain on University Avenue."[72] Pritzker observed that from the very beginning of the founding of New Mount Sinai Hospital in 1953 research remained a coveted objective: "It's almost forgotten that the hospital had a research department with a small dedicated space on the 12th floor perhaps 3,000 sq ft and 2–3 researchers, funded fully from hospital resources. The research department was envisioned, built and operationally organized by Drs. Bernard S. Liebel and Harold Pritzker. By 1966, a small amount of new research space had been disencumbered for the young academic physicians and surgeons, Jerry Bain, Paul Walfish, Irving Koven and Robert Ruderman."[73]

Once in the new building in 1974, "the atmosphere for teaching and clinical research," said Pritzker, "was buzzing with energy. For the first time in the faculty's history a critical mass of young physicians with training from all over North America had come together within 1–2 years to begin their careers mentored by a cadre of enthusiastic teachers who were only 10–15 years older. Mount Sinai, equipped for the time with splendid education facilities, set out to be the best teaching hospital for undergraduate students and the most attractive hospital for residents. These latter programs had multidisciplinary components. By the end of the 1970's this goal had been achieved and other organizations were palpably envious."[74]

Then the hospital progressed to a proper research institute, and in 1975 the Mount Sinai Institute was registered as a charitable foundation, the purpose of which was "to assist Mount Sinai Hospital in its research program."[75] In 1976 the hospital formed a Research Advisory Committee, with eighteen to twenty projects in course every year, privileging gerontology and immunology. Obstetrician Sidney Tobin was the acting director, and Lou Siminovitch, George Connell, and John Hamilton, all campus heavyweights, served as external advisers.[76] By the 1979–80 session, the staff had bulked up: there were now 157 clerks, interns, residents, and fellows. The hospital's medical-dental staff of 306 all had teaching appointments at U of T. So a critical mass was forming.

In the 1979–80 session the board created a Scientific Advisory Committee to further the drawing up of research applications; by this point forty-two research projects were in course at the hospital. A promised million-dollar gift from the estate of Harold Tanenbaum resulted in naming the research facility after the donor.[77] (Pritzker said that owing to "financial difficulties" only $250,000 was actually donated and that "the name was quietly dropped after a few years.") Tobin, chair of the Research Advisory Committee, said, "The Hospital from its inception has been cognizant of the fact that to obtain excellence in patient care and clinical teaching, a successful research programme is necessary. Therefore the Hospital has strived over the years to achieve excellence in research."[78]

In the 1980–1 session an Office of Research Administration was set up.[79] It began looking for targets of opportunity, and, as the location of a fourth unit in Toronto for cardiovascular surgery was up for grabs, the hospital made a strong play for it – with emphasis on the "considerable degree of cooperation [that] already exists" with TGH[80] – losing out, however, to Sunnybrook. There was a thought that Bernie Goldman might be appointed to cardiovascular surgery at the Sinai and somehow bridge open-heart surgery between the General and the Sinai, but Goldman ended up running the open-heart surgery program at Sunnybrook instead (see p. 557).[81]

A new era began for research at MSH in 1985 when Lou Siminovitch became inaugural director of research at the Mount Sinai Institute. Much of this story concerns molecular medicine and is told in chapter 28. But Siminovitch did lay down certain principles that applied not just to molecular biology but to research at the hospital in general, in the wet labs and animal facilities on the hospital's eighth and ninth floors, where the director had, as Siminovitch said in February 1985, "complete control over budget, space and people." He insisted that half the space be allocated to basic science, the rest to clinical research. Research at the institute would not be organized, he said, on a departmental basis but programmatically. Alan Bernstein, Robert Kerbel, and John Roder were already on board as directors of their specific divisions.[82]

What was behind this intense drive for research, this upgrading of a shoestring community hospital into a research behemoth? Kenneth Pritzker, who had a ringside seat at the dinner table of his father Harold, founder of the Department of Pathology, said it "was definitely the Board of Governors, absolutely. The Board had this ambition, and it's not often talked about explicitly, but there were two drivers. One was to provide the very best care; and the other was a projection of the Jewish community and the good the Jewish community could do for the general community. That was very much a driver, and probably still is a driver."[83]

*Some of the Mount Sinai Departments*

The hospital departments themselves, quite separate from the Research Institute, also ginned up research. (This story is told throughout this book rather than merely in the following several pages.)

In the 1967–8 session, Stanley Greben founded the hospital Department of Psychiatry, establishing a Mount Sinai tradition of emphasis on psychotherapy.

Under Greben, in the 1970–1 session, the department organized a Youth Clinic at the New Mount Sinai Hospital.[84] Later chairs such as Joel Sadavoy (in 1993) and Molyn Leszcz (in 2006) were also much inclined to psychotherapy. Yet the great break in this psychotherapy stream at the Sinai was the appointment of Mary Seeman in 1985 as psychiatrist-in-chief. Seeman made fundamental contributions to the literature on schizophrenia, where she pioneered the study of gender differences and became an international figure.[85]

In the 1967–8 session, the hospital Department of Radiology became a teaching department as Bernard J. Shapiro, radiologist-in-chief, was appointed to the university faculty.[86] Shapiro was one of the foundation figures in Toronto radiology. Born in Montreal in 1920, he earned an MD from McGill in 1943, served in the Canadian Army Medical Corps, then finished radiology training and worked at the Jewish General Hospital in Montreal. After a brief sojourn at the University of Western Ontario, he arrived in Toronto in 1955 as radiologist-in-chief at the New Mount Sinai Hospital, where he stayed abreast of the technology wave then sweeping radiology. He acquired for the Sinai one of the first gamma cameras in Canada and in 1971 became a founding member of the Canadian Association of Nuclear Medicine. One of his students wrote at the time of his death in 1996, "The residents he referred for training with the luminaries in various fields of diagnosis and intervention returned to help establish diagnostic imaging as a diverse, powerful specialty. Many of us who came under Bernie's influence as medical students or interns were attracted to diagnostic imaging as a career by absorbing his enthusiasm and vision."[87] Ken Pritzker added, "Bernie was a great enthusiast for multidisciplinary teaching, rather exceptional in the 1970's. We had weekly rounds where those of us interested in musculoskeletal disease, Bernie, Allan Gross in Surgery, Joe Houpt in Rheumatology, Jose Jiminez in Rehabilitation Medicine and myself in Pathology participated. We taught each other and our students around discussion of specific current cases."[88]

When Shapiro stepped down as chief in 1980, George Wortzman replaced him. Wortzman faced immediately the problem of "staff ... involved with private outside interests on a non-pooled basis," and several members left the department as Wortzman steered the group, which had just acquired a CT scanner, increasingly in the direction of research.[89]

The large Department of Medicine became a teaching department in the 1962–3 session. In the following year, Mitchell Kohan, who as previous chief had led the department into the university, retired and was succeeded by Barney Berris. At this point, several clinicians active in research were already on staff, most notable of whom was probably Victor Feinman, who organized a liver clinic for the study of infectious hepatitis. "We had the foundation of an outstanding medical department. I was very grateful to all of these doctors, who carried the ball for six years until additional staff could be appointed," Berris later said.[90]

Berris made some significant appointments in the hospital's Department of Medicine. In 1971 he lured Allan Adelman from the General to begin catheterization in heart disease. In 1972 they added Jerald Bain, an endocrinologist from the Western, and Noe Zamel, a full-time researcher who started a pulmonary function lab at Mount Sinai and who, while previously at the University of Nebraska, was noted for "flow volume curve" research in small-airway obstruction.[91] (At Mount Sinai, Zamel proceeded to find his flow volume curves unhelpful in diagnosing obstructive sleep apnea, however useful in routinely evaluating pulmonary function.[92]) In 1973 Jack Colman was appointed to supervise the coronary care unit and Arnie Aberman joined the staff to co-direct the Intensive Care Unit. Berris, Colman, and Aberman shared the same office because the new hospital had not yet opened. Berris said, "Some days we felt like the Marx brothers coming in and going out of the office door. The three of us took the situation lightly and we became good friends."[93]

In 1974 Alexander ("Sandy") Logan, a nephrologist, joined the internists, according to Berris "the first non-Jewish doctor in the Department of Medicine and was later followed by many others."[94]

The Department of Medicine at Mount Sinai developed its own three-year training program for residents, accredited by the Royal College. "Some of the top graduating students came to train at Mount Sinai," said Berris, "because they wanted to learn from the new staff doctors we were hiring." Berris had no trouble making new appointments, he said. "They were excited by the challenge of building their specialty in a new academic department." He noted, "Hospital administrators and the board of directors were determined that Mount Sinai should become a major research centre." But what they needed was funding. Berris created a Department of Medicine Research Fund to which grateful former patients contributed.[95]

The stories of the involvement of the Department of Medicine at Sinai with tropical diseases and with the Centre for Cardiovascular Research are told elsewhere in this volume.

In the 1963–4 session the Department of Surgery at the Sinai, under David R. Bohnen, who had just been appointed surgeon-in-chief in 1961, joined the faculty teaching program. A number of staff on the teaching unit of thirty-two beds received university appointments.[96] Of the department's various achievements, high on the list would be Allan Gross's 1972 knee transplantation operation, acknowledged by the American Hospital Association as "among the ten most important recent advances in medicine" (see pp. 156–157).[97] Just as a footnote, as Bernie Langer recalls, Bohnen "was the first Jewish guy taken on in the Gallie Course in Toronto. Before that, everybody had to go somewhere else. And Bohnen became chief of surgery at Mount Sinai rather quickly. He was not allowed to stay on staff at Toronto General very long." Bernie Langer was the first Jew given a regular staff appointment in surgery at the General.[98]

The Department of Surgery at the Sinai contributed to surgical education when in September 1998 the doors of the surgical skills centre (Centre for Surgical Education and Research) opened under the direction of Carol Hutchison, "largely due to the generosity of US Surgical Corporation which has donated $1.5 million over the first five years of the Centre's operation."[99] Pritzker said, "This was an accomplishment of the Chief of Surgery, Zane Cohen, who lobbied his mentor Bernie Langer and MSH equally in the competition for this centre." Surgery residents and medical students were able to practice making incisions. External reviewers who visited the hospital in 2007 found this centre to be one of the jewels of the Department of Surgery: "a very impressive facility with high and low fidelity simulators, some of which are very innovative."[100]

Of the department's innovative Division of Orthopaedic Surgery, led by Allan Gross: in 1988–9 Robert Bell moved from St Michael's to the Sinai, where he was joined by Fred Langer and Andrei Czitrom "in establishing an orthopaedic oncology unit, the first of its kind in Canada."[101]

There are some stories to tell of the Sinai's Department of Pathology. In 1938 Harold Pritzker established a laboratory in the old hospital at 100 Yorkville Avenue. Pritzker was among the pioneers of Jewish medicine in Toronto. He was born in Cleveland in 1909 and came as a child to Toronto, attending the Williamson Road Public School and Malvern Collegiate Institute. He earned an arts degree in biological and medical sciences in 1931 at U of T and a medical degree in 1934, a classmate of Vera Peters. Unsurprisingly, he "returned to the city of his birth" at Cleveland's Mount Sinai Hospital to take his internship (given that Jews were not accepted in Toronto hospitals), decided on pathology, and spent the next two years training at St Luke's Hospital in Cleveland. Pritzker returned to Toronto in 1937 "to be the first pathologist at the original Mount Sinai Hospital on Yorkville Avenue." He was given two rooms in the basement and shortly developed a laboratory. "For lab equipment," said his son Ken in an interview, "he went over to the local Woolworth's and bought dishes and things like that for $50, this was the kind of budget they had." Yet they did autopsies in the little lab, and it was outstanding to the extent that, as his Faculty Council eulogist put it, "soon his talents were sought by other hospitals." The position at the Yorkville Avenue hospital was unsalaried – the hospital offered something to every Jewish physician who asked – and to keep body and soul together, Pritzker had a family practice in the basement of his house and also secured a staff position as the first pathologist at the Oshawa General Hospital.

During the war he organized laboratory services at the Oshawa General Hospital and at St Mary's Hospital, the later Scarborough General Hospital. With the opening of the New Mount Sinai Hospital in 1953, Pritzker became their full-time laboratory director. In the new pathology labs they began accepting residents, simple enough in those days because residents were hospital-based, not university-based. Pathology became a university department in 1963 as the other hospital departments began to affiliate with the faculty.

The contributions of many other scientists and clinicians from the Mount Sinai – such as endocrinologists Paul Walfish and Bernard Zinman – are scattered throughout this volume. The story of the hospital in its growth from a starveling community facility on Yorkville Avenue to an international scientific powerhouse at 600 University Avenue is actually quite astonishing and continues in chapter 28, "Molecular Medicine."

## Women's College Hospital

The Union of those who love on behalf of those who suffer.

Women's College Hospital, 1915

When the Faculty of Medicine was re-established in 1887, it was as an exclusively male institution, which it remained for nearly two decades. Women were not admitted until 1906. (For further details on women in the faculty see chapter 3.)

*Early Days*

Women's College Hospital traces its origins to the establishment in 1883 of the Woman's Medical College in Toronto, renamed the Ontario Medical College for Women (OMCW) in 1895 after amalgamating with a rival school in Kingston. Although it did not itself grant degrees, the college qualified students to sit the medical examinations at Trinity (with which it was loosely affiliated), Victoria, and the U of T; clinical instruction was provided through special arrangements with the General, HSC, and St Michael's. "Although special attention was given to ensuring that the curriculum provided was identical to that offered in medical schools for men," the college emphasized training in gynecology, obstetrics, and "the diseases of children."

A midwifery service, in which trainees "provided women in the community with pre- and post-natal care and attended home births," was established in 1891, and in 1898 a Dispensary for Women was set up in the college building on Sumach Street in Toronto's east end by Ida Lynd, Jennie Gray, and Susanna Boyle. Here trainees "received instruction in dispensing and pharmacy,"[102] while senior medical students "assisted in clinic activities." The Dispensary proved popular, especially with less affluent women: fees were reduced or waived for those who could not afford them. "Medical advice was given free of charge and medicaments dispensed for only a 'nominal' fee."[103]

In 1972 Geraldine Maloney, a former chief of obstetrics and gynecology at Women's College Hospital, commented on the value of the Dispensary for both medical women and the community. Prior to its existence, she said, "[t]here were no facilities for women physicians to treat patients other than in their offices or the patients' homes. There were no clinics where patients, unable to pay, could consult a woman physician and, above all, no facilities for women medical students to see patients or gain any practical experience."[104]

By the early 1900s enrolment at the OMCW began to decline as co-educational medical programs started to appear in American and Canadian universities. In 1905 its directors proposed the creation of a Faculty of Medicine for Women at the University of Toronto, but this plan was rejected, the university instead announcing that the Faculty of Medicine would now admit female students. In the spring of 1906, therefore, the college closed its doors and its students transferred to U of T. The midwifery service was lost with the closure of the college, but the Dispensary survived,[105] moving in February 1908 to the corner of Parliament and Queen Streets.

During this period two groups of women came together to advance the creation of a women's hospital. A committee of physicians led by Emma Skinner-Gordon joined forces with a group of philanthropic women and adopted the name "Women's College Hospital Committee" in memory of the college in which the Dispensary had been formed.[106] Their mandate: "To provide for women, medical and surgical care by physicians and surgeons of their own sex; to furnish opportunities for female medical graduates to continue their studies in all branches of medicine; to afford facilities for clinical instruction to women medical students and to train nurses in the care of the sick."[107]

In October 1911 the group bought a building on Seaton Street, also in the east end of the city, and the new seven-bed Women's College Hospital and Dispensary opened its doors on 10 November 1911 with Skinner-Gordon as medical director. (Ironically, the hospital's first patient was male, a six-year old boy.) Its founding staff consisted of the eleven women doctors who had been on the staff of the OMCW when it closed in 1906,[108] plus Jane Sproule, newly returned to Toronto after becoming Canada's first woman specialist with British qualifications in otolaryngology. Sproule (later Sproule-Manson – see p. 549) began the hospital's first specialty service, an ear, nose, and throat clinic.[109]

Among those who continued on the active staff at WCH were Ida Lynd and Jennie Gray Wildman, founding directors of the Dispensary. Both were early graduates of the original Woman's Medical College. Lynd (MB from Trinity in 1890), the second woman to practice medicine in Toronto, was the college's instructor in materia medica. She went on to become the hospital's first chief of medicine from 1920 to 1926 and remained in practice for more than fifty years, dying in 1943 at the age of eighty-six.[110] Wildman (MD and CM from Trinity in 1892), who taught anatomy and gynecology at the OMCW, became the first head of gynecology at WCH, 1920–6.[111]

In keeping with the college's original focus on obstetrical care, the hospital's first baby was born on 25 December 1911. As WCH's first head nurse, Clara Dixon, recalled, a woman was left on their doorstep by her husband on Christmas Eve, "well on in labour and soon ready for delivery. The hospital was not ready for obstetrical work, had no place for babies." Isabella Wood arrived "by horse and buggy" and took charge, reminding the staff "that the first Christmas Baby had no bed." A bassinet was hastily improvised from a clothes basket, and the child arrived at "3AM on Christmas day ... The birth of the hospital's first baby was quite a challenge, but everything went fine with the confinement, and we have never stopped having babies since."[112] Wood, a 1903 graduate of the college, was connected with St Michael's and Toronto Western as well as WCH during her fifty-year medical career and "was widely known for her work among mothers and children."[113]

The seven-bed facility on Seaton Street quickly became inadequate, and again Skinner-Gordon and Mrs Annie Rutherford, president of the hospital board from 1909 to 1923, organized a fundraising campaign for a larger facility.[114] In 1915 WCH moved to a site on Rusholme Road in the west end, accommodating twenty-five adult beds and ten infant cots. A nursing school and residence was established the same year in a rented building nearby.[115] Along with its new quarters, the hospital selected a motto: "The Union of those who love on behalf of those who suffer." During the war the number of patients continued to increase, and by November 1918 another property had been purchased and a new wing was ready for use. Before any patients were admitted, however, the facility was temporarily commandeered by the city to manage the 1919 influenza epidemic. Following this crisis, the wing opened with an increased capacity of fifty-two beds and twenty-five infant cots.[116]

In addition to directing the Seaton Street hospital, Skinner-Gordon was head of pediatrics there and at Rusholme Road, retiring in 1936. Described in her 1949 obituary as a humanitarian with an interest in youth, she also "organized a small group of incorrigible boys into a religious and educational club" in 1898, founded the Merton Street Gospel Mission, "and was an enthusiastic member of the Women's Christian Temperance Union."[117]

Even before the move to Rusholme Road, WCH was beginning to develop specific clinical services and departments. As previously noted, an ear, nose, and throat clinic was opened in 1911,[118] and in 1914 Margaret McCallum-Johnston became the first chief of the Department of Anaesthesia. A 1900 graduate of the OMCW, McCallum became the first woman to obtain an internship in a Canadian hospital (at the Hospital for Sick Children) and in 1903 joined the staff of the Women's Dispensary. The following year she married Samuel Johnston, "who was in fact the first full-time anesthetist in Canada (contrary to reports that Dr. Margaret was) at the Toronto General Hospital" and introduced her to the specialty.[119] McCallum-Johnston continued to head the department until 1925 and remained a member of the active medical staff until her retirement in 1930.[120] Hannah Reid (MB from OMCW in 1905) became her assistant in 1914 and succeeded her as chief of anesthesia in 1926. In addition she opened a private practice in obstetrics which she maintained until 1950.[121]

Obstetrics and gynecology were of course among the hospital's key clinical services from the beginning. As in other hospitals and in the Faculty of

Medicine itself, these were initially treated as separate disciplines (see chapter 21), with Rowena Hume as the first chief of obstetrics and Jennie Gray Wildman as chief of gynecology.[122] After graduating from the OMCW (MD and CM in 1899) Hume undertook postgraduate studies in England and the United States before returning to the college as an instructor in pathology and bacteriology and member of the Dispensary. In addition to her position at WCH, she was a lecturer in bacteriology at the university's School of Household Science and an early pioneer of family planning. When the Hamilton Planned Parenthood Society was formed in 1930, she made weekly visits for a year when no other physician would do so. She was still running a private practice from her Toronto home at the age of eighty-nine when she was murdered by a transient worker whom she had employed to do odd jobs.[123]

Previously gynecology had been the traditional "medical" variety. Surgical gynecology was launched soon after the establishment of WCH by Jennie Smillie, the first woman to perform major gynecological procedures in Canada.[124] Smillie began her medical education with the last class of the OMCW, completing her MD in 1909 at U of T. Unable to obtain an internship or surgical training in Toronto, she took a residency and six months' training in surgery at the Quakers' Women's Hospital in Philadelphia and later took additional postgraduate work in New York and London. Returning to Toronto in 1911 to find that no hospital would grant surgical privileges to a woman, Smillie performed her first laparotomy on the patient's kitchen table – "at noon, so the light was good."[125] A leading figure in the establishment and evolution of Women's College, she was associate chief of gynecology until 1942 and remained on its staff until 1948, "doing mostly abdominal and gynecological surgery."[126] Following her retirement, Smillie married her childhood sweetheart, Alex Robertson (by now a widower), at the age of seventy, "and they had a happy 10 years together before his death."[127]

In 1926 obstetrics and gynecology were combined into a single department headed until 1947 by Marion Grant Kerr. The daughter of a physician, Kerr graduated with an MB from the Faculty of Medicine in 1919; the yearbook noted, "In spite of being Scotch, she can see jokes and give feeds ... Success will attend her."[128] She interned at the General and undertook postgraduate training in 1929 at the Rotunda Hospital, Dublin, and the Royal Infirmary, Glasgow, and again in 1934 in Vienna and Budapest. The growth of the obstetrical service during her tenure is illustrated by the fact that when she joined the hospital staff "there were only six public obstetrical beds. This number was increased to 23 in 1935 and still more when the new building on Grenville St. was opened on Jan. 4, 1936."[129]

In 1915 Minerva Reid became the inaugural chief of surgery at WCH (earning an MD and CM from OMCW in 1905). She took over a brother's private practice in Tillsonburg for a few years while he undertook postgraduate studies abroad, then proceeded to London and Dublin herself in 1911, acquiring surgical and medical credentials there. During World War I she served as an assistant to surgeon Fred Starr and headed the surgical service at WCH until 1925. Minerva was a younger sister of anesthetist/obstetrician Hannah Reid, with whom she often worked. Reid remained on the active staff of the hospital until 1938, although she continued a private practice until 1955. In addition to her clinical activities, she served on the Toronto Board of Education from 1928 to 1932 and in 1944 headed a committee of Toronto women to press for the speedy construction of Sunnybrook Hospital to replace the antiquated veterans' facilities at the Christie Street Hospital.[130]

With the 1919 expansion of WCH, an X-ray department was established by Elizabeth Stewart.[131] A graduate of the second co-educational class in medicine at U of T in 1911, she interned at Women's Hospital in Philadelphia, then returned to Toronto as a member of the medical staff of WCH in 1913. In 1918–19 she undertook specialty training in radiology at Lennox Hill Hospital in New York and at Johns Hopkins in Baltimore, "possibly because all the other hospitals were acquiring departments and she wanted to keep Women's College abreast of the times."[132] Upon her return Stewart became Canada's first career radiologist and one of only four physicians doing all the X-ray work in Toronto. In 1923 she was joined by Helen Bell-Milburn, who had likewise studied radiology in New York and had worked as a radiotherapist at the General in 1922–3. Milburne went on to become the hospital's breast specialist and head of the outpatient department.[133] Both women retired in 1955 as the department moved into new quarters on the second floor of the Grenville Street hospital.[134]

Around 1919–20 a pathology department was launched by Vivian Laughlen, followed by a venereal-disease clinic administered by Edna Mary Guest and "sponsored by the recently established Provincial Board of Health and the city of Toronto."[135] Guest was one of three women who graduated with 150 men from the faculty in 1910, and she went on to have a remarkable and varied career. Following postgraduate work at Harvard and internship at the Women's and Children's Hospital in Boston, she worked from 1912 to 1915 as a medical missionary, professor of anatomy, and assistant in surgery at the Women's Medical College in Ludhiana, India, then served in several hospital units during the First World War, finishing up in charge of the base hospital on the Western Front in France in 1918–19. (For this work she was later, in 1935, awarded an OBE by King George V.[136]) Upon returning to Toronto after the war, Guest established a private practice in the Medical Arts Building in addition to her work at WCH, where she went on to become the hospital's second chief of surgery from 1926 to 1931 and officiated at the opening of the Grenville Street hospital shortly before her retirement in 1936.

In 1924 Jane Sproule-Manson returned to WCH, joining the active staff as chief of the ear, nose, and throat department, a position she held until her retirement in 1940.[137] She had been appointed an assistant in the Department of Otolaryngology at the General in 1912, and during the First World War she served for two years at the London Hospital before returning to her position in Toronto. According to the 1993 history of the hospital, Sproule-Manson "worked diligently to promote the study of epidemiology and made health and community medicine a priority for Women's College Hospital."

*Towards a Modern Hospital*

In 1924 its name was officially changed from Women's College Hospital and Dispensary to just Women's College Hospital.[138] In the late 1920s, two houses on large lots were purchased at Grenville Street and Surrey Place. These buildings served as the hospital's new outpatient clinic[139] and, more significantly, were deliberately chosen for their proximity to the University of Toronto. Surgeon-in-chief Jessie Gray, the first woman to become a Fellow of the Royal College of Surgeons of Canada, later remarked on WCH's goal of becoming a teaching hospital. "The men at the University, of course, knew nothing about this and probably would have laughed heartily had they known. But a group of determined women is a force to be reckoned with."[140]

The goal of teaching-hospital status, however, proved contentious. The Board of Governors in the interwar period was forward-thinking, encouraging "staff members to gain advanced qualifications," and actively promoted the move to the Grenville site. Some of the staff, including radiologist Elizabeth Stewart and otolaryngologist Jane Sproule-Manson, were also "dedicated to the ... association of the hospital with a teaching institution." But others, for "equally valid" reasons, did not.[141] In 1935 and again in 1947, the majority of the medical staff voted against affiliation. Opponents of this measure recognized that WCH "would ... have to give up some of its autonomy and permit the University of Toronto to approve policies and appointments. This was not an acceptable trade-off for many of the women who remembered the days when they could not gain a staff appointment at any hospital." Most significantly, appointment to the faculty required fellowship status in the Royal College of Physicians and Surgeons of Canada, though very few women had yet attained this level of postgraduate specialty training.[142] (Surgeons Jessie Gray and Marjorie Davis, physician Jean Davey, and ob-gyn Geraldine Maloney were among the first to do so, during the Second World War.[143] Davey, born in Hamilton, Ontario, in 1909 and a medical graduate of the U of T in 1936, was, according to a standard source, "the first Canadian woman doctor to enter the Canadian armed forces. ... [As] Senior Medical Officer and squadron leader RCAF, 1939–45, [she was] responsible for the medical aspects of the women's division."[144]) The older staff members realized that "men would have to be hired in order to satisfy the University's requirements for professors,"[145] a step they were not (yet) prepared to take.

Meanwhile in 1928 the hospital's Board of Governors, under the direction of its chair, the powerful Florence (Mrs Archibald) Huestis, launched a campaign to raise $750,000 for the new hospital. "Mrs Huestis persevered even during the Depression years to secure funding from the general public, the business community and the Board of Control of Toronto. Their campaign slogan, 'How Long Shall They Be Turned Away?' captured people's imagination and in 1934 with the Prime Minister R. B. Bennett officiating, the cornerstone for the first building of today's Women's College Hospital was laid." On 22 February 1936 (following a month's postponement out of respect for the death of King George V on 20 January), the hospital was officially opened by Governor General Lord Tweedsmuir. "The new hospital was ten stories tall with 140 beds and 45 cots. It had a well-equipped laboratory and an X-Ray Department. The ninth floor was fully outfitted with up-to-date operating rooms and the tenth floor had obstetrical delivery and labor rooms."[146]

With the outbreak of war, opportunities for women in medicine in both military and civilian life began to expand. Jessie Catherine Gray,[147] a 1934 medical graduate of U of T, had been a kind of supernova as a medical student, arriving at the faculty with a BA in hand (as well as the Moss Scholarship for "all-round competence"[148]) and plunging herself into tennis, hockey, and Daffydil; she was a class officer in every year, editor of the *University of Toronto Medical Journal*, and, someone noted in black ink in the margin of her entry in the yearbook *Torontonensis*, "head of year."[149] Her professional career was marked by so many "firsts" that she would become known as Canada's "First Lady of Surgery":[150] the first woman to win the gold medal for highest standing in her graduating class, the first accepted into the Gallie Course in surgery, the first to obtain a master of surgery degree at the University of Toronto (1939),[151] the first to hold a surgical residency at the General Hospital (1940–1), and the first "to earn the fellowship degree in the Royal College of Physicians and Surgeons of Canada as a surgical specialist."[152]

Gray's acceptance into the surgical program was all the more remarkable given Gallie's low opinion of female surgeons at the time: in 1941–2, he ranked women alongside the "medically unfit" and "casual applicants" during the wartime absence of the stalwart young men usually in his program.[153] Along with Marjorie Davis (the second woman to hold a surgical residency at TGH[154]), she remained there during the war, studying the effect of the sulfa drugs in peritonitis among her other duties.[155] By 1945 Gallie's attitude towards women in surgery may have softened somewhat, given that he reported, "The two young ladies have given assistance of the highest order both in the matter of teaching and in the routine operative and clinical work of the hospital."[156]

In addition to her wartime position at TGH, Gray joined the staff of WCH in July 1941 as associate surgeon-in-chief and in 1942 was appointed a clinical instructor in the Faculty of Medicine. She was appointed surgeon-in-chief at Women's College Hospital in 1946 and remained in this position until her retirement in 1964. In 1954 she was one of nine women physicians (and the sole Canadian) awarded an Elizabeth Blackwell Citation from the New York Infirmary in celebration of the hundredth anniversary of women in medicine,[157] and in 1973 she received a Toronto Civic Award of Merit "for her career as a distinguished public servant."[158] Along with Florence McConney, its inaugural director, she helped establish Canada's first Cancer Detection Clinic at WCH in 1948; although not a cancer specialist, Gray's "surgical judgements and techniques were so outstanding that she was called one of the four top cancer surgeons in North America."[159] In 1957 the Department of Surgery was accredited for undergraduate teaching in the Faculty of Medicine, and by the 1959–60 session, second-year surgery clinics were being conducted by Gray along with Marjorie Davis and Olive Ibberson.[160] Following her death in 1978, a memorial fund was set up in her name, resulting in the establishment of the Jessie Gray Colorectal Unit in 1982, a service for the early detection of cancers of the colon and rectum.

Wartime opportunities played an even greater role in the career of Jean Davey.[161] The daughter of a Hamilton physician, she graduated in medicine at Toronto in 1936 and joined the staff of WCH in 1939. She had been about to embark on postgraduate study in England when these plans were derailed by the outbreak of World War II. Instead she became the first woman doctor to enter the Canadian Armed Forces. From 1941 to 1945 she served as senior medical officer of the Royal Canadian Air Force, with the rank of squadron leader, and was responsible for medical care in the Women's Division. In recognition of her wartime contributions she was awarded the Order of the British Empire in 1943.

In 1945, with the end of the war, Davey became the first Canadian woman to obtain the Royal College of Physicians and Surgeons of Canada in medicine by examination. She returned to WCH as associate chief of medicine and in 1950 succeeded Florence McConney[162] as chief. In 1958 university teaching status was extended to the hospital's Department of Medicine, and undergraduate lectures began that fall under Davey, Joan Vale, and Marguerite Hill in "a closed teaching unit of 40 beds."[163] The university affiliation made Davey the first woman to head a Department of Medicine in a Canadian teaching hospital. When she died in 1980, a rose garden was established in front of the hospital in honour of her interest in rose gardening and "as a loving tribute to her professional skills, compassion, and ability to inspire and teach students."[164]

### Hilliard

The best-known figure at WCH during the post-war years, however, was Marion Hilliard, who led the Department of Obstetrics and Gynaecology from 1947 until 1956.[165] Anna Marion Hilliard was born in Morrisburg, Ontario, in 1902, the third of five children in what a eulogist described as "a family whose heritage was one of leadership and courage based on firm conviction."[166] A 1924 arts graduate of Toronto's Victoria College, she entered the faculty and graduated with an MD in 1927, distinguishing herself both scholastically and as an athlete. In October 1927, the Faculty Council stated, "Medicine is honoured in having the most outstanding woman athlete at the University as a graduate of '27.

While Miss Marion Hilliard particularly excels at hockey, she also takes part in tennis tournaments, and plays interfaculty basketball, Star left wing of the intercollegiate hockey team for the past five years, Captain 1924 and 1927."[167] She then spent a year abroad training in obstetrics and gynecology at the Queen Charlotte Lying-in Hospital in London and the Rotunda Hospital, Dublin, becoming the third woman to obtain the LRCP (London) and MRCP (London). Following her return to Toronto, she was appointed to the staff of WCH as assistant to Marion Kerr, chief of obstetrics and gynecology.

In the mid-1940s Hilliard began to work with Eva Mader MacDonald (sometimes McDonald) and William L. Robinson of the Banting Institute, professor of pathology and the hospital's consulting pathologist, on a simplified test for cervical cancer (based on "the work of [Georgios] Papanicolaou and others" but requiring only regular pathological methods rather than a "trained cytologist and the necessary laboratory"). Their new "cervical scrapings test" was developed in 1947, and in 1950 Hilliard reported on its introduction and early results in the *Canadian Medical Association Journal*.[168] (MacDonald herself is an interesting figure. Born in Nova Scotia in 1902, she decided to study medicine after helping her father treat burn victims from the explosion in 1917 in the Halifax harbor. She was director of laboratories at WCH from 1945 to 1952.[169])

The introduction of this valuable screening test was followed closely by another cancer initiative in which she played an important role. "After much work and lobbying for money,"[170] Hilliard opened Canada's first Cancer Detection Clinic in April 1948. Florence McConney, the clinic's inaugural director, modelled the facility on the Strang Cancer Prevention Clinic at New York's Memorial Hospital. One dignitary praised this innovation at the clinic's official opening, declaring, "Ignorance is cancer's greatest friend, knowledge is its most potent enemy."[171] Interest in this service was immense: according to a biographer, "So many women came on their own initiative or by referral from doctors all over Canada ... that in five months blueprints were drawn up for alterations ... to provide expanded quarters."[172] By May 1949 the clinic had "examined 429 patients" and the waiting list had swelled to 1,700 women.[173] A few months later, WCH's efforts were recognized by the Ontario Cancer Treatment and Research Foundation with an award of $1,000 "for laboratory and clinical cancer research."[174] By 1954 it had seen its ten thousandth patient.[175]

Hilliard succeeded Marion Kerr as chief of the Department of Obstetrics and Gynaecology in 1947 and became one of the most notable figures in the history of the specialty in Canada; in one biography she was said to have "made the largest impact on the community due to her strong and vital personality ... During her 27 years [at WCH], her department gained a world-wide reputation."[176] This was justly deserved: in 1953, the *Canadian Medical Association Journal* reported, 2,800 babies – "more than 10% of babies born in Toronto" – were delivered there "without a single maternal death."[177]

*University Affiliation*

During her tenure, Hilliard set about her cherished goal of affiliation with the University of Toronto as a teaching hospital. At a meeting of the Medical Advisory Committee on 20 September 1951, she proposed the issue and received enough encouragement to pursue this objective. On the faculty side she found two crucial sympathizers: Joseph MacFarlane, dean of the faculty, who supported the proposal although "he made some demanding requirements," and Douglas Cannell, chair of obstetrics and gynecology.[178]

Chief among the dean's requirements was that heads of teaching departments hold fellowships in the Royal College, a qualification that no one in her department possessed. She was highly qualified according to pre-war standards – in addition to her British credentials, she had taken further postgraduate studies on infertility at the Poliklinik in Budapest in 1934 – and easily able to obtain Royal College certification in her specialty, which she applied for and received in April 1946. But Hilliard (like most doctors of her generation) was ineligible to take the rigorous fellowship exam without further postgraduate study.[179] She was nevertheless determined to see her department attain teaching status and in 1955 recruited Geraldine Maloney from TGH as associate chief "in charge of the teaching program" on the understanding that Maloney would be her successor.[180] As Maloney later put it, "Dr. Hilliard's stature and the unselfish singlemindedness of her purpose is evidenced by the fact that to achieve her objective she retired as Head of her department in 1956 in order to meet the university requirements regarding the qualifications of that office."[181] The agreement "between the Governors of the University of Toronto and Women's College Hospital" permitting students in the Faculty of Medicine "to take clinical instruction at the Hospital in Obstetrics and Gynaecology" was signed on 15 February 1956.[182] That fall, third-year undergraduates were to begin training there under "Drs. Marion Hilliard, Geraldine Maloney, Sheila Hill, and Henrietta Banting."[183]

Hilliard retired the following year, announcing her intention to the WCH Board on 4 March: "I believe the time is exactly right for me to do this … The affiliation of the Obstetrics and Gynaecology Department with the University of Toronto has been a realization of my dreams."[184]

Hilliard's determination to achieve teaching status for her department spearheaded the affiliation of other departments, surgery in 1957 and medicine in 1959. The entire hospital was affiliated in 1961, when WCH proudly described itself as "a fully accredited teaching hospital with 279 adult beds and 103 infant bassinets, representing all the branches of medicine staffed by women physicians and surgeons."[185]

In the history of women's health care in Canada, these efforts were of great importance. It was also a not inconsiderable achievement for Hilliard to write a best-selling advice manual to women, *A Woman Doctor Looks at Love and Life*, that

Doubleday in New York published in 1956. The book was translated into numerous languages, went through several editions, and, together with her other writings, reached an enormous public. It contained deeply personal notes, such as the news that she had, in her professional capacity, delivered a baby fathered by a man who had jilted her for another woman. Hilliard wrote, "Even at the instant that I delivered the child that might have been mine, I was moved through my anguish to feel, 'This is worth while. What you are doing now is the most worth-while occupation on earth.'"[186]

Geraldine Maloney, who led the department between 1957 and 1966,[187] completed her MD at Toronto in 1937 and did postgraduate work at St Michael's Hospital and in London. In 1942 she joined the Royal Canadian Army Medical Corps, spending most of her time posted in London and rising to chief of medical services for women with the rank of major by the end of the war. In 1945 she passed the Royal College Fellowship examination in obstetrics and gynecology and was on the medical staff at the General before her appointment to WCH. During her tenure the department became increasingly involved in medical education, including the postgraduate training of interns and residents as well as "clinical teaching to third and fourth year students."[188] As her close friend and colleague Marjorie Davis put it, "Medicine was her one great passion."[189]

The full accreditation of WCH coincided with the hospital's fiftieth anniversary, as noted in a *Canadian Medical Association Journal* editorial of February 1961: "The Women's College Hospital of Toronto is the only hospital in this country staffed by women for women patients, and indeed is one of but three such institutions on the North American continent."[190] That some men were later added to the active staff does not alter the hospital's historic roots as staffed for women by women.

*Obstetrics, Gynecology, Perinatology*

Obstetrics and gynecology, already one of the hospital's leading departments, evolved into a powerhouse during this era. The 1962 consultants' report concluded that "this Hospital has a great deal to offer the obstetrical patient,"[191] and although it did not recommend an actual increase in bed capacity, it "urged that this service be accentuated in an effort to maintain the department at its present level and make it the most modern obstetrical service available in Canada."[192] When Geraldine Maloney stepped down as chief in 1966, there were still no suitably qualified female ob-gyns available, and Walter Hannah became the hospital's first male department head. (He would hold this position for the next two decades, becoming in addition the university chair of obstetrics and gynecology in 1981.)

Under Hannah's leadership, the department began an ambitious program in basic research with the recruitment in July 1967 of James W. Goodwin and John E. Milligan, who were the first members of the department to have undertaken postgraduate research fellowships at Oxford under fetal physiology pioneer Geoffrey Dawes.[193] They were tasked with "setting up, in the new wing, laboratory facilities for an intensive programme of research in the physiology of the foetus. This hospital," Hannah reported in 1967, "will be one of the very few areas in Canada where this kind of work will be done – work which is of fundamental and far-reaching importance in our understanding of the complexities of intra-uterine life."[194] In addition to launching a "large animal research program" (carried out initially in a laboratory at Ontario Research Foundation on Queen's Park Crescent[195] and later in the new facilities at WCH), they established the first purpose-built Perinatal Intensive Care Unit in Canada.[196] Goodwin designed the unit – or, more accurately, redesigned it after learning that it was not adjacent to the obstetrical area in the initial plans – and later praised the hospital's leadership for "downing tools" and letting him do it properly.[197] Goodwin was also responsible, along with two colleagues, for devising "[a] simple scoring technique for the antepartum identification of the fetus at risk" and testing it in 936 obstetrical cases at the hospital.[198]

The new perinatal unit opened in the latter half of 1970, coinciding with the recruitment of Ann Llewellyn as full-time head of the department's Division of Paediatrics, which "has added a new dimension to the quality of care we can now provide our newborn infants."[199] WCH's PICU went on to achieve "worldwide advances in the health and survival of infants born prematurely" and was augmented in 1981 with the establishment of Canada's first Regional High-Risk Perinatal Unit. In 1979 Andrew T. Shennan, who had become its neonatal director four years earlier, along with Milligan and chief obstetric resident Peter K. Yeung, reported proudly on the successful delivery and survival of quadruplets in a thirty-two-year-old woman who "had taken no drugs prior to conception that might have resulted in a multiple pregnancy."[200] The positive outcome of this case was attributed to "several aspects of the combined obstetric-neonatal approach to perinatal care," including early diagnosis, close monitoring, and "elective delivery by cesarian section" in order to maximize the survival of the four infants after "persistent twin-to-twin transfusion" was suspected.[201] In 1983 the use of a "natural surfactant preparation" for the prevention of respiratory distress syndrome (RDS) in premature infants was tested by Shennan and Milligan under the direction of Goran Enhorning, a professor of ob-gyn at Toronto who was of Swedish origin, trained at the Karolinska Institute, and had been studying the problem of RDS for twenty years.[202] This trial proved successful and led to the widespread use of surfactant in preterm infants.[203]

By the 1990s, the hospital was well established as a leading centre for perinatology, with its 1993 history stating, "This program is now, and will continue to be of high priority to Women's College Hospital." A strong multidisciplinary research component was established in the form of a university-supported Perinatal Clinical Epidemiology Unit (PCEU) in 1989 under the direction of Mary Hannah and Arne Ohlsson, and the following year the neonatal and follow-up service (formerly a division of pediatrics within the Department of Obstetrics and Gynaecology) became a separate Department of Newborn and Developmental Paediatrics with Andrew Shennan as chief.[204]

While ob-gyn and maternal-fetal medicine thus enjoyed particular prominence during these years, the hospital's other departments and programs also continued to flourish.

### Medicine

The leading figure in the Department of Medicine at WCH during most of this era was F. Marguerite Hill.[205] After graduating with her MA in psychology from the University of Toronto in 1941, she became one of the few women psychologists serving overseas with the Canadian Women's Army Corps. She subsequently entered the Faculty of Medicine, graduated as the gold medalist in 1952, and undertook specialty training in internal medicine. In 1957, during Ray Farquharson's tenure as professor of medicine, she became the first woman to hold the position of chief resident at the Toronto General Hospital. According to Farquharson's daughter, Helen "Nell" Farquharson, a medical student at the time, "We were all appalled."

> Interviewer: "Why?"
> "Oh, you know, it just seemed sort of strange to have, there never had been a girl, a woman on staff."[206]

The following year Hill joined the Department of Medicine at WCH, where along with its chief, Jean Davey, she helped create a strong clinical and teaching unit. In 1965 she succeeded Davey as physician-in-chief (thereby becoming the second woman to hold this position in a U of T teaching hospital) and in 1968 was promoted to full professorship in the Faculty of Medicine. Her philosophy of medical training was patient-centred: "My main concern is that the art of medicine will continue to be as vital as the science of medicine. I want my doctor to have a good and updated base of scientific knowledge ... but I would rather have care and compassion at my bedside than a computer."[207]

### Surgery

Following Jessie Gray's retirement in 1964, the Department of Surgery was led until 1976 by Marjorie Davis (another first-generation Royal College Fellow) and until 1988 by Robert D. Henderson. Bob Henderson was born in Scotland in 1936 and studied medicine at the University of Edinburgh (MB in 1959). After interning at the University of Alberta Hospital in Edmonton – and participating in the flying doctor service in Northern Alberta – he came to Toronto in 1962, obtained his surgical training in the Gallie Course, and became a RCPS Fellow in 1966. Henderson gravitated to Griff Pearson in the new subspecialty of thoracic surgery, helping Pearson perfect an esophageal operation described elsewhere (pp. 167–168), and himself writing a classic textbook, *The Esophagus: Reflux and Primary Motor Disorders*.[208] In the words of his colleague and successor Lavina Lickley, "He became acknowledged both in Canada and internationally as one of the most important authorities on benign esophageal disease. He set up the first esophageal motility laboratory at the Toronto General Hospital. As surgeon-in-chief at Women's College he was said to be "much sought after, and the morning after he was taken ill for the last time [dying of cancer in 1988 at fifty-two] our Chief Resident summed up what we were all thinking when he said, 'It is so awful to think that I will be the last person to scrub with Dr. Henderson and to be able to learn from him.'"[209]

### Family Medicine

In 1954 a group of general practitioners was organized under the leadership of Bette Stephenson into a Department of General Practice,[210] "the first such department ... within a departmentally structured hospital in Toronto."[211] Later renamed the Department of Family Medicine, it was headed by Stephenson until 1964, and in 1966 under Marjorie C. Swanson it was reconfigured as part of the university Department of Medicine (see p. 602). In 1969 it became part of the Department of Family and Community Medicine (DFCM) at the University of Toronto. In 1993 the hospital's Family Practice Health Centre's philosophy was described as treating "each patient as an individual with unique feelings and needs while at the same time recognizing that she or he is also a member of a family unit. By emphasizing education, open communication and feedback between the patient and physician, patients learn to take responsibility for their health care."[212] (A 1964 graduate of the faculty, Stephenson went on to become the first woman president of the Ontario Medical Association in 1970–1 and the Canadian Medical Association in 1973–4, followed by a career as an Ontario legislator from 1974 to 1985.)

Hollister King, the family-physician-in-chief at WCH between 1982 and 1992, was responsible for founding the Teaching Practices Program at the DFCM; at the time of her death in April 1996, this initiative had expanded to include thirty-five "community-based faculty."[213] As of 2008, it had expanded to more than seventy faculty in approximately thirty community practices in rural and northern Ontario and provided 25 percent of the core family medicine training for all second-year residents.[214]

### Dermatology

Dermatology at WCH evolved into a unique resource over nearly half a century through the efforts of one remarkable woman, Ricky Kanee Schachter.[215] According to a grandson, young Ricky Kanee entered medical school over her father's admonition that "she would be taking up a place for a man" and the dean's [MacFarlane's] warning that her "'two congenital anomalies' – being a woman and being Jewish – ensured she wouldn't succeed."[216] After graduating in 1943, Schachter (who had married biochemist Benjamin Schachter in 1942) undertook postgraduate training in dermatology at Columbia University and joined the staff of WCH in 1946 as the founding head of its dermatology service, becoming "the first woman to head an academic division of dermatology in Canada" and remaining its chief until her retirement in 1985. In 1961, as WCH attained teaching hospital status, she was appointed as associate professor in the Faculty of Medicine.

A highlight of Schachter's career was her establishment in April 1976 of the Psoriasis Education and Research Centre (PERC) at WCH, "the first one of its kind on the continent," with funding from the Atkinson Charitable Foundation, federal research grants, and the hospital.[217] In 1992 she commented that PERC had been designed as an outpatient service "because we really believed that we needed to be treating patients in a vertical position rather than a horizontal position." The centre was the first to emphasize self-care in managing chronic skin diseases, "using the three-pronged approach of treatment, education, and research." By the early 1990s, the program had "helped patients from all over the world," including a child from Philadelphia who was enabled to "lead a near-normal life" as a result of her treatments there.[218] In the meantime the Division of Dermatology as a whole had become "so comprehensive that in 1983/84 the TGH moved its skin disease patient beds to WCH,"[219] where medical staff from both hospitals cared for patients in a new twenty-five-bed unit.[220] A fund was established on her retirement in 1985, and in July 1991 it was used to endow the new Ricky Kanee Schachter Dermatology Centre at the hospital. Building on the services she had established, the new centre provided "a unique facility for treating patients with skin diseases."[221]

Schachter was the recipient of many awards during her lifetime, including induction into the Order of Canada in 1998. Yet she was remembered most for her commitment to her patients as people whose "illness just wasn't on the skin" and for her ability to strike "a balance between her career and family."[222] Dean Catharine Whiteside noted in her September 2007 memorial that Schachter "was an advocate for women in academic medicine both as a mentor and a role model … She had an unquestionable passion for women's rights, but what set her apart from many others, was that this tenacity was carefully balanced alongside a tremendous kindness, generosity, and deep commitment to her colleagues, her patients, and always to her family."[223]

## Women's Programs

The preventive approach to women's cancers which originated with the introduction of cervical screening and the Cancer Detection Clinic in the late 1940s was expanded following the hospital's affiliation with U of T. The 1962 consultants' report on services at WCH said that although its "work ... could be done in the Princess Margaret Hospital," nonetheless "there is a particular value in having this service done by women in a women's hospital and we believe that its contribution is so great that it would be a mistake to discontinue this clinic."[224] A 1964 editorial in the *Canadian Medical Association Journal* likewise emphasized the importance and popularity of the Cancer Detection Clinic, still "working in cramped quarters in a house near the hospital," in calling for support for the WCH building campaign.[225] Between 1958 and her retirement in 1971 the clinic was directed by Lady Henrietta (Ball) Banting,[226] widow of the co-discoverer of insulin. She had completed a master's degree in medical research at U of T in 1937, and shortly after her husband's death she entered the medical school, graduating in the wartime class of 1945. In 1957 Banting, who had taken postgraduate ob-gyn training in England, joined the staff of WCH as its first "Hilliard Fellow." "Under her guidance," the *Canadian Medical Association Journal* reported in its 1977 obituary, "the clinic became known as one of the top centres of its kind." Banting also served as a director of the Canadian Cancer Society and "was a lifelong advocate of ... women in medicine," urging young women to enter medicine rather than nursing.[227]

In 1963, under the leadership of M. Elizabeth Forbes, chief of radiology between 1955 and 1975, WCH became the first hospital in Ontario to use mammography for the detection of breast cancer.[228] The Department of Radiology received a grant of $6,000 from the Ontario Cancer Treatment and Research Foundation to fund this initiative.[229] Following Banting's death in 1977, the Henrietta Banting Breast Centre was established in her honour "to provide compassionate, multidisciplinary care for patients with breast disease" along with specialized education and research programs. Breast cancer specialist Lavina Lickley became the centre's co-director in charge of research in 1985[230] (and WCH's surgeon-in-chief from 1988 to 2000);[231] under her leadership the centre was one of twelve facilities across Canada chosen in 1992 to participate in a study investigating the effectiveness of tamoxifen in preventing breast cancer in high-risk women.[232] Lickley herself is a survivor of the disease (though she prefers the term "thriver").[233]

A number of other initiatives focused on women at WCH during the 1970s and 1980s. The Bay Centre for Birth Control, founded by Jadwiga Iwanowska in March 1973, "was the first hospital-supported street centre to make contraception widely available to thousands of clients." Iwanowska was succeeded as medical director in 1980 by Marion Powell,[234] who was also active in family planning education with the University of Toronto's Population Unit – "You can count on the fingers of one hand the number of outstanding sex educators in Canada," she said in 1975, "there's missionary work to be done in this field"[235] – and was instrumental in establishing a Regional Women's Health Centre at WCH in 1988. This facility provided educational and support services for women at all stages of life, including single mothers and individuals dealing with premenstrual syndrome, menopause, and infertility.[236] In response to public concern about acute and follow-up treatment for rape victims, the hospital set up Ontario's first regional Sexual Assault Care Centre in 1984, a unique multidisciplinary resource.[237] And in 1987, Howard Book, chief of the hospital's Department of Psychiatry (a unit dating back to 1954), launched the Brief Psychotherapy Centre for Women, designed to provide "holistic treatment of women's psychological difficulties."[238]

In 1989 WCH expressed an interest in "setting up a Women's Health Programme of international stature" and was seeking a "linkage with another institution."[239] In 1995 the hospital joined forces with the University of Toronto to form the Centre for Research in Women's Health (CRWH), with Heather Maclean, a former chair of the Department of Nutritional Sciences as director.[240] By 2003, CRWH had more than 250 partners, "including universities, hospitals and health centres, funding agencies, corporations, and community-based national and international organizations from across Canada and around the world."[241]

The hospital's later merger with Sunnybrook Health Sciences Centre, and subsequent de-merger, will not be considered here.

## Afterthought

It was from the cauldron of discrimination and prejudice that Toronto was able to draw the glistening new talent that women and Jews brought to medicine and science and that Mount Sinai Hospital and Women's College Hospital arrayed in research and patient care. Yet women and Jews were not the only groups that had been marginalized and stifled: one thinks of the hostile reception the Italians met with their arrival, the South Asians derided with ethnic slurs, and the Chinese segregated in their various "Chinatowns" of Metro Toronto. The new talent brought to medicine in the 1950s and after was stunning, overthrowing the dominance of the Protestant denizens of rural Ontario that populated earlier chapters and strengthening the faculty immeasurably in its drive for international recognition. The success of this drive was owed to the end of gender discrimination and to the talents that surged in Toronto's ethnic communities. It is a story of the triumph of brilliance and drive over prejudice and narrow-mindedness and of the human spirit over provincial pokiness.

Occupational therapy in Canada had been developed essentially by Canadians and following the American schools. Physiotherapy in Canada followed the pattern of the English physiotherapist. For years you could not teach Physiotherapy unless you were trained in England or at least had been trained by a graduate of an English school. There was very little communication or feeling between the two.[1]

Helen LeVesconte, 1975

The rehabilitation sector in Toronto came to include physical therapy, occupational therapy, speech-language pathology, and physiatry. Each has its own story.

### The Origins of Physical Therapy

Physical therapy, known at the time as physiotherapy, began in Toronto during the First World War. It followed the English model of the Chartered Society of Physiotherapists, formed in 1894, with an emphasis on diagnosis and massage. It was only later that physical therapists, desirous of enhancing their standing – and of maximizing their ability to do good – embarked upon the diagnosis and treatment of mechanical disorders.

In 1917 the Military Hospitals Commission established a six-month program, using Hart House as its temporary base, called the Military School of Orthopaedic Surgery and Physiotherapy, to train physiotherapists. Thousands of injured veterans were returning to Canada in need of rehabilitation treatment that as yet had not been created. Under the direction of Lt. Col. Robert Wilson, a radiologist, "The Hart House Course" was divided into three sections, namely, massage and electrotherapy, gymnastics, and muscle function training. Its mandate was, as the official history of physical therapy in Toronto explains, "to educate students to rehabilitate veterans with disabilities so they could once again re-sume their useful place within society." In two years, "250 people completed the six-month course and been assigned to military hospitals across Canada." Play-fair McMurrich from the faculty lectured on anatomy;[2] the classes lasted until 1919 and produced 250 "Hart House Graduates."[3]

Enid Finley, a young woman from a wealthy Montreal family who had stud-ied massage at Heidelberg and also at the Philadelphia Orthopaedic Institute, was on staff, having moved from Montreal to Toronto to head the Massage and Treatment Department at Hart House. A tragedy in her personal life had, how-ever, an unexpected outcome for the physiotherapy program in Toronto. She had been married to the brilliant young surgeon at the children's hospital, Law-rence Bruce Robertson, who pioneered battlefield blood transfusion. When he died in 1923 at age thirty-eight, she was cast loose as a widow with two small children. As Robert Kerr and Douglas Waugh tell the story, "While still in her widow's weeds, Mrs. Robertson arrived at [Duncan] Graham's office, looking for the office of the Toronto Academy of Medicine, to which she wanted to do-nate her late husband's medical books. Duncan gallantly took her in tow and guided her to the Academy offices. On his return he remarked ... on the young widow's remarkable attractiveness." Enid, with considerable family resources available, spent the next three years travelling with her children in Europe. But as they approached school age she brought them back to Toronto and "im-mersed herself in the promotion of a university School of Physiotherapy." And then, guess what? She began encountering Graham at social gatherings and one thing led to another, and she and Graham were wed at St Andrew's Pres-byterian Church in 1929.[4] Thereafter, the Toronto physiotherapy program had a powerful ally.

In July 1919, the Hart House Course wrapped up and the program moved to a couple of tents on the lawn of St Andrew's Military Hospital, located on a Rosedale estate. This was supposed to be the end of the military school, but the McMurrichs, Duncan Graham, and Colonel Wilson "were not prepared to accept that this would spell the end of physiotherapy at the University." Mean-while, the Canadian Association of Massage and Remedial Gymnastics had come into being (with a dominion charter in March 1920, it became in that year the Canadian Physiotherapy Association), which would control the certifying of physiotherapy. On the advisory board were Duncan Graham, W.E. Gallie, and Clarence Starr, among others.[5]

A fundamental change in the position of physiotherapy in the university oc-curred in March 1920 when a Faculty of Medicine committee, headed by Alex-ander Primrose, recommended that physiotherapy join the faculty: "Adequate provision must be made for this important department."[6] In November 1920 D.J. Gibb Wishart, the otolaryngologist and chairman of the Medical Advisory Board of TGH, wrote Mrs L. Bruce-Robertson asking if they might have "a per-manent massage course in Toronto University."[7]

In 1925 the government of Ontario adopted a Drugless Practitioners Act, which included "masseurs" as drugless practitioners. "They were strictly forbidden to diagnose and prescribe, thus establishing physiotherapists as ancillary workers in the health field." But the act did secure a place for "massage" "as a distinct occupation in the health sector." In these years a number of distinct professional courses arose, especially for women, all leading to a diploma or a certificate.[8]

In the1926–7 session, Harry Arthur Cates of the Department of Anatomy began teaching in physiotherapy with a course in kinesiology to students from the School of Vocational Therapy and from the class in physical training of the Faculty of Household Science."[9] The official history of physical therapy at the University of Toronto observes that, unlike Britain, where physiotherapists were educated in the hospitals (and the system produced workers on the ground, not academics), in Canada "the venue for the education of physiotherapists ... was the university setting." "Canada is recognized as a leader in the establishment of academic physical therapy education."[10] In April 1929 a physiotherapy committee recommended to the president "that a two-year Diploma course in Physio-therapy be established to commence in September 1929." The physiotherapy students were to do academic work together with the occupational therapists, "under the direction of the Committee on University Extension." The first headquarters was at the Schoenberger house at 184 College Street and included twelve students. "Dr. William Gardiner, who taught some of the Physiotherapy courses at the Toronto General Hospital, was named supervisor of the course." Miss C.A. Kaulbach was the first day-to-day supervisor, followed in 1930 by Miss Lillian Pollard, who had trained as a physiotherapist at St Thomas's Hospital in London. "She was a proper, straight-backed Englishwoman who believed that, when a physician entered a patient's room, the physiotherapist should rise."[11] The faculty advisory committee included Duncan Graham, who, as mentioned, had fortuitously married Enid Finley Bruce-Robertson, a mainstay of the program. In 1931 the university granted its first diploma in physical therapy.[12]

During the Depression, enrolment in physiotherapy courses dropped way off but Mrs Graham helped out financially and Duncan Graham persuaded President Cody not to cancel the program. There was a demand for graduates. As one scholar observes, "In 1931, 27 percent of Ontario hospitals ... had physical therapy departments."[13]

Some knowledge of physical therapy was deemed useful for medical students, and in the 1933–4 session, physical therapy became a sub-department of therapeutics in the Faculty of Medicine, alongside anesthesia. "This ... marks a real step in advance," said President Cody. "Under the guidance of scientifically trained persons massage and physical manipulation can be taught and practised in closest alliance with the regular medical profession."[14]

Thus, in the 1930s two streams in physical therapy were organized, one for the medical students and graduates, the other for a physical therapy program taught to non-MDs, as with the program in occupational therapy, in the Department of University Extension.

By 1934–5 the Sub-department of Physical Therapy, part of the Department of Therapeutics, was under the direction of William J. Gardiner, head of the Department of Physical Therapy of the Toronto General Hospital. (In 1928 Duncan Graham had brought Gardiner, two years post-MD who had no training in physical medicine, to teach the subject at the General; in 1932 Gardiner qualified as a member of the Royal College of Physicians of London and was the first physician in physical medicine to occupy a university post in Toronto and possibly in Canada.) In the 1937–8 session, the Committee on Curriculum recommended increasing the number of hours of instruction given to the medical students, given "the increasing popularity of various empirical forms of Physiotherapy." Under Gardiner in the Department of Therapeutics, "the teaching of Physiotherapy has been established on a scientific basis and each student is given an opportunity to acquire both theoretical and practical training in the essentials."[15] Every year the medical stream of physical therapy became more imposing. It was called physiatry in the 1940s and after and undertaken solely by physicians.

In 1938–9 the Sub-department of Physiotherapy doubled the time for its teaching, and each group was divided in two. "This has made the hours of teaching four times greater than previously given. The department is indebted to Miss R[ebecca] Shilton, Chief Instructor in Physiotherapy, University of Toronto, who has given freely of her time."[16] (It was Enid Graham who convinced Shilton to move to Toronto from Montreal. As chief instructor, she taught medical gymnastics and massage alongside Florence Woodcock.[17])

Physical therapy practiced by physicians received a powerful boost in 1945 with the establishment by Harry Botterell and Albin Jousse of Lyndhurst Lodge as North America's first spinal rehabilitation centre. This story has been outlined in chapter 5, but here the focus is physical therapy, and Botterell's discovery of the horrid conditions at the Christie Street Department of the Veterans Affairs Hospital in Toronto (officially, the Dominion Orthopedic Hospital).[18] Botterell recruited Jousse as medical director of the new facility, which was established as a rehabilitation centre rather than a hospital. Spinal-injury rehabilitation in North America thus began in 1945 at Lyndhurst Lodge and with it a major avenue for physical therapists. (Charles Godfrey points out that previously spinal patients had received chronic care at the Queen Elizabeth Hospital in the Parkdale district of Toronto.[19]) Their 1946 report concluded, "The treatment of paraplegic patients depends for its success upon the enthusiastic cooperation of the patient and all those attending him." It was a dynamic note on which to begin the rehabilitation of a population that had been badly served.[20]

As for the nonmedical stream intended to produce physiotherapists, said the President's Report in 1935, "As in former years, instruction has been given to students in the course in Physiotherapy of the Department of University Extension."[21] In 1946 physical therapy classes were moved, along with occupational therapy classes, to "the huts," wartime structures transferred from Little Norway Exhibition Park to where Massey College stands today. They were drafty and unsatisfactory. Both programs were ready for transfer to the Faculty of Medicine.

### The Origins of Occupational Therapy

Like the physical therapists, the occupational therapists (OTs) initially began with a narrow program of activity: bringing mechanical skills to mental patients. Then with time, the OTs moved away from teaching patients mechanical skills to a wider field of functional assessment and cognitive therapy in association with psychological specialists.[22]

Occupational therapy in Toronto began during the First World War with the young women of the Voluntary Aid Detachment trained by the St John's Ambulance at the Spadina Military Hospital on Spadina Crescent and in the basement of the Mining Building. They were called "Ward Aides." Professor Herbert E.T. Haultain of the engineering department, apparently motivated by the patriotic duty to look after the "re-establishment" of wounded young men, saw to the organization; Professor Alexander Bott of the Department of Psychology introduced "exercise" into the program. (Bott apparently used to say, "I created Occupational Therapy."[23]) In 1920 the Ward Aides became the Ontario Society for Occupational Therapy (OSOT).[24]

Thus it was that in 1918 the Council of the Faculty of Applied Science and Engineering established a program of training for occupational therapists.[25] Although the faculty did not as yet have a department of occupational therapy, the whole concept was very much in the air when, in January 1924, Dean Primrose, who was president for years of the organization, talked to the Ontario Society for Occupational Therapy. "The aim of [occupational therapy] is to provide suitable occupation for sick folk who are suffering from long and tedious illness … to convert [their] hours of idleness into those of activity in some useful occupation; [this] is sufficient often to transform an individual from a permanent invalid to a useful citizen."[26]

In 1926 OSOT "succeeded in obtaining the creation of a two-year course,"[27] under the Department of University Extension. Primrose had pushed for it. Two years later, in 1928, the U of T granted its first diploma in OT.[28] It was Harry Cates who, in association with Kathleen McMurrich, gave the anatomy lectures to the "36 students taking the course in the first year and 20 in the second year."[29]

Meanwhile, in 1921 a Department of Rehabilitation and Physical Medicine (Department of Rehabilitation Medicine) was established at TGH at the instigation of Goldwin William Howland, a member of the Department of Medicine. It is widely unknown that the Toronto General Hospital was, in the words in 1923 of hospital Superintendent Chestnut J. Decker, "the first civilian hospital on the continent to adopt Occupational Therapy." He added, "It is now a recognized fact that success in the treatment of a great many cases is dependent largely upon the attitude of mind of the patients." The hospital's occupational therapy department "has interested patients in various activities in which the patient displays a deep interest, thereby diverting the mind from the bodily ailment."[30]

Howland had earned his medical degree in 1912 and, a Member of the Royal Society of Physicians, had trained at Queen Square in London.[31] (He was the founder of the neurology division of the Department of Medicine, and a photograph in the early 1920s shows the occupational therapists encouraging handicrafts among female patients in a section of the Neurological Ward.)

Early on, OT established itself in the treatment of psychiatric illness as well as neurologic. In the 1934–5 session, Helen LeVesconte, the occupational therapy consultant in the provincial asylum service, in charge of this work at the Toronto Psychiatric Hospital (TPH), was appointed to the OT staff in the Department of University Extension.[32] OT work in "mental hygiene" was deemed greatly improved. Students in the program would serve two-month rotations at TPH and other Ontario Hospitals and indeed take a further postgraduate internship for psychiatric or general hospital work.[33]

**Combined Course: The Division of Physical and Occupational Therapy**

A fundamental shift occurred on 1 July 1950 as the Faculty of Medicine took over the courses of physical therapy and occupational therapy for nonphysicians. On 2 March 1949 at a meeting of the heads of departments, the resolution was passed "that the Faculty of Medicine assume the responsibility for the administration and teaching of the courses in Physical Therapy and Occupational Therapy, provided that the two courses be combined into one and that the Faculty of Medicine has full control of administration and establishment of a curriculum."[34] At an April 1949 meeting of the Faculty Council, the issue was hashed out. Hardolph Wasteneys, chair of biochemistry, had reservations: "He felt that it was in the position of a technical course ... He thought this was bad for the future of the university." Harry Botterell, who had a great interest in spinal rehabilitation, approved: "He stressed particularly the need of well trained personnel in the rehabilitation of paraplegics."[35]

Agreement was obtained that, starting in the fall of 1950, there would be "a new combined course" in a three-year program in the Division of Physical and Occupational Therapy, qualifying students for a diploma in physical and occupational therapy. The program would entail eight months of clinical practice. Botterell chaired the organizing committee. Dean MacFarlane brought Andrew Zinovieff, a rheumatologist and consultant in physical medicine from the United Oxford Hospital system. MacFarlane had apparently met Zinovieff during the war and was impressed by him. "He will have the responsibility of directing this pioneer effort," MacFarlane said.[36] Added the dean the following year, "A much greater number enrolled than was expected, 110 students being accepted in September." He noted, "One of the specially successful features of the new course has been the series of lecture-demonstrations in Medicine and Surgery arranged at the Toronto General Hospital." To take pressure off TGH they would use the whole building at 6 Devonshire Place. Alterations were being done during the summer and would "include a room for electro-therapy teaching, complete with muscle stimulators."[37] The first graduates of the program emerged in the middle of a polio epidemic and were badly needed.[38]

Why in the Faculty of Medicine and not elsewhere in the university? Later Jan Steiner said that "historically when the decision was taken to remove Physical Therapy and Occupational Therapy from the Department of Extension those programmes requested to be placed within the Faculty of Medicine ... [They] require levels of training closer to that given to medical students than for example dentists and pharmacists."[39] This issue of why the female-dominated rehabilitation specialists needed to be in the (male-dominated) faculty surfaced on other occasions as well and was for years a thorn in the side of rehabilitation.

In June 1953 Zinovieff returned to England because, said veteran occupational therapist Helen LeVesconte in an interview, Mrs Zinovieff was very unhappy in Toronto.[40] Botterell's collaborator Albin Jousse became director of the division and would remain until 1972. There were now expanded practical training programs at both TGH and TWH.[41]

A chronic problem was too few occupational therapists going into the psychiatric hospitals. "It is of some concern," said Jousse, "that only six or seven sought employment in the psychiatric field, where the need for Occupational Therapy is required." The administration resolved (in 1953–4) to start admitting some male students next session (yet did not actually happen until the 1960–1 session).[42]

There were other problems too: the Toronto Division was stretched increasingly thin with teaching both on campus and at the Université de Montréal, whither staff were often seconded. And the steady flow of instructors from the United Kingdom, whence most of them were recruited, had started to slacken.[43]

### Division of Rehabilitation Medicine

As for the patient whose illness is not fatal we find increasing interest in the concept of rehabilitation, by which is meant the employment of all possible methods to produce restoration of function as rapidly as possible ... For this reason there has been serious discussion of the advisability of establishing a separate division of rehabilitation medicine to encompass all the disciplines which might be involved in such an endeavour.[44]

K.J.R. Wightman, June 1959

Rehabilitation was in the air. On 3 April 1959, the Faculty Council received Kager Wightman's report, on behalf of the Sub-Committee on Physical Medicine and Rehabilitation, that "a separate Department or Division of Rehabilitation Medicine in the University should be developed." The head would lead the Division of Physical Therapy and Rehabilitation Medicine at the Toronto General Hospital. "The concept of rehabilitation has become much broader; the requirements for the service ... are expanding, and the need for an increased number of trained personnel in the field is already apparent."[45] In the 1959–60 session, the division was thus renamed the Division of Rehabilitation Medicine and had responsibility as well for speech pathology and audiology and for the small number of physicians wishing training in physical medicine, also called physiatry.[46]

Meanwhile, in 1957 the National Hospital Insurance and Diagnostic Services Act made physical therapy an insured service; provinces and federal government would cost-share 50/50. The Ontario Hospital Services Commission introduced in 1963 the Private Physiotherapy Plan to pay for outpatient services (so patients wouldn't clog hospital beds waiting for physiotherapy).[47] Now doctors were able to charge for physiotherapy procedures and physiotherapists began private practices. In some cases physiotherapists worked in doctors' offices.

A central player in these early rehab days was the energetic Charles Godfrey. Born in 1917 in the United States, Godfrey had started out as a physiotherapist, registering for practice in 1942. After five years in the Royal Canadian Air Force, he decided to study medicine in Toronto and graduated in 1953. Thereupon, he earned a liberal arts degree, with a particular interest in medical history, obtaining a bachelor's degree from the University of Toronto in 1962 and a master's in 1975. He qualified for the Royal College's certification in physical medicine and rehabilitation in 1959. An industrious researcher and public speaker, Godfrey was invited to visiting professorships literally all over the world, from the University of Surakarta in Java, to the Union of Afghan Mujahid Doctors in Peshawar, Pakistan. (He was also a provincial Member of Parliament in Ontario from 1975 to 1976.) In Toronto, he had academic appointments at Sunnybrook (director of physical medicine and rehab in the late 1950s); the Wellesley Hospital (in the same positions, 1960s); and the Princess Margaret Hospital (director of rehab from 1972 to 1990); he also held consulting appointments at the other teaching hospitals and thus was the public academic face of rehabilitation.

In September 1960 a long-term thirty-bed Active Treatment Unit, funded by the Ontario Division of the Canadian Arthritis and Rheumatism Society, opened at the Queen Elizabeth Hospital for arthritis patients "who are admitted after having been studied in a teaching hospital."[48] (There was also an acute rheumatology service at Sunnybrook under Wallace Graham, with a research unit under Almon Fletcher.) This marked the beginning of the integration of the Queen Elizabeth Hospital, established in 1873, then located on Dunn Avenue, into academic medicine. In the 1962–3 session Lyndhurst Lodge, which under

Jousse had been used for training physical and occupational therapists, became affiliated with the university's training system.[49]

In 1967, Terence Kavanagh, a physical medicine specialist who earned his medical degree in 1953 from Manchester, became medical director of the Toronto Rehabilitation Centre on Rumsey Road near Sunnybrook Hospital. The following year Kavanagh founded one of the first cardiac rehabilitation programs in Canada. Kavanagh is remembered, together with Roy Shephard, professor of applied physiology in the Faculty of Medicine, for enrolling a number of what were then called "cardiac cripples" in the Boston Marathon in 1985 – and having the satisfaction of watching them succeed. He also followed over 12,000 men referred to his outpatient cardiac program between 1968 and 1994, discovering that exercise capacity exerted "a major long-term influence" on their prognosis.[50]

In 1962–63 the division moved from the huts to "Old Red 'Skule House'" once used by engineers, which has survived in the collective rehabilitation memory as horrible. Then in 1966 the division's peregrinations came to an end with a move to a renovated warehouse owned by the university at 256 McCaul Street, where it would stay for the next thirty-five years[51] (and which turned out to be as unsatisfactory as previous accommodations in view of the booming demand for rehabilitation therapists).

In the mid-1960s the same pressures began to exert themselves on rehabilitation that sooner or later affect all diploma programs: to upgrade to a higher academic level, in this case to a bachelor's degree program.[52] McGill had paved the way here, but soon Toronto would follow. Leadership changes took place within the division as well: in 1966–7 Helen LeVesconte, who had led occupational therapy for many years, retired, succeeded by Isobel Robinson; Lillian Pollard, in charge of physical therapy since the Second World War, also retired, succeeded by Ruth Bradshaw (from England).[53] In charge of the hospital programs were physiatrists Charles Godfrey at the Wellesley, William O. Geisler and Geoffrey Secord at Lyndhurst Lodge, Jose Jiminez at Mount Sinai, and John S. Crawford and orthopod Alan M. Wiley at the Western. Research publication in the division was dominated, as had been true for many years, by Godfrey.

Interestingly, the opening gun in persuading the physiotherapists to do research themselves, rather than just to cooperate with MDs, was fired in 1963 by Phyllis Carlton, a physiotherapist at the Wellesley Hospital. She pointed out in a much cited article that it was possible for physiotherapists to undertake important research on their own: "It must be remembered that these [cooperative] studies will be the property of the doctor, and, if valuable, lost to our profession as far as publication is concerned." Physiotherapists in England in the mid-1950s, she said, had provided a research template, and now it was up to the Toronto physiotherapists to press ahead with such useful questions as "physiological effects of ice" and "the most advantageous temperature of a hydropool in treatment of Multiple Sclerosis." The Toronto branch of the Canadian

Physiotherapy Association, she said, had organized a Research Committee (the committee then changed its name to "Clinical Studies" because apparently too many members found it intimidating). It was, Carlton argued, important to increase the awareness of the medical profession that "[w]e are not technicians."[54]

In these years rehabilitation medicine was plagued by problems. The Independent Planning Committee found the physiatry branch in 1969 to be overwhelmed by service demands. "The time and energy of the physiatrist is engulfed by primary service demands and research and teaching are pushed to the periphery." Many more physiatrists were needed. "The most serious deficiency facing the Division is the almost total lack of beds available in the hospitals under the direction and control of the medical staff of the Division." The teaching of medical students was called almost impossible and "gravely hampers" the teaching of physical and occupational therapists. "Without beds, the approval of a teaching programme by the Royal College of Physicians and Surgeons is granted only on a limited basis." Relief was in view with a special twenty-five-bed unit coming soon at Sunnybrook and the affiliation there with the family practice unit. "It is hoped that the Ontario Health Services Commission will establish a large, say, 100-bed unit in Rehabilitation Medicine in what is now New Mount Sinai Hospital when that building ceases to be used as a general hospital on completion of Mount Sinai Hospital in 1972."[55] (This would move the Queen Elizabeth Hospital from Dunn Avenue to University Avenue to join the other "hospital row" denizens.) These events came to pass, though not quite as quickly as hoped.

Physiatry itself became greatly diminished. Charles Godfrey, who could look back on a half century of experience, commented, "By the end of the century, the PM&R [physical medicine and rehabilitation] man was no longer necessary to the other specialists so he entered the geriatric field, where once again he would be working with physio and occupational therapists (not necessarily a male-dominated situation)." A very few, such as spinal-cord-injury specialist William Geisler, "remained at the side of the neurosurgeon, as did a few other PM&R specialists who maintained their presence on other speciality teams."[56] Yet grosso modo the physical therapy specialist began to go the way of the hydrotherapy specialists of the nineteenth-century spas.

### Separate Bachelor's Degrees in Physical Therapy and Occupational Therapy, Department of Rehabilitation Medicine

In March 1971 the university Senate ruled that beginning September the diploma course in physical and occupational therapy should be divided into two separate courses and each "elevated to a three-year degree course following a preliminary year in Arts and Science." Simultaneously, the Division of Rehabilitation Medicine, formerly part of the Department of Therapeutics under Jousse, became an independent department under John Crawford.[57] Physical therapy and occupational therapy became divisions in the new department. Why was the upgrade needed? Crawford told the long-range planners in February 1975, "Previously these were diploma programmes. As these fields have progressed into the active aspects of health delivery a degree was required to make them more responsible members of the health delivery programme."[58] The spring convocation of 1974 saw the first bachelor's degrees conferred in these fields.

In the mid-1970s, diploma upgrading as well became highly desired. In 1975 Woodsworth College, the undergraduate college oriented towards adult students, offered a degree completion option for a BSc in physical therapy and a BSc in occupational therapy. The physical therapy and occupational therapy faculty began upgrading their own degrees so that they could take part in university committees[59] – and, more importantly, be equipped to undertake research activities.

In 1973 surfaced a theme that sooner or later affected the various units staffed heavily by females: the attempt to chase physical and occupational therapy out of the Faculty of Medicine. In November, John Crawford mentioned to Jan Steiner in passing that "[h]e was indeed quite enthusiastic about the possibility that part or all of this programme may be moved to a Community College … He warned, of course, about the political difficulties involved … particularly since the ladies in his department violently object to any depreciation of the programme. Dr. Crawford himself, however, favoured the idea that the University should concentrate on the education of teachers of Physical & Occupational Therapy, rather than the education of practitioners of the art."[60] Crawford backtracked quickly, however, on this suggestion. Associate Dean Robin Hunter talked with him later in November and learned that the suggestion of leaving the faculty "has met with strenuous objection from his staff … He made what I felt to be a cogent point … that at this time it might be very undiplomatic indeed for the University of Toronto to be seen as getting rid of Health Care Delivery workers of any kind without a very rigorous and painstaking approach to the matter."[61]

Steiner himself, perhaps acting as devil's advocate, asked representatives of rehabilitation why they actually needed to be in a medical faculty rather than in a community college. The answer was that they needed anatomy, in addition to practice in working with other members of the health care team.[62] Again in 1975 it was orthopedic surgeon W. Robert Harris, chair of the long-range planners, who insisted "that the undergraduate programmes in Physical Therapy and Occupational Therapy may be inappropriately placed in the Medical School setting."[63]

Then finally there appeared beds! In December 1974 the plans came together to give the Department of Rehabilitation the beds it had so long sought. Led by Dean Holmes at the Faculty of Medicine, the General, Mount Sinai, and the Queen Elizabeth Hospital proposed to the Ministry of Health that the building at 550 University (formerly New Mount Sinai Hospital) be converted to a long-term rehabilitation unit; fifty beds of which would be under the supervision of the physiatrist-in-chief of the General and the Queen Elizabeth Hospital, who would have a full-time appointment in the Department of Rehabilitation Medicine. Overall control of the hospital would be under the chairman of the Department of Rehabilitation Medicine (but administered by the board of Queen Elizabeth Hospital), where "a teaching programme exclusively oriented to the care of chronically ill and elderly patients" will be situated.[64] This marked a fundamental step forward in the history of the rehabilitation sector.

What limped behind now was research. The department lacked virtually everything needed. Crawford told the long-range planners in February 1975, "It is a new venture. Grants are just beginning."[65] In 1983 the Self-Study said, the department "has started from scratch both as a residency program and in its research program. It also inherited the mantle of the 'Heat and Massage' group that haunts it to this day." In both divisions (PT and OT), "[m]any of the staff are on contractual limited term appointments: 'five years and out.' ... The CLTA situation is killing the department."[66]

For the rehabilitation department there was a kind of research high point, or low point, in 1983, when Dean Lowy came for a visit on 26 January. "The entire department was asked to assemble in the large ground floor room at 256 McCaul." "Dean Lowy told us that we were not behaving as a university department because we were conducting a very limited amount of research." The department responded. "We took Dean Lowy's message to heart and shaped up ... It was a watershed event. Molly Verrier spearheaded the change, with help of John Brown of the Faculty of Medicine."[67]

Molly Verrier was the big agent of change in rehab. She had earned a diploma in physical and occupational therapy from the University of Toronto in 1970, then a master's degree in health science from McMaster University in 1977. In 1978 she was appointed assistant professor in the Division of Physical Therapy of the University of Toronto, becoming in 1981 a collaborative investigator at the Playfair Neuroscience Unit at the Western, where she rose to the rank of clinical scientist by 1988, her major interest rehabilitation from spinal cord injuries, stroke, and traumatic brain injury.

In 1983 John Crawford retired; Joe Marotta, the associate dean of clinical affairs, became acting chair, shortly to be replaced by Morris ("Mickey") Milner at the Hugh MacMillan Medical Centre, who had a PhD in biomedical engineering and had participated in the design of useful devices such as prosthetic hands for children.[68] Milner oversaw a large upgrading of the credentials of the occupational therapists: He said in 1987, "Within a span of approximately 5 years, the Division has progressed from having faculty primarily at the Bachelors and Masters levels ... to faculty now primarily either holding Ph.D.s or in the midst of Ph.D. training." He noted that Robin Schaffer, and her colleague Helene Polatajko at the University of Western Ontario – soon to be at Toronto – were "the first occupational therapists in Canada to have received MRC funding."[69]

One bright light in the research tunnel was the cross-appointment in 1987 of Geoffrey Fernie, director of research at West Park Hospital who also held appointments in the Department of Surgery and Institute of Biomedical Engineering. (West Park itself was founded in 1904 by Sir William Gage as the Toronto Free Hospital for Consumptive Poor and, becoming a convalescent and rehabilitation hospital in the 1960s after the decline of tuberculosis, was renamed West Park Hospital in 1976.) Fernie invented assistive devices for the elderly and disabled, including the "Toilevator," a mechanism installed under toilets to aid people who have difficulty lifting themselves.[70] In 1973 Fernie was asked by the Division of Orthopaedics in the university Department of Surgery to get rehabilitation going. He later said, "Orthopedic surgeons at that time felt they were advancing surgery, but that the rehabilitation part was lagging." Fernie said his role was to "advance rehabilitation for the Department of Surgery, helping patients return to their daily lives after surgery." Fernie led research in engineering and computer science in rehab. Under his leadership, by 2009 Toronto had "the largest rehabilitation engineering research group in the world." Fernie himself became vice president of research in 2003 at the Toronto Rehabilitation Institute.[71]

As for teaching, the Divisions Physical Therapy and Occupational Therapy both developed a new curriculum, crafted on "the McMaster model" of problem-based learning, which passed in the Governing Council in 1985.[72] In 1986 Pat Faris replaced a retiring Ruth Bradshaw as acting director of the Division of Physical Therapy.[73] Thus a whole new team came on board.

It was no secret that the rehabilitation sector had been treated as a stepchild within the faculty, the parental indulgence going to such mainline departments as medicine, surgery, and pediatrics. This was to change in the late 1980s. In 1987 the Faculty Education Committee "discussed some of the divisions/departments with apparently lesser priority in the Faculty such as Occupational Therapy, Physical Therapy, their increasing importance in the health care system and their ambition to more academic pursuits as well as maintaining excellent clinical training for students, and the impact of increased enrollment in their programs."[74]

This academic upgrading went hand in hand with a rising demand for physical and occupational therapists. As Dean Dirks said in October 1988, "There is a shortfall of professionals in the [rehabilitation] community, particularly in the fields of Physical Therapy, Occupational Therapy and Speech Pathology ... There is a need for a proposal which will lead to an improved funding situation to enhance faculty and facilities." We're working on it, he said.[75]

The year 1988 saw another leadership change: Marotta succeeded Milner as acting chair of the department, and Molly Verrier, whose research was in neurophysiology, became director of the Division of Physical Therapy. Verrier later wrote, "In August of 1988 when I took over as the new Director of the program, we were two years into the new curriculum ... One of the main issues that the Directors of Physiotherapy of the clinical facilities wanted to discuss was the creating of Status Appointments for individuals who were doing significant teaching ... with very little recognition. Therefore, 26 status appointments were created in the first year ... Five graduate student teaching assistant positions were also created." It was obvious from the tone of the account that Verrier really was a new broom, but she conceded as weaknesses of the division its "small faculty complement," the "lack of a graduate programme," and lack of "research infrastructure."[76]

Ever since 1981, when Molly Verrier chaired a graduate planning committee, the two divisions had ardently aspired to a graduate program but were rebuffed by the School of Graduate Studies.[77] In 1989 Don Cowan succeeded Marotta as acting chair and recommended to Dean Dirks that the department's application for a graduate program should again be turned back because not enough of the staff qualified for SGS membership. Cowan said that Associate Dean Laszlo Endrenyi at SGS "feels there are insufficient staff to mount a graduate department ... at the moment."[78]

Disaggregation loomed. External assessors in 1981 recommended that physiotherapy, occupational therapy, and physiatry continue in the same department but that speech pathology be spun off into a separate department.[79] In 1986 the decision was made as of July 1987 to remove physiatry from the General and other downtown teaching hospitals and to concentrate it in a northern cluster at Sunnybrook and Lyndhurst hospitals and the Hugh MacMillan Centre and a southern cluster at Queen Elizabeth and Mount Sinai Hospitals. This was part of a downsizing of physiatry driven by Associate Dean Joseph Marotta, who was determined to slash weak programs.[80]

In 1989 Dean Dirks established a task force to decide what to do with the various disparate components of the Department of Rehabilitation Medicine. The first decision was to transfer the Division of Physiatry to the Department of Medicine. This was done in 1990.[81] (Physiatry remained a small division in medicine with a four-year clinical residency leading to the fellowship of the Royal College of Physicians. In the 1984–5 session, for example, there were around twelve postgraduates in the program.[82])

The second decision was to convert the other divisions into free-standing departments. "The Task Force concluded that ... the best interests of each division [OT, PT, and speech pathology] would be served by staying with the Faculty of Medicine and seeking departmental status. In the long-term, the divisions envisage a more independent but allied role within the University. To this end, all three divisions have embarked on a plan of recruiting talented, bright faculty with strong academic qualifications." The new departments were to have a research and funding focus.[83]

It was on 20 June 1991 that the report of the Faculty of Medicine Task Force on Physical Therapy and Occupational Therapy was handed down: Don Cowan was acting chair; the drafters were Molly Verrier from physical therapy and

Judy Friedland from occupational therapy. The report recommended that the two divisions achieve departmental status and remain within the clinical sector of the Faculty of Medicine. "While the Department of Rehabilitation Medicine may have served the diploma programs well, it has, in recent years become problematic for the separate BSc (Occupational Therapy) and BSc (Physical Therapy) programs." Accreditation teams were "appalled by the inadequate resources base." The bill of particulars was shocking: "The University of Toronto educates the largest number of Occupational Therapy students and the second largest number of Physical Therapy students in all of Canada. Yet the student/ faculty ratios for each Division are among the worst in the country [the student/ faculty ratio at McMaster University was 8:1 for physical therapy, 28:1 at U of T]. Although the programs at the University of Toronto are the oldest, they are the last to have a graduate program." The report continued, "The physical plant for the Divisions is inadequate. They have been housed, 'temporarily,' in a converted warehouse since 1968. Most faculty do not have enclosed office space ... There is no study space or lounge for the 500 undergraduates and classroom space is inadequate and poorly equipped."[84]

The circumstances described in the report were so dismal that physical therapy and occupational therapy became, after decades of neglect, a top priority of the faculty. In July 1990, Dirks decided to make them the number one funding priority in the faculty's five-year capital plan.[85] Until the physical and occupational therapists could be made into separate departments, they were placed under the guardianship of the Department of Medicine.[86]

### Department of Occupational Therapy (Again)

In July 1991 Judy Friedland succeeded Robin Schaffer as director of the Division of Occupational Therapy. When the Department of Occupational Therapy was created in July 1993, Friedland was acting chair; a year later, she was appointed as chair. She served until June 1999, when she told Dean Aberman she did not wish to be reappointed and was succeeded by Helene Polatajko from the University of Western Ontario.

Friedland described events during her chairmanship:[87] "By the start of the 1990s it was clear that there was an urgent need to prepare faculty for the research that had been sorely lacking. The first step had to be the development of the faculty members so that they would be in a better position to undertake research. Continuing the approach taken by Milner, new hires came on with their PhDs in hand while former faculty members enrolled in PhD programs in cognate departments."[88] By the end of Friedland's term in office, the department boasted the highest number of PhD-qualified faculty in the country.[89]

Research activities increased as faculty qualifications grew. A copy of the department's Report of Scholarly Activity for 1996–8 was sent to Fred Lowy, now rector and vice chancellor of Concordia University, with a comment on his role in having provoked the increased focus on research activity following his visit a decade earlier. Lowy acknowledged the change, saying, "It is indeed something for which you may be justifiably proud. It is amazing what you have accomplished." The external review noted the improvement, stating that "current levels of research funding would place the department on a level similar to the top three to four occupational therapy programs in Canada." That the faculty's new level of research activity was just beginning was recognized in their statement that "[t]he department appears well placed to increase this research funding over the next few years." The department's research activities were now focused in five areas: the science of occupation, factors affecting community participation, the experience and impact of disability, assistive technology, and learning and education in health professions.[90]

The number of tenured and tenure-stream faculty increased during this period and the department entered into a period of stability. Core faculty were supported by a large cohort of clinicians in the community both for teaching and fieldwork placements. The status-appointee process was formalized, and by 1999, some 123 members of the clinical community were listed in this capacity. Promotions now became a focus in the department, with the first promotion to full professor occurring in 2000.[91] Among those promoted was Angela Colantonio at the Toronto Rehabilitation Institute, whose work on long-term outcomes of traumatic brain injuries, including her educational dramatic production *After the Crash*, had won international recognition. She found, for example, that women with traumatic brain injuries experienced significantly more menstrual irregularities than women without.[92]

Meanwhile, major structural changes were also taking place. The Departmental Task Force, initiated under Dean Dirks in 1989, had examined the options for an appropriate structure for the divisions. Though occupational therapy and physical therapy had effectively separated with the establishment of their respective degree programs in 1971, the two divisions had been left within the Department of Rehabilitation Medicine and were subject to the department's decision-making structure. The task force met sporadically until 1991 when it determined that departmental status would provide the much-needed independence and secure a more appropriate place within the Faculty of Medicine. A proposal for departmental status for occupational therapy and physical therapy was prepared by Friedland and Verrier and approved by Faculty Council on 17 September 1992. In a subsequent motion, the Department of Rehabilitation Medicine was closed.[93]

With departmental status in hand, occupational therapy was free to establish its own agenda for development. It revamped its curriculum structure and content. The proposal for a "2+2+" (two years of undergraduate study plus two years of OT) leading to a BScOT, approved in the spring of 1994 by the Governing Council, made it a second-entry program and positioned the department for its planned move to a master's entry-level program[94]. The proposal for the master's program in occupational therapy, prepared by a task force chaired by Friedland, was approved by the School of Graduate Studies and submitted to the Ontario Council of Graduate Studies (OCGS) in March 2000. The new program accepted its first students in 2001.

A new problem-based learning curriculum was approved in 1994. In addition to changing the approach to teaching and learning, the new curriculum increased the research focus so that all students undertook a major research project under supervision. External reviewers remarked on the new stature of the department whereby the changes had "produced an academic department in addition to a professional school." They further noted that the "organization, structure and faculty in the Department of Occupational Therapy at the University of Toronto put it amongst the top 10–15 universities [with occupational therapy programs] in the world."[95]

There was further good news. In 2003 the rehabilitation departments were relocated from the "sub-standard space at 256 McCaul Street" to the "newly renovated Rehabilitation Sciences Building at 500 University." A new entry-level master's in occupational therapy (MScOT) was established in 2001 under Helene Polatajko as chair. The undergraduate program was phased out. The OT department responded rather pridefully to an external review: "All of the graduate students are involved in research projects." Dean Naylor said in his response, "I completely agree with the reviewers that the move of the Rehabilitation Science sector to newly renovated space has revitalized the Department of Occupational therapy and the sector in general."[96]

There are few stories in the faculty more dramatic than the decline and rebirth of occupational therapy as an agency for training and research.

### Department of Physical Therapy

On 1 July 1993 the Department of Physical Therapy was created, with Molly Verrier as acting chair; she became chair the following year. As the rehabilitation sector history observes, "In accepting this appointment, Molly gave up her clinician scientist role at the Playfair Neuroscience Unit and moved her lab to 256 McCaul – a first for Physical Therapy." It was noted, "Physical therapy at last had its own strong voice, and stood on equal ground with other university departments." Verrier became speaker of the Faculty Council of the Faculty of Medicine.[97]

Around 1998 a new evidence-based curriculum was introduced into physical therapy, which required "eight case-based ... seminar rooms" that they did not at the moment have. External reviewers in 1999 found that there was a real space crisis. But the students were very enthusiastic. "The Physical Therapy Department enjoys a fine reputation within Canada and beyond the country ... The research component holds enormous promise which will undoubtedly come to fruition if funding to support new space and more faculty is obtained."[98]

## Rehabilitation Moves Forward

In 1993 the Departments of Occupational Therapy and Physical Therapy joined hands to propose a master's (MSc) program in rehabilitation sciences, approved by the Academic Board in December 1993.[99] By April 1995 the new Graduate Department of Rehabilitation Science was a reality, with Molly Verrier as chair. In the two rehabilitation departments, future accents lay on upgrading: just as diploma programs had once been turned into undergraduate degree programs, in the late 1990s the undergraduate programs were to be abolished in favour of entry-level master's programs, the MScOT and the MScPT, implemented in 2001. As the faculty's Strategic Directions and Academic Plan specified for 2000–4, there was to be a doctoral stream program in rehabilitation science, launched in 2002.[100] This development was compared to introducing advanced degrees in other once devalued female-dominated fields such as nursing and speech pathology.[101]

Rehabilitation moved forward in other ways as well. In summer 1996 the Health Services Restructuring Commission completed an initial report on "restructuring the Metropolitan Hospitals." Among the proposed initiatives was "the amalgamation of Hillcrest Hospital and Queen Elizabeth Hospital to become a fully-affiliated Teaching and Research Rehabilitation Centre."[102] In June 1997 the Rehabilitation Institute of Toronto (RIT) was decided as the name of the new fully affiliated institution.[103] In November 1998 the Rehabilitation Institute of Toronto (a product of the merger of Hillcrest Hospital and Queen Elizabeth Hospital) combined with Lyndhurst Hospital and the Toronto Rehabilitation Centre to form the Toronto Rehabilitation Institute (TRI).[104]

The new organization simply screamed "research." In November 2000, Jack Williams of the Department of Public Health Sciences was appointed vice president of research of TRI. "Upon his arrival at the Toronto Rehabilitation Institute in November, his first task will be to develop a strategic plan for research and identify research priorities. Next on his agenda will be recruiting the organization's first Research Chair, filling current research vacancies, and securing the funds to support research endeavours."[105]

In 2001 the rehabilitation sector, including the Graduate Department of Rehabilitation Science, the Department of Occupational Therapy, the Department of Physical Therapy, and the Department of Speech-Language Pathology, began the move to their new quarters at 500 University Avenue, the former site of the New Mount Sinai Hospital. The move was completed by October 2002. It was a way station on a long odyssey towards professionalization and academic respectability that both physical therapy and occupational therapy had undertaken following the First World War and was completed, with the acceptance of PhD programs, in the new century. It is an unfortunate comment on the faculty that both of these female-led fields arrived in the charmed circle of research so many years after medicine and surgery and the rest of the male-dominated academic panoply of medicine. Yet they made the voyage surely and with panache.

## Speech-Language Pathology

The first stirrings of interest in speech pathology in Toronto appeared in the 1954–5 session as Jousse was said to be contemplating a "training course for workers in audiology and speech pathology."[106] He rather dawdled in the contemplation, for it was only in the fall of 1958 that "[t]he Faculty is offering this autumn for the first time a two year diploma course in Speech Pathology and Audiology ... Those at present engaged as therapists have had their training in the United States or Great Britain."[107] Speech pathology thus started out as a diploma program to train therapists in speech disorders particularly for patients with stroke, stuttering, and laryngeal speech. This put it on an even level with the fellow disciplines of physical and occupational therapy; the Senate approved its diploma program in 1957.

When in 1958–9 the faculty sought authorization for the establishment of a Division of Rehabilitation Medicine, speech pathology and audiology were to be included, with Charles Godfrey as the medical director.[108] It was the first in English Canada.

There were several scientific landmarks. In the 1960–1 session, the division organized a Speech Clinic at the Princess Margaret Hospital, staffed by volunteers who had sustained a laryngectomy, "concerned with teaching oesophageal speech to patients who have suffered functional and anatomical impairment of the body as a consequence of the ravages of cancer."[109] The hospital division at TGH was also quite active, specializing in patients with neurogenic speech, language, or swallowing disorders; those disorders because of laryngeal cancer; and "patients with disorders of the voice."[110]

In 1967 the unit moved to the Old Zion Church at 88 College Street. In 1973 Crawford, head of rehabilitation medicine, persuaded the dean to drop "Audiology" from the name of the division, which henceforth became the Division of Speech Pathology, Department of Rehabilitation Medicine. (Audiology joined the Department of Otolaryngology.) Jean Ward became director of the Division of Speech Pathology, William Franks the medical coordinator.[111]

The female-dominated Division of Speech Pathology turned out to be no less endangered than any of the other such divisions of the faculty. Around October 1974 Crawford fought against efforts to drop the proposed master's program in speech pathology "in favour of the Master's Programme at the University of Western Ontario." Crawford opposed this on the grounds that the school system in Ontario very much needed speech pathology graduates. If the speech pathology program were discontinued, "I suspect that the only aspect of communication taught in this University, of any value, will end up in the Department of Linguistics of the Faculty of Arts and Science. Frankly I believe that this would be a black mark in our Faculty and would result in rather poor publicity for the Faculty of Medicine."[112]

Thus the diploma program was saved, and in 1978 the diploma converted to a master's degree (MHSc) in the Graduate Department of Speech Pathology, recognizing the field as a distinct academic discipline.[113] Yet so unhappy were the accommodations at 88 College Street, previously a day-care centre for the Department of Psychiatry, that during the 1980s the division repeatedly faced closure.

In 1982 the Division of Speech Pathology was detached from the Department of Rehabilitation Medicine at the suggestion of an external reviewer. In fall 1982 Dean Lowy set up a task force under Joe Marotta to advise him on best arrangements for the division. Opinion was divided on whether the division should be an independent department or a division in the Department of Otolaryngology, "with the understanding that it become a Division of Communication Disorders in association with the Audiology group that now exists within that Department." Dean Lowy and Peter Alberti at otolaryngology were in favour because, as Alberti put it, the concept of "communication disorders" was so powerful. The Faculty Council voted for the transfer.[114] Yet the decision was delayed. As Lowy said, "Because of the extreme reluctance of members of the Division of Speech Pathology to accept this administrative arrangement, no steps have been taken to implement it, and the matter is undergoing further examination."[115] The division later returned to the Department of Rehabilitation Medicine, and in November 1989 the first students to participate in the "extended Speech Pathology Program" graduated.[116]

These years were marked by a tug of war between the division and the faculty. The division wanted to convert itself into a Centre for Communication Disorders; the faculty was rather cool to this project in the absence of an internationally recognized leadership figure.[117] Jean Ward-Walker led the division from 1972 to 1983, Margaret L. Stoicheff from 1983 to 1989. Under Paula Square-Storer, chair from 1989 to 2001, the division gained departmental status in 1992 as the rest of the remnants of the former Department of Rehabilitation Medicine became departments in their own right. In 1995 a research degree, the MSc, was inaugurated.

In 1995 the name of the discipline was changed from "speech pathology" to "speech-language pathology" to include language disorders resulting from developmental delays or head injuries, as well as speech disorders. A PhD program began in 1996. By 2000 the new Department of Speech-Language Pathology had 118 faculty, of whom 8 were full-time. The department's two research concentrations were speech motor control and developmental language disorders, and they were adding a third, hearing sciences, through collaborations with Department of Otolaryngology.[118]

Jean Ward-Walker later said, "In looking back, my predominant recollection of the program is that of struggle and a fight for survival." One associate dean told them in a meeting in the dean's Conference Room, "You will be eliminated." It was essential for them to replace the former diploma with a master's degree, yet they had endless difficulty making this happen, a consequence in part of the division's not entirely tranquil relations with rehabilitation medicine, Ward-Walker said. Nonetheless, "[r]ecollections of struggles aside, it is enormously gratifying to see the advances which have been made by the discipline of speech pathology within the University." In 1993 the department left the hated Old Church at 88 College Street for new quarters in the Tanz Neuroscience Building.[119] (And the History of Medicine Program moved into the Old Church.)

For the generation of W.E. Gallie, such concepts as "family medicine" and "community risk" did not belong to the core knowledge of medicine. The founders of the faculty tended to be somatic reductionists, and anything that did not involve tissue changes was probably not worth teaching the medical students, however sensitive the founding generation might have been to the "whole patient." Yet in the 1970s and after, several factors drove such softer concepts as family and prevention onto the radar. Mushrooming medical costs made cash-strapped ministries much keener to supplant specialist care with less costly primary care. As well, many began asking, with Hippocrates, not what kind of illness the patient has, but what kind of patient has the illness, the social and personal factors in health and disease, in other words. Firm alliances were built between family medicine and social medicine, which is why both appear together in this chapter.

### Department of Family and Community Medicine

It is perfectly appropriate for a family physician to adopt a "wait and see approach," rather than launching into a series of expensive and invasive investigations ... Much illness that presents to family physicians is either transient and self-limiting in nature, or has a psychological basis and responds favorably to reassurance by the physician. In contrast, consultant specialists generally adopt an "investigate and rule out" approach, using all of the power and technology of biomedical science at their disposal.[1]

Eliot Phillipson, Chair of Medicine, 2004

*Family Medicine Avant la Lettre*

With the advent of the divisional system in the Departments of Medicine, Surgery, and Paediatrics after the 1960s, Toronto became ever more oriented towards turning out specialists. Yet that was not what the population needed, nor what the province wanted. Family physicians, the latter-day descendants of the general practitioner, were desired and steps had to be taken for their production. A Department of Family and Community Medicine was needed.

Let us step back a pace. In years gone by, medical students in Toronto did not receive adequate preparation for clinical practice. Most students could forget about internships. William Gallie remembered of the period around 1900 that there were only eleven internships at the General, four at HSC, and two at St Michael's. "The remainder of our year of 106 either did without internships or sought them in some other city. Our provision for the practical training of a general practitioner was minimal."[2]

The vast majority of these graduates in 1900 went on to become general practitioners (GPs), the backbone of medicine. Specialists were relatively few. Yet after the First World War the rise of specialism took hold in earnest and many more young medical graduates, relishing the prestige and the income that specialized knowledge conferred, went on to train in the postgraduate programs of the faculty. At the Toronto General Hospital, beds were allocated by specialty, the GPs treating the outpatients. The success of the Royal College of Physicians and Surgeons of Canada, founded in 1929 for the certification of specialists, was stunning. The share of physicians in Canada doing general practice declined from 67 percent in 1955 to 52 percent a decade later. "There was very little pride in admitting one was 'just a GP,'" writes medical historian Jack Leitch. "The GP, who frequently had been described as the backbone of the profession was ... in danger of becoming the coccyx."[3]

In 1954 the College of General Practice of Canada was established, with W. Victor Johnston of Lucknow, Ontario – a 1923 graduate of the University of Toronto – as its founding director. (He had grown up on a farm near Donnybrook, Ontario, and chose at his graduation motto, "Be sure you're right; then go ahead."[4]) The college was intent on advancing the postgraduate training of family doctors, as GPs were starting to be called.

Some postgraduate training for family physicians was required, as Kenneth Clute discovered, in a survey of family practice in Nova Scotia and Ontario published in 1963: the level of general practice was abysmal. Regarding ongoing medical education, for example, Clute described one older practitioner, "who received the Canadian Medical Association Journal but regarded it as of no value, listed no books, and attended one local medical society meeting per year but no conventions, postgraduate courses, or hospital staff meetings. He 'never' read textbooks, read journals 'occasionally,' and regarded both as of 'no value.' The yearly meeting of the local medical society consisted of business and one paper on a general medical topic ... The only source of information that he considered of great value was the publications of the pharmaceutical companies."[5] Once upon a time, said Clute, it didn't matter if the general practitioner stayed up on the latest developments because there were so few. In the "medicine of more than twenty-five years ago … there were no sulphonamides, no antibiotics, no antihistamines, no ACTH or cortisone, and no hypertensive drugs."[6] Now, things were different.

In 1948 the Postgraduate Commission of the faculty established a "mixed" residency "to prepare candidates for careers in general practice." By the 1950–1 session this was up and running: "A special internship for limited numbers of men who intend going into general practice has been instituted as a joint effort of the Hospital for Sick Children and the Toronto General Hospital," Dean MacFarlane explained in 1951. "65 per cent of the present class indicated their intention of going into general practice."[7] Robert C. Dickson, an internist at the Wellesley with an interest in psychological medicine, was apparently the spark plug of this "GP course." Dickson later told Jack Leitch, the historian of the Department of Family and Community Medicine, "The program in Family Practice … was a very loose arrangement in which medicine and psychiatry were provided at the Wellesley, Surgery and Obstetrics sometimes at the Wellesley and sometimes at the Toronto General."[8] Cosbie called this "the first planned internship for general practice offered in Canada."[9] This early program for training GPs was successful for many years, but by the late 1960s the specialist residences were draining off its recruits.[10]

In the late 1940s the faculty also offered refresher courses, or Continuing Medical Education as it was later called, for family physicians. One such course, offered at Sunnybrook, was "attended by some 300 doctors."[11] By 1969, over 2,500 Ontario physicians signed up for continuing and postgraduate education in the faculty of one kind or another: 20 percent were house staff, almost all others "doctors in practice who registered for short intramural refresher courses in various special and general fields."[12] Thus, family physicians were intent upon staying abreast.

As these events were taking place in training, Wightman began adding family practitioners to his Department of Medicine. At the national level, a series of conferences in the early 1960s put on the table the idea of family medicine as an academic theme, something to which the medical students should be exposed. The Family Practice College proposed a two-year postgraduate training program in university hospitals, launching a pilot project in 1966 at Calgary General Hospital.[13] An intellectual substructure was thus moving into place.

But this burgeoning of family medicine soon became seen as a danger by the internists. In 1967 Wightman deplored the centrifugal tendencies threatening to tear the Department of Medicine apart: "On the other hand the Department is also in danger of attrition from the 'general' side." The family doctors were all setting up clinics "which would afford students an opportunity to see the nature of general practice." These clinics have developed under aegis of Department of Medicine. "However, we are already beginning to hear that they should be separate departments." In the last year the department had made twenty-two staff appointments "to men working in the Outpatients Department and General Practice Clinics in the various teaching hospitals."[14]

### Founding the Department of Family and Community Medicine

Reginald Perkin and Fred Fallis were the founders of family medicine in Toronto. "Reg" Perkin, as he preferred to be known, completed his medical degree at Toronto in 1954, then opened a family practice in Mississauga, a suburb of Toronto, in 1956. In 1962 he started building this small practice into a group practice with seven other family physicians. Perkin taught family medicine at U of T and headed the Family Practice Unit at Toronto Western Hospital from 1966 to 1971; in 1969 he became the inaugural head of the university Department of Family and Community Medicine. Later, he headed the Family Practice Units at Queensway General and Mississauga Hospital and served as executive director of the College of Family Physicians of Canada from 1985 to 1996.

Fred Fallis was born in Vancouver in 1921, earned a bachelor's degree from the University of Toronto in 1942, then served with the RCAF as a pilot and afterwards as an officer in the Department of External Affairs. He graduated with an MD at Toronto in 1953. After interning, he worked in the outpatient department of the General and its Venereal Disease Clinic. He was also a staff doctor at the Addiction Research Foundation and had a private practice in North Toronto before becoming in 1966 head of TGH's General Practice Clinic.

These family practice units were situated in the teaching hospitals under the aegis of the Department of Medicine. Others opened in 1966 at Women's College Hospital under Marjorie C. Swanson and at the Wellesley under Arthur Squires and Lorne P. Laing. Sunnybrook's clinic was established in 1967 under Douglas Johnson; there were others in 1969 at St Michael's and in 1970 at the New Mount Sinai Hospital.

The next step was this: in 1967 a series of important meetings was held in Toronto envisioning the establishment of a Department of Family Medicine in the faculty. On 28 February, Associate Dean Kergin brought Perkin, Laing, and Fallis together at Sunnybrook Hospital to "discus the place of Family Practice in the Faculty of Medicine and the teaching of this subject both at the undergraduate and graduate levels." Again in July, Kergin convened a group of family doctors active in the teaching hospitals to discuss future postgraduate training programs. This group constituted itself on the spot as the Ad Hoc Committee to Consider Postgraduate Training for General Practice, and, at the suggestion of Dean Chute, who attended the meeting, the group recommended to the executive committee of the faculty (called the Committee on Curriculum and Examinations) that a Department of General Practice be formed in the faculty. An implementation committee, called the "Feasibility Committee" under Irwin Hilliard, was then struck to bring about the founding of such a department.

In March 1968 Fallis suggested to Hilliard that the new department be called "Family and Community Medicine," a name that carried the day.

At a February 1969 meeting of the Committee on Curriculum and Examinations, Dean Chute said that "the Ontario Deans met recently with the Minister of Health," at which time a need to train more family doctors emerged. Chute said that the faculty must decide whether it needed a separate Department of Family Practice. "There are a number of well qualified staff within the Department of Medicine who might form the nucleus of such a department." Roderick Gordon, the head of anesthesia, moved that such a department be founded. Wightman agreed that, if they wanted more people in general practice, they needed a separate department. "He felt that the people in his department whose responsibility this has been are now in a position to function as a separate department." The committee discussed whether such a program should be four years, or would less do? McCulloch said that a questionnaire showed staff and students were in favour. "A suggested aim was 100 places a year." The motion carried.[15] These were the first birth pangs within the faculty.

At a meeting of the senior committee several weeks later it became apparent how far plans had progressed in the hospitals. Douglas Johnson said there was some urgency about it "since one hospital, namely Sunnybrook, is to have a major emphasis on Community Medicine, and Department Heads there find it difficult to proceed with planning residency programmes, recruitment of staff etc until the degree of their involvement with Family Practice is known." At the Western they had already dedicated six beds for GPs. "This serves as an important working model to illustrate how various members of the profession work together as a team." Several members emphasized the preventive medicine component of family practice. Fallis questioned the name that the faculty had proposed, "Department of Family Practice." He wanted a broader emphasis to "bring the University and Community into closer relation." An amendment therefore passed stipulating "that the name be changed to the Department of Family and Community Medicine." This distinctive ideological emphasis, therefore, on "the community" was present from the beginning.[16] The emphasis was, it must be said, shared entirely by the students: in 1969 the faculty's Independent Planning Committee wanted Sunnybrook drawn into training family doctors. "This conclusion is reinforced by the knowledge that some 45% of the members of the current final year in the medical school have indicated a wish to study family practice medicine."[17]

Meanwhile, at the Ministry of Health the drums were beating on behalf of family practice. At a meeting of the provincial Senior Co-ordinating Committee in September 1969, the question was raised "whether the production of family practitioners is being neglected. It was suggested this should be given careful consideration when discussing priorities."[18] (Apparently at this meeting the Ministry of Health submitted a document suggesting an increase in the production of family doctors.) At a later meeting, the Senior Co-ordinating Committee wanted to know "the role of each hospital in relation to other hospitals as well as to the community. Facilities will be shared to the greatest extent possible in order to ensure that public money has been wisely spent ... Ambulatory care facilities will be emphasized." The Ontario Hospital Services Committee was said to want "emphasis on family physicians," including "[m]ethods of delivering health care other than on an in-patient basis, especially ambulatory services, including family practice units and home care programs."[19]

In February 1969 the Faculty Council accepted the recommendation of the Feasibility Committee that a new department with the name Family and Community Medicine be created. In spring of 1969 the DFCM opened as "the birth of the first new clinical department in the Faculty of Medicine in modern times."[20] Under Reg Perkin, it was the first in Canada.[21]

In June 1970 the enrolment of the residents for the two-year program began, twenty-four first-year and six second-year. Thirty-five teaching practices were available to these residents. In 1970 Fred Fallis succeeded Perkin as chair of the department.

*Research*

As the dean announced in 1969 that the Senate had just approved the new body, he said, "It is expected that the new department will encourage larger numbers of students to accept the challenge of this type of medical practice."[22] The phrase "challenge" was a tip-off to a kind of culture clash between the founders of the DFCM and the rest of the faculty. Family medicine with its doctrine of community involvement was as close to a movement as it gets in medicine. Most medical specialties are not ideological movements, in the sense of the drive for female suffrage. Family medicine was. In the late 1960s it still had a wisp of the 1960s clinging to it, and external reviewers even as late as 2000 said, "The Department members continue to feel that generalists are part of the 'counter-culture.'" (Interestingly, Dean Naylor agreed with this assessment in his response: "The Department ... has, as the reviewers put it, a 'counter-culture' self-perception that lends itself to alienation from the rest of the Faculty."[23] By 2000 investigators from the DFCM had accepted their role as researchers, congruent with the rest of the faculty, but at the beginning, the firebrands of the DFCM had little interest in quantitative research and lots of interest in community action.

The mission of the new department was the training of family physicians by family physicians, not research in the classic sense or as the rest of the faculty understood the term. Family medicine itself was being elevated to a specialty, with its own "content, attitudes and skills," as Leitch put it. This was an important difference between the family doctors and the internists: family doctors had a different philosophy of care. "Research was to be directed towards medical problems in family practice, toward better methods of training of family physicians and the study of patterns of health care delivery."[24]

The issue of research raised its head from the very beginning. In the 1966–7 session, Fallis at TGH was working on Pap smears, Perkin at TWH is working on urinary tract infections, and the Family Practice Unit at the Wellesley was studying smoking and health.[25] Yet in an increasingly research-oriented faculty, the question how much research the family physicians were – or were not – doing proved greatly vexatious.

*Growth*

The family medicine residency program that began in July 1970 was widely represented in the community, as opposed to being concentrated in the teaching hospitals. The twenty-four first-year and six second-year residents who completed the first year of the program in June 1971 were distributed among thirty-five teaching practices and several new programs in community health centres and hospitals, such as the Gerrard-Broadview Clinic of St Michael's.[26] In April 1973 the government directed "that 50% of the output of Ontario Medical Schools should be in the area of Family Medicine." So all signals were set for growth.

By the mid-1970s the DFCM was experiencing growth pains. Paediatrics was a bottleneck. In 1974 the Department of Paediatrics aired its woes to the long-range planners: "The massive increase in numbers in the Family and Community Medicine 2nd year programme has made it impossible to provide their paediatric training at HSC. Yet 30% of the patients they encounter will be in the paediatric age group and it is our feeling that at least 4 months of their training should be provided by paediatricians."[27]

Some of the established departments found their noses out of joint at the nursling's rapid growth. An onsite survey team that visited late in 1974 noted "the major 'problems' that result when a young, aggressive department is introduced into an established faculty." The volunteer senior family physicians who sprang in to help with training often did not have university appointments. Certification is one of the foundation stones of academic life, and family medicine's apparent willingness to brush by it was troubling. Other departments were fearful that family medicine was eating their lunch. Were all internships to be converted into family practice residencies? The teaching hospitals had tended to fling their family practice units into cramped and undesirable quarters. Laments about the General and the Western were especially penetrating. And the obstetrical rotations at several hospitals were disasters, giving the residents little hands-on experience.

A more fundamental problem was the lack of supervision: there simply was not enough senior staff available in the hospitals to give adequate teaching. Women's College and Mount Sinai in particular lacked "active family physician teachers." As well, a quarter of total teaching time was devoted to internal medicine. Yet, the site visitors found, "internal medicine applied in family practice is different from that practiced by the consultant." The curriculum did not really reflect this reality.[28] The long-range planners brooded in June 1975, "This department represents one of the major problem areas both programmatically and structurally."[29]

Two different models of care were clashing here, that of hospital care and that of community care. At a tension-filled meeting of the long-range planners in February 1976, Fallis said, "It is inappropriate to apply the absolute standards of individual clinical disciplines to his department. It is the aim of the department to produce the best practitioner possible within the time and resources available, but it is obvious that such individuals will not be trained to the same level of competence as specialists in any given discipline." Douglas Johnson added that the family practice trainees needed "role models" different from those in internal medicine: "Ideally in each teaching hospital there should be a small cluster of beds recognized as a viable teaching unit, in which residents would see a role model of the family physician having responsibility for a totality of patient care." Fallis "expressed the hope that this committee might make a recommendation [that] attempts be made to ensure that family physicians can serve as a role model. This would enable them to keep up their skills and give the resident a perspective on the role he will need to fulfill in practice."[30] The new department thus strove sharply to differentiate itself from the traditional disciplines. (The traditional disciplines, in turn, bridled at this presumption of moral superiority in doctor-patient relations and were sceptical about family medicine's claim "to have special lessons to teach undergraduates." As Bob Harris, head of the long-range planners, put it, "The Department's teaching objectives for undergraduates are not unique to it but are responsibilities of all clinical departments."[31]

Despite resistance within the faculty, health care economics alone were travelling in the direction of family medicine. In February 1977 the powerful Long-Range Planning Committee heard Robert Ehrlich in the Department of Paediatrics tell them that just now physicians were "too expensive," that family doctors referred patients too often to "consultants," meaning that the family physicians themselves lacked the self-confidence and training to deal with problems of any complexity, and that "[d]octors and acute care hospital beds [were] the most expensive part of the health care system." How to circumnavigate these obstacles? Ehrlich said that the faculty must actively support a two-year Family Practice Program (and that paramedics – meaning non-MDs – could do yeoman service in the context of group practices).[32] This was not what the barons of the faculty – still suspicious of the "suddenly" founded Department of Family and Community Medicine – necessarily wanted to hear. But it was the wave of the future.

Shortly after these events, the department found itself buffeted by pressure from an unexpected quarter: the ministry wanted it to decentralize and move teaching to the peripheral hospitals. This insistence was most unwelcome, and the department felt there was no way of maintaining quality education in outlying community hospitals. In March 1978 the DFCM responded to this thrust: "It is really quite unrealistic to assume that specialist physicians in community hospitals whose prime concern must be the provision of patient care, could provide a comparable learning experience for a resident without adequate university recognition and funding."[33]

The pressure was thus on the department to articulate a convincing concept of what they were about and why they should have departmental status in the big teaching hospitals. In March 1980, Fred Fallis explained to Dean Holmes the vision of family medicine, in words that might be engraved in marble on the entryway to any family practice clinic: "We see our department putting forward on behalf of the Faculty a particular point of view which always needs to be represented in the life sciences. This view is that while universities should continue to emphasize excellence to the point of elitism in fundamental research and scholarship, the contemporary function of the University also include commitment to ... excellence in the applied arts and the satisfaction of human need ... It is the function of the University to house both these points of view and to encourage the productive tension between them." He continued, "The uniqueness of our discipline lies in its focus of application. It is the academic study of the art of the possible in personal medical care by the physician and his health team who have primary responsibility over time for the care of a set of patients and families."[34]

Family medicine truly was the concept of the good old GP brought back to life: the kindly family doctor who followed his patients over the arc of their lives and provided psychological support through his very presence (often because, in the pre-antibiotic days, he had nothing else to offer). Except that there were some differences: family medicine tended to be practiced in groups and not by the kindly old doctor making house calls in his Model-T. And the new family physicians were socially much more sensitive than the kindly old doc, who had studied anatomy in medical school rather than psychology. But even so.

*Research (More Trouble)*

Fallis also articulated a vision of family practice research. In his letter to Holmes of March 1980 he said, "Our 'art of the possible' implies a continuing study of the best methods of keeping the primary health care team's knowledge up to date, integrated and available to the problem at hand. We see a need to study life's normal benchmarks in order to modify therapeutic plans according to what is possible and best for each patient."[35]

What was the actual role of research in the new department? It should have been considerable, given that in 1967 Stanley T. Bain and William Spaulding wrote one of the classic contributions on the natural history of symptoms, a certain base on which to build.[36] Yet the department remained tentative about research for many years. To be sure, in 1979 the department began to require one major research project from each resident.[37]

Yet older members were unconvinced. At a meeting in April 1980 of the DFCM executive committee, the department's resistance to research became evident. Fallis was supposed to meet with the Faculty Research Committee. Drs Earl Dunn and John Hilditch registered their concerns with him: "Our first priority is teaching which requires a good deal of time. The Medical Research Council suggests that a researcher should devote 75% of his time to research! [exclamation mark in original] It was noted that across Canada no large number of Family Practice research projects have been funded and there is little relationship with MRC. Dr Dunn remarked ... that the amount of time expected to be devoted to research under present arrangements interferes with credible teaching practice ... The major task at the present time is to develop the community and patient base, and to put this base at the disposal of reasonable research."[38] So, in at least some quarters of the new department, the faculty's customary emphasis on research was received with a scornful flick of the wrist: family doctors played by different rules.

When in July 1991 Walter Rosser succeeded Wilfred Palmer as chair of the DFCM, research came back onto the radar. In 1995 Rosser implemented the Research Scholar Program in the DFCM under the guidance of Yves Talbot.[39] (By 2005 there were sixteen Research Scholars with 40–80 percent of their time protected.) The guiding theme for the research program was the "3 E's": effective practice, equity, and educational research.

It was thus under Walt Rosser that the department achieved a breakthrough into research. An external review in 2000 said, "Under his leadership, the DFCM has carved out funds to provide dedicated time for faculty who wish to undertake a research career." The reviewers found "a palpable sense of genuine excitement about research among young and mid-level faculty," thus ending the nimbus about research that had dogged the department in its early days.[40]

Dean David Naylor later underlined the distinctive research contribution of family medicine: "No other department has the same number of patients flowing through its members' clinical practices. No other department is in the same position to do high volume clinical research of a nature that could fundamentally change decision making on the front lines of clinical service provision."[41]

What kind of research was distinctive to family medicine? An example: Did it really matter if patients had a family doctor? Maybe the attentions of the emergency department would work just as well? Using the 1994 National Population Health Survey, Warren McIsaac and Yves Talbot at the Family Healthcare Research Unit of Mount Sinai Hospital determined in 2001 that it made a big difference. The higher the level of regular care by a family doctor, the greater the likelihood of "receiving preventive services." "Those without regular doctors ... were less likely to have ever had their blood pressure checked ... Women reporting some or no care were less likely to have had mammography within 2 years or to have ever had Pap smears."[42] This was among the earliest of the epidemiological studies that started to come from the Department of Family and Community Medicine.

The Faculty Plan for 2000–4 spelled out the department's research ambitions in detail. The DFCM had 603 faculty, of whom 59 were full-time. The department wanted to increase the numbers in all of their academic programs. "Develop PhD research clinician programs in collaboration with Health Administration." The plan noted, "Through the 1990's the Department focused on building the strongest academic Family and Community Medicine department in the world."[43] The next decade, the planners said, would see international sharing, "with particular focus on developing countries."[44]

### "The Largest Single Group Being Trained in Canada"

Under the leadership of Wilfred Palmer from 1981 to 1991, the growth in family medicine was enormous. Palmer, a McGill graduate of 1954 who had trained as an internist, was chief of family medicine at the General as well as departmental chair at a time when expansion seemed almost overwhelming. In 1983 the Self-Study group said, "This is now the largest single group being trained in Canada when compared with other specialties. There are ... 650 people writing certification examinations this year." At TGH a big new Family and Community Medicine Centre had just been built.[45] The 1981 decision of the College of Family Physicians of Canada to change the training needed for qualification from a one-year rotating internship to a two-year family practice residency aroused much anger. But Perkin said, "In the view of the [Family Practice] College the family practice training programme offers a better preparation for practice than the rotating internship and should be the standard for practice in this country."[46]

In 1990 the Ministry of Health decided that some postgraduate training was required to receive a license to practice medicine. Previously, a one-year internship would confer that right, but now one would either have to complete a two-year residency in family medicine to qualify as a family doctor (with membership in the Canadian College of Family Practice) or take a longer specialist residency to qualify for membership in the Royal College of Physicians and Surgeons. Because half of all graduating physicians in Ontario tended to choose family medicine, this greatly increased the number of postgraduate "PGY" slots the ministry would have to fund. It also reduced the flexibility of medical students and graduate doctors in choosing a career: They would have to decide in their third year what specialty they wished to enter. Dean Aberman explained, "Once they're in it, there's no flexibility, because those 600 [specialty] positions are divided up into a certain amount in internal medicine, surgery, etc. at that point."[47]

In 1993 the new two-year training requirement for family medicine went into effect, the culmination of a long campaign by the Ministry of Health to train physicians for community practice. Said John Provan, associate dean for postgraduate medical education, in 1993, "There is a perception by the Ministry of Health that we teach people to practice medicine as if they were all practicing in downtown teaching hospitals, when in fact, the majority of our trainees are going to work in smaller cities … The perception is that physicians who have trained in the downtown teaching hospitals … will do the investigation [of something like colon cancer] because they've seen it done in Toronto." The Ministry of Health and College of Physicians and Surgeons had decided that all "people who have obtained their MD must have two more years of training before the [college] will give them a license to practice in Ontario." The Ministry of Health wanted them to train at hospitals outside of Toronto. But Provan had a problem with this: "Once we start expanding into hospitals that are outside the fully affiliated downtown teaching hospitals, the supervision becomes much more difficult."[48]

A review in 2000 found the DFCM, "by virtue of its research and academic profile, a contender for the preeminent department of family medicine in North America." The reviewers praised a department, founded in the 1970s "with residency teaching as its only focus," for an undergraduate teaching commitment second only to that of the Department of Medicine. Given the enthusiasm and community focus of the staff, undergraduates wanted "an expansion of their role." The only confusion the reviewers found concerned the "core competencies" of the program's graduates. Were they to be proficient in obstetrics? Pediatrics? Inpatient family medicine? Yet there was a saving grace: "This situation should be seen in the context of uncommon confusion and upheaval in the organization of health care services the world over." So in Toronto the department was not doing so badly.[49]

## Community Health/Public Health

Some individuals have told us that graduate education in Community Health is moribund; our job was to administer the last rites … We unanimously reject these negative viewpoints. They are unwarranted and inaccurate. In the context of the Canadian experience with all aspects of graduate studies in Community Health, the University of Toronto's program commands resources which are not matched elsewhere in the nation … All of these developments, taken together, constitute a firm basis for pride in the past and optimism for the future.[50]

Advisory Committee on MSc and PhD Studies in Community Health, 1978

The narrative of the School of Hygiene and the Connaught Laboratories will not be followed further in this volume, given that several excellent accounts of events already exist.[51] The School of Hygiene was abolished in 1975.

### Department of Health Administration

The School of Hygiene had a Department of Health Administration. With the dismantling of the school, the department became part of the Faculty of Medicine. John E. Hastings, its acting chair, acknowledged that previously "research has not had as high a priority in the department as the provision of programs and courses," but its focus was changing. As of June 1975 it had twenty-two full-time academic staff, twelve with their primary appointment in the department, and twenty-seven part-time academic members.[52]

Following Hastings's appointment as associate dean in charge of the new Division of Community Health, the search for a new department head continued, apparently as "a high priority" for which the current financial constraints did not apply. Asked about the balance between service and research, Hastings said the candidate needed "to be credible to the School of Graduate Studies" but that "service orientation" was also "an important feature."[53] In 1976 the search committee selected Eugene Vayda as its first choice,[54] and he was successfully recruited to the position.

An American physician from Cleveland, Ohio, Vayda was a 1951 medical graduate of Case Western Reserve University in his hometown and practiced internal medicine for nearly a decade before moving into medical administration. In 1963 he gave up full-time clinical work to assume the directorship of the Cleveland Community Health Foundation. One of a number of American physicians increasingly concerned about the direction of medical care administration, in 1969 Vayda became a fellow in Public Health at Yale, where some faculty members from the new McMaster medical school in Hamilton were also studying. The Canadian contingent persuaded Vayda to accept a position in the Department of Clinical Epidemiology at McMaster, working on a program to apply epidemiologic principles to medical decision-making. Yet ultimately his interest in the organization and structure of health services won out, and in 1976 he moved to Toronto to accept the chair in health administration.[55] Vayda served in this position until 1981, when he succeeded Hastings as the associate dean of the community health division.

In keeping with the goal of increasing research, J.I. Williams was appointed director of the new Health Care Research Unit in the area of community health in late 1976, and a decade later the unit was under the directorship of Cameron Voelker.

After Vayda became associate dean, Theodore Goldberg took over the chair of the department in 1983, serving in this capacity until 1987. Goldberg had received his PhD in political economy at U of T, with Hastings serving as an examiner on his committee. After two decades in the United States, including work in the private sector and as a professor at Wayne State University in Detroit, Goldberg returned to Toronto to become chair. An important factor in his appointment was his front-line experience in the field of public health and health care, as well as his record as an advocate, researcher, and teacher in the North American group health movement.[56]

Peggy Leatt was named department chair and principal investigator for the Hospital Management Research Unit in 1987, holding these positions until being seconded to the post of president and CEO of the Health Service Restructuring Commission in September 1998.[57]

During her tenure in 1994 the Department of Health Administration created a "modular program" in which instruction was clustered once a month from Wednesday evening through all day Thursday, Friday, and Saturday, thus enabling students to continue working as well as furthering their education. An external review of the department in 1998 noted that applications "have doubled in the last few years and the school has acquired a very positive national and international reputation." The University of Toronto's program is "one of the leading centres in graduate health administration in North America."[58]

Leatt returned in 2000 from her nineteen-month position with the Restructuring Commission to be named the first Liberty Health Chair in Health Management Strategies, which provides placement within both the medical and law faculties. The Liberty Health Chair is the first endowed chair in health management strategies in Canada, funded by the leading health benefit management company in the country with a matching endowment by the university.[59]

### Preventive Medicine and Biostatistics

Among the three departments in the new Division of Community Health, preventive medicine and biostatistics evolved from the merger of three departments in the School of Hygiene: epidemiology and biostatistics, environmental health, and preventive medicine.

Following this reorganization Richard Osborn, a member of the former Department of Preventive Medicine, became chair of the larger combined unit. Osborn stepped down at the end of his five-year term in 1980, and Mary Jane Ashley served as acting chair during 1980–1 and was then appointed for a full term. Ashley completed all of her professional education at U of T, including her MD in 1963, DPH in 1967, and MSc in epidemiology in 1972. She was hired as an assistant professor in epidemiology and biostatistics at the School of Hygiene in 1974, the year before it was abolished. Ashley began her career doing epidemiological research on tuberculosis (the subject of her thesis was on recent trends in morbidity and mortality from the disease in Ontario) but later moved into tobacco and alcohol research, with a particular focus on policy. She was reappointed for a second five-year term in 1986, leading the Department of Preventive Medicine and Biostatistics for a full decade until 1991.[60]

The creation of several externally funded research units within the department enabled it to grow in size and strength. In the mid-1970s, as the restructured Department of Preventive Medicine and Biostatistics was itself being established, negotiations began with the National Cancer Institute of Canada (NCIC) to relocate its epidemiological unit to the department. NCIC agreed to pay for renovating the space and supporting the unit on an ongoing basis.[61] By autumn 1977 it was conducting trials, and the relationship between institute and university had strengthened by October 1979 to the point that it was then being referred to as the "NCIC – Epidemiology Unit."[62] Other independently funded research initiatives followed, including the epidemiological units of the Ontario Cancer Treatment and Research Foundation and the Ontario Foundation for Diseases of the Liver, later called the Canadian Liver Foundation. In the 1980s the department also established an AIDS research unit led by Ted Myers, as the disease began to reach full-blown epidemic proportions.[63]

The main criticism in the 1983 Self-Study was that it was "rather strange that the department does not have a program in clinical prevention." The Faculty of Medicine had adequate talent for such a program, and one had already been established in the Department of Health Administration. In response, Dean Lowy struck a Task Force on Clinical Epidemiology in 1985, headed by John Evans, "to develop a plan for a Faculty program in this area."[64] Its negotiations resulted in the creation in 1988 of a clinical epidemiology program in the Graduate Department of Community Health headed by Claire Bombardier. It had two training streams, a diploma in clinical epidemiology and a master's program, and approval had been received to begin a doctoral stream as well.[65] Although the focus on clinical epidemiology developed under Bombardier, her appointments were in the Departments of Medicine and Health Administration, thus leaving the epidemiologists in the Department of Preventive Medicine and Biostatistics to focus on public health issues in epidemiology.[66]

A significant program developed during Ashley's tenure was the Centre for Health Promotion (CHP). Noticing an interest in health promotion in the corridor talk, she chaired a committee with representatives from both preventive medicine and biostatistics and behavioural sciences and developed a proposal which resulted in the creation of the CHP. John Hastings, in his second stint as associate dean, fully supported the plan and secured a tenure-stream position for a director. The CHP was approved by Faculty Council in May 1990, and that fall Irving Rootman was appointed as its director and a professor in the Department of Preventive Medicine and Biostatistics. In December 1994 he was reappointed for a further five-year term.[67] In 1996 the importance of the unit was recognized when the World Health Organization designated it as one of six WHO Collaborating Centres in Health Promotion.[68]

Anthony Miller became chair of the department between 1992 and 1996. Miller had a long history of pioneering epidemiological analyses. He was based at the National Cancer Institute of Canada's Epidemiology Unit at the University of Toronto, and in 1981 he led a group of epidemiologists in developing a protocol for breast screening for cancer.[69] In 1982 a team studying cervical cancer in British Columbia of which he, in Toronto, was the senior (last named) author, found that a goodly portion of the cases of cervical dysplasia and carcinoma in situ regressed spontaneously, without ever progressing to invasive cancer, though progression was more common in older women.[70] In 1989 a team including Miller cast doubt upon the notion that smoking caused breast cancer.[71] The same year Miller headed the writing committee of the National Workshop on Screening for Cancer of the Cervix, held in Ottawa, which recommended in

1991 that Canadian women be given "the protection of regular cervical cytology screening" every three years from eighteen onwards.[72]

### Department of Behavioural Science

Unlike preventive medicine, the Department of Behavioural Science originated solely within the Faculty of Medicine. In 1967 Dean Chute stated, "The Faculty has ... recognized the need to give the student a better understanding of the individual and the community, and has endorsed the development of a division of behavioural science to cover this need in our plan of education."[73] The resulting department was established "for the primary purpose of introducing social and psychological aspects of health care into medical education."[74]

Initially behavioural science was a division in the Department of Paediatrics (which had been headed by Chute prior to his elevation to the deanery). Robin Badgley accepted appointment as director "on the understanding that a department would be formed."[75] Under his leadership, "the momentum of interest in the fusion of behavioural science and medicine" grew sharply both in Canada and internationally.[76]

Early in 1970 a subcommittee of the Committee on Curriculum and Examinations considering the establishment of this department reported back approvingly: "The multidisciplinary approach to teaching is inherent in the new curriculum ... Staff may be more readily attracted to a setting such as the proposed Department." Yet the committee showed some hesitancy about establishing a formal department, and the proposal was tabled for a year for the development of a curriculum.[77] By the end of the year, however, the committee reversed its previous decision after learning from Harry Bain, the head of pediatrics, that the unit had "in fact been operating much as an autonomous Department with a budget from the Dean." It was now in its second year of existence and had recruited staff.[78] On the basis of this endorsement the governing body, at that time the Senate, approved the creation of a Department of Behavioural Science within the Faculty of Medicine.

Upon its establishment in 1971 the department already included two full-time and five part-time members, seventeen sessional lecturers, and vibrant student participation. The *Dean's Report* emphasized that behavioural science was an "emerging field ... in which there is as yet little consensus about curriculum or the direction of research activities." The departmental staff were involved in many research projects, but Badgley authored the majority of the publications.[79]

With the dissolution of the School of Hygiene four years later, Badgley proposed the creation of a Department of Social Medicine to the Long-Range Planning and Assessment Committee (LRPAC). He did not want behavioural science to be included with other "community" departments, stating that it viewed itself more as a "basic science department relating basic problems to clinical areas."[80] Questions regarding the future of behavioural science continued as the Faculty of Medicine absorbed the School of Hygiene and restructured its departments.

Committee member Robert Harris, an orthopedic surgeon, recommended despite Badgley's protests that the department should be transferred to the community health division.[81]

Even as this plan was carried out, some people, including Harris, questioned whether behavioural science had "sufficient uniqueness to warrant continuation of departmental status ... It is adjusting to a role in a Faculty of Medicine with which it is not always in full agreement. This can develop into what might be called 'constructive tension.'"[82] Despite these concerns, the Self-Study group said in 1983, "The biggest strength of this department is that it is lively and active. It teaches and it talks and it does research work. It has become the centre in Canada for behavioural science in the medical area."[83] Any academic department should be thrilled to have such an accolade.

In November 1977, two years after the move, Stephen Griew became chair. Griew came to Toronto from Murdoch University in Western Australia, where he had been vice chancellor since 1972.[84]

From this department emerged the high-profile work of Ruth Cooperstock on benzodiazepines and addiction in women. Cooperstock, a sociologist, was educated at Sarah Lawrence College in New York and worked as a researcher at Columbia and the National Opinion Research Center. In 1955 she immigrated to Saskatchewan as a psychiatric researcher in the Department of Public Health. In 1964 the Cooperstocks moved to Toronto, where in 1966 she gained a post at the Addiction Research Foundation as a scientist in their epidemiology and social policy research department. There she documented "the 2:1 ratio of women to men in ... psychotropic drugs" as a sign of "the higher rates for women of neurotic illness, symptoms of both physical and mental discomfort, and help-seeking and drug-taking behaviour."[85]

Cooperstock was appointed to the Department of Behavioural Science in 1981, where, in the words of her eulogist Eugene Vayda, she "studied tranquilizer use and became a world expert in this field. She identified the disproportionate prescription and consequent overuse of minor tranquilizers, particularly the benzodiazepines, by women and wrote many papers and several books on this subject ... More recently she identified the untoward effects of these psychotropic drugs on the aged."[86]

Child psychiatrist Quentin Rae-Grant became chair of Behavioural Science in 1984[87] and was in turn succeeded by Harvey Skinner in 1987. By this time the department numbered several constituent research units, including aging and health, children's health, and physician behaviour, with a fourth, the Centre for Health Promotion, established jointly with the Department of Preventive Medicine and Biostatistics in 1990.[88]

*Graduate Department of Community Health*

The three departments comprising the faculty's Division of Community Health in 1975 – the Department of Preventive Medicine and Biostatistics, the

Department of Health Administration, and the Department of Behavioural Science – were mirrored in the new Graduate Department of Community Health in the School of Graduate Studies (SGS), ratified by the Governing Council the same year.[89]

Upon his appointment as the division's associate dean, John Hastings moved immediately to replace most of the diplomas offered by the former School of Hygiene with master of health sciences degrees. Some of the programs, which varied in quality, likewise needed to be upgraded: in hospital administration, there were roughly ten applicants annually, "about one-half of whom" were qualified, whereas in the DPH program "the quality of applicants is more varied" because many of its candidates were foreign students "from developing countries whose qualifications are more difficult to assess."

Hastings was not alone in driving these changes. The provincial Ministry of Health was calling for "greater emphasis on practice and less on administration," and the Royal College had recently broadened its specialization in public health to community medicine "with a potential for a number of streams."[90] In addition, since the 1960s the alumni of the hospital administration program, an increasingly influential group, had been lobbying the School of Hygiene to create professional master's degrees and were doing so more vigorously with the creation of the Division of Community Health. With the support of the Society of Graduates in Hospital Administration, the faculty obtained a grant from the US-based W.K. Kellogg Foundation "to study the educational needs of health and hospital administration."[91]

The resulting task force report proposed the establishment of a master of public health degree, which the SGS rejected.[92] From the ensuing back-and-forth, there emerged in 1979 the master of health sciences (MHSc), "a generic degree favored by the University of Toronto's leadership," according to historian Paul Bator. "The new degree gave respectability to the professional graduate degree. Hastings deemed the new programs as intellectually rigorous as the old-fashioned classical graduate studies requiring primary research and the writing of a thesis."[93]

After Eugene Vayda succeeded Hastings as associate dean of the division in 1981, its academic MSc and PhD programs were strengthened and the clinical epidemiology program was brought in under Claire Bombardier and Allan Detsky.[94] Efforts to strengthen the graduate programs continued. In 1990 Dean John Dirks expounded on the importance of the MHSc and MSc/PhD programs in community health, with their almost 300 graduate students: "Our graduates are necessary to the functioning of the health system and they are the major reason for the size and structure of this sector, the unique equivalent of a School of Public Health in English-speaking Canada."[95]

A Graduate Department of Health Administration was created in 1998. The Centre for Health Promotion, founded in 1990, was moved to it the same year, and soon thereafter, the programs in clinical epidemiology and health care research were transferred there as well. These developments, the faculty's Academic Plan for 2000–4 commented, "significantly strengthened what constitutes Canada's only 'school' of public health."[96]

*Department of Health Policy, Management and Evaluation*

The Department of Health Administration underwent a restructuring of its own. These changes were led by Vivek Goel, who had joined the Department of Preventative Medicine and Biostatistics in 1991 before being appointed chair of the Department of Health Administration for a five-year term in February 1999.[97] Goel completed his MD at McGill in 1984; then, after interning at St Joseph's Health Centre in Toronto and spending a year in general practice, he enrolled in the faculty's graduate health administration program in clinical economics under Allan Detsky, obtaining his MHSc in 1988 and a second master of science degree in biostatistics (health decision sciences) in 1990 at the conclusion of a research year at the Harvard School of Public Health.[98] After returning to Toronto, Goel joined the Clinical Epidemiology Unit at Sunnybrook.

Under Goel's leadership, the Program in Clinical Epidemiology and the Health Care Research Unit merged into the Department of Health Administration in 2000. According to David Naylor, former director of the team at Sunnybrook, Goel was perfectly positioned to bring the clinical epidemiology program fully into the department.[99] Following the merger, program director Tina Smith chaired a task force to determine a suitable name for the reconstituted department. A referendum was held among faculty members in February 2001 to decide between "Health Strategies" and "Health Policy, Management and Evaluation," and the latter won by an overwhelming majority of both primary and cross-appointed faculty. The new designation was officially approved by the Governing Council and went into effect in July 2001.[100]

Here is one exception to this book's determination to draw a line on events at 2000. In 2008, owing to the generosity of private donors, the Dalla Lana School of Public Health was created. This completed a circle that began in 1975 with the abolition of the old School of Hygiene. The hygienists of yore once again had a venue in which to pursue their own ideals of prevention and community health that, they were proud to say, diverged somewhat from the "medical model."

# 25  Hospitals

The teaching hospitals of Toronto were part and parcel of the academic health science complex. "The academic programs of the Faculty of Medicine are greatly enhanced by the affiliated teaching hospitals," as the faculty's "Strategic Directions" report put it in 1993.[1] Although a history of each hospital would take this book too far afield, their contributions to the faculty's larger mission are important. The Mount Sinai Hospital and Women's College Hospital are discussed in chapter 22 and the psychiatric hospitals in chapter 14. This chapter is given over to the Toronto General Hospital, St Michael's Hospital, the Toronto Western Hospital, and Sunnybrook Hospital.

## Toronto General Hospital

Patients in sufficient numbers remain the one indispensible resource of a medical school.[2]
Independent Planning Committee, Faculty of Medicine, 1969

Even though this book is in no sense a history of the Toronto General Hospital – several excellent ones already exist – it is impossible to understand the story of the faculty without knowing the vicissitudes of the faculty's once main clinical arm, the "Big House," as it was sometimes called, or "TGH." Among the oldest hospitals in North America, the General was founded in 1819 as a legacy of the War of "1812–14," in which Canada of course fought on the side of the British. Hospital functions commenced in 1829 and, after various vicissitudes, in 1854 the hospital was erected at its Gerrard Street site in the east end.[3] Thanks to Joseph Flavelle, the meat-packing magnate who was chair of the Board of Governors, in 1913 a splendid new building in central Toronto at the corner of College Street and University Avenue was constructed. The Ontario government, the City of Toronto, the university, and private donors such as John Eaton, owner of a flagship department store that bore his name, all contributed substantial sums. The institution that historian Michael Bliss has called "the most modern, best equipped hospital in Canada, one of the best in the world,"[4] thus took form. Martin Friedland, historian of the University of Toronto, has termed the General a "first-class hospital building to match its medical school."[5]

Let's cast a brief backward glance. In 1889–90, a year after the medical school opened, the Calendar of the U of T medical faculty had several pages on the hospital: "The hospital has now 350 beds." Clinical teaching: "Regular clinical lectures are given daily over patients brought from the wards to the large theatre by the Professors of clinical medicine and clinical surgery to the students of the third and fourth years." "Six assistants [interns] are appointed annually, and hold their positions for one year. They will be selected from the graduates every spring." They rotated among the various services.[6] Students learned surgery from viewing operations on Saturday afternoons in a 600-seat theatre. "The facilities afforded the students situated in all parts of the room for witnessing operations in all their details are unusually good," said the hospital.[7]

Physicians in the hospitals received virtually no compensation for teaching. In the public wards, which became the de facto teaching wards, care was basically free, at the cost of the city. In the private wards the patients paid the hospital and their physicians' fees but were not examined by the medical students and were free from the distractions of instruction. In 1905 John N.E. Brown, who had just taken office as superintendent, acknowledged rather ruefully the reality of "the unselfish service and skill of the various men who have served on the staff from time to time. But while this is true, it is to be regretted that from a scientific standpoint, little of permanent character has been accomplished." The unremunerated staff were simply too busy with their private practices, he said.[8]

The hospital had a few interns, but for the most, internship was rare to nonexistent in Toronto. In the 1890s the General had six "resident assistants," who were appointed annually and held their posts for a year. They were chosen every spring from the medical graduates and rotated in two-month shifts through the surgical wards, the medical wards, obstetrics in the Burnside, the eye and ear department, the gynecological and infectious diseases wards, the pharmacy ("Dispensary"), and the pathology department.[9] In 1906 TGH's first laboratory was set up for blood and urine tests. In 1912 the Wassermann test for syphilis was introduced.[10]

In 1906 the hospital decreed that staffers at the General were not allowed to admit patients to other hospitals: "Members of the Staff of the Toronto General Hospital be not permitted to belong to the active staff of any other General Hospital."[11] As historian James Connor points out, this reorganization caused a realization among physicians "that the medical community had split into 'haves' and 'have nots.' Specialist practitioners who held formal appointments at the University of Toronto as well as the Toronto General Hospital had become a super-elite within the fraternity. Those who held hospital appointments in the city's other hospitals occupied a lower rung; those who did not hold any hospital privileges ... ran the risk of being pushed to the margins of the profession."[12] The "two-tier" system was to become problematical over the years. In 1936 the retiring chairman of the TGH board Mark Irish told President Cody that unhappiness about the "closed" hospital – closed to nonacademic physicians in Toronto who could not admit and care for their own patients – was building in the medical community and that if the Private Pavilion did not turn enough of a profit to support the public wards, the city of Toronto, motivated by the fury of the excluded physicians, would refuse to further subsidize the hospital: "I do not hear the thousand Medical men who are out of Hospital affiliation chorusing consent to their Taxes being diverted to deficits created in Institutions from which they are rigorously excluded ... The demand will be for Public Beds to which any reputable Physician may follow his Patient. This may be hampering to Science, but, in the last analysis, Public Hospitals are for the treatment and cure of the Sick Poor, and are so viewed by an overwhelming majority of Taxpayers."[13]

In 1908 a reorganization created departments of medicine, surgery, obstetrics, gynecology, and ophthalmology; otology, rhinology, and laryngology were combined. Medicine and surgery were divided into three services each.

On 19 June 1913 the Toronto General Hospital moved into new quarters at the corner of College Street and University Avenue. President Falconer said, "The opening of the new General Hospital in June was an event of the first importance to this University, which contributed to its erection and which has the privilege of the clinical facilities afforded by its wards ... In recent years much has been done in the University for the development of the work in medicine by the erection and equipment of laboratories for the training of students in, and for the investigation of, the pure sciences preliminary to the study of medicine. This foundation has now been crowned by the new hospital."[14] The spanking new hospital was popularly called "the New General." "For several days after the opening, the Hospital was thrown open to the public, and it is estimated that not less than one hundred and fifty thousand persons viewed the institutional wards and other departments." Three ambulances helped empty out the wards of the old Gerrard Street hospital.[15]

The history of the General after 1913 was one of steady growth. In 1930 the public wards were much expanded "by extending the pavilions of the main building. A new private ward pavilion has been erected on University Avenue to provide for 350 patients ... replete with modern equipment and devices for the care of the sick. The entire hospital now contains 1,200 beds."[16]

From the viewpoint of academic medicine, the next milestone in the history of TGH came in 1947 with the changing of the guard: both William Gallie, the head of surgery, and Duncan Graham, the head of medicine, retired. Gallie, on the teaching staff of the faculty since 1908 and dean from 1936 to 1946, was replaced by his student Robert Janes; Graham, in the Eaton Chair for twenty-eight years and the first full-time professor of medicine in the British Empire, was succeeded by his student Ray Farquharson. Janes and Farquharson steered their large departments, the flagships of Canadian medicine, into the turbulence of the post-war years, when for the first time science and research began to supplant clinical training as the departmental missions.

The post-war emphasis on research had both positive and negative features. On the negative side, it gave the hospital a poor reputation among clerks and interns, who felt themselves ignored by the giants of medicine and surgery whose eyes were fixed upon distant horizons. In 1970, of forty-two clerkship places available, TGH was the first choice for only thirty. For the rather dowdy and scientifically unglamorous Wellesley Hospital, by contrast, fifty-six medical students campaigned for the thirty available clerkships. Interns had a history of avoiding the General because of the volumes of "scut work" said to be dumped on them. Said one critic, "TGH, until a few years ago, had its interns performing such worthwhile tasks as pasting lab results in the charts."[17]

On the positive side, the General became an international locomotive of research, forming in 1974 a Research Committee that directed millions of dollars to the development of "appropriate physical and clinical research space within the hospital."[18] TGH was late in organizing a Research Institute, and research in the 1970s remained at the departmental and divisional levels. Yet in medicine and surgery in the 1970s the numbers of "research-oriented staff" increased remarkably.[19] In 1978 the board of the hospital decided it would need around 80,000 square feet of research space, in a facility "sufficient to meet the needs of all researchers in the TGH and conceivably provide some space also for basic scientists associated with multidisciplinary programs."[20] By the end of 1984 the TGH board had made two decisions: one, to appoint a vice president and director of research at the hospital, the first of whom was scientist-administrator Donald S. Layne. The second decision was to commit $10 million for a new research facility. In December 1984 Layne told the faculty, "Largely through the initiative of a group of clinicians at the Toronto General Hospital, it was brought to the attention of the Board of Trustees that the hospital lacked certain features to give it the research stature usually associated with a large hospital in a major medical school, ie no physical plant or focus for research, and no single individual speaking for research at the higher decision-making levels." The board's Programme Advisory Committee made several basic decisions. "It was decided that space would not be assigned on a departmental basis, but a series of programmes would be identified which would be given hospital sanction." Layne had been in contact with Siminovitch at the Mount Sinai Research Institute, which to some extent provided a model. Yet there were fundamental differences: "[Layne's] mandate was to strengthen the existing research endeavour through the provision of adequate facilities, to co-ordinate existing activities and to facilitate the development of programmes identified as areas of concentration." Siminovitch by contrast had to "bring in outstanding scientists to form groups."[21]

In the fall of 1985, the seven-story Max Bell Research Centre and the Charlie Conacher Research Wing in renovated space in the old College Street wing opened; these together constituted the TGH Research Facility.[22] These facilities put a short-term, though alas not a long-term, end to the griping about shortages of research space. (As for clinical care, in 1979 the hospital's Eaton Wing with its 400 beds opened, built on the site of the 1913 Private Patients' Pavilion, the nurses' residence, and the Burnside obstetrical unit.[23])

Driven by W. Vickery Stoughton, the dynamic president and CEO of the Toronto General Hospital who had come up from Boston where he was chief executive officer of the Peter Bent Brigham Hospital, in 1985 discussions began about merging the General and the Toronto Western Hospital into a single entity, the Toronto Hospital. The members of the clinical departments of the two hospitals were massively unhappy about the merger, yet the hospitals' leadership and the Dean's Office were enthusiastic. Joe Marotta, as associate dean, organized a committee to oversee academic and clinical implications of the merger.[24] Lowy as dean backed the merger as "offer[ing] more opportunities, among them the opportunity to create a relationship between the Research Institute of the merged hospital and the University which would be an improvement over existing arrangements."[25] The merger itself was consummated in 1985 with Alan Hudson of the General as the chief executive officer of the new unit.

The merger headlined a concern that had wormed at the medical community for a century: fear and suspicion of the power of the "General." The faculty had eight teaching hospitals but somehow, it seemed to others, the General had taken more than its share. An external review of the Department of Ophthalmology in 1987 captured this begrudging suspiciousness: "[Fear is expressed at other teaching hospitals] that the Toronto General–Western amalgam may get an unfair total piece of the resources and equipment allocations, which confers upon the latter competitive and economic advantages over the other hospitals. We believe that such concerns are highly prejudicial to the academic mission of the Department."[26]

During Hudson's tenure as its CEO, The Toronto Hospital merged with the Princess Margaret Hospital in 1999 to form the University Health Network; its three "sites" reverted to their original names.[27] According to David Naylor, the creation of UHN "was tied to leadership transitions at PMH, friendships among the directors of the two institutions, and the logic of co-location once PMH moved to University Health Network." The Health Services Restructuring Commission "did not mandate that decision."[28] The University Health Network came to include several massive centres in its "focus of care" – the Krembil Neuroscience Centre at the Toronto Western Hospital; the Medical and Community Care unit at the General, as well as the PMH Cancer Program, the Peter Munk Cardiac Centre, the Surgical and Critical Care unit, and the Multi-Organ Transplant Program. By 2008 these and other programs at the three hospitals included over 1,300 clinicians and scientists with research funding of $55 million.[29] This was quite an extraordinary odyssey from Gerrard Street a century previously.

## Toronto Western Hospital

There is considerable research strength at the Western Hospital which seems to have been achieved by a deliberate policy of "protecting" scientists from other demands on their time, in particular, from service responsibilities.[30]

Report by George Connell, Ernest McCulloch, and Louis Siminovitch, 1973

The Toronto Western Hospital was founded in 1896 on Bathurst Street in the western section of Toronto as "new areas were spreading rapidly out towards High Park." William R. Feasby said in his history of the faculty, "To serve this area, doctors of the region had formed themselves into a founding committee; each man put up $1,000 and so a new hospital had its origin … Its founders and directors recognized the importance of university teaching affiliation, and in 1911 applied to the Faculty Council to become an affiliated hospital for teaching of undergraduate students."[31] In 1912 the new hospital, with its 250 teaching beds, began the clinical instruction of undergraduates in medicine, easing the shortage of teaching beds that had arisen at the General with hordes of students in the operating rooms and clustered in the wards.[32] This "proved a boon to the students, as it means that with the Toronto General, St Michael's, the Hospital for Sick Children and the Western Hospital more than a thousand beds will be available for clinical teaching."[33]

In 1936 the Western undertook a major reorganization, in which medicine under Herbert K. Detweiler, surgery under Thomas A.J. Duff, gynecology and obstetrics under Robert Watson Wesley, and pathology under George Shanks all became teaching departments.[34] In the Department of Medicine, Duncan Graham said, "A teaching staff, the majority of whom had received training at the Toronto General Hospital, was appointed. In order that the staff might be able to devote more time to hospital work, the Western Hospital agreed to remunerate the Physician-in-Chief and one junior member of the staff. Unfortunately the training programme … was interrupted by the war."[35]

By 1945, over half of the hospital's 515 beds were dedicated to teaching.[36] At the same time, the university agreed with the hospital (and with St Michael's) that all new hospital appointments would "be made after consultation with and on the advice of the respective university departments. Each new appointment … will carry with it appropriate university rank." Both the Western and St Michael's therewith obtained "full membership in the federation of teaching hospitals associated with the University."[37]

In the 1958–9 session, the Western acquired a dedicated research unit, named after donor William E. Coutts.[38] For practical purposes, this was the beginning of the Research Institute at the Western.

*Departments and Divisions at the Western: Some Stories*

The story of medicine at the Western, or at any other single teaching hospital, cannot be told because the tableau in this volume is already vast enough. But a couple of events might be highlighted.

The Department of Medicine led the research bandwagon at the Western. In the 1949–50 session, W. Hurst Brown succeeded Herbert Detweiler as physician-in-chief.[39] Brown was known for building up research at TWH. In the 1961–2 session Irwin M. Hilliard, a Toronto-trained internist who had been the first professor of medicine at the University of Saskatchewan, returned to Toronto to succeed Brown.[40] In Hilliard's department respiratory disease was a prominent object of study. In 1970–1, the Department of Medicine in the Western and the National Sanitarium Association jointly set up a research institute with immunological aspects of respiratory disease as the major focus. It was officially launched in 1974 as the Gage Research Institute (because it was in the Gage building) with Irvin Broder its director.[41] (In January 1996 the Gage Research Institute was merged with the Occupational and Environmental Health Unit to create the Gage Occupational and Environmental Health Unit, at 223 College Street, its director remaining Linn Holness of the Department of Preventive Medicine.[42])

Psychiatry at the Western had a history of strength. In the 1952–3 session, still a division of the Department of Medicine, psychiatry at the Western became part of the campus Department of Psychiatry's training program.[43] In the 1967–8 session the hospital Division of Psychiatry under Alan J. Preston received departmental status, joining the campus Department of Psychiatry.[44] Shortly thereafter, the Western added a Mental Health Centre. It also organized a special psychiatric consultation program to the Renal Transplant Unit and to the Arthritis and Rheumatology Unit.[45] In 1970–1 a Drug Abuse Clinic was founded at the Western.[46]

In scientific terms, the most prominent member of the Department of Psychiatry was Harvey Moldofsky, who in 1978 discovered the efficacy of pimozide in Tourette's syndrome.[47] And in 1982, together with Gregory Brown of McMaster University, Moldofsky proposed a dopaminergic hypothesis of Tourette's.[48] Moldofsky established a Tourette's clinic and in 1993 became the founding director of the university's Centre for Sleep and Chronobiology.

As for surgery, in 1924 the twenty-five-bed surgical service at TWH was reorganized, with Henry A. Beatty as chief and "granted University standing as Assistant Professor of Clinical Surgery."[49] As mentioned earlier, in 1936 the surgical services at the Western were reorganized with Duff as surgeon-in-chief; four other surgeons had university appointments and plans were completed to offer clinical teaching in surgery.[50] In 1940 the Gallie Course was extended to the Western so that trainees rotated among the four hospitals: the Western, St Michael's, the children's hospital, and the General.[51]

Robert C. Laird replaced Duff as surgeon-in-chief in 1945–6, and when Laird retired in 1965–6, Donald Wilson succeeded him. Wilson became university head of the Department of Surgery and profiled, in events related elsewhere in this volume, cardiovascular surgery at the hospital.

In the large reorganization of surgical services attending the merger of the General and the Western, in the late 1980s the trauma program was moved from the General to the Western division under the leadership of Darrell Ogilvie-Harris. "The intent is to run a first-class Trauma Program of limited dimensions so that the Western Division is not over-run by the victims of trauma."[52]

Neurosurgery had figured at the Western ever since William Keith's arrival in 1936. Keith, who undertook neurosurgery at both HSC and the Western, attracted John Silversides to the Western in 1950 to organize a neurological service. Together, Keith and Silversides built, as Ross Fleming put it, "a combined neuroscience unit which was a model of close cooperation between neurology and neurosurgery." Fleming joined them at TWH in 1956, becoming division head in 1965.[53] Subsequent events in neurosurgery at the Western are discussed elsewhere in this volume.

Radiology became a teaching department at the Western in 1948–9 with the appointment of William Cecil Kruger.[54] The department was led from 1951 until his retirement in 1986 by Louis Ralph Harnick, whom radiology colleague Brian Holmes described as "a people person, a true extrovert who was happiest in the company of friends and colleagues." Lou Harnick was later elected president of the Ontario Medical Association, the first Jew to hold that office, as Holmes remarks. "It was during this time the OMA saw the need to construct its own headquarters, but was intimidated by the financial implications. Due to Dr. Harnick's eloquent persuasion a commitment was made, and he became known far and wide as 'what's-a-million-Harnick.'"[55] (On the not entirely happy story of radiology at the Western under Harnick, however, see chapter 20.)

## St Michael's Hospital

The nuns of the Sisters of St Joseph opened the hospital in May 1892, their "own rooms near the patients." According to the *Toronto Star*, "The happiest days were when the sisters were in charge of the large 80-bed public wards where the neediest patients were cared for and where," said Sister Irene McDonald in an interview many years later, "the rewards were greatest." Writing in June 1998 of the nuns' finally moving out of St Michael's and uptown to a retirement home, the *Star* added, "The culture the nuns brought to the hospital was one of efficiency, self-discipline, respect for authority – both church and hospital – good housekeeping and prudent management. They were also the ones to find the hospital's signature statue of St. Michael blackened and abandoned in a Queen St. second-hand store."[56]

Almost from the beginning of the faculty's relaunch in the late 1880s, St Michael's with its eighty beds was one of the teaching hospitals. The 1894–5 Calendar of the faculty showed the big guns of the faculty also as "members of the staff of St. Michael's Hospital": Irving Cameron, Alexander McPhedran, John Amyot, and others.[57] The integration of St Michael's into the faculty was eased by Robert Joseph Dwyer, chief physician of the hospital, who graduated in medicine from U of T in 1892, the year the hospital was established. He became a lecturer in the faculty and applied for an associate professorship in 1900 (but was swatted down).[58] He then studied in Europe, in 1902 receiving membership in the Royal College of Physicians of London. The same year he returned to join the staff of the hospital, also receiving a regular faculty appointment.[59]

By 1904–5 the number of beds at the hospital had increased to 160, and the affiliated faculty included numerous physicians, surgeons, obstetricians, and others. There were also, as at the General, four "resident assistants," or interns, appointed from the graduating class.[60] In 1908 St Michael's became a fully affiliated teaching hospital. Dean Clarke said, "Fortunately the authorities of St Michael's Hospital are willing that the University should use its very valuable clinical material for instruction. There will be two services in Medicine and two in Surgery under the direction of University professors."[61]

Teaching facilities at SMH grew apace with the development of academic life in the city. In the 1927–8 session, the hospital built a "new students' laboratory … It will be completely equipped next session, and it is hoped its facilities will aid materially the teaching strength of this department."[62] By 1945 teaching beds at SMH numbered 375 out of almost 700 total beds.[63] Of these teaching beds, around 200 were on the "medical public wards" (and included 36 beds for "neuropsychiatry").[64]

In the 1946–7 session the same agreement was negotiated with the faculty as described earlier for the Western: all new appointments in all hospital departments would be negotiated directly between hospital and faculty, and all staff would have university ranks.[65]

Research was always a sensitive matter at St Michael's because many staffers perceived themselves in the shadow of the Toronto General Hospital and wanted to make sure they were not marginalized. In the 1960s a "Research Society" was founded to foster investigation. When in 1974 SMH prepared its statement to the Petch committee that was organizing material for the Ontario government's Task Force on Health Research Requirements, they wrote, "Research at Saint Michael's Hospital is mostly of a programmatic nature. Most of the investigators are entrepreneurs who disregard departmental boundary lines seeking collaboration with experts in other departments and other institutions in order to get the job done." As an example they give the Lipid Research Clinic Project, which embraced institutions as far away as Soviet Russia and included eight campus departments.[66]

By the late 1970s the hospital had a scientific advisory committee and a finance committee for research fundraising. They had no Canadian government funds, and half their research budget came from a big grant from the National Institutes of Health in the United States for the hospital's lipids research program. SMH established a Research Institute in 1994.[67]

Research at St Michael's took a big leap forward in 2000 with the appointment of Arthur Slutsky of the university Department of Medicine as the vice president of research.[68]

For all the talk in the Toronto Academic Health Sciences Complex about "integration," St Michael's valued its independence. In 2003, at the time of an external review of the Department of Medicine, Robert Hyland, physician-in-chief at SMH, said that many clinicians in the hospital would resist centralizing attempts: "There was strong feeling amongst the Division Heads that St Mikes has benefitted from its independence and that any other structure [such as strengthening university division heads] would run the risk of tipping the balance of power towards University Avenue."[69]

In the story of the teaching hospitals there is thus this constant underlying tension between strengthening the power of the University Avenue hospitals, closely identified with the Faculty of Medicine, and the more peripheral institutions such as the Western and St Michael's, subject to a continuing perceived assault upon their autonomy from the Big House and its allies in the Dean's Office. The reality of this conflict was quite different, with the dean and the departmental chairs trying to establish their control over the academic programs of the big University Avenue hospitals and research institutes. But in politics, perceptions count for a great deal.

This volume cannot attempt a systematic review of all the departments and divisions at St Michael's; that awaits a comprehensive hospital history. But a few high points might be mentioned. (Many other achievements are found throughout the clinical chapters of this volume.)

The history of surgery at St Michael's illustrates well the pivot from teaching to science that occurred in much of academic medicine in Toronto. Until the 1970s, the chief surgeons were often beloved and distinguished individuals but not plugged into the international stream of science. To be sure, surgical training at SMH was bound into the Gallie Course in 1939–40, becoming part of the rotations.[70] Yet only in the late 1960s did the hospital Department of Surgery begin discussing the appointment of non-practicing surgeon-scientists. Surgeon Donald Currie, giving an update on the department's plans in 1969, said that a number of retirements were coming up. "In addition to the proposed number of eight clinical surgeons in the next five years, we would be most anxious to have nonpractising surgeons who would be willing to devote all of their time to surgical research. We would be anxious to have four or five of these scientist-surgeons."[71] This sounded a new note.

The big problem in expanding surgical research at SMH was not lack of will but a shortage of space. The hospital was even willing to rent expensive outside laboratory and office space, "essential if we are to attract new Staff," as neurosurgeon William J. Horsey told William Drucker, head of the university department, in 1969. The hospital department was moving the number of geographic full-time staff in surgery up from five in 1969 to eleven in 1974 and of fellows from two to seven. "A Fellow is almost indispensable for a person whose activities in research are part time."[72]

Important contributions were not long in coming. In 1988 Alan Hudson conducted the world's first nerve transplant. Ralph Manktelow pioneered muscle transplantation (see p. 173). (Both in turn were hired away to the General.)

In 2004 Ori Rotstein was appointed chief surgeon at the hospital. Rotstein, the son of a surgeon who had to train in the United States because of the Jewish exclusion in Canada, had quickly cottoned to research when he became a staff surgeon at the Western in 1985, then at the General in 1988. He rose through the research ranks to run the Surgical-Scientist Program and in 2001 became director of the Institute of Medical Science in the faculty. An innovative translational researcher and chest surgeon, his lab was interested in ischemia in the lung, and Rotstein pioneered the use of hypertonic saline in preventing lung injury.[73] He said in an interview, "Of all the things I've done, I think I was most proud of that. So it was kind of fun. Unfortunately, because hypertonic saline is not a commercial product, we were never able to go the commercialization route to make a drug." Yet the Canadian army, he said, had adopted its use.

Rotstein came to St Michael's after Arthur Slutsky, vice president of research, recruited him. He had been at the Division of General Surgery at TGH for the previous seven years and was "kind of looking for something else to do." He put his hand to the task, as Richard Reznick put it, "of expanding the academic profile of the surgery department"; it was the same mission that Bob Hyland had taken on as chief of medicine. Hyland had recruited forty new clinicians; off the mark Rotstein hired twelve "surgeon-scientists, many repatriated from the US."[74] Slutsky told Rotstein, "I want you to build up the academic activities in the Department of Surgery. That was the mandate I had. And from the minute I stepped in the recruitment has been unbelievable."

Rotstein wanted to recruit Subodh Verma, a cardiac surgeon. "Verma is a phenom, so every institution in the country is trying to recruit this guy. So Art and I, one Sunday afternoon, Richard Weisel and Subodh went over to Art's house, we had lunch, we signed the deal there, and it included a Canada Research Chair. So you know this was like, as much as you can get, a blank cheque in the Canadian health care system to build a research group, that's what Art provided."[75]

Rotstein's arrival thus infused surgery at St Michael's with a new excitement. SMH was further enriched in 1998 when the Hospital Restructuring Commission closed the Wellesley Hospital, transferring its medical staff and programs to St. Michael's. According to David Naylor, the merger proved "something of a reverse takeover" as "the heads of medicine, surgery and family medicine from the Wellesley all ended up with those jobs in the combined institution."[76]

SMH's open-heart surgery program, founded in 1958, was undertaken independently of the TGH program because of antipathy between SMH surgeon Clare Baker and Bill Bigelow, who was said to have prevented many residents from training at SMH.[77] The distinguished St Michael's cardiac program is discussed on pp. 100–102. There was something of a hiatus then with the departure of the early cardiac surgeons. When Lee Errett was recruited as head of surgery at SMH in 1994, he re-established the cardiovascular clinical and research program, with support of benefactor Terrence Donnelly.

The Department of Surgery at St Michael's is forever connected with the name of Alan Hudson, who with the help of plastic surgeon Susan E. Mackinnon performed the world's first peripheral nerve transplant there in 1988 – the sciatic nerve. In May 1988 an eight-year-old boy's sciatic nerve was severed by a propeller in a boating accident. When in September a sixteen-year-old girl died from a stroke in London, Ontario, her sciatic nerve was harvested, then rushed to Toronto where Hudson and Mackinnon transplanted it under an operating microscope. With the passage of two years the lad was able feel a pinprick in the sole of his foot for the first time since the accident.[78] Born in Cape Town, South Africa, in 1938, Hudson earned his MD degree at the University of Cape Town in 1960, trained in neurosurgery in the United Kingdom, and immigrated to Canada, passing his medical licensing exam in 1965. He joined the neurosurgical staff of St Michael's in 1970, founding a peripheral nerve injury clinic in 1980 which by the late 1980s was receiving patients from all over the world. In these years St Michael's neurosurgical division was, in Martin McKneally's judgment, "regarded by the residents as the best place to learn neurosurgery."[79]

In 1989 Hudson migrated to the Toronto General Hospital as surgeon-in-chief.[80] In the 1990–1 session he became president and CEO of the Toronto Hospital.

In urologic surgery at SMH, Vincent Colapinto was a star. Born in Toronto in 1928, he received his medical degree from Toronto in 1952, then trained in general surgery from 1955 to 1958; he fellowed in urologic surgery for two more years. Colapinto joined the staff of SMH in 1961 and went on to start the hospital's dialysis unit in 1968; he performed the first kidney transplant at St Michael's in 1971.[81] In research, he and Ron McCallum in radiology wrote the monograph *Urological Radiology of the Adult Male Lower Urinary Tract* (1976) that, as his eulogist Norman W. Struthers says, "established him as a leader in the management of urethral stricture." He served as urologist-in-chief at the hospital from 1982 until his death in 1985.[82]

Of particular interest in the history of obstetrics and gynecology at St Michael's is that Ewan Stuart Macdonald, who joined the department in 1947 after serving in the Royal Canadian Navy during the war, was the son of Lucy Maud Montgomery, author of the Canadian classic – and international bestseller – *Anne of Green Gables*. Macdonald himself was said to be, appropriately, "an avid reader and a lifelong student of the English language. He was a severe critic of those who played fast and loose with proper grammatical construction and [readers of] his correspondence were treated to the beauty of a disciplined but flowing prose which was a delight to the senses and to the mind."[83] The comment is interesting because many members of the faculty in those days were beautiful writers, and the sturdy and workmanlike offering from their pens will remain a pleasure for future historians of the faculty to discover.

In oncology, St Michael's had two strong areas, the Breast Clinic, involved in a massive screening program, and a neurosurgical unit that in the 1980s had, as James Waddell, surgeon-in-chief (himself an orthopedic surgeon), pointed out, "the largest number of brain tumours of any neurosurgical unit in Canada." Also, using the mouse model, the SMH neurosurgeons were heavily involved in brain tumour research.[84]

What else? In 1967 Michael Shea in the Department of Ophthalmology pioneered cryosurgery on retinal tears without detachment.[85] And David Jenkins, the founding director of the Clinical Nutrition and Risk Factor Modification Centre, developed in 1981 his "glycemic index," a measure of the rapidity with which carbohydrates release glucose into the bloodstream (see also p. 445).[86] Jenkins, who had done research on diabetes at Oxford, moved to Canada in 1980. Foods with a high glycemic index, he showed, led to high insulin levels, which in turn were linked to diabetes. Out of his collaboration with industry came grocery-chain Loblaws's "Too Good To Be True" and "Blue Menu" products.[87] In a randomly controlled trial published in the *Journal of the American Medical Association* in 2008, Jenkins demonstrated that in type 2 diabetes, a low-glycemic diet reduced the glycemic index better than did a high-cereal fibre diet.[88]

The Centre for Faculty Development at SMH opened in 2002 with psychiatrist Ivan Silver as director and cosponsored by the faculty's continuing education office. The centre's mission was to enhance instructional skills in continuing medical education. In 2005 Silver was appointed associate dean of continuing education.[89]

Located in a rather gritty piece of east-end real estate in Toronto, St Michael's had always prided itself on its work with the disadvantaged and down-and-out, especially in its Inner City Health Research Unit. In 1969 Murray Cathcart became inaugural chief of the hospital's socially committed Department of Family and Community Medicine. Phil Berger followed him as chief in 1997, simultaneously becoming medical director of the Inner City Health Program.[90] The following year, 1998, Donald Wasylenki, chief psychiatrist at SMH, became the inaugural holder of a dedicated chair in inner-city health, held jointly between the hospital and the university.[91] "The thing that is woven into the fabric of the institution is the inner-city hospital mentality," said Rotstein, "and that came from the CEO [Jeff Lozon] all the way down. It's just a place where you feel like you're part of it. There's a warmth here that isn't at a lot of other places."[92]

When he arrived from Mount Sinai as vice president of research, Art Slutsky was pleased to encounter once again this distinctive culture (he had scrubbed in with Sam Lichtenstein and Tom Salerno in 1990 at the time of their trial showing warm cardioplegia superior to the hypothermic variety in open-heart surgery[93]). "The hospital started in 1892 to take care of the poor in downtown Toronto, and it's been doing that ever since. It has the most incredible culture of caring that I've seen in any hospital, and it all comes from the Sisters of St. Joseph. Remember, I'm not Catholic, but boy, that culture of caring is remarkable. You can't go a week in this institution without hearing about culture and caring." The hospital picked inner-city health research as a priority area and by 2009 had "one of the top three strongest programs in inner-city health research in the world, doing research on homelessness."[94]

### Sunnybrook Hospital

Sunnybrook Veterans Hospital was officially opened in 1948, though D Wing was already accepting patients in 1946. The hospital continued to be run by Veterans Affairs until the University of Toronto began to manage it in 1966, thus making it the first university teaching hospital, properly understood. Yet teaching had gone on at Sunnybrook almost from the start.

Just after the Second World War both the Christie Street and Sunnybrook Veterans Hospitals began accepting interns, integrating their training in 1946–7 "where possible with the various training programs of the University teaching hospitals ... It will provide, through university affiliation, for a continued maintenance of a high standard of treatment for the veterans."[95] The Faculty of Medicine recommended all staff appointments at Sunnybrook but collaborated with the Department of Veterans Affairs at Christie Street.[96]

The federal government was also cooperative in opening Sunnybrook to the faculty for training of residents. In the 1948–9 session, the Department of Veterans Affairs made the Neuropsychiatric Unit of Sunnybrook available for postgraduate psychiatry training.[97] (An actual hospital Department of Psychiatry at Sunnybrook would be founded only in 1967–8 under Wilfred E. Boothroyd.[98])

Most of the major university departments were in place at Sunnybrook before the university took over the hospital. In the 1948–9 session, Desmond T. Burke, a Queen's University graduate of 1932, was appointed associate in radiology, thus making the Sunnybrook department a university teaching department.[99] In the 1951–2 session the campus Department of Medicine established a hospital department at Sunnybrook under Ian Macdonald. The resident veterans' population lent itself splendidly to long-term studies, and in the 1951–2 session Harold Rykert and Donald Moran at Sunnybrook undertook a sustained investigation of atherosclerosis.[100] In 1958 Alan W. Harrison founded the Division of General Surgery, "with a mandate to establish an academic postgraduate surgical program."[101]

Other departments were established at the time of the takeover in 1966. Otolaryngology, for example, arrived at Sunnybrook in the 1966–7 session, as Percy Ireland, who had retired downtown, became chief.[102]

As the number of veterans at Sunnybrook began to decline in the 1960s, and as Medicare loomed, it was decided to develop Sunnybrook as a teaching hospital. John Evans, the young cardiologist who ultimately ended up as U of T president in 1972, was said to have first called attention in the early 1960s to a faculty future at Sunnybrook when he served as secretary to a committee of the Board of Governors.[103] The faculty then formed a working group consisting of Evans, Fred Kergin, and urologist Carl Aberhart, who had a strong interest in the rehabilitation of spinal patients and introduced tidal irrigation of paraplegics' bladders. The working group was to consider making Sunnybrook a teaching hospital "at a time when the University was looking for more places for teaching purposes because of the decrease in indigent patients. The committee advised that Sunnybrook should become a university hospital." Lots of negotiation followed. It was agreed that the Board of Governors would acquire Sunnybrook on condition that veterans had first access to the 630 active treatment beds. "The University took possession of Sunnybrook in October, 1966 for the sum of one silver dollar."[104]

Martin Friedland in his history of the University of Toronto says that, as an additional consideration, the university wanted to develop Sunnybrook in order to forestall York University from establishing a second medical school in the Toronto region.[105] The second medical school for southern Ontario in fact went to McMaster University, where Evans was inaugural dean. On this development, David Naylor commented that it is "hard not to see some irony in the enthusiasm for a second campus at Sunnybrook." John Evans, a leading proponent of that plan, was wooed away to McMaster in large part because of "the failure of the medical school and university to support that idea."[106]

The acquisition of Sunnybrook did not excite universal jubilation. General surgeon Robert Mustard protested against funding Sunnybrook, given the cuts that the other teaching hospitals must sustain. Yet Dean Chute remained committed to the enterprise, stressing "the need for developing the requirements for research and educational space in terms of an integrated programme in order to make it effective and at the same time economically feasible."[107] From the beginning the Sunnybrook staff wished the institution to have "a strong research component," as they told members of the Faculty Council's Sub-committee on Science Policy, who conducted a site visit in January 1973. Yet the site visitors said, "Their research objectives do not seem to have been thought out in any detail." Sunnybrook had a research committee, but "[t]he committee does not seem to have spent much time thinking and arriving at a consensus of their research objectives." This is unsurprising given that in the early 1970s the faculty in general was struggling with the concept of a research culture and what one did to acquire one. But Sunnybrook was aware that the hospital required research space of its own because the distance to the Medical Sciences Building downtown made doing research there "almost prohibitively difficult." The Sunnybrook clinicians wanted to recruit people with a "strong research interest" immediately. But there was no space for labs and the tiny animal care facility was "horribly inadequate." "To meet these problems," said the site visitors, "the staff believe that it is important to create some additional laboratory space *now*, contiguous to the animal building." And as the faculty's first university hospital, they wanted funds from the Dean's Office at once.[108]

The ministry thought to relieve Sunnybrook's thirst for development funds by merging it with another hospital, and in 1987 a merger with the Wellesley Hospital was considered and then rejected in favour of closing the Wellesley. A merger with Women's College Hospital was then achieved in 1999 (though mandated earlier)ending in 2006. It was thus only in 1989 that the Ministry of Health permitted Sunnybrook to proceed with its own development plan, which included, as Dean John Dirks put it, "a very substantial research facility. The hospital is interested in enhancing its development, perhaps by fulfilling the academic plans envisaged in the merger."[109]

The Sunnybrook Research Institute (SRI) was thus formed in 1989 with the appointment of R. Mark Henkelman as vice president of research, "with a mandate to turn Sunnybrook into a research hospital."[110] Henkelman, a well-known medical imager in the Department of Medical Biophysics (who introduced magnetic resonance imaging to Canada), came up from Princess Margaret Hospital to lead a team colloquially known as the "Group of Seven" in establishing SRI as a pioneering centre for imaging research.[111] Henkelman raised the level of external funding from about $1 million per year to $30 million a year within the next ten years and built a 10,000-square-metre research facility to support a team of around forty principal investigators (including David Naylor, the future dean of medicine and university president).[112]

*Research at Sunnybrook*

In 1973 a team of heavyweights from the downtown campus, including Lou Siminovitch, dean-to-be Brian Holmes, and Ernest McCulloch, visited Sunnybrook to assess the research situation. They found a hospital filled with aspirations but little practical idea of how to get going. First of all, space for research was lacking. The campus Medical Sciences Building was a half hour's drive away, but Sunnybrook itself had no dedicated research space, and the animal facility, in demand particularly for the surgeons' research, was "horribly inadequate for its function." This lack of space "makes it difficult to attract anyone to the Hospital … who has a strong research interest." Moreover, the current staff, "very occupied by their clinical responsibilities, spend only a limited time at their research ... There is no real research leader among the group."[113] Yet the spirit was willing: "The one philosophy for which there is a consensus within the hospital [is that] Sunnybrook should eventually contain a major research facility."

Despite the visitors' superior airs, Sunnybrook had in fact already compiled something of a research record.

After James Dauphinee became chair of the Department of Pathological Chemistry in 1947, he created one of the first clinical investigation units in Canada at Sunnybrook in 1951, which he supervised until 1966.[114]

The Department of Medicine at Sunnybrook had its own budget and was largely autonomous of the university department. In 1965–6 John Paterson became chief of medicine at Sunnybrook, replaced then by Don Cowan in 1974 as physician-in-chief, just as John W. Norris, Vladimir Hachinski, and John G. Edmeads opened the MacLachlan Stroke Unit, the first in Canada.[115] (Edmeads, a neurologist and big international authority on headaches, became physician-in-chief in 1994.) It is interesting that when in 2007 Wendy Levinson became university head of the Department of Medicine, she also became physician-in-chief at Sunnybrook.

Over the decades, the Department of Surgery at Sunnybrook became a major dynamo, led initially in the late 1950s by urologist Carl Aberhart. The department was later headed by such distinguished figures as orthopedic surgeon Marvin Tile (1985–98) and cardiac surgeon Bernard Goldman (1998–2001). Scientific contributions from Sunnybrook surgeons included orthopedic surgeon Joseph Schatzker's description of internal fixation of the fractured neck of the femur in 1986 (together with Stuart Goodman at Stanford: Schatzker was, at the time, at the Wellesley Hospital)[116] and Marvin Tile and George Pennal's 1980 classification of pelvic fractures, or pelvic "disruption," widely used among radiologists.[117]

Before the recruitment in 1975 of Robert McMurtry as director of the trauma program and the emergency department at Sunnybrook, the university had no trauma program. Sunnybrook's was said to be the first in Canada. In the 1986–7 session, a trauma residency position was given to Sunnybrook, the first of a hoped-for series of positions concentrating on trauma.[118] In 1986 as well, the emergency department initiated its P.A.R.T.Y. program, for Prevent Alcohol and Risk Related Trauma in Youth, which, the hospital claimed, was "world renowned." (On the neurosciences at Sunnybrook see chapter 14.)

The Department of Medical Biophysics at Sunnybrook, founded in the late 1980s as an offshoot of the downtown department at the Ontario Cancer Institute, was highly productive in research. Jorge Filmus, a PhD from the University of Buenos Aires, was interested in cancers of the digestive tract.[119] In 1991 Robert Kerbel came up from the Lunenfeld Research Institute to run Sunnybrook's molecular and cellular biology program; he and his successor Dan Dumont made several important findings in tumour angiogenesis. In 2000 Kerbel and colleagues demonstrated in preclinical studies that low-dose chemotherapy plus anti-angiogenic drugs delay tumour growth.[120] In 2005 a team including Dumont, Kerbel, and postdoctoral fellow Yuval Shaked found that a simple blood test could indicate how well anti-angiogenic therapy was working.[121]

Imaging research has remained a key focus of activity since the SRI's creation under Henkelman's leadership, such as how to visualize the vasculature of a tumour in the liver beneath the resolution power of ultrasound. In 2000 Peter N. Burns at Sunnybrook and Stephanie Wilson in the Department of Medical Imaging at TGH proposed a technique called pulse inversion imaging as an improved technique of bubble-specific imaging to extend the power of ultrasonography.[122]

Sunnybrook researchers figured prominently in establishing the International Digital Mammography Development Group in 1993.[123] In 2000 the group, including Martin Yaffe, Roberta Jong, and Donald Plewes of SRI, established the desirability of monitor systems permitting "flexibility and easy, quick access to differently processed versions" of digital mammograms, a technology still under development.[124] In 2005 the Sunnybrook researchers participated as the only Canadian team in the multi-site Digital Mammography Screening Trial (DMIST). This comparative study of digital and film mammography confirmed that digital screening was significantly more accurate among women under fifty, those with dense breasts, and pre- and perimenopausal women.[125] Two years earlier, they had become the world's first investigators to use intravenous contrast material in digital mammography to help identify lesions in dense breast tissue.[126]

### Cardiovascular Surgery at Sunnybrook

This story has an early beginning. In the early 1950s Bill Bigelow performed at Sunnybrook the first closed mitral valvotomies in Toronto and the second in Canada. Only later did he undertake the operation at TGH.[127] Then there was a long hiatus.

In 1971 the interhospital coordinating committee (IHCC) for Cardiovascular Surgery, chaired by Bigelow, recommended unanimously an open-heart surgical unit for Sunnybrook Hospital. They reasoned, "There is every reason to expect that the scope of surgery for coronary artery disease will continue to increase" and that another surgical team would soon be required. They focused on Sunnybrook because the hospital already had "an established cardiological service and catheter laboratory," and the planning authorities would greet the establishment of a unit serving the northern suburbs. "It is also a possible site for a second medical school."[128]

There was, however, a hook, as the teaching hospitals of University Avenue batted at the newcomer: they didn't want Sunnybrook training residents in cardiovascular surgery. William Drucker, professor of surgery, told Dean Chute, "[We] are seriously concerned regarding the implication to our graduate program in surgery were such a unit to be established. Until such time as there is documented evidence of the need for increased output of cardiac trainees from this department, we shall continue to harbour this concern."[129]

So Sunnybrook yearned in vain for cardiac surgery for a decade. When in 1979 Ramsay Gunton, now at the University of Western Ontario, conducted a site visit at the Division of Cardiology at Sunnybrook, he said, "I am firmly convinced that the lack of open heart surgery has created a serious morale problem at this hospital. It would be … a magnificent boost to clinical cardiovascular disease and research to open a cardiovascular surgical unit at Sunnybrook Hospital."[130]

The concept of a heart surgery unit at Sunnybrook started to be actively weighed. At a meeting of the Cardiovascular Surgery Task Force in July 1982, Don Cowan made a strong case that Sunnybrook should have the fourth cardiovascular unit being contemplated for Toronto: "Such a unit would be of central importance in providing educational and research experience for trainees in a range of other disciplines." He added, "It was recognized that the unit was not required for the training of cardiovascular surgeons, nevertheless … it was essential for the provision of a full training experience to cardiology and internal medicine residents." Also, there were concerns about Sunnybrook being regarded as a "'second class institution' … because of the lack of cardiovascular surgery facilities." (The Sunnybrook proposal was competing against a joint proposal from the General and Mount Sinai hospitals.)[131]

The following month, in August 1982, the committee recommended situating the new unit at Sunnybrook and not at Mount Sinai Hospital. Sunnybrook already had large catheter and pacemaker labs. Also, "[o]ver the years there has been a moral commitment to the hospital to provide a cardiovascular unit. Should this not materialize it is conceivable that a considerable number of staff may leave." Finally, a crisis in morale was building at the hospital: "A decision not to locate the unit at Sunnybrook Hospital would inevitably have a considerable effect on morale. The hospital suffers to some extent from geographical isolation, and unless having a good range of tertiary care units it will have difficulty attracting scientists; without major programmes it may have difficulty retaining even the existing staff."[132]

By the beginning of 1983, a crisis in open-heart surgery was growing. "Heart patients in Metro Toronto are waiting too long for open-heart surgery and some will die unless services are expanded," blared the *Globe and Mail* in January. The Toronto District Health Council had recommended that Sunnybrook become the fourth area hospital for open-heart surgery, after the General, the Western, and St Michael's. Current waiting lists were two to three months, but, the council said, the wait time should be a maximum of one month "after tests are completed to allow the patient and family time to prepare for the surgery."[133]

Time passed. Bigelow apparently "postponed" Sunnybrook's plans to have an open-heart unit. Meanwhile, the crisis worsened. "Metro Triage" was established in the late 1980s to ease the waiting-list crisis.[134] Bernard Goldman, who served as co-director of the Metro Toronto Triage Registry, recalled the crisis, "There was the issue of patients leaving the country, of patients seeking compensation from the government, while others were being sent from Windsor. Waiting lists were meaningless, we had no triage system. Ultimately, David Naylor created a triage system. David was extremely important."[135]

And so the Sunnybrook surgeons won out. In November 1989 Bernie Goldman and Stephen Fremes (who had finished medicine at U of T in 1979, passing his Royal College Fellowship in 1987) opened the cardiac surgical unit at Sunnybrook.[136] "We were heavily funded by the Ministry," said Goldman. "Martin Barkin was the CEO, and he and I had gone right from nursery school through medical school [Barkin graduated with an MD in 1960], so there was a personal element to his support." Goldman had also worked closely at the General with Ron Baigrie, the chief of cardiology.[137]

Thus all the pieces came together at Sunnybrook. The Sunnybrook heart surgeons recruited their own anesthetists. "We had our own ICU, we had our own operating room, totally dedicated, and everyone pissed off: 'Oh, heart surgery just uses all the blood in the bank, they use up all the clotting factor' – all these things that had bedeviled us for thirty years downtown that we had gotten over." Goldman continued, "We had to establish ourselves as safe and competent … We started operating November 27, 1980, and by March or April we had done 167 cases without a death. We were off and running."[138]

Goldman headed cardiovascular surgery at Sunnybrook from 1989 to 1998 and was surgeon-in-chief from 1998 to 2001. A thoughtful man with a scholarly bent, he is one of the more underappreciated figures in the history of cardiac surgery in Toronto, probably because of Sunnybrook's isolation from the heroes downtown.

There is an interesting footnote to this story. In 1992 the provincial Ministry of Health founded the Institute for Clinical Evaluative Sciences (ICES), a non-profit research organization, as an autonomous agency physically located at Sunnybrook. David Naylor, who had an active interest in scientifically assessing the outcomes of cardiac surgery, headed it. In 1994 Naylor co-designed and co-authored the report on the large-scale "Warm heart trial" with a team of investigators including heart surgeons Samuel Lichtenstein at St Michael's Hospital and Stephen Fremes at Sunnybrook, which found that "warm heart surgery may be preferable to hypothermic techniques for isolated coronary bypass surgery";[139] in 2004 he was part of a team led by Fremes and Nimesh Desai that established that radial artery grafts are preferable to saphenous veins grafts in bypass surgery.[140] ICES undertook several such cool assessments of procedures universally assumed to be meritorious and universally beneficial.[141]

**A Powerful Partnership**

The common denominator of the stories of these general hospitals is that they were all teaching hospitals of a single medical school – the University of Toronto – and that the Faculty of Medicine arrayed them all as a chain of locomotives to pull together. This applied a concentration of horsepower to the resolution of scientific questions that is otherwise unknown in North America.

For a faculty so committed to the department structure, the onrush of new ideas was like a one-two punch in the head. The faculty responded by creating new units outside the departments to sort and measure this avalanche of innovation. This volume cannot consider all of these small divisions and "extra-departmental units," yet some are worth particular mention.

### Centre for Studies in Medical Education–Wilson Centre

The Wilson Centre now aims to be the most important research centre in healthcare education and practice in the world.[1]

Brian Hodges, Director Wilson Centre, 2008

In the 1960s, interest quickened in how to teach medical students and how to convey and manage new knowledge. This eventuated in research in medical education. In October 1966 an "Academic Service Unit: Testing Service" was created in the faculty under J.F. Flowers, to score and analyse medical students' test results. Simultaneously, in 1967, with the aid of a grant from the Commonwealth Fund of New York, an Educational Research Unit was established "to assist Faculty in improving their teaching and to study the effective uses of many of the newer instructional devices, including television."[2] In the summer of 1967 the testing unit was transferred to the research unit with Flowers the director of the combined operation.[3] This was the beginning of educational research in the faculty.

In the meantime, George Connell became associate dean of basic sciences and enlarged the brief of this unit, appointing as director in 1969–70 Arthur Irving Rothman, a psychologist with a background in educational measurement who had joined the unit in 1968. The unit was "intended to function mainly in a service role" and carried out studies sampling student opinion and introducing (and scoring) the multiple-choice examinations so hated by a generation of medical students ("C: both B and A"; "D: none of the above"). In the 1969–70 session, the name was changed from Educational Research Unit to Division of Studies in Medical Education because of "a shift towards service to the educational system, with research playing a supporting role."[4] The unit developed examinations for medical undergraduates as well as the "practice examination" the students took prior to the Medical Council of Canada qualifying exams.[5] (As was said later, "The quality of this service is sufficient that some dozen medical faculties in Canada make use of the Toronto 'practice examination.'"[6])

Yet in the mid-1970s the unit fell into internal squabbling and the faculty considered abolishing it. Educator Niall Byrne joined it and defended the division against suggestions of the long-range planners that it might be left by the wayside: Byrne told them that "in his opinion the Division makes a valuable contribution, not across the Faculty but in specific instances for specific people."[7] Yet however welcome educational research might have been in future years, in the mid-1970s the faculty was said to "continue to regard the division with some suspicion and resentment."[8]

In 1984 the unit was hit with a quite negative review. Still, the review maintained, "There is a need for a separate medical education unit ... simply [because] the largest Faculty of Medicine in Canada in the nation's foremost university cannot afford to ignore and downplay, or appear to do so, an area of study in which it has played the pioneering role."[9]

After the review, in 1984–5 Edward M. Sellers became acting director while a new director was sought. In 1986 Sellers became director. The division's status was changed in 1987 to a "Centre" in order to permit the unit to apply to the School of Graduate Studies for formal standing and in line with Dean Lowy's plan that the Centre for Studies in Medical Education (CSME) become the academic focus "for educational research and expertise in undergraduate, postgraduate, and continuing medical education."[10] A number of changes were made, including over fifty cross-appointments of academic faculty. The CSME staff started meeting and holding educational rounds. In 1988 a new master's program in medical/health professional education was established in conjunction with the Ontario Institute for Studies in Education (OISE). In 1989 a CSME Research Day was initiated.

Big change lay ahead when in 1987 Richard Reznick, who had trained in surgery in Toronto and then earned a master's degree in surgical education at the University of Southern Illinois, returned to Toronto to direct the Department of Surgery's undergraduate education committee. He was the first surgeon to have formal training in education. In 1988 Reznick initiated a surgeon-educator program at the centre as part of the OISE collaboration. He said that at the beginning, they had "just a dream and hot dogs and beer ... the enticement we provided for young residents to come to a meeting to learn about training opportunities in education." Sixteen years later, they had graduated twenty-five surgeons at the master's level.[11]

In 1990 Niall Byrne became acting director, succeeded in 1995–6 by Reznick. Simultaneously, the CSME shifted from its somewhat grubby quarters in the FitzGerald Building to brand-new offices in the Toronto Hospital as the Centre for Research in Education, "intended to serve as the focal point for education research in the Faculty." Its objectives were to look at education in the faculty in the widest possible sense.[12] The centre was named the Donald R. Wilson Centre for Research in Education at the University Health Network in 2003, after Don Wilson, the head of cardiovascular surgery at the Western for many years, then head of the Department of Surgery, who in 1990 as president of Associate Medical Services had launched Educating Future Physicians for Ontario (EFPO).

In October 2002, Reznick stepped down as director to become professor of surgery and head of the department. Glenn Regehr succeeded him as acting chair, and in July 2003, Brian Hodges, vice chair of education in the Department of Psychiatry, was appointed director of the Wilson Centre. Hodges went to work with ferocious energy: Total grant funding increased from $5.5 million in 2003 to $13 million in 2007. Research publications of the centre's scientists grew from eighteen in 2003 to fifty-two in 2007.[13] This success might not have occurred had the centre been enveloped within the department structure.

### Banting and Best Diabetes Centre

As a memorial to Charles Best, who expired in March 1978 a week after hearing that his eldest son had died of a heart attack, in the fall of that year Edward A. Sellers proposed to Dean Brian Holmes a diabetes centre in Best's honour.[14] Sellers and Best had been close friends. It was to be an extra-departmental unit (EDU), reporting directly to the dean. Sellers was the first director. Simultaneously, the Charles H. Best Chair of Medical Research was created.

In a eulogy in 1985, Charles Hollenberg characterized Sellers as "a quiet, almost shy man [with] great determination," He said of Sellers's role, "Dr. Sellers conceived of the development of a diabetes centre at the University of Toronto, that would be named in honour of Banting and Best and that would encourage the development of research, education and patient care in this field both locally and nationally." Hollenberg continued, "This Centre is now a flourishing academic unit backed by a substantial endowment and shortly to occupy its own laboratories."[15]

At the beginning, the centre was somewhat in search of a role. Sellers told a meeting in the Dean's Office in January 1979, "The concept of the Centre is one of co-ordination and promotion rather than the creation of a physical facility." The centre did not have enough money to sponsor research. Hollenberg said, "The Centre's role might be to identify 4 or 5 new research programmes both basic and clinically applied in areas in which the Faculty should be moving, and to identify the resources required to get the programme going."[16]

Yet lots was happening on campus in diabetes research at a university that, Sellers told Dean Lowy in April 1980, did not yet have a centre or institute with "world-wide recognition." "The objective of the Banting and Best Diabetes Centre is just that – to develop a comprehensive Centre of international renown. This objective has not yet been achieved as yet, but is not an idle dream. The artificial pancreas project (a delivery system for insulin) at the Research Institute of the Hospital for Sick Children is first-rate; the work of Mladen Vranic on counter-regulatory hormones and exercise is widely quoted." David Jenkins from Oxford and London will soon join them to "develop a nutrition group devoted to diabetic research." The first Charles H. Best Chair of Medical Research would head another such group. But funding was required.[17] Financial support arrived from the Marion Hamilton Estate Bequest, the R. Samuel McLaughlin Foundation, and the Province of Ontario. The centre was thus was able to stretch its wings.

From 1981 to 1993 Charles Hollenberg was the director and simultaneously the inaugural Charles H. Best Professor of Medical Research. Hollenberg gave the centre visibility. In 1985 the centre contracted with the General Hospital to house its administrative offices in the former College Wing and its laboratories on the fourth floor of the Max Bell Research Centre.

Two years after Hollenberg became director of the Ontario Cancer Treatment and Research Foundation, in 1993 endocrinologist Bernard Zinman took over the directorship of the Banting and Best Diabetes Centre (BBDC). He made sure the centre was considered open to the university community. An external review in 1997 was laudatory: "The open faculty policy is a major strength of the BBDC. It has clearly created an atmosphere in which all faculty members interested in diabetes research … can participate … Having a defined physical space within the Toronto Hospital for the Core Laboratory … provides a clear identity for the BBDC."[18] It is rather interesting, eighty years after the discovery of insulin, that the insulin story continued to have enormous drawing power as one of the central events in the history of modern medicine. But between the Toronto General Hospital and the faculty, the story of insulin at the University of Toronto remained up for grabs. Bernard Schimmer at the Department of Medical Research said that "the Toronto General Hospital, the Endocrine Division, campaigned to set up a Banting and Best Diabetes Centre, which they did, and at one point they wanted to take over the Department [of Medical Research], merge it into that, and focus research back to diabetes research. We were not interested in that. There's been a lot of interest in name-association with Banting and Best. The hospital has an interest, we have the Department. The Department of Physiology continues to have an interest as well."[19] Many at the faculty had an interest in the insulin legacy.

## University of Toronto Joint Centre for Bioethics

Confronted with new ethical issues, in the 1980s the hospitals began opening their own ethics programs. As early as 1985 the idea arose within the School of Graduate Studies of organizing a University Ethics Centre that would combine research with the practical problem-resolution being done in the hospitals. Jim Till chaired a Feasibility Committee. Yet Charles Hollenberg, chair of medicine, threw cold water on the idea as impractical, and development of a joint ethics centre was put on hold.[20]

But many people were interested in combining research and practice in bioethics, and in 1986–7 the decision was made to move forward through the Consultation/Liaison Division of the Toronto General Hospital.[21] In 1990 the new Centre for Bioethics opened. "Today, issues in medical ethics span life's stages from genetic counseling to the post mortem recovery of organs that can save living patients," said Fred Lowy, the inaugural director, at the opening ceremony on 23 October, an occasion at which Brian Dickson, chief justice of Canada, and President George Connell were present.[22] John Evans, past U of T president, chaired the centre's Board of Advisors. Simultaneously, clinical ethics units were being established in the teaching hospitals, which led in 1995 to renaming the centre the Joint Centre for Bioethics (JCB), including the Hospital for Sick Children, Mount Sinai Hospital, Sunnybrook, and the Toronto Hospital.

Fred Lowy would step down in June 1995. Whom to choose as new director? In April 1995, Jim Till, on the executive committee of the new centre, told Dean Aberman they expected the new director to symbolize collaboration between faculty and hospitals: "It would be particularly appropriate if the acting director were not a member of the Faculty of Medicine, to emphasize the fact that the present Bioethics program is indeed a collaborative academic program, involving the Faculties of Arts & Science, Law, and Nursing, as well as Medicine."[23] Yet in November the faculty settled on Peter Singer of the Department of Medicine to carry the JCB through the next five years of growth, and in this they were not disappointed.

In 1997 Singer became the inaugural holder of the Sun Life Chair in Bioethics; the chair originated in a $1 million donation the company had made to the university under a matching grant program in 1995. Under Singer, the UTJCB experienced dynamic growth, bringing in the other teaching hospitals and launching a number of research programs. Naylor said in 2000, "During the past five years, the UTJCB has become one of the leading bioethics centres in the world. It is among the very few centres that have been able to pull together a broad range of disciplines and span the spectrum of bioethics from theory to practice. We are not aware of any other bioethics centre in the world that spans a major university and 8 large teaching hospitals."[24] A master of health science (MHSc) degree in bioethics was created.

In July 2006, Ross Upshur, of the Department of Family and Community Medicine, succeeded Singer, who Dean Whiteside said was "completing a spectacular ten years as the Director of the Joint Centre for Bioethics. Over the past decade, Prof Singer has demonstrated outstanding academic leadership and enabled the Joint Centre to reach international recognition for graduate education and research in bioethics." Whiteside called Singer "Canada's pre-eminent scholar in global bioethics."[25]

## Department of Art as Applied to Medicine

The Art as Applied to Medicine course teaches students to make drawings, but to think like scientists.[26]

Nancy Joy, 1974

Talk about new ideas! The idea that female illustrators could make a contribution to a medical faculty was certainly novel in 1925, when Maria T. Wishart was appointed as "artiste" in a room in the Anatomy Building. She had been a student of the famous medical illustrator Max Brödel at Johns Hopkins. The new service was said to have been very successful, with drawings and "coloured wax models."[27] By the 1929–30 session they had constructed a proper studio in the Banting Institute "with excellent lighting and adequate equipment" for the Art Service.[28]

In the Art Service Wishart usually had several collaborators, invariably female, who evidently had also been trained under Brödel at Hopkins. Yet Brödel's death in 1941 created a new opportunity for Toronto. Dean Gallie said in 1945, "With the death of Prof. Brödel ... that school has lost its pre-eminence and our Faculty decided that the time was ripe for the establishment of a school here. A Department of Art as Applied to Medicine has accordingly been organized" that would train artists in medical illustration and assist other departments with drawings. The three-year course would include anatomy, pathology, and drawing, eventuating in a diploma. In December 1944 the Faculty Council approved the motion "that a department of the Faculty of Medicine called 'Art as Applied to Medicine,' [AAM] be established and that this department be administered under the Faculty of Medicine in a manner similar to other departments."[29] This, then, was the birth of this unusual department, rare in a faculty of medicine.

The new department offered a diploma. A medical audience had been primed by the war for illustration. Dean MacFarlane, in charge of Canada's medical forces during the war, commented in 1946, "The medical men returning from overseas had learned the value of Visual Education, and were eager to record their work in writing and illustration."[30]

A new era in teaching medical illustration at Toronto began in 1962 when Wishart retired, succeeded by Nancy Joy, then at the University of Manitoba and a previous collaborator in Toronto with J.C.B. Grant.[31] Shortly thereafter, AAM moved from its cramped quarters in the Banting Institute to a lovelier space on McCaul Street with better light. An academic triumph followed in the 1967–8 session as the AAM department won the right to offer the degree of bachelor of science, art as applied to medicine, "conferred for the first time at the 1968 Commencement on June 10."[32] As a regular academic program, no longer a diploma program, the department spun off its medical art services division in 1969 and devoted itself entirely to teaching.[33]

The little program was on a roll. Nancy Joy pointed to a "growing demand for medical artists. In 1968 … there were four practicing medical artists in Toronto. In 1974 there are 28."[34]

Then the roll came to an end as the faculty attempted to abolish the program. At a meeting of the long-range planners in December 1974, Ernest McCulloch suggested that maybe AAM should be at Ryerson Polytechnic Institute. Joy pointed out that AAM has to be based in a medical school. "The Art as Applied to Medicine course teaches students to make drawings, but to think like scientists."[35] It is quite interesting that the same fate nearly befell the Department of Art as Applied to Medicine that threatened the other female-dominated subjects. Influential barons of the faculty attempted to banish them. In 1975 a report of the long-range planners called Art as Applied to Medicine "Inappropriate for Faculty of Medicine; transfer to … Ryerson."[36]

To their credit, members of the Faculty Council rose hotly to the defence of AAM: when the issue came up several months after the long-range planners' report, neuroscientist John Scott said it was "the only centre in Canada for training medical illustrators; there is a shortage of them; and the course has a good [international] reputation."[37] Despite Dean Holmes's argument that the Department of Art as Applied to Medicine should be abolished for budgetary reasons, in November 1975 Nancy Joy defended it passionately before the Faculty Council, and the council voted in a secret ballot 64-31 to save it.[38]

In 1989 Linda Pauwels-Wilson succeeded Nancy Joy, initially as acting chair then the following year as chair, just in time to fight off yet another attempt at abolition! In February 1990 Dean Dirks wrote Vice-Provost A. Richard Ten Cate that AAM was an obvious candidate for abolition: "It is generally conceded to be a high-quality program, unique nationally, but of low priority to the Faculty of Medicine. The Faculty has attempted to terminate this program on two occasions in the past, but has been blocked by Faculty Council." They could try to cut it again, but it "will require considerable political will on the part of the Faculty and the Provost."[39] Dirks then backed off an actual closure, deciding to end its "department" status and transfer Pauwels-Wilson and colleagues to the Department of Surgery.[40] In December 1990 AAM joined the Department of Surgery as the Division of Biomedical Communications. Linda Pauwels-Wilson gave a sigh of relief. "Medical illustration is not integral to patient care and management but it is invaluable in learning and communication," she said.[41]

The story actually has a happy end. In 1994 art as applied to medicine was converted from a bachelor's program to a master's, conferring the degree of master of science biomedical communication (MScBMC).[42] The program reached out beyond medical illustration to medical procedure simulations and 3-D biomedical animation, a program they offered together with Sheridan College. As Dean Naylor noted proudly in 2003, "Biomedical Communications is the only program of its kind in Canada and one of six accredited programs in the world."[43]

## History of Medicine

We have attempted to sort through the records in the Dean's Office ... This has not been a highly rewarding activity.[44]

Irving Fritz, chair, BBDMR, 1975

There is actually nothing new about the history of medicine. In fact it is probably the oldest of the medical specialties, given that physicians have always been interested in their own history. But medical history done in a professional manner, by trained historians rather than by curious physicians, is relatively new.

Medical history as a discipline began at the University of Toronto in 1924 with the appointment of internist John T. Fotheringham, then sixty-four, to a chair in the history of medicine.[45] When Fotheringham stepped down in 1931, Jabez H. Elliott, fifty-eight, a tuberculosis specialist and something of a polymath with wide intellectual interests, succeeded him.[46] Elliott finished medical studies in 1897 and will probably be remembered more for his clinical acumen than his historical scholarship. He had a reputation as a very astute diagnostician, and *Epistaxis* waxed poetically of him in 1921, "E is for Elliott, on T.B. a wizard, / Who knows at a glance the state of your gizzard." Elliott lectured on a vast range of topics until his death during the 1942–3 session, after which medical history was deleted from the curriculum.[47]

There the history of medicine rested until 1976 when Pauline Mazumdar, an English pathologist and immunologist with a PhD in history of medicine from Johns Hopkins University, accepted a chair in medical history that had been endowed by the private foundation Associated Medical Services and named after the founder of the foundation, the neuropathologist Jason A. Hannah. In contrast to her predecessors in the faculty, Mazumdar was not only a distinguished scientific figure but enjoyed a noted international reputation in medical history. With the acceptance of the appointment, she became the most eminent medical historian in Canada.

And she had her work cut out for her! The medical students seemed to have no interest in understanding themselves as part of a great therapeutic and scientific river of time. Frustrated at this ignorance, immunologist Hardi Cinader wrote Associate Dean Bill Francombe in 1981 about how the faculty had failed "to provide a framework in which they can understand research as ... a bridge between the past and the future." What was needed, he said, was a brief course "which will convey to the students the historic sequence of the major discoveries, from Harvey to Jenner, and the gradual transformation of homeopathic medicine to contemporary medicine."[48] Many professional historians may wince at the idea that they are supposed to teach "great man history." Many professional clinicians may wonder idly who Harvey and Jenner are.

After Mazumdar stepped down from the chair, it was assumed in 1991 by the author of the present volume.

# 27 Student Life and Learning

We're Medicals of Varsity, There's no better faculty. Fill once again the foaming mug, To the Meds of U. of T. – SO Let's shout to Alma Mater, She who taught us all we know, PAINS FLY, GERMS DIE, WHEN WE CRY, MEDS OF OLD TORONTO![1]

Medical Song (1939)

## Setting the Stage

In the beginning, students learned clinical medicine on the wards and in the surgical amphitheatre of the Toronto General Hospital. "Students shall enter by the rear door under the theatre, and remain in the theatre or students' waiting-room until required by the medical officer of the day either in the theatre or the wards," stipulated the hospital in 1891. "No students (except clinical clerks) will be allowed in any other part of the Hospital." It was also not permitted to spit tobacco on the floor. When, under the supervision of a physician, they were permitted to visit patients, they were told to "stand in an orderly manner around the patient." They should not "at any time sit or stand on the beds."[2] Were the medical students so badly in need of socialization?

It was not by accident that the course was steadily lengthened. The course began in 1887 at four years following high school. In 1899 a fifth year was added following a decision of the Ontario Medical Council.[3] After the First World War, a sixth year was added on. Why was it becoming longer? So much more to learn?

The course became longer partly because of a nonmedical consideration: the faculty's decision that that students should spend a good deal of the first two years acquiring some general knowledge about language, culture, and society. Why? Because it's necessary to have doctors who speak French? No. It was because the faculty saw these physicians in training as future community leaders and wanted them properly outfitted for this role. Today, people do not necessarily expect their physicians to become civic personalities, although they are not displeased if they do so. But today the whole social role of medicine has changed. In the past, one of the goals of medical education was to prepare doctors to serve as community notables, to be able to inspire others as models of rectitude and civic-mindedness. This ambition produced much purple prose. During the Clarke deanship, just before the First World War there evidently occurred "a most notable amelioration in the character and conduct of the student body, a happy consummation long devoutly wished, at length brought about almost entirely by [the dean's] noble example and remarkable influence amongst the undergraduates."[4] Splendid.

In 1957 Gallie recalled what being a student had been like around 1900: "We had a four-year course based on a minimum entrance requirement of junior matriculation." This meant basically the minimum high-school leaving certificate, and all who possessed it had the right to enter medical studies at the University of Toronto. Gallie continued, "The first two years were spent in Queen's Park [the main campus, in the Biology Building] and were devoted to anatomy, physiology, histology, physics and chemistry … the last two years were spent at the old School at Gerrard and Sumach." Gallie recalled wryly the "endless lectures on medicine, surgery, gynaecology, obstetrics, forensic medicine, eye, ear nose and throat and all the rest of it. Each day we spent an hour or so on the wards, arranged in small groups about the beds, receiving instructions in physical examination, diagnosis and treatment from our clinicians … The presence of a hundred or more students in an operating room, without gowns or masks, had not struck the surgeons as causing risk to the patient. Only rarely did we have an opportunity to take a history or make a physical examination or do the clinical investigation so essential to diagnosis. When we graduated with our bachelor's degree we certainly did not know much."[5] Lamenting how little the students knew was to become a standard professorial complaint over the years, an academicism resembling gripes about grammatical errors in student papers.

In 1919–20 the new six-year curriculum was introduced, except for the returning veterans, who qualified for the five-year period of study. There were so many in the first year of the six-year program – all Ontario high-school graduates were still eligible to enroll – that the faculty felt mobbed. Primrose said, "Indeed, the congestion was such that it will be necessary to limit numbers as soon as possible, as there are not in Toronto sufficiently large clinical faculties to train in the final years [such numbers]."[6] The class that graduated in 1924 was the last class admitted under the five-year system. Henceforth, all undergraduates in medicine would study for six years: two in premedical studies, four in the study of basic sciences and clinical diagnosis and treatment.

Dean Primrose told the medical graduates in 1924 that the demands of science were extending the curriculum. He and his colleagues in their day had studied only four years, "and in a former period, still more remote, the apprentice system was in vogue, while the University in the main merely made provision for didactic lectures, conducted examinations and conferred degrees … The advance in science, in all its branches, in the last quarter of a century, has been tremendous … To keep abreast of the times, it is imperative to devote more time to pure science on the one hand and to the study of the clinical application of scientific truth on the other." And so the purpose of a medical education was to produce mini-scientists? Not at all, said Primrose. They were educating family physicians, but "each patient treated by the doctor, in his daily routine of work, presents a problem in scientific research, and so it comes about that the student in medicine must become saturated with research methods both in the foundation sciences of medicine and in the scientific investigation of disease at the bedside."[7]

The lengthening of the curriculum from four years in 1887 to six in 1919 – and the internal upheavals in the teaching hospitals that put Duncan Graham at the helm in medicine, Clarence Starr in surgery, and Alan Brown in pediatrics – transformed the undergraduate experience. Gallie said, "It introduced the student into the wards and outpatient departments for much longer periods … In this way he was given responsibilities in the diagnosis and treatment of patients. He became, in fact, an apprentice while still an undergraduate."[8]

The first two years of the new six-year program concluded with a quite difficult exam, intended to weed out the less qualified. In 1926 the yearbook noted, "When the dust and smoke of the eliminations due to the exams had cleared away, there were found to be many missing." (Many of these students had seen combat in the World War and were fond of military images.) The good news for the third-years was that now real medical studies began. "We turned our thoughts to Anatomy. This seemed so much nearer heaven than Physics, that we reveled in it."[9]

Then there were combined arts and medicine courses, beginning in the 1902–3 session with the course in "Biological and Physical Science"; in 1909–10 another such course leading to a combined arts and medical degree called "Physiological and Biochemical Science" was instituted; it eventuated in a BA degree in four years and MB degree in seven.[10] These were part of an ongoing effort, which continues even today, to give medical students a good grounding in the basic sciences as an incentive to go on and do research.

The faculty's desire to recruit first-class students, with a science background in the Faculty of Arts if possible, resulted in a kind of egalitarianism about fees. To maintain the stream of poor farm boys, fees must remain low. The faculty's fees, at $163 a year in 1925, were the third lowest in Canada (only Queen's and Laval charged less). At a December 1925 meeting, the Faculty Council opposed a prospective fee increase on the grounds that "students who have not sufficient funds to meet such an increase, but who have the mental capacity, would be prevented from taking a medical course." Moreover, a fee increase "would result in an increase in the number of students with recently acquired wealth, but no inherited brains."[11]

It is quite charming to see this egalitarianism persist over the years. In 1939 Gallie deplored raising the fees "owing to the reduction of the annual government grant to the university." The cost of medical education, he said, is now three times what it was thirty years ago. "Had the cost been anything like as much in the early part of this century very few of the present professors could have entered medicine. The result is that a smaller and smaller proportion of the bright boys from farm and village are coming up to the university, much to the disadvantage of the profession."[12]

*Rowdy Lot, But Cultivated ...*

The medical students ("Meds") in these years were something of a rowdy lot, partly because they were fully grown men and often military veterans. In 1920 a writer known as "GM" (Gordon Murray?) poetized in *Epistaxis*, the satirical student publication,

> "You may educate the Art's Men,
> You may even culture School,
> You may fine them till they're broke, then
> You may make them stick to rule.
> But the Meds, they scorn their penalty,
> They'll pay their fines (perhaps),
> But as long as they're a Faculty
> They'll always have their scraps."[13]

The Meds were constantly fighting with brigades from other faculties of the university and with little thought might smash things up a bit – in a way that would later have been inconceivable. "Many are the tales that could be told of the basement of the Medical Building," said the scribes of the class of 1926. "When the water was shut off, and the police had arrived, there was hardly a window left intact ... The 'Powers that Be' imposed a heavy fine, but we had had our fun."[14] The "Medettes," as the female medical students were called, appeared somewhat less rowdy but still were not wimps. Grace Baker, who graduated in 1923, chose as her motto, "She does not say what I expect, but I'm the better pleased."[15]

At the end of the First World War the moral theme sounded with renewed vigor: physicians must be cultivated citizens and not merely technically competent professionals. Dean Clarke said in June 1919, in anticipation of the six-year curriculum to be introduced in the autumn, "The changes made in the curriculum will enable students to acquire a broader culture ... Six years may seem a long time to remain at College, but those who have acquaintance with the history of medicine are fully convinced that it is not possible to graduate a cultured and practical physician or surgeon in less time."[16] President Falconer said hopefully, "It seems probable that this course ... [will] turn out a broadly educated as well as an expert medical man."[17] In 1926 he dilated upon liberal arts education for the Meds:

> The propinquity of the medical departments to those of the Faculty of Arts has made possible the experiment in medical education which has been tried during the past six years. In the first three years of the medical course options from the Arts departments are included in order that the student may get some tincture of a different quality of liberal education ... for a modern medical course conducted by men of genuine scientific spirit does liberalise the mind. The greatest problem in our higher education seems to me to be how we shall prepare the professional man to fill a fuller and larger place in society, how we are to broaden his human interests. The experience of the past leads us to believe that this can be done by giving him more than the mere rudiments of a liberal education before he enters upon the special professional studies.[18]

As seen, the faculty believed that it was training not just physicians but community leaders. The conception of the physician in those days was as a local notable, a person who would not only heal the sick but set high moral standards also for the community. The problem with this conception was that the average beginning medical student was a late adolescent with a high school degree who was not really convincing as a community leader. The ideal of the physician as moral and social beacon could only work if the young doctors were given a substantial education in the humanities – history, a foreign language, literature – as well as in the study of histiocytes. Hence, for several decades, the first two years of a medical education were given to premedical studies, in which the humanities would figure strongly. The faculty were encouraged in this by the aspiration of the university's new president, Henry John Cody (1932–45), to combine science and the humanities. In 1934 Cody said, "The sciences and the humanities must never become strangers to each other. Natural science has rolled like a flood into school and university. Its attractiveness is so great as well nigh to be all-absorbing; its applications to life are so real and immediate as almost to exclude all other forms of mental exercise."[19] The desire to get the humanities on board, by convincing the Faculty of Arts to mount special courses for the Meds, was thus supported from the very top.

In the 1930s and 1940s, the time of the great pivots from teaching to research, and from the United Kingdom to the United States, was as yet far distant. The Toronto faculty prided itself on adopting the small-group and one-on-one training that, as so much else, had been brought over from Britain. It was indeed this attachment to the time-intensive apprenticeship system that made the faculty somewhat resistant to taking time for research. They would rather be shaping young doctors, a not wholly ignoble motive. Barney Berris described the clinical training he encountered around 1942 as a medical student

> For practice in what we were taught in our lectures, our class was divided into groups of ten. The groups were distributed amongst the teaching hospitals, where we were taught history-taking and physical examination on patients in the hospital public wards ... The next step was to learn the symptoms and signs of common diseases ... One or two students were assigned to a patient. We were asked to take a complete history, do a physical examination, record our findings, and list the possible diagnoses. We then had to decide which diagnosis we thought was correct ... Our training in the basic clinical skills was excellent and was modeled after the British system. Later, when I went to the United States for post-graduate work, I discovered that our training in this area was better than theirs.

But only in the second-to-last year were they allowed to "be involved in patients' investigation or treatment with the staff doctors."[20]

This intensity of training produced superior clinicians: that was a Toronto tradition.

*After Graduation*

Final exams finished, the young medical graduates could enter practice immediately or take an internship. Most chose internship (for the class of 1922 over 80 percent; for the class of 1925, under the six-year course, over 90 percent[21]).

In Toronto, the prospects of internship were not rosy. Of the 1920s, Dean Joseph MacFarlane later recalled, "When I finished my undergraduate course a little more than thirty years ago [in 1922], forty percent of a large class left immediately for the United States. The reason — there were insufficient hospital internships in this country, and few opportunities for intensive postgraduate training."[22]

Yet for those who got internships at the General, it wasn't such a bad deal. Surgeon Fred Dewar recalled, "Everybody liked interning. We had a doctors' dining room, in which members of the staff would come up occasionally ... We could meet all our friends and discuss the various problems of being an interne. We had a pool-table, tennis courts. We were laundered and fed. Our beds and rooms in which we lived were cared for by maids. We really lived like kings, even though there wasn't a dime." And the nurses? "We took them out, we danced in their Residence and many of us married nurses as a result of this. This is completely altered today."[23]

In 1938 Gallie described how the final-year undergraduates (sixth-year) spent the surgical rotation of their clerkship: "The students report at their wards at 8:30 a.m. and take up the following duties: the taking of all histories as assigned to them in rotation by the intern and the making of the physical examinations and conducting the clinical investigation as far as they are able." Then routine dressings, assisting at operations on their own patients, making rounds, and "tak[ing] a short course of instruction from the operating room nurse on operating room technique." Then comes noon, which is devoted to a "theatre clinic" in the Toronto General Hospital, where patients in medicine, gynecology, or surgery are demonstrated. In the afternoon more of the same, except that at 5:00 p.m. the day is not over: "From then till next morning, the students are on call for whatever emergencies come to their division. Every night students will be found in the emergency Department observing and assisting in the accident cases and other emergencies that may arrive and they are sometimes there most of the night."[24] Many readers will say, "Plus ça change ...," and indeed they would be right.

Postgraduate education was just getting going in the 1920s. "The primary object of the curriculum of study is to provide the most efficient training possible for the general Practitioner in Medicine," said Dean Primrose in 1924. But graduate work too "is constantly on the increase. Year by year an increasing number come to this University for work in special Departments." Also, there were many extension lectures: 139 demonstrations and "papers" "provided in the Province of Ontario, exclusive of Toronto."[25] But such efforts were embryonic. At this point, the Faculty of Medicine was still devoted almost entirely to the preparation of physicians for general practice.

### Fun and Sport

If ever I get out of here; I'll specialize in pimples, In liver, stomach, toes and ear. And making ladies' dimples.[26]
        Aaron Glassberg-Volpe, graduated MB from the University of Toronto, 1920

The Medical Society, founded in 1888,[27] was made up of graduates and undergraduates of the faculty; after 1895 it was under the honorary presidency of the dean.[28] Its purpose was "to supply magazines and periodicals for the reading room" and to be generally helpful to the medical students. "Our Hallow'en concert and elections for the Dinner Committee was a great success. The 'Newsboy's Quartette' ... made quite a hit ... while the Dean, with his usual kindness and thoughtfulness, had supplied a most enjoyable feast," was the drill for 1902.[29]

Among the earliest achievements of the Medical Society was the "first annual At Home," organized in 1905. "This happy event replaced the dinner which for seventeen years had stood as the only social function of the students in medicine. Mr. Duncan Graham, a man of gift and graces, presided over the innovation."[30] It is interesting to see the mores of their parents perpetuate themselves in the world of the Meds. The very British term "at home," meaning a dinner party, is unknown in the United States. Rather than having beer and pizza, self-understood for later generations of Meds, these medical students donned formalwear and planned dinner evenings of which their parents would have been proud (had the parents lived in upper-middle-class Toronto – but many of the parents were farmers and would have found the new urban whirl into which their sons and daughters plunged baffling though desirable).

## Daffydil

"Daffydil" was the annual student theatrical production, which began in 1897 as a skit night, in which each class performed competitively its own skit; it evolved after World War II, and much vulgarity on the part of the students, into a musical. The very first Daffydil night in 1897 "took the form of a Punch and Judy show in which paper dolls were designed to represent the various professors"; it was held in the lecture theatre of the old Medical College at Gerrard and Sackville Streets. Only students were admitted. After several years' suspension, in 1912 the first renewed performance was held in Convocation Hall, with student Don Alexander Warren the first chairman (Warren ended up practicing in Hamilton). Obstetrician Herman Van Wyck was musical director and Dean Clarke played violin in the orchestra.[31]

This 1912 revival apparently occurred when the Medical Society "conceived the idea that the Meds were not sufficiently demonstrating their proud position as leaders in University life ... since they were allowing the 'despised' Arts to 'put something over' on them in the shape of a funny night, viz, 'Mock Parliament,' for which the said Meds had no equal or superior ... 'Daffydil Night' was the prescription handed out ... The work the first year was arduous and often the Daffydil Committee were tempted to admit defeat, but spurred on by the encouragement, personal and financial, of a fun-loving Dean (Dr CK Clarke) they finally produced in a sparsely filled Convocation Hall, with gratis admission, the first Daffydil Night."[32]

Next year Daffydil Night was skipped, then revived in 1914, with a big silver cup, donated by the faculty "to be awarded to that year producing the funniest and cleverest 15 minute skit." Thereafter Daffydil was a huge success, with such classes as 1T7 (class of 1917) winning for presenting "The Ancient Order of Presbyterians," which caused great amusement. The first freshman victory, of 2T0 (class of 1920), was won with "The Minstrelettes." In 1923 *Epistaxis* opined, "If it continues to be well received ... no doubt the custom will go on in the future and in after years will become a tradition."[33]

After the war, Daffydil soared. In 1921, "Daffydil night this year was conducted almost entirely by fourth year men, which probably accounted in no small degree for its tremendous success. An enthusiastic and hard-working committee took charge and Convocation Hall, as of old, was a scene of great activity for a few days. Owing to its immense popularity, Daffydil was produced on two successive nights, and our year stunt, cleverly composed by Ross Jewell, though it did not win the cup, was considered, by all, original and witty."[34]

Daffydil also provided occasion for socializing, as the Meds scanned the audience. "Over a little to one side are a flock of sweet young things, some one whispered 'nurses.' Is it possible?" asked one observer, tongue in cheek.[35]

The female medical students styled themselves "Medettes," and in the 1923 Daffydil, the "Medettes" strode jointly upon the stage for the first time, giving "Twinkle, Twinkle, Little Stars," featuring Queen Cathrine [*sic*], King Henry VIII, and so on. The staff also had a presentation, "At the Gates of Heaven," starring Roscoe Graham and John Oille, among other faculty members.[36] In 1925 the Medettes presented "Memories of a Medette," with Marion Hilliard playing "Varsity's Ace." Scene I was "Her graduation night," scene II, "What she saw in the flames."[37]

Daffydil rituals began to evolve. In 1925 approached "the time for which the Daffydil Committee plot and plan and where intimate glimpses of members of the staff are portrayed ... to the consternation of several and the amusement of many." As the different classes grouped themselves about Convocation Hall, "the programme is composed of acts put on by the men of the various years, and the Medical women who indulge a skit of their own which is usually a feature event." Following the performance is the Daffydil banquet, "for the Daffydil Committee, representatives from the Faculty and the members of the best act who are also presented with the Daffydil Cup which becomes the property of their year if won three successive times."[38]

Thus did Daffydil become an intimate part of the student world. By 1936 the demand for seats had become so great that Daffydil went over to a three-night stand. Participating in it was hugely popular among the medical students and featured many later giants of the faculty, such as Vera Peters, who played starring roles in four of her five years.

A sophomoric side of undergraduate humour was not unknown to Daffydil. In 1912 the Medical Society began editing a sort of joke-book program called *Epistaxis*, or "nose bleed," for the evening. The 1939 edition, for example, had a skit on breaking wind. The sketches became increasingly "piercing," as faculty historian W.R. Feasby puts it, and in 1939 the Faculty Council closed Daffydil down as "a disgrace." Upon a petition by the students in 1945, Dean MacFarlane reinstituted Daffydil on the condition that "the level of humour and entertainment is such that no offence is given."[39] *Epistaxis* was now retitled *Nose Bleed*, and the 1946 edition announced that all had been scrubbed clean:

> "'Be clean,' said the Caput, 'be highbrow, select,
> For that is the way you will win our respect.
> Too long have your skit nights been loaded with spice,
> Now is the time to be clean and be nice.
> We warn you, my dears, that we will get haughty
> Should skits, songs or programme turn out to be naughty.'"[40]

The product, accordingly, was much more musical revue than skit night – and Daffydil retained in the years ahead the character of a musical. Also, the competition among the classes that had added spice to be saltiest was abolished. Nor did the Medettes have any longer a section of their own. The title *Epistaxis* was later restored, but the flysheet, for better or worse, lacked the essays and jokes of yesteryear.

Social events increased in number. Of the Medical Society it was said in 1925, "It assumes entire responsibility for the major functions of the Faculty – Medical-At-Home and Daffydil Night at Convocation Hall." It also has a Medical Sick Benefit Fund for ailing students and organizes all student elections. In 1925 it revived the "Medical Faculty Banquet, "after it had been in abeyance for some years."[41]

The medical At-Home shifted in 1925 from the King Edward Hotel to the Royal York Hotel or to Hart House, "when those halls so accustomed to heavy tread respond on this occasion to lighter steps and the walls re-echo soft voices as the Meds' fair friends go gaily chattering past." Herbert Hyland, later a prominent neurologist, was among the organizers.[42]

These medical At-Homes became known as "the premier social event in Toronto," at least for the medical students. In 1935, for example, the At-Home, held at the Royal York – Toronto's swankiest hotel – saw the dinner dance conducted in the form of a "'Social Clinic' to treat ailing students who had that dread malaise known as 'Duck's Disease,' the etiology of this disease is attributed to overwork in the medical course."[43]

*Athletics*

And athletics! How many of the biographies in preceding chapters contain sports participation. The men and women of the faculty were all over the hockey rink and rugby field. The class of 1926 had nineteen "T" letter holders.[44] Arthur Ham, for example – later one of the faculty's most eminent scientists – "has shown more preference for a racquet than a probe. He has been Varsity tennis champion for the past two years and among the best at squash." Herbert Hyland was captain of "Senior Meds rugby … Prince of good fellows and personality plus."[45] Margaret Burridge captained "a champion basketball team."[46] Marion Hilliard will be remembered as head of obstetrics at Women's College Hospital and originator of a technique for the early diagnosis of cervical cancer though not necessarily to her fellow classmates of "Medical 2T7." "Marion has been one of the outstanding among the women athletes at the University. While she particularly excels at hockey, she also takes part in tennis tournaments, and plays interfaculty basketball. Star left wing of the intercollegiate hockey team for the past five years."[47] Much later, the tendency arose in the culture of medical students to concentrate feverishly on their studies to the exclusion of all other outside interests. It is therefore of interest to see among this generation of students, many of whom went on to become brilliant scientists and clinicians, that they had time to balance body and spirit.

In the 1923–4 session, the Medical Athletic Association fielded twenty different teams for interfaculty contests. "In addition to this, the second Track Meet and the first Assault-At-Arms were held." (Assault-at-arms meant public displays of skill at arms.) Meds won championships in tennis, basketball, and hockey. "On the University teams medical students fill a large and enviable place. They hold more U of T colours than any other college or faculty. Fifteen men of the graduating class of 2T4 hold first University colours. This is probably the largest number ever held by any graduating class." In 1926 the Meds were everywhere: eleven of them in senior rugby, four in hockey, five in basketball, three in water polo, and five in assault-at-arms, with plenty of trophy cups to show for success.[48]

The women's teams were especially splendid. The Faculty Council noted in 1930, "Although a great advance was made during the year in athletics, it remained for the women of the Faculty to bring home an inter-faculty championship. In spite of the comparatively small number of women enrolled in Medicine, they took an active and leading part in athletics and entered teams in practically every interfaculty series. After giving an excellent account of themselves in Swimming, Baseball and Basketball, the women of the faculty after a long hard grind won the cup cymbolic [sic] of the Interfaculty Ladies Hockey Championship."[49] In 1935, "[t]he women undergraduates, 70 in number, had their own organization, financed similarly to the men's ... Several first 'T's' were awarded to medettes this year." Thirty women took part.[50] (Yet the Medettes were not universally triumphant: in the 1933–4 session, the Medical Women's Athletic Association retreated from baseball: "The baseball team was composed chiefly of girls from the Public Health course, so it was decided that in future the sports would be limited to tennis, basketball, badminton and hockey."[51])

In a campus environment that was often far from congenial, the Medical Society thus offered in sport impetus to physical restoration and in Daffydil a recoupment of the mind. In 1945 John M. Stephenson, president of the Medical Society (who ended up practicing in Moncton), said, "It is my hope that the Society may fill a place which has been glaringly empty since the founding of this School, that is, as a promoter of medical citizenship and of affection for the School." Medical graduates here "have few kind words to say for Toronto University except in argument."[52]

Yet it wasn't so bad to be a med student in those days. Fred Dewar, later head of orthopedic surgery, entered medical school in 1930, right at the beginning of the Depression. "Hart House was open and functioning with its gym and its pool," he later said in an interview. "There were rowing teams with a coach that you could go and work out with. There were tennis courts that you could play on. You could play soccer or football. You could get involved in literary societies, you could get involved with the Varsity. There were a million things to do. The girls' residences had been put on the campus at the corner of Hoskins and

St George and they were a beehive of activity and there would be little parties and people playing the piano and singsongs, little bits of food here and there."[53]

It wasn't such a martyr's path.

### "Our Best Students Are Excellent; Our Poorest Students Are Numerous and Extremely Poor"

The wave of ex-servicemen who flooded into medicine after the First World War touched off much agonizing about the low quality of the medical students; it was a faculty bellyaching that would last until after the imposition of strict entrance standards decades later.[54] This began in the Office of the President. In 1920, Falconer said, "The standard of Junior Matriculation for entrance is too low." The president said that it should be raised to Honour Matriculation "in at least three subjects." "It seems probable that this course … [will] turn out a broadly educated as well as an expert medical man."[55] When the Faculty Council met in October 1920, "Professor Wishart reported that the Committee on Curriculum and Examinations [the senior committee] are considering the question of raising the standard of entrance into the Faculty of Medicine and have appointed a sub-committee to go into the whole problem."[56] This was the opening gun in a long battle to raise the quality of the medical students.

It was a battle only because the entire issue of open admission to medicine was politically very sensitive. Yet voices began to demand the raising of admission standards. A succession of barriers thought to be politically defensible was thrown up.

The first barrier was insisting on higher high school matriculation credentials. After the war the entrance standard was increased to honour matriculation. But this hadn't stemmed the tide. We're going to have to think about further raising standards, said Dean FitzGerald in 1932, because excess numbers were applying. "Limitation of the number of students admitted into medicine is carried out in the majority of universities in Canada and the United States. It has become necessary because a far larger number seek admission than the facilities of institutions can accommodate." These large numbers especially militate against "close personal contact between students and members of the teaching staff."[57] In the Department of Medicine, for example, it was said in 1932, "Owing to the longer stay in hospital of patients and the large number of students, the same patients are used so often for clinical instruction that patient, student and clinical instructor lose interest. Students of at least two, and often three different years, are allotted to the same patients." In the Department of Surgery, "the provision of adequate training is almost impossible on account of over-taxing the endurance of the patients by repeated examinations by individual students, as well as by repeated clinics in groups on the same patient." Further, "[t]he size of student groups in the operating room sometimes … threatens strict asepsis."[58]

The problem worsened. The secondary school population almost doubled from 40,000 in 1921 to 75,000 in 1930. In those years, the number of pupils in secondary schools writing honour matriculation exams in Ontario increased from around 1,500 to over 12,000. And of those students who chose medicine, fully a third (39 percent in 1930) failed their first medical year![59] The medical schools were clearly about to be overwhelmed – with poor students.

Thus the desperate faculty petitioned the university for limiting to eighty the number of students admitted to the medical course. Said the Faculty Council in 1932, "This [restriction], with the addition of 20 graduates in Arts of the B & M Course, and men entering the Fourth Year ad eundem [granting of academic standing to students from another university] from the other Provinces, would yield in each of the clinical years about 100 students." The numbers of American students applying for admission to Toronto increased steadily (from 217 in 1927 to 415 in 1931), but unless one of their parents was a Toronto medical graduate, they hadn't a chance. And only under special circumstances were a few Canadians admitted from other provinces – those that didn't have medical schools.[60] Of course this was a recipe for parochialism, but the taxpayers were thought not to care so much.

John Gerald FitzGerald as dean after 1932 was strenuous on the subject of limiting class size. In October of that year he said that "decidedly fewer physicians and surgeons … will be able to serve the community efficiently in future. [A report] reveals an unwieldy growth of the medical school of recent years." He was referring to a story in the *Globe and Mail*, which said this trend "has produced an impracticable crowding of many classrooms and laboratories … Comment by the head of one of the medical departments … indicates that medical students are acquiring a lazy mental attitude." (This professor was apparently Velyien Henderson, head of the Department of Pharmacology.) FitzGerald recommended cutting the first-year class from 150 to 100. The students would be selected on the basis of their marks in the first premedical year.[61] As the Depression ground on and the university grants became ever less, FitzGerald returned again and again to the need for smaller classes, if only to shift money to research.[62] All comers with the honours matriculation had to be taken! In 1933 FitzGerald was vehement about the first year: "No less than 167 were enrolled. The highest figure in a decade." This includes nineteen students repeating the year, which the faculty were particularly alarmed about. "Why should universities in this province continue, at great expense, to train more physicians than are currently needed? There seems at present to be a world-wide oversupply and overproduction of physicians."[63]

But open admission proved a difficult concept to discard because it was politically popular; FitzGerald's impatience rose. In 1935 he wrote, "The present methods of admission to this Faculty, without limitation or selection, cannot, by any stretch of the imagination, be regarded as adequate or satisfactory. This situation surely calls for drastic revision. We have too many medical undergraduates, and the obstacles in the way of their rejection or elimination constitute a case for reform." Last year, he said, there had been over 800 undergraduates in medicine. This was far too many to school properly.[64]

Thus, a second barrier went up. In February 1935 E. Stanley Ryerson, the faculty secretary, said that admission from the first year to subsequent years would be strictly curtailed. "In order to secure standing at the annual examination in the first year, a candidate must have obtained at least fifty per cent in each subject of the course." Entrance to the second medical year will be based on academic standing in first year, as well as "the personality, aptitude and character of the student," health, and physical condition.[65] It's interesting to see the faculty trying to creak the door slowly shut – first raising high school marks, then barring advancement within the program – without coming right out and saying that the faculty would impose an elitist admission policy.

So massive did faculty unhappiness with the poor quality of the students become that in 1936 a "special committee" was struck to study the curriculum.[66] In an effort to reduce advancement of first-year students into the upper years, the grading became ever stricter. In 1937 Gallie (now dean) said, "It has long been felt that students who are unsuited to the long and arduous training required by modern medicine should be dropped from the course at the earliest possible moment and given an opportunity to select, before it is too late, some other vocation." So the curriculum in the first year had been divided into three groups: first group, French or German; second group, biology, chemistry, and physics; third group: history of science and civilization. "To obtain standing at the end of the year, the student must obtain at least fifty per cent in each subject and an average of sixty per cent in the group composed of Biology, Chemistry and Physics. As a result of the raising of standards in the first year, it is hoped that the weak students will be detected at once and started in other directions."

Moreover, at the end of the first year, all students would take the Aptitude Test of the American Association of Medical Colleges, "designed to discover whether the students have those qualities which would enable them to face a rigorous six-year course, to become good doctors afterwards and to occupy that place in the life of the country which a medical degree from this University suggests that they should occupy."[67]

The gates creaked even closer shut. Regarding the three natural science subjects, Gallie said in 1938, "There will be no supplemental [make-up] exams. This has clearly reduced the number progressing to second year. But we made the unhappy discovery last year that there was no way to prevent those whom we wished to eliminate from re-registering the following year. So, the first year was larger than ever." Therefore, now they were providing that those who fail the first year may not re-register.[68]

In 1938 the special curricular reform committee delivered a devastating critique of the consequences of overcrowding. "The Committee feels very strongly that the teachers of all years, but particularly those of the senior years, have been greatly handicapped by the large number of students, and still more by the large percentage of inferior students. When ... some 40 out of the 135 students of the fourth year ... have repeated some one year or have come over from the B & M course owing to deficiencies, a great inert mass is imposed upon the senior teachers ... We do well by our weaker students but we are not doing enough for the better ones, and even the better students are more concerned with acquiring information for the purpose of passing examinations than in studying whole individuals in health or disease."[69]

In fairness, the curriculum itself was calculated to grind curiosity from these young minds. Here is Kager Wightman, later head of medicine, on the biology course he was obliged to take in the first year, "which I found largely incomprehensible. Dr Bailey was a very scholarly man and we all realized, at least I realized it, that what he was giving us was really terribly important but somehow or other it didn't get across." Bailey's colleague Dr Benstead "used to write his lectures on the blackboard – they had blackboards that would slide up and down, you know, and he would write his in the most beautiful handwriting, and as he talked he would write it all and then shove up the blackboard and then start on the next one, and if you wanted to, you could copy this all down. He wrote a book called 'The Anatomy of the Rabbit' so we had to dissect a rabbit."[70]

The aforementioned 1938 report was not just about the poor quality of the students but also the poor quality of the curriculum: overly laden with facts and curiosity-crushing. The words of the drafters will ring in the heads of all medical readers of this volume who went through the faculty in the years before the introduction of the problem-based learning curriculum in the 1990s: "Each teacher feels the importance of his own subject ... His natural tendency, therefore, is to endeavour ... to impart as great a wealth as possible of factual detail – a wealth which the student has difficulty in assimilating and much of which he sheds from memory as soon as the examination is over ... Too intensive an effort to keep abreast of modern research is likely to leave the student with an imperfect background of the fundamentals of the subject, confused by a mass of uncoordinated details, too dazed and too harassed to develop any interest beyond that of preparing for examinations."[71]

Surely it was time for curricular reform.

*Reforming the Curriculum*

Reforming the medical curriculum became almost a cottage industry after the 1930s as the faculty was unable to resolve the contradiction between giving individual departments blocks of time to teach whatever they thought best and the need to reduce the sheer number of facts flung at the often obtunded students in endless hours of lectures. This began in the 1936–7 session, with a committee report that said "the time-table was too full and that matters might be improved by a general reduction by each of the departments of the number of hours pre-scribed ... for laboratories and lectures." We have adopted the report, said the dean, and will try to implement it. But it was controversial, and anatomy, the most time-hungry of the basic sciences, strongly resisted decreasing the hours.[72]

The faculty's first ever curriculum reform committee proposed in 1938 some practical changes to the clinical years, years four to six. Gallie said that previ-ously, "[e]ach Department has tended to elaborate its courses to the fullest pos-sible extent, and with this object has sought the largest attainable share of the student's time. The result is that the curriculum has become overloaded in con-tent, and overcrowded in time. The student has no time for individual study and reading ... His one duty he feels, and is practically made to feel, is to com-mit to memory a certain mass of information; and, having discharged this at an examination, to replace it as completely as possible by another. The Faculty is convinced that the results of this system are not good." Now the Curriculum Committee made the same criticism of the clinical years as of the primary years. They were going to have big cutbacks in the hours dedicated to bacteriology, pathological chemistry, and radiology.[73]

In the 1943–4 session, the suggestion was offered of limiting class size at in-take, given that internal brakes on advancing from the preclinical to the clinical years had failed. Gallie said in 1944 that the temporary wartime increase to 150 in the freshman year was unsatisfactory. "This is too many to allow of proper training in the clinical years. Further, the quality of the matriculants in the lower third of the class ... is so low that there is no possibility of their getting through the difficult medical course creditably. It is certain, therefore, that with the re-turn of normal times the Faculty will recommend that a limit of 100 be placed on admissions."[74]

### The Second World War and Its Consequences

World wars tend to have big consequences for medical education. The First World War saw the curriculum jump to six years; the Second World War saw medical education intensify.

As war erupted in September 1939 it was clear that the faculty would have to increase the production of physicians. With the same patriotic fervor that greeted hostilities in 1914, both med students and staff rushed to enlist anew. The dean told the president four days after war was declared, "It was agreed that it would be unwise to encourage Medical students to enlist in other units than the CAMC [Canadian Army Medical Corps], having in mind the shortage of young officers that occurred in the later years of the last war."[75]

How could they speed up medical training, given that the volume of ma-terial to be mastered remained the same? Lengthen the session! The faculty decided to extend the period of medical training by beginning the session in August rather than September and finishing the year at the end of June rather than mid-May. They also reduced the internship from a one-year rotation to eight months. Said Dean Gallie in 1941, "The continuance of four and a half months' holidays in war-time is not justifiable and would leave both Faculty and students open to criticism of slackness in the national war effort." Thus the medical course will last, starting next May, only a little over five years instead of seven, including internship. They also suspended the biological and medical sciences honour course and virtually all of the students were transferring to medicine.[76]

In 1944 the Curriculum Committee proposed a formal two-year "premedical" course of thirty weeks each and a four-year medical course of thirty-six weeks each. "The new medical course ... is designed to give the student, in the early part of his university career, some of the elements of a liberal education as well as the necessary training in the basic sciences. To this end there have been incorporated in the two premedical years certain subjects from the humanities, selected in the hope that the cultural horizon of the medical student may be widened and that he may thus be made more fit to assume those numerous extra-professional responsibilities which, in any community, fall on the shoulders of the doctor." The new curriculum would come into effect in 1945–6 and passage from it into the medical program would be carefully gated.

In the first and second premedical years, the course choices were divided between obligatory and elective. Obligatory were chemistry, English, and physics, plus either history or philosophy, and one of anthropology, botany, foreign language, or mathematics. The curriculum planners collaborated with arts faculty to design a special set of premedical courses, neither the honours courses of arts nor the "pass" courses.[77] (Today, humanists among medical educators can only dream of requiring that the students have preparation in English, anthropology, or history!)

The Calendar for 1945–6 made clear that this humanizing of the medical students occurred not in the larger context of making them more sensitive clinicians, as drives medical humanities today, but in the context of the doctor-as-gentleman, a theme present in medical education since the First World War: "The medical course which came into operation for the first time in the session 1945–1946 is designed to give the student ... some of the elements of a liberal education ... in the hope that the cultural horizon of the medical student may be widened and that he may thus be made more fit to assume those numerous extra-professional responsibilities which, in any community, fall on the shoulders of the doctor."[78]

Just as his predecessors, President Sidney Smith too waxed enthusiastic about bringing arts into the medical curriculum: "Undoubtedly the infusion into the medical course of additional subjects from the fields of the humanities and the social sciences will produce graduates who have not only professional proficiency, but also a better appreciation of the society in which they will practise ... Moreover, the opening of new windows through which the young doctor may view contemporary civilization will restore in considerable degree his warrant to membership in a learned profession." Clearly, from the medical humanities so much was expected that it is amazing today we can do without it.[79]

## The Toronto Model of Teaching

The patient was the big teacher. That was the modus operandi of the day.[80]

Donald Cowan, 2009

The end of the Second World War saw a last attempt to hang onto the British model that had guided the faculty for the previous three-quarters of a century. There was haste to ditch the classes of 200 students per year that military needs compelled and to cap the class size at 100. But the entire discourse was shifting southwards. In March 1946 the Faculty Council said this cap was necessary "if we are to maintain our position among the Class A Medical schools of America and turn out properly qualified graduates." Note that classes at Harvard are 125, Columbia 115, and Hopkins 72. "Several of these are in very large cities with numerous first class hospitals and with enormous endowments, yet they deliberately keep the number of students down to certain limits on the grounds that they could not handle more efficiently."[81]

Thus there was a Toronto model of teaching, thought comparable to the best US schools though it had stemmed from the United Kingdom. It is interesting that this Toronto model of teaching – with its close student-professor relationships – was so revered that even university president Sidney Smith, a nonphysician, held to it. He said in 1954 on the subject of class size, "A first-class medical school is in a sense self-limiting as to size [160 is current class]. There is a point beyond which it should not enroll more students, even if it is given sufficient financial support to do so ... Personal communication between the students and the senior members of the staff would become too attenuated. It must be possible for every student to have a real, and not merely a formal, contact with the eminent doctors who are heads of the teaching departments."[82]

In 1958 Farquharson described the careful clinical instruction at the bedside then fundamental to medical education in Toronto. "An attempt is made in the early part of the second year to bridge the gap between clinical work on the one hand and anatomy and physiology on the other ... From the first day on the wards they record their examination of the patient's appearance and discuss its relation to his general symptoms. As they gradually acquire routine methods of physical examination they learn to enquire systematically into the particular symptoms that may arise from disorders of each particular system. Great stress is placed on the accurate description of each symptom and its significance. As [nineteenth-century Scottish physician] Dr John Brown said, 'Symptoms are the voice of nature.' Nothing in medical education is more important than to learn to recognize them clearly and interpret them correctly."

In the third year, said Farquharson, the students divided into small clinical groups that stay on one ward with one teacher for eight weeks, giving the students opportunity to follow the patients whose histories he or she has taken. "It is gratifying to find how often these patients confide in the third year clerks." Then in the final year, students receive more responsibility. "On two mornings a week he attends the medical out-patients department where he has a room to himself to see new patients and follow those whose histories he has taken previously, just as he would in private practice ... Should the patient be admitted to hospital, he [the patient] is sent to the ward on which the student is a member of the clinical team composed of three staff men, one assistant resident, one interne and two students. Here he acts as an assistant interne and takes part in all the activities and discussions of the ward."

Arcane acronyms and abbreviations were shunned (today's readers can only smile). Farquharson continued, "Practice in giving a well organized description of the patient's case in clear, concise, ordinary English words is considered an important feature of medical education. It gives the student a clearer view of each problem. It helps him in talking to his patients and their friends." Farquharson noted the importance of getting the family on board. "Good treatment is frequently a matter of explanation in clear simple terms and of persuasion to follow a given regimen. To do it well requires endless thought and practice."[83] This, then, was the Toronto system, borrowed from "the Mother land" and nurtured with a distinctive Canadian attentiveness to close contact between teacher and student. Can it be any wonder that these teachers shuddered as they saw the American research behemoth approaching?

*Social Change*

After the Second World War, Canada began to change as a society, more urban and more mercantile than agricultural. These changes started to be reflected in medical school admissions: the farm boys from whose Scottish ranks the faculty seemed mainly recruited before the war started to be pushed aside. Indeed, Sidney Smith said in 1947, "Steps must be taken to ensure that the cost of medical education shall not prevent the registration of talented young persons from rural districts."[84] In September 1948 the Admissions Committee decided to give some preference to farm boys. In admissions, "[w]hile matriculation standing was of the greatest importance some effort was also made to give a certain advantage to candidates from rural areas."[85] A layered admissions policy was adopted. In 1949, some 55 percent of all applicants were admitted, 61 percent of those who applied from small cities and towns of Ontario. The successful candidates were overwhelmingly from Ontario. This displeased Ray Farquharson, who "felt very strongly that we should admit some students to the clinical years from the United States, Great Britain, and other countries, otherwise we would tend to become more and more provincial."[86]

In 1956–7, a Committee on Admissions was struck, which formulated explicit rules for admission. The desirable outcome was roughly two-thirds of the students from pre-medicine, one-third from other degree courses, "thus allowing an intake of students," as the report by Associate Dean Jan Steiner later put it, "from other Universities and other countries ... It was hoped that this would prevent what Dr. Farquharson the then Professor of Medicine, called 'the danger of becoming too provincial in character.'"[87]

By the early 1950s, urbanization was clearly shifting candidates for admission to the cities. In the 1951–2 session, 57 percent of medical students came from Metro Toronto.[88] Urbanization increased the number of hospitals and therewith the number of internship positions, forcing fewer medical graduates to train in the United States. In 1951, of the graduating class of 170, only 20 sought internships in the United States. MacFarlane attributed this to the "large numbers of hospitals in the great industrial centres." He noted, "This is much more favourable than twenty years ago when 30 to 40 per cent of Toronto graduates immediately sought internships outside Canada."[89]

Yet the faculty did not lose its fondness for students from small towns, if only to ensure that some medical graduates would return to these towns to practice. In September 1971, Steiner and Dean Chute held a press conference to assure the public that 88 percent of the medical admissions last year were Ontario residents and 95 percent would be that year. Steiner said that in medical admissions, preference was given first to those who had done well in the first two years of the science course at U of T, then to "students from towns with less than 5,000 people, and students who previously had been rejected but had remained at university and 'redeemed themselves.' Preference is given students from small towns because that is where doctors are needed, Steiner said."[90]

*The Moral Curriculum Again*

Physicians as community leaders was a subject to which MacFarlane returned as a dog to a bone. He conceded in 1952 that humanities classes were anything but popular among the students. Yet "[t]he teachers in the upper years of the professional course have noted the improvement in ability to write papers and a greater facility in discussion. [In university forums] our students ... speak with a clarity and confidence which has been gratifying and even surprising to their teachers."[91] Leaders were those able to speak strongly and convincingly (rather than simply to flash PowerPoint slides).

It was in these years that MacFarlane's efforts to teach "moral values" to students, in the view that they would be the community leaders of tomorrow, reached their acme. This was the virtue of the British system of close personal relationships between teachers and students, that moral wisdom was conveyed at the same time as clinical knowledge. The knowledge explosion must be reflected in an increasingly complex curriculum, said MacFarlane in 1955. Yet the most comprehensive of lesson plans would fail "if at some stage, preferably throughout the entire course, the student is not impressed with the importance of sound moral values ... This maintenance of moral values, this constant striving for the first-rate, encompasses principles that are best taught by example rather than precept."[92]

This whole subject of the curriculum as a source of moral guidance came to an end with MacFarlane's stepping down as dean in 1960. It went away at around the same time that the faculty's systematic anti-Semitism disappeared, and one wonders if there was a connection. Both themes today are deeply démodé and perhaps for similar reasons: they reflect a constricted moral outlook that assigns special social privilege to those with the right genes and the right educational training. Duncan Graham's appearance at the home of a senior faculty member one evening to rail against the appointment of the Jew Hollenberg may have gone hand and hand with his and his colleagues' elevation of those with medical training to the status of "community leaders."[93]

*The Block Curriculum (and Its Discontents)*

In the 1960–1 session, Bill Oille, an internist and senior member of the Department of Medicine, became coordinator of a special committee on the curriculum.[94] Three years later the Oille committee recommended major changes. First of all, in the premedical course, the changes would bring it closer to the general course in science. Two humanities were, however, preserved in each of the two premedical years.[95] Second, in the preclinical years of the medical course the Oille committee recommended the adoption of "block" teaching: sixteen weeks devoted, for example, to anatomy; a second block devoted to biochemistry and physiology; a third block to history taking and physical examination.[96]

In the 1967–8 session the new "block" curriculum began to be implemented. Unhappiness was the response among departments that had not been given large enough blocks. The Department of Ophthalmology complained that their teaching had been squeezed to "a two-week interval in Period III." The new curriculum required numerous small-group discussions. "This has been found to be a strain on the department, since these learning experiences occur during busy clinics and heavy commitments to service." In conclusion, "[t]he overall experience with the new curriculum has not been happy."[97] Similar complaints came from the Department of Pathology: "Little can be said of the new undergraduate curriculum in Medicine. Confusion and doubt, would perhaps, be the two most appropriate epithets at this time."[98] A year later, "[t]he student who ends with a good understanding of pathology could be said to have gained it in spite of the curriculum."[99]

The surgeons' noses were also out of joint. "Of ... concern is the discovery that certain topics are no longer included in the curriculum and that individuals highly qualified to teach have not been asked to do so. Such subjects as soft tissue wound healing, the burned patient, and the broad subject of max-illo facial injuries are not discussed. This problem will be a recurring one as the knowledge explosion continues. Coverage of all knowledge is out, but a continuing assessment of content is very much in."[100]

And anesthesia! Arthur J. Dunn, head of the hospital Department of Anesthesia at St Michael's, was very upset at the proposal to remove the two-week clerkship in anesthesia, evidently in favour of expanding the Department of Family and Community Medicine: "This 2-week exposure is the sole planned and predictable exposure of clerks to the knowledge and skills appropriate to life threatening situations. These will arise in most doctors' careers no matter how great their commitment to social work." The sneering note anticipated what would become the new curriculum of the 1990s – problem-based learning – and affirmed the general practitioner as a doctor trained to save lives: "I cannot over-emphasize the absolute necessity of being able to show the student ... how to establish airways, maintain ventilation, manage fluid and transfusion therapy, use properly the most potent drugs in Medicine, and continually assess and adjust the condition of unconscious patients. The imperfect state of these skills in the general medical population can be readily determined by travel in less populated areas of this vast country."[101]

The response of the radiation oncologists illuminates beautifully the tension between a curriculum consisting of "basics" and one composed of useful knowledge. The radiotherapists sounded a particularly vexed note about an undergraduate program heavy in subjects the students would soon forget such as biochemistry and void of those they would soon need, such as cancer care. "The University of Toronto shares with most other universities the distinction of being in the 'disaster area' as far as the undergraduate education is concerned." The curriculum organizers had managed, said the radiation oncologists, to stagger together "four or five formal lectures given at a time just preceding his or her vital examinations. It is not surprising that these lectures were poorly attended, and that the lecturers lost heart." Otherwise the students had only the crumbs of misinformation their teachers recalled from a distant past whose "selective memories remembered the complications rather than the benefits to mankind." If students were permitted to spend a bit more time at Princess Margaret Hospital, the radiation oncologists argued, "[t]hey would be equipped with a real understanding of the nature and management of cancer, which they do not get in the fragmented and often indifferent teaching as now practiced. It should be appreciated that much of cancer care is, in reality, the management of a chronic disease, no different from, and more successful than that practiced in psychiatry, rheumatic disease, cardiology and respiratory disease. The concept of 'cancer cure' is a myth and relates to the simplistic view promoted by the excisional concept and the cancer society's belief that 'the cure is just around the corner.'" Alas, by the time the students reach Princess Margaret Hospital "it is too late to influence their choice of a career ... had they known about oncology earlier they might well have chosen it as their life's work, particularly when they appreciate that oncology is the general practice of cancer – and general practice is the current fashion."[102] Thus, an eloquent lament about a giant blind spot in undergraduate teaching, one with immense clinical consequences (for more, see chapter 13).

The negative reaction of the faculty to a block curriculum heavy in basic sciences emphasizes perfectly the conflict that exists in any system of medical education between educating medical students in science and training them in disease management. In understanding why, twenty years later, the faculty was willing to abandon the block curriculum and go over to a very different system that was a kind of third way, problem-based learning, this steady erosion of support from old-line departments must be kept in mind.

### The Social Curriculum

After the war the idea gathered force that physicians in training must know how to treat patients in the community and not just in the wards of tertiary teaching hospitals. This ideal culminated in the foundation of the Department of Family and Community Medicine in 1969 (see chapter 24). But it germinated in the faculty long before. In the 1951–2 session, social worker Elizabeth Clarkson, trained in Glasgow, came on staff part-time in the Departments of Medicine and Public Health to introduce some third- and fourth-year students to the homes of patients attending the Toronto General Hospital "to study environmental and social factors." Support for this project came from the Rockefeller Foundation.[103]

This notion of community involvement remained almost inaudible, whispered but occasionally in the research-oriented faculty. In the 1971–2 session, a subcommittee of the Ontario Council of Health dealing with future arrangements for health education recommended shifting undergraduate medical education from hospital to "the community."[104] One of the recommendations of the "Mustard Report" of 1972 – which endorsed a huge increase in class size – was educating medical students in "community centres" as well as in teaching hospitals.[105] But as yet, few were listening.

Or rather, the entire culture was listening. The late 1960s and 1970s saw student interest in "science" at low ebb, their interest in community involvement at high tide. The increasingly research-oriented faculty did not experience this as good news. At a 1973 meeting of the Faculty Council's Sub-committee on Science Policy, Eliot Phillipson in the Department of Medicine said there was "a decreasing interest in science, and in a scientific approach to medicine among medical students." The subcommittee, aware of swimming against the tide, therefore added to its brief, "To keep under review the general scientific climate in the Faculty, to examine particularly the scientific element in medical education, and the recruitment of students for scientific careers in medicine."[106]

   In an interview in March 1978 with the science policy thinkers, Charlie Hollenberg mused about the failure to interest many undergraduates in research
careers. He "established that the Department has not been as successful as it
might wish in recruiting interns and residents into research. This appears to
be a general problem across Canada." Hollenberg said exposure to research
should start "by encouraging students to complete a degree before entry [into
medical school]."[107] The disconnect between the communitarian aspirations of
the students and the research hopes of the barons was striking.

*Changing the Final Year and the Internship*

In 1958 the College of Physicians and Surgeons of Ontario required an internship as a precondition for licensing. For Toronto at least, the requirement was
pointless. MacFarlane had earlier said, "A student who spends four years in
a medical course is scarcely ready for practice; [this] has been recognized for
many years, and 99 per cent of the graduates have immediately undertaken a
year of internship."[108]

   Yet a strong desire was abroad to pump up clinical exposure in the final year
of medicine, and in the 1964–5 session, Wightman moved to convert the "junior
internship" of the final year into a clerkship, "designed to integrate theory and
practice in a protected and closely supervised setting."[109] Thus the old junior
internship, a postgraduate post, was abolished, replaced by a clerkship that all
final-year students would serve before moving onto a regular internship that
might or might not mark the beginning of a residency. In the 1967–8 session, the
new clinical clerkship was established, which now lasted twelve months (and
therefore would require some financial support for the students).[110]

*Limiting Admissions*

In the fall of 1962, for the first time students with good high school grades were
prevented from enrolling in the first premedical year on the grounds that there
was no space for them: seventy high school graduates with grade 13 averages
of over 65 percent were turned away. Said the dean, "This is not satisfactory,
and a decision will have to be made about the number of students who take the
premedical course prior to the first professional year."[111] By September 1965 the
dean was thinking of dropping the premedical course "in favour of the first two
years of the course in General Science."[112] In September 1966, the Faculty Council voted "[t]hat all students wishing to enter the 1st professional year, including
those students from the premedical course, must apply for admission and enter
into competition for available places in the first professional year." This was the
beginning of the end of the two-year premedical program.[113]

   In 1962 as well the premedical program in the Faculty of Arts was restored
called the biological and medical sciences course (the premedical program

properly understood was in the Faculty of Medicine). After completion of the first year, the students might move into medicine.[114] "B & M" was later stopped because the overall arts and science curriculum changed and specialty programs were discontinued.

### Academies: Early History

Among the most significant developments in undergraduate life and teaching was the decentralizing of the curriculum into hospital-based "academies," where significant parts of the preclinical and clinical instruction would take place and the students have a kind of "home base." This move towards decentralization was inevitable, given pressures to increase class size and the faculty's fondness for the system of small-group instruction in an English apprenticeship setting.

The roots of this decentralization reach far back in time, indeed to the 1955–6 term, when the dean mused about assigning students "to one of the three general teaching hospitals where the staff would be responsible for all their clinical instruction except in … Pediatrics."[115] This came to nothing but marks the initial appearance of this rhetoric.

In the mid-1960s, with pressures from the province and the Board of Governors to increase class size to 250, the talk about academies began in earnest. At the same time, increasing the class size brought the faculty face to face with the challenge of bigness, an affront to an almost hundred-year-old British-inspired system of small classes and close personal relationship between student and teacher. Dean Hamilton insisted, "In the clinical sciences the student must have a direct and individual relationship with his teacher just as he must with the patient he is studying. This means that the ratio of clinical teachers to students is very high, in fact, greater than one to one."[116]

In 1964 the decision to increase the class size to 250 was reached. The special committee of the Board of Governors on the Faculty of Medicine, created in 1963 and reporting in 1964, wished to encourage parallel programs in clinical teaching at the General, the Western, and St Michael's. The smaller teaching hospitals would be associated with teaching in one of the big three. Instruction in the basic sciences, by contrast, would be centralized in the new medical building already being planned, the Medical Sciences Building.[117]

In November the committee report on the "Future Development of the Faculty of Medicine" was laid out in detail, recommending "the creation of several clinical schools, where the academic programme of the last two years of the undergraduate course would be given in parallel. Breaking up a class of 250 students into smaller units and providing continuity of association with one major hospital and its teaching staff would overcome the problem of the large class rotating through many hospitals. The prolonged association of a student with one institution would permit him to develop a greater sense of identification with that institute and a more intimate, because prolonged, relationship with the staff. The optimum atmosphere for good teaching would thereby be established."[118] Each clinical school would be supervised by an assistant or associate dean.[119] The report imposed upon St Michael's and the Western in particular the need for more teaching space, research space, and additional full-time staff: "It will mean in time that there will be, in terms of full-time staff, approximately one for each member of the graduating class of students."[120] In one elaboration of this scheme, a fourth academy would be added at Sunnybrook, which had just become the university teaching hospital. (HSC would provide pediatric teaching to several of the academies.)[121]

But then that was the end of it. In March 1967 Dean Chute told the Joint Hospitals Committee, "The original suggestion of four separate hospital schools is not being considered seriously at present."[122]

In the early 1970s the academies idea flickered briefly back to life when in September 1971 the Ministry of Health commissioned a "Role Study" of the Toronto teaching hospitals to determine if eliminating duplication of services might save money. The Role Study report recommended "the formation of four semi-autonomous clinical schools."[123] In September 1972 the Faculty Council grappled with "The Task Force on Future Arrangements for Health Education ('The Mustard Report')," including a proposed expansion of the first-year class to 350 students in "four semi-autonomous clinical satellites for education and service."[124] This, too, came to nothing.

*Growth*

Growth was the main accent after the war's end. The residents of Ontario became ever more numerous and their medical demands more insistent with the advent of a provincial health plan. More doctors were needed. The faculty's resistance to increased class size started to waver in the 1950s as a consequence, as Sidney Smith put it, "of the seriously declining ratio of physicians to population which is beginning to be evident in Canada." If additional teaching beds could be arranged, in 1957 the faculty was said willing to add on an additional hundred students.[125]

As well, to make scientific progress the faculty absolutely had to grow, but there was no room for more labs or offices. Everything was chock-a-block. Simultaneously, as mentioned, the Province of Ontario agonized about a doctors' crisis: the population was outpacing the supply of physicians. Thus on 31 October 1964, a grand bargain was reached. The province announced that it would pump up faculty funding if the faculty would agree to increase the size of the first-year class by 75 students, from 175 to 250. This was part of a larger provincial scheme to fund a new medical school in Hamilton at McMaster University and to renovate the medical school at Queen's. Implicit in the deal was the ministry's apparent promise of a new Medical Sciences Building to the University of Toronto.[126] Grand bargain or not, the faculty opposed increasing the class size for "fear of slipping standards," as Bissell said. The decision to increase the size of the first-year class to 250 was taken not by the faculty but by the Board of Governors.[127]

Growing to 250 meant not just expanding basic science facilities. The extra students would also need more bedside teaching. Led by chairman Henry Borden, the U of T Board of Governors eyed Sunnybrook Hospital, hitherto a veterans facility and after 1966 the first university hospital of the Faculty of Medicine (see chapter 25).[128] And growth there was. In October 1969 the Independent Planners said enrolment was increasing 43 percent! In session 1969–70 they were admitting 175 to the first medical year; this will be increased to 200 for the second medical year by intake of 25 students from the course in biological and medical science. By September 1972 enrolment in the first medical year will hit 250 students. "Thus by September 1974, the total number of students in the Professional Course in Medicine will be 1000."[129]

These words were uttered with a kind of awe as though watching a piece of a great glacier crash into the sea. People could see the British system slipping away.

### The Undergraduate Curriculum: Problem-Based Learning

The faculty really was caught between a rock and a hard place. The rock was a science-heavy curriculum. Kager Wightman reminisced about the 1930s when he was a medical student: Charles Best "believed that everything should be taught by the guy who knew most about it, so we were exposed to a bunch of people who had special interests and who were doing research ... and most of them I felt tried to teach us far too much because they were so interested in their subjects." Wightman tried later on "to persuade Dr Best to change his method," but he didn't.[130] Later years had the same problem. Dean Fred Lowy said of the 1960s and 1970s, "Students felt that the curriculum was too highly structured and was oriented more to factual transfer than to knowledge integration and problem solving ... The expectations of some teachers were unrealistic; for example, [the students] pointed out ... that several of the undergraduate course syllabi were highly sought after by final year specialty residents due to the depth and detail of information included." The department-controlled curriculum was thus inevitably fact-laden, and this realization, Lowy said, led to a task force in 1982–3 under Assistant Dean Edward M. Sellers to revise the curriculum.[131]

The hard place was risking that the students would bypass the demanding science-based medical specialties in favour of community involvement.

The unraveling of the hated block curriculum began in April 1976 as the Faculty Council received the recommendations of a Curriculum Renewal Task Force headed by Bill Francombe of the Department of Medicine. The main recommendation was that "[t]he Faculty return to a four year curriculum, with the introduction of clinical experience earlier than at present, and with a steady increase in clinical activity during the four years" – first year: basis science; second: bridging year; third: "almost entirely clinical but with some central teaching"; fourth: "similar to the existing clinical clerkship."[132]

Instead, a very different outcome occurred. Edward M. Sellers was the lead figure here. The son of the distinguished pharmacologist Edward A. Sellers, Edward M. was a 1965 U of T graduate who himself had become a professor of pharmacology and was now associate dean. Sometime in 1982 or early 1983, Dean Fred Lowy placed him in charge of yet another curriculum review committee. At an April 1983 meeting of the Committee of Clinical Chairmen, Sellers explained that, in regard to the vexed undergraduate curriculum, "[a] large number of problem areas were identified, a few examples being: fact overload, the examination system which reinforces fact overload, [lack of] critical appraisal as an aid to problem solving, and communication within a complex curriculum." Sellers's committee had asked the department chairs for comments. The results indicated huge dissatisfaction among the professors as well; for example, "Students appear to be 'turned off' during the course of the programme. One solution might be to reduce the first two years to essentials, and start the clerkship in the third year." Sellers's committee, the Undergraduate Medical Curriculum Committee, was going to "develop a proposal for curriculum renewal."[133]

In 1985 the merger of the General Hospital and the Western was progressing apace. Lowy put Sellers in charge of a committee to assess the consequences for undergraduate medical education of the merger. It was this somewhat technical sounding committee that made the fundamental recommendations for a "hospital based curriculum" that produced problem-based learning (PBL).

On 24 October 1986 the committee reported. Its recommendations:

One, "decreased scheduling time" and "radical reduction in the number of lectures (to one to two hours per day)."

Two, "case-based learning" which will "take place mainly in small groups and will involve consideration of carefully constructed and focused cases … Case-based learning and the problem-solving that is associated with it requires knowledge of basic concepts and principles." "[The teaching] will be organized according to body systems."

Three, "The Toronto Hospital tutorial system": "A hospital based tutorial system will be a major innovative feature of the new program. Tutorial groups of 4 to 6 students will meet weekly for two hours with their respective faculty tutors." "The diminished structure in the program will transfer significant responsibility for learning to the students." [The Toronto Hospital terminology is interesting here. That PBL was developed at McMaster University is never mentioned.]

There were other points about clinical experience beginning early, numerous electives, much interdisciplinarity, and ongoing feedback to students rather than grades, but the previous is the gist.

There was one final point to bring the hospitals on board, and that was to emphasize the capital role of the hospital: "The Hospital and its academic departments will assume responsibility for planning and implementation of the program including formative student assessments and the ongoing monitoring of teaching."[134]

Lowy played a substantial role in the evolution of these events. In 1986 he said that there were major problems in the undergraduate curriculum.

> My own assessment is that our education programs are for the most part adequate, but some are stagnant. They lack excitement and innovation. ...Higher priority for the undergraduate medical program is appropriate because educating physicians is the fundamental (though not the only) reason our Faculty exists. ...We have let some of our programs stagnate. Much of our medical curriculum has remained unchanged for 15 years..... All of our didactic teaching suggests we believe that transmission of the facts known in 1986 is sufficient to produce the physician, the researchers, the leader ... These students want to be challenged by problem and issues, not only the rote learning of facts...I believe we should set for ourselves the goal of destructuring 50 percent of our currently scheduled lecture and seminar time in the medical curriculum in order to allow time for educational experiences that encourage students to think in depth about problems.[135]

Getting a change of this magnitude through the faculty required much manoeuvring, which will not be discussed here. In November 1989, following the Self-Study, a task force for curriculum renewal was launched, chaired by Ken Shumak of the Department of Medicine, who was designated associate dean for undergraduate medical education as well as chair of the Curriculum Renewal Task Force. The brief of the task force was this: "increased small group teaching, lengthening of the clerkship, earlier clinical exposure and problem-based learning."[136] The Self-Study of January 1990 itself was scathing about the prevailing climate of undergraduate medical education at U of T. The Department of Pharmacology's take was, "The culture in the medical school should be one in which students were expected to reflect on problems, to discuss issues, to question 'facts.' ... [But] many undergraduate medical students who are admitted to the MD programme after two years of university are unable to separate concepts from facts. They are (or become) 'fact junkies.'"[137] (The comment was an interesting one. But in fact, fewer and fewer were the medical applicants without a previous undergraduate degree: in 1993–4 only 35 percent. By contrast 13 percent of the applicants had a master's degree or higher.[138])

Meanwhile, the old block curriculum was coming under withering fire. Robert Haslam, chair of the Department of Paediatrics, was upset about the overweening departmental control of the curriculum. He said in 1990, "There is a strong feeling that the medical school needs to break down its 'turfdoms.' It must move toward self-learning and problem-solving instead of focusing on the number of teaching hours allotted to each department. The curriculum should be more globally planned, with one central committee empowered to plan the entire curriculum and allocate time on the basis of an overall view of the content required to produce doctors for the 1990s ... Such a change would mean a loss of control by departmental chairmen."[139]

What tipped the old block curriculum into oblivion was a visit in late winter 1990 of the Accreditation Survey Team. The team expressed doubts about the current curriculum, which "continues to be heavily didactic, overloaded and repetitive; there is a clear need for more self-directed learning, problem-solving." The Survey Team was curious "why the Faculty did not have a comprehensive curriculum renewal following the Accreditation Visit of 1983." "While endorsing our present Curriculum Renewal process," said Dean John Dirks, "they sought considerable assurance that would lead to a new curriculum and to a successful implementation." Dirks assured them this would happen by the time of the interim visit two years later. He was confident that Ken Shumak and the Curriculum Renewal Task Force would achieve this goal.[140] By July 1990 Dirks was notifying Provost Joan Foley that substantial renovations would be necessary within the Medical Sciences Building to accommodate the new curriculum: "[N]ot only these facilities, but also our style of instruction are outmoded ... [Dirks was] in favour of self-directed, small group, problem-based learning. Extensive renovations of current facilities will be necessary."[141]

In April 1991 Shumak presented the new curriculum and the academies (about which more shortly) to the Committee of Clinical Chairs. Many more committee meetings followed, but by September 1991 the new curriculum was a done deal, to be introduced in September 1992.[142]

The PBL curriculum required enormous changes. In December 1991, Alvin Newman of the Department of Medicine was appointed director of curriculum development, chairing the Committee of Course Directors, which planned the new curriculum. "While this activity has been taking place, the Problem-Based Learning Faculty Development Group, chaired by Dr Robert Cohen of the Department of Surgery has been working on a series of workshops to train the 124 Faculty members who will be acting as tutors in the small group learning sessions." All the different pieces of the new curriculum, such as "Metabolism and Nutrition" and "Fundamentals of Medical Practice," had course directors of their own. The first eighty-two weeks were the pre-clerkship, including six such courses. "Each course integrates basic science, clinical science and community health concepts and includes Problem Based Learning experiences ... One half day of each week is dedicated to clinical medicine, so that students have much earlier exposure to the hospital/clinical environment." Also, students were in the community for one half day each week. The second eighteen months of the new curriculum were the clerkship.[143]

The new curriculum was thus the culmination of a half century of development in the faculty: the growing dissatisfaction with the fact-heavy teaching after the Second World War, the unhappy attempt of the "block" curriculum to modify it, the student revolt of the 1960s that scorned structure and insisted on spontaneity in learning, the gathering commitment to the community, and the crashing realization, coming from all sides, of the bankruptcy of the old curriculum.

The innovations were a big success. The students' work weeks were organized around solving specific problems in small groups and working up the basic and clinical science for each problem on their own in the library with only the occasional lectures, in contrast to the previous drill of sitting passively in the large lecture halls and soaking up the material. A year after the introduction of the new curriculum, Christopher Jamieson, director of undergraduate education in the Department of Surgery, said, "Within a few weeks the students were discussing how to manage clinical problems and were learning the skills of history taking and physical examination. They did not attend many lectures but instead worked in groups with their tutor. Each week there was a new case which was the subject for their problem-based learning. They spent many hours in the library researching their assignments for the group."[144] (In 1993 the Ministry of Health negotiated with the faculty a reduction in the size of the first-year class from 252 to 177;[145] although the purpose was to reduce the number of doctors, this had the effect of making the curriculum roll-out more manageable.)

The method of examination changed too. The Department of Surgery introduced into the faculty in the 1992–3 session a structured exam, taking the clinical clerks at the end of their surgery rotation from one station to the next, as opposed to the previous oral exam. The new exam was called an "Oskey," or OSCE, meaning an objective structured clinical examination.[146] When the first cohort of students in the new curriculum graduated in the spring of 1995, they performed as well as their predecessors in the final clerkship year and were just as successful in the Medical Council of Canada examinations[147] (a 2.9 percent failure rate, as opposed to a 4.5 percent failure rate for all sixteen medical schools[148]). So the new curriculum was indeed a success.

How about marking? Should there be numeric grades or pass/fail? The faculty had already tried pass/fail in the mid-1970s, then abandoned it. A tense shoot-out eventuated in the Faculty Council in May 1997, as psychiatrist Brian Hodges, later director of the Wilson Centre, argued for pass/fail on the grounds that it would reduce student stress and make them more collaborative and less competitive. Internist Eliot Phillipson, by contrast, argued for maintaining numerical marks on the grounds that "excellence [is] the overriding criterion of this University, and that excellence should be incorporated in our educational programs." He was dubious about the stress-reduction argument and said "that in every human endeavour, there was some degree of stress and that the emphasis should be on how to cope with it."[149] Phillipson lost. In January 1998, the Faculty Council recommended replacing "the current alpha-numeric grading system with an Honours/Pass/Fail grading system." This was perhaps the final turn away from the marks-driven old system.[150]

The excitement about the social dimensions of the new curriculum – about the patient's subjective experience and insertion in society – was huge. But the curriculum planners were less interested in other aspects of medicine, such as the administration of anesthesia. Said an external review of the Department of Anaesthesia in 1992, "More than 30 staff have volunteered for the 96-hour commitment to be tutors in the new curriculum, but their offers do not appear to have been accepted by the university administration ... No department members have been appointed to important roles in sections developing the problem based discussion topics."[151]

The new curriculum was also perceived as downgrading the importance of basic science, an understanding of which is the gateway to research. In December 1998 Phillipson kicked back against the de-emphasis on basic science education that he saw in the PBL curriculum and against the emphasis on psychosocial factors, as well as the "perceived failure of the 'biomedical model' to fully explain and eradicate disease." There had been a big decline in use of basic scientists as PBL tutors and in clerkship teaching, he said. A driving force of PBL was to diminish "irrelevant" facts from the basic sciences in the curriculum. Yet doctors have to know some basic science because in coming years genetics and molecular biology would transform medicine. Phillipson, the respirologist, said that just as you have to know sodium excretion to understand diuretics, "an understanding of the functions of the oncogenes and tumor suppressor genes will be necessary in assessing the clinical significance of 'cancer gene' mutations." Downgrading basic science meant, he said, "a return to a pre-Flexnerian model of medical education, in which clinical medicine lacked a strong scientific underpinning." He dwelt on science because "we believe that medical education is indeed an education and not merely a form of trade school job training." Phillipson also felt that trends in PBL violate "the provostial mandate that all teaching in the University should be rooted in and built upon our strengths in research ... We should ensure our medical students direct exposure to the vast and exciting research enterprise that is to be found in the basic science departments." This was very much a throwing down of the gauntlet to the new curriculum from the science- and research-oriented side of the faculty.[152]

Unhappiness with PBL from some basic science departments such as pharmacology was massive. External reviewers in 1999 found that that department "seems to have lost out very seriously in the transition to the PBL-based curriculum ... It is apparent to the reviewers that the Department of Pharmacology controls relatively little of its input into the undergraduate medical curriculum." The department did not have the time to impart to the first- and second-year students "the basic concepts of pharmacology." The students had instead a smattering of lectures. Of the fifteen areas of pharmacology that the students identified as important, a survey found that "there were only three areas where

50% or more of the students indicated that they felt that the topic had been covered well during their pre-clerkship experience ... Only 2% of all of the students surveyed felt that the PBL approach would be either their first or second choice for learning pharmacology."[153]

The physiologists felt equally shut out of the tutorials that constituted the core of PBL. They complained to external reviewers in 1999 that the small-group sessions "deter basic scientists from participating because they feel that they lack the clinical knowledge required to provide adequate guidance through the cases ... The fact that clinicians do not feel any similar anxiety about their knowledge of modern basic medical science suggests that the cases themselves may overemphasize clinical skills during the earlier stages of medical education."[154]

A committee reviewing Arnie Aberman's deanship in March 1999 concluded that, amidst the many strengths of Aberman's tenure, the basic science education in the new curriculum was inadequate: "Although the quantity of basic science teaching in the curriculum may be adequate overall, the content and delivery should be re-examined."[155]

The Faculty of Medicine's Academic Plan for 2000–4 demonstrated uneasiness with the large increases in medical school enrolment to produce primary care doctors: "There is growing awareness that the omnibus role of the school in producing an undifferentiated graduate may be increasingly at variance with the research intensitivity of the Faculty ... The incredible and growing richness of the scientific environment in which the medical school is imbedded, the tight linkages with world-class teaching hospitals and their research institutes, and the remarkably diverse urban environment of the Greater Toronto Area, all argue that it is appropriate for Toronto to begin a process of 'differentiation.'"[156]

The new curriculum also found critics in the Department of Surgery, where hands-on training in a master-student relationship harkened back decades. Chair of surgery Richard Reznick was deeply uneasy about the orientation of the new program towards social problems as a basis for training future surgeons. "I think it is weird that we don't have any other models that will compete with problem-based learning," he once said.[157] He argued that the concept of "surgical principles," a unit that he taught, was no substitute for experience and emphasized that surgeons are trained by doing not by watching. They have to "be in the same situation over and over and over again," he said.[158] Francis D. Moore, professor of surgery at Harvard, had once said, "One cannot learn to play the piano by going to concerts."[159] Reznick questioned the new regime's emphasis on educating family doctors. The bottom line for Reznick was this: "Early exposure to junior medical students is critical if we are to continue to attract the best and the brightest to surgery."[160]

The whole story of the new curriculum puts in sharp relief the tension in the faculty between the traditional Toronto ways of doing things, with their emphasis on apprenticeship training and preparation for science, and the more recent emphasis on community involvement and social issues. It is interesting that the

Departments of Medicine and Surgery, long-time fortresses of the research dis-position, were first to bear arms publicly against the new concept.

### The Academies: Final Success

Hand in hand with the story of the new curriculum goes the story of the acad-emies and their final success. The concept of reviving the academies germi-nated as the new curriculum was being discussed,[161] and in April 1991, when the new curriculum was presented to the Committee on Clinical Chairs, a role for the academies was taken for granted. So the idea had clearly been brewing that these decentralized teaching units might cradle the tutorials and seminars of the innovative new program. By December 1992 the Faculty Council had ap-proved the academies as the "home bases" for the pre-clerkship component. "Following the pre-clerkship, students will have an opportunity to select the academy in which they will complete their clerkship."[162]

There were to be four academies, named after giants of the faculty: the Peters Academy at Mount Sinai/Women's College; the Boyd Academy at Sunnybrook/ Hospital for Sick Children; the Wightman Academy at the Toronto Hospital; and the FitzGerald Academy at St Michael's/Wellesley. The names of the direc-tors were announced in April 1994, effective in July.[163] Students would be ran-domly assigned to one academy for their first two (pre-clerkship) years, then be able to choose another for the duration of their last two (clerkship) years. (In 1996 some 44 percent stayed at the same academy.[164]) In July 1998 the Peters Academy at Women's College was deleted as that hospital merged (temporar-ily as it turned out) with Sunnybrook (Mount Sinai joined the Wightman Acad-emy at the Toronto Hospital).[165] And there were naming issues to sort out: the Wightman Academy became the "Wightman–Berris Academy" (Barney Berris having been the distinguished head of medicine at Mount Sinai), and the Boyd Academy at Sunnybrook became the "Peters–Boyd Academy." With the dis-solution of the Wellesley Hospital, the FitzGerald Academy existed solely at St Michael's.[166]

Despite the enthusiasm surrounding their launch, the academies immedi-ately experienced problems in getting members of clinical departments to teach for them. In 2000 Dean David Naylor struck a committee headed by Associate Deans Catharine Whiteside and Murray Urowitz to figure out why this should be difficult. At the same time the Department of Medicine asked St Michael's cardiologist Duncan Stewart to take a look at recruitment issues. The two re-ports converged in part on the classic tension between science-based research and community-based care. Phillipson explained, "In broad terms, several factors appear to contribute to the growing disenchantment of some clinical faculty members for teaching." One was a shift in the teaching format from systems-based to problem-based: "The new format provides fewer opportu-nities for specialists to teach in their field of expertise, requiring instead that they function as 'non-expert' tutors in a broader range of disciplines." Second, the preparation time required to be a tutor was greater than that required for a classroom lecturer (as it does not require, say, a nephrologist hours on end to prepare a lecture on acid-base physiology for first-year medical students). Finally, the PBL "package" demanded "a much more concentrated commitment of time on the part of the teacher than did the previous weekly bedside clinics and seminars." Thus many clinical teachers were concentrating their efforts at the postgraduate level, "where the content is well-aligned with their expertise and the timetable is more accommodating to their busy schedules."[167] The massive pivot from education to research, so evident in many other aspects of the life of the faculty, had been momentarily arrested in undergraduate education.

## The Medical Alumni Association

In a world in which so much is changing so rapidly the need for continuity and for the preservation of traditions is great … The presence of a strong Medical Alumni Association on the campus is one of the safeguards of these traditions.[168]

Dean Fred Lowy, 1983

This chapter cannot be closed without some mention of the history of the Medical Alumni Association (MAA), founded in 1897 with Dean Richard A. Reeve as its first president.[169] As Ruth Kurdyak, its much beloved secretary, later said, "When the Alumni Association was established in the early days of this medical school its mandate was to assist students through bursary and loan programs to attain graduation."[170] In 1947 the MAA was incorporated as a charitable organization,[171] and in the 1947–8 session it seemed to come to life, with bursaries and scholarships; the association also arranged "an annual dinner … on the eve of graduation to the students of the final year. On this occasion the alumni are hosts to the members of the graduating class as well as the graduates of 50 years ago. The 1948 dinner was held in the same week as the meeting of the Canadian Medical Association. There was a very large attendance of members of the alumni from all over Canada."[172] (These alumni dinners turned out to be ample sources for what a sociologist might call the intergenerational transfer of knowledge. Alumnus Eric Grief, class of 9T1 (1991), recalls, "During my convocation week, I attended the Alumni graduation dinner where I met graduates from the class of 4T1. One fellow told me a piece of advice that stuck, 'Take Good Notes!' Boy, was he right."[173]

In the 1953–4 session, the MAA received office space in the Medical Building with their own secretary,[174] an allocation they retained with the move in the late 1960s to the Medical Sciences Building, where, under Kurdyak, the association sought to increase its contacts with undergraduates. In the late 1980s, Jay Raisen, past president of the Medical Society, said, "This school is so large, and one of the problems is that it is very easy to lose yourself in the crowd, either intentionally or unintentionally. The more personal contact there is between students and alumni … the more people start to feel the sense that they are a part of something."[175] This effort to help the undergraduates feel grounded paid off in an increase in membership: in 1990 the MAA had about 9,000 members.[176]

Especially poignant were the fiftieth reunions of medical classes. In June 1984 the class of 3T4 celebrated at the commencement. The first evening the 50 surviving graduates of the original 104 members of the class of 3T4 were feted by the Medical Alumni Association in the Great Hall of Hart House; on the second evening they were toasted by the Toronto mayor, Arthur Eggleton, on the occasion of the bicentennial celebration of the province of Ontario.

On that first evening, Harold Cranfield, a graduate of 3T4, answered the toast: some things had changed. "In our day, we studied TB, Polio, Typhoid, Smallpox and Diphtheria by treating patients with it. 8T4 finds these in books 'as history.' So, count your blessings for now, perforated peptic ulcer, schizophrenia and even pneumonia can be treated because of our generation of doctors." Loved ones sat beamingly at these graduations in 1934 and 1984: "We were students in the Great Depression! Our parents made untold, uncomplaining sacrifice. They spoke of us to others as, 'My son the doctor,' with a ring of pride in their voice."[177]

The parents still speak with pride, but it is, increasingly, of "My daughter the doctor."

We feel that we are trying something unique in Canada.[1]

Louis Siminovitch, 1969

Genetics has changed medical research comparable to the Parisian Clinical School's introduction around 1800 of the anatomical-clinical method, which remained the basic motor of medical progress for the next hundred years. The anatomical-clinical method involved reasoning back and forth from premorbid signs and symptoms to postmortem anatomical findings in order to describe the major diseases. Molecular medicine moves the frame from the autopsy suite to the interior of the cell: What is happening with the DNA in disease? How does communication within the cell take place in illness and in health? The anatomical-clinical method led directly to few cures, just as genetics has yet to guide us to a cornucopia of therapeutic new molecules. Yet these are early days, and when the Department of Molecular and Medical Genetics of the University of Toronto writes, "We are on the threshold of discovering how genes control the development of simple and complex organisms, how genetic alterations lead to cancer," it is not mere hype.[2] Molecular medicine opens the way to the future.

### Genetics in Toronto: Prehistory

Genetic studies in Toronto began in the 1930s, when Norma Ford Walker worked on human genetics in the Department of Zoology.[3] Born Norma Ford in St Thomas, Ontario, in 1893, Walker earned her PhD at the University of Toronto in zoology in 1923; she had an academic career in the Department of Zoology, serving finally as professor of human genetics from 1949 to 1958 (and as acting dean of women at Victoria College, from 1931 to 1934). This was said to be the first genetics professorship in any Canadian university. She is remembered for her anthropological investigations of the Dionne quintuplets, who were born in a northern Ontario farmhouse in 1934. (Walker noted that "they shared such rare characteristics as an incomplete separation of the second and third toes and they all had the same blood type," and the same palm patterns, "revealing further evidence that they were a monozygotic set."[4])

Encouraged by Alan Brown, Walker began consulting in 1940 at the children's hospital on human genetics. In 1951 she founded the Department of Genetics in the newly built hospital, said to be "the first hospital in the world to include a department of genetics in its building plans."[5] In several publications in the mid-1950s with Nobelist Oliver Smithies, who was then at the Connaught Labs, she showed that some previously unknown differences in normal plasma proteins were inherited.[6] Around 1960 the HSC Department of Pathology began a chromosome laboratory under Patrick Conen. Walker's biographer Fiona Miller says that through the HSC association, "Ford Walker gained access to extraordinary cases of disease and disability, notably monozygotic twins with discordant anomalies and rare childhood diseases." She attributes to Walker a special Toronto school of "dermatoglyphics," the study of genetically influenced dermal patterns.[7] What survived, however, from the Walker era was not so much dermatoglyphics but the use of quantitative measurements as a diagnostic tool that she and her student Margaret Thompson pioneered (e.g., the Walker index for Down syndrome).

Genetic studies continued at HSC under Thompson, who by the 1966–7 session was chief of the hospital's Division of Genetics.[8] These two female scholars thus established the initial beachhead of genetics in Toronto. It has not been lost on other observers that the early geneticists in Toronto tended to be women, and Alice Miller, the foremost student of the early history of genetics in Toronto and in Canada generally, writes, "Women dominated this field in Toronto because it was available for their exploitation, and because they were prepared – precisely because they could not anticipate great scientific careers – to embark on work that was of dubious merit."[9] The rule of women would, however, shortly falter under the rod of a large, fierce man.

### Siminovitch

The story of Toronto research is the story of Lou. It really is. If he hadn't been there, it wouldn't have happened. Or something else would have happened, but it wouldn't have had that shine to it.[10]

Jim Friesen, 2009

Louis Siminovitch established the study of molecular biology – the molecular structures, including genes, that underlie biological processes – at the University of Toronto and in much of Canada. So the story begins with him.

Siminovitch was born in Montreal in 1920 of a poor family of Jewish immigrants from Bessarabia, on the border between Romania and Russia. "My parents were extremely family-directed," he later said, and under their encouragement he taught himself mathematics. He did very well on the general entrance exam for McGill, "allowing [him] to meet the unofficial relatively stiff entrance standards for Jewish students to McGill University."[11] Helped by numerous bursaries and awards, he earned a bachelor's degree in science from McGill University in 1941 and a PhD in physical chemistry in 1944. Siminovitch learned three things, he said, as a graduate student. One, "I learnt to do research." His supervisor was busy with his own laboratory, "and so I learnt to be independent." Second, "I learnt the importance of collegiality" in dealing with his collaborators and other graduates students in the same lab. Finally, "I experienced for the first time the joys, excitement, and self-fulfillment of discovery." It was that excitement that Siminovitch succeeded in communicating to subsequent generations of Canadian scientists. As James Till said of him later, "His predominant trait as a scientist is his power as a catalyst. Because of his enthusiasm, foresight, wisdom and sound judgement, new investigators are inspired to tackle problems of central importance, and established investigators are encouraged to look critically at the excellence and originality of their work."[12]

While a graduate student in Montreal during the war, Siminovitch got to know Louis Rapkine, a French biochemist then scientific head of the Free French Forces. Rapkine invited Siminovitch to join his lab at the Institut Pasteur after the war. In 1947, on a Royal Society fellowship, Siminovitch and his new bride Elinore travelled to Paris, to Rapkine's lab just equipped by the Rockefeller Foundation. At the Pasteur Institute, Siminovitch quickly found his way to the labs of future Nobelists Jacques Monod and André Lwoff. Until this point, Siminovitch knew nothing about genetics, bacteria, or viruses. But he had landed well: "The Lwoff-Monod laboratory happened to be one of two outstanding world centers for this kind of work." The California Institute of Technology ("CalTech")in Pasadena under Max Delbrück was the other.

Working with Lwoff from 1949 until his return to Canada in 1953, Siminovitch became involved in the research for which Lwoff later won a Nobel Prize. Lwoff had set out to show why, in some cases, viruses that replicated in bacterial cells were able to coexist with the bacteria rather than killing them. Lwoff intensified the study of such bacterial viruses, especially the lysogenic variety (viral DNA is integrated in the chromosome of the bacterium). This research, Siminovitch said, "provided some of the framework for the eventual development of understanding of regulation in bacteria and viruses and for the later spectacular successes in molecular biology."[13] In 1950 Lwoff, Siminovitch, and another collaborator found out how to increase the frequency with which the bacterium B megatherium made virus. They exposed the bacteria to ultraviolet radiation in order to induce the production of viruses and found that this worked in many bacteria. Moreover, this capacity to produce virus was heritable, determined by a bacterial gene.[14] (Their work showed that the virus inserts its DNA into that of the host bacterium, and when the host replicates, the DNA of the virus is included.) This research led directly, as Till later pointed out, "to our current understanding of the molecular mechanisms regulating gene expression in microorganisms." Moreover, the study of such lysogenic bacteria "has formed the intellectual framework for much of the work relating animal viruses to human cancer."[15]

During Siminovitch's six years in Paris, he learned a lot about how scientific discovery works. "The Pasteur laboratory of the fifties," he later wrote, "represents an extraordinary entity which will never be repeated. It was small but not too small; of course, it included a group of first-rate scientists of various backgrounds; almost everyone in it was engaged in full-time scientific activity; there was a frequent infusion and turnover of excellent scientists from abroad; there was a warm feeling of comradeship and thus a free exchange of ideas and information ... Even the lunch tables were centres of animated discussion and excitement, the discussion ranging through politics through theatre, geography and literature."[16] Most of all, said Siminovitch, "I learnt about the power of genetics as a discipline."[17] Much of Siminovitch's subsequent activity in Toronto may be understood as an effort to recreate in some way this idyll.

After these years of spectacular excitement in Paris, the return to Toronto in 1953 marked the beginning of his scientific independence. Why Toronto rather than the scientifically more luminous Montreal? Siminovitch found in Toronto a post in the lab of Angus Graham, a Scottish microbiologist who had come to Connaught in 1947 and was virtually the only scientist in Canada then working with bacterial viruses. It was Graham who arranged for Siminovitch a fellowship from the National Cancer Institute of Canada. Graham introduced Siminovitch to Hal Warwick, then head of the NCIC, and even though Siminovitch was not doing cancer research he was sufficiently impressive that Warwick said, "Yes, we'll bet on this man." Back on the Connaught "Farm," Graham told Siminovitch, "Do what you want."[18] Out of this collaboration came the introduction to Canada of work on "somatic cells" in culture, which means studying cells such as those in humans.[19]

A parenthesis on why somatic cell research was then considered important: Allan Okey, chair of pharmacology, said of Siminovitch's somatic cell work, "Lou was one of the people to see that somatic cells in culture could be extraordinarily powerful tools for asking all kinds of questions." Okey mused, "The people who are gene-jockeying [today] probably can answer a lot of the questions much more efficiently and rapidly than using the classic kinds of somatic cell genetics."[20]

Siminovitch decided that he didn't want to continue in Toronto the Paris work with bacteria but instead shifted over to somatic cells, and there was only one lab in Toronto growing animal cells, Ray Parker's. (Raymond C. Parker was a Nova Scotian cancer scientist trained at Yale and the Rockefeller Institute who returned to Canada, to Connaught, in 1941.) Siminovitch went to Parker and said, "Will you show me how to grow cells?" Siminovitch made a scientific breakthrough in 1955. Parker and everybody else were growing cells on a solid substrate, which made taking a sample difficult. Siminovitch figured out the technique of growing cells in suspension.[21] (The scientific interest in Toronto in this discovery, he said, was "zero.") As well, Siminovitch started collaborating with Klaus Rothfels, a cytogeneticist at U of T, and discovered a new method for analysing the chromosome composition (karyotyping) of mammalian cells.[22]

In 1956 Ham asked Siminovitch, whom he knew from Siminovitch's cancer fellowship, to join him in the Division of Biological Research at the just founded Ontario Cancer Institute, even though Siminovitch's research was completely unrelated to cancer. "Using our methods," said Siminovitch, "we were able for the first time to show that animal [cell] cultures could become contaminated in the laboratory by cells from other cultures," a finding of some importance in laboratory practice.

It was at the Ontario Cancer Institute that Siminovitch began his contributions to molecular biology, in the perfervid atmosphere of the Sherbourne Street building that recalled the Lwoff lab in Paris. Siminovitch's seminal paper in these years appeared in 1970. He and collaborators succeeded in isolating temperature-sensitive mutants of cultured mouse and hamster cells. This is important because it showed the possibility of isolating diploid cell mutants, laying the foundation of the field of somatic cell genetics.[23] Siminovitch thus played a major role in the development of molecular medicine in Toronto. Jim Friesen later said, in an interview, "Lou's real forte was an eminence grise behind biomedical research in Canada for half a century – pushing it, massaging it, recommending that this should happen, trying to make sure that that happened, getting the right people, pushing the right people in the right path."[24] This is not generally known.

## Department of Medical Cell Biology

Genetics has now reached maturity as a science and it forms an important foundation stone in medical education, research, and treatment. Human genetics in particular has a special relationship to medicine which is analogous to the relationship of human anatomy.[25]

Lou Siminovitch, 1965

In October 1966 Siminovitch was appointed chair of the Cell Biology Group, the forerunner of the coming department.[26] This was a big new initiative. In 1967 Chute said, "The Faculty has taken note of the major advances in the field of molecular biology, and has recommended the formation of a division of cell biology in Medicine to ensure an adequate presentation of this subject to the student."[27] At the time of its founding, the department had a mandate to offer an "umbrella" for genetics, immunology, and microbiology. The responsibility for the latter was given up quickly to the Department of Medical Microbiology.

In 1969 the new department was founded as the Department of Medical Cell Biology, an undergraduate teaching unit of the Department of Medical Biophysics and a research unit under the direction of Siminovitch, with genetics and immunology the principal components. Siminovitch took with him to the Medical Sciences Building the group of researchers at OCI who had been working on bacterial genetics. Yet the scientists in the Department of Medical Cell Biology remained part of the graduate teaching program of the Department of Medical Biophysics. The new department, shorn of budget and appointment authority, moved into the Medical Sciences Building in the fall of 1969.

Siminovitch said that the other basic science departments were not exactly delirious with joy at the foundation of this upstart, possibly because they felt Siminovitch's contempt for some of the leadership, which was palpable. Siminovitch later said in an interview, "They all felt, 'Why do we need genetics and immunology?' They didn't even know what the words meant. And we were taking space away. They were not doing any of this modern stuff, none of them. They didn't know what the word modern molecular biology was. I'm not sure they knew what the word genetics meant. Some of them said, 'Genetics is not going to cure any disease.'"[28] (But there was a national group called the "Young Turks," including John Evans, Fraser Mustard, and Jack Laidlaw at Toronto and Charlie Hollenberg at McGill, who were very interested indeed. They wanted to get Francis Crick to come out to Banff and talk to them but Crick couldn't come so they asked Siminovitch, who gave the talk, "and Farquharson sat beside me, and he was just glowing," said Siminovitch.[29])

In the new department there were two immunologists, the Viennese émigré Bernhard ("Hardi") Cinader and McGill graduate Brian J. Underdown; there were two "cell biologists," Siminovitch and Bishnu Dat Sanwal (a graduate of the Federal Institute of Technology in Zurich, who then left for the University of Western Ontario, returning in 1978 to write a report on his former department), and several geneticists whose major interest was bacterial phage genetics. Technically, Siminovitch was a "cell biologist," for his interest was not in human genetics but somatic cell genetics (as opposed to molecular genetics, a distinction that today is meaningless but then involved lower forms of life). Thus, at the beginning the department was divided between immunology and genetics, and each group had to instruct the medical students in its lore.

It was a hodgepodge of a department. After an evaluation in 1972 by Charles Scriver of McGill and the Montreal Children's Hospital, it was named the Department of Medical Genetics, to include clinical genetics, population genetics, and developmental biology. (Scriver, striving to be diplomatic, found "somatic cell genetics" somewhat overrepresented.[30]) Said a 1978 assessment, "The department developed two thrusts: in molecular genetics at the Medical Sciences Building and in applied genetics at the Research Institute of the Hospital for

Sick Children." The department had nine full-time posts for genetics and two and a half for immunology; Cinader guided the immunology group. The genetics and immunology groups, said the review, had little in common. "There is a significant dependence by the genetics groups upon the leadership of Dr Siminovitch. The members of the faculty look to him as a father-figure and consider themselves part of his 'family.' The immunology group functions essentially as an independent entity."[31]

On the occasion of the site visit in 1978, Sanwal, one of the reviewers, asked, "How could such discordant subgroups with differing academic loyalties be held together under one Department?" He had the impression that the HSC nucleus cared little for its association with the campus department, and the immunologists cared little for either. "It was very clear to me that the whole Medical Genetics Department was held in one piece because of the authority, presence and prestige of only one person, namely, the chairman of the Department, Dr. Siminovitch."[32]

One 1978 reviewer, Samuel Freedman, a McGill internist, was even more scathing about the lack of intellectual fraternity between the geneticists and the immunologists: "There is no apparent relationship at any level between the immunology group and the medical genetics group ... except that they are housed in the same geographic area."[33]

The major part of the PhD program was, as Siminovitch said, "conducted under the aegis of the Department of Medical Biophysics. Because of the excellent collaboration between these two departments, this program has worked very well." Yet medical genetics would be wanting its own graduate program.[34] Margaret Thompson was apparently unhappy that so little basic human genetics was taught to the medical undergraduates. Siminovitch shrugged and said they were building to strength. "One cannot expect to cover all the areas." How about the relationship between medical genetics and immunology? Siminovitch said "the relationship is one of a common budget only, otherwise they function as two separate entities."[35] The long-range planners recommended the creation of a separate Department of Immunology (see chapter 17).[36]

When Siminovitch stepped down in 1979 he left as one legacy the "Phage Morphogenesis Group," including Helios Murialdo, Marv Gold, and Andy Becker. (A bacteriophage is a virus that lyses bacteria. This research was important partly because it foreshadowed recombinant DNA work.) They were among the earliest systems biologists, trying to figure out, as Friesen put it, "what are the pieces and how do they come together and what are the pathways of the assembly. I think they were very successful. They were very smart guys."[37]

Friesen took over the chair in 1981, and in 1986 the Department of Medical Genetics became a formal division through cross-appointed faculty members within the Department of Medical Biophysics, representing the research interests of the faculty as separate from the OCI headquarters of medical biophysics.

This was a small department with high morale and huge research funding. They considered themselves among the elite scientists of the faculty and at one point rejected a merger with biochemistry on the grounds that the biochemists were not quite up to snuff. The title of the department itself, however, was a handicap, suggesting that their main brief was somehow traditional genetics, while their chief interest by the 1980s had become such issues in molecular medicine as protein folding and "complex genome structure and function."[38]

The centre of gravity of the department began to shift away from OCI towards the Medical Sciences Building, the Hospital for Sick Children, and the Mount Sinai Research Institute. The department increased greatly in size, to become the "dominant graduate program in Medical Biophysics," as Robert A. Phillips, chair of medical biophysics and a somatic cell researcher at the HSC institute, put it in 1986.

James Donald Friesen, one of the dons of molecular biology, was born in Rosthern, Saskatchewan, in 1935. After a BA and MA in physics at the University of Saskatchewan, he followed a kind of "pipeline" that Harold Johns had established from the West to Toronto, to take a PhD in the Department of Medical Biophysics. He was Lou Siminovitch's first student, finishing in 1962.

"When I arrived," Friesen said in an interview, "there were actually a whole bunch of us, who had undergraduate or in some cases graduate degrees in physics, and we knew nothing about biology – not one thing. So they gave us a list of about five courses and said, 'If you take these courses and do all right in them, we'll take that as sort of a qualification, and then you're in. One of them was Arthur Ham's Histology course, and I learned more biology faster from that book [his histology textbook] than any other place." Friesen thus became "biologized," he said.

Friesen spent the next two years as a postdoctoral fellow at the Institute of Microbiology of the University of Copenhagen. Out of this Danish collaboration, Friesen became in 1976 the first scientist in Canada to clone a gene, using Lambda phage on E. coli.[39] After stints at Kansas State University (in physics) and York University in Toronto (in biology), in 1981 Friesen accepted the chair in medical genetics at Toronto, where he would stay for six years before becoming director of the Research Institute of the children's hospital in 1987. Siminovitch characterized Jim Friesen and Cecil Yip at Banting and Best as scientists who are "givers," which, said Siminovitch, "is certainly not the typical attitude in Europe … Their objectives have always been clear: striving for the best in every context in which they have been involved, nearly always for the benefit of others rather than themselves. They have kept their focus on quality and integrity." Siminovitch mentioned Friesen's role in advancing genomics in Ontario, first in a provincial Challenge Fund, then in Genome Ontario and Genome Canada. "From this he personally profits little, if at all. These activities are all unheralded and perhaps even unappreciated by some. But both men are wonderful examples of leaders who are givers."[40]

In 1987 Paul Sadowski, a 1963 medical graduate of U of T with a doctoral degree in pathology as well, succeeded Friesen as chair of the Department of Medical Genetics. Under Sadowski (who was provisionally chair of both departments), in 1996 the Department of Microbiology and the graduate portion of the Department of Medical Genetics were amalgamated into the new Department of Medical Genetics and Microbiology.[41] In 1999 Brenda Andrews succeeded Sadowski as chair of the new department.

Some name changing went on. In 1990 the School of Graduate Studies gave the Department of Medical Genetics their own graduate program – separate from medical biophysics – under the name of the Department of Molecular and Medical Genetics. Thus at the beginning of the 1990s there were two departments of medical genetics: the graduate department was called Molecular and Medical Genetics. The undergraduate department was called Medical Genetics.

All these moving parts are characteristic of a young science trying to crystallize its identity. In 1996 the Department of Medical Genetics acquired a small number of campus-based microbiologists. (The other microbiologists joined the Department of Laboratory Medicine and Pathobiology.) The undergraduate Department of Medical Genetics was therefore renamed the Department of Medical Genetics and Microbiology, while the name of the graduate department remained unchanged as Molecular and Medical Genetics. This confusing terminology drove everyone crazy. "A single name for the Department would avoid much of this confusion," said a faculty report. In 2006 therefore, department chair Howard Lipshitz (chair of both the undergraduate and the graduate departments) polled the members about what name they would like. The most popular choice was "Molecular Genetics," endorsed by 35 percent of those who voted. More voting. Molecular Genetics was still on top. Lipshitz said, "This vote indicates that the faculty members in our Department recognize that the one thing that unites them is the fact that essentially all of them use molecular genetic approaches." Lipshitz therefore recommended in March 2007 "that our name be changed to 'Department of Molecular Genetics' and that this be both our undergraduate and graduate name."[42] The recommendation was accepted.

External reviewers in 1998 said of molecular and medical genetics, "The Department sees the training of graduate students as one of their most important missions, and the establishment of an independent graduate program in 1990 has been a great success." Paul Sadowski, the chair, added, "Having a broad-based department with strengths in so many different areas (protein structure to human genetics) makes us virtually unique among North American genetics departments. A strong campus-based focus [in the Medical Sciences Building] coupled with unique strengths in two Hospital Institutes [HSC and Mount Sinai] provides us with a competitive advantage as we approach the post-genome era."[43]

An external review in 2003 of the Department of Medical Genetics and Microbiology found that of the seventy-five faculty, a third were housed at the

Medical Sciences Building, others at the Samuel Lunenfeld Research Institute, the Hospital for Sick Children Research Institute, or the Banting and Best Department of Medical Research. Some were full-time, some were status-only. "Grant capture" had doubled to $44 million per year. "The Department is arguably the best biomedical research department in the country and … is poised to be one of the best in the world."

This snapshot of "MGM" in 2003 found a tilting of the scientific centre of gravity away from the campus basic science departments and towards the hospitals and their big Research Institutes. To be sure, the individual scholars were excellent, "some of the very best in Canada and many are international stars." Yet, "[w]ith the development of research training programs [at the hospitals and the Centre for Cellular and Biomolecular Research, CCBR, also called the Donnelly Centre after a donor], there is a danger that departmental loyalties will be diminished. This potential division of loyalties is even more acute in situations where members are hospital based."[44]

### Department of Molecular Genetics at the Children's Hospital

A very important fraction of the admissions to the Hospital for Sick Children (around 30%) bear lesions attributable to genetic causes.[45]

Department of Medical Genetics, 1974

Sometime in the late 1960s Siminovitch got a phone call from Harry Bain, head of pediatrics at HSC, who said "I want you to come over here and start genetics at Sick Kids." Since the retirement of Ford Walker in 1962, the division had rather drifted.[46] In 1970 Siminovitch became geneticist-in-chief, turning the division into the Department of Medical Genetics and greatly expanding the service and the research. He tapped Manuel Buchwald as point person in the lab and Ron Worton for cytogenetics, at the time conducted in the Department of Pathology (Worton, then at Yale, wanted to return to Toronto and knew little about cytogenetics, Siminovitch said, but worked it up); Linda Stevens was also recruited for cytogenetics lab.[47] Peggy Thompson remained as the PhD geneticist, her primary appointment in zoology.

What was the rationale for such a department? Siminovitch said in 1974, "In biological science, genetics serves as a ground base discipline, much in the same way that mathematics is basic to physics and chemistry." But this also has clinical importance, "a recognition that an increasing proportion of diseases have a genetic etiology." Thirty percent of the admissions to HSC "bear lesions attributable to genetic causes." Yet genetics also played a role in several disorders that usually do not become apparent until adult life, such as diabetes and cardiovascular conditions. This then was the difference between genetics in clinical medicine and classic one-gene-one-disease genetics. Siminovitch said, "It is important to emphasize that the role of genetics in clinical medicine differs …

from that of other clinical departments, in that its major impact is in prevention of disease."[48]

Accordingly, the new campus Department of Medical Genetics that Siminovitch was founding – at the same time as the hospital department at HSC – had two thrusts: (1) "to fill a recognized gap in one important area of biology – molecular genetics" (this would all be centred in the Medical Sciences Building); and (2) human genetics, where they were very involved with the genetics of cystic fibrosis and metabolic disease, under Andrew Sass-Kortsak. This would all be at HSC.[49] The people that Siminovitch recruited for this department would constitute the second generation of molecular biologists in Canada: Ron Worton, Roy Gravel, Manuel Buchwald, and Rod McInnes.

Thus Siminovitch set to work. At the cytogenetics lab, he envisaged initiating an amniocentesis program with cell-culture techniques, making possible cytogenetic diagnosis for a host of genetic diseases.[50] In 1970 the Prenatal Diagnosis Program was founded. In 1975 Noreen Rudd, a pediatrician-geneticist, became head of the Genetics Clinic, or "the syndrome fiefdom," as Siminovitch referred to it. She was joined later by fellow pediatricians Helen Hughes and Rosanna Weksberg. "As a result of these developments, genetic counseling at the HSC improved by leaps and bounds," he said.[51]

Genetic services multiplied at the University Avenue hospitals. In 1971 a group led by obstetrician Terence A. Doran at the General initiated an amniocentesis service. Andrew Sass-Kortsak had established in 1974 a Metabolic Genetics Unit in the Department of Paediatrics, and this group too was merged with the Department of Medical Genetics. Ditto for a carrier detection program for Tay-Sachs disease initiated by J. Alexander Lowden.[52] Just two blocks away from the Hospital for Sick Children was Surrey Place Centre, a multidisciplinary facility for children with intellectual disabilities, established in 1966. From the outset it incorporated genetic services, including a cytogenetics laboratory. In 1970 Joseph Berg was appointed director of genetic services and research, and in 1975 the centre joined the Toronto Prenatal Genetic Diagnosis Program.[53]

Under Siminovitch the focus of the hospital medical genetics department was somatic cell genetics, which had been his life's work. The arrival of Roy Gravel in the early 1980s changed this, as his group cloned six different genes responsible for metabolic diseases. Gravel was one of the rising stars in the department and at the HSC Research Institute.[54] He earned his BA and master's at McGill and a PhD at Yale University on metabolism in fungi. While at Yale, he received an MRC (Medical Research Council of Canada) Fellowship to study human genetics, then came to Toronto in 1974 as an assistant professor with a lab at the children's hospital. In 1986 Gravel and lab colleagues isolated the cDNA clones that coded for one of the subunits of a mutant enzyme (hexosaminidase B) involved in Tay-Sachs disease, an often fatal metabolic disorder in children.[55] Two years later, in 1988, they identified "a single-base mutation in a cloned fragment of the HEXA gene from an Ashkenazi Jewish patient."[56] (Jews of East European origin are especially liable to Tay-Sachs disease.) From Toronto, Gravel moved first to the Research Institute of the Children's Hospital in Montreal and McGill University, then to the University of Calgary.

In 1985 Ron Worton succeeded Siminovitch as geneticist-in-chief at HSC. Worton had earned his bachelor's and master's degrees at the University of Manitoba, then received a PhD in medical biophysics from the U of T in 1969. As a student of Till's, Worton made in 1969 the first effort to fractionate the stem cells that Till and McCulloch had discovered to see if individual precursors of the stem cells might be identified.[57] (They couldn't be.) Worton joined the Research Institute of HSC as a research scientist in 1971 and remained there until replacing Siminovitch as head of the hospital genetics department. Worton phased out the somatic cell work of the department to concentrate on cloning the gene responsible for Duchenne muscular dystrophy; the discovery of the gene that coded for dystrophin was achieved in 1986.[58] (In 1988 Worton co-founded the Canadian Genetic Diseases Network with Charles Scriver, Michael Hayden, and Lap-Chee Tsui, the beginning of Canada's national efforts in genome research.[59] In 1992 he headed the Canadian Genome Project and in 1996 left U of T for a post as director of research at the Ottawa General Hospital.) Friesen called this research "a brilliant example of positional cloning. Using genetics, you figure out the closest way you can to where that gene probably is, and then you just use various molecular techniques to jump and hop and walk along the chromosome until you find it. And Ron Worton had a brilliant idea [see later] to get the Duchenne muscular dystrophy gene."[60]

In the meantime, the field of genetics became dramatically transformed in the 1980s by the advent of recombinant DNA technology (gene splicing) to isolate and examine the portions of DNA that caused genetic disease. "The entire professional staff in research," said Worton, "undertook to retrain in molecular technology, and began to develop the approaches to genetic disease that brought highly visible successes," such as the cloning of the various genes mentioned farther on.[61] In 1982 Worton himself took the Cold Spring Harbor cloning course and in 1984 he and co-workers identified the genetic abnormality in Duchenne muscular dystrophy: a genetic translocation splitting the block of genes encoding ribosomal RNA on the short arm of chromosome 21. It became possible to produce ribosomal RNA gene probes to identify patients with this abnormality at the translocation site.[62]

In 1986 Worton created a Division of Clinical Genetics under Joe Clarke, shared by the Departments of Genetics and Paediatrics, to manage patient care. One responsibility of the division was the prenatal diagnosis program, along with a genetic metabolic diseases program; its Lysosomal Disease Laboratory conducted carrier screening in the Jewish community for Tay-Sachs disease. The division's Intermediate Metabolism Laboratory, Worton said, "is essentially unique in the world, receiving blood and skin samples from around the world for diagnosis of such conditions as lactic academia." A Cytogenetics Laboratory of the division, founded in 1970 with the opening of the Elm Street Wing, examined chromosome breaks in such illnesses as fragile-X syndrome, a common cause of mental disability, and undertook chromosomal analysis (karyotyping) on samples of amniotic fluid or postnatal blood.

In 1985 research programs began examining the DNA of individual patients for defective genes, and in 1988 a DNA Diagnostic Laboratory was established in the division for gene analysis at the DNA level. For such diseases as Duchenne muscular dystrophy and cystic fibrosis (that hospital staff had cloned), it permitted the defective gene to be located directly. "With direct gene analysis," said Worton, "most carriers can now be accurately identified in families with a previously affected child, and an 8–10 week male fetus with the defective gene can be easily distinguished from one whose gene is normal." This ability, of course, spared the family agonizing uncertainty. Peter Ray was the founding director.[63]

### It Was a Big Deal

By 1990 the Department of Genetics at HSC had a full-time medical and scientific staff of eighteen, all members of various university departments. They were in the first line science-driven, not task-oriented. "Traditionally, the major strength of the Department has been its research programs," said Worton. "The philosophy of the Department has been to hire researchers whose primary credential is excellence in research, without insisting on any particular research emphasis. Research is technology-driven and it is assumed that the best researchers will have at their disposal the most up-to-date technology and that in the environment of the Hospital for Sick Children they will apply that technology to the most pressing problems in paediatric genetics." Worton observed that this philosophy had paid off, given that the Department of Genetics had been rated "as one of the two leading centers for genetic disease research in the world."[64]

What had the pay-off been? By 1990 Worton and Peter Ray had, as mentioned, cloned the gene responsible for Duchenne muscular dystrophy; Roy Gravel and Donald Mahuran had cloned the gene for Tay-Sachs disease; Lap-Chee Tsui and Manuel Buchwald had cloned the gene for cystic fibrosis. John Dick had elaborated mouse models that would eventuate in the discovery of cancer stem cells for leukemia; and Maria Musarella, cross-appointed to the Department of Ophthalmology, had mapped several eye disease genes. Worton stated modestly, "Several of these research accomplishments have brought international recognition to the Department and to the individual scientists involved in the research."[65] To this list might be added Diane Wilson Cox's adumbration in 1993 of the gene for Wilson's disease,[66] or Jeffrey Wrana's discovery in 1996, together with his wife Liliana Attisano in the Department of Anatomy and Cell Biology, of the gene MADR2 implicated in colon cancer.[67] (Attisano herself, earlier in anatomy, later in biochemistry, discovered in 2004 a possible signalling pathway in the genesis of cancer.[68]) Friesen said, exaggerating only slightly, "Something like 90 percent of all the human diseases that were cloned in the world were cloned at Sick Kids."[69]

When in 1989 Lap-Chee Tsui found the cystic fibrosis gene, it was really a big deal. Copies of the journal *Science* announcing the finding arrived at HSC. Okey recalled, "There were three big articles in there and a cover story and all, and I just happened to be walking down the hall having got my mail. Lap-Chee was coming through the same hall and I asked for his autograph. That seems like a strange thing, to ask a colleague to autograph the magazine, but we took a lot of pride in that, I think, across all of Canada."[70]

In November 1990, when Tsui appeared on the podium to address the American Society of Human Genetics, according to the reporter, "the 3,000 participants gave him a standing ovation that went on and on and on. They finally stopped when Dr. Tsui leaned into the microphone and asked with his quiet modesty, 'Do you want to hear this talk or not?'" The discovery has been called "one of the most significant events in the history of human genetics."[71]

Tsui began his research at HSC in 1981, then in 1985, together with Manuel Buchwald – and with the help of scientists from Collaborative Research Incorporated in Boston – established that the cystic fibrosis gene was located on chromosome 7. In 1987 Tsui's lab had further localized the gene to a location on chromosome 7. Tsui was now working in close collaboration with Jack Riordan, director of HSC's cystic fibrosis program, and Francis Collins of the Howard Hughes Medical Institute at the University of Michigan. Tsui's lab "began 'walking' along the chromosome to find the gene. To walk they would use the end of one piece of the chromosome to identify the adjacent piece. They repeated this procedure over and over until they reached the region close to the CF gene." Collins's lab at Michigan accelerated this procure by "jumping" along the chromosome, and Riordan's lab compared cells from non-affected and affected individuals. By March 1989 the investigators had a "candidate" gene that in fact turned out to be the real CF gene, a mere difference of a three base pair deletion in the DNA. Said Johanna Rommens in the CF program, "It was a big worry for many weeks that such a subtle difference could cause the disease."[72]

After the discovery leaked to the press there was a media storm. Rommens said, "People kept calling to confirm the findings. But it was a nice feeling. Everyone from the different labs on this floor dropped by to congratulate us or to ask if they could do anything to help. Dr. Worton answered our phones all day." Mila Mulroney, wife of Canadian prime minister Brian Mulroney, held a thousand-dollar-a-plate dinner for them in Ottawa for 500 guests. "I think it's appropriate that the discovery happened here [at HSC]," said Riordan."[73]

The hospital had a big footprint. By 1990 veterans of the cytogenetics laboratory were heading cancer cytogenetics programs, and their technologists were "populating laboratories, throughout Ontario and in the US." Likewise with the diagnostic laboratory. The research training program had produced thirty-eight

PhD scientists. "These individuals are now in academic positions or further training positions all over the world."[74]

When the Royal College of Physicians and Surgeons of Canada adopted medical genetics as a free-standing specialty in 1989, it put great new pressure on Toronto – and on HSC – to serve as a training centre. Teresa Costa became the first director of the training program. When Worton was asked at a five-year review in December 1990 how he maintained a "cohesive group" under the conditions of extreme overcrowding that then prevailed at the hospital, he replied, in the summary of the secretary of a meeting, "Crowded conditions may stimulate interaction. As well, he encourages research which he feels is worthwhile even if it might be seen as risky or demanding."[75] (It is interesting that Tsui later told Dean John Dirks, "I almost decided to take an offer from a US biotechnology company." But he decided to stay because he liked the academic environment and felt comfortable in Toronto.[76])

### Research Institute of HSC

Many of HSC's scientific accomplishments came from investigators in the hospital's Research Institute, which under Manuel Buchwald in the 1990s became an enormous operation, dwarfing the faculty's basic science departments. Buchwald was born in Lima, Peru, in 1940. He graduated with a bachelor's degree from Dartmouth College in 1962 and received a PhD in biochemistry from Brandeis University in 1967. He came to Toronto as a postdoctoral fellow in the Department of Medical Cell Biology and in 1970 was appointed staff geneticist at the Research Institute of HSC, where he served as assistant director in 1982, then in 1986–7 succeeded Aser Rothstein as acting director. In 1995 Buchwald again became acting director, then director in 1996. He was a member of the research team under Tsui that identified the cystic fibrosis gene in 1989; in 1992 his lab discovered that there were at least four Fanconi anemia genes on chromosome 9.[77]

In 1996 Buchwald established a Research Training Centre at the institute, and it is a measure of the international visibility of the institute that half of the trainees would come from outside of Canada.[78] This was the first of the hospital research training centres, of which a number more followed elsewhere.[79]

In the new century the Research Institute developed strength in a number of areas. One example among many: Stephen Scherer was a member of the Program in Genetics and Genomic Biology of the institute. Born in Windsor in 1964, Scherer earned a bachelor's degree in biology at the University of Waterloo in 1987 and a PhD in medical biophysics at the University of Toronto in 1995. He then enjoyed several prestigious research grants. In 2001 he became a senior scientist in the Department of Genetics at HSC and associate director of the Research Institute the following year. In 2002 as well he became director of the Centre for Applied Genomics. In 1998 Scherer and neurologist Berge Minassian discovered a gene called EPM2A for Lafora disease, a severe form of adolescent-onset epilepsy.[80] (In 2003 Minassian and Scherer discovered a second gene associated with the disease, NHLRC1.[81]) A team led by Scherer isolated in 1996 the genomic segments on chromosome 7 (which was becoming known as the "Canadian chromosome" because of the number of genes that Canadian investigators were finding on it) of a terrible cause of a childhood disfigurement called holoprosencephaly. The gene in question was called "sonic hedgehog" (SHH), an almost whimsical term to give to a strip of DNA that could produce such unhappy results in children.[82]

Thus, Toronto became a world centre for molecular medicine in the 1990s because of the presence of the Research Institute at the children's hospital; the faculty's basic science departments, contrary to their fears, were greatly strengthened by the cross-appointment of most of these scientists to the university.

### Samuel Lunenfeld Research Institute

In 1975 Mount Sinai Hospital founded a research institute of its own.[83] In the 1979–80 session the hospital created an Office of Research Administration and a Scientific Advisory Committee. The project sprang from Mount Sinai's underlying commitment to world-class research, sustained by donations from the community. In 1985 Lou Siminovitch was appointed scientific director.

Siminovitch was key in recruiting good people. He courted Arthur Slutsky, a McMaster medical graduate who had just finished a fellowship in pulmonary critical care at the Peter Bent Brigham Hospital in Boston. Slutsky said of his first meeting with Siminovitch, "I liked what I saw. He was a very straightforward guy, good sense of humour, clearly had a vision of where he wanted to go. He said, 'This is going to be a great place!'"[84]

Siminovitch steered the institute in the direction of molecular medicine. "They had a major budget from their Foundation," Siminovitch said, "and I decided that they were spreading it around among people doing what I would call half-assed research. So when I had my meeting with the Select Committee, I said, 'I'm taking that away after one year.' It was a million dollars' worth of support."[85]

Very early, the hospital administrators asked Siminovitch, "What it would take to make the research institute here world famous?"

Siminovitch answered, "Fifty thousand square feet of space, and two million dollars."

Irving Gerstein said, "OK, we'll get it."[86] The estate of Samuel Lunenfeld, after whom the Research Institute was named, became a major contributor.[87]

Siminovitch recruited five key people to run the institute's various divisions: Alan Bernstein for developmental biology, Robert Kerbel for cancer biology, John Roder for the immunology division, and Janet Rossant and Tony Pawson to complete the leadership in molecular biology. Slutsky said of these five,

"They were spectacular. And they were young at the time, right?" Siminovitch had a real eye for talent.[88]

Thus Alan Bernstein, a student of Till and McCulloch from the Ontario Cancer Institute, was Siminovitch's first recruit. Born in Toronto in 1947, Bernstein earned a bachelor's degree from the U of T in 1968 and a PhD in medical biophysics in 1972. Following postdoctoral research at the Imperial Cancer Research Fund Laboratories in London, in 1973 he came on staff in the Division of Biological Research at OCI, becoming professor of medical biophysics in 1984. He progressed to the Mount Sinai Research Institute in 1985 to head the Division of Molecular and Developmental Biology. His research contributions at the Lunenfeld included specifying in 1989, together with Yaacov Ben David, the molecular basis of erythroleukemia induced by the Friend virus, a subject to which he had previously contributed (see farther on).[89]

Another important hire was Janet Rossant, who belonged to the ever dwindling number of academics recruited from the United Kingdom. Born in Chatham, England, in 1950, she received a BA from Oxford in 1972 and a PhD in embryology from Cambridge in 1976. At Cambridge, she was a student of Richard Gardner, one of the first scientists to genetically alter a mouse. The following year, in 1977, she was recruited to the biology department of Brock University in St Catharines, Ontario, while simultaneously teaching pathology at McMaster University. After starting to collaborate with Alan Bernstein, in 1985 she joined the Research Institute of Mount Sinai Hospital as senior scientist and several years later was also appointed to the university's Department of Medical Genetics. In 2005, as stated, she crossed University Avenue to lead the HSC Research Institute. Working in a general hospital, she developed an interest in clinical issues, and at the Centre for Modelling Human Disease at the Lunenfeld, her lab generated random mutations in mice, then screened them for symptoms of disease. This work brought Rossant to an interest in creating mutant mice from stem cells (see farther on).[90]

The other crucial appointment to the Division of Molecular and Developmental Biology at the Lunenfeld was Tony Pawson, who is one of Toronto's major scientists. Anthony J. Pawson, like Rossant, was British, born in Maidstone in 1952 with a bachelor's degree from Cambridge in 1973. He trained in molecular biology at the Imperial Cancer Research Fund in London, where he met Alan Bernstein. Pawson received a PhD from King's College, London University, in 1976. From 1976 to 1980 he was a postdoctoral fellow at the University of California at Berkeley investigating retroviral oncogenes. In 1981 he joined the University of British Columbia and in 1985 moved to Toronto to the Sinai's Research Institute. Pawson pioneered the study of intracellular signalling within cells, one of the ideas being that a disease such as cancer represents a breakdown in some signalling pathway. In particular, Pawson proposed the idea that signalling proteins have a singular adapter structure and that the binding of these adapters, which carry a module that he called the "SH2 domain," to specific domains that contain phosphotyrosine induces a cascade of intracellular events that regulates cell growth and differentiation, including the growth of cancer cells. This idea had a profound impact on the international research community. Pawson first laid out the concept of the SH2 domain in 1986, based on research at the University of British Columbia but written just after coming to Toronto in collaboration with two other investigators.[91] When in 2008 he won a Kyoto Prize, the award stated, "The human body consists of about 60 trillion cells, and its life is maintained by the organic activity of cells based on the correct transduction of signals ... Cancer, diabetes, autoimmune system disorders, and other diseases are all caused by malfunction of the intracellular signal transduction. Through his work from the mid-1980s to the early 1990s, Pawson made new discoveries about the mechanism of signal transduction within cells and went on to develop a new concept of intracellular signal transduction."[92]

Leading the cancer division was Robert Kerbel, whose subject was tumour angiogenesis and targeting drugs to cut off the blood supply of tumours (anti-angiogenesis); he was involved with the clinical investigation of Avastin (bevacizumab) and its mechanism of action as an anti-angiogenic agent.[93] He also investigated "metronomic chemotherapy," giving chemotherapy at closely spaced intervals.[94] Born in Toronto in 1945, Kerbel earned a BA in life sciences from the University of Toronto in 1968 and a PhD in microbiology and immunology from Queen's in 1972. After fellowing at the Chester Beatty Research Institute in London from 1972 to 1974, Kerbel worked as a research scholar at the National Cancer Institute of Canada from 1975 to 1981, then joined the Department of Pathology at Queen's University until summoned to Toronto. After leaving Lunenfeld, in 1991 Kerbel became senior scientist in molecular and cellular biology at the Sunnybrook Research Institute.

Still other divisions of the Lunenfeld Institute made significant appointments as well, such as Andras Nagy, who completed a PhD in genetics in Budapest in 1979, then later joined the campus Department of Medical Genetics and Microbiology and the Lunenfeld Institute. Nagy discovered knockout vascular endothelial growth factor in 1996 and Canada's first two human embryonic stem cell lines in 2005.

Fittingly, Lou Siminovitch's daughter Katherine Siminovitch went into molecular biology; at the Lunenfeld Institute in 1987 she started closing in on the location on the X chromosome of the Wiskott-Aldrich syndrome gene, an immunodeficiency syndrome characterized by eczema and repeated infections; she and co-workers identified in 1995 the exact gene mutation.[95]

On Lou Siminovitch's retirement in 1994, Bernstein became the director of the Research Institute before moving to Ottawa in 2002 as the inaugural president of the Canadian Institutes of Health Research. Pawson was appointed director of the Lunenfeld Institute in Bernstein's place. A measure of the institute's importance was its inclusion in a list of international "citation-impact institutions" for 2002–6. It came in twentieth in a list of twenty-five, the only Canadian institute on the list (and ahead of the Max Planck Society, the Scripps Research Institute, and Yale University).[96]

"Did you ever have any political difficulties in dealing with the hospital here?" an interviewer asked Siminovitch.
"No, no. They love me here."
Interviewer: "I'll bet they do!" (laughing)
"Well, because they became famous, and they've never had anything like that happen before."[97]

### Ontario Cancer Institute/Princess Margaret Hospital

By the late 1970s, among the generation following Siminovitch there were new stars in the biology division at the Ontario Cancer Institute: Alan Bernstein, Victor Ling, Tak Mak, and Ronnie Buick.[98]

Alan Bernstein, as seen, joined the division in 1973 and together with Tak Mak studied viral components of leukemia. In McCulloch's estimation, "His success in research and his powerful personality gave Bernstein much influence at the Ontario Cancer Institute."[99]

Victor Ling was the first OCI scientist "with dedicated training in molecular biology," as McCulloch puts it.[100] A 1969 PhD in biochemistry from the University of British Columbia whom Till had brought to OCI in 1971, Ling ended up discovering the genetics of multi-drug resistance. The story is this: in cancer treatment, patients often become resistant to the different agents they are being given; this is called "multi-drug resistance," and it occurs in laboratory cell lines as well. In 1986 Victor Ling and collaborators found that all these resistant cell lines had in common "the increased expression of P-glycoprotein," a protein that Ling had discovered in 1974. In back-to-back articles in *Nature* in 1985, Ling and collaborators developed monoclonal antibodies specific for P-glycoprotein in order to see where it abounded. (Monoclonal antibodies are specific for one invader; they are made by identical immune cells that, themselves, are all clones of a single parent cell.) The glycoprotein was little found in "drug-sensitive cells."[101] They also cloned at the same time the "mammalian gene" that coded for P-glycoprotein.[102] As they amplified their findings the next year, "[t]he level of P-glycoprotein expression correlates with the degree of drug resistance in a variety of different cell types." Further, the development of resistance was not the result of mutation but of gene amplification.[103] This finding had great potential significance for cancer chemotherapy, in that patients expressing lots of P-glycoprotein might be unresponsive to conventional cancer chemotherapies and could be spared the side effects.

Ronald Buick, a Scot with graduate training in biochemistry at the University of Wisconsin, was recruited to OCI by McCulloch in 1976. In 1979 he applied himself to the problem of "the clonogenic assay for leukemic blast cells," important because one would want to know whether such cells were stem cells. They were, and the vigor of their self-renewal capacity turned out to be related to their responsiveness to chemotherapy (low self-renewal equals successful induction of remission).[104]

Of the four successors to Siminovitch, Tak Wah Mak is probably best known internationally, for his discovery of how T-cells work. In 1983, he cloned the T-cell receptor and published on it in 1984.[105] The T-cell receptor enables the T-cells to lock onto their targets. Mak was born in Canton, Republic of China, in 1946; he studied for a bachelor's at the University of Wisconsin in 1967 and a PhD at the University of Alberta in 1972. His career in Toronto at OCI began as a postdoctoral fellow in 1972.

As McCulloch tells the story, "Early in 1983 an excited Tak Mak came into [my] office, announcing that he had found the holy grail of immunology" – the gene "encoding the antigen receptor on T-lymphocytes." (He had been denied a National Cancer Institute of Canada grant for this research.) The finding was reported in *Nature* in March 1984: "We have cloned and sequenced a human mRNA specific for mammalian T-lymphoid cells."[106]

The impact? Around the time of his discovery there was a National Cancer Institute site visit at OCI: "Mak made a description of his finding the opening … of his presentation to the panel. There was an immediate sensation, because the immunologists in the visiting group saw the importance of the discovery. It is probable that no other way of announcing the finding would have had such an immediate and widespread response … For the first time, a press conference was held to announce the finding." In 1992 the Amgen Company financed an institute at OCI with Mak as the director, knocking out individual genes in mice to study T-cell development. Other genes were discovered. The Amgen Institute at OCI was a very big deal.

*Stem Cell Research*

Readers will recall from chapter 5 McCulloch and Till's original discovery of stem cells in the early 1960s. They irradiated mice to destroy their blood-forming tissues and then injected the mice with marrow cells from healthy donors. McCulloch, speaking of himself and Till in the third person, briefly described the results: "After 10 days [the investigators] examined the spleens of the irradiated recipients and found the spleens contained visible lumps that could be counted easily. The lumps proved to be colonies, each derived from a single cell from the injected marrow." These single cells had given rise to all main types of blood cells, red cells, white cells, and platelets. The spleen lumps were called "colonies," and the colony-forming unit (CFU) was a hemopoietic stem cell. This technique became for years the standard for analysing stem cells in hematology and was known as "the Till-McCulloch assay."[107]

Yet the search for stem cells became urgent when other researchers discovered that many leukemias began in the hemopoietic stem cells. These stem cells would thus, said McCulloch, "be the correct targets for treatment." It also became apparent that stem cells were not limited to blood formation and blood cancers. "Rather the cells of many cancers, perhaps all cancers, were observed to be organized like hemopoiesis." Thus it was possible that cancerous stem cells caused most cancers.[108] This realization ignited a tsunami of stem cell research around the world. It also focused minds powerfully at the University of Toronto.

Among the most notable of the post–Till and McCulloch generation of stem cell researchers was John Dick at the Toronto General Research Institute, who identified and characterized the different kinds of leukemia stem cells. A Manitoban, in this story already rich with Westerners, born in 1957, Dick grew up on a Mennonite farm; after attending a one-room schoolhouse, he went to Winnipeg to become in 1974 an X-ray technician. After sharing a house with university students studying biology, he himself decided upon an academic course and ended with a PhD in microbiology and biochemistry from the University of Manitoba in 1984. Dick fellowed with Bernstein at OCI between 1984 and 1986, who guided him towards the leukemias; after joining the Department of Molecular and Medical Genetics at U of T in 1987, in 1991 he came to the Research Institute of HSC as a senior scientist.

In 1994 Dick identified the first leukemia stem cell, after transplanting into SCID mice ("severe combined immuno-deficient") cells from human acute myeloid leukemia. The researchers fractionated the leukemia cells in the mice and found a progenitor cell, or stem cell, that in other SCID mice could produce large numbers of colony-forming progenitors.[109] This work initiated cancer stem cell research. In 2001 Dick discovered that there were short-term repopulating and long-term repopulating stem cells, providing an explanation of why leukemias often returned after long remissions.[110] Remaining within the leukemia model, Dick achieved great recognition with his discovery that, just as in normal blood-forming systems, leukemias are arrayed as cellular hierarchies, composed of stems cells and more differentiated cells alike. This "hierarchical model of oncogenesis" returned to older concepts of cancer as "differentiation gone awry." In support of this concept, in 1989 he showed that human leukemias could be transplanted into immunodeficient mice.[111] This greatly enabled their study. He then showed in 1994 that only a small group of the leukemic cells gave rise to leukemias upon transplantation and that these had a distinctive surface marker (CD34+CD38-).[112] These concepts had an international impact as they were applied by others in solid tumour biology (and by Peter Dirks in Toronto).

Interviewed by a journalist in 2006, Dick said, "Science, like any other human endeavour, can be a slave to fashion. From 1975 to 1995, the research world was captivated by the wonder of genes and molecular biology. Cell biology had fallen by the wayside, and stem cell research was carried on by a fairly small club of people." Now the spotlight turned to Canada. Max Wicha, director of cancer research at the University of Michigan, said of the Toronto researchers, "They have been the pioneers and they are the clear leaders. There have been meetings all over the world. People are really jumping into this."[113]

The discovery of cancer stem cells meant that much previous cancer research may have been pursuing false leads. Said the journalist, "Billions of dollars and decades of research may have targeted the wrong cells to cure the disease." In Dick's modest office at OCI, "[t]he only symbols of his success are the 19 bottles of champagne lined up like soldiers along his window ledge. Since researchers often celebrate the publication of big discoveries with a bit of bubbly, his bottles tell the story."[114]

One of John Dick's students, in a sense, was a neurosurgeon at HSC, Peter Dirks, Dean John Dirks's son. Peter Dirks discovered stem cells in brain cancer. Peter studied medicine at Queen's University, graduating in 1989. In 1990 he began training in neurosurgery and also completed in 1998 a PhD thesis in cellular and molecular pathology as Jim Rutka's first graduate student. His research interest was genes that stop cell growth in brain tumours. In 1998 he joined the neurosurgical staff at HSC and often had to tell parents they might lose a child to a brain tumour. "It catches you sometimes, you know, when you see a patient who reminds you of one of our own," said Dirks, who had three daughters.

"I started to turn to John Dick's work," he said, "because I thought … 'I've got to think outside all of the research that's going on in brain tumours.'"

Dirks knocked on John Dick's door. The first time, they spoke for an hour. "I was green," said Dirks, "and I felt privileged that he would spend that kind of time with a nobody. He was inspirational."[115]

Dirks managed to get private funding for a small lab. The work of several researchers in Calgary convinced him that epidermal growth factor could be used to make brain cells reproduce. Using a growth factor cocktail on surgically removed tumours, Dirks, together with neurosurgical colleague Sheila Singh, established in 2003 in a historic article in *Cancer Research* the existence of cancer stem cells in human brain tumours. The tumour stem cells were only a fraction of the total cells in the tumour and carried the identifying protein CD133. "The data suggest that the tumors originate from tumor cells that express CD133, as this fraction exclusively had the ability to proliferate, self-renew, and differentiate."[116] In a 2004 article in *Nature*, this research reached a broader audience. He and Singh wrote, "The identification of brain tumour initiating cells provides insights into human brain tumour pathogenesis giving strong support for the CSC [cancer stem cell] hypothesis as the basis for many solid tumours, and establishes a previously unidentified cellular target [CD133+ cells] for more effective cancer therapies."[117] The significance of this work, Dirks said, is that "[w]e have recently demonstrated that brain tumours … are organized as a functional hierarchy with growth dependent on relatively rare cells that have stem cell properties."[118]

In her work at Mount Sinai, Janet Rossant, collaborating with Till's student Alan Bernstein, reinforced the Toronto tradition of stem cell research with her discovery of mammalian blastocyst stem cells. (The blastocyst is the mammalian conceptus in an early stage of development.) She and co-workers found that "early differentiation of the mammalian embryo leads to the development of two distinct lineages – the inner cell mass (ICM) and the trophectoderm. While both types of tissues produced 'immortal cell lines,' only the inner cells mass was pluripotent, capable of giving rise to all the tissues of the fetus," whereas the cells of the trophoblast gave rise only to the trophoblast cell layers of the placenta. Yet in a certain environment, the gene Oct4 could push embryonic stem cells towards the trophoblast phenotype. "Stem cell potential in the early embryo thus appears to depend on a combination of the levels of expression of key intrinsic regulators and the appropriate extrinsic environmental factors," she concluded.[119] Based on the number of papers and citations, Rossant in 2004 was seen as the number two embryonic stem cell researcher in the world.[120]

There were other stem cell discoveries in Toronto. For the work of Cindi Morshead on neural stems cells in the Division of Anatomy see chapter 15. In 1999 A. Keith Stewart and co-workers at The Toronto Hospital, together with a number of American centres, tried purging the myeloma cells from the stem cell harvest in the treatment of multiple myeloma.[121]

In 2001, a year before coming to Toronto, Freda Miller at McGill discovered the existence of "multipotent adult stem cells" in the dermis of mammalian skin.[122] Miller was born in Calgary in 1957, enrolled as an undergraduate at the University of Saskatchewan, and earned a PhD at the University of Calgary in 1984. She fellowed at the Scripps Foundation in La Jolla, California, from 1985 to 1988, then joined the Department of Anatomy and Cell Biology at the University of Alberta from 1988 to 1992. She worked at the Montreal Neurological Institute from 1993 to 1999, was a CIHR senior scientist, then in 2002 came to Toronto to HSC's Program in Developmental Biology; in 2007 she reported that such "skin-derived precursors," or SKPs, as "neural crest-related precursors" might have the potential of helping to repair spinal cord injury.[123]

Jumping ahead for a second, the individual stem cell discoveries occurring across the faculty were impressive but uncoordinated, representing the efforts of individual scholars rather than "one unified initiative," as an academic health network document put it in 2010. To hook these forces together, in January 2008 the faculty initiated the Toronto Stem Cell Initiative (TSCI), a collaboration among labs conducting stem cell research. The goal was "to carry out stem cell research at all stages from basic biology to translational and clinical research on stem cell-based therapies."[124]

### Molecular Medicine in the Faculty of Medicine

There's no line, really, between cell biology and biochemistry and molecular biology and genetics – it's all one big ball now. Everybody does it anyway. You can't really tell the difference any more among basic science departments in the medical school. The names are irrelevant, except for their undergraduate teaching.[125]

Jim Friesen, 2009

For the faculty as a whole, the new molecular era began on 9 February 1977, at 12:00 noon, when Bun McCulloch, who with Till had discovered stem cells a decade previously, told the Long-Range Planning Committee what he thought the future held in store: "Molecular, cellular, genetic." "During the next decade," he said, "our medical school must recognize and be an active participant in: new horizons ... including molecular cloning and genetic engineering, cellular communications based on recognition proteins and ... genetic mapping." McCulloch said these new horizons had various implications for the faculty: "A new attitude about 'science' and 'research' must be developed in both students and clinical faculty. A high priority must be given to developing teaching hospitals into laboratories of health care delivery."[126]

But there was more on McCulloch's plate. "Since new horizons do not fit into strict departmental moulds," he said, "new groupings of investigators are needed." Unfortunately, all the staff in the faculty's basic science departments had tenure and would be most unwilling to contemplate "new groupings." But already the hospital Research Institutes were visible on the horizon. "There should be more emphasis on molecular genetics," he added. And, finally, "[f]aculty hiring policy must take into account present age distribution of our faculty," meaning young blood was needed.[127]

McCulloch suggested that the faculty as a whole was really not quite up to speed when it came to world-class research and that the Research Institutes had pioneered the early decades. For all the suspiciousness of the basic science department towards the institutes, it was the Research Institutes of the big hospitals that had brought molecular medicine to Toronto.

Why was molecular biology so important to the faculty as a whole, in contrast to a handful of arcane scientists in their wet labs? Jim Friesen explained in 1986 that molecular biology provides the common language of the basic sciences, in a journalist's paraphrase: "Investigators versed in molecular biology can fit into almost any basic science department ... A scientist could work out of a department of physiology or pharmacology as readily as a department of biochemistry or genetics if, for instance, his or her main concern is the interaction of molecules with receptors." Friesen said, "Traditionally we have been thinking along departmental lines, but when you start to look at problems of developmental biology – these genetic diseases know no such boundaries." Friesen put emphasis on the technology of manipulating DNA, crucial in neurobiology, developmental biology, and protein engineering, "the three major areas for development." "Once a gene is purified it can be treated as a chemical substance. It is then possible to analyse and study it by various biochemical methods. The results of such analysis can reveal how the cell responds to signals controlled by its DNA."[128]

By 1980 there was enough ferment in the molecular end of the basic sciences to raise the question: Should microbiology, genetics, and immunology in the faculty be merged in a single department? The discussion is interesting because it shows a faculty where knowledge had traditionally been poured into rigid concrete forms, the departmental system, struggling with an onrush of new and unconventional knowledge. In 1980 Keith Dorrington, associate dean of basic sciences, asked a few select colleagues to reflect on the following: the present Departments of Medical Microbiology (the traditional faculty department, the successor of the Department of Bacteriology) and Microbiology and Parasitology (an inheritance from the School of Hygiene) were about to merge, he said. A number of important chairmanships were becoming empty. This would be a propitious moment to reconfigure the department structure, given that a multidisciplinary program in immunology was underway and another in molecular and cell biology was in advanced planning. "This Program will also include areas (eg Microbial Genetics) which have formally been part of the teaching load of Microbiology and Parasitology."[129] So the time to move was now.

Yet movement was slow and it was only in February 1987 that Hollenberg reported on the planning group assigned to the Biology of Development in the faculty's complement review. The faculty, he said, must become much more deeply involved in developmental biology. Needed was a program of "strength in cell and molecular biology ... although a major gap was apparent in the field of whole organism genetics, particularly at the molecular level. [His committee] noted also that the area of cellular interaction during development, which involved the phenomenon of pattern formation, is under-developed." Hollenberg's committee recommended "that two research groups be formed: (1) [one for] study of animal genetics at the cellular and molecular levels, using rapidly reproducing organisms; (2) a group to study cell interactions and pattern formation."[130] Out of these proposals came a Committee on Clinical Genetics. In February 1988 the committee, chaired by Ronald Worton, told Dean Dirks that the medical faculty needed a "program in molecular and genetic medicine," apart from the Department of Medical Genetics.[131]

At the same time, in January 1988 Lap-Chee Tsui at HSC was writing Dean Dirks complaining of severe deficiencies in the faculty's approach to human genetics. "This area is clearly the next big challenge in medical and basic genetic research. While the rest of the world is gearing up to have a serious look at the human genome, I would like to see some major commitment from the University so that Toronto would not be left in the cold in the next decade." Tsui reproached the faculty for a lack of follow-up. "There have been a number of major discoveries in human diseases in Toronto in the past few years. Unfortunately, none of the Toronto groups have been able to take advantage of the early lead and maintain the initial momentum." The main problem involved was a lack of "good post-doctoral fellows and graduate students ... I really fail to see a pouring [sic] number of postdoctoral applicants knocking at our doors or students coming with great enthusiasms. In fact, we have difficulty recruiting qualified and experienced postdoctoral fellows."

Why were there so few good graduate students? For one thing, Tsui said, the material rewards in the field were inadequate. "Why would one like to take such an unrewarding job? One of my students actually told me that he would not see himself working as hard and getting as little (pay) as I; he quit after obtaining a master's degree and ended up studying law. He was my best student." For another, there were so few foreign graduate students in the Department of Medical Genetics: "We have almost 90 graduate students but only 10 are from other countries. This is extremely unusual, if we compare our department with other major universities ... The foreign students are discouraged by an excessively high tuition."[132]

In response to this and similar laments, Jeremy Carver, associate dean of basic sciences, attempted early in 1990 to bring a campus group together in molecular structure: "We are currently searching for a full Professor in Protein Crystallography, to be located in the Biochemistry Department; we have two positions in Protein Engineering that are currently being filled in the Medical Genetics Department; and we have active discussion going on in the Basic Science Sector around the question of creating a Structural Biology Department. I am attempting to coordinate the growth of molecular structure activities in the hospital institutes as part of my current job." Also, OCI intended to "play a major role in these developments ... I am not aware of any similar initiative world-wide."[133]

So things did finally start to move at the level of the faculty. In March 1999 the Department of Medicine began preparing a subspecialty in "Molecular Medicine."[134] By September 2000 the program was up and running. Trainees would enter it following three years of the core internal medicine scheme. Phillipson said, "Unlike traditional Medical Genetics, which focuses largely on single-gene disorders (such as muscular dystrophy and cystic fibrosis), the program in Genetic Medicine will focus on multigenic adult disorders, such as diabetes, coronary artery disease, cancer, and dementia. These disorders are thought to result from an interaction between an individual's genetic predisposition to disease and the environmental risk factors to which the individual is exposed."[135]

The rise of molecular biology in the Research Institutes changed the traditional pecking order. Those with scientific training were starting to look down on medical training. Previously, it had often been possible to become a scientist only by first becoming a physician. Yet external reviewers of the Department of Medicine said in 2003, "Clinician scientists ... expressed concern about the balance of power of the Research Institute Directors and the Departmental Chair. Clinical scientists are unsure they are as valued as PhD scientists by the Research Institute Directors. For example, they expressed concern that PhD scientists would garner more resources than Clinician Scientists when it came to space and long-term salary support." Traditionally, in a teaching hospital, the MD was the prestigious degree and the PhDs tumbled along behind the men in the white coats. The rise of molecular biology essentially devalued clinical knowledge and exalted pure basic research. Phillipson's response as head of medicine was rather defensive: "The clinician-scientists involved in basic scientific research are particularly vulnerable in hospitals in which the Research

Institute Directors do not understand or value the role of the clinician-scientist. For this reason, it is critically important that the Chair be committed to, and be a strong advocate for, this group, given that of the 102 clinician-scientists in the Department [as of June 2003], over half are involved in basic research at the cellular and molecular levels."[136]

### McLaughlin Centre for Molecular Medicine

An important link between the faculty and the hospital research institutes was formed in 2001 with the creation of the McLaughlin Centre for Molecular Medicine (MCMM) to promote "the application of molecular discovery to clinical care." Made possible by a $50 million bequest from the McLaughlin Foundation and matching funds from the Ontario Innovation Trust, the centre was "a joint initiative of the University of Toronto and four partner hospital institutions, University Health Network, Hospital for Sick Children, Mount Sinai Hospital and Sunnybrook Health Sciences Centre." During the first decade of its existence, MCMM invested in a variety of projects, including the McLaughlin-Rotman Centre for Global Health and the faculty's MD/PhD program.[137] In 2010 it began a new phase as the "McLaughlin Centre" under the leadership of geneticist Stephen Scherer and a tighter focus on genomic medicine.[138]

### Terrence Donnelly Centre for Cellular and Biomolecular Research

Cecil Yip and I, that was our building. We got the money, we told the stories, and all that stuff. Our idea was that it would be BBDMR writ large.[139]

Jim Friesen, 2009

In the molecular medicine story, the Donnelly Centre for Cellular and Biomolecular Research – CCBR – was the faculty's answer to the hospital Research Institutes. The Donnelly Centre was also physically magnificent, which the institutes weren't. It featured a glass skywalk, six floors above the ground, connecting physically the centre with the Medical Sciences Building and connecting symbolically the old world of basic science research in established departments with the new interdisciplinary world. Peter Lewis, vice-dean of research, said in 2009, "If Toronto's global pre-eminence in fields such as stem-cell, cardiac and cancer research has flowered ... it is due primarily to the cross-pollination of disciplines." Robert Bell, head of the University Health Network, added, "This interdisciplinary aspect is something that gets engendered by architecture."[140]

This interdisciplinarity was envisaged from the very beginning of the Donnelly Centre, although the CCBR was not yet named after Donnelly. The "Strategic Directions" academic plan of 2000 noted, "The creation of CCBR represents primarily the 'basic' end of a continuum of health research." "Creation of CCBR is the top priority research initiative, not only of the Faculty but also of the

University. With researchers from the biological sciences side by side with researchers [from other disciplines], CCBR represents a new approach to bio-medicine. By placing a selected group of faculty members ... for a fixed but renewable period of time in a totally research-oriented environment not unlike that of a Howard Hughes Medical Research Institute, CCBR will create a paradigm for research that truly transcends department structures."[141]

How did CCBR come into being, in a faculty so long without a new building? Former chair of the Banting and Best Department David MacLennan said, "Jim [Friesen] is a visionary thinker. He saw that with the removal of the technological barrier in genomics, he decided he was going to recruit in the area of genomics, but that he was going to have people cross-reacting, interacting." Former Canadian prime minister Jean Chrétien had just launched the Canadian Foundation for Innovation (CFI). "So there were Jim and Cecil that inherited this [BBDMR interdisciplinary] culture, and they saw the potential for putting this into 13 floors. Rather than a 4-story Best Institute, they would carry it over to a 13-story CCBR. That was how they sold the idea that got the CFI money, Jim hired the nucleus of the people that would go over there." And money, such a limiting factor in the 1980s, was no longer an issue. "You could find money through the Canada Research Chairs. There were many ways that you could create positions. He created the nucleus of the group that filled this building, and really interacted in the way that we had done 20 years earlier. They were now doing it in this building. The floors were full of people who were all excited about what they could do with the genome, and they were using the technology back and forth – the proteomics and the structural genomics, and all these things blossomed at that time."[142] Thus, there is an organic continuity between the Banting and Best Department of Medical Research and the Donnelly Centre. A basic difference, however, is that BBDMR in its salad days under Charles Best was isolated and insular, whereas the Donnelly Centre under Brenda Andrews reached out broadly to the world of science, with collaborations in every direction.[143]

CCBR cost a lot of money. Rob Prichard, president of the university, and David Naylor, dean of the faculty, were instrumental in raising it. Friesen recalled visiting the Canadian Foundation for Innovation with Prichard: "Rob stood up and did his spiel, and everybody said, 'Oh, yes!' and he really supported us." Naylor helped plug a huge budget gap between what CFI was willing to contribute and what was needed. "David cobbled together interest from the Faculty and Pharmacy and Engineering to participate in this building, and have a few people in there eventually, and of course, contribute to the money. There was still a shortfall, so then Terry Donnelly came along with his thirteen million bucks, and David was of course very helpful there."[144]

In May 2001, the federal Canadian Foundation for Innovation agreed to support the centre and by October Cecil Yip and Jim Friesen, who had both led the Banting and Best Department of Medical Research, signed on as interim co-directors of the CCBR. The interim executive committee fairly breathed interdisciplinarity, and included Michael Sefton of the Institute for Biomaterials and Biomechanical Engineering; Mel Silverman in the Department of Medicine; Brenda Andrews, head of the Department of Medical Genetics and Immunology; Peter Lewis, Department of Biochemistry; Rob MacGregor, Faculty of Pharmacy; and Pekka Sinervo, vice-dean of the Faculty of Arts and Science.[145] By March 2004, the CCBR, the first new Faculty of Medicine building since 1968, was being billed as a joint project of the Faculties of Medicine, Applied Science and Engineering, and Pharmacy.[146] In November 2004 the faculty celebrated Terrence Donnelly's donation that permitted the completion of all ten laboratory floors.[147] In honour of his philanthropy, the centre was named the Terrence Donnelly Centre for Cellular and Biomolecular Research. That month there was a grand opening, and the forty to forty-five faculty began moving in shortly thereafter.

In 2004 Brenda Andrews, former chair of the Department of Medical Genetics, was appointed the centre's inaugural director and chair of the BBDMR.

Brenda Andrews, from Clinton, Ontario, studied zoology as an undergraduate at the University of Toronto and received a PhD in medical biophysics from U of T in 1986, then worked on yeast genetics at the University of California San Francisco with Ira Herskowitz. In 1991 she returned to the Department of Medical Biophysics in Toronto, becoming chair in 1999. Her scientific interests revolved around "functional genomics," mapping the interactions within the cells. In 2004 she co-headed an international "global mapping of the yeast genetic interaction network."[148]

A landmark article on yeast in *Science* in 2010 helped open up the subject. Andrews's lab and Charlie Boone's lab looked at 5.4 million gene-gene pairs in order to generate "genetic interaction profiles" for three-quarters of the genes in the budding yeast. This means they had grouped the genes responsible for protein folding, for secretion and vesicle transport, for DNA replication and repair, and so forth. The authors said that "genetic interaction maps provide a model for understanding the link between genotype and phenotype and for outlining the general principles of complex genetic interaction networks, which play a key role in governing inherited phenotypes, including human disease."[149] In this remarkable research, and in other similar projects across the globe, lay the promise of throwing open the genome and marching into it to find the roots of illness.[150] "Nobody has made a map of these genetic interactions," said Andrews. "This research has provided us with a functional view of the cell."[151]

# 29   The Deans

**Deans of the Faculty of Medicine, University of Toronto**

William Thomas Aikins, 1887–93
Uzziel Ogden, 1893–6
Richard Andrews Reeve, 1896–1908
Charles Kirk Clarke, 1908–20
Alexander Primrose, 1920–32
John Gerald FitzGerald, 1932–6
William Edward Gallie, 1936–46
Joseph Arthur MacFarlane, 1946–61
John Drennan Hamilton, 1961–6
Andrew Lawrence Chute, 1966–73
Richard Brian Holmes, 1973–80
Frederick Hans Lowy, 1980–7
John Herbert Dirks, 1987–91
G. Harvey Anderson (acting dean), 1992
Arnold Aberman, 1992–9
Christopher David Naylor, 1999–2005
Catharine Isobel Whiteside, 2005–present

It is a universal maxim among academic administrators that Medicine is the most difficult of all the faculties. In discussions of the nature of the complex university, someone will eventually say "that's the university with a medical faculty"; and the result is good-natured laughter, such as follows a joke about mothers-in-law.[1]

Claude Bissell, President of the University of Toronto, 1973

**Early Deans**

Previous chapters have sketched in the early history of the faculty's governance and that will not be repeated here. By the time of the First World War the Faculty of Medicine of the University of Toronto was the largest in the British Empire with the exception of Edinburgh, the model to which all the British colonies aspired in those days.[2] Toronto's was a faculty that then offered no postgraduate preparation of any kind – the term "postgraduate" meaning post-medical-degree. Gallie said of the time when he graduated from the school in 1903 that there was no provision for the training of specialists (or of family doctors either, for that matter, as in the whole city there were only seventeen internships). Gallie recalled, "No attempt whatever was made to train an internist or a surgeon or any kind of specialist. Such training had to be acquired elsewhere."[3]

Under these circumstances, a full-time deanship would have been meaningless, there was so little to administer. The early deans all retained their chairs and performed their functions on a part-time basis. This undifferentiated state changed significantly after the First World War with the reorganization of the Departments of Medicine, Surgery, and Paediatrics. With Duncan Graham, Clarence Starr, and Alan Brown in charge, postgraduate training came to the fore. Gallie noted, "Whereas formerly there was really no graduate training worthy of the name, the clinical departments now began a system which permitted our graduates to obtain adequate training in whatever direction they wished to go." Soon the two other teaching hospitals – St Michael's and the Western – noticed these changes and proceeded to reorganize themselves. "Before long they had moved into magnificent new buildings and had adopted a system of staffing very similar to that at the General."[4]

On Dean Charles K. Clarke's watch (1908–20) some new offices appeared. Archibald Macallum was "instrumental in the establishment of the Ph.D. degree [achieved in 1897] that he saw as a research degree requiring a thesis."[5] In 1915 Macallum chaired a PhD advisory Board of Graduate Studies. In December 1918 E. Stanley Ryerson, who had been assistant secretary of the faculty since 1908, succeeded Alexander Primrose as secretary of the faculty.[6]

When Alexander Primrose took over from Clarke as dean in 1920, the post of dean had become somewhat more demanding. In the 1921–2 session, a School of Graduate Studies was founded under the leadership of anatomist J. Playfair McMurrich. President Falconer said, "When the organization is complete, this body will assume administrative control of the curriculum of study leading to the higher degrees in Medicine." The faculty now had a three-year graduate curriculum, leading to the MD or ChM (Master of Surgery) degrees. "This means a student who wishes to qualify as a surgeon or a physician and practice as a specialist, is able to obtain a thorough training." The faculty also had short graduate courses in medicine, surgery, and obstetrics and gynecology.[7]

What is now called continuing medical education was just arriving in the 1920s and that had to be administered as well. In the 1925–6 session the "extension" lectures (to graduate community physicians) were expanding. Also, in cooperation with the Ontario Medical Association, the faculty had scheduled lectures and demonstrations throughout the province. The Sun Life Assurance Company had donated $30,000 to the Canadian Medical Association to carry on similar activities throughout Canada, and under this CMA scheme, in 1925–6 the Toronto faculty staged eighty-six lectures.[8]

And then there was the medical library, said in 1926 to be in a "calamitous state." In 1927 the faculty, together with the Academy of Medicine, organized a medical reading room in the main library.[9]

Under Primrose's tenure, the basic medical degree was upgraded from an MB to an MD. In September 1928 the Faculty Council learned that Board of Governors had approved a resolution that the degree in medicine is the doctor of medicine – MD. Those with previous MB degrees could convert to MD for a fee.[10] This was a decision to which the faculty had aspired for many years. In 1898 J.E. Graham had moved in the Faculty Council that the MD degree be granted on graduation, but, said Primrose, "the Senate would have none of it."[11] Why was this decision finally taken? Work in the United States was at stake. As Dean MacFarlane explained in 1955, "Our graduates, particularly in the United States, were having some difficulty in convincing their local societies that an M.B. denoted an adequate education in a good school." Yet older medical graduates were proud of their MBs, and refused the automatic upgrades to "MD" that the faculty offered. MacFarlane continued, "It was interesting to note on the occasion of the Medical Convocation in June [1955] … when according to custom, the University offered the M.D. to those members of the class of 1905 who had not availed themselves of the opportunity of procuring it for a nominal fee, that a large number of that class declined the degree on the grounds that it now has ceased to be any special mark of distinction, wisdom or attainment when it is given at the end of a basic course."[12]

Graduate certification received a large upgrading in November 1929, when the Royal College of Physicians and Surgeons of Canada was organized. Honours were divided between McGill and U of T: John C. Meakins of McGill was president; Duncan Graham became vice president of the medical division, Fred N.G. Starr of the surgical division.[13] (Another change in the direction of nationwide certification: in the 1934–5 session, the College of Physicians and Surgeons of Ontario ceased to conduct examinations of undergraduates and would henceforth require the certificate of the Medical Council of Canada.[14])

The end of the Primrose deanship in 1932, therefore, brought with it a host of changes in medical organization in Toronto and in Canada. Changes in the U of T undergraduate program have been discussed in another chapter ("Student Life and Learning," chapter 27).

*FitzGerald (1932–6) and Gallie (1936–46)*

Work was beginning to pile up in the deanery. In January 1932 Gerry FitzGerald became dean, and simultaneously E. Stanley Ryerson, who since 1908 had served as assistant secretary, then as secretary, was appointed assistant dean. (He continued as secretary.) President Falconer appeared at Faculty Council to explain the creation of the post of permanent assistant dean: We've decided to limit the tenure of dean to three years, he said. (This was not implemented.) "The policy is to have a permanent Assistant Dean raising it to a higher position, covering added duties that have hitherto been performed by the Secretary."[15]

As of 1 July 1936, Edward Gallie, professor of surgery, succeeded FitzGerald, who went on to become director of the International Health Division of the Rockefeller Foundation. Gallie thus inaugurated what some look back on as a kind of collegial golden era, the dean as unos inter pares, one among equals, and much beloved.

Research started to arrive in the decanal portfolio. In 1937 an Associate Committee on Medical Research was established under the National Research Council to encourage medical research in Canada. Fred Banting was its first chair (it would play a big role in wartime research).[16]

National organizations began to figure as well in the dean's jobs. In the 1942–3 session, the Association of Canadian Medical Schools was founded. It would convene during the annual meeting of the Medical Council of Canada.[17] Thus complexities compounded. As Gallie put it upon stepping down in 1946, "This Faculty has grown so large and the business of managing it has become so complicated and onerous that it is no longer possible for the head of one of the departments to administer its general business and, at a the same time, give the personal leadership required by his own department."[18]

*The Beginnings of Postgraduate Training*

Perhaps the thorniest challenge Gallie faced in his deanship was postgraduate training, recent medical graduates becoming house officers in the big teaching hospitals for the sake of learning a specialty. "Postgraduate studies" in the faculty had a special meaning: further study after receiving the undergraduate medical degree was called "postgraduate." Elsewhere in the university, an undergraduate degree would lead to "graduate" studies. This little conceit goes back to the early days of the faculty. In the summer of 1904, the first "summer Post-Graduate Course" was offered,[19] and over the following decades various departments participated in a dribble of what would now be called continuing medical education.

As the Second World War ended, Gallie had to deal with the large number of recent medical graduates who had served in the armed forces and now were demanding postgraduate training. In "Plans for the Rehabilitation of Medical

Officers upon Demobilization," Gallie said "There will be a broad increase in the senior intern appointments available in each of the four University hospitals. As this will naturally reduce the number of patients per intern ... these interns will receive refresher courses ... so that they will be prepared for the examinations for Fellowship in the Royal College ... In addition the Faculty is committed to a general programme of postgraduate teaching."[20]

Gallie used the term "residency" in quotation marks, so unfamiliar did he find it, and said in retrospect, "The most important advance in postgraduate training ... has been the introduction of the system in all our hospitals whereby our graduates are stepped up year after year until ... they finally reach a 'residency.' This is an internship that most of us alumni [writing in 1953] know nothing about. It is a post in which the resident physician, or surgeon ... has been gradually raised to a position of responsibility similar to that of a junior member of the Attending Staff. He has charge, under moderate supervision, of diagnosis and treatment, and he has regular duties in the teaching of students and in the training of interns. Naturally it is from this group that candidates for permanent staff appointments are chosen."[21]

The colleagues agreed postgraduate training was needed. Neurosurgeon Ken McKenzie spun it partly as an exercise in what would later be called "branding." The influence of the University of Toronto on the education of doctors in Canada had been waning, he said, because of all the provincial medical schools that were springing up across the country. "All this has gradually brought about a dilution of University of Toronto graduates in Provinces other than Ontario and a consequent lessening of U. of T. influence on Medical Practice in Canada." The time is right to attract postgraduate students, he thought, and through them, put a stamp on medical practice in Canada. "In the past, many have continuously sought this instruction in other countries especially in the United States. Well organized and progressive post-graduate instruction in the U. of T. would and could attract many students from the world at large. It is desirable for this University to play an increasingly larger part in the international exchange of medical knowledge and further enhance a reputation already well established."[22] What McKenzie was proposing here was a kind of reputation enhancement that is pursued quite vigorously today, in the certain knowledge that top reputations win top students and top scientists.

Thus in February 1946 the barons of the faculty met with Gallie to decide plans for postgraduate study in the faculty. They devised a "Proposal regarding the establishment of a graduate school in the Faculty of Medicine, University of Toronto." This would enroll postgraduates taking the course for the master of surgery degree, the four diploma programs (public health, industrial hygiene, psychiatry, and radiology), and students wishing to qualify for the examinations of the Royal Colleges of Medicine and of Surgery, the Royal Colleges of the United Kingdom, and the advisory boards of the medical specialties in the United States. They also agreed that regular postgraduate courses in pathology, anatomy, and physiology should be organized specially for the interns.[23] (Here is a key in understanding some of these terms unfamiliar to today's readers: a "junior internship" = PGY1; senior internship = PGY 2,3; assistant resident = PGY4; resident = PGY 5.[24])

The need for postgraduate training in medicine was felt in the university as a whole. In June 1947 President Sidney Smith re-emphasized its importance: "Special encouragement should be given to plans for the offering of refresher and postgraduate courses. There is a pressing need in Canada for an outstanding graduate centre. Such a centre would serve the general practitioner as well as the specialist. Without any institutional conceit it must be stated that the responsibility is ours."[25] The selection of new interns for postgraduate training catalyzed cooperation between faculty and hospitals. In December 1947 the new dean, Joseph MacFarlane, said, not just apropos selecting interns for the hospitals of the Department of Veterans Affairs but for the teaching hospitals in general, "I have talked this matter over with the Professor of Surgery and it is hoped that after the first of July we will receive most of our new internes from a joint select[ion] board with representatives from all the teaching hospitals. We would seek people who had had at least the [surgery] rotation and preferably their senior year." Janes, the professor of surgery, added, "So far as surgery is concerned the program is already underway and they have agreed that they will refer applications to Joint Committee of the committees of the teaching hospitals. The group will be considered as a whole."[26]

Should the faculty itself grant a graduate degree after the completion of a residency in addition to certification by the Royal Colleges? The psychiatry diploma came to mind. The colleagues considered this: "It was the feeling … that any degree should be of a very high caliber, and granted following certification or the obtaining of fellowship. It would be unwise for a man who had received a diploma in the university to run the risk of failing to attain his fellowship."[27]

As for funding, it soon became apparent that sending trainees abroad for a final buffing was expensive. In February 1949 Dean MacFarlane consulted with Charles Wilkinson of the Kellogg Foundation about supporting the faculty's fledgling postgraduate program. MacFarlane especially wanted funds for travel for trainees at the end of their residencies: "[We need] the 'finishing off' of certain well trained men whom it is the intention of the University to appoint to positions on the staff. Living as we do with one foot so to speak in the United States and the other in Great Britain, and gradually building up our own facilities as a postgraduate centre, we [want] our own graduates who expect to be teachers in this school to spend some time abroad studying."[28]

In 1950 a Committee on Post-Graduate Studies was created to coordinate postgraduate training and continuing medical education; Robert C. Dickson, a 1934 U of T graduate, was chair.[29] Yet there were problems for the new committee. One was the steady increase in demands for postgraduate training that a committee found difficult to administer. Another was the numerous medical meetings at which colleagues spoke without any faculty efforts to give a sense of direction or control the quality of the meetings. A special committee of the Faculty Council considered these issues in 1954 and drew up recommendations in 1955.[30] Thus a Division of Postgraduate Studies came onto the horizon, as the offering by 1955 was becoming substantial: "Some fifty-odd teachers contributed to the teaching programme, and it is estimated that in this way 150 doctors have the benefit of these day-long teaching seminars each month during the fall and winter."[31]

In January 1955 the Faculty Council struck a special committee on postgraduate education.[32] Following the May recommendation of this committee, in February 1956 the Board of Governors established a new Division of Postgraduate Medical Education. It had "two main groups of doctors," the postgraduate trainees plus the practicing doctors in their home communities who had "only a limited time for formal postgraduate instruction" and who want "refresher courses." "Another main contribution of the Faculty is the programme of Decentralized (Travelling) Clinics which have been functioning successfully since the 1951–1952 session. These involve close cooperation between the Faculty and different Medical Societies in Ontario and in effect bring university type clinics to the home areas of many doctors throughout the Province."[33] The head of the new division, Ian MacDonald, would be the director of postgraduate medical education and assistant to the dean. There would also be a Board of Postgraduate Studies, a calendar, and a separate budget.[34] This was the first new office created in the deanery since its inception in 1887.

Ranald Ian MacDonald himself was a faculty utility hitter. In the 1946–7 session he was appointed medical director of both the Toronto veterans hospitals, Christie Street and Sunnybrook, as Farquharson retired from the post.[35] This was the beginning of MacDonald's long career in the faculty that ended with him as associate dean for postgraduate affairs in the 1960s. MacDonald was Nova Scotian in origin. After gaining a medical degree from Dalhousie University in 1930, he began his junior internship at the Toronto General Hospital. Duncan Graham identified him as a comer and brought him into the Department of Medicine. MacDonald then studied neurology at Queen Square in London, returned to Halifax, and landed in 1936 as a staffer at the General. He served during the war, then, as noted earlier, passed through the Christie Street and Sunnybrook Hospitals en route back to the General. His colleague and friend Fred Kergin said, as MacDonald stepped down as associate dean of postgraduate education in 1969, that he would be remembered for "his dry humour, and ... his forthright common sense. In the terminology of a fellow angler, he casts a straight line."[36]

The new division had to pay its own way. The intramural continuing education program was a money-spinner that generated funds for other activities. But the extramural program needed support from such organizations as the Kellogg Foundation for the first five years, then the Ontario Medical Association, the Ontario Heart Foundation, and the Ontario Cancer Treatment and Research Foundation.[37]

### Joseph MacFarlane, 1946–61

He was terribly good looking, and impressive in that way, a very good lecturer, a very kindly person.[38]

Helen LeVesconte, 1975

In 1946 Joseph MacFarlane succeeded Gallie as dean of medicine. He was the faculty's first full-time dean and would guide it for the next fourteen years as it began a period of almost uninterrupted growth from the war's end for the sixty years to come. MacFarlane was born on a farm in Lanark County, Ontario, in 1893 and grew up "in the atmosphere of late Victorian rural Ontario," as his colleague Ian MacDonald later said. After completing the junior matriculation there, he moved with his family to open up virgin land in Saskatchewan, settling in a township named Nokomis because, as one journalist said, "someone in the family was reading Hiawatha." He attended the University of Saskatchewan, earned a bachelor's degree in 1916, and won the Rhodes Scholarship allocated to that province. Yet instead of studying in England, he enlisted as a stretcher-bearer and spent three years with the 11th Canadian Field Ambulance. After returning to Canada, he enrolled in medicine at the University of Toronto and chaired the Daffydil committee in 1920–1, the year before he graduated;[39] his motto for the yearbook was, "A man so various that he seemed to be, Not one, but all mankind's epitome." MacFarlane then trained in surgery in Toronto and, picking up his Rhodes Scholarship again, returned to England for further work. He thereupon joined the surgical staff of the General in 1926 and spent the next years as a senior demonstrator in surgery and in private practice.

In patriotism, he was truly a man of his times. When the Second World War broke out, MacFarlane re-enlisted in the Canadian army, was invalided home in 1940, and became consulting surgeon to the Canadian Army Overseas with the rank of brigadier. MacDonald said, "He brought a combination of personal qualities and professional experience which enabled him to exert a profound influence on the organization and quality of surgical services for Canadian troops." In 1945 he served briefly as head of surgery at the Christie Street Hospital before accepting the deanship.[40] It was evident even in Europe that MacFarlane had a kind of magnetic attractiveness as a medical leader. Recalled Fred Dewar, a field surgeon at one of the Canadian casualty clearing stations, of the ability of the commanding officers to produce heparin or whatever was needed, "That was another joy of the Canadian Army, if you could convince the powers-that-be what your interest was and what you were trying to do, they would move hell and high water to get you the materials and things to do it, and that depended almost entirely on Dr MacFarlane – Brigadier MacFarlane – who would look after us like children."[41]

MacFarlane was evidently chosen dean because of his "high reputation as an imaginative leader and competent administrator," as MacDonald puts it.[42] In a medical culture dominated by veterans, he was an obvious choice. As a brigadier he had been accustomed to leadership and took on the job apparently unfazed that many members of his executive committee, called the Curriculum and Examination Committee, had been his professors. President Bissell credited MacFarlane with "sens[ing] the changes in the offing, the break-up of the old standard mechanized curriculum, the emphasis on medicine as part of a united social effort, the need to shatter the encrusted economics of the profession." MacFarlane greeted change, said Bissell.[43]

It was also helpful to MacFarlane, Bissell continued, that the Faculty of Medicine was something of a darling of the university's Board of Governors. "Medicine aroused the board's interest most easily. In part, it was social – a doctor with a university appointment and a large practice was likely to be one of the few academics that a governor would know; he might be a member of the same club in the city or a fishing partner in the wilderness." Members of the board were also likely to serve as trustees of teaching hospitals "and saw the constant pull between patient care and instruction and research; in hospitals, too, they were no doubt fascinated by the complexities of medical finance, which had its own dense jargon." There could, Bissell said, "be no doubt about the value of a medical education. It provided the leadership and the intelligence in the fight against disease."[44] Coming out of the gate after the war, the faculty therefore had several pluses going for it.

Under MacFarlane, the duties of the dean increased. Dealing with department heads over appointments and salaries was one. As John Hamilton, who succeeded MacFarlane in 1960 as dean, later said of MacFarlane's tenure, "The appointment of a full time Dean reflected the growing complexity of the University and the necessity for the President to delegate some of his responsibilities, most notably the power to recommend new appointments and the power to allocate funds." Previously, the individual department heads had negotiated directly with the president for funds, and the president interviewed candidates for department headships and appointed them himself. Hamilton said, MacFarlane "made the Deanship the focal point for Faculty administration."[45] There would be no more going to the president.

Academic rank has always been a sore point in medical faculties, as senior clinicians are the functional equivalents of professors in arts and science but before the 1960s did not have the title "professor." In the 1947–8 session, MacFarlane re-established the rank of associate professor in several clinical departments and replaced the terms "Senior" and "Junior Demonstrator" with "Clinical Teacher." "The establishment of the rank of Associate Professor for senior clinicians allows for the promotion to Faculty rank of many able and experienced younger men. Their services will be invaluable in the rapidly increasing committee work in a large faculty organization."[46] (In 1965 a committee of the Faculty Council recommended at the department level the following titles: professor and chairman (the head of a university department), professor and head (the head of a hospital department), associate professor, and assistant professor.[47] This scheme is not always followed in the present volume, where "head" and "chair" are used interchangeably; "chief" denotes the leader of a hospital department.)

In research, MacFarlane at least diverted the gaze of his faculty, largely intent upon teaching and service, in the direction of investigation. Fifteen years afterwards, as MacFarlane finally laid his office aside in 1961 – he was the longest-tenured dean – he said, quoting an anonymous American colleague, "There has been more medical research carried on in the past fifteen years than in all the previous history of medicine. [This] indicates how important a part research must play in the everyday life of a modern medical school."[48] It was just the beginning.

MacFarlane ended his deanship on a bit of a nativist note. In June 1960 he said that one third of the newly registered physicians in Ontario in the years 1954–9 were "qualified in schools outside Canada." Was it not now time to look at Canadian candidates, in view of the fact that many more applied to medicine than were accepted? "It seems inevitable that in the next five years there will be many more good Canadian applicants than there are places available in the country."[49] It is amusing to look back and think that, today, among the ranks of Canada's future doctors would excel precisely the students who themselves, or whose parents, were born outside the country. Today, these new Canadians, and not the farm boys of Ontario, would be the wave of the future.

In retrospect, Joseph MacFarlane was one of the great deans of the faculty. He was able to lead an academic staff – who conceived of their roles mainly as teachers and educators – through a door marked "Research." And he administered his domain with wisdom and judgment. At the end of his tenure, quoting the *British Medical Journal*, he reflected about what made for a good dean. "He must himself remain a student, although so much a senior. He must learn along with the school … He will not forget the stimulus of the unexpected. He will be interested in medical education in itself, realizing, as Emerson said, that the secret of education lies in respecting the student. Above all, he must be able to appreciate the point of view of the young, to make due allowances for their follies and extravagances, to encourage their good endeavours and try to forecast their future."[50] These lines were written in 1956, before the role of dean became daunting in its complexity. Yet their wisdom resonates even today: one of the primary missions of a medical school is training doctors to care for and heal the taxpayers, and responsibility for the successful achievement of this mission stops at the desk of the dean.

## John Hamilton, 1961–6

John Drennan Hamilton, who became dean in 1961, was recruited from the Department of Pathology. Born in Revelstoke, British Columbia, in 1911, Hamilton received a medical degree from the University of Toronto in 1935, then interned at the Toronto General Hospital. He was a demonstrator for several years in the Department of Pathology. From 1937 to 1939 he studied at Cambridge University, thereafter spending a year at Johns Hopkins. After military service, Hamilton served briefly as assistant professor of pathology at McGill, then headed the pathology department at Queen's University from 1946 to 1951, when he came to Toronto as pathologist-in-chief at the General and head of the campus Department of Pathology.

Hamilton turned up the rheostat even farther on research. In the 1960s money available for research – though not alas the space to do it in – grew by leaps and bounds. Hamilton said, "The total spent on research in the past academic year [1961–2] exceeds, by a small margin, the budget of the Faculty."[51] On Dean Hamilton's watch, the first of many space and funding crises reached a head. In fact it would be possible to write the history of the faculty over the last half century as a continuous lament over funding and space. A sample lament came from the Department of Anaesthesia in 1964–5: "The difficulties of carrying out a satisfactory teaching programme based on total reliance on part-time staff, who are hard pressed to meet their commitments for services to patients, the growing inadequacy of space and facilities for the prosecution of basic and clinical research and the lack of financial support for research projects within the department, are demoralizing."[52]

To make scientific progress, the faculty absolutely had to grow, but there was no room for more labs or offices. Everything was chock-a-block and the faculty had too little space to take advantage of all the new federal funding for medical research.[53] Simultaneously, the province of Ontario agonized about a doctors' crisis as the population was outpacing the supply of physicians. Henry Borden, chair of the university Board of Governors, went to Premier John Robarts to solicit support for a new Medical Sciences Building.[54] Thus, on 31 October 1964, a grand bargain was reached. The province announced that it would pump up faculty funding if the faculty would agree to increase the size of the first-year class by 75 students, from 175 to 250. This was part of a larger provincial scheme to fund a new medical school in Hamilton at McMaster University and to renovate the medical school at Queen's.[55] Shortly thereafter, the dean made clear to the faculty that the decision to increase class size to 250 had been reached by the Board of Governors (and there would be no push-back). How to cope with it? De-centralization was the answer: We've already made the fourth year hospital-based and we have money to do so for the third year as well, he noted.[56]

Immediately after the announcement, a users committee was struck to specify details for the new Medical Sciences Building that had already been conceived but not funded or laid out in detail. A second users committee went to work on the Banting Building, also bulging at the seams and desperately in need of new lab space and room for animal quarters[57] (under existing conditions there was, for example, no isolation room and the sick animals infected the healthy). As seen, there was a separate but equally weighty deal: the faculty agreed to make Sunnybrook Hospital a university affiliate. Both the Medical Sciences Building and Sunnybrook were to be up and running by 1969, when the new students were expected. "This has been a year of planning and uncertainty," Wightman said of these events. "The winds of change are reaching gale force, which may mean that some good things will be blown away with the bad. Nonetheless there is tremendous feeling of imminent progress and improvement."[58] Wightman was right. This was the start of the big expansion in medical education and facilities in Ontario, and later across Canada, that took place during the 1960s.

On Hamilton's watch, the logic of centralizing lectures in the basic sciences and simultaneously decentralizing clinical instruction and research in the teaching hospitals was worked out, following the recommendation of a special committee of the Board of Governors in 1964 that he chaired. Hamilton said, "Such a bipolar development is considered the only one possible for this Faculty of Medicine with its three major hospitals, one of the largest undergraduate schools in North America, and the most highly developed programme in Canada for the training of graduate and postgraduate students."[59]

For the Faculty Council, the changes in basic organization since the early 1920s had been trivial. In November 1965 the Committee on Structure and Organization recommended the establishment of six new standing committees and renaming the Committee on Curriculum and Examinations the Senior Committee, with the dean as chair.[60] The committee said that "there was a great need for reorganization of the administration of the Faculty aimed primarily at greater efficiency and better communication at all levels." Why did it matter? "This Faculty has the potentiality of becoming a great medical school."

How was this greatness to be achieved? Walls between disciplines were to be lowered, for one thing. The Faculty Council report in 1965 did not yet use the term "interdisciplinary," yet the dean must be able to ensure that in research and teaching "the Faculty ... can act as a unified body." Also, the faculty was underfunded and desperately needed more money from the central administration. The committee was thrilled that the Board of Governors had recommended moving ahead with the construction of a new Medical Sciences Building that would relieve the aching space problems. Thank God there was going to be a new associate dean for student affairs, and another new committee was needed to look at the convulsion taking place in public funding of medical services and at the Ontario Hospital Commission. Finally, the Faculty Council laid great emphasis upon the constitution of a Research Committee (see p. 287).[61]

So the logic of expanding the deanery was ineluctable: the more functions, the more help needed in the Dean's Office. In January 1964 William R. Feasby, a medical editor and 1937 graduate of the faculty, was appointed executive assistant to the dean, bringing about "major improvements in dealing with the university budget and research funds."[62] In 1965 Hamilton set up a tier of associate deans: Edward A. Sellers (basic science); Ian MacDonald (postgraduate medical education); Jan W. Steiner (student affairs – replacing William Spaulding who decamped for McMaster University); and Fred G. Kergin (in charge of integrating Sunnybrook).[63] Thus the apparatus the deans needed to manage complexity was growing rapidly.

## Lawrence Chute, 1966–73

The traditional medical school organization was laid down when its sole function was to train undergraduate medical students. Today, medical centres are multimillion dollar enterprises in which expenditures for research, graduate education and residency training far exceed expenditures for undergraduate education. The first four years of medical education is today but one of many programs in the medical center, and it no longer commands the prime time of the full-time faculty.[64]

Lawrence Chute, 1967–8

Andrew Lawrence ("Lawrie") Chute, who became dean of medicine in 1966, was recruited from the Department of Paediatrics, where he had been professor of pediatrics since 1952 (see p. 252).

During Chute's term of office, external relations took on an unprecedented importance. The faculty, hitherto devoted to undergraduate medical education, would have to negotiate with the teaching hospitals, the federal government, and the province over "the health-sciences centre." This would eat up large amounts of decanal energy (see pp. 306–315).

A second new issue in the decanal portfolio in the late 1960s was student unrest. Under the impact of student demands for a greater role in university governance, in the fall of 1968 the Faculty Council appointed an Ad Hoc Committee under surgeon Robert I. Mitchell to consider "Decision-making Processes in the Faculty of Medicine." At the same time, university governance as a whole was in upheaval, and a Presidential Commission on the Government of the University of Toronto was meeting. Both bodies ended up conceding greater student and staff participation, though to differing degrees. In June 1969 the Ad Hoc Committee submitted its report, recommending complex reforms.[65] The Faculty Council ended up being restructured: its 165 members now would be elected by constituency, including 34 ex officio members and 30 students. There will be "a semi-annual Faculty Assembly to receive reports from Council."[66]

Mainly of interest here, however, are Chute's own ideas about faculty governance, given that those prevailed. "[Dean Chute] believed it to be a departmental organization rather than a structure composed of the basic science departments and several hospitals. He expressed a preference for general

Faculty committees rather than committees whose members represent hospitals. The former preserves the concept of a medical school which is primarily an academic community." Chute also rejected egalitarian democracy: "The University is only a limited form of democracy. It cannot legislate knowledge and excellence." He therefore wanted the maintenance of a tradition of strong department chairs: "Department Chairmen have been appointed to contribute to the establishment of an excellent medical school."[67]

In retrospect, the storms of the student revolt were much ado about nothing. Members of the Faculty of Medicine never developed a lively interest in the Faculty Council, and the whole matter really passed into desuetude as the struggle to achieve even a quorum preoccupied further meetings of the council.

In the 1969–70 session Kager Wightman succeeded Ian MacDonald as associate dean of the postgraduate division. The job had become huge: the faculty now had over 1,000 interns, fellows, and residents, in 10 hospitals, under 13 university departments in addition to a large postgraduate medical education program.[68] In the winter of 1969 the Independent Planning Committee began meeting, chaired by Robert I. Harris. Though most of its plans were ultimately not implemented, its constant meetings through the first half of the 1970s provided a further decanal distraction.

### Brian Holmes, 1973–80

Holmes came to the Dean's Office in 1973 from the chair of radiology, and further information about his life may be found in that chapter (see p. 508). Holmes conducted a major reorganization of the deanery. He said in September 1973, "A review of the existing structure led to the concept of areas of responsibility and autonomy, not based on a pyramidal hierarchical structure, but on a cabinet system with portfolios. Each Associate Dean would hold one or more portfolios." Two of the portfolios related to "resources": associate dean of basic sciences, where George Connell, appointed in the 1971–2 session, replaced Sellers who had stepped down several years earlier; and associate dean of clinical sciences, where psychiatry chair Robin Hunter would inaugurate the portfolio. There would be three portfolios relating to "programmes and cross departmental lines": in future this would be organized as: (1) associate dean of postgraduate education and continuing education; (2) associate dean of undergraduate affairs; and (3) a new position, associate dean of research affairs. Among other new posts, Holmes was contemplating an associate dean of community affairs and associate dean of planning and operations. It would be too much to follow the changing incumbents of these many portfolios. The point is that the deanery was tenaciously pushing back against being crushed by the faculty's increasing size. Change would have to be administered and it would take a "cabinet system," as Holmes called it, to do the administering.[69]

Then Holmes had to wrestle with the faculty's "goals." Under the old-style deans such as MacFarlane the goal was just muddling through the evil of the day. MacFarlane apparently never anticipated such management concepts as objectives. But these concepts crept increasingly into the daily life of the Dean's Office. Apparently in response to a query from Vice President Connell and Provost Donald Chant, Holmes was asked late in 1975 to articulate the goals of the faculty for the 1980s. It is interesting what he did with the request. First, he responded with a point that had been in everyone's mind for decades: "Canada, in view of its population and resources, should have at least one medical school of world stature; that this medical school [U of T], because of its resources, its financial situation, and its setting, was probably in the best position of any in Canada to achieve world stature." How to make that happen? Holmes said, "In order to introduce significant changes, it would be necessary to state the goals clearly and precisely to ensure they are understood by everyone, and to get as full a commitment to them as possible throughout the Faculty." Thus, goal-oriented future talk originated not from outside management consultants, as one might be inclined to think, but from the very barons of the faculty themselves.[70]

Later, in 1977, Holmes devised still further administrative changes: an assistant dean of institutional affairs (hospitals); an assistant dean of continuing education; and an associate dean of academic affairs. As well, Holmes finally got the Senior Committee up and running.[71]

Was he just shifting the deck chairs? Not exactly. Behind this blizzard of portfolios lay the systematic transfer of power from the Faculty Council to the Dean's Office. Research, for example, had been in the hands of the Science Policy Committee, a committee of the Faculty Council. With the creation of an associate dean of research or a decanal Research Committee chaired by Aser Rothstein (which was Holmes's provisional concept), research shifted from legislative to executive control.[72] Hollenberg, a bear for tough executive authority, was thoroughly behind this move: "It is essential for the Dean to have the capability, with proper advice, of introducing new research developments in selected areas." The dean needed a research advisory committee.[73]

Holmes initiated another apparently technical administrative change of huge practical significance: having an external review of a department at the end of the chairman's term. Although ostensibly designed for "input" to the new search committee, it gave the dean substantial control over the briefing of the search committee, thus moulding the selection of the new departmental chair to suit the dean's wishes.[74] In this period the Faculty Council expressed great unhappiness about the erosion of its powers and in 1979 rejected the draft report of a Task Force on Faculty Governance chaired by anatomy chair Jim Thompson.[75]

### Fred Lowy, 1980–7

In retrospect, Fred Lowy was one of the great deans of the faculty. And the interesting thing is he knew he could do it. A member of the search committee that hired Lowy (and who wishes to remain anonymous) remembers from Lowy's big interview, "I don't think Fred Lowy was at the top of the list to begin with. During his interview, I remember him, he was at the end of the table, and he leaned over the table, and he said – remember he'd come from Montreal – 'In my wildest dreams, I never thought I'd be a candidate for this position. But you know what, I really want it, I really want to do this, and I think that I can do a good job.'"[76] And he did.

Three months after taking office in July 1980, he told the Faculty Council at his first appearance that his goal was clear: "Move the Faculty toward world stature in the 1980's."[77]

How to achieve this goal? He said later, "When I became Dean six years ago [1980], it was apparent that the primary need of the Faculty at that point was to strengthen our research activities."[78] To this end, in 1981 Lowy installed Keith Dorrington (who had been assistant dean of basic sciences) as associate dean of research, the first in that portfolio. By 1983 the Faculty Research Committee had concluded, "The faculty does not have an efficient mechanism for strategic planning in research"[79] (see also p. 299 in chapter 11).

Lowy was impatient with elaborate "mission statements" for the faculty. He said the medical school had basically two missions, training physicians and inculcating research. At a meeting of the Committee of Basic Science Chairman in March 1983 Lowy discussed the Faculty Mission Statement: "The objectives themselves are largely motherhood statements." He said the faculty essentially had two broad missions: "(1) To produce a substantial number of competent health care professionals; (2) Given the unique collection of tertiary care treatment facilities and the large concentration of biomedical scientists, the Faculty has an obligation to use these resources to mount graduate programmes and research programmes which are at the cutting edge of the field and among the best in Canada, and which are able to compete internationally."

But, Lowy said, in times of stringency the missions may be in conflict, for example, "in terms of the proportion of family practitioners to be trained vis-à-vis specialists." So, Lowy said, priorities are important: "The current mission statement attempts to project a sense of where the Faculty should be going. To this end it is proposed that priority should be given to scientific excellence and the education of people who will be leaders in the field, in contrast to placing as first priority the objective of simply training excellent physicians. It is assumed, however, that this medical school will do both."[80]

Research is well and good. But what were the faculty research priorities to be? In 1984 the research committee was reorganized, to be co-chaired by the associate dean of research and by one of the hospital research directors (in 1985 it was Donald Layne at TGH). By 1985 the research committee had worked out the faculty priorities: (1) neurobiology (hence the decanal post in neurosciences); (2) immunology and transplantation; (3) clinical epidemiology (from this sector David Naylor emerged as leader, then dean of medicine, then university president; a task force under John Evans had recommended policies and structures); (4) developmental and regulatory biology (here Alan Bernstein, Irving Fritz, and Jim Friesen were the movers); (5) molecular genetics and biology.[81] What the research committee sketched out in 1985 turned out to be the wave of the future.

To make the Dean's Office more efficient, Lowy divided the assistant and associate deans into two groups: those with "divisional" responsibilities (running departments) and those with "programmatic" responsibilities (education, etc.). When the faculty's administrative and development officers were added in, by 1984 the total in the Dean's Office was twelve administrators, including William Tatton as associate dean for neurosciences development, a post added that year.[82] (The argument was that the faculty had once appointed an associate dean for Sunnybrook development to integrate this veterans hospital into the faculty, so dedicating a portfolio to a substantive field did not seem like such a stretch.[83])

Lowy and Hollenberg drove forward the concept of long-term planning cycles, where the Department of Surgery had already led the way. In 1983 Hollenberg argued for a three-year cycle at the departmental level. Lowy seconded the idea: "The existence of such plans would strengthen the position of individual departments and of the Faculty as a whole in negotiations with the Central Administration."[84]

Part of planning was agreement across departments within a sector about hiring, called "complement planning." In the winter of 1986 anatomist Keith Moore, then associate dean of basic sciences, succeeded "for the first time in the faculty's history" in bringing together the basic science chairs in a joint planning effort around tenure complement. "They have agreed on mechanisms for interdepartmental review and decision-making on both specific appointments and recruitment policy." Complement planning was already in effect in the community health sector, under Eugene Vayda, associate dean of community health.[85] In April 1986 the basic science chairs had to work out the sector's academic strengths for future appointments. Moore proposed four areas: neurobiology (chair Harold Atwood); developmental biology (Martin Hollenberg); regulatory biology (David MacLennan); and application of new technology to the study of disease (Jim Friesen). Each group should be planning three to six appointments "for a total of approximately 24 positions."[86] In September Moore said that these planning reports "would be used when requesting new tenure-stream positions from Simcoe Hall." The report of the Neurobiology Planning Group in particular had been useful in planning for the new Centre for Neurodegenerative Disease.[87]

When George Connell, former head of biochemistry, became university president in 1984, there was a strong synergy between him and Lowy. Both were intent on boosting research. Connell's "renewal" document in 1987 called for reballasting the university onto a firm research platform. "Our objective, individually and collectively, should be to find our ways to the pinnacle of Parnassus. To reach the pinnacle a university must have a strong sense of corporate direction and a willingness to endure a substantial measure of pain."[88] When Lowy's deanship ended in 1987, this had pretty well been its overriding theme.

## John Dirks, 1987–91

John Herbert Dirks was the first dean of medicine who was neither a U of T graduate nor a member of the faculty (Lowy was a McGill graduate but had previously chaired the psychiatry department at Toronto). Dirks was hired away from the University of British Columbia (UBC), where he had been professor and head of medicine. Born in Winnipeg in 1933, he had graduated with an MD from the University of Manitoba in 1957. He trained in medicine at McGill from 1960 to 1962, then was a Medical Research Council fellow and visiting scientist at NIH from 1962 to 1965. He served as a nephrologist at McGill from 1965 until joining the Department of Medicine at UBC in 1976 as professor and head. Dirks was accustomed to the world of elite medicine and made clear his expectations to the colleagues. In an appearance at the faculty's education committee in October 1987 just after taking office, he offered, "Perhaps we should develop a tighter academic environment, e.g. Massey College [a campus think-tank]." It must have irritated the members to hear that "[t]he Arts and Science Faculty regard themselves as more intellectual and academic." The good news, said Dirks, was that Connell's "Renewal" promised better funding. After Dirks left the meeting, the committee members scoffed at several of his points.[89] Faculty pride in its research record clearly had been bruised.

The great pivot from the United Kingdom to the United States, already evident in the careers of Bernie Langer and Charlie Hollenberg, swung farther under Dirks, who preferred the more American style of McGill that he had come to know in his years there. He said in an interview that he attended McGill because Toronto was "very passive." "Attendance at grand rounds here was always sporadic," he said. "It was much better at McGill." Dirks contrasted the General with the Peter Bent Brigham Hospital in Boston, "where the leaders of cardiology were always in the front row."

Dirks also found past leadership in Toronto lacking in dynamism. "Until Hollenberg came [from McGill] they didn't have a builder here." Yet Toronto was "one of the unique situations in the world," he said, with all the University Avenue hospitals. "McGill's pediatric hospital was fifteen blocks away." Dirks revealed his admiration for Langer, Hollenberg, and Siminovitch, "the people who actually built things."

Dirks was attracted to Toronto because it was the hospitals that "could gather the money. They could move outside the departmental structure. Siminovitch could build at Mount Sinai." Dirks noted how jealous the basic science departments were of the hospital research institutes. "But over the long view the University was very fortunate: the research institutes were the foundation stone for the university community."[90]

In 1989, Dirks established an Office of International Relations, reporting directly to the dean.[91] This was an unsurprising move in view of his own global interests, and it is not startling that after he left the deanery in 1991 he became dean-rector of the Aga Khan University in Pakistan and chaired the International Society of Nephrology Commission for the Global Advancement of Nephrology, a worldwide organization with the mission of preventing chronic kidney disease. In 1983 Dirks joined the Medical Advisory Board of the Gairdner Foundation and in 1993 became president and scientific director of the foundation, propelling the Gairdner Awards into international prominence.

"When I was Dean, U of T had no money," Dirks said in an interview. "We were under pressure. The loss of accreditation would have been embarrassing." He realized that the Faculty of Medicine was being strangled by years of budget cuts. He said in 1990, "the current funding situation makes it difficult for the medical school to fulfill its mandate in the health care system, but the responsibility to do so is tremendous. How will we respond?" he asked.[92] In February 1989 Dirks hired the faculty's first professional fundraiser.[93] This was clearly the wave of the future.

These promising beginnings were unfortunately interrupted in a controversy in November 1991 over the dismissal of some nonacademic staff from the faculty, and Dirks stepped down.

### Harvey Anderson, Acting Dean, 1992

"When I assumed the position of Acting Dean in January," wrote Harvey Anderson later in 1992, "there was, both within the Faculty and within the central University administration, a sense of urgency that we tackle our problems."[94] Acting deans are usually associated with trimming the sails and waiting for the next full-time dean to catch the wind. This was not the case with the year that Harvey Anderson was in office. Anderson, a PhD nutritionist, had been chair of the Department of Nutrition (see pp. 444–445) and was one of the faculty all-around hitters, most recently associate dean of research and chair of the Faculty Research Committee, available for ad hoc leadership posts as they arose. This was a big one.

As Anderson took office, there was an urgent need to act on a budget plan, which would entitle the faculty to provostial funds. But no such plan was ready, so in May 1992 Anderson struck a committee for each of the three sectors – basic science, clinical science, and community health – to "examine budget, governance and strategic planning." "By the time that my term as Acting Dean is completed I would hope that the Faculty will have developed not only a workable budget and be in the implementation stage of curriculum renewal, but also have started to develop a strategic plan," he said.[95] In the fall of 1992, under Anderson, the Faculty Budget Committee put in place the first long-term budget plan, incorporating the severe cuts imposed by the province.

Anderson made changes in decision-making machinery: "Instead of the Decanal Team bearing full responsibility, we have adopted a process of extensive consultation and consensus building. The Executive Committee [all the deans plus executive chairs for the three sectors; in the financial crisis, the associate deans were eliminated] is responsible for identifying issues and suggesting policies. These ideas are then presented at the All Chairs meetings for further discussion … or approval. Thus, in our new administrative structure, the Chairs have assumed a much larger role in the decision making process." On the subject of academic matters Anderson said that the agenda committee of the Faculty Council considers these recommendations and passes them on. "Overall, we have taken major steps towards improved accountability throughout the Faculty. The new management structure ensures that we have the means to capture a broad-range of opinion and perspective which are imperative to effective decision making."[96] The stage was set for Arnie Aberman to stride upon.

### Arnold Aberman, 1992–9

Aberman became dean in 1992. Born in Montreal in 1943, he earned an MD from McGill University in 1967, then trained in medicine at the Royal Victoria Hospital in Montreal and Albert Einstein College of Medicine in the Bronx, New York. He specialized in pulmonary disease and shock, coming to Mount Sinai in 1973 and serving until 1989 as director of the Intensive Care Unit. Aberman rose very rapidly – indeed with preternatural speed – as an administrator. In 1977 he became physician-in-chief at Mount Sinai, at age thirty-four the youngest physician-in-chief among the Toronto teaching hospitals. In 1989 he became physician-in-chief of the newly created Toronto Hospital and presided over the merging of the twelve divisions of the Department of Medicine. In the same year he received the Eaton Professorship and during his tenure merged the six hospital-based departments of medicine into a single integrated university-based Department of Medicine with a single central budget. He was known for his fierce energy and organizing ability. "A little jumping jack," said Nell Farquharson. "You could pass his door, he had two phones to his ears and he was talking alternately to two people at the same time!"[97]

Under Aberman, events happened across a broad front. In the early 1990s the university was buzzing about "strategic directions" as for the first time this vast organization tried planning for change. Beginning in February 1992, Aberman led the "strategic directions" discussion for the Faculty of Medicine with its 4,000-plus academic faculty members. The single most important leadership issue was clear. As the strategic report that came out in November 1993 said, "Ten years ago, the Faculty could have been characterized as campus based with Clinical Departments situated in the teaching hospitals. Now basic science research activities have spread to hospital-based research institutes and community health activity is spreading across the broader health sciences complex."[98]

The faculty had, in other words, to reach out to the teaching hospitals and to the community as never before.

Simultaneously, Aberman had to manage internal events. In June 1993, the faculty received a new constitution. Aberman said,

> An important principle of our new Constitution is the separation of Faculty academic management (as represented by the Deans and Chairs) and Faculty governance (as represented by Faculty Council and its Speaker). In our previous constitution important standing committees of Council, eg the Undergraduate Medical Education Committee … were chaired by the Associate Deans responsible for those programs. Thus … Faculty governance was not independent of Faculty academic management. It was difficult for Faculty Council to assess properly proposals emanating from the Dean, when its key committees were chaired by representatives of the Dean. This lead to the appearance, if not the reality, that academic management (the Dean) had too much influence on governance (Faculty Council).

Under the new Constitution chairs of Faculty Council committees are elected by the Faculty Council. "Governance and academic management are now separated."[99]

There had been a University of Toronto Presidential Commission on the Health Sciences (the "Leyerle Commission"), which recommended in June 1993 in its final report "an increase in interaction and coordination among the health sciences … and a widening of the focus of activities concerning the determinants of health."[100] This set the stage for reaching out to the other health care faculties, such as nursing, pharmacy, and dentistry, to mount interfaculty programs.

Aberman made dramatic changes in the dean's corridor. He abolished the "sectoral" associate deans (basic, clinical, etc.). From now on, the department chairs reported directly to him and would come together in regular monthly meetings. "This new organization," he said, "has resulted in greater cohesion of the faculty." There was better communication and a "significant increase in academic collaboration."[101] Aberman restored other associate deans and appointed a vice-dean of research and a vice-dean of education. Reporting to the vice-dean of education would be the associate deans for continuing education, postgraduate medical education, student affairs, and undergraduate medical education. This was high time because big events were happening on the education front. In September 1993, Aberman reach an agreement with the Ministry of Health in which the first-year class was reduced in size from 252 to 177. But there were corresponding reductions in first-year resident (PGY1) slots as well.[102]

The backstory was this: in the early 1990s the province, upset about rising health care costs, wished to reduce the number of physicians, in the belief that reducing access to doctors would reduce costs. This meant reducing the size of the medical class in all the province's medical schools. Aberman recounted events from 1993: "When the government came to the five deans about this reduction, the other schools said they did not want to do it." But the University of Toronto, he said, "saw this as an opportunity." The U of T wanted to reduce its class size anyway, so "[w]hen all was said and done, we negotiated with the government to decrease our class by 75 spots, from 252 to 177." Yet Aberman also negotiated with the government not to reduce the operating grant. "We never in our wildest dreams thought that we could decrease from 250 to 175, because we thought we'd lose our budget, but we thought this was a terrific opportunity for us to reset the faculty ... That's how we reached that number. It was the desire of the government in Ontario, but it fit our strategic plan, so I'm quite happy to say we did it quite willingly."[103]

Yet Aberman had pared significantly the dean's corridor in the Medical Sciences Building.[104] Reporting to the dean himself were the thirty departmental chairs, the faculty administrative officer, and the fundraiser. Reporting to the vice-dean of research were twenty-four extra-departmental units, the free-standing centres and institutes that were beginning to populate the campus in an effort to break out of the rigid department structure.

As dean, Aberman restructured the finances of the faculty, with its 4,000 faculty members and an operating budget of over $100 million, turning a $2 million deficit into a $5 million surplus. And he did this by realizing savings, merging eight academic departments – pathology, microbiology, and clinical biochemistry went into the Department of Laboratory Medicine, for example – and trimming the size of the central administration. Meanwhile, he helped increase the faculty's research budget to over $200 million annually, making it among the largest in North America.

Aberman had to administer the sequelae of a major report by Richard Ten Cate, dentistry dean and vice-provost of health sciences, on faculty governance. In response, in the 1991–2 session, the faculty formed two Working Groups, both chaired by John Leyerle, former dean of the School of Graduate Studies. Working Group A studied health science education outside the Faculty of Medicine, which would lead to new undergraduate "non-professional health science programs." Working Group B studied changes needed in Faculty of Medicine and the teaching hospitals (the "Health Sciences Complex") needed "to achieve the vision of the Ten Cate Report." In January 1994, Aberman began the reorganization of the health sciences on the basis of Leyerle's working groups: (1) He acceded to the creation of the post of vice-provost of relations with health care institutions, which Aberman himself would fill in addition to being dean (the post of vice-provost of health sciences was abolished). (2) A provostial adviser on "Population Health" was to be appointed. (3) A Council of Health Science Deans was to be established to advise the provost.[105]

Thus Aberman had to coordinate programs among the health faculties. In January 1996, an Interprofessional Education Implementation Committee (IPE) among the health science faculties of U of T was formed to work on interdisciplinary offerings.[106]

When David Naylor took over as dean in July 1999, he assessed the strengths of the Aberman team: "They dealt effectively with unprecedented fiscal pressures by reducing layers of administration, streamlining overheads, selectively allocating budget cuts, and restructuring departments. The departmentalized organization of the Faculty was strengthened."[107] Aberman was not a researcher but an administrator and leader. And in those days the faculty needed leadership.

### David Naylor, 1999–2005

At lunch with David Naylor, I once casually remarked that the job of being dean must be exhausting. Naylor shrugged coolly and said, "I don't feel exhausted." It was a key to his style.

Christopher David Naylor was born in Woodstock, Ontario, in 1954 and studied arts at U of T, for two years. He was admitted to the medical program at the end of his second year, and graduated MD in 1978. Yet his upward course in medicine was interrupted by a four-year stint as a Rhodes Scholar at Oxford in the Department of Social and Administrative Studies, where he received a DPhil in 1983. Naylor thereupon trained in internal medicine at the University of Western Ontario, ending in 1983–5 as chief medical resident at Victoria Hospital in London, Ontario. Naylor's swerve towards epidemiology began with a year as a fellow of the Medical Research Council in clinical epidemiology, spent in 1987–8 at The Toronto Hospital. In 1990 Naylor joined the Clinical Epidemiology Unit at Sunnybrook as director; it was folded into the Institute for Clinical Evaluative Sciences (ICES) in 1992, of which he became the chief executive officer. In 1999 he became dean of medicine at U of T (and in 2005 president of the university).

At ICES Naylor took part in several important studies. It was actually Naylor who wrote finis to one of the great Toronto medical sagas: cold-heart surgery. In 1994, in an article in the *Lancet*, he and coworkers compared outcomes in cold- and warm-heart surgery – and found no difference. The investigators concluded, "Warm heart surgery is a safe and effective alternative to conventional hypothermic techniques for patients undergoing coronary bypass surgery."[108] In 1999 he and lead author David Alter determined that, even under Canada's supposedly universal health care system, patients who live in poorer neighbourhoods have a higher rate of mortality in heart attacks and experience greater difficulty in accessing services. The study, based on almost 52,000 heart attack patients tracked between April 1994 and March 1997, was published in the *New England Journal of Medicine*, the flagship journal of North American medicine.[109]

As Naylor began his deanship, it was, to paraphrase Dickens, the best of times, the worst of times. The financial challenges that Dirks and Aberman had faced had not gone away. From 1987–8 to 2001–2, provincial operating grants per university student in Ontario fell 33 percent in constant dollar terms and were in 2002 lowest of all Canadian provinces. In the previous six years, Ontario's per-university-student funding declined by 3 percent, whereas the average state funding in the United States rose by 37 percent.[110]

Meanwhile, demands were rising. The provostial White Paper "Raising Our Sights" of January 1999 had emphasized the "research-intensive nature of the faculty" and, as Naylor put it, initiated new funding demands in the area of "inter-departmental, inter-institutional and inter-faculty collaboration."[111] There was also an explosion of interest in the health sciences among undergraduates. Naylor said, "Scholars in the Faculty of Medicine are being called upon to do an ever-increasing amount of teaching in other professional programs and especially in Arts and Science. In lockstep, the related graduate programs within the Faculty are expanding steadily. These are very positive developments." But they must be funded. On the bright side, the faculty had lots of new sources of income, for example, from practice plan income and outside grants to hospital budget support. "The emergence of the CIHR [Canadian Institutes of Health Research] could provide an unprecedented level of support for all our research enterprises. These observations suggest a pressing need for a new capital plan that will give the Faculty of Medicine room to grow and develop." Therefore, "[t]he bottom line is simple: The Faculty is in an excellent position move forward rapidly … The next few years should be an exciting period of renewal!"[112]

Naylor drew the decanal team on board, in four administrative clusters within the faculty: clinical medicine, basic science, community health, and rehabilitation science. He created a new portfolio, associate dean of interfaculty and graduate affairs, which Catharine Whiteside agreed to administer, simply because the devolution of the School of Graduate Studies had shifted much work onto faculty departments with graduate units.[113] New decanal portfolios were created for legal affairs and public policy matters.[114] To manage this sprawling "Dean's Corridor," Naylor created a kind of inner circle, or "Dean's Group," led by the dean and including the dean's executive and the chairs from the faculty's four sectors.[115]

The Strategic Plan for 2000–4 that the faculty worked out in response to the White Paper placed great emphasis on "international leadership" in order to "challenge the boundaries of health research, creating knowledge from 'genes to populations' and from 'molecules to communities.'" The plan stated baldly, "The Faculty of Medicine at the University of Toronto is Canada's pre-eminent School of Medicine and one of the leading Faculties in the world. It ranks second worldwide to Harvard Medical School in peer review publications, and places among the top North American schools in attracting research funding."

Thus, just a medical school? Not at all! The plan said, "The Faculty of Medicine is much more than a medical school as it comprises departments of basic science, community health, and rehabilitation, in addition to clinical science." The Health Sciences Complex included as well eight teaching hospitals. Indeed, the hospitals had raced ahead of the faculty, for in 2000 there were forty-six hospital-based endowed chairs and only twenty-five university-based chairs.[116]

The plan offered a snapshot of the duchy that Naylor now had to lead: "4,790 academic faculty spanning the University campus and affiliated teaching hospitals and agencies. These faculty members represent one of the largest pools of intellectual and academic talent in North America." Of these 1,812 are full-time. Of the full-time, 206 are tenured or tenure-stream. Most of the total faculty are paid through the teaching hospitals, the clinical practice plans, or other sources, not by the university.[117]

The funding picture started to brighten. In June 2000 the CIHR was officially launched, with a budget of $402 million in 2000–1 and soon to become much larger. Toronto's Alan Bernstein was president of the organization, which numbered thirteen separate "institutes," classified by discipline.[118] In 2000, as Peter Lewis, vice-dean of research, later put it, the "total research funding trendline" took a dramatic turn upwards.[119] To give a sense of order of magnitude, in 1978 the total annual funding for research available to the faculty was $431,000; in the 2001–2 session, in terms of funds administered by the university and the teaching hospitals, it was $346 million.[120]

Added to this federal money came the many donations from the university fundraising drive. By January 2004 the U of T fundraising campaign, started in 1997, had raised $1 billion, of which $230 million was for the Faculty of Medicine. The number of endowed chairs at the university had increased to 175. "In addition, over 80 joint chairs were created with the teaching hospitals … An endowment of nearly $500M for student aid has been created, making the University of Toronto the first Canadian university to guarantee financial accessibility to all qualified students. More than 107,000 donors contributed to the campaign – 45,000 of them for the first time. Nearly sixty-six percent of donations came from individuals and eighteen percent from corporations. The remainder came from foundations and organizations."[121] These were really spectacular results and the envy of many other institutions.

Under Naylor, the vexing practice plans were finally tamed. In May 2002, a provostial Task Force on Clinical Faculty laid down explicit principles for them: "Competitive and financially unrestricted private practice is incompatible with academic goals. Group practices with distributed earnings to support the academic mission are the norm to ensure academic productivity." There were to be explicit academic job descriptions, to let individuals know the performance standards under which they would be judged. And the plans "must have economic mechanisms that support and reward academic activity."[122] It was now clear that all staff physicians in teaching settings were putting their shoulders in some manner to the research and education wheel, not just making money.

This task force eventuated in a Memorandum of Agreement, dated 31 January 2003 and signed by President Robert Birgenau, covering a number of other points not discussed in this volume.[123] In December 2004 the whole package was accepted by the Governing Council, "end[ing] more than a quarter-century of ambiguity about the status of clinical faculty, passing a new clinical faculty policy that sets out a taxonomy for academic appointments of clinical faculty, clarifies access to perquisites and a dispute resolution mechanism for clinical colleagues."[124]

Naylor stepped down from the deanship in 2005 to accept the presidency of the university. The tenure of Dean Catharine Whiteside, which began in 2005 and continues at this writing, will not be considered here except to note that she is the first female dean – and the only dean of medicine at the University of Toronto ever to have been reappointed to a second term!

The Edinburgh and Toronto faculties are two of the wisest in the world. I think that is significant.[1]

Clarence Starr, Professor of Surgery, University of Toronto, 1923

Some things never change. In 1923 the faculty was mindful of its place in the world, but its world was the Commonwealth. Today as well faculty rankings are avidly scanned to see where the faculty ranks in the pecking order, but its world is the globe. "We are truly a global player," Dean Whiteside told the faculty in May 2009. "Toronto's global reach in discovery, translation, and advanced training should never be underestimated ... We are one of the top ranked institutions in health and life sciences in North America and globally."[2]

The story started in 1887 with the faculty as a magnet for farm boys from rural Ontario. The story finds its provisional end at the beginning of the new millennium with Toronto as a global "life-science" capital. Enthused a journalist in 2008, apropos a rush in building hospital Research Institutes, "Toronto is witnessing a health-care building boom the likes of which it hasn't seen in decades." In the new lab building of the children's hospital, the labs would front onto the street. Said Janet Rossant, chief of research at HSC, "You'll be looking at the scientists scribbling on a whiteboard, or drinking a cup of coffee and waving their hands as they get excited about a project."[3]

There was a lot to wave hands about. According to Robert Bell, president and CEO of the University Health Network, in 2008, "The University of Toronto and its affiliated hospitals generate more published health research than any of its publicly funded counterparts in North America."[4]

Lured by the glittering lifestyle of Metro Toronto – in contrast to the "hogtown" of yore – and by the faculty's reputation, students came flocking into the residency programs. In 2009, for the second year in a row, the faculty filled all of its 367 residency positions in the first round of the annual Canadian residency matching program (CaRMS), the only medical school in Canada to do so. A second round of balloting was not necessary. Said Sarita Verma, vice-dean of postgraduate medical education, "This is no mean feat, given the competitive recruitment environment across Canada. These students can pick from anywhere in the country and they want to come here. It's not just that people want to live in Toronto. We have the perfect recipe: a great program, incredible faculty, fantastic applicants and the best environment in which to learn, with both research-oriented hospitals and community hospitals as partners." She noted that since 2000, the faculty had increased its intake of residents in specialties by 31 percent and in family medicine positions by 70 percent.[5]

As these students and trainees have gone out into the world, they have left a big footprint. Dean Whiteside said in 2009, "Since the early 1980s the University of Toronto has trained close to 50% of the family physicians in Ontario and 25% of all the specialist physicians in Canada."[6]

By the beginning of the new millennium, the Faculty of Medicine of the University of Toronto was the largest in Canada and ranked academically towards the top of the list in North America. In the 2007–8 session the total expenditure on research alone within TAHSN (Toronto Academic Health Sciences Network) was about a billion dollars a year.[7] The university faculty numbered over 5,000. The twenty-six departments offered seventy-five specialty training programs leading to certification by the Royal College.[8]

When Art Slutsky, vice-president of research at St Michael's Hospital, enlists outside scientists for the hospital, he doesn't say, "Here are our people at St Michael's." He tells them, "Look at the city, you can collaborate. All these people are a 20-minute walk away."[9]

Why has the Faculty of Medicine of the University of Toronto been so successful? Throughout the book one can see one factor: the university marching together, as a single medical school, with the eight great teaching hospitals. But there's more. And it goes back to the wars of the twentieth century. As two external reviewers of the university Department of Surgery noted in 2002, "The collegiality is striking at the University of Toronto in relationships between department heads and departments."[10]

There is something very Canadian about this, an easy "clubability" that arose with those who served as medical officers in the two world wars and were accustomed to collegial solidarity rather than individual advancement. Other countries fought in the war, too, of course, but I as a historian have never seen anything comparable to the sense of patriotic duty that infused the young medical officers of 1914 and 1939. After demobilization they continued to be comrades as well as colleagues. And this tradition was handed on in such places as the boardrooms of the banks and the coffee rooms of the departments of the Faculty of Medicine.

By the new millennium, memories of the war had faded. Yet this collegiality remained, and there was perhaps no better expression of it than the willingness of full-time clinical faculty in all the teaching hospitals to enter voluntarily into group practice plans that, as a decanal document put it in 2006, "distribute earnings to support the joint (university and hospital) institutional academic mission and the scholarly activity of the faculty members." Dean Whiteside noted the importance of "a collegial relationship" among department chairs, the hospital division heads, and the elected practice plan leaders in "establishing the most successful clinical academic enterprise in Canada."[11]

But there is something more to this story than just being agreeable, for if success boiled down to jolly getting along, the Boy Scouts would rule the world. There is a steelier element than mere niceness and it is called leadership. This faculty has thrived in the world of science and research because it has had several generations of strong leaders, men and women who were not arrogant or bullies, and who did not come across as titans, yet who were in some way titans because they stood head and shoulders above the others.

There are two clearly defined generations of such leaders, and while comparisons are always odious – the faculty had hundreds of important and distinguished figures – nonetheless at the end of this long odyssey, two groups of men stand out. And they are alas all men, although future historians may well celebrate the leadership of the current dean Cathy Whiteside. It is striking that the two generations are as different from each other as cheese and chalk, though both had the ability to inspire others, which is the essence of leadership.

The main figures in the first leadership generation of the years from 1930 to 1960 were all from small towns, mostly in Ontario. W.E. Gallie stemmed from Barrie; Joe MacFarlane was born on a farm in Lanark County; Ray Farquharson came from Claude, Ontario; and Kager Wightman from Sandwich, Ontario. Nobody has ever heard of any of these places, with the possible exception of Barrie (which nobody outside of Ontario has ever heard of). Charles Best grew up in a small town in Maine, with deep roots in Canada's Maritimes. These five men had the ability to lash the wagon train forward, but with the exception of Best, it was not the research wagon train. They influenced their generation by providing models of the learned, thoughtful clinician and scholar, the physician as diligent investigator yet broadly learned academic – and caring colleague. All were wonderful colleagues and treasured by their contemporaries as models of what young physicians should become. They laid the foundation of a faculty that was to become one of the top twenty or so in the world. This was no mean achievement.

The second leadership generation is still with us for the most part at this writing. Again, comparisons are difficult because in the last thirty years this faculty has spun off so many memorable figures whose presence fills these pages. Yet in terms of their ability to inspire others, in their profile of what the clinician-scientist and academic leader should represent, they too loom above their colleagues.

Yet how different they are from the first generation. They are all city boys. Fred Lowy, Lou Siminovitch, and Arnie Aberman all grew up in Montreal! Charlie Hollenberg came from Winnipeg and Bernie Langer from Toronto. Strikingly, all are Jews, and this in a faculty that until the beginning of the 1960s was markedly anti-Semitic. They had, unlike the first generation, no unifying vision of how they wanted young doctors to be formed, but they had a vision of science. They knew the clinic and the lab and how to get from basic and translational research to discoveries that would benefit humankind. It is not that they themselves were pioneering investigators, because leaders rarely commit themselves to the single-minded intensity required for scientific breakthroughs. But they knew how to inspire others to such breakthroughs. And if the Faculty of Medicine of the University of Toronto has become an international heavyweight, it owes more to their influence than that of any other individuals.

If any single lesson emerges from this book, it is the importance of such leaders in building institutions and inspiring those that people them. So the take-home message for public policy is, how does one continue to cultivate such leadership figures? How must one structure the life of a faculty such as this, so that gifted leaders continue to rise up from the huddled masses in the labs and the clinics and become deans and heads and professors? As I look back at their individual biographies, I am somewhat puzzled, to tell the truth. That the second generation is entirely of Jewish origin tells us something of the importance of struggling against prejudice – for all of them experienced it at various points. It is hard to distil the magic leadership formula in a bottle and sell it in a drugstore. But as I look out at the faculty today and see the energetic young men and women from the far-flung corners of the world – in 2006, 54 percent of students in the university as a whole were from "visible minorities"[12] – I know that the next historian who takes up the story of this faculty will have a lot to say about people who experienced early challenges not because of their religion but because of the colour of their skin.

The take-home message is that large investments of taxpayer money plus a judicious research strategy – clinician-scientist programs and close collaboration with the hospitals – have made the University of Toronto one of the world's best. All this research contributed useful knowledge for the improvement of the human condition. As Dean Whiteside said in 2010, "We believe that, in creating new knowledge and applying that new knowledge, our contributions will not only improve the health of Canadians but will have impact on the health of individuals globally."[13]

# Acknowledgments

A project such as this has debts. Some concern support. The Faculty of Medicine made available funds for conducting the research. Other debts concern the investment of time and energy required to dig out the story from the archives and libraries, and it must be said that the University of Toronto Archives have done their utmost to yield a great volume of documents. Among the researchers who helped search this material were Heather Dichter, Daniel Peleschuk, Jonathan Ruelens, and Ellen Tulchinsky. Susan Bélanger has functioned as chief coordinating officer, and it is fair to say that without her able and thoughtful assistance the task would have taken decades rather than mere years.

I am indebted to a number of faculty members who have offered critical feedback on portions of the book or indeed on the entirety of it: Arnold Aberman, Peter Alberti, Mary Jane Ashley, Harold Atwood, Edna Becker, Michael Bliss, Robert Byrick, Peter Carlen, Richard Cobbold, John Court, Donald Cowan, Bernard Cummings, Ross Fleming, Judith Friedland, Charles Godfrey, David Goldbloom, Bernard Goldman, Jack Laidlaw, Bernard Langer, David MacLennan, David Naylor, Allan Okey, Marian Packham, Gordon Potts, Kenneth Pritzker, Michael Ratcliffe, Reinhardt Reithmeier, Knox Ritchie, Stephen Scherer, Bernard Schimmer, Louis Siminovitch, James Till, Mladen Vranic, and Catharine Whiteside.

Edward Shorter<br>
December 2011

# Notes

**Abbreviations in Photo Captions and References**

AO: Archives of Ontario, Toronto

HMP: History of Medicine Program, Faculty of Medicine, University of Toronto, Picture collection

HSC: Hospital for Sick Children, Toronto

MSH: Mount Sinai Hospital

TGH: Toronto General Hospital

MSH: Sunnybrook Hospital/Health Sciences Centre

TTH: The Toronto Hospital (product of 1986 merger between the Toronto General and Toronto Western Hospitals)

UHN: University Health Network (product of 1999 merger between TTH and the Princess Margaret Hospital)

UTA: University of Toronto Archives

WCH: Women's College Hospital

## Note on Sources

The story of the Faculty of Medicine and its academic hospital partners has been drawn extensively from primary sources found in the archives and libraries of the Toronto Academic Health Sciences Network, and from first-person interviews. Additional information has been provided from the private archives of the Dean of Medicine, from various university and hospital departments, and from individuals involved in the history of medicine in Toronto.

Internal reports and newsletters produced by the university and its hospital affiliates also proved invaluable for chronicling developments and for filling in many of the human interest stories. Particularly useful publications include the University of Toronto's yearbook *Torontonensis*; the medical students' comic magazine *Epistaxis*; faculty newsletters and magazines (*MedEmail, Tablet,*

*UToronto Medicine*); and departmental bulletins such as the Department of Medicine's *MediNews* and the Department of Surgery's *Surgical Spotlight.*

## 1 Introduction

> At this writing (early 2013), the Toronto Academic Health Science Network consists of nine fully affiliated research hospitals: Baycrest; Centre for Addiction and Mental Health (College Street, Queen Street sites); Holland Bloorview Kids Rehabilitation Hospital; Hospital for Sick Children; Mount Sinai Hospital; St. Michael's Hospital; Sunnybrook Health Sciences Centre; University Health Network (consisting of the Toronto General Hospital, Princess Margaret Hospital, Toronto Western Hospital, and Toronto Rehabilitation Institute) and Women's College Hospital. In addition it includes 19 community hospitals and clinical care sites. However, the composition of the network (and thus the number of affiliates) has varied historically. The terminology used throughout the volume reflects this changing landscape. (University of Toronto, Faculty of Medicine, *Dean's Report* 2011–2, 3, 9)

1  See David Crawford, "Histories of Canadian Hospitals and Schools of Nursing," http://internatlibs.mcgill.ca/hospitals/hospital-histories.htm; accessed 12 Oct. 2012; the seminal work here is James T.H. Connor, "Hospital History in Canada and the United States," *Canadian Bulletin of Medical History* 7 (1990): 93–104.

2  See Murray L. Barr, *A Century of Medicine at Western* (London, Ontario: University of Western Ontario, 1977); John W. Scott, *The History of the Faculty of Medicine of the University of Alberta, 1913–1963* (Edmonton: University of Alberta, 1963).

3  See, however, Alice Miller, "A Blueprint for Defining Health: Making Medical Genetics in Canada, c. 1935–1975" (PhD diss., Graduate Programme in History, York University, 2000); yet Miller's excellent study comparing Toronto and London, Ontario, goes only to the mid-1970s.

4  Knox Ritchie interview with Susan Bélanger, 19 Mar. 2010.

5  Barnet Berris, *Medicine: My Story* (Toronto: University of Toronto Press, 2001), 72–3.

6  James Till interview with Edward Shorter, 26 Nov. 2009.

7  W.G. Bigelow, *Cold Hearts: The Story of Hypothermia and the Pacemaker in Heart Surgery* (Toronto: McClelland and Stewart, 1984), 9.

8  Catharine Whiteside, "Message from the Dean," *MedEmail*, 5 Apr. 2006.

## 2 At the Corner of College and University

1  Townsend Ludington, ed., *The Fourteenth Chronicle: Letters and Diaries of John Dos Passos* (Boston: Gambit, 1973), 100–1.

2  Abraham Flexner, *Medical Education in the United States and Canada: A Report to the Carnegie Foundation for the Advancement of Teaching* (New York: Carnegie Foundation, 1910; bulletin no. 4), 323.

3 University of Toronto, Faculty of Medicine, *Report of the Dean* [hereafter *Dean's Report*], 1949–50, 3.

4 Fred Lowy, interview, *Tablet* 3, no. 2 (Fall 1987): 6.

5 Quoted from *Annual Report, Department of Medicine, 1966/67*, cited in Hill, "History of the Department of Medicine," MS, 1977, p. 28; Department of Medicine Archive.

6 "Strategic Directions for the Faculty of Medicine," Nov. 1993; Dean's Archive.

7 Wendy Levinson, *MediNews* (Department of Medicine newsletter), Dec. 2004, 1; http://www.deptmedicine.utoronto.ca/Medinews.htm.

8 Faculty of Medicine, University of Toronto, *Academic Plan, 2004–2010: International Leadership in Health Research and Education*, 98,. http://www.facmed.utoronto.ca/ Assets/FacMed+Digital+Assets/Faculty+of+Medicine+1/FacMed+Digital+Assets/ about/2010plan.pdf?method=1

9 Eliot Phillipson, *MediNews*, May 2000, 2.

10 Louis Siminovitch to David Naylor, undated letter, 2007 or 2008; I am grateful to Professor Siminovitch for a copy.

11 *Dean's Report* 1953–4, 3.

12 Jack Laidlaw personal communication, 30 Sept. 2010.

13 R.M.H. Pinkerton, head of ophthalmology, Queen's University, to Dean Brian Holmes, 22 Nov. 1979; UTA A1985/0026/004 (026).

14 Faculty Council minutes, 24 June 1969, 336; UTA A1993/0025/007.

15 Ibid.

16 L.E. Ferris, P.A. Singer, and C.D. Naylor, "Better Governance in Academic Health Sciences Centres: Moving Beyond the Olivieri/Apotex Affair in Toronto," *Journal of Medical Ethics* 30 (2004): 25–9, 26.

17 Robert Byrick, personal communication, 28 Oct. 2010.

18 William Boyd, *Textbook of Pathology: Structure and Function in Disease*, 8th ed. (Philadelphia: Lea & Febiger, 1970), vi.

## 3  An Afternoon in October 1903

1 [Alexander Primrose], "Ceremonies in Connection with the Opening of the New Medical Building, Toronto, October 1st, 1903," 36; UTA A1979/0023/1001 (2). Loudon also mentioned the United States in the same sentence, yet the "Mother Land" meant England.

2 John P.M. Court, "An Erosion of Imagination: Unfulfilled Plans for a University Botanical Gardens and Taddle Creek, 1850 to 1884," *Ontario History* 95, no. 2 (2003): 174, 186n37.

3 Michael Bliss, *William Osler: A Life in Medicine* (Toronto: University of Toronto Press, 1999), 463.

4 [Alexander Primrose], "Ceremonies in Connection with the Opening of the New Laboratories, Erected for the Faculty of Medicine of the University of Toronto" [1903], 15–16; UTA A1979/0023/1001 (02). Bowditch did not actually come to Toronto, and his talk was read by a deputy.

5  This account is based on a series of anonymous accounts, evidently authored by Alexander Primrose, secretary of the faculty, entitled "History of the Faculty of Medicine" and now in UTA A79/0023/1001(01). On his typing of material from the secretary's office, see Primrose remarks, Faculty Council, 8 Jan. 1932, 284; UTA A1986/0027/020.

6  Faculty Council, 2 Oct. 1914, 1536; UTA A1986/0027/017. Sources diverge on the beginning of Reeve's tenure at Toronto General Hospital. I accept 1872, the date given in the obituary in *BMJ* 1 (15 Feb. 1909): 202.

7  "Richard Andrews Reeve," Faculty Council, 4 Apr. 1919, 92; UTA 1986/0027/018.

8  I.H. Cameron and J.T. Fotheringham, "The Inauguration of New Medical Laboratories," *University of Toronto Monthly* 4 (Oct. 1903): 10–25, 13.

9  Ibid., 21.

10  [Primrose], "Ceremonies in Connection with the Opening of the New Laboratories," 7.

11  W.R. Feasby, "A Short History of the University of Toronto Medical Faculty, Part VI: The New Era: 1903–1914," *Medical Graduate* 28, no. 1 (Fall 1983): 14–17, 14. On the floor plan, see A.B. Macallum, "The New Medical Buildings of the University of Toronto," *Science*, n.s., 17 (22 May 1903): 813–17.

12  University of Toronto, *President's Report*[hereafter *President's Report* 1965–6, 69.

13  [Primrose], "Ceremonies in Connection with the Opening of the New Laboratories," 9.

14  Ibid.

15  Ibid., 31–2.

16  "German System Not Followed in Medical Faculty," *Toronto Daily Star*, 30 Jan. 1923.

17  *Torontonensis*, University of Toronto yearbook (1903), 129, 141.

18  Ibid., 138.

19  See Charles Godfrey, *Aikins of the U of T Medical Faculty* (Madoc, ON: Codam, 1998).

20  R.I. Harris, "Alexander Primrose, 1861–1944," *Canadian Journal of Surgery* 1 (1958): 183–8.

21  Primrose remarks, Faculty Council, 8 Jan. 1932, 282; UTA A1986/0027/020.

22  Faculty Council, 8 Jan. 1932, 281; UTA A1986/0027/020; see also *President's Report* 1931–2, 1–2. On Primrose's career, see Eulogy, Faculty Council, 6 Apr. 1944, 327–9; UTA A1986/0027/023 (02).

23  Faculty Council, 5 Feb. 1932, 316; UTA A1986/0027/020.

24  Cameron and Fotheringham, "Inauguration of New Medical Laboratories," 25.

25  Dean A.L. Chute, *Dean's Report* 1967–8, 3–4.

26  James H. Richardson to President James Loudon, 27 June 1899; UTA A79/0023/1001(01).

27  J.T.H. Connor, *Doing Good: The Life of Toronto's General Hospital* (Toronto: University of Toronto Press, 2000), 65.

28  William Canniff, *The Medical Profession in Upper Canada, 1753–1850* (Toronto: Briggs, 1894, repr., Hannah Institute for the History of Medicine, 1980), 61–2, 100–1, 534–6.

29  Richardson to Loudon, 27 June 1899.

30  For details, see Richardson to Loudon, 27 June 1899. Information on Nicol from *MedEmail* (Faculty of Medicine newsletter), 7 June 2004.

31  For a careful description of this early period see Canniff, *Medical Profession in Upper Canada*, and Jabez H. Elliott, "The Medical Faculty of the University of Toronto: Its Early History and Development," *Messenger of the Theta Kappa Psi Medical Fraternity* 34 (1937): 87–93.

32  For details see Canniff, *Medical Profession in Upper Canada*, and A.B. McKillop, *Matters of Mind: The University in Ontario, 1791–1951* (Toronto: University of Toronto Press, 1994), 57–62.

33  Charles Morris Godfrey, "The Evolution of Medical Education in Ontario" (master's thesis, Institute for the History and Philosophy of Science and Technology, 1974), 35.

34  *Annual Announcement of the Toronto School of Medicine, in Affiliation with The University of Toronto and The University of Victoria College … 1878–1879* (Toronto: Guardian, 1878).

35  "History of the Medical Faculty," *Torontonensis* (1904), 109.

36  R.D. Gidney and W.P.J. Millar, "The Reorientation of Medical Education in Late Nineteenth-century Ontario: The Proprietary Medical Schools and the Founding of the Faculty of Medicine at the University of Toronto," *Journal of the History of Medicine and Allied Sciences* 49 (1994): 52–78, 54.

37  *Torontonensis* (1909), 174.

38  Lykke de la Cour and Rose Sheinin, "The Ontario Medical College for Women, 1883–1906: Lessons from Gender-Separatism in Medical Education," *Canadian Woman Studies* 7, no. 3 (1984): 73–7.

39  See the brief biography in "100th Anniversary of Women at U of T," UTA A1994/0012/05.

40  Based on Martin L. Friedland, *The University of Toronto: A History* (Toronto: University of Toronto Press, 2002), 205; Godfrey, "Evolution of Medical Education," 117–20; "History, Ontario Medical College for Women," *Torontonensis* (1906), 189; *Torontonensis* (1907), 168.

41  *Torontonensis* (1909), 174.

42  *Torontonensis* (1907), 168.

43  Alexander Primrose (?), "Historical Sketch of Medical Faculty," *Torontonensis* (1903), 123–4.

44  Marianne P. Fedunkiw, *Rockefeller Foundation Funding and Medical Education in Toronto, Montreal, and Halifax* (Montreal: McGill-Queen's University Press, 2005), 16.

45  [Alexander Primrose], "History of the Faculty of Medicine (cont'd)," UTA A1979/0023/1001(01), 2.

46  Sandra F. McRae, "A.B. Macallum and Physiology at the University of Toronto," in *Physiology in the American Context*, ed. Gerald L. Geison (Bethesda, MD: American Physiological Society, 1987), 97–114, 101.

47  Primrose (?),"Historical Sketch of Medical Faculty," 124.

48  McRae, "A.B. Macallum," 101.

49  David R. Keane, "Aikins, William Thomas," in *Dictionary of Canadian Biography Online*, vol. 12, *1891–1900*; http://www.biographi.ca.

50  See ibid.

51  Charles W. Harris, "William Thomas Aikins," *Canadian Journal of Surgery* 5 (1962): 131–7, 137.

52  See, for example, Helen M. Dingwall, *A History of Scottish Medicine: Themes and Influences* (Edinburgh: Edinburgh University Press, 2003); and Matthew H. Kaufman, *Medical Teaching in Edinburgh during the 18th and 19th Centuries* (Edinburgh: Royal College of Surgeons of Edinburgh, 2003).

53  Godfrey, *Aikins of the U of T*, 279.

54  Flexner, *Medical Education in the United States and Canada*, 323.

55  Friedland, *University of Toronto: A History*, 132.

56  Pauline M.H. Mazumdar, "Anatomy, Physiology and Surgery: Physiology Teaching in Early Nineteenth-Century London," *Canadian Bulletin of Medical History* 4 (1987): 119–43, 138.

57  John P.M. Court, "Recruiting a Scientific Enigma: Ramsay Wright at the University of Toronto and Its Reconstituted Medical School, 1874–1912," *Historical Studies in Education* 22, no. 1 (Spring 2010): 61–81.

58  Gidney and Millar, "Reorientation of Medical Education," 65.

59  Cameron and Fotheringham, "Inauguration of New Medical Laboratories," 23.

60  Elrid Gordon Young, *The Development of Biochemistry in Canada* (Toronto: University of Toronto Press, 1976), 6.

61  A.B. Macallum, "The Development of Physiology and Biochemistry in Canada," in *Royal Society of Canada, Fifty Years Retrospect, Anniversary Volume 1882–1932* (Ottawa: Royal Society of Canada, [1932]), 163–5.

62  "J.B.L. [John Beresforde Leathes]," *Obituary Notices of Fellows of the Royal Society* 1 (Dec. 1934): 287–91, 288.

63  McRae, "A.B. Macallum," 101.

64  John P.M. Court, "Introducing Darwinism to Toronto's Post-1887 Reconstituted Medical School," *Canadian Bulletin of Medical History*.28 (2011), 191–212, 204–5. *The Maritime Medical News* 1, no. 5 (July 1889) to 4, no. 9 (Sept. 1892). The deception was dropped by altering the text beginning with the next edition, 4, no. 10 (Oct. 1892).

65  Faculty of Medicine, *Calendar*, 1892–3, 12.

66  *Calendar*, 1894–5, 107.

67  Ibid., 106.

68  "Class of '03 Medicine," *Torontonensis* (1903), 128.

69  *Torontonensis* (1902), 115.

70 William Edward Gallie, "The University of Toronto Medical School: Fifty Years' Growth," *Medical Graduate* 111 (1956–7): 6–13, 7.

71 "Class of '03 Medicine," 128.

72 Alexander Primrose, "Memorandum Prepared by the Faculty of Medicine of the University of Toronto as a Memorial to be Presented to the University Commission Lately Appointed by the Government of Ontario to Deal with Certain Matters Concerning the University of Toronto," 27 Nov. 1905, 4, 18–19; UTA A1979/0023/1001(02).

## 4 Getting Going

1 Obstetrician Kennedy C. McIlwraith, testifying at a provincial hearing. "Hospital Teaching Remains Efficient," *Globe*, 12 Jan. 1923.

2 *President's Report* 1933–4, 19.

3 "Class of '05: Annual Bulletin," no. 3 (July 1909), 1 (copy in UTA).

4 "Death Notice," *JAMA* 33 (15 July 1899): 175.

5 H. Barrie Fairley, "Recollections of the Toronto General Hospital and the University of Toronto, 1955–1969," in *A Commemorative History of the Department of Anaesthesia,* ed. Robert J. Byrick (Toronto: Department of Anaesthesia, 2004), 109–35, 110–11.

6 Toronto General Hospital [hereafter TGH], *Annual Report* 1905, 23.

7 Ibid., 23–4.

8 Alexander Primrose biographical file, UTA A1973/0026/368 (86), unsourced clipping of 15 Dec. 1926.

9 "Dean Primrose Gives Past. Pres. and Future of Medical Faculty," *Varsity*, 18 Feb. 1921.

10 *President's Report* 1934–5, 33–4, and standard biographical sources.

11 Alexander McPhedran eulogy, Faculty Council, 1 Feb. 1935; UTA A1986/0027/021.

12 Gallie, "Fifty Years' Growth," 10.

13 Ibid., 7.

14 University of Toronto, Faculty of Medicine, *Tablet*, 1989 (quarterly tabloid; copy in UTA).

15 "Dr Duncan Graham," undated; Faculty Council, session 1972–3; UTA A1993/0025/007.

16 Arthur H. Squires, "Too Much a Scientist?" *CMAJ* 141 (15 Nov. 1989): 1066–7; the book was Robert B. Kerr and Douglas Waugh, *Duncan Graham: Medical Reformer and Educator* (Toronto: Dundurn Press, 1989).

17 Faculty Council, 31 May 1923, 122; UTA A1986/0027/018.

18 Ibid.

19 Michael Bliss, personal communication, 18 Aug. 2010.

20 "Department of Medicine"; UTA A1979/0023/002, 3.

21 This account of William Goldie's role in Duncan Graham's appointment is taken from "First Full-Time Professor of Medicine," *Tablet*, Summer 1989, 10.

22 These details in "Duncan Graham to University President Sidney Smith," 22 Feb. 1946; Department of Medicine Archive.
23 Faculty Council, 16 Sept. 1932.
24 Wightman, *Dean's Report* 1968–9, 71.
25 Draft agreement of 12 Jan. 1946, between Flora McCrea, Lady Eaton, and the T. Eaton Co. Limited and the Governors of the University of Toronto; Department of Medicine Archive.
26 Duncan Graham to Sydney Smith, 22 Feb. 1946.
27 Decker to Chairman, Board of Trustees, TGH, 27 Jan. 1932; University Health Network Archives [hereafter UHN Archives], TGH Fonds, sub-series 2.1: Reports to Board of Trustees, Box 13, File 2.1.7. Superintendent's Report 1931.
28 See the anonymous editorial, hostile to Graham, in *Canadian Journal of Medicine and Surgery*, 53 (1923), 201–21.
29 *President's Report* 1919–20, 9.
30 Robert Falconer to "Dear Sir," 19 Oct. 1921; Department of Medicine Archive.
31 Duncan Graham, "Focal Infection," *CMAJ* 25 (Oct. 1931): 422–4, 423.
32 "William Goldie," Faculty Council, 2 Feb. 1929, 110–12.
33 *Torontonensis* (1915), 163; "Historical File," Department of Medicine Archive.
34 *Prophylaxis* [formerly *Epistaxis*] (1947), 7.
35 James Goodwin interview with Edward Shorter, 10 Sept. 2009, 23.
36 *Torontonensis* (1913), 139.
37 Gallie, "Fifty Years' Growth," 10.
38 Godfrey, *Aikins of the U of T.*
39 Some details from a eulogy at retirement, "Irving Heward Cameron," Faculty Council, 28 Oct. 1920, 300–2; UTA A1986/0027/018.
40 On the dating of these events, see Faculty of Medicine *Calendar* 1913–14, 24–5.
41 Anonymous eulogy, Faculty Council, 6 Apr. 1934.
42 C.W. Harris, "Irving Heward Cameron (1855–1933)," *Canadian Journal of Surgery* 8 (1965): 131–6, 133.
43 Ibid., 135.
44 Faculty Council, 6 Oct. 1933.
45 George A. Peters, "Transplantation of Ureters into Rectum by an Extraperitoneal Method for Exstrophy of Bladder, and a New Operation for Procidentia Recti in the Same Patient," *British Medical Journal* [*BMJ*] 1 (22 June 1901): 1538–42.
46 W.E. Gallie, "George Armstrong Peters (As I Remember Him)," *Canadian Journal of Surgery* 2 (1959): 119–22, 120.
47 George Armstrong Peters obituary, *BMJ* 1 (4 May 1907), 1095.
48 Gallie, "Fifty Years' Growth," 8.
49 George A. Peters, "A Demonstration of a New and Original Method of Making Casts," *BMJ* 2 (3 Sept. 1898): 621–4.
50 Gallie, "Peters," 119.
51 Ibid., 121.

52 "University of Toronto Department of Surgery and Clinical Surgery," 16 Feb. 1920; UTA A1979/0023/002.

53 Faculty Council, 31 Dec. 1919, 138; UTA A1986/0027/018; Newton Albert Powell, the professor of medical jurisprudence, had discussed possible Rockefeller aid to Canadian medical education with George E. Vincent of the Foundation; UTA A1986/0027/018.

54 Fedunkiw, *Rockefeller*, 47.

55 "University of Toronto Department of Surgery and Clinical Surgery," 16 Feb. 1920; UTA A1979/0023/002.

56 Faculty Council, 1 Mar. 1920, 168–9.

57 "Clarence Leslie Starr," Faculty Council, 2 Feb. 1929; UTA A1986/0027/020.

58 Faculty Council, 27 May 1921, 391; UTA A1986/0027/018.

59 Editorial, *Canadian Journal of Medicine and Surgery* 53 (1923): 201–21, 202–3.

60 On these rather stormy events, see Fedunkiw, *Rockefeller*, 63–80.

61 *President's Report* 1922–3, 15–16.

62 "CL Starr Urges Fair Trial for Reorganization," *Toronto Daily Star*, 12 Jan. 1923.

63 "German System Not Followed in Medical Faculty," *Toronto Daily Star*, 30 Jan. 1923.

64 *Report of Special Committee Appointed by the Legislature to Inquire into the Organization and Administration of the University of Toronto* (Toronto: Legislative Assembly of Ontario, 1923).

65 Faculty Council, 2 Feb. 1929, 109.

66 *Torontonensis* (1909), 187.

67 On Robertson's life, see Robert Craig Brown, "Robertson, Lawrence Bruce," in *Dictionary of Canadian Biography Online*, vol. 15, *1921–1930*; http://www.biographi.ca; Peter H. Pinkerton, "Canada's Transfusion Pioneer: Lawrence Bruce Robertson," *Transfusion* 41 (2001): 283–6.

68 Lawrence Bruce Robertson, "Blood Transfusion," *CMAJ* 4 (1914): 501–7.

69 L. Bruce Robertson, "The Transfusion of Whole Blood: A Suggestion for Its More Frequent Employment in War Surgery," *BMJ* 2 (8 July 1916): 38–40, 38.

70 Brown, "Robertson, Lawrence Bruce."

71 Bruce Robertson, "Blood Transfusion in Haemorrhagic Disease of the Newborn," *BMJ* 1 (28 May 1921): 791.

72 Bruce Robertson, "Blood Transfusion in Severe Burns in Infants and Young Children," *CMAJ* 11 (1921): 744–50.

73 G. Kerr Cross, "Report on Blood Transfusion Work Seen in the Hospital for Sick Children, Toronto, Canada," *British Journal of Children's Diseases* 21 (1924): 173–82, 182.

74 *Essays in Surgery Presented to Dr WE Gallie on the Occasion of His Retirement from the Chair of Surgery in the University of Toronto* (Toronto: University of Toronto Press, 1950), xiii.

75 Joseph MacFarlane, "Dr WE Gallie"; UTA A1976/0054/018 (14).

76 *Surgical Spotlight* [Department of Surgery newsletter] Summer 2007, 8.
77 W.E. Gallie and D.E. Robertson, "The Repair of Bone," *British Journal of Surgery* 7 (1919): 211–61.
78 See W.E. Gallie and A.B. LeMesurier, "The Use of Living Sutures in Operative Surgery," *CMAJ* 11 (1921): 504–13.
79 W.E. Gallie and A.B. LeMesurier, "A Clinical and Experimental Study of the Free Transplantation of Fascia and Tendon," *Journal of Bone and Joint Surgery* 4 (1922): 600–12, 612.
80 "World-Noted Surgeon Dr. W. E. Gallie Dies," *Toronto Daily Star*, 26 Sept. 1959.
81 W.E. Gallie and A.B. LeMesurier, "Living Sutures in the Treatment of Hernia," *CMAJ* 13 (1923): 469–80, 480.
82 Bigelow, *Cold Hearts*, 20.
83 *Dean's Report* 1931–2, 36.
84 Ibid., 35–37.
85 *Dean's Report* 1934–5, 40–41.
86 William Gallie, "Report of Undergraduate Teaching, Department of Surgery, Jan 1938"; UTA A1989/0030/001.
87 W.G. Bigelow, "Donald Walter Gordon Murray," In Memoriam, Faculty Council, date not given; UTA A1993/0025/007, meetings 1974–5. Murray died 7 Jan. 1986.
88 *Epistaxis* (March 1920), 3.
89 Shelley McKellar, *Surgical Limits: The Life of Gordon Murray* (Toronto: University of Toronto Press, 2003), 25–30.
90 Ibid.
91 For a scholarly account of the heparin story, see J.A. Marcum, "The Development of Heparin in Toronto," *Journal of the History of Medicine* 52 (1997): 310–37.
92 W.G. Bigelow, *Mysterious Heparin: The Key to Open Heart Surgery* (Toronto: McGraw-Hill, 1990), 58.
93 *Dean's Report* 1934–5, 41.
94 *Dean's Report* 1935–6, 42.
95 D.W.G. Murray, L.B. Jaques, T.S. Perrett, and C.H. Best, "Heparin and the Thrombosis of Veins Following Injury," *Surgery* 2 (1937): 163–87. See also D.W.G. Murray and C.H. Best, "Heparin and Thrombosis: The Present Situation," *JAMA* 110 (8 Jan. 1938): 118–19.
96 *President's Report* 1936–7, 7, 67.
97 *Dean's Report* 1937–8, 50.
98 Ibid.
99 Gordon Murray, "Heparin in Thrombosis and Blood Vessel Surgery," *Surgery, Gynecology & Obstetrics* 72 (1941): 340–4; the paper had been presented in October 1940.
100 Berris, *Medicine: My Story*, 24.
101 *Dean's Report* 1938–9, 55–6.
102 Bigelow, *Mysterious Heparin*, 108.
103 Susan E. Bélanger, *Continuing the Banting Legacy: The Banting Research Foundation, 1925–1995: 70 Years of Medical Research in Canada* (Toronto: Banting Research Foundation, 1995), 40.

104 Faculty Council, 17 Sept. 1920, 275; UTA 1986/0027/018.

105 *Epistaxis* (1926), 17.

106 Michael Bliss, *The Discovery of Insulin: 25th Anniversary Edition* (Chicago: University of Chicago Press, 2007; originally published in 1982 by University of Toronto Press), 53, citing Banting's 1922 account of the discovery of insulin, Thomas Fisher Rare Book Library, University of Toronto, MS. COLL. 76 (Banting papers), box 37, folder 2. This document, written in response to Col. Albert Gooderham's request that each of the co-discoverers write an account of the discovery of insulin, has been published along with Best's and Collip's statements with an introduction by Michael Bliss as "Banting's, Best's and Collip's Accounts of the Discovery of Insulin," *Bulletin of the History of Medicine* 56 (1982): 554–68.

107 Macleod's account of these events, written September 1922, "History of the Researches Leading to the Discovery of Insulin," together with some addenda, may be found at UTA A1979/0007/008(01).

108 Bliss, *Discovery of Insulin*, 46–7, 54–5.

109 Ibid., 56–7 and 253n39; Banting, 1922 account. Sources disagree on the exact date of his return to Toronto, but Bliss thinks it more likely that the meetings with Macleod resumed in May, which agrees with Macleod's "History of the Researches."

110 Mladen Vranic, "The Physiology Department, University of Toronto, 1887–1921," in *The Discovery of Insulin at the University of Toronto: An Exhibition Commemorating the 75th Anniversary*, ed. Katharine Martyn (Toronto: University of Toronto Library, 1996), 9–12.

111 Macleod, "History of the Researches."

112 Bliss, *Discovery of Insulin*, 63.

113 Mark Jurdjevic and Caitlin Tillman, "E.C. Noble in June 1921, and His Account of the Discovery of Insulin," *Bulletin of the History of Medicine* 78 (2004): 864–75. This source also reveals that although Best spent most of the summer working with Banting, Noble filled in during the latter half of June while Best was away training with the militia.

114 Bliss, *Discovery of Insulin*, 58 and 254n47.

115 Henry B.M. Best, *Margaret and Charley: The Personal Story of Dr. Charles Best, the Co-Discoverer of Insulin* (Toronto: Dundurn Group, 2003), 47.

116 Banting, 1922 account.

117 Bliss, *Discovery of Insulin*, 68–73.

118 Macleod to Banting, 23 Aug. 1921, Fisher Library, MS COLL 76, box 62, folder 4. Emphasis as in original.

119 Bliss, *Discovery of Insulin*, 68.

120 Ibid., 78–9.

121 Macleod, "History of the Researches."

122 Bliss, *Discovery of Insulin*, 82–4.

123 Banting, 1922 account.

124 Macleod, "History of the Researches."

125 Bliss, *Discovery of Insulin*, 90–1 and 104–8, 108.

126 F.G. Banting and C.H. Best, "The Internal Secretion of the Pancreas," *Journal of Laboratory and Clinical Medicine* 7 (1922): 251–66, 265.

127 Bliss, *Discovery of Insulin.*, 98.

128 Alison Li, *J.B. Collip and the Development of Medical Research in Canada: Extracts and Enterprise* (Montreal: McGill-Queen's University Press, 2003), xii.

129 Macleod, "History of the Researches."

130 H. Best, *Margaret and Charley*, 60.

131 *Epistaxis* (1921), 20.

132 Macleod, "History of the Researches."

133 Charles Best talk at Canadian National Exhibition, 19 Aug. 1977; reprinted in *Quoddy Tides* (Eastport, ME), 14 Oct. 1977, 21–3.

134 Bliss, *Discovery of Insulin*, 112–20, 118.

135 Banting, 1922 account.

136 Sir Frederick Banting, "The Story of the Discovery of Insulin," Fisher Library, MS COLL 76, box 1, folders 9–13; also quoted in Bliss, *Discovery of Insulin*, 118.

137 C.H. Best, typescript letter to Sir Henry Dale, 22 Feb. 1954, 5, Fisher Library, MS COLL 235 (William R. Feasby Papers), box 3, folder 5.

138 H. Best, *Margaret and Charley*, 65.

139 F.G. Banting, C.H. Best, J.B. Collip, W.R. Campbell, and A.A. Fletcher, "Pancreatic Extracts in the Treatment of Diabetes Mellitus," *CMAJ* 12 (Mar. 1922): 141–6.

140 *Toronto Daily Star*, 22 Mar. 1922, clipping in Fisher Library, MS COLL 76, Banting scrapbook 1, box 1, p. 3.

141 Bliss, *Discovery of Insulin*, 125, 127–8.

142 Ibid., 129–34, 129. (Bliss notes at p. 130 that such failures were not uncommon in the early development of biologicals; purifying the hormone thyroxin, for example, took "years of effort and hundreds of thousands of dollars.")

143 Ibid., 131–41.

144 Hill, "History of the Department of Medicine," 5.

145 Decker to Chairman, Board of Trustees, TGH, 27 Jan 1932; UHN AR, TGH Fonds, sub-series 2.1: Reports to Board of Trustees, box 13, file 2.1.7.; Superintendent's Report 1931.

146 Connor, *Doing Good*, 209.

147 J.J.R. Macleod and W.R. Campbell, *Insulin: Its Use in the Treatment of Diabetes, Part I – Physiology, Part II – Clinical Section* (Baltimore: Williams & Wilkins, 1925), viii.

148 W.R. Campbell, "Some Aspects of the Management of the Diabetic Patient," *Canadian Public Health Journal* 28 (1937): 318–26.

149 Bigelow, *Mysterious Heparin*, 45.

150 Bliss, *Discovery of Insulin*.

151 Ibid., 196–200, 197.

152 Macleod to Col. Albert Gooderham, 20 Sept. 1922, attached to David Campbell to G.E. Hall, 11 Jan. 1949; UTA A1979/0007/008(01). A copy of the letter was found in the papers of Macleod's sister-in-law after her death.

153 J.J.R. Macleod, "History of the Researches Leading to the Discovery of Insulin," copy updated by Macleod in May 1923; UTA A1979/0007/008(01).

154 Bliss, *Discovery of Insulin*, 229–31.

155 John James Rickard Macleod, *Carbohydrate Metabolism and Insulin* (London: Longmans, 1926).

156 S.K. [Seymour Kanowitch], "The Insulin Committee," UTA A1983/0036/11 (2); the Banting letter was attached to this document.

157 Seymour Kanowitch, "The Banting Research Foundation," 26 July 1978; UTA A1983/0036/011 (06).

158 "Special Report by the Honorary Secretaries of the Banting Research Foundation," Mar. 1946; UTA A1983/0036/011 (06).

159 Faculty of Medicine *Calendar*, 1889–90, 11.

160 William Oldright tribute, Faculty Council, 2 Dec 1910; UTA A1986/0027.

161 For an account of Sheard's life that does not give details of his academic career, see Heather MacDougall, "Sheard, Charles," in *Dictionary of Canadian Biography Online*, vol. 15, *1921–1930*; http://www.biographi.ca.

162 For the dating of these early chairs, which largely existed in the absence of departments, I rely upon Faculty of Medicine *Calendar*, 1913–14, 27–8.

163 Paul A. Bator with Andrew J. Rhodes, *Within Reach of Everyone: A History of the University of Toronto School of Hygiene and the Connaught Laboratories*, vol. 1, *1927 to 1955* (Ottawa: Canadian Public Health Association, 1990), 13.

164 Donald T. Fraser, Various Departments Postgrad Training, 12 Dec. 1945, UTA A1988/0010/001(07).

165 James FitzGerald, *What Disturbs Our Blood: A Son's Quest to Redeem the Past* (Toronto: Random House, 2010), 202–3.

166 These details of FitzGerald's early life are from C.B. Farrar, "I Remember JG FitzGerald," *American Journal of Psychiatry* 120 (1963): 49–52.

167 Italian psychiatrist Ugo Cerletti, quoted on his experiences in the years following World War I in Edward Shorter, *A History of Psychiatry from the Era of the Asylum to the Age of Prozac* (New York: John Wiley & Sons, 1995), 218.

168 Christopher J. Rutty, "Personality, Politics, and Canadian Public Health: The Origins of the Connaught Medical Research Laboratories, University of Toronto, 1888–1917," in *Essays in Honour of Michael Bliss: Figuring the Social*, ed. E.A. Heaman et al. (Toronto: University of Toronto Press, 2008), 273–303, 283.

169 FitzGerald, *What Disturbs*, 217–24, 217 and 220.

170 Farrar, "JG FitzGerald," 49.

171 FitzGerald, *What Disturbs*, 222, 234–5.

172 James FitzGerald interview in Canadian Medical Hall of Fame, "Dr. John Gerald FitzGerald" (videotaped documentary, 2004), available at http://www.cdnmedhall.org/dr-john-gerald-fitzgerald, accessed 3 May 2009).

173 James FitzGerald, "The Troubled Healer," *University of Toronto Magazine*, Spring 2002, 86–93.

174 Robert D. Defries, *The First Forty Years, 1914–1955: Connaught Medical Research Laboratories, University of Toronto* (Toronto: University of Toronto Press, 1968), 5.

175 Bator and Rhodes, *Within Reach,* 1:18.

176 "Can Prevent Deaths from Diphtheria," *Globe,* 20 Dec. 1920.

177 Defries, *First Forty Years,* 63–6.

178 FitzGerald, *What Disturbs,* 263.

179 Bator and Rhodes, *Within Reach,* 1:13, 15.

180 FitzGerald, *What Disturbs,* 267.

181 Bator and Rhodes, *Within Reach,* 1:28.

182 *President's Report* 1923–4, 14–15.

183 *Dean's Report* 1923–4, 7.

184 FitzGerald, *What Disturbs,* 291.

185 Ibid., 304.

186 *President's Report* 1923–4, 14–15.

187 "Obituary: Robert Davies Defries," *Canadian Journal of Public Health* 66 (1975): 510–12; Bator and Rhodes, *Within Reach,* 1:15, 21; Defries, *First Forty Years,* 9, 20–1.

188 "Obituary: Robert Davies Defries," 511; Bator and Rhodes, *Within Reach,* 1:118.

189 1955 Winners, Albert Lasker Public Service Award, http://www.laskerfoundation. org/awards/1955_p_description.htm#defries.

190 FitzGerald, *What Disturbs,* 232–3.

191 *Torontonensis* (1911), 162.

192 Bator and Rhodes, *Within Reach,* 1:15, 21.

193 "Obituary: Robert Davies Defries," 511.

194 FitzGerald, *What Disturbs,* 233.

195 Donald Thomas Fraser, Faculty Council, 1 Oct. 1954, 15–16; UTA A1986/0027/ 026.

196 D.T. Fraser et al., "Tetanus Toxoid and Its Use for Active Immunization," *American Journal of Public Health* 33 (1943): 1107–14.

197 Bator and Rhodes, *Within Reach,* 1:51.

198 Ibid., 71.

199 Ibid., 122.

200 "Speech to the Senate on Passing of DT Fraser, Oct 1954"; UTA A1976/0054/018(9). John MacFarlane was eulogist.

201 Bator and Rhodes, *Within Reach,* 1:38.

202 *Torontonensis* (1921), 134.

203 FitzGerald, *What Disturbs,* 340.

204 Paul A. Bator, *Within Reach of Everyone: A History of the University of Toronto School of Hygiene and Connaught Laboratories Limited,* vol. 2, *1955 to 1975, with an Update to the 1990s* (Ottawa: Canadian Public Health Association, 1995), 43.

205 FitzGerald, *What Disturbs,* 341.

206 Bator and Rhodes, *Within Reach,* 1:38 and 191nn33–4.

207 Ibid., 1:38.

208 Defries, *First Forty Years,* 102.

209 Bator and Rhodes, *Within Reach*, 1:126.

210 For details of Charles Best's illness, see H. Best, *Margaret and Charley*, 389–97.

211 Name of eulogist not given. "Charles Herbert Best," Faculty Council Minutes, Sept. 1977–May 1978, 269; UTA A1993/0025/009.

212 George R. Minot and William P. Murphy, "Treatment of Pernicious Anemia by a Special Diet," *JAMA* 87 (1926): 470–6.

213 E.W. McHenry, E.S. Mills, and R.F. Farquharson, "The Treatment of Pernicious Anaemia by the Intramuscular Administration of Liver Extract," *CMAJ* 28 (1933): 123–32, 132; see also Defries, *First Forty Years*, 121–3.

214 William Henry Howell and [Luther] Emmett Holt, "Two New Factors in Blood Coagulation – Heparin and Pro-Antithrombin," *American Journal of Physiology* 47 (1918): 328–41. See also Charles H. Best, "Preparation of Heparin and Its Use in the First Clinical Cases," *Circulation* 19 (1959): 79–86; Jay McLean, "The Discovery of Heparin," *Circulation* 19 (1959): 75–8.

215 Defries, *First Forty Years*, 123–5.

216 D.Y. Solandt and C.H. Best, "Heparin and Coronary Thrombosis in Experimental Animals," *Lancet* 2 (16 July 1938): 130–2, 131; see also Charles H. Best, "Heparin and Thrombosis," *BMJ* 2 (12 Nov. 1938): 977–82.

217 D.Y. Solandt, Reginald Nassim, and C.H. Best, "Production and Prevention of Cardiac Mural Thrombosis in Dogs," *Lancet* 234 (9 Sept. 1939): 592–5.

218 Defries, *First Forty Years*, 120–1; R.B. Kerr, C.H. Best, W.R. Campbell, and A.A. Fletcher, "Protamine Insulin," *CMAJ* 34 (1936): 400–1; see also W.R. Campbell, A.A. Fletcher, and R.B. Kerr, "Protamine Insulin in the Treatment of Diabetes Mellitus," *American Journal of the Medical Sciences* 192 (1936): 589–600.

219 R.B. Kerr and C.H. Best, "The Effects of Protamine Insulin and Related Compounds in Normal and Depancreatized Dogs," *American Journal of the Medical Sciences* 194 (1937): 149–59.

220 Ibid., 112–19.

221 "To Human Race," *Hamilton Spectator*, 15 Dec. 1938.

222 FitzGerald, *What Disturbs*, 344.

223 Bator and Rhodes, *Within Reach*, 1:46.

224 FitzGerald, *What Disturbs*, 344–5.

225 Bator and Rhodes, *Within Reach*, 1:38.

226 Defries, *First Forty Years*, 114.

227 Bator and Rhodes, *Within Reach*, 1:122.

228 Ibid., 38.

229 Ibid., 122.

230 Ibid., 42–6.

231 *Dean's Report* 1932–3, 18.

232 Bator and Rhodes, *Within Reach*, 1:52–3.

233 Bator, *Within Reach*, 2:81.

234 Jane Lewis, "The Prevention of Diphtheria in Canada and Britain, 1914–1945," *Journal of Social History* 20 (1986): 163–86, 165.

235  Christopher J. Rutty, "Connaught and the Defeat of Diphtheria," *Conntact* 9 (Feb. 1996): 11; http://www.healthheritageresearch.com/Diphtheria-conn9602.html.

236  Bator and Rhodes, *Within Reach*, 1:52–3.

237  Mary A. Ross and Neil E. McKinnon, "The Efficiency of Toxoid in Controlling Diphtheria," *Canadian Public Health Journal* 22 (1931): 333–41, 341. See also N.E. McKinnon, Mary A. Ross, and R.D. Defries, "Reduction in Diphtheria in 36,000 Toronto School Children as a Result of an Immunization Campaign," *Canadian Public Health Journal* 22 (1931): 217–23; J.G. FitzGerald, R.D. Defries, D.T. Fraser, P.J. Moloney, and N.E. McKinnon, "Experiences with Diphtheria Toxoid in Canada," *American Journal of Public Health* 22 (1932): 25–8.

238  FitzGerald, *What Disturbs*, 290.

239  Ibid., 291; Lewis, "Prevention of Diphtheria," 163–86.

240  James FitzGerald interview with Edward Shorter, 9 Apr. 2009.

241  FitzGerald, *What Disturbs*, 321.

242  Ibid., 348–9.

243  Ibid., 353.

244  FitzGerald interview with Edward Shorter, 7 Apr. 2009.

245  John F. FitzGerald remarks, Faculty Council, Jan. 8, 1932, 288; UTA A1986/0027/020.

246  FitzGerald, *What Disturbs*, 327, 366–7.

247  FitzGerald interview, 7 Apr. 2009.

248  FitzGerald, *What Disturbs*, 372–4.

249  FitzGerald, "Troubled Healer," 93.

250  It was told briefly by Friedland, *University of Toronto: A History*, 291.

251  Catharine Whiteside, "Dean's Message," *MedEmail*, 12 Nov. 2008.

252  Alexander Primrose, remarks, Faculty Council, 8 Jan. 1932, 287; UTA A1986/0027/020.

253  K.J.R. Wightman to A.L. Chute, 29 Apr. 1969; Department of Medicine Archive.

254  Editorial, *Globe and Mail*, 18 Aug. 1937 (a manually copied typescript is in Department of Medicine Archive).

255  William Goldie to Cody, 5 July 1944; Department of Medicine Archive.

256  For these details see Graham to Smith, 22 Feb. 1946.

## 5  Big Deeds

1  Goodwin interview, 10 Sept. 2009, 22.

2  "New Medical Arts Building," [Toronto] *Globe*, 18 May 1928, 18.

3  Kellogg Questionnaire, 13 Dec. 1945; UTA A1986/0028/011.

4  *President's Report* 1954–5, 23.

5  *Dean's Report* 1948–9, 18.

6  See presentation of Wilbur Howard Harris at the Academy of Medicine meeting of 21 June 1914 and the comment of Wallace Scott in the discussion. "Academy of Medicine," proceedings, *Dominion Medical Monthly* 43 (1914): 13–14.

7  The Starr detail is from anonymous, "Some Notes on the History of Neurosurgery in Toronto," 1958; UTA A1976/0054/18 (13).
8  E.H. Botterell, "Dr Kenneth George McKenzie: An Appreciation," *CMAJ* 91 (17 Oct. 1964): 880–1.
9  *Dean's Report* 1923–4, 9.
10  Thomas P. Morley, "Biographical Sketch of Kenneth G. McKenzie (1892–1964)," *Journal of Neurosurgery* 93 (2000): 518–25, see 522.
11  E. Harry Botterell, "Kenneth George McKenzie," *Surgical Neurology* 17 (1982): 81–9.
12  Anonymous, "Some Notes on the History of Neurosurgery."
13  Charles G. Drake, "Perspectives from Dr. Charles Drake: Early Training in Toronto," *Canadian Journal of Neurological Sciences* 26 (1999): 331–3.
14  Kenneth G. McKenzie, "The Surgical Treatment of Spasmodic Torticollis," *Clinical Neurosurgery* 2 (1955): 37–43, 37, 42–43.
15  Morley, "Biographical Sketch McKenzie , 523.
16  J. Max Findlay, "Neurosurgery at the Toronto General Hospital, 1924–1990: Part 1," *Canadian Journal of Neurological Sciences* 21 (1994): 146–58, see 147.
17  Kenneth G. McKenzie and Lorne D. Proctor, "Bilateral Frontal Lobe Leucotomy in the Treatment of Mental Disease," *CMAJ* 55 (1946): 433–41, 436, 440.
18  Dean AR 1944–5, 31.
19  Morley, "Biographical Sketch of Kenneth G. McKenzie," 518–25.
20  *Dean's Report* 1929–30, 11.
21  *Dean's Report* 1937–8, 49–50.
22  Ronald R. Tasker, "E. Harry Botterell," *Surgical Neurology* 21 (1984): 215–17, 215.
23  John Russell Silver, *History of the Treatment of Spinal Injuries* (New York: Kluwer, 2003), 137.
24  Findlay, "Neurosurgery at the Toronto General Hospital," 151.
25  Silver, History of the Treatment of Spinal Injuries., 138.
26  *Dean's Report* 1944–5, 36.
27  Findlay, "Neurosurgery at the Toronto General Hospital," 152.
28  Silver, *History of the Treatment*, 142.
29  Quoted in Geoffrey Reaume, *Lyndhurst: Canada's First Rehabilitation Centre for People with Spinal Cord Injuries, 1945–1998* (Montreal: McGill-Queen's University Press, 2007), 42.
30  *Dean's Report* 1945–6, 37.
31  T.P. Morley, "Botterell the Leader," *Canadian Journal of Neurological Sciences* 26 (1999): 233–4.
32  F. Gentili, "EH Botterell's Contributions to Cerebrovascular Surgery," *Canadian Journal of Neurological Sciences* 26 (1999): 243–4, 243.
33  E.H. Botterell, W.M. Lougheed, J.W. Scott, and S.L. Vandewater, "Hypothermia, and Interruption of Carotid, or Carotid and Vertebral Circulation, in the Surgical Management of Intracranial Aneurysms," *Journal of Neurosurgery* 13 (1956): 1–42.
34  Gentili, "Botterell's Contributions , 4.

35  J.F. Ross Fleming, "Botterell the Teacher," *Canadian Journal of Neurological Sciences,* 26 (1999), 235–6.

36  Findlay, "Neurosurgery at the Toronto General Hospital," 155.

37  J. Max Findlay and William S. Tucker, "William John Horsey, M.D., F.R.C.S.C.: Neurosurgeon to St. Michael's Hospital, Toronto," *Canadian Journal of Neurological Sciences* 20 (1993): 254–5.

38  H. Hamlin, W.H. Sweet, and W.M. Lougheed, "Surgical Reconstruction of Occluded Cervical Carotid Artery: Report of a Successful Case with 4-year Follow Up," *Journal of Neurosurgery* 15 (1958): 427–37, see 431.

39  See on this J. Max Findlay, "William M. Lougheed and the Development of Vascular Neurosurgery at the Toronto General Hospital," *Canadian Journal of Neurological Sciences* 20 (1993): 337–40, 339.

40  "Ingenuity, Innovation and Intuition: Remembering Bill Lougheed," *Surgical Spotlight* [U of T Department of Surgery], Spring 2005, 13–14.

41  W.M. Lougheed and D.S. Kahn, "Circumvention of Anoxia during Arrest of Cerebral Circulation for Intracranial Surgery," *Journal of Neurosurgery* 12 (1955): 226–55.

42  Botterell et al., "Hypothermia, and Interruption of Carotid, or Carotid and Vertebral Circulation," 1–42.

43  Ibid., 2–3.

44  Findlay, "William M. Lougheed," 338.

45  David Naylor, personal communication to Edward Shorter, 7 Jan. 2013.

46  Ronald R. Tasker, "One Man's Recollection of 50 Years of Functional and Stereotactic Neurosurgery," *Neurosurgery* 55 (2004): 968–76.

47  H.J. Hoffman, "An Odyssey of a Pediatric Neurosurgeon," *Child's Nervous System* 14 (1998): 207–9, 207.

48  Robin P. Humphreys, "The History of Pediatric Neurosurgery," in *Principles and Practice of Pediatric Neurosurgery,* 2nd ed., ed. A. Leland Albright et al. (New York: Thieme, 2008), 3–11, 7.

49  Robin Humphreys, "A Sixty Year History of the Division of Neurosurgery at the Hospital for Sick Children," http://www.surg.med.utoronto.ca/NEURO/sickkids.html. See also Robin Humphreys, "The History of Neurosurgery at the Hospital for Sick Children in Toronto," *Neurosurgery* 61 (2007): 612–25.

50  *Dean's Report* 1934–5, 41.

51  *Dean's Report* 1944–5, 36.

52  Harold J. Hoffman, "Dr. William S. Keith," *Child's Nervous System* 3 (1987): 195–6.

53  Ross Fleming, "William Strathearn Keith," *Canadian Journal of Neurological Sciences* 15 (1988): 165–6.

54  [Harold Hoffman], "Dr. Edward Bruce Hendrick," *The Neurotransmitter* [Hospital for Sick Children, Division of Neurosurgery newsletter] 6 (Winter 2002): 4.

55  Ibid.

56  Findlay, "Neurosurgery at the Toronto General Hospital," 156. Humphreys makes 1956 the date for Hendrick becoming the first full-time neurosurgeon, as A.W.

Farmer, then surgeon-in-chief at HSC, set up the specialty divisions within the Department of Surgery.

57 "The Harold J Hoffman/Shoppers Drug Mart Chair in Paediatric Neurosurgery," *The Neurotransmitter* 5 (Summer 2000): 2.

58 "Dr Harold Hoffman, 72: Neurosurgeon Was World-Famous," *Toronto Star*, 27 Dec. 2008.

59 James T. Rutka, "Celebrating the Life of Dr. Harold J Hoffman, 1932–2004," *Surgical Spotlight* [Department of Surgery, University of Toronto], Winter 2004–5, 11–12.

60 Ibid.

61 E.B. Hendrick, D.C.F. Harwood-Nash, and A.R. Hudson, "Head Injuries in Children: A Survey of 4465 Consecutive Cases at the HSC," *Clinical Neurosurgery* 11 (1964): 46–64.

62 D.C. Harwood-Nash and C.R. Fitz, *Neuroradiology in Infants and Children* (St Louis: Mosby, 1973).

63 Michael S. Huckman, "Derek F. C. Harwood-Nash," *American Journal of Neuroradiology* 18 (1997): 1803–2812, 1808.

64 Bernard S. Goldman and Susan Bélanger, eds., *Heart Surgery in Canada: Memoirs, Anecdotes, History and Perspective* (Philadelphia: Xlibris, 2005), 96.

65 Gordon Murray, F.R. Wilkinson, and R. MacKenzie, "Reconstruction of the Valves of the Heart," *CMAJ* 38 (1938): 317–19.

66 G.D.W. Murray, L.B. Jaques, T.S. Perrett, and C.H. Best, "Heparin and the Thrombosis of Veins Following Injury," *Surgery* 2 (1937), 163–87. The investigators induced experimental injuries in dogs.

67 D.Y. Solandt, Reginald Nassim, and Charles H. Best, "Production and Prevention of Cardiac Mural Thrombosis in Dogs," *Lancet* 2 (9 Sept. 1939): 592–5. Murray and Best's 1938 article showed no particular clinical benefit: "Heparin and Thrombosis: The Present Situation," *JAMA* 110 (8 Jan. 1938): 118–19.

68 Gordon Murray, "Heparin in Thrombosis and Blood Vessel Surgery," *Surgery, Gynecology & Obstetrics* 72 (1941): 340–4, 344.

69 Bigelow, *Mysterious Heparin*, 108–9.

70 Alfred Blalock and Helen B. Taussig, "The Surgical Treatment of Malformations of the Heart in which There Is Pulmonary Stenosis or Pulmonary Atresia," *JAMA* 128 (19 May 1945): 189–202.

71 Gordon Murray, "The Tetralogy of Fallot and Its Surgical Treatment," *BMJ* 2 (6 Dec. 1947): 905–6.

72 Ronald J. Baird, "Cardiac Surgery in Toronto – A Memoir," in Goldman and Bélanger, *Heart Surgery in Canada*, 102–13, 103.

73 Gordon Murray, "The Pathophysiology of the Cause of Death from Coronary Thrombosis," *Annals of Surgery* 126 (1947): 523–34. The Matas comment is in the discussion, p. 534.

74 R.O. Heimbecker, C. Chen, N. Hamilton, and D.W.G. Murray, "Surgery for Massive Myocardial Infarction: An Experimental Study of Emergency Infarctectomy,"

*Surgery* 61 (1967): 51–8. On these and similar approaches, see B.B. Milstein, "Exploring Surgical Treatment for Myocardial Infarction," *British Heart Journal* 32 (1970): 421–6.

75 W. Thalhimer, "Experimental Exchange Transfusions for Reducing Azotemia: Use of Artificial Kidney for This Purpose," *Proceedings of the Society for Experimental Biology and Medicine* 37 (1938): 641–3; William Thalhimer, D.Y. Solandt, and Charles H. Best, "Experimental Exchange Transfusion Using Purified Heparin," *Lancet* 2 (3 Sept. 1938): 554–6. See also Bigelow, *Mysterious Heparin*, 124.

76 Gordon Murray, Edmund Delorme, and Newell Thomas, "Development of an Artificial Kidney," *Archives of Surgery* 55 (1947): 505–22. See also Gordon Murray, Edmund Delorme, and Newell Thomas, "Artificial Kidney," *JAMA* 137 (28 Aug. 1948): 1596–9.

77 Gordon Murray, Edmund Delorme, and Newell Thomas, "Artificial Kidney," *BMJ* 2 (22 Oct. 1949): 887–91.

78 McKellar, *Surgical Limits*, 92–5.

79 Gordon Murray, "Homologous Aortic-Valve-Segment Transplants As Surgical Treatment for Aortic and Mitral Insufficiency," *Angiology* 7 (1956): 466–71, 470.

80 Raymond O. Heimbecker, "Heart Valves 1955," *Canadian Journal of Cardiology* 10 (1994): 571–2.

81 Baird, "Cardiac Surgery in Toronto, 104.

82 For details, see McKellar, *Surgical Limits*.

83 Bigelow, *Mysterious Heparin*, 78.

84 Donald Wilson interview with Edward Shorter, 17 Oct. 2009.

85 Berris, *Medicine: My Story*, 24.

86 Wilson interview, 17 Oct. 2009.

87 W.G. Bigelow, "Intellectual Humility in Medical Practice and Research," *Surgery* 65 (1969): 1–9, 5.

88 That is, the class of 1938. This rendering of the year of graduation is a University of Toronto tradition.

89 *Torontonensis* (1938), 99.

90 Bigelow, *Cold Hearts*, 35.

91 McKellar, *Surgical Limits*, 102.

92 Goldman and Bélanger, *Heart Surgery in Canada*, 137.

93 Ruth Mather, *The Doctor's Office: A Secretary's Memoir* (Scarborough: Abbeyfield, 1998), 66. This little gem of a memoir has remained largely undiscovered, despite the richness of the insights into cardiology practice in the 1950s and 1960s.

94 W.G. Bigelow to R.M. Janes, 22 Feb. 1955; UTA A1989/0030/002.

95 W.G. Bigelow to W. Drucker, 14 Oct. 1966; attached is a document, "Cardiovascular Division, Toronto General Hospital," that reviews the historic development of the division, see 1–2; UTA A1989/0030/002.

96 W.G. Bigelow to F.G. Kergin, 18 Sept. 1957, plus attachment, "Requirements for Cardiovascular Surgery, Toronto General Hospital"; UTA A1989/0030/002. On McFayden see Bigelow, *Cold Hearts*, 121.

97  Bigelow, *Cold Hearts*, 123, 126.

98  W.F. Greenwood, A.D. McKelvey, J.K. Wilson, and W.G. Bigelow, "The Results of Surgical Treatment of Mitral Stenosis," *Proceedings of the Royal College of Physicians and Surgeons of Canada*, 3–4 Oct. 1952, 10–11; W.G. Bigelow, W.F. Greenwood, A.D. McKelvey, and J.K. Wilson, "The Surgical Treatment of Mitral Stenosis," *CMAJ* 69 (1953): 588–97.

99  Harold N. Segall, *Pioneers of Cardiology in Canada, 1820–1970: The Genesis of Canadian Cardiology* (Willowdale, Ontario: Hounslow, 1988), 399–404.

100  W.G. Bigelow, J.C. Callaghan, and J.A. Hopps, "General Hypothermia for Experimental Intracardiac Surgery: The Use of Electrophrenic Respirations, an Artificial Pacemaker for Cardiac Standstill, and Radio-Frequency Rewarming in General Hypothermia," *Annals of Surgery* 132 (1950): 531–7; W.G. Bigelow, W.K. Lindsay, R.C. Harrison, R.A. Gordon, and W.F. Greenwood, "Oxygen Transport and Utilization in Dogs at Low Body Temperatures," *American Journal of Physiology* 160 (1950): 125–37.

101  F. John Lewis and Mansur Taufic, "Closure of Atrial Septal Defect with the Aid of Hypothermia; Experimental Accomplishments and the Report of One Successful Case," *Surgery*, 33 (1953), 52–59.

102  F.G. Pearson interview with Edward Shorter, 2 Feb. 2009.

103  W.G. Bigelow, W.T. Mustard, and J.G. Evans, "Some Physiologic Concepts of Hypothermia and Their Applications to Cardiac Surgery," *Journal of Thoracic Surgery* 28 (1954): 463–80.

104  Baird, "Cardiac Surgery in Toronto," 107.

105  S.V. Lichtenstein, T.A. Salerno, and A.S. Slutsky, "Pro: Warm Continuous Cardioplegia Is Preferable to Intermittent Hypothermic Cardioplegia for Myocardial Protection during Cardiopulmonary Bypass," *Journal of Cardiothoracic Anesthesia* 4 (1990): 279–81.

106  Wilfred G. Bigelow, "The Pacemaker Story: A Cold Heart Spinoff," *Pace* 10 (1987): 142–50, 142; this is a condensed account of the version in Bigelow, *Cold Hearts*.

107  Bigelow, Callaghan and Hopps, "General Hypothermia", 535.

108  J.C. Callaghan and W.G. Bigelow, "An Electrical Artificial Pacemaker for Standstill of the Heart," *Annals of Surgery* 134 (1951): 8–17, 17.

109  W.G. Bigelow note to F. Kergin, Oct. 1956; UTA A1989/0030/002.

110  W.G. Bigelow to W. Drucker, 14 Oct. 1966, attachment "Cardiovascular Division, Toronto General Hospital"; UTA A1989/0030/002.

111  Raymond O. Heimbecker, "A Medical Milestone – Canada's First Adult Open-Heart Operation," Goldman and Bélanger, *Heart Surgery in Canada*, 115–19, 117.

112  See Peter Allen letter, *Surgical Spotlight*, Winter 2005, 17.

113  Heimbecker, "Medical Milestone,"., 118–19.

114  "The Heart of the Matter" [interview], www.simcoe.com/article139812, 30 June 2009.

115  Segall, *Pioneers of Cardiology*, s.v. "James Alastair Key," 404–6.

116 R.W. Gunton, W. Paul, and R.O. Heimbecker, "Appraisal of Left Heart Catheterization and Dye Dilution Technics in the Diagnosis of Mitral Valve Disease," *Clinical Research* 6 (1958): 218–19.

117 Baird, "Cardiac Surgery in Toronto," 109.

118 Williams obituary of Bigelow, *Transactions of the Meeting of the American Surgical Association* 124 (2006): 302.

119 R.O. Heimbecker, R.J. Baird, T.Z. Lajos, A.T. Varga, and W.F. Greenwood, "Homograft Replacement of the Human Mitral Valve: A Preliminary Report," *CMAJ* 86 (5 May 1962): 805–9.

120 Goldman and Bélanger, *Heart Surgery in Canada*, 100–1.

121 Arthur Vineberg, "Development of an Anastomosis between the Coronary Vessels and a Transplanted Internal Mammary Artery," *CMAJ* 55 (1946): 117–19.

122 R.J. Baird et al., "A Modification of the Internal Mammary Implant Operation," *Annals of RCPS Canada* 1 (1968): 23.

123 "Details of Heart Transplant Reported," *JAMA*, 202 (18 Dec. 1967): 23–24.

124 "Animal Heart Transplants Tried Here," *Globe and Mail*, 4 Dec. 1967.

125 Daniel J. DeBardino, "The History and Development of Cardiac Transplantation," *Texas Heart Institute Journal*, 26 (1999): 198–205, 203.

126 W.R. Drucker, memo to Members, Cardiovascular Surgical Division, University of Toronto, 10 May 1968; UTA A1989/0030/002.

127 Denton A. Cooley et al., "Transplantation of the Human Heart," *JAMA* 205 (12 Aug. 1968): 479–86.

128 Bernard Goldman, interview with Edward Shorter, 4 Feb. 2009.

129 "Bricklayer Satisfactory in 1st Toronto Heart Switch," *Globe and Mail*, 21 Oct. 1968; "Heart, Kidneys, Corneas of Man Implanted in 4," *Globe and Mail*, 30 Oct. 1968; Baird, "Cardiac Surgery in Toronto," 111.

130 W. G. Bigelow, D. R. Wilson, C. B. Baker, "Heart Transplantation, University of Toronto," *Laval Médical* 41 (1970): 170–3, 170.

131 Baird, "Heart Surgery in Toronto," 111.

132 Clare Baker, Lee Errett, and Bernard Goldman, "St. Michael's Hospital," in Goldman and Bélanger, *Heart Surgery in Canada*, 132–6, 134.

133 Ibid, 133–34.

134 Ibid., 134.

135 Baird, "Cardiac Surgery in Toronto," 111.

136 Segall, *Pioneers of Cardiology*, s.v. "James Key," 405.

137 Bigelow, *Cold Hearts*, 172–3.

138 S.V. Lichtenstein, T.A. Salerno, and A.S. Slutsky, "Warm Continuous Cardioplegia Versus Intermittent Hypothermic Protection during Cardiopulmonary Bypass," *Journal of Cardiothoracic Anesthesia* 4 (1990): 279–81, 281.

139 Baker, Errett, and Goldman, "St Michael's Hospital,", 135.

140 The Warm Heart Investigators, "Randomised Trial of Normothermic Versus Hypothermic Coronary Bypass Surgery," *Lancet* 343 (5 Mar. 1994): 559–63, 563.

141 Goldman and Bélanger, *Heart Surgery in Canada*, 132–6.

142 Stephen Westaby with Cecil Bosher, *Landmarks in Cardiac Surgery* (Oxford: Isis Medical Media, 1997), 129.

143 George A. Trusler, "Reflections on Bill Mustard and the Early Days at the Hospital for Sick Children, Toronto," in Goldman and Bélanger, *Heart Surgery in Canada*, 140–51.

144 Segall, *Pioneers of Cardiology*, 398–9. With his background in orthopedics, Mustard did not confine himself entirely to the heart. Ron Baird said in an obituary, "In 1952, he developed the iliopsoas muscle transfer operation for polio victims who could not stand or walk. The operation was accepted internationally and known as 'the Mustard procedure.'" (Faculty Council meeting, 25 Jan. 1988; UTA A1996/0007/001). W.T. Mustard, "Iliopsoas Transfer for Weakness of the Hip Abductors: A Preliminary Report," *Journal of Bone and Joint Surgery*, n.s., 34, no. 2 (1952): section a: 647–80.

145 Segall, *Pioneers of Cardiology*, s.v. "John Keith," 269.

146 W.T. Mustard, "The Operation for Closure of Patent Ductus Arteriosus," *CMAJ* 57 (Oct. 1947): 340–1.

147 W.T. Mustard and John Fraser, "Replacement Transfusion in Erythroblastosis Fetalis," *CMAJ* 59 (1948): 378–9.

148 W.T. Mustard, A.L. Chute, and E.H. Simmons, "Further Observations on Experimental Extracorporeal Circulation," *Surgery* 12 (1952): 803–10.

149 Marilyn Dunlop, *Bill Mustard: Surgical Pioneer* (Toronto: Dundurn Press, 1989), 54.

150 W.T. Mustard and A.L. Chute, "Experimental Intracardiac Surgery with Extracorporeal Circulation," *Surgery* 30 (1951): 684–8.

151 John H. Gibbon Jr., "The Maintenance of Life during Experimental Occlusion of the Pulmonary Artery Followed by Survival," *Surgery, Gynecology & Obstetrics* 69 (1939): 602–14.

152 See W.T. Mustard, A.L. Chute, J.D. Keith, A. Sirek, R.D. Rowe, and P. Vlad, "A Surgical Approach to Transposition of the Great Vessels with Extracorporeal Circuit," *Surgery* 36 (1954): 39–51, 39; W.T. Mustard and J.A. Thomson, "Clinical Experience with the Artificial Heart Lung Preparation," *CMAJ* 76 (15 Feb. 1957): 265–9, 266, case 1.

153 "Toronto-Made Machine Enabled Babes to Live during Heart Surgery," *Toronto Daily Star*, 8 June 1952.

154 Mustard et al., "Surgical Approach to Transposition," 39–51.

155 Trusler, "Reflections on Bill Mustard," 146.

156 W.T. Mustard, "Mortality in Congenital Cardiovascular Surgery," *CMAJ* 72 (15 May 1955): 740–4.

157 Mustard and Thomson, "Clinical Experience," 268.

158 W.T. Mustard, J.D. Keith, G.A. Trusler, R. Fowler, and L. Kidd, "The Surgical Management of Transposition of the Great Vessels," *Journal of Thoracic and Cardiovascular Surgery* 48 (1964): 953–8; W.T. Mustard, "Successful Two-stage Correction of Transposition of the Great Vessels," *Surgery* 55 (1964): 469–72.

159 Trusler, "Reflections on Bill Mustard," 148–9.

160  Segall, *Pioneers of Cardiology*, s.v. "John D. Keith," 272.

161  A.J. Rhodes et al., "Studies on Poliomyelitis in Ontario, II: Isolation of the Coxsackie Virus in Association with Poliomyelitis Virus: A Preliminary Report," *Canadian Journal of Public Health* 41 (1950): 51–9; "III: Further Observations on the Association of Coxsackie and Poliomyelitis Viruses," *Canadian Journal of Public Health* 41 (1950): 183–8; see also Nelles Silverthorne et al., "Studies on Poliomyelitis in Ontario, IV: Further Observations on the Spread of Poliomyelitis and Coxsackie Infections in Small Communities," *CMAJ* 64 (1951): 309–63.

162  Bator, *Within Reach*, 2:35.

163  Christopher J. Rutty, "'Herculean Efforts': Connaught and the Canadian Polio Vaccine Story" (1996), www.healthheritageresearch.com/Polio-Contact9606.html

164  Hart E. Van Riper, "Progress in the Control of Paralytic Poliomyelitis through Vaccination," *Canadian Journal of Public Health* 46 (1955): 425–36, 426.

165  Rutty, "Herculean Efforts."

166  The Ontario Cancer Institute included the Princess Margaret Hospital. Its academic members belonged to the university department of Medical Biophysics. Further details on cancer treatment and research in Toronto are provided in chapter 13.

167  Lou Siminovitch, *Reflections on a Life in Science* (Toronto: self-published, 2003), 54, 197.

168  E.A. McCulloch, *The Ontario Cancer Institute: Successes and Reverses at Sherbourne Street* (Montreal: McGill-Queen's University Press, 2003), 29.

169  Joe Sornberger, "Canadians Till and McCulloch Proved Existence of Stem Cells," *Stem Cell Network News Magazine* 3, no. 1 (2004): 1–6.

170  Till interview, 26 Nov. 2009.

171  R.B.L. Gwatkin, J.E. Till, G.F. Whitmore, L. Siminovitch, and F.A. Graham, "Multiplication of Animals Cells in Suspension Measured by Colony Counts," *Proceedings of the National Academy of Sciences* 43 (1957): 451–7.

172  McCulloch describes in *Ontario Cancer Institute*, 7, three such procedures in 1958. The outcomes were poor, with only one temporary remission, and the idea was abandoned after only an oral report at a meeting.

173  "Obituary Dr. Ernest McCulloch," *Toronto Star*, 21 Jan. 2011, GT1.

174  J.E. Till and E.A. McCulloch, "A Direct Measurement of the Radiation Sensitivity of Normal Mouse Bone Marrow Cells," *Radiation Research* 14 (1961): 213–22.

175  A.J. Becker, E.A. McCulloch, and J.E. Till, "Cytological Demonstration of the Clonal Nature of Spleen Colonies Derived from Transplanted Mouse Narrow Cells," *Nature* 197 (1963): 452–4.

176  L. Siminovitch, E.A. McCulloch, and J.E. Till, "The Distribution of Colony-forming Units among Spleen Colonies," *Journal of Cellular and Comparative Physiology* 62 (1963): 327–36.

177  *Dean's Report* 1961–2, 32. Till noted, however, that the term "stem cells" had been "around since the beginning of the 1900s." A.F. Howatson was a PhD researcher whose role in the story was more peripheral.

178 McCullough, *Ontario Cancer Institute*, 60.
179 Megan Ogilvie et al., "Nobel Buzz Surrounds Toronto Scientists," www.health-zone.ca, 3 Oct. 2009; journalist's paraphrase.
180 Joseph MacFarlane, "Empire Club, Jan 13, 1955"; UTA A1976/0054/018 (10), 12.

## 6 Surgery

1 Richard Reznick, "Chair's Column," *Surgical Spotlight*, Winter 2004–5, 3.
2 F.P. Dewar interview by Valerie Schatzker, 22 June 1976, at the York Club, p. 18'; Dean's Archive.
3 Faculty Council, 6 Dec. 1929, 264; UTA A1986/0027/020.
4 *Dean's Report* 1933–4, 41.
5 *Dean's Report* 1938–9, 53–4.
6 *Dean's Report* 1951–2, 53.
7 LRPAC [Long Range Planning and Assessment Committee] Minutes, 15 May 1974, 3; UTA A1979/0010/006.
8 Department of Surgery, *Annual Report* 1989–90, 4–5.
9 "Surgical Skills Lab Expansion," *Surgical Spotlight*, Fall 2007, 19.
10 Bernard Langer, personal communication, 25 Aug. 2010.
11 Richard Reznick, "Chair's Column," *Surgical Spotlight*, Winter 2008, 3–4, 4.
12 *Dean's Report* 1937–8, 47–8.
13 The dating of this is based on Gallie's remark in 1938 that "[t]his postgraduate course has now been in action for eight years." *Dean's Report* 1938–9, 35.
14 *Dean's Report* 1938–9, 53–4.
15 *Dean's Report* 1939–40, 56–7.
16 Ibid., 57.
17 *Dean's Report* 1941–2, 30.
18 W.E. Gallie to R.M. Gorssline, 3 Mar. 1941; UTA A1989/0030/001.
19 Bernard Langer, personal communication, 25 Aug. 2010.
20 *Dean's Report* 1943–4, 36.
21 *Torontonensis* (1910), 152.
22 Eulogy, Faculty Council, 6 Feb. 1948.
23 Goldwin Howland, Walter R. Campbell, and Ernest J. Maltby, "Dysinsulinism: Convulsions and Coma Due to Islet Cell Tumor of the Pancreas; Operation and Cure," *Transactions of the American Neurological Association* 55 (1929): 551–6; the case was also published in *JAMA* 93 (31 Aug. 1929): 674–9; see also Sebastian G. De La Fuente and Theodore N. Pappas, "Roscoe Reid Graham (1890 to 1948)," *Current Surgery* 59 (2002): 428–9. Graham himself later published the case in Walter R. Campbell, Roscoe R. Graham, and William L. Robinson, "Islet Cells Tumors of the Pancreas," *American Journal of the Medical Sciences* 188 (1939): 445–54; see case 1, p. 446.
24 Roscoe R. Graham, "The Surgeon's Problem in Duodenal Ulcer," *American Journal of Surgery* 40 (1938): 102–17, 117.

25  Berris, *Medicine: My Story*, 23.
26  [TGH] *Monitor*, Winter 1985–6, 6.
27  Helen ("Nell") Farquharson interview with Edward Shorter, 21 July 2009, 11.
28  Bigelow, *Cold Hearts*, 19.
29  Harold Wookey, Clifford Ash, W. Keith Welsh, and R.A. Mustard, "The Treatment of Oral Cancer by a Combination of Radiotherapy and Surgery," *Annals of Surgery* 134 (1951): 529–38, 530.
30  Bigelow, *Cold Hearts*, 19.
31  W.E. Gallie and A.L. LeMesurier, "Recurring Dislocation of the Shoulder," *Journal of Bone and Joint Surgery* 30B (1948): 9–18; the research was first presented as a lecture in 1947.
32  "Salute to Great Doctor," *Globe and Mail*, 20 Dec. 1950, 6.
33  Wilson interview, 17 Oct. 2009.
34  W.E. Gallie, "Edinburgh and London Revisited"; undated record of a visit in June 1955; UTA A1989/0030/001.
35  J.G. Goodwin, "Note" [2009], 2; undated brief MS in the form of a personal communication.
36  *President's Report* 1945–6, 35.
37  W.E. Gallie in *President's Report* 1944–5, 26.
38  McKellar, *Surgical Limits*, 81.
39  Robert M. Janes, "Surgery in the Treatment of Pulmonary Tuberculosis," *CMAJ* 33 (1935): 389–92.
40  F.G. Pearson, "Adventures in Surgery," *Journal of Thoracic and Cardiovascular Surgery* 100 (1990): 639–51, 640.
41  *Dean 's Report*, 1929–30, 12.
42  A.P. Naef, "The Mid-century Revolution in Thoracic and Cardiovascular Surgery: Part 2: Prelude to 20th Century Cardio-thoracic Surgery," *Interactive Cardiovascular and Thoracic Surgery* 2 (2003): 431–49, 437.
43  F.G. Kergin, "Robert Meredith Janes," *CMAJ* 95 (24 Dec. 1966): 1399–1400; F. G. Kergin, "Robert Meredith Janes," [Toronto] *Academy of Medicine Bulletin* 40 (1967): 71–2.
44  Pearson, "Adventures in Surgery," 640.
45  *Dean's Report* 1947–8, 44.
46  R.J. Delaney, "Dr Robert Meredith Janes," *Canadian Journal of Surgery* 12 (1969): 2–11, 2.
47  W.G.C. [Cosbie], "Dr Norman Strahan Shenstone," *CMAJ* 102 (23 May 1970): 1112–13.
48  W.K.W., "Norman S Shenstone," [Toronto] *Academy of Medicine Bulletin* 43 (1970): 139–40.
49  *Dean's Report* 1940–1, 34.
50  *Dean's Report* 1945–6, 35–6.
51  *Dean's Report* 1948–9, 45.
52  *Dean's Report* 1950–1, 51.

53  Bernard Langer personal communication, 25 Aug. 2010.

54  "Post-Graduate Training," minutes, 18 Dec. 1947; UTA A1993/0025/4.

55  *Dean's Report* 1947–8, 44.

56  *Dean's Report* 1948–9, 44.

57  *Dean's Report* 1947–8, 44.

58  *Dean's Report* 1949–50, 50.

59  R.J. Baird and F.G. Pearson, "Frederick G Kergin," *Canadian Journal of Surgery* 16 (1973): 65–6.

60  Dewar interview by Schatzker, 22 June 1976, p. 32.

61  *Dean's Report* 1949–50, 51.

62  Ibid., 66.

63  Pearson interview, 2 Feb. 2009.

64  F.G. Kergin, D.M. Bean, and W. Paul, "Anoxia during Intra-thoracic Operations," *Journal of Thoracic Surgery* 17 (1948): 709–11.

65  Bigelow, *Cold Hearts*, 111.

66  Peter Beaconsfield, H.S. Coulthard, and F.G. Kergin, "Treatment of Pulmonary Tuberculosis by Thoracoplasty in Patients Over 50 Years of Age," *Thorax* 9 (1954): 211–15.

67  Frederick G. Kergin and Hugh S. Coulthard, "The Surgical Treatment of Pulmonary Tuberculosis," *Surgical Clinics of North America* 34 (1954): 931–49.

68  Pearson, "Adventures in Surgery," 641.

69  F.G. Pearson, "Frederick Gordon Kergin," *Canadian Journal of Surgery* 18 (1975): 109–10.

70  *Dean's Report* 1961–2, 82.

71  *Dean's Report* 1960–1, 79–81. Research results were already at this point being reported for "General Surgery." But the actual division does not seem to have been created until 1966–7.

72  *Dean's Report* 1962–3, 86.

73  *Dean's Report* 1967–8, 135.

74  *Dean's Report* 1965–6, 107.

75  Bernard Langer personal communication, 25 Aug. 2010.

76  Bernard Langer, Eulogy of Robert A. Mustard, Faculty Council, 19 Apr. 1985; UTA A1993/0025/09; *Torontonensis* (1938), 105; *Surgical Spotlight*, Summer 2006, 13–14.

77  Anonymous obituarist, "Owen Vernon Gray," Faculty Council, undated, 1972–3 session; UTA A1993/0025/007.

78  *Dean's Report* 1969–70, 159.

79  *Dean's Report* 1970–1, 167.

80  Bernard Langer interview with Edward Shorter, 20 Oct. 2009, 4.

81  *Dean's Report* 1969–70, 158–60.

82  *Dean's Report* 1970–1, 168.

83  F.G. Pearson, "Goals and Objectives – Department of Surgery, 1978–1988," March 1983; Dean's Archive.

84  Ibid.

85  Ibid.
86  Wilson interview, 17 Oct. 2009.
87  Ibid.
88  Department of Surgery, External Review, 1981; Dean's Archive.
89  External review committee, Department of Surgery, 1991; Dean's Archive.
90  The exact figure was 102 in 1987; "Department of Surgery, On-Site Review," 18–20 Feb. 1987; Dean's Archive.
91  Bernard Langer personal communication, 25 Aug. 2010.
92  Langer interview, 20 Oct. 2009.
93  Ibid.
94  Bernard Langer, "The Clinician Scientist – Preserving an Endangered Species," Gallie Lecture, RCPSC Halifax, Sept. 1996.
95  Langer interview, 20 Oct. 2009.
96  Ibid.
97  Ori Rotstein interview with Edward Shorter, 9 Apr. 2009.
98  Langer interview, 20 Oct. 2009.
99  Dept of Surgery, *Annual Report* 1988–9, 4–5.
100  Langer, "Clinician Scientist." See also Bernard L. Langer, "The Surgical Scientist Program at the University of Toronto: A Model for Training Clinician Investigators," *Clinical and Investigative Medicine* 20 (1997): 257–8.
101  See Bernard Langer to Arnie Aberman, 19 Apr. 1994; Bernard Langer private archive.
102  Timothy J. Ley and Leon E. Rosenberg, "The Physician-Scientist Career Pipeline: Build It and They Will Come," *JAMA* 294 (21 Sept. 2005): 1343–51.
103  Richard Reznick, "Chair's Column," *Surgery Newsletter*, Nov. 2002, 1; Dept of Surgery, *Annual Report* 2001–2, 4.
104  "Transdisciplinary Research to Help the Underdog," *Surgical Spotlight*, Winter 2003–4, 6–7.
105  Rotstein interview, 9 Apr. 2009.
106  Bernard Langer personal communication, 25 Aug. 2010.
107  "Professor John Wedge Steps Down at U of T," HSC, *The Neurotransmitter*, Summer 2002.
108  Dept of Surgery, *Annual Report* 1993–4, 9, 13.
109  Dept of Surgery, *Annual Report* 2006–7, 5.
110  Richard Reznick, "Chair's Column," *Surgical Spotlight*, Winter 2004–5, 3.
111  Richard Reznick, "Chair's Column,", Department of Surgery, *Surgery Newsletter* , Nov 2002, 1–2.
112  Dept of Surgery, *Annual Report*, 2007–8, 6.
113  Martin McNeally," Editor's Column," *Surgical Spotlight*, Summer 2004, 4.
114  Dept of Surgery, *Annual Report* 2006–7, 4.
115  Dept of Surgery, *Annual Report* 2007–8, 8.
116  Dept of Surgery, *Annual Report* 2006–7, 5.

117 Jonathan L. Meakins and Garth L. Warnock, "The External Review Report of the University of Toronto Department of Surgery, Oct 4–5, 2007," 6, 9; http://www. surg.med.utoronto.ca/newsletter/Surgery_External_Reviewers_Report_2007.pdf.

118 Dept of Surgery, *Annual Report* 2004–5, 116.

119 Richard Reznick, "Chair's Column," *Surgical Spotlight*, Spring 2007, 3.

120 Reznick, "Chair's Column," *Surgical Spotlight*, Spring–Summer 2008, 3.

## 7  The Surgical Subspecialties

1 Bernard Langer, personal communication, 18 Sept. 2010.

2 *Dean's Report* 1929–30, 11.

3 *Dean's Report* 1932–3, 37.

4 Ibid., 38.

5 Wilson interview, 17 Oct. 2009.

6 John H. Dirks to A.R. Ten Cate, 23 Feb. 1990; UTA A1996/0011/18 (4).

7 *President's Report* 1944–5, 31.

8 Richard Reznick, "General Surgery in Peril?" *Surgical Spotlight*, Winter 2009.

9 E.B. Tovee, "A Report of the Interhospital Co-ordinating Committee of the Division of General Surgery, University of Toronto," September 1968; UTA A1989/0030/002.

10 Bernard Langer, "Citation for Dr Bruce Tovee," Faculty Council, 29 May 1989; UTA A1996/0007/003.

11 Bernard Langer, personal communication, 18 Sept. 2010.

12 Dept of Surgery, *Annual Report* 1990–1, 2, 12.

13 Dept of Surgery, *Annual Report* 1991–2, 13.

14 Dept of Surgery, *Annual Report* 1998–9, 22.

15 Melvin S. Henderson, "Orthopaedic Surgery: An Historical Review," *University of Toronto Medical Bulletin*, 6 Apr. 1936, 1.

16 Quoted in Noah Schiff, "'The Sweetest of All Charities': The Toronto Hospital for Sick Children's Medical and Public Appeal, 1875–1905" (master's thesis, Department of History, University of Toronto, 1999), 104–5.

17 Faculty Council, 19 June 1903; UTA A1986/0027/016.

18 Seyed B. Mostofi, *Who's Who in Orthopedics* (London: Springer, 2005), 126.

19 Dewar interview by Schatzker, 22 June 1976, p. 37.

20 *Dean's Report* 1939–40, 57.

21 Dewar interview by Schatzker, 22 June 1976, p. 62–3.

22 Wilson interview, 17 Oct. 2009.

23 Mostofi, *Who's Who in Orthopedics*, 213.

24 W.G. Cosbie, *The Toronto General Hospital, 1819–1965: A Chronicle* (Toronto: Macmillan, 1975), 285, 325–6.

25 Dewar interview by Schatzker, 22 June 1976, p. 67–8.

26 Ibid., 87–8.

27 Dept of Surgery, *Annual Report* 1990–1, 17.

28 Dewar interview by Schatzker, 22 June 1976, p. 105.

29 Melvin J. Glimcher to F.P. Dewar, 18 Sept. 1967; UTA A1989/0030/001.

30 R.M. Letts and W.P. Bobechko, "Fusion of the Scoliotic Spine in Young Children," *Clinical Orthopaedics and Related Research* 101 (1974): 136–45.

31 Robert N. Hensinger, "Walter P Bobechko (1933–2007)," *Pediatric Orthopedics* 27 (2007): 723. See W.P. Bobechko, "The Toronto Brace for Legg-Perthes Disease," *Clinical Orthopaedics and Related Research* 102 (July–Aug. 1974): 115–17.

32 M.A. Herbert and W.P. Bobechko, "Paraspinal Muscle Stimulation for the Treatment of Idiopathic Scoliosis in Children," *Orthopedics* 10 (1987): 1125–32; M.A. Herbert and W.P. Bobechko, "Scoliosis Treatment in Children Using a Programmable, Totally Implantable Muscle Stimulator (ESI)," *IEEE Transactions on Biomedical Engineering* 36 (1989): 801–2.

33 "Medicine: Bionic Back," *Time*, 12 Apr. 1982.

34 Hensinger, "Bobechko," 723.

35 D.L. MacIntosh, "Hemiarthroplasty of the Knee Using a Space Occupying Prosthesis for Painful Varus and Valgus Deformities," *Journal of Bone and Joint Surgery* 40A (1958): 1431.

36 R.D. Galway, A. Beaupré, and D.L. MacIntosh, "Pivot Shift: A Clinical Sign of Symptomatic Anterior Cruciate Insufficiency," *Journal of Bone and Joint Surgery* 54B (1972): 763–4.

37 D.L. MacIntosh and T.A. Darish, "Lateral Substitution Reconstruction," *Journal of Bone and Joint Surgery* 58B (1976): 142.

38 J.P. Kostuik, "Anterior Cruciate Reconstruction by the Macintosh Techniques," *Journal of Bone and Joint Surgery* 59B (1977): 511.

39 Robert W. Jackson, "History of Arthroscopy," in *Operative Arthroscopy*, 3rd ed., ed. John B. McGinty (Philadelphia: Lippincott, 2003), 3–8, 6–7.

40 Richard Hoffer, "Dr Robert Jackson," *Sports Illustrated*, 19 Sept. 1994.

41 Robert W. Jackson and D.J. Dandy, *Arthroscopy of the Knee* (New York: Grune and Stratton, 1976).

42 "In Remembrance: Robert W. Jackson," *MedEmail*, 27 Jan. 2010.

43 Richard Reznick, "Chair's Column," *Surgery Newsletter*, Fall 2003, 2.

44 John Wedge, "Robert Bruce Salter," *Journal of Pediatric Orthopaedics* 30 (2010): 631–2, 631.

45 Robert B. Salter, "Innominate Osteotomy in the Treatment of Congenital Dislocation and Subluxation of the Hip," *Journal of Bone and Joint Surgery* (British ed.) 43B (1961): 518–39; the findings were presented at a conference in 1960.

46 Robert B. Salter and W. Robert Harris, "Injuries Involving the Epiphyseal Plate," *Journal of Bone and Joint Surgery* 45 (1963): 587–622.

47 Robert B. Salter, *Textbook of Disorders and Injuries of the Musculoskeletal System: An Introduction to Orthopaedics* (Baltimore: Williams & Wilkins, 1970); Reznick, "Chair's Column," *Surgical Spotlight*, Fall 2006, 6.

48 Robert B. Salter, "The Philosophy and Nature of Surgical Research," *Canadian Journal of Surgery* 23 (1980): 349–54.

49  Richard Reznick," On The Shoulders of Giants," *Surgical Spotlight*, Fall 2006, 5–6.

50  A.E. Gross, E.A. Silverstein, J. Falk, R. Falk, and F. Langer, "The Allotransplantation of Partial Joints in the Treatment of Osteoarthritis of the Knee," *Clinical Orthopaedics and Related Research* 108 (May 1975): 7–14.

51  A.G.P. McDermott, F. Langer, K.P.H. Pritzker, and A.E. Gross, "Fresh Small-fragment Osteochondral Allografts: Long-term Follow Up Study on First 100 Cases," *Clinical Orthopaedics and Related Research* 197 (1985): 96–102, 102.

52  TGH *Annual Report* 1985–6, 78–9.

53  The Toronto Hospital, *Annual Report* [hereafter TTH *Annual Report*] 1988–9, 143–4.

54  Dept of Surgery, *Annual Report* 1991–2, 19.

55  Dept of Surgery, *Annual Report* 1994–5, 26.

56  Ibid.

57  Dept of Surgery, *Annual Report* 2007–8, 12.

58  Hollenberg report, 17 July 1973, 6–8; UTA A1986/0028/004 (002).

59  Goldman and Bélanger, *Heart Surgery in Canada*, 101.

60  Baird, "Cardiac Surgery in Toronto," 113.

61  Ronald J. Baird, "Videos Reassure Patients," *Tablet*, Winter 1984, 3.

62  Ibid.

63  "TGH Doctor Implants Nuclear Heart Pacemaker," *Monitor*[TGH], 1 Nov. 1973, 1–2.

64  TGH *Annual* Report 1956, inside front cover.

65  Segall, *Pioneers of Cardiology*, 403.

66  W.G. Bigelow to F.G. Kergin, 16 Dec. 1964; UTA A1989/0030/002.

67  "The New and Expanding Centre for Cardiovascular Research Is … Centred at the General," TTH *Annual Report* 1990–1, 3.

68  "Heart at Work," *Toronto Star*, 20 Sept. 1994, A24.

69  Dept of Surgery, *Annual Report* 1987–8, 6.

70  Dept of Surgery, *Annual Report* 1994–5, 14.

71  Jean F. Morin and K. Wayne Johnston, "Improvement after Successful Percutaneous Transluminal Dilation Treatment of Occlusive Peripheral Arterial Disease," *Surgery, Gynecology & Obstetrics* 16 (1986): 453–7; see also Baird, "Cardiac Surgery in Toronto," 112; Dept of Surgery, *Annual Report* 1992–3, 188; *Surgical Spotlight*, Summer 2009, 13–14.

72  TGH *Annual Report* 1983–4, 14.

73  L.L. Mickleborough et al., "Balloon Electric Shock Ablation: Effects on Ventricular Structure, Function, and Electrophysiology," *Journal of Thoracic and Cardiovascular Surgery* 97 (1989): 135–46; an article in *Monitor* called attention to the six patients and to the role of cardiologist Eugene Downar in this research. "TG Doctors Pioneer Procedure," [TGH]*Monitor*, Spring/Summer 1989, 6–7.

74  Lynda Mickleborough, Hiroshi Maruyama, Peter Liu, and Shanas Mohamed, "Results of Left Ventricular Aneurysmectomy with a Tailored Scar Excision and Primary Closure Technique," *Journal of Thoracic and Cardiovascular Surgery* 107 (1994): 690–8.

75  TTH AR 1987–8, 192.
76  Note in *Surgical Spotlight*, Fall 2004, 6.
77  Ren-Ke Li, Zhi-Qiang Jia, Richard D. Weisel, Donald AG Mickle, Molly K Mohabeer, Vivek Rao, and Joan Ivanov, "Cardiomyocyte Transplantation Improves Heart Function," *Annals of Thoracic Surgery* 62 (1996): 654–60.
78  Shinji Tomita, Ren-Ke Li, Richard D. Weisel, Donald A.G. Mickle, Eung-Joong Kim, Tetsuro Sakai, and Zhi-Qiang Jia, "Autologous Transplantation of Bone Marrow Cells Improves Damaged Heart Function," *Circulation* 100 (1999): II-247–56.
79  Shafie Fazel, Massimo Cimini, Liwen Chen et al., "'Cardioprotective C-Kit+ Cells Are from the Bone Marrow and Regulate the Myocardial Balance of Angiogenic Cytokines," *Journal of Clinical Investigation* 116 (2006): 1865–77, 1875.
80  V. Rao, C.M. Feindel, R.D. Weisel, P. Boylen, and G. Cohen, "Donor Blood Perfusion Improves Myocardial Recovery after Heart Transplantation," *Journal of Heart and Lung Transplantation* 16 (1999): 667–73.
81  *Surgical Spotlight*, Spring–Summer 2008.
82  Baird," Cardiac Surgery in Toronto," 111.
83  Tirone E. David, Glorianne C. Ropchan, and Jagdish Butany, "Aortic Valve Replacement with Stentless Porcine Aortic Bioprostheses," *Journal of Cardiac Surgery* 3 (1988): 501–5.
84  Jagdish Butany, Mauro de Sa, Christopher M. Feindel, and Tirone E. David, "The Toronto SPV Bioprosthesis: Review of Morphological Findings in Eight Valves," *Seminars in Thoracic and Cardiovascular Surgery* 11, no. 4, supplement 1 (1999): 157–62.
85  Tirone E. David and Christopher M. Feindel, "An Aortic Valve-Sparing Operation for Patients with Aortic Incompetence and Aneurysm of the Ascending Aorta," *Journal of Thoracic and Cardiovascular Surgery* 103 (1992): 617–22.
86  Tirone E. David, Christopher M. Feindel, and Joanne Bos, "Repair of the Aortic Valve in Patients with Aortic Insufficiency and Aortic Root Aneurysm," *Journal of Thoracic and Cardiovascular Surgery* 109 (1995): 345–51.
87  Dept of Surgery, *Annual Report* 2007–8, 12.
88  Segall, *Pioneers of Cardiology*, s.v. "G.A. Trusler," 409; Goldman and Bélanger, *Heart Surgery in Canada*, 158.
89  See, for example, G.A. Trusler, C.A.F. Moes, and B.S.L. Kidd, "Repair of Ventricular Septal Defect with Aortic Insufficiency," *Journal of Thoracic and Cardiovascular Surgery* 66 (1973): 394–403. For a retrospective on this work see George A. Trusler, William G. Williams, Jeffrey F. Smallhorn, and Robert M. Freedom, "Late Results after Repair of Aortic Insufficiency Associated with Ventricular Septal Defect," *Journal of Thoracic and Cardiovascular Surgery* 103 (1992): 276–81.
90  William G. Williams, E. Douglas Wigle, Harry Rakowski, Jeffrey Smallhorn, Jacques LeBlanc, and George A. Trusler, "Results of Surgery for Hypertrophic Obstructive Cardiomyopathy," *Circulation* 76 (1987): V-104–8.
91  Dept of Surgery, *Annual Report* 1991–2, 32.

92  Profile of Glen Van Arsdell, http://www.sickkids.ca/AboutSickKids/Directory/People/V/Glen-Van-Arsdell.html.

93  Martin McKneally interview with Edward Shorter, 2 Feb. 2009.

94  Thomas R. J. Todd, *Breathless: A Transplant Surgeon's Journal* (Renfrew, ON: General Store Publishing House, [2007]), 70–1.

95  Norman S. Shenstone and Robert M. Janes, "Experiences in Pulmonary Lobectomy," *CMAJ* 27 (1932): 138–45; the paper was first read at a meeting in 1930.

96  H. Wookey, "The Surgical Treatment of Carcinoma of the Pharynx and Upper Esophagus," *Surgery, Gynecology & Obstetrics* 75 (1942): 499–506.

97  Harold Wookey, "The Surgical Treatment of Carcinoma of the Hypopharynx and the Oesophagus," *British Journal of Surgery* 35 (1948): 249–66.

98  Pearson, "Adventures in Surgery," 644.

99  Norman C. Delarue and Evarts A. Graham, "Alveolar Cell Carcinoma of the Lung (Pulmonary Adenomatosis, Jagzietke) – a Multicentric Tumor of Epithelial Origin," *Journal of Thoracic Surgery* 18 (1949): 237–51.

100 Norman C. Delarue, "Reconsideration of Some Significant Aspects of the Cigarette Smoking-Lung Cancer Controversy," *CMAJ* 89 (21 Dec. 1962): 1277–83. See also Norman C. Delarue et al., "Bronchiolo-Alveolar Carcinoma: A Reappraisal after 24 Years," *Cancer* 29 (1972): 90–7.

101 Robin P. Humphreys, "The Modernization of Pediatric Neurosurgery," *Child Nervous System* 20 (2004): 18–22, 21.

102 Douglas Waugh, "Norm Delarue Took on the Tobacco Industry Long Before It Was the Fashionable Thing to Do," *CMAJ* 150 (1 Jan. 1994): 64.

103 Pearson, "Adventures in Surgery," 644.

104 Stuart Vandewater, "The Toronto General Hospital, 1952–1953: A Personal Experience," in *A Commemorative History of the Department of Anaesthesia, University of Toronto*, ed. Robert Byrick (Toronto: Department of Anesthesia, 2004), 101–7, 103–4.

105 Pearson, "Adventures in Surgery," 644.

106 Ibid., 639.

107 Ibid., 642.

108 Pearson interview, [TGH]*Monitor*, Summer 1989, 10.

109 Pearson interview, 2 Feb. 2009.

110 Owen Gray, "Memorandum of Interview with Dr. FG Pearson, June 26, 1969"; UTA A1989/0030 (001).

111 *Dean's Report* 1966–7, 199.

112 Pearson interview, 2 Feb. 2009.

113 Dept of Surgery, *Annual Report* 1974–7, 14.

114 Pearson interview, 2 Feb. 2009.

115 F.G. Pearson, "Mediastinoscopy: A Method of Biopsy in the Superior Mediastinum," *Canadian Journal of Surgery* 6 (1963): 423–9; see also F.G. Pearson, N.C. Delarue, R. Ilves, T.R.J. Todd, and J.D. Cooper, "Significance of Positive Superior

Mediastinal Nodes Identified at Mediastinoscopy in Patients with Resectable Cancer of the Lung," *Journal of Thoracic and Cardiovascular Surgery* 83 (1982): 1–11.

116 See I. Boerma and Clarence Crafoord, discussion, in F.G. Pearson, "Mediastinoscopy: A Method of Biopsy in the Superior Mediastinum," *Journal of Thoracic and Cardiovascular Surgery* 49 (1965): 11–21, 21.

117 Pearson, "Mediastinoscopy," *Journal of Thoracic and Cardiovascular Surgery*, 19.

118 F.G. Pearson, B. Langer, and R.D. Henderson, "Gastroplasty and Belsey Hiatus Hernia Repair: An Operation for the Management of Peptic Stricture with Acquired Short Esophagus," *Journal of Thoracic and Cardiovascular Surgery* 61 (1971): 50–63; F. Griffith Pearson, "Complications and Pitfalls: Belsey and Collis-Belsey Antireflux Repairs," *Chest Surgery Clinics of North America* 7 (1997): 513–31.

119 Pearson, Langer, and Henderson, "Gastroplasty and Belsey Hiatus Hernia Repair," 50, 63.

120 Joel D. Cooper, "Lifetime Achievement Award: F Griffith Pearson," *Journal of Thoracic and Cardiovascular Surgery* 132 (2006): 453–4.

121 Ibid.

122 Todd, *Breathless*, 5.

123 Joel D. Cooper, F.G. Pearson, G.A. Patterson, T.R.J. Todd, R.J. Ginsberg, M. Goldberg, and W.A.P. DeMajo, "Technique of Successful Lung Transplantation in Humans," *Journal of Thoracic and Cardiovascular Surgery* 93 (1987): 173–81, 174.

124 Pearson interview, 2 Feb. 2009.

125 Toronto Lung Transplant Group [led by Joel D. Cooper], "Sequential Bilateral Lung Transplantation for Paraquat Poisoning," *Journal of Thoracic and Cardiovascular Surgery* 89 (1985): 734–42; see also [TGH] *Monitor*, Spring 1983, 8–9.

126 Todd, *Breathless*, 68.

127 Pearson interview, 2 Feb. 2009.

128 TGH *Annual Report* 1983–4, 1, 15.

129 Cooper et al., "Technique of Successful Lung Transplantation."

130 J.H. Dark, G.A. Patterson, G A., A.N. Al-Jilaihawi, H. Hsu, T. Egan, and J.D. Cooper, "Experimental En Bloc Double-Lung Transplantation," *Annals of Thoracic Surgery* 42 (1986): 394–8.

131 "First Double-lung Transplant Recipient Dies," *CMAJ* 164 (29 May 2001): 1610.

132 Thomas R.J. Todd, Jean Perron, Timothy L. Winton, and Shafique H. Keshavjee, "Simultaneous Single-lung Transplantation and Lung Volume Reduction," *Annals of Thoracic Surgery* 63 (1997): 1468–70.

133 R. Goldstein, T. Todd, G. Guyatt, S. Keshavjee, T. Dolmage, S. van Rooy, B. Krip, F. Maltais, P. LeBlanc, S. Pakhale, and T. Waddell, "Influence of Lung Volume Reduction Surgery (LVRS) on Health Related Quality of Life in Patients with Chronic Obstructive Pulmonary Disease," *Thorax* 58 (2003): 405–10.

134 J.D. Cooper et al., "Bilateral Pneumectomy (Volume Reduction) for Chronic Obstructive Pulmonary Disease," *Journal of Thoracic and Cardiovascular Surgery* 109 (1995): 106–19.

135 "Sunday Profile: Shaf Keshavjee," *Toronto Star*, 21 Feb. 2010, IN 1–2.

136 Novalung press release, 14 Feb. 2007.

137 "Sunday Profile," *Toronto Star*, 21 Feb. 2010; Marcello Cypel, Jonathan C. Yeung, Mingyao Liu et al, "Normothermic Ex Vivo Lung Perfusion in Clinical Lung Transplantation," *New England Journal of Medicine* 364 (14 Apr 2011), 1431–40.

138 H.W. Wookey, "The Surgical Treatment of Carcinoma of the Hypopharynx and Oesophagus," *British Journal of Surgery* 35 (1948): 249–66.

139 A.B. LeMesurier, *Hare-lips and Their Treatment* (Baltimore: Williams & Wilkins, 1962).

140 J.H. Couch, *Surgery of the Hand* (Toronto: University of Toronto Press, 1944).

141 *Dean's Report* 1932–3, 38.

142 *Torontonensis* (1926), 109.

143 W.K. Lindsay, "History of the University of Toronto Plastic Surgery Training Program," *Annals of Plastic Surgery* 22 (1989): 182–3.

144 *Dean's Report* 1944–5, 33, 36.

145 *Torontonensis* (1945), 92.

146 Dept of Surgery, *Annual Report* 1988–9, 24.

147 Pearson, "Goals and Objectives – Department of Surgery, 1978–1988," 8.

148 Ralph T. Manktelow and Nancy H. McKee, "Free Muscle Transplantation to Provide Active Finger Flexion," *Journal of Hand Surgery* 3 (1978): 416–26.

149 [TGH]*Monitor*, Spring 1984, 3.

150 TGH *Annual Report* 1982–3, 9.

151 Ronald M. Zuker and Ralph T. Manktelow, "A Smile for the Möbius Syndrome Patient," *Annals of Plastic Surgery* 22 (1989): 188–94.

152 Ralph T. Manktelow and Ronald Zuker, "Introduction" [to special issue], *Operative Techniques in Plastic and Reconstructive Surgery* 6 (1999): 151.

153 Jeffrey C. Posnick, M.M. Al-Qattan, and R.M. Zuker, "Large Vascular Malformation of the Face Undergoing Resection with Facial Nerve Preservation in Infancy," *Annals of Plastic Surgery* 30 (1993): 67–70.

154 R.A. Newton, "Surgical Tattooing for Port-wine Stain," *Canadian Journal of Otolaryngology* 2 (1973): 251–3.

155 Susan E. MacKinnon and Alan R. Hudson, "Clinical Application of Peripheral Nerve Transplantation," *Journal of Plastic and Reconstructive Surgery* 8 (1992): 695–8.

156 Dept of Surgery, *Annual Report* 1991–2, 22–4.

157 Dept of Surgery, *Annual Report* 1993–4, 3, 209.

158 *Surgical Spotlight*, Fall 2006, 7–8.

159 TTH *Annual Report* 1988–9, 152.

160 TGH *Annual Report* 1914, 7. It is possible that the clinic was founded a year or two previously as I have not seen the organizational tables for 1911–13.

161 *Dean's Report* 1937–8, 52; *Dean's Report* 1945–6, 36.

162 *Dean's Report* 1933–4, 42.

163 D.R. Mitchell, "A Preliminary Report on Sulphanilamide as a Urinary Antiseptic," *CMAJ* 39 (1938): 22–6.

164 *Dean's Report* 1937–8, 51; D.R. Mitchell, P.H. Greey, and C.C. Lucas, "Sulphanilamide in the Treatment of Cystitis and Pyelitis," *CMAJ* 40 (1939): 336–42.

165 Pearl Summerfeldt and D.R. Mitchell, "Treatment of Urinary Infections in Children with Sulfanilamide," *Journal of Urology* 41 (1939): 59–63.
166 Cosbie, *Toronto General Hospital,* 337–8.
167 "Cancer, Smoking and the Bladder," *Time,* 26 Mar. 1965. See W.K. Kerr, M. Barkin, P.E. Levers, S.K.-C. Woo, and Z. Menczyk, "The Effect of Cigarette Smoking on Bladder Carcinogens in Man," *CMAJ* 93 (1965): 1–7.
168 *Dean's Report* 1948–9, 44.
169 *Torontonensis* (1942), 111 (for April class).
170 *Dean's Report* 1956–7, 59.
171 "Charles J Robson," Faculty Council, 1986–8; UTA A1995/0004/004.
172 Dept of Surgery, *Annual Report* 1974–7, 15; *Tablet,* Summer 1989, 4.
173 A. Morales, D. Eidinger, and A.W. Bruce, "Intracavitary Bacillus Calmette-Guerin in the Treatment of Superficial Bladder Tumors," *Journal of Urology* 116 (1976): 180–3.
174 TGH *Annual Report* 1983–4, 1.
175 Pearson, "Goals and Objectives – Department of Surgery, 1978–1988," 9.
176 Dept of Surgery, *Annual Report* 1987–8, 14.
177 TTH *Annual Report* 1988–9, 153.
178 Dept of Surgery, *Annual Report* 1992–3, 30.
179 Joao L. Pippi Salle et al., "Urethral Lengthening with Anterior Bladder Wall flap (Pippi Salle Procedure): Modifications and Extended Indications of the Technique," *Journal of Urology* 158 (1997): 585–90.
180 Dept of Surgery, *Annual Report* 1999–2000, 45.
181 TGH *Annual Report* 1985–6, 69–70.
182 C.M. Morshead et al., "Neural Stem Cells in the Adult Mammalian Forebrain: A Relatively Quiescent Subpopulation of Subependymal Cells," *Neuron* 13 (1994): 1071–82.
183 Langer interview, 20 Oct. 2009, 18.
184 "Surgery Expands Clinical Excellence to Multiorgan Transplants," *Tablet,* Fall 1985, 3.
185 Martin Hollenberg to Bernard Langer, 31 July 1989; UTA A96/0011/023 (10).
186 Langer interview, 20 Oct. 2009, 21.
187 *Tablet,* Fall 1985.
188 Langer to D. Dupreau, Imperial Oil, 24 Nov 1986; UTA A1994/0012/002.
189 Dept of Surgery, *Annual Report* 1989–90, 2, 130.
190 TTH *Annual Report* 1990–1, 7.
191 Ibid., 8–9.
192 "External Review: The Multi-Organ Transplant Program," 1997; Dean's Archive. The "Proposal for a Department of Immunology and Transplantation" (2007) (Dean's Archive) gives the date as 1995.
193 G. Levy, P. Burra, A. Cavallari et al., "Improved Clinical Outcomes for Liver Transplant Recipients Using Cyclosporine Monitoring Based in 2-HR Post-dose Levels (C2)," *Transplantation* 73 (2002): 953–9.

194 Peter Lewis, *Synopsis of Research Activities in the Faculty of Medicine, University of Toronto, and its Affiliated Teaching Hospitals, April 2004–March 2005* (17 Aug 2006) (Office of the Dean), 81.

195 "External Review: The Multi-Organ Transplant Program"; Dean's Archive.

196 Quoted in "A Proposal to Establish a Department of Immunology and Transplantation" (2007), 54; Dean's Archive.

197 *MedEmail*, 30 Mar. 2009.

## 8  Medicine

1 Faculty of Medicine, Self-Study, Feb. 1983; UTA F016/030/031.

2 *Dean's Report* 1938–9, 27; Duncan Graham, W.P. Warner, J.A. Dauphinee, and R.C. Dickson, "The Treatment of Pneumococcal Pneumonia with Dagenan (M&B 693)," *CMAJ* 40 (1939): 325–32.

3 Dewar interview by Schatzker, 22 June 1976, p. 33; Dean's Archive.

4 John A. Oille, "My Experiences in Medicine," *CMAJ* 91 (17 Oct. 1964): 855–60, 860.

5 *Dean's Report* 1960–1, 36.

6 Berris, *Medicine: My Story*, 98.

7 Ibid., 99.

8 *Torontonensis* (1922), 153.

9 J.C. Laidlaw, "Ray Fletcher Farquharson – a Memoir," 2 Apr. 2007, MS. I am grateful to Dr Laidlaw for making a copy available to me.

10 Cosbie, *Toronto General Hospital*, 264.

11 Ray F. Farquharson and Duncan Graham, "Liver Therapy in the Treatment of Subacute Combined Degeneration of the Cord," *CMAJ* 23 (1930): 237–44.

12 George R. Minot and William P. Murphy, "Treatment of Pernicious Anemia by a Special Diet," *JAMA* 87 (14 Aug. 1926): 470–6.

13 E.W. McHenry, E.S. Mills, and R.F. Farquharson, "The Treatment of Pernicious Anaemia by the Intramuscular Administration of Liver Extract," *CMAJ* 28 (1933): 123–32.

14 Donald Cowan, personal communication, 22 July 2010.

15 Ibid., 10 June 2010.

16 R.F. Farquharson and Duncan Graham, "Cases of Simmonds' Disease," *Transactions of the Association of American Physicians* 46 (1931): 150–61.

17 R.F. Farquharson and H.H. Hyland, "Anorexia Nervosa: A Metabolic Disorder of Psychologic Origin," *JAMA* 111 (17 Sept. 1938): 1085–92; R.F. Farquharson and H.H. Hyland, "Simmonds' Disease: Clinical and Pathological Observations on Four Cases," *Transactions of the American Clinical and Climatological Association* 54 (1938): 106–23.

18 R.F. Farquharson and H.H. Hyland, "Anorexia Nervosa: The Course of 15 Patients Treated from 20 to 30 Years Previously," *CMAJ* 94 (1966): 411–19.

19 Helen Farquharson interview, 21 July 2009.

20 Jack Laidlaw, personal communication, 30 Sept. 2010.

21 Quoted in Laidlaw, "Ray Fletcher Farquharson – a Memoir," 10.

22 Helen Farquharson interview, 21 July 2009, 12–13.

23 Laidlaw, "Ray Fletcher Farquharson – a Memoir."

24 Helen Farquharson interview, 21 July 2009, 27.

25 *Dean's Report* 1952–3, 23.

26 R.F. Farquharson, "Concepts of Medical Education in Canada As They Relate to Cardiovascular Teaching," Fifth Conference of Cardiovascular Training Grant Program Directors, Williamsburg, VA, 7–8 June 1958; UTA A1976/0054/18 (13).

27 Berris, *Medicine: My Story*, 75.

28 Hill, "History of the Department of Medicine," 17, quoting from Department of Medicine, *Annual Report* 1960–1.

29 Berris, *Medicine: My Story*, 100.

30 Keith John Roy Wightman, interview with Valerie Schatzker, 7 Jan. 1977, transcript at UTA B1977-0037.

31 The date given in Wightman's CV is 1953, yet other evidence points to 1950.

32 John M. Finlay, "Keith John Roy Wightman," Faculty Council, 13 Apr. 1978; Sept. 1977–May 1978, 266; UTA A1993/0025/009.

33 *Dean's Report* 1969–70, 72.

34 *Dean's Report* 1968–9, 71.

35 Finlay, "Keith John Roy Wightman,"13 April 1978.

36 Wightman interview, 7 Jan. 1977.

37 Donald Cowan, "Kager," undated talk. I am grateful to Dr Cowan for sharing with me a copy of this document.

38 This section on Wightman is based on a number of documents in his personal file at the University of Toronto Archives, including the interview by Valerie Schatzker, 7 Jan. 1977. See also *Dean's Report* 1950–1, 22.

39 Helen Farquharson interview, 21 July 2009, 7.

40 *Dean's Report* 1959–60, 76.

41 *Dean's Report* 1958–9, 67.

42 Wightman in Dept of Medicine, *Annual Report*, 1968–9; quoted in Hill, "History of the Department of Medicine," 36–8.

43 University of Toronto, Faculty of Medicine, *Report of the Independent Planning Committee, constituted by the Faculty Council of the Faculty of Medicine* (Toronto, 1 Oct. 1969) [hereafter Independent Planning Committee *Report* (1969), 84]. Copies of the report are available at UTA and in the Gerstein Science Information Centre, University of Toronto.

44 *Dean's Report* 1948–9, 4, 32; *Dean's Report* 1950–1, 36. Jack Laidlaw established another such unit de novo in 1956 at the General, as stated in his CV (Laidlaw private archive).

45 Jack Laidlaw interview with Edward Shorter, 8 Apr. 2009.

46 *Dean's Report* 1954–5, 25.

47 *Dean's Report* 1952–3, 6.

48 J.C. Laidlaw, E.R. Yendt, and A.G. Gornall, "Hypertension Caused by Renal Artery Occlusion Simulating Primary Aldosteronism," *Metabolism* 9 (1960): 612–23;

see also J.C. Laidlaw, E.R. Yendt, C.E. Bird, and A.G. Gornall, "Hypertension Due to Renal Artery Occlusion Simulating Primary Aldosteronism," *CMAJ* 90 (25 Jan. 1964): 321–5.

49  D.J.A. Sutherland, J.L. Ruse, and J.C. Laidlaw, "Hypertension, Increased Aldosterone Secretion and Low Plasma Renin Activity Relieved by Dexamethasone," *CMAJ* 95 (1966): 1109–19.

50  John Eager Howard, Morgan Berthrong, David M. Gould, and Edmund R. Yendt, "Hypertension Resulting from Unilateral Renal Vascular Disease and Its Relief by Nephrectomy," *Bulletin of the Johns Hopkins Hospital* 94 (1954): 51–75.

51  D.A. Garcia and E.R. Yendt, "Temporary Remission of Hypercalcemia in Hyperparathyroidism Induced by Corticosteroids," *CMAJ* 99 (30 Nov. 1968): 1047–50.

52  *Dean's Report* 1963–4, 43.

53  *Dean's Report* 1965–6, 44.

54  *Dean's Report* 1966–7, 43–4.

55  *Dean's Report* 1967–8, 55.

56  *Dean's Report* 1968–9, 71.

57  Ibid., 72.

58  Ibid., 73.

59  *Dean's Report* 1967–8, 56.

60  K.J.R. Wightman, Dept. of Medicine, *Annual Report* 1969," 6.

61  *Dean's Report* 1968–9, 73.

62  See John Hamilton to A.L. Chute, 4 Feb. 1969; Dept of Medicine Archive.

63  K.J.R. Wightman to C.T. Bissell, 5 Feb. 1969; Dept of Medicine Archive.

64  Donald Cowan, personal communication, 22 July 2010.

65  A.L. Chute to John David Eaton, 31 Mar. 1969; Dept of Medicine Archive.

66  Michelle ("Mimi") Hollenberg interview with Edward Shorter, 6 Apr. 2009.

67  Donald Cowan interview with Edward Shorter, 4 Feb. 2009.

68  Eliot Phillipson, *MediNews*, May 2007, 3.

69  See Robert G. Petersdorf to Brian Holmes, 8 Jan. 1980; UTA A1985/0026/004 (016); the visit took place in December 1979. Petersdorf was evidently sending a draft of his own impressions to Holmes for Holmes to edit, together with the drafts of the other two visitors, into a final report.

70  Mimi Hollenberg interview, 4 Feb. 2009.

71  Charles Hollenberg interview, in Canadian Medical Hall of Fame video, http://www.cdnmedhall.org/dr-charles-h-hollenberg.

72  John Evans interview, in Canadian Medical Hall of Fame Hollenberg video.

73  Eliot Phillipson, *MediNews*, May 2003, 2.

74  Berris, *Medicine: My Story*, 102.

75  *Dean's Report* 1971–2, 88.

76  *Dean's Report* 1970–1, 75.

77  *Dean's Report* 1971–2, 89.

78  Lee Goldman and Lorne Tyrrell, "External Review – Department of Medicine, University of Toronto," 30 Sept.–1 Oct. 2003; Dean's Archive.

79  *Dean's Report* 1970–1, 75.

80 Department of Medicine contribution to the Petch committee: H.E. Petch, Chairman, *Brief on Health Research from the Faculty of Medicine, University of Toronto to the Ontario Government Task Force on Health Research Requirements* (16 Dec. 1974), vol. 3, p. 1; in Gerstein Science Information Centre under call no. R 749 T635.

81 Eliot Phillipson, *MediNews,* June 2007, 1.

82 Undated document, "Organization of Research in Clinical Departments: Department of Medicine – Dr. CH Hollenberg," in Science Policy Committee file following minutes of 2 Mar. 1978 but not identified as part of those minutes; UTA A1993/0025/008.

83 LRPAC Minutes, 19 Feb. 1975, 4; UTA A1979/0010/006.

84 Gerard Burrow, [briefing document for external reviewers, untitled]; in External Review, 1985; Dean's Archive

85 Donald Cowan et al. to F.H. Lowy, 20 Mar. 1986; part of External Review, Department of Medicine, 1985; Dean's Archive.

86 Gerard N. Burrow to F.H. Lowy, 13 Mar. 1986; attached to External Review, Department of Medicine, 1985; Dean's Archive.

87 Ibid.

88 Burrow, [briefing document for external reviewers, untitled].

89 Cowan et al. to Lowy, 20 Mar. 1986. I am also grateful for a personal communication from Eliot Phillipson on this subject, 3 Mar. 2011.

90 "Report of the External Review, Department of Medicine," 1985; Dean's Archive.

91 TGH *Annual Report* 1986–7, 204.

92 Research Program Advisory Committee minutes, 3 Nov. 1987; UTA A1996/0011/022 (4).

93 Gerard Burrow, "Interview," *Monitor,* Winter 1988, 11.

94 Arnie Aberman, personal communication, 21 July 2010.

95 Eliot Phillipson, personal communication, 3 Mar. 2011.

96 Louis Siminovitch interview with Edward Shorter, 16 Dec. 2008.

97 Berris, *Medicine: My Story,* 104.

98 Helen Farquharson interview, 21 July 2009.

99 Eliot Phillipson, *MediNews,* May 2003, 3.

100 Eliot Phillipson, *MediNews,* Sept. 2001, 1–2.

101 Eliot Phillipson, *MediNews,* June 1998, 4.

102 Jack Laidlaw, personal communication, 30 Sept. 2010.

103 Eliot Phillipson, *MediNews,* Nov. 1997, 1–2.

104 Ibid., 2–4.

105 Eliot Phillipson, *MediNews,* May 2007, 3.

106 Wendy Levinson, *MediNews,* Feb. 2006, 1–2.

107 Eliot Phillipson, *MediNews,* June 1997, 2.

108 Ibid.

109 Eliot Phillipson, *MediNews,* Sept. 1997, 2.

110 Eliot Phillipson, personal communication, 3 Mar. 2011.

111 Eliot Phillipson, *MediNews,* June 1998, 1–2.

112 Goldman and Tyrrell, "External Review – Dept of Medicine."
113 Eliot Phillipson, *MediNews*, June 1997, 3–4.
114 Eliot Phillipson, *MediNews*, Mar. 1997, 4–5.
115 *Dean's Report* 1929–30, 14.
116 See "Medical Department," *Varsity*, 3 Feb. 1891, 166; E.C. Séguin, "Lectures on Some Points in the Treatment and Management of Neuroses: Delivered before the Medical Society of the University of Toronto, March 11–12, 1890," *New York Medical Journal*; repr. New York: Appleton, 1890. I am grateful to John Court for these references.
117 "The Sub-committee [on the merger with Trinity] recommend that the Department be reorganized and that the teaching be apportioned between Prof. JM McCallum and Dr. J[ohn] T[aylor] Fotheringham, Prof McCallum to lecture on Materia Medica, Pharmacology and a portion of Therapeutics, the remainder of the subject of Therapeutics to be given by Dr. Fotheringham in addition to his duties in Clinical Medicine. As soon as the University is in a position to pay for a Professor of Pharmacology it is recommended that the department be reorganized." UTA A79/0023/1001(2).
118 Faculty Council, 6 Apr. 1900; UTA A1986/0027/016.
119 Duncan Graham, Recommendations for Appointment, 1920–1; Dept of Medicine Archive, no date.
120 *Dean's Report* 1929–30, 14.
121 *Dean's Report* 1934–5, 21.
122 *President's Report* 1934, 8.
123 *Dean's Report* 1937–8, 11.
124 *Dean's Report* 1939–40, 61.
125 *Dean's Report* 1953–4, 36.
126 Cosbie, *Toronto General Hospital*, 244.
127 *Dean's Report* 1950–1, 55.
128 *Dean's Report* 1952–3, 57.
129 J.A. MacFarlane, *Dean's Report* 1960–1, 3.
130 *Dean's Report* 1957–8, 66.
131 *Dean's Report* 1961–2, 88; Wightman wrote the report for the Department of Therapeutics in that session, a new head of therapeutics not yet having been appointed.
132 Ramsay Gunton, *Dean's Report* 1965–6, 116–17.

## 9  The Medical Subspecialties

1 *MediNews*, June 2009, 1–2.
2 Eliot Phillipson, *MediNews*, Mar. 1998, 2–3.
3 J.A. MacFarlane, "The Medical School in a Canadian Community," *CMAJ* 73 (15 July 1955): 117–20, 188.
4 Eliot Phillipson, *MediNews*, May 2003, 2.
5 *Dean's Report* 1966–7, 43.

6  Ibid.
7  *Dean's Report* 1968–9, 74.
8  Robert G. Petersdorf to Brian Holmes, 8 Jan. 1980; UTA A1985/0026/004/(016); the visit took place in December 1979.
9  External review, Department of Medicine, 1986, attached to Frederick H. Lowy to G.N. Burrow, 31 Jan. 1986; UTA A1994/0012/014.
10  Wendy Levinson, *MediNews*, Nov. 2007, 1–2.
11  W.R. Campbell to K.J.R. Wightman, 2 July 1963; Department of Medicine Archive.
12  *Epistaxis* (1921), 20.
13  *Torontonensis* (1903), 157.
14  Biographical details on Oille from Segall, *Pioneers of Cardiology*, 69–71.
15  *Dean's Report* 1961–2, 6.
16  "Andrew Robertson Gordon," Faculty Council, 2 Feb. 1917; UTA A1986/0027/018.
17  Details on Jamieson's life from Segall, *Pioneers of Cardiology*, 80–1; *Torontonensis* (1910), 157.
18  Ibid., 87.
19  *Torontonensis* (1921), 131.
20  "John Hepburn," Faculty Council, 8 June 1956; UTA A1986/0027/026.
21  J. Hepburn and R.A. Jamieson, "The Prognostic Significance of Several Common Electrocardiographic Abnormalities," *American Heart Journal* 1 (1926): 623–8, 628. On John Hepburn's colourful life, see Segall, *Pioneers of Cardiology*, 87–91.
22  H.E. Rykert and J. Hepburn, "Electrocardiographic Abnormalities Characteristic of Certain Cases of Arterial Hypertension," *American Heart Journal* 10 (1935): 942–52.
23  *Epistaxis* (1934), 19.
24  Berris, *Medicine: My Story*, 63, 76–7.
25  H.E. Rykert, "Penicillin in Subacute Bacterial Endocarditis," *CMAJ* 55 (1946): 543–7.
26  Department of Medicine, *Annual Report* 1945–6, 3–4.
27  McKellar, *Surgical Limits*, 45.
28  Bigelow, *Mysterious Heparin*, 109; Greenwood's paper was unpublished.
29  Max M. Gorelick, Susan C.M. Lenkel, Raymond O. Heimbecker, and Ramsay W. Gunton, "Estimation of Mitral Regurgitation by Injection of Dye into the Left Ventricle with Simultaneous Left Atrial Sampling: A Clinical Study of Sixty Confirmed Cases," *American Journal of Cardiology* 10 (1962): 62–9.
30  Bigelow, *Cold Hearts*, 129.
31  Segall, *Pioneers of Cardiology*, s.v. "William Bigelow," 403.
32  K.W.G. Brown, R.L. MacMillan, N. Forbath, F. Mel'grano, and J.W. Scott, "Coronary Unit: An Intensive-Care Centre for Acute Myocardial Infarction," *Lancet* 2 (17 Aug. 1963): 349–52.
33  Sandra Martin, obituary for Robert Laidlaw MacMillan, *Globe and Mail*, 14 Sept. 2007, S9.
34  Ibid.
35  Segall, *Pioneers of Cardiology*, 201.

36  Segall, *Pioneers of Cardiology*, s.v. "William F. Greenwood," 280; *Dean's Report* 1955–6, 29.
37  John Morch, response of Division of Cardiology to Petch committee, 6–7.
38  E. Douglas Wigle, "The Diagnosis of Hypertrophic Cardiomyopathy," *Heart* 86 (2001): 709–14.
39  Ramsay Gunton, "External Review of Cardiology at the University of Toronto," Sept. 1979, attached to John E. Morch memo, 2 Nov. 1979; UTA A1985/0026/004 (016).
40  Faculty Research Committee, minutes, 21 May 1987; UTA A1996/011/022(4).
41  Research Program Advisory Committee minutes, 3 Nov. 1987; UTA A1996/0011/0022 (4).
42  Michael J. Sole to Peter McLaughlin, 9 Sept. 1988; UTA A1996/011/022(4).
43  Executive Summary [of a proposal for The Toronto Hospital Heart Institute], 4 Apr. 1989; UTA A1996/011/022(4).
44  William Sibbald and Tejdip Singh, "Critical Care in Canada: The North American Difference," *Critical Care Clinics* 13 (1997): 347–62.
45  Fairley, "Recollections of the Toronto General Hospital," 122–3.
46  *Dean's Report* 1958–9, 32.
47  H.O. Barber, R.A. Chambers, H.B. Fairley, and C.R. Woolf, "A Respiratory Unit: The Toronto General Hospital Unit for the Treatment of Severe Respiratory Insufficiency," *CMAJ* 81 (15 July 1959): 97–101.
48  Berris, *Medicine: My Story*, 76.
49  UTA A1986/0028/001, 2 June 1967.
50  J.M. Nelems, J. Duffin, F.X. Glynn, J. Brebner, A.A. Scott, and J.D. Cooper, "Extracorporeal Membrane Oxygenator Support for Human Lung Transplantation," *Journal of Thoracic Cardiovascular Surgery* 76 (1978): 28–32.
51  E.B. Phillipson, response of Respirology Division to Research Committee of the Department of Medicine, for Petch committee, 25–6.
52  Hollenberg report, 17 July 1973, 6; UTA A1986/0028/004 (002).
53  N.R. Anthonisen, "Report on University of Toronto Department of Medicine Program in Pulmonary Disease," 5 July 1979; UTA A1985/0026/004 (016).
54  Eliot Phillipson, personal communication, 3 Mar. 2011.
55  TGH *Annual Report* 1984–5, 86–9.
56  Yuji Takasaki, D. Orr, J. Popkin, R. Rutherford, P. Liu, and T. Douglas Bradley, "Effect of Nasal Continuous Positive Airway Pressure on Sleep Apnea in Congestive Heart Failure," *American Review of Respiratory Disease* 140 (1989): 1578–84.
57  T.D. Bradley and J.S. Floras, "Sleep Apnea and Heart Failure: Part I: Obstructive Sleep Apnea," *Circulation* 107 (2003): 1671–8.
58  V. Marco Ranieri, P.M. Suter, C. Tortorella, R. De Tullio, J.M. Dayer, A. Brienza, F. Bruno, and Arthur S. Slutsky, "Effect of Mechanical Ventilation on Inflammatory Mediators in Patients with Acute Respiratory Distress Syndrome," *JAMA* 281 (7 July 1999): 54–61. Quote from Niall D. Ferguson and Arthur S. Slutsky, "Point: Counterpoint: High-frequency Ventilation Is/Is Not the Optimal Physiological

Approach to Ventilate ARDS Patients," *Journal of Applied Physiology* 104 (2008): 1230–5, 1230. Slutsky called attention to the consequences of mechanical ventilation in "Lung Injury Caused by Mechanical Ventilation," *Chest* 116 (1999): 9S–15S.

59 Lorraine N. Tremblay, Debra Miatto, Qutayba Hamid, Anand Govindarajan, and Arthur S. Slutsky, "Injurious Ventilation Induces Widespread Pulmonary Epithelial Expression of Tumor Necrosis Factor-alpha and Interleukin-6 Messenger RNA," *Critical Care Medicine* 30 (2002): 1693–700.

60 *Dean's Report* 1933–4, 23.

61 R.A. Cleghorn, E.W. McHenry, G.A. McVicar, and D.W. Overend, "Experimental and Clinical Studies on Adrenal Insufficiency," *CMAJ* 37 (1937): 48–52; see also R.A. Cleghorn, J.L.A. Fowler, J.S. Wenzel, and A.P.W. Clarke, "The Desoxycortisone Acetate Requirement of the Adrenalectomized Dog," *Endocrinology* 29 (1941): 535–44.

62 R.A. Cleghorn, "Recognition and Treatment of Addison's Disease," *CMAJ* 44 (1941): 581–6, 586; the paper was delivered in 1940. See also *Dean's Report* 1938–9, 25.

63 *Dean's Report* 1948–9, 4, 32.

64 Cosbie, *Toronto General Hospital*, 300.

65 J.C. Laidlaw, "Nature of the Circulating Thyroid Hormone," *Nature* 164 (26 Nov. 1949): 927–8.

66 Laidlaw interview, 8 Apr. 2009.

67 Ibid.

68 D. Fraser and J.C. Laidlaw, "Treatment of Hypophosphatasia with Cortisone," *Lancet* 1 (1956): 553.

69 Laidlaw, Yendt, and Gornall, "Hypertension Caused by Renal Artery Occlusion," 612–23.

70 Sutherland, Ruse, and Laidlaw, "Hypertension, Increased Aldosterone Secretion," 1109.

71 Amir K. Hanna, Bernard Zinman, A.F. Nakhooda, H.L. Minuk, E.F. Stokes, A.M. Albisser, B.S. Leibel, and E.B. Marliss, "Insulin, Glucagon, and Amino Acids during Glycemic Control by the Artificial Pancreas in Diabetic Man," *Metabolism* 29 (1980): 321–32. For early work see A.M. Albisser, B.S. Leibel, T.G. Ewart, Z. Davidovac, C.K. Botz, and W. Zingg, "An Artificial Endocrine Pancreas," *Diabetes* 23 (1974): 389–96.

72 The Diabetes Control and Complications Trial Research Group [Zinman chaired the writing committee], "The Effect of Intensive Treatment of Diabetes on the Development and Progression of Long-Term Complications in Insulin-Dependent Diabetes Mellitus," *New England Journal of Medicine* 329 (30 Sept. 1993): 977–86; on a follow-up morbidity study see the Diabetes Control and Complications Trial Study Research Group [Zinman chaired the writing committee], "Intensive Diabetes Treatment and Cardiovascular Disease in Patients with Type I Diabetes," *New England Journal of Medicine* 353 (22 Dec. 2005): 2643–53.

73  William D. Wilson and Calvin Ezrin, "Three Types of Chromophil Cells of the Adenohypophysis," *American Journal of Pathology* 30 (1954): 891–9.

74  "Historical File," Department of Medicine Archive, 3–4. See J.G. Edmeads, R.E. Mathews, N.T. McPhedran, and C. Ezrin, "Diarrhea Caused by Pancreatic Islet Cell Tumours," *CMAJ* 86 (1962): 847–51.

75  Robert Volpé, Douglas L. Schatz, Aileen Scott, Joseph A. Peller, Joan M. Vale, Calvin Ezrin, and MacAllister Johnston, "Radioactive Iodine in the Treatment of Hyperthyroidism: Experience at the Toronto General Hospital, 1950–58, Part I," *CMAJ* 83 (31 Dec. 1960): 1407–13; this was the first of three parts.

76  Ibid.; Robert Volpé, Douglas L. Schatz, Aileen Scott, Joseph A. Peller, Joan M. Vale, Calvin Ezrin, and MacAllister Johnston, "Radioactive Iodine in the Treatment of Hyperthyroidism: Experience at the Toronto General Hospital, 1950–58, Part II," *CMAJ* 84 (14 Jan. 1961): 84–7.

77  Robert Volpé, Merrill Edmonds, Lamk Lamki, Peter V. Clarke, and Vas V. Row, "The Pathogenesis of Graves' Disease: A Disorder of Delayed Hypersensitivity?" *Mayo Clinic Proceedings* 47 (1972): 824–34, 832.

78  Terry F. Davies, "Growing an Interest in Autoimmune Thyroid Disease: An Interview with Robert Volpé," *Endocrinology and Metabolism Clinics of North America* 29 (2000): 431–42, 441.

79  Paul G. Walfish, Murray Miskin, Irving B. Rosen, and Harry T.G. Strawbridge, "Application of Special Diagnostic Techniques in the Management of Nodular Goiter," *CMAJ* 115 (3 July 1976): 35–40.

80  I.R. Hart and J.W. Meakin, "Report on the University of Toronto Training Program in Endocrinology," April 1979; UTA A1985/0026/004 (016).

81  TGH *Annual Report* 1915, 9.

82  Mentioned in *Dean's Report* 1933–4, 43.

83  *Torontonensis* (1924), 129.

84  *Dean's Report* 1954–5, 26.

85  *Dean's Report* 1948–9, 19.

86  John R. Bingham, Franz J. Ingelfinger, and Reginald H. Smithwick, "The Effects of Sympathectomy on the Motility of the Human Gastrointestinal and Biliary Tracts," *Gastroenterology* 15 (1950): 6–17.

87  Stanley J. Dudrick, "History of Parenteral Nutrition," *Journal of the American College of Nutrition* 28 (2009): 243–51; Dudrick does not mention Jeejeebhoy's work.

88  K.N. Jeejeebhoy et al., "Total Parenteral Nutrition at Home for 23 Months, Without Complication, and with Good Rehabilitation," *Gastroenterology* 65 (1973): 811–20, 812.

89  Langer interview, 20 Oct. 2009, 22.

90  G. Forstner, response of Gastroenterology Division to Research Committee of Department of Medicine, for Petch committee, 13–14.

91  L.S. Valberg, "Residency Training Program in Gastroenterology, University of Toronto," no date [1979]; UTA A1985/0026/004 (016).

92  C. Hollenberg, "Personnel Requirements, Department of Medicine, 1974–76"; UTA A1979/0010/006.

93  TTH *Annual Report* 1987–8, 136–7.

94  Sharif B. Missiha, Mario Ostrowski, and E. Jenny Heathcote, "Disease Progression in Chronic Hepatitis C: Modifiable and Nonmodifiable Factors," *Gastroenterology* 134 (2008): 1699–714.

95  Charles H. Hollenberg, eulogy, "Dr M. Lenczner," Faculty Council, 13 Dec. 1976; UTA A1993/0025/009.

96  See Charles Hollenberg memo of 17 July 1973, UTA A1986/0028/004 (002).

97  Hillar Vellend, personal communication, 27 Jan. 2010.

98  "Review, Division of Infectious Diseases, Department of Medicine," no date [1979]; no author stated; UTA A1985/0026/004 (01):6.

99  TGH *Annual Report* 1984–5, 105.

100  TGH *Annual Report* 1986–7, 256–8.

101  See, for example, Kai Hübel, David C. Dale, and W. Conrad Liles, "Therapeutic Use of Cytokines to Modulate Phagocyte Function for the Treatment of Infectious Diseases," *Journal of Infectious Diseases* 185 (2002): 1490–501.

102  The MaRS Discovery District, located on the southwest corner of College Street and University Avenue, is a not-for-profit corporation launched in 2000 to commercialize publicly-funded research. The facility incorporates (as its Heritage Building) the preserved façade of the Toronto General Hospital's College Wing. http://www.marsdd.com/aboutmars.

103  *MediNews*, Dec. 2006, 4.

104  Donald Cowan, personal communication, 22 July 2010.

105  *Dean's Report* 1966–7, 44–5.

106  According to TGH *Annual Report* 1984–5, 977, "fifteen years ago."

107  M.B. Goldstein, response of Nephrology Division to Research Committee of the Department of Medicine, for Petch committee, 20–1.

108  Jack Rubin, Dimitrios G. Oreopoulos, Gordon Blair, Lionel D.J. Chisholm, Eric Meema, and George A. de Veber, "Chronic Peritoneal Dialysis in the Management of Diabetics with Terminal Renal Failure," *Nephron* 19 (1977): 265–70.

109  Ahmad Alfaiw, Stephen Vas, and Dimitrios Oreopoulos, "Peritonitis in Patients on Automated Peritoneal Dialysis," in *Automated Peritoneal Dialysis: Contributions to Nephrology*, vol. 129, ed. C. Ronco et al. (Basel, Switzerland: Karger, 1999), 213–28, 213.

110  Stephen I. Vas, "Peritonitis during CAPD: A Mixed Bag," *Peritoneal Dialysis International* 1 (1981): page numbers not included in download.

111  Douglas R. Wilson to Mortimer Levy, 8 Mar. 1979; UTA A1985/0026/004/016.

112  Mortimer Levy, "University of Toronto Nephrology Program: A Mini-Review Based on a Visit March 15, 1979"; UTA A1985/0026/004 (016).

113  See Carl J. Cardella et al., "Rejection Episodes and Lymphocyte Responses in Patients Treated with Rabbit Antithymocyte Sera," *Transplantation Proceedings* 16

(1984): 1089–92; Carl J. Cardella, "Plasma Exchange and Renal Transplantation," *Journal of Clinical Apheresis* 2 (1985): 405–9.

114 TGH *Annual Report* 1982–3, 10.

115 TGH *Annual Report* 1984–5, 61, 97–8.

116 Ibid., 97–8.

117 TGH *Annual Report* 1985–6, 1, 134–6.

118 "External Review: Multi-Organ Transplantation Program," 1992; Dean's Archive.

119 The first edition was M.L. Halperin and Marc B. Goldstein, *Fluids, Electrolyte, and Acid-Base Emergencies* (Philadelphia: Saunders, 1988).

120 TTH *Annual Report* 1988–9, 106–10.

121 *MediNews*, Nov. 2000.

122 See, for example, A. Almon Fletcher and J. Wallace Graham, "Complications of Diabetes Mellitus with Special Reference to Cause and Prevention," *CMAJ* 41 (1939): 566–70. "It would appear wise to protect diabetic patients as far as possible from repeated infection, to keep them free of focal infection" (570).

123 A.A. Fletcher and Duncan Graham, "The Large Bowel in Chronic Arthritis," *Journal of the Medical Sciences* 179 (1930): 91–3.

124 See K.M. Graham, "Origins and Early Beginnings of the Canadian Arthritis Society and the First Rheumatic Disease Units in Canada," *Journal of Rheumatology* 27 (2000): 1592–8.

125 Ibid., 1593.

126 "An Interview with Dr. Hugh Smythe," *Journal of the Canadian Rheumatology Association* 9 (1999): 6–8.

127 *Dean's Report* 1940–1, 18. J.W. Graham and A.A. Fletcher, "Gold Therapy in Rheumatoid Arthritis," *CMAJ* 49 (1943): 483–7.

128 Wallace Graham, "The Fibrositis Syndrome," *Bulletin on Rheumatic Diseases* 3 (1953): 51–2; see George S. Young, a Toronto family physician, giving a talk, "Fibrositis as a Cause of Pain and Disability," at a meeting of the Ontario Medical Association, 28 May 1931; *CMAJ* 24 (1931): 718. On the history of fibrositis as a concept see Edward Shorter, *From Paralysis to Fatigue: A History of Psychosomatic Illness in the Modern Era* (New York: Free Press, 1992), 311–12.

129 Wallace Graham and James B. Roberts, "Intravenous Colchicine in the Management of Gouty Arthritis," *Annals of Rheumatic Disease* 12 (1953): 16–19.

130 "James Wallace Graham," Faculty Council, 25 Jan. 1963, 234–7; UTA A1986/0027/027.

131 This dating is supplied by K.M. Graham, "Origins and Early Beginnings," 1594.

132 M.A. Ogryzlo and Wallace Graham, "Reiter's Syndrome: Effect of Pituitary Adrenocorticotropic Hormone (ACTH) and Cortisone," *JAMA* 144 (9 Dec. 1950): 1239–43.

133 M.A. Ogryzlo, "The L.E. (Lupus Erythematosus) Cell Reaction," *CMAJ* 75 (15 Dec. 1956): 980–93.

134 M.A. Ogryzlo and H.A. Smythe, "Systemic Lupus Erythematosus and Syndromes Possibly Related," *Pediatrics* 19 (1957): 1109–23.
135 Hugh Smythe, "Tender Points: Evolution of Concepts of the Fibrositis/Fibromyalgia Syndrome," *American Journal of Medicine* 81, supplement 3A (1986): 2–6.
136 Almon Fletcher to K.J.R. Wightman, 10 June 1963; Dept of Medicine Archive.
137 Wallace Graham and John Digby, U of T Rheumatic Diseases Unit, Queen Elizabeth Hospital Division, First Annual Report, 1 Oct. 1960–30 June 1961; UTA A1976/0054/14 (R).
138 Duncan A. Gordon, Murray B. Urowitz, and Hugh A. Smythe, "MA Ogryzlo," Faculty Council, 13 June 1977; UTA A1993/0025/(009).
139 Louis G. Johnson, E.R. Yendt, L. Shulman, and A.S. Russell, "Report of the On-Site Visit to the RDU, University of Toronto," 12 Aug. 1977; UTA A1985/0026/004 (019).
140 Eliot Phillipson interview with Edward Shorter, 12 Apr. 2011.
141 *Dean's Report* 1970–1, 75.
142 TGH *Annual Report* 1984–5, 111.
143 TGH *Annual Report* 1985–6, 119.
144 For example, V. Goel, R.B. Deber, and A.S. Detsky, "Nonionic Contrast Media: A Bargain for Some, A Burden for Many," *CMAJ* 143 (1990): 480–1.
145 See Lowy to M.J. Ashley et al., 26 Mar. 1985; UTA A1994/0012 (06); Committee of Clinical Chairs meeting, 27 Jan. 1987; UTA A1993/0025/01.
146 "As Brilliant as House: But Nicer," *Globe and Mail*, 20 Nov. 2009.
147 Phillipson interview, 12 Apr. 2011.
148 Ibid.

## 10  The Children's Hospital

1 Hospital for Sick Children, *Annual Report* [hereafter HSC *Annual Report*] 1906, 8.
2 On the hospital's origins and history see Abelardo A. Retureta et al., "The Hospital for Sick Children, Toronto," *International Pediatrics* 15 (2000): 179–85; C.P. Shah, Helen E. Reid, and W.E. Zingg, "A Century of Care: A Future of Caring," *CMAJ* 113 (1975): 485–6; and Schiff, "'The Sweetest of all Charities.'" Biographies of Elizabeth Wyllie (McMaster) and John Ross Robertson appear in the *Dictionary of Canadian Biography Online*. See also Judith Young, "A Divine Mission: Elizabeth McMaster and the Hospital for Sick Children, Toronto, 1875–92," *Canadian Bulletin of Medical History* 11 (1994): 71–90.
3 HSC *Annual Report* 1887, 10
4 HSC *Annual Report* 1915, 23.
5 HSC *Annual Report* 1906, 6.
6 HSC *Annual Report* 1887, n.p.
7 Faculty of Medicine, *Calendar* 1892–3 , 156.
8 Shah, Reid, and Zingg, "Century of Care."
9 See Faculty Council, 6 Apr. 1900; UTA A1986/0027/016.
10 "Allen MacKenzie Baines," Faculty Council, 7 Apr. 1922, 453; UTA A1986/0027/018.

11  "Dr. Allen MacKenzie Baines," obituary, *CMAJ* 12 (1922): 192.

12  See *President's Report* 1921–2, 14; earlier dates for Machell and Baines come from the *Calendar* of the Faculty of Medicine.

13  Faculty of Medicine *Calendar*, 1904–5, 80.

14  The reorganization is mentioned in "New Head Surgeon," *Toronto Telegram*, 20 Aug. 1921.

15  Gallie, "Fifty Years' Growth," 10.

16  *Torontonensis* (1909), 158.

17  Allison B. Foster Kingsmill, *Dr. Alan Brown: Portrait of a Tyrant* (Toronto: Fitzhenry and Whiteside, 1995), 39.

18  Ibid., 50–1.

19  J. Harry Ebbs, "Alan Brown, the Man," *CMAJ* 113 (20 Sept. 1975): 557.

20  *Epistaxis* (1926), 18.

21  Berris, *Medicine: My Story*, 26.

22  "Department of Medicine" [1920]; UTA A1979/0023/002.

23  "Tuitional Extension"; HSC *Annual Report* 1919, 4.

24  "Department of Medicine" [1920]; UTA A1979/0023/002.

25  "Larger Theatre for Lectures"; HSC *Annual Report* 1920, 5.

26  "Chemical Research Laboratory"; HSC *Annual Report* 1920, 5.

27  HSC *Annual Report* 1920, 2.

28  J.H. Ebbs, "The History of the Canadian Paediatric Society," *CMAJ* 78 (1957): 662–4.

29  *Epistaxis* (1927), 16.

30  *Dean's Report* 1935–6, 28.

31  Alan Moncrieff, "The London Letter," *CMAJ* 47 (1942): 587–8.

32  University of Toronto, *Medical Bulletin* 4 (1923): 2.

33  *Dean's Report* 1936–7, 31.

34  *Dean's Report* 1937–8, 32.

35  *Torontonensis* (1914), 117.

36  *Torontonensis* (1916), 117.

37  On Courtney see Ebbs, "Alan Brown," 557.

38  *Dean's Report* 1926–7, 8.

39  Paul Danby, "1920s Mush Burps Money," *Toronto Star*, 28 May 1998.

40  Frederick F. Tisdall, T.G.H. Drake, and Alan Brown, "A New Cereal Mixture Containing Vitamins and Mineral Elements," *American Journal of Diseases of Children* 40 (1930): 791–9, 799.

41  Alan Brown, T.G.H. Drake, and J.H. Ebbs, "Dr. Fred F. Tisdall, an Appreciation," *CMAJ* 61 (1949): 86.

42  John Ross and Alan Brown, "Poisonings Common in Children," Symposium on Common Poisonings, *Canadian Public Health Journal* 26 (1935): 237–43.

43  John R. Ross and Colin C. Lucas, "A New Method for the Determination of Minute Amounts of Lead in Urine," *Journal of Biological Chemistry* 3 (1935): 285–97.

44  "In Memoriam, John Ross," *American Academy of Pediatrics, AAP News* 11 (1995): 22.

45 Louis Eisenberg, "History of Inhalation Therapy Equipment," *International Anesthesiology Clinics* 4 (1966): 549–62.

46 *Popular Science Monthly*, Sept. 1929, included a photo.

47 *Dean's Report* 1933–4, 25.

48 James H. Maxwell, "The Iron Lung: Halfway Technology or Necessary Step?" *Milbank Quarterly* 64 (1986): 30–8.

49 *Dean's Report* 1938–9, 35.

50 Christopher J. Rutty, "The Middle-Class Plague: Epidemic Polio and the Canadian State, 1936–37," *Canadian Bulletin of Medical History* 13 (1996): 277–314, 293.

51 F.F. Tisdall, A. Brown, R.D. Defries, M.A. Ross, and A.H. Sellers, "Zinc Sulphate Nasal Spray in the Prophylaxis of Poliomyelitis," *Canadian Public Health Journal* 28 (1937): 531–7.

52 Rutty, "Middle-Class Plague," 294.

53 Ibid., 295.

54 Ibid., 297.

55 Ibid., 298.

56 *Dean's Report* 1937–8, 52.

57 Rutty, "Middle-Class Plague," 300.

58 "Women Hail Gain in Paralysis Fight," *New York Times*, 7 Jan. 1940, 3.

59 Rutty, "Middle-Class Plague," 301.

60 Department of Paediatrics, "History of the Department of Paediatrics," http://www.paeds.utoronto.ca/about/history.htm.

61 Ibid.

62 *Dean's Report* 1950–1, 6; the report, written in June 1951, said the conference would be taking place the coming October.

63 A.J. Rhodes, L. McClelland, and W.L. Donohue, "Laboratory Studies on Poliomyelitis, Toronto, 1947," *CMAJ* 60 (1949): 359–63; Nelles Silverthorne, A.J. Rhodes, M. Patricia Armstrong, F.H. Wilson et al., "Studies on Poliomyelitis in Ontario," *CMAJ* 61 (1949): 241–50. This work continued through the early 1950s.

64 *Dean's Report* 1950–1, 31.

65 "Dr. Alan Brown, Pediatrician, 73," *New York Times*, 9 Sept. 1960, 29.

66 *Dean's Report* 1948–9, 28.

67 "Obituaries: Alan Brown," and "Dr. Alan Brown: An Appreciation," *CMAJ* 83 (1960), 730.

68 Carlotta Hacker, *The Indomitable Lady Doctors* (Toronto and Vancouver: Clarke, Irwin, 1974), 118–22. On Pearl Smith Chute see the brief biography in "100th Anniversary of Women at U of T," UTA A1994/0012/05.

69 Biographical details from *Toronto Telegram*, 27 Oct. 1952; *Toronto Daily Star*, 12 Sept. 1952.

70 *Dean's Report* 1956–7, 39; *President's Report* 1956–7, 56.

71 *Dean's Report* 1961–2, 56–57.

72 *Dean's Report* 1957–8, 42.

73 *Dean's Report* 1958–9, 46.

74 *Dean's Report* 1962–3, 59.

75 *Dean's Report* 1963–4, 64.

76 *Dean's Report* 1964–5, 68.

77 *Torontonensis* (1944), 135.

78 "Enterprise," *Globe and Mail*, 27 Feb. 1969.

79 Obituary, *Toronto Star*, 7 Dec. 2001.

80 On this litany of complaints, see Department of Paediatrics Presentation to the LRPAC, Nov. 1974, 7; attached to W.R. Harris to LRPAC, 21 Nov. 1974; UTA A1979/0010/006.

81 Charlotte Gray, "Profile: Harry Bain," *CMAJ* 129 (15 Sept. 1983): 614.

82 Department of Paediatrics Presentation to the LRPAC, Nov. 1974, 4.

83 Ibid., 7.

84 Allan B. Okey interview with Edward Shorter, 19 Nov. 2005, 5.

85 Faculty of Medicine, Self-Study, Feb. 1983, 79–80; UTA F016/030/031.

86 "History of the Department of Paediatrics," http://www.paeds.utoronto.ca/about/history.htm.

87 Robert H.A. Haslam, "Robert Haslam: An Autobiography from a Canadian Perspective," *Journal of Child Neurology* 20 (2006): 547–52, 547.

88 Donald Medearis, Jr., "Report of an External Review of the Department of Pediatrics, University of Toronto and the Hospital for Sick Children, Feb. 12, 1991"; attached to External Review, Department of Pediatrics, 1991; Dean's Archive.

89 Faculty of Medicine, Self-Study, Jan. 1990, 116; UTA A1996/0011/0018 (6).

90 Faculty of Medicine, *Tablet*, Sept. 1991, 2–3.

91 "The Hospital for Sick Children: The Perfect Setting; Pediatric Care Finds Its Jerusalem," *Globe and Mail*, 25 Jan. 1993, C3.

92 "The Hospital for Sick Children: A Miracle Renewed," *Globe and Mail*, 25 Jan. 1993, C3.

93 Dept of Surgery, *Annual Report* 1995–6, 45.

94 *New York Times*, 30 July 1995, E13.

95 Information on Hugh O'Brodovich is drawn from his 1 Feb. 2005 CV from HSC and his profile at Stanford, http://pediatrics.stanford.edu/faculty/chair.html.

96 HSC, Division of Respiratory Medicine, http://www.sickkids.ca/RespiratoryMedicine/Who-we-are/Our-history/index.html.

97 H. O'Brodovich, V. Hannam, M. Seear, and J.B.M. Mullen, "Amiloride Impairs Lung Water Clearance in Newborn Guinea Pigs," *Journal of Applied Physiology* 68 (1990): 1758–62.

98 Ibid.

99 "External Review, Department of Pediatrics," 2000; Dean's Archive.

100 O'Brodovich profile at Stanford.

101 Department of Paediatrics Presentation to the LRPAC, Nov. 1974, 10–11.

102 Independent Planning Committee *Report* (1969), 52–3.

103 Self-Study, Feb. 1983, 81.

104 "Rules Finally Passed by the Committee, 11th December, 1878," HSC *Annual Report* 1887, 8.

105  HSC *Annual Report* 1906, 16.

106  HSC *Annual Report* 1908, 7.

107  HSC *Annual Report* 1908.

108  HSC, Division of Neonatology, "Our History," http://www.sickkids.ca/neonatology/index.html, accessed 8 Apr. 2010. (This source gives the number of cubicles as twenty-eight however, whereas the hospital's 1915 *Annual Report*, p. 4, says, "There are 40 in the baby wing.")

109  HSC *Annual Report* 1915, 4.

110  Peter M. Dunn, "Dr Alfred Hart (1888–1954) of Toronto and Exsanguination Transfusion of the Newborn," *Archives of Disease in Childhood* 69 (1993): 95–6, 96.

111  A.P. Hart, "Familial Icterus Gravis of the New-Born and Its Treatment," *CMAJ* 15 (1925): 1008–11.

112  "Dr. Alfred Hart, 66, Transfusion Pioneer," *New York Times*, 5 Sept. 1954, 51.

113  Paul R. Swyer and G.C.W. James, "A Case of Unilateral Pulmonary Emphysema," *Thorax* 8 (1953): 133–6.

114  M.D. Papadopoulos and P.R. Swyer, "Assisted Ventilation in Terminal Hyaline Membrane Disease," *Archives of Disease in Childhood* 39 (1964): 481–4.

115  L.S. Linsao, H. Levison, and P.R. Swyer, "Negative Pressure Artificial Respiration: Use in Treatment of Respiratory Distress Syndrome of the Newborn," *CMAJ* 102 (28 Mar. 1970): 602–5.

116  *Dean's Report* 1970–1, 107.

117  Paul R. Swyer, *The Intensive Care of the Newly Born: Physiological Principles and Practice* (Basel, Switzerland: Karger, 1975).

118  *Living Lessons: Three Stories from the Medical Profession About Quality of Life for the Last Stages of Life* (GlaxoSmithKline Foundation and Canadian Hospice Palliative Care Association, n.d.), http://www.living-lessons.org/resources/secured/PhysicianStoriesEN.pdf.

119  Keith Tanswell, email communication, 18 Mar. 2010; Tanswell CV; U of T, Department of Paediatrics, Division of Neonatology History, http://www.paeds.utoronto.ca/division/neon.htm.

120  Dept of Paediatrics *Annual Report* [1999–2000, 3–4.

121  John D. Keith, "The Prognosis in Rheumatic Heart Disease," *CMAJ* 45 (1941): 119–27.

122  Vera Rose, "John Dow Keith," *Canadian Journal of Cardiology* 5 (1989): xi–xii.

123  Keith personal memoir, in Segall, *Pioneers of Cardiology*, 269.

124  Ibid., 270.

125  Trusler, "Reflections on Bill Mustard," 143.

126  J.D. Keith, R.D. Rowe, and P. Vlad, *Heart Disease in Infancy and Childhood* (New York: Macmillan, 1958); subsequent editions were published in 1967 and 1978.

127  Rose, "John Dow Keith."

128  Robert F. Freedom, "Richard D Rowe, MD (1923–1988)," *American Journal of Cardiology* 62 (1988): 957–8, 958.

129 Lee N. Benson and Robert H. Anderson, "The Paediatric Cardiology Hall of Fame: Robert Mark Freedom MD, FRCPC, FACC, O. Ont," *Cardiology in the Young* 15 (2005): 206–12, 210.

130 Freedom, "Richard D Rowe, MD," 957.

131 Ibid.

132 R.M. Freedom, S.-J. Yoo, H. Mikailan, and W.G. Williams, eds., *The Natural and Modified History of Congenital Heart Disease* (New York: Futura, 2004).

133 HSC/Dept of Paediatrics, *Annual Report* 2000–1, 4.

134 Michael Bliss, *Discovery of Insulin*, 161.

135 HSC, Division of Endocrinology, "Endocrinology: History," http://www.sickkids.ca/Endocrinology/Who-we-are/History/index.html.

136 *Dean's Report* 1954–5, 37; *Dean's Report* 1956–7, 41.

137 Obituaries of Sass-Kortsak in the *Globe and Mail*, 13 Oct. 1986, A11, and *CMAJ* 136 (1 Jan. 1987): 70; HSC, Research Institute, "The Andrew Sass-Kortsak Award," http://www.sickkids.ca/research/abouttheinstitute/milestones/55th_anniversary/did-you-know/andrew-sass-kortsak-award.html

138 *Dean's Report* 1966–7, 78.

139 HSC, "Endocrinology: History."

140 A. Zipursky, "Editorial: A History of Pediatric Hematology/Oncology in Canada," *Pediatric Hematology and Oncology* 8 (1991): iii–viii, iv.

141 Ibid., iii–viii; the dating of McClure's appointment is from Deans Report 1967–8, 86.

142 *Dean's Report* 1971–2, 122–3.

143 Ibid., 123.

144 See J. Douglas Snedden, "Proposal" [for a Bone Marrow Transplantation Unit] to Chairman, Dean's Committee, 23 Jan. 1980; UTA A1985/0026/06/03.

145 Dept of Paediatrics, *Annual Report* 2001–2, 26.

146 "William Goldie," Faculty Council, 2 Feb. 1929, 110–11.

147 George Alfred McNaughton, In Memoriam, Faculty Council minutes, 27 Jan. 1967, 259–61.

148 *Dean's Report* 1968–9, 107.

149 *Dean's Report* 1970–1, 108.

150 "Review, Division of Infectious Diseases, Department of Medicine" [1979]; no author.

151 *Dean's Report* 1966–7, 79.

152 *Dean's Report* 1968–9, 109.

153 *Dean's Report* 1970–1, 108.

154 *Dean's Report* 1971–2, 124.

155 Dept of Paediatrics *Annual Report* 2000–1, 34.

156 *Torontonensis* (1907), 151.

157 Dept of Medicine, Division of Neurology, "History of Neurology in Toronto," http://www.neurology.utoronto.ca/index.php/about-us/history-of-neurology

158 *Dean's Report* 1938–9, 35.

159 "John Stobo Prichard," Faculty Council, 23 Feb. 1987; UTA A1995/004/04.

160 Gabrielle deVeber statement of research interests, *Neuroscience Newsletter* (University of Toronto Program in Neuroscience), July 2005, 1–2.

161 HSC *Annual Report* 2005–6, 14.

162 On early days in radiology at HSC and the Rolph era see Edward Shorter, *A Century of Radiology in Toronto* (Toronto and Dayton, OH: Wall & Emerson, 1995), 23–8.

163 *Dean's Report* 1948–9, 43.

164 Shorter, *Century of Radiology*, 82.

165 Ibid.

166 Ibid., 84–5.

167 Derek C. Harwood-Nash, E. Bruce Hendrick, and Alan R. Hudson, "The Significance of Skull Fractures in Children: A Study of 1,187 Patients," *Radiology* 101 (1971): 151–6.

168 Michael S. Huckman, "In Memory: Derek FC Harwood Nash," *American Journal of Neuroradiology* 18 (1997): 1803–12, 1808.

169 Self-Study, Feb. 1983, 100; UTA F016/030.031.

170 Robin Humphreys, "Editorial Comment: Are the Machines Taking Over?", *The Neurotransmitter*], Winter 2002, 1–3.

171 Department of Surgery, 16 Feb. 1920, 3; UTA A1979/0023/002 (02).

172 *Torontonensis* (1907), 186.

173 Eulogy, Faculty Council, 6 Apr. 1944; UTA A1986/0027/023 (02).

174 *Tablet*, Spring 1990, 8.

175 *Torontonensis* (1910), 160.

176 W.K. Lindsay, "Arthur Baker LeMesurier," eulogy, Faculty Council, 22 Feb. 1982; UTA A1993/0025/009.

177 "Robert Marshall Wansbrough," Faculty Council, 8 June 1956, 275–7; UTA A1986/0027/026.

178 Robin Humphreys, *Sick Kids Newsletter* 7, no. 2 (Winter 2003): 2.

179 Kergin, in *Dean's Report* 1965–6, 106.

180 Robin Humphreys, *The Neurotransmitter* [HSC], Winter 2003, 2.

181 Ibid., 2.

182 "Star Finds Herbie Quinones Jr. Healthy at 30," *Toronto Star*, 5 Dec. 2009.

183 See, for instance, the hospital's website, http://www.sickkids.ca, accessed 8 Apr. 2010, which renders its name as "SickKids®," as does the current building signage. Annual reports for the Department of Paediatrics identify the facility as "The Hospital for Sick Children" up to 2006–7, adopting the "SickKids" name and the trademarked motto "Healthier Children. A Better World" the following year.

184 Faculty Council, 28 Sept. 1981; UTA A1993/0028/009.

185 "New Technique Gives Hope Polio Vaccine Not Far Away – Chute," *Toronto Daily Star*, 23 Sept. 1952.

186 "Institute to Co-ordinate Research Set Up by Sick Children's Hospital," *Globe and Mail*, 1 Dec. 1953, 15.

187 "Enlarging Research Is Plan at Hospital for Sick Children," *Toronto Daily Star*, 1 Dec. 1953.
188 *Dean's Report* 1965–6, 106.
189 *Dean's Report* 1956–7, 40.
190 *Dean's Report* 1961–2, 57; *Dean's Report* 1962–3, 77.
191 *Dean's Report* 1961–2, 57.
192 *Dean's Report* 1964–5, 69.
193 Faculty Council, 28 Sept. 1981; UTA A1993/0025/09.
194 Aser Rothstein, "Nonlogical Factors in Research: Chance and Serendipity," *Biochemistry and Cell Biology* 64 (1986): 1055–65.
195 Okey interview, 19 Nov. 2009.
196 *Tablet*, Summer 1985, 12.
197 Aser Rothstein to Senior Staff, 24 Apr. 1972; UTA A1983/0007/005.
198 LRPAC Minutes, 27 Nov. 1974; UTA A1979/0010/006.
199 Science Policy Committee, minutes, 9 Dec. 1976; UTA A1993/0025/008.
200 Rothstein in Faculty Council, 28 Sept. 1981; UTA A1993/0028/009.
201 Louis Siminovitch to David Naylor, undated copy, 2007 or 2008; Siminovitch private archive.
202 External Review 1991; Dean's Archive.
203 M.J. Glimcher to F.P. Dewar, 18 Sept. 1967; UTA A1989/0030/001.
204 "External Review: Bloorview Children's Hospital 1985"; Dean's Archive.
205 *MedEmail*, 18 Feb. 2002.
206 Dept of Paediatrics, *Annual Report* 2005–6, 116.
207 *Dean's Report* 1969–70, 99.
208 Martin Mifsud, Ishan Al-Temen, William Sauter et al., "Variety Village Electromechanical Hand for Amputees Under Two Years of Age," *Journal of the Association of Children's Prosthetic-Orthotic Clinics* 22 (3): 41.
209 W.F. Sauter, R. Dakpa, E. Hamilton, E. Milner and H.,R. Galway "Prosthesis with Electric Elbow and Hand for a Three-year-old Multiply Handicapped Child," *Prosthetics and Orthotics International* 9 (1985): 105–8.

## 11 Research

1 Gallie, "Fifty Years' Growth," 12.
2 Claude Bissell, *Halfway Up Parnassus: A Personal Account of the University of Toronto, 1932–1971* (Toronto: University of Toronto Press, 1974), 72–3, 92.
3 Stanley Joel Reiser, "Human Experimentation and the Convergence of Medical Research and Patient Care," *Annals of the American Academy of Political and Social Science* 437 (May 1978): 8–18, 15.
4 Primrose, "Memorandum Prepared by the Faculty of Medicine," 18–19; UTA A1979/0023/1001(2).
5 *President's Report* 1913–14, 22.
6 See its first report in the *President's Report* 1913–14, 21–4.

7  *President's Report* 1925–6, 25–6.

8  *Dean's Report* 1936–7, 9.

9  President's Report 1946–7, 11, 31.

10  *Dean's Report* 1950–1, 6.

11  Document "Faculty of Medicine: Research," 15 Mar. 1947; attached to J.A. MacFarlane to Sidney Smith, 28 May 1947; UTA A1983/0036/11 (10).

12  Meeting of Special Sub-Committee of Committee on Post-Graduate Studies for Consideration of Concrete Plans for Post-Graduate Education, 19 Feb. 1946; UTA A1993/0025/004.

13  *Dean's Report* 1948–9, 32.

14  *Dean's Report* 1950–1, 13, 40.

15  Bissell, *Halfway Up Parnassus*, 36–7.

16  John Hamilton and W.A. Oille, "Brief to the Royal Commission on Health Services, presented on behalf of the Faculty of Medicine, University of Toronto," Apr. 1962, 8 (MS at University of Toronto Library).

17  Faculty Council, 6 Feb. 1959, 66; UTA A1986/0027/027.

18  Ibid.

19  Faculty Council, 3 Apr. 1959, 77–8; UTA A1986/0027/027.

20  *President's Report* 1960–1, 43.

21  Colin Bayliss, interview, Faculty of Medicine, *Tablet*, Fall 1988, 7.

22  *President's Report* 1961–2, 40.

23  *Dean's Report* 1963–4, 3–4.

24  Ibid.

25  Joseph MacFarlane, speech to Senate, 8 Mar. 1957; UTA A1976/0054/018 (12).

26  Faculty Council, 31 Jan. 1964; UTA A1986/028/008 (003).

27  Faculty of Medicine, University of Toronto, "Report of the Special Committee on the Structure and Organization of the Faculty," 1 Nov. 1965, 69; UTA A1993/0025/007; also at A1986/0028/008 (003).

28  Daniel Cappon to John Hamilton, 31 Jan. 1964; UTA A1986/0028/008 (003).

29  Special Committee on the Structure and Organization of the Faculty (1965), 69; UTA A1993/0025/007; also at A1986/0028/008 (003).

30  Ibid.

31  *President's Report* 1965–6, 69–70.

32  Lowell T. Coggeshall, *Planning for Medical Progress Through Education* (Evanston, IL: Association of American Medical Colleges, 1965), 97–9.

33  Bissell, *Halfway Up Parnassus*, 103–4.

34  Friedland, *University of Toronto: A History*, 507.

35  Review Committee, 4 Dec. 1968, 184; UTA A1993/0025/007 (06).

36  Howard E. Petch, *Health Research Requirements Task Force Report*, ([Toronto: Ministry of Health], 1976), viii. Petch was the president of the University of Victoria in British Columbia, formerly vice president of academics, University of Waterloo.

37  A.L. Chute to Chairmen of Departments, 13 Oct.1967; attached to Joint Hospitals Committee, Minutes, 20 Oct. 1967; Archives of Ontario, RG 10/6/0/1911/1916/box #183.

38  *Dean's Report* 1967–8, 56.

39  Faculty Council, 24 Sept. 1973; UTA A1993/0025/007.
40  Kenneth Pritzker interview with Edward Shorter, 20 Oct. 2009.
41  Petch *Report* (1976), xi–xiv.
42  Bissell, *Halfway Up Parnassus*, 106.
43  J.C. Laidlaw to J.D. Hamilton, 10 Mar. 1964; UTA A1986/0028/008 (003).
44  Committee on Curriculum and Examinations, 12 Sept. 1966, 204; UTA A1993/0025/007. A note said this was being communicated to the Faculty Council only "for information," since the IMS would report to SGS.
45  McCulloch, *Ontario Cancer Institute*, 63.
46  Faculty Council, 27 Jan. 1967, 257; UTA A1993/0025/007.
47  *Dean's Report* 1966–7, 3–4.
48  Ibid., 43; *Dean's Report* 1967–8, 55.
49  Laidlaw interview, 8 Apr. 2009.
50  LRPAC Minutes, 18 Feb. 1976; UTA A1979/0010 (005).
51  IMS report, 17 Feb. 1976; UTA A1986/0028/004 (001).
52  *Dean's Report* 1968–9, 69.
53  IMS report, 17 Feb. 1976; UTA A1986/0028/004 (001).
54  John Leyerle to Roger de C. Nantel, 26 Nov. 1983; Till Papers, UTA, B2005/003/006(02).
55  Committee of Clinical Chairs,[hereafter Clinical chairs] 12 Nov. 1974; UTA A1993/0025/006.
56  Daniel Roncari presentation, Clinical chairs, 19 May 1981; UTA A1993/0025 (1). Roncari was director from 1980 to 1983.
57  Daniel A.K. Roncari, Robert B. Salter, James E. Till, and Frederick H. Lowy, "Is the Clinician-Scientist Really Vanishing? Encouraging Results from a Canadian Institute of Medical Science," *CMAJ* 130 (15 Apr. 1984): 977–9.
58  Rotstein interview, 9 Apr. 2009.
59  See E.M. Sellers to William Francombe, 12 June 1981; UTA A1987/0035 (/001).
60  Rotstein interview, 9 Apr. 2009.
61  Five-year Review of the MD/PhD Program; UTA A1996/0011/0022 (7).
62  Faculty of Medicine, University of Toronto, *Strategic Directions and Academic Plan: International Leadership in Health Research and Education [hereafter Plan 2001–4]*; http://www.facmed.utoronto.ca/Assets/FacMed+Digital+Assets/faculty+of+Medicine+1/FacMed+Digital+Assets/about/academicplan/pdf?method=1 Academic Plan 2000–4, 45–6.
63  Science Policy Sub-committee, Minutes, 18 Dec. 1972; UTA A1993/0025/008.
64  Science Policy Sub-committee, Minutes, 4 Dec. 1973; UTA A1993/0025/008.
65  Science Policy Committee, Minutes, 13 May 1974; UTA A1993/0025/008; the sub-committee had in the meantime declared itself a committee; UTA A1993/0025/008.
66  Senior Advisory Committee meeting of 6 Nov. 1978; UTA A1993/0025/4.
67  Science Policy Committee, Minutes, 26 Apr. 1979; UTA A1993/0025/008.
68  All of the above from Hollenberg, undated document, "Organization of Research in Clinical Departments: Department of Medicine – Dr. CH Hollenberg," in Science Policy Committee file following minutes of 2 Mar. 1978, but not identified as part of those minutes; UTA A1993/0025/008.

69 "Report of Long-Range Planning and Assessment Committee to Dean RB Holmes, Nov. 30, 1977, Re: Research"; UTA A1993/0025/0038.
70 *Tablet*, Fall 1987, 6–7.
71 "Meeting of the Faculty Education Committee," 25 Sept. 1987; UTA A1995/0004/005
72 "Meeting of the Committee of Basic Science Chairmen" [hereafter Basic Science chairs], 7 June 1985; UTA A1993/0025/01.
73 *Tablet*, Winter 1986, 2.
74 Arthur Slutsky interview with Edward Shorter, 7 Apr. 2009.
75 Ibid.
76 Basic Science chairs, 14 Dec. 1982; UTA A1993/0025/01.
77 Basic Science chairs, 8 Feb. 1983; UTA A1993/0025/01.
78 Basic Science chairs, 8 Mar. 1983; UTA A1993/0025/01.
79 Clinical chairs, 15 Feb. 1983; UTA A1993/0025/01.
80 Faculty Council Minutes, 24 Oct. 1983; UTA A1993/0025/09
81 Ibid.
82 Ibid.
83 *Tablet*, Spring 1985, 7.
84 Ibid.
85 Basic Science chairs, 13 Feb. 1987; UTA A1993/0025/01.
86 *MedEmail*, 6 June 2005.
87 Cowan interview, 4 Feb. 2009.

## 12 An Academic Health Sciences Complex

1 J.D. Hamilton to R.I. Mitchell, 20 Aug. 1969; UTA A1979/0061/001.
2 L.E. Ferris, P.A. Singer, and C.D. Naylor, "Better Governance in Academic Health Sciences Centres: Moving Beyond the Olivieri/Apotex Affair in Toronto," *Journal of Medical Ethics* 30 (2004): 25–9.
3 On various US models, see Bryan J. Weiner et al., "Organizational Models for Medical School – Clinical Enterprise Relationships," *Academic Medicine* 76 (2001): 113–24.
4 John Hamilton and R.M. Janes, "Brief to the Royal Commission on Health Services presented on behalf of the Teaching Hospitals of the University of Toronto," Apr. 1962, 5; in University of Toronto Library.
5 Gallie, "Fifty Years' Growth," 7.
6 Connor, *Doing Good*, 171–2.
7 TGH *Annual Report* 1906, 59–60.
8 *President's Report* 1907–8, 13; President Falconer evidently let the various deans write the section of the report for their faculty.
9 Connor, *Doing Good*, 177–80.
10 Cosbie, *Toronto General Hospital*, 147.
11 *President's Report* 1911–12, 9.
12 Petch committee (1974), see section on TGH, 1.
13 *Dean's Report* 1934–5, 39–40.

14 "Post-Graduate Training," minutes, 18 Dec. 1947; UTA A1993/0025/004.

15 *Dean's Report* 1958–9, 3.

16 *President's Report* 1963–4, 52.

17 Review Committee, minutes, 4 Dec. 1968; UTA A1993/0025/007 (06); N. Tait McPhedran, *Canadian Medical Schools: Two Centuries of Medical History, 1822 to 1992* (Montreal: Harvest House, 1993), 85.

18 "The Medical Sciences Centre-University Controlled Teaching Hospital concept appeals to all the Deans of the Faculties of Medicine." (John B. Neilson to Mathew Dymond, 15 July 1964, Archives of Ontario [hereafter AO], RG 10-6-0-1911, #183).

19 *President's Report* 1965–6, 70. On the Senior Co-ordinating Committee see Petch *Report*(1976), viii.

20 Dr B.L.P. Brosseau to Dr J.B. Neilson, 7 July 1965; AO RG 10-6-0-1916, #183.

21 13 Dec. 1966: at meeting of Committee on Curriculum and Examinations, UTA A1986/0028/008/003.

22 Meeting of Committee on Curriculum and Examinations, 12 Sept. 1966, 202; UTA A1993/0025/007.

23 "Report to the Meeting of the Chairmen of the Boards and the Administrators of Teaching Hospitals," 12 Aug. 1966; AO RG 10-6-0-1916, #183.

24 Meeting of Senior Co-ordinating Committee, 26 Aug. 1969; these events were explained at a subsequent meeting of the SCC on 25 Sept. 1969; UTA A1993/0025/5. The Senior Co-ordinating Committee was established by the province in 1966, chaired by the deputy minister of health; following its dissolution in 1972, its responsibilities were assumed by the Health Science Education Committee – see Petch *Report* , (1976), viii.

25 K.J. Rea, *The Prosperous Years: The Economic History of Ontario, 1939–1975* (Toronto: University of Toronto Press, 1985), 116–17.

26 Ibid., 124–5.

27 Ibid., 126.

28 For details see *Dean's Report* 1968–9, 3–4.

29 12 Dec. 1967 memo from G.W. Reid, Director, Research and Planning Branch of MOH, to K.C. Charron, Deputy Minister of Health; AO RG 10-6-0-1911, #183.

30 Hospital Planning Committee of the MOH, "Planning – Health Sciences Capital Programmes," 21 Dec. 1967; AO RG 10-6-0-1911, #183.

31 Ontario Hospital Services Commission (OHSC) meeting of 13 Oct. 1967; AO RG 10-6-0-1916, #183.

32 10 July 1968: MOH memo from K.C. Charron, Deputy Minister, to M.E. Dymond, Minister of Health; AO RG 10-6-0-1916, #183.

33 Review Committee, minutes, 4 Dec. 1968; UTA A1993/0025/007 (06).

34 Ibid.

35 Faculty Council, 11 Dec. 1968, 95, 97.

36 "Proposals on the Organization of the University Hospital System"; date received in the MOH: 23 Dec. 1968; AO RG 10-6-0-1916, #183.

37  Independent Planning Committee *Report* (1969); a brief summary is found in [Faculty of Medicine] *Synapse*, 11 Dec. 1969, 2–3.

38  Ibid., 11, 19.

39  Ibid., 155–6.

40  15 June 1971: OHSC interoffice memo headed "Toronto Health Sciences Complex," from Mrs V. MacDonald, consultant, Special Facility Planning to File, cc D.N. Teasdale; AO RG 10-6-0-1916, #183.

41  OHSC, "Toronto Health Sciences Complex," revised Sept. 1971; AO RG 10-6-0-1916, #183.

42  Northern Ontario School of Medicine, "About NOSM: Innovative Education for a Healthier North," http://www.nosm.ca/about_us/default.aspx.

43  Joint Hospitals Committee, minutes, 17 Mar. 1967, 2.

44  "Meeting of the Senior Co-ordinating Committee with the University of Toronto Health Science Centre and Affiliated Hospitals," 25 Sept. 1969; UTA A1993/0025/5.

45  Ibid.

46  J.D. Wallace to TGH Board of Trustees, 4 Mar. 1970; UHN Archives, TGH Fonds, sub-series 2.1: Reports to Board of Trustees, box 13, file 2.1.8.

47  Executive Director's Report to Trustees, May 1970; UHN Archives, TGH Fonds, sub-series 2.1: Reports to Board of Trustees, box 13, file 2.1.8.

48  K.J.R. Wightman, "Report of the Department of Medicine," May 1969, 2; Department of Medicine Archive.

49  Eliot Phillipson, *MediNews*, Nov. 2001, 1.

50  J. D. Wallace to TGH Board of Trustees 1970.

51  *President's Report* 1969–70, vol. II, 7–8.

52  21 Oct. 1971: MOH: "Proposed role study for the Toronto Health Sciences Complex"; AO RG 10-6-0-1916, #183.

53  Hamilton memo, 8 Dec. 1972; UTA A1979/0010/001/6.15.72; the reference here is apparently to earlier events.

54  John Hamilton to Dean A.L. Chute, 24 Apr. 1972; UTA A1979/0010/001/6.15.72.

55  "Report on Sub-Committee on Obstetrics and Gynacology [*sic*], Tri-Hospitals Complex," attached to Hamilton to W.J. Hannah, 4 Aug. 1972; UTA A1979/0010/001/6.15.72.

56  See the outraged letters that Bruce Tovee and J.A. McNab directed at Holmes (UTA A1979/0010/001; McNab to Holmes, 11 Sept. 1972; Tovee to Holmes, 24 Aug. 1972; also Emergency Services Subcommittee – Tri Hospital Complex, meeting of 26 July 1972; UTA A1979/0010/001 (6.15.72).

57  Faculty Council, 24 Sept. 1973; UTA A1993/0025/007.

58  See "Plan," attached to Hollenberg to Hamilton, 11 Jan. 1973; UTA A1979/0010/001 (6.15.72).

59  Hamilton memo, re "QP Hospitals, re FCM," 19 Jan. 1973; UTA A1979/0010/001 (/6.15.72).

60  Faculty Council, 24 Sept. 1973; UTA A1993/0025/007.

61  *Medisphere* (Faculty of Medicine newsletter), Nov. 1977, 1–2.

62  Hamilton to Holmes, 2 Apr. 1973; UTA A1979/0010/001 (6.15.72)
63  Louis Siminovitch, chair, Science Policy Sub-committee of the LRPAC, 14 May 1973; UTA B1979/0051/04.
64  Petch *Report*(1976), 70, 73.
65  Agreement between the Governing Council of the University of Toronto and the Sisters of St. Joseph, 1 July 1979; UTA A1994/0012 (004).
66  Faculty Council, 27 Apr. 1981; UTA A1993/0025/009.
67  Lowy, Midterm Report, 1984, 10–11.
68  Faculty Council, 16 June 1981; UTA A1993/0025/001.
69  Lowy, Midterm Report, 1984, 11.
70  Committee of Clinical chairs, 21 Apr. 1981; UTA A1993/0025/1; for further details see Faculty Council, 22 Feb. 1982, appendix II.
71  See Faculty Council, 22 Feb. 1982; UTA A1993/0025/009.
72  F.H. Lowy to A. Hudson, 27 Sept. 1984; UTA A1994/0012/007. Lowy enclosed a copy of his memo of 20 Sept. 1983 to all the teaching hospitals.
73  Faculty Council, 22 Feb. 1982; UTA A1993/0025/009.
74  Senior Advisory Committee minutes, 25 May 1982; UTA A1993/0025/004.
75  Lowy, Midterm Report, 1984, 11.
76  Clinical chairs, 21 Jan. 1986; UTA A1993/0025/001.
77  Clinical chairs, 22 Apr. 1986; UTA A1993/0025/001.
78  Ibid.
79  *Tablet*, Fall 1986, 14.
80  Clinical chairs, 16 Sept. 1986; UTA A1993/0025/001.
81  Faculty of Medicine, Self-Study, Jan. 1990, 14; UTA A1996/0011/0018 (6).
82  Ibid., 80
83  B. Langer to John Dirks, 17 Aug. 1990; UTA A1996/0011/023 (14).
84  Dept of Surgery, *Annual Report*1991–2, 18.
85  Ad Hoc Survey Team, "Report of the Limited Survey of the University of Toronto, Faculty of Medicine, May 11–14, 1992 Prepared for the Committee on Accreditation of Canadian Medical Schools and the Liaison Committee on Medical Education," Dean's Archive.
86  *MedEmail*, 10 Sept. 2001; on this alphabet soup of liaison organizations, see also *MedEmail*, 8 Dec. 2003; 22 Mar. 2004; 26 Apr. 2004.
87  Eliot Phillipson, "Chair's Column," *MediNews*, Dec. 2002, 1.

## 13  Cancer Care

1  D.H. Cowan, *Closing the Circles: A History of the Governance of Cancer Control in Ontario* (Toronto: Cancer Care Ontario, 2004), 3.
2  *President's Report* 1933–4, 16.
3  *Dean's Report* 1944–5, 11.
4  *Dean's Report* 1946–7, 5.
5  Cowan, *Closing the Circles*, 7.

6 On these events, see Cowan, *Closing the Circles*, 7; Ontario Cancer Institute (OCI), *Annual Report* 1959, 8f.

7 Donald Cowan interview with Edward Shorter, 4 Feb. 2009.

8 R.S. Bush, "Dr. Clifford L Ash," Faculty Council, 27 Apr. 1981; UTA A1993/0025/009.

9 OCI *Annual Report* 1959, 8.

10 Bernard Cummings, personal communication, 19 Nov. 2010.

11 James Till, "Harold Elford Johns"; Till Papers, UTA B2005/031/ 004 (019).

12 *Tablet*, Summer 1985.

13 McCulloch, *Ontario Cancer Institute*, 86–7.

14 Bernard J. Cummings interview with Edward Shorter, 22 Oct. 2009.

15 L. Siminovitch, *Reflections*, 54, 72–3.

16 McCulloch, *Ontario Cancer Institute*, 36–7.

17 "Dr. Ernest McCulloch," University Health Network Research news release, 21 Jan. 2011, http://www.uhnres.utoronto.ca/news/php/readarticle.php?id=31327 .

18 Cummings interview, 22 Oct. 2009.

19 L. Siminovitch, *Reflections*, 48.

20 L. Siminovitch interview, 16 Dec. 2008.

21 Ibid.

22 McCulloch, *Ontario Cancer Institute*, 17–18.

23 Ibid., 20.

24 Ibid., 44.

25 E.A. McCulloch, A.F. Howatson, L. Siminovitch, A.A. Axelrad, and A.W. Ham, "A Cytopathic Agent from a Mammary Tumour in a C3H Mouse that Produces Tumours in Swiss Mice and Hamsters," *Nature* 183 (30 May 1959): 1535–6.

26 [Ernest McCulloch], eulogy, "Alan Ming-Ta Wu," Faculty Council, 16 Mar. 1981; UTA A1993/0025/009.

27 McCulloch, *Ontario Cancer Institute*, 67, 108.

28 Ibid., 99; Cowan, *Closing the Circles*, 4.

29 Dept of Surgery, *Annual Report* 1993–4, 3–4, 46.

30 Cowan interview, 4 Feb. 2009.

31 Donald Cowan, personal communication, 10 June 2010.

32 On Warwick see Shorter, *Century of Radiology*, 48.

33 James Innes and W.D. Rider, "Multiple Myelomatosis Treated with a Combination of Urethane and an Oral Nitrogen Mustard," *Blood* 10 (1955): 252–8.

34 Cowan interview, 4 Feb. 2009.

35 McCulloch, *Ontario Cancer Institute*, 42–3.

36 D.E. Bergsagel memo, 31 Oct. 1979; UTA A1985/0026/004/(016).

37 Ian F. Tannock et al., "Chemotherapy with Mitoxantrone Plus Prednisone or Prednisone Alone for Symptomatic Hormone-resistant Prostate Cancer: A Canadian Randomized Trial with Palliative End Points," *Journal of Clinical Oncology* 14 (1996): 1756–64.

38  Ian F. Tannock, 'Eradication of a Disease: How We Cured Symptomless Prostate Cancer," *Lancet* 359 (13 Apr. 2002): 1341–2.
39  Bernard Cummings, personal communication, 19 Nov. 2010.
40  McCulloch, *Ontario Cancer Institute*, 129.
41  R.S. Bush, M. Gospodarowicz, J. Sturgeon, and R. Alison, "Radiation Therapy of Localized Non-Hodgkin's Lymphoma," *Cancer Treatment Reports* 61 (1977): 1129–36.
42  Simon B. Sutcliffe, Mary K. Gospodarowicz, Raymond S. Bush, Thomas C. Brown, Theresa Chua, Helen A. Bean, Roy M. Clark, Alon Dembo, Peter J. Fitzpatrick, and M. Vera Peters, "Role of Radiation Therapy in Localized Non-Hodgkin's Lymphoma," *Radiotherapy and Oncology* 4 (1985): 211–23.
43  "Minutes of Review – Chief of Medicine, The Princess Margaret Hospital," 8 June 1982, 4; Dean's Archive.
44  Ibid., 11.
45  Ibid., 14.
46  Cowan, *Closing the Circles*, 11.
47  McCulloch, *Ontario Cancer Institute*, 143–7.
48  Faculty Council, 24 Oct. 1988, 5–8.
49  Dept of Surgery, *Annual Report* 1989–90, 2.
50  *FAXulty of Medicine*, 10 June 1996 [faxed newsletter distributed to members of the Faculty of Medicine; superseded by *MedEmail*; copies in the author's archive].
51  McCulloch, *Ontario Cancer Institute*, 149–55.
52  Planning Directorate and the Interdepartmental Division of Oncology, "Draft Proposal to Establish a Department of Radiation Oncology, Faculty of Medicine, University of Toronto," 10 Jan. 1991, 2; attached to Committee of Clinical Chairmen, minutes, 15 Jan. 1991; UTA A1996/0007/002.
53  A.B. Miller, G.R. Howe, and C. Wall, "The National Study of Breast Cancer Screening: Protocol for a Canadian Randomized Controlled Trial of Screening for Breast Cancer in Women," *Clinical and Investigative Medicine* 4 (1981): 227–58.
54  N.F. Boyd, J.W. Byng, R.A. Jong, E.K. Fishell, L.E. Little, A.B. Miller, G.A. Lockwood, D.L. Tritchler, and M.J. Yaffe, "Quantitative Classification of Mammographic Densities and Breast Cancer Risk: Results from the Canadian National Breast Screening Study," *Journal of the National Cancer Institute* 87 (1995): 670–5.
55  *FAXulty of Medicine*, 28 Nov. 1994.
56  See Ellie Tesher column, *Toronto Star*, 4 Mar. 1996, A2.
57  *FAXulty of Medicine*, 4 Nov. 1996.
58  *FAXulty of Medicine*, 3 Sept. 1996.
59  Cowan, *Closing the Circles*, 13.
60  Donald Cowan, personal communication, 10 June 2010.
61  Cowan, *Closing the Circles*, 15.
62  UHN *Annual Report* 1998–9, 12.
63  Cowan, *Closing the Circles*, 1, 5–6, 18.

64  Ibid., 6. Leslee J. Thompson and Murray T. Martin, "Integration of Cancer Services in Ontario: The Story of Getting It Done," *Healthcare Quarterly* 7 (2004): 42–8.
65  Cowan interview, 4 Feb. 2009.
66  Ibid.
67  *Dean's Report* 1934–5, 40.
68  Cowan interview, 4 Feb. 2009.
69  Ibid.
70  Dept of Surgery *Annual Report* 1989–90, 2.
71  Dept of Surgery *Annual Report* 1990–1, 2.
72  Dept of Surgery *Annual Report* 1992–3, 37.
73  Dept of Surgery *Annual Report* 1993–4, 46.
74  Ibid., 3–4, 46.
75  Dept of Surgery *Annual Report* 1994–5, 4, 44.
76  Martin McKneally, *Surgical Spotlight*, Spring 2005, 18.
77  Dept of Surgery *Annual Report* 1995–6, 3.
78  Dept of Surgery *Annual Report* 1997–8, 43–4.
79  Dept of Surgery *Annual Report* 1998–9, 49.
80  *MedEmail*, 15 Oct. 2001.
81  McKneally, *Surgical Spotlight*, Summer 2005, 14.
82  *Dean's Report* 1955–6, 29–30.
83  Donald Cowan, personal communication, 10 June 2010.
84  E.A. McCulloch to L. Loach, 24 Mar. 1966; UTA B1991/0004/04 (04).
85  Hill, "History of the Department of Medicine," 16.
86  John Crookston, "University of Toronto Training Program in Clinical Hematology" [1979]; UTA A1985/0026/004 (016).
87  Helen Farquharson interview, 21 July 2009.
88  Cowan interview, 4 Feb. 2009.
89  Langer interview, 20 Oct. 2009, 6.
90  Cowan interview, 4 Feb. 2009.
91  D.H. Cowan and D.E. Bergsagel, response of Hematology-Oncology Division to Research Committee of the Department of Medicine, for Petch committee, 16–17.
92  Charles Hollenberg report, 17 July 1973, 9; UTA A1986/0028/004 (002).
93  ca. 1975–6: Draft Report to LCME Steering Committee; UTA A1979/0010/005.
94  TGH *Annual Report* 1984–5, 94.
95  TGH *Annual Report* 1985–6, 3, 123.
96  "Proposal for a Bone Marrow Transplant Center for Adult Patients at the Ontario Cancer Institute" [1979], UTA A1985/0026/006 (03.
97  D. Amato, D.H. Cowan, and E.A. McCulloch, "Separation of Immunocompetent Cells from Human and Mouse Hemopoietic Cell Suspensions by Velocity Sedimentation," *Blood* 39 (1972): 472–80, 478.
98  Cowan interview, 4 Feb. 2009.
99  H. Abu-Zahr, D. Amato, M.T. Aye, D.E. Bergsagel, A.M. Clarysse, D.H. Cowan, V.L. Fornasier, R. Hasselback, N.N. Iscove, E.A. McCulloch, H. Messner, R.G.

Miller, R.A. Phillips, A.H. Ragab, W.D. Rider, and J.S. Senn, "Bone Marrow Transplantation in Patients with Acute Leukaemia," *Series Haematologica* 5 (1972): 189–204.

100 Undated memo "Clinical Marrow Transplantation Programme"; Till Papers, UTA B1991/0004/05 (27).

101 TGH *Annual Report* 1986–7, 243.

102 TTH *Annual Report* 1991–2, 11.

103 TTH *Annual Report* 1987–8, 109, 144; see also TGH *Annual Report* 1984–5, 164–5.

104 J.W. Meakin, "JM Darte Memoriam," Faculty Council, 1976; UTA A1993/0025/007. Date of council meeting unknown. Darte died 28 Dec. 1975.

105 McCulloch, *Ontario Cancer Institute*, 7.

106 Robert Harris, "Progress Report," 2 June 1975; UTA A1979/0010/005.

107 Kathleen J. Pritchard to B.M. Thall, 13 Feb. 1985; UTA A1994/0012/010.

108 Bernard Cummings, personal communication, 19 Nov. 2010.

109 Hill, "History of the Department of Medicine," 51.

110 Donald Cowan, personal communication, 10 June 2010.

111 "Oncology Unit Opens at Toronto General," TGH *Monitor*, 15 July 1978, 1.

112 Pearson, "Goals and Objectives – Department of Surgery, 1978–1988," 34.

113 TGH *Annual Report* 1984–5, 61.

114 Ibid., 179–80.

115 TGH *Annual Report* 1985–6, 200–3.

116 Kathleen J. Pritchard to B.M. Thall, 13 Feb. 1985; UTA A1994/0012/010.

117 The report was attached to Clinical chairs, 12 June 1985, UTA A1994/0012/009.

118 Clinical chairs, 23 Oct. 1985; UTA A1993/0025/001.

119 A Cancer Cytogenetic Laboratory was founded in 1986 at the Banting Institute, made possible by a three-year government grant. Clinical chairs, 16 Sept. 1986; UTA A1993/0025/12.

120 Clinical chairs, 17 June 1986; UTA A1993/0025/001.

121 *Tablet*, Fall 1990, 2.

122 See J.E. Till to C.H. Hollenberg, 20 Oct. 1992, turning down Hollenberg's inquiry about Till serving as a possible director of such a division; Till Papers, UTA B2005/0031/014(10).

123 Cummings interview, 22 Oct. 2009.

124 Plan 2000–4.

125 Cummings interview, 22 Oct. 2009.

126 "Planning is proceeding regarding designation of site groups in preparation for the planned move to University Ave"; Dept of Surgery *Annual Report* 1990–1, 2.

127 Cummings interview, 22 Oct. 2009.

128 Ibid.

129 M. Vera Peters, "A Study of Survivals in Hodgkin's Disease Treated Radiologically," *American Journal of Roentgenology and Radium Therapy* 63 (1950): 299–311; M. Vera Peters and K.C.H. Middlemiss, "A Study of Hodgkin's Disease Treated By Irradiation," *American Journal of Roentgenology* 79 (1958): 114–21.

130 On Peters's contributions, see D.H. Cowan, "Vera Peters and the Curability of Hodgkin Disease," *Current Oncology* 15 (2008): 206–10; and D.H. Cowan, "Vera Peters and the Conservative Management of Early-stage Breast Cancer," *Current Oncology* 17 (2010): 50–4.

131 M.V. Peters, "Cutting the 'Gordian Knot' in Early Breast Cancer," *Annals of the Royal College of Physicians and Surgeons of Canada* 8 (1975): 186–92, 191–2; see also M.V. Peters, "Wedge Resection With and Without Radiation in Early Breast Cancer," *International Journal of Radiation Oncology* 2 (1977): 1151–6.

132 Donald Cowan, personal communication, 10 June 2010.

133 Ibid.

134 Innes and Rider, "Multiple Myelomatosis," 252–6.

135 See Shorter, *Century of Radiology*, 47.

136 Douglas P. Bryce and W.D. Rider, "Pre-operative Irradiation in the Treatment of Advanced Laryngeal Carcinoma," *Laryngoscope* 81 (1971): 1481–90; see also W.D. Rider and Douglas P. Bryce, "Evolution in Management of Laryngeal Cancer at the University of Toronto: 'A Love Story,'" *Journal of Otolaryngology* 11 (1982): 151–4.

137 Cummings interview, 22 Oct. 2009. The paper was Douglas P. Bryce and W.D. Rider, "Pre-operative Irradiation in the Treatment of Advanced Laryngeal Carcinoma," *Laryngoscope* 81 (1971): 1481–90.

138 Ibid.

139 B.J. Cummings, W.D. Rider, A.R. Harwood et al., "Combined Radical Radiation Therapy and Chemotherapy for Primary Squamous Cell Carcinoma of the Anal Canal," *Cancer Treatment Reports* 66 (1982): 489–92.

140 W.D. Rider, "Quinquennial Review of Radiation Oncology at Ontario Cancer Institute/Princess Margaret Hospital," 20 May 1982; Dean's Archive.

141 Minutes of the Meeting of the Staff of the Department of Medical Biophysics, 3 June 1960; UTA A1983/0007/004.

142 E.M. Sellers to I. Quirt, memo, 9 Aug. 1984; UTA A1994/0012/010.

143 Minutes of Review – Chief of Radiation Oncology, the Princess Margaret Hospital, 7 June 1982, 3; Dean's Archive.

144 Ibid., 10.

145 Bernard Cummings, personal communication, 19 Nov. 2010.

146 Minutes of Review, 7 June 1982, 14.

147 Cummings interview, 22 Oct. 2009.

148 Planning Directorate and the Interdepartmental Division of Oncology, "Draft Proposal to Establish a Department of Radiation Oncology, Faculty of Medicine, University of Toronto," 10 Jan. 1991, 4; attached to Committee of Clinical Chairs, minutes, 15 Jan. 1991; UTA A1996/0007/002.

149 Burnett Thall, "Faculty of Medicine Task Force, First Meeting Comments," 16 Aug. 1984; UTA A1994/0012/010.

150 "Task Force on Oncology: Final Report," May 1985; attached to Burnett M. Thall to Frederick H. Lowy, 29 Apr. 1985; UTA A1994/0012/010.

151 Planning Directorate, 3.

152 Ibid., 5–6.

153 Clinical chairs, 15 Jan. 1991, 1.

154 UTA A1996/0007/002.

155 Cummings interview, 22 Oct. 2009.

156 Ibid.

157 Bernard Cummings, personal communication, 23 Dec. 2010.

158 *MedEmail*, 5 May 2003.

159 M. James Phillips, "Pathology Comment on Models for Oncology," 7 Nov. 1984; attached to Oncology Task Force Minutes, 8 Nov. 1984; UTA A1994/0012/010.

160 External Review, Department of Radiation Oncology, 2000, Dean's Response, 26 Mar. 2001.

161 Cummings interview, 22 Oct. 2009.


## 14 Neuroscience and Psychiatry

1 Thomas E. Brown, "'Living with God's Afflicted': A History of the Provincial Lunatic Asylum at Toronto, 1830–1911" (doctoral dissertation, Queen's University, 1980), chap 2.

2 Quoted in Henry Hurd, ed., *The Institutional Care of the Insane in the United States and Canada* (4 vols., Baltimore: Johns Hopkins Press, 1916–17), 4, 135.

3 I am grateful to John Court for this fact and for his valuable editorial suggestions for this chapter.

4 Note, "Psychological Medicine in Toronto," *Journal of Insanity*, Oct. 1882, 266–7.

5 Barbara R. Craig, "Clark, Daniel," in *Dictionary of Canadian Biography Online*, vol. 14, *1911–1920*; http://www.biographi.ca.

6 Brown, *Provincial Lunatic Asylum*, 271n79.

7 This dating is provided by Faculty of Medicine Calendar, 1913–14, 28. On Beemer's death see *Dean's Report* 1934–5, 10. Helpful details have been supplied by John Court at the Center for Addiction and Mental Health (CAMH) Archives, drawing upon TPH [Toronto Psychiatric Hospital] fonds, file 1–25.

8 Cyril Greenland, "Origins of the Toronto Psychiatric Hospital," in *TPH: History and Memoires of the Toronto Psychiatric Hospital, 1925–1966*, ed. Edward Shorter (Toronto: Wall & Emerson, 1996), 19–58, 21.

9 Charles K. Clarke, "The New Department of Psychiatry," *The University Monthly* 8, no. 4 (1908): 139–41. See also Charles K. Clarke, "The Psychiatric Clinics of Germany," *Bulletin of the Toronto Hospital for the Insane* 1 (Jan. 1908): 3–37.

10 John R. Wherrett, "History of Neurology in Toronto," 1993 MS, 36.

11 Charles K. Clarke, "Psychiatric Treatment," in *Military Hospitals Commission Canada: Special Bulletin, April 1916*, ed. J.A. Lougheed (Ottawa: MHCC, 1916), 99–102.

12 See Ian Dowbiggin, "Clarke, Charles Kirk," in *Dictionary of Canadian Biography Online*, vol. 15, *1921–1930*; http://www.biographi.ca.

13 On Hincks's life see Charles G. Roland, *Clarence Hincks: Mental Health Crusader* (Toronto: Hannah Institute & Dundurn Press, 1990).

14 Editorial, "Canadian National Committee for Mental Hygiene," *CMAJ* 8 (June 1918): 551–4.

15 Faculty Council, 1 Mar. 1920, 173; UTA A1986/0027/018.

16 See Shorter, *TPH: History and Memories of the Toronto Psychiatric Hospital*, 25–27.

17 Faculty Council, 9 Mar. 1920, 248; UTA A1986/0027/018.

18 Faculty Council, 3 Dec. 1920, 328; UTA A1986/0027/018.

19 On Farrar's life see Edward Shorter, "CB Farrar: A Life," in Shorter, *TPH: History and Memories of the Toronto Psychiatric Hospital*, 59–96.

20 *Dean's Report* 1931–2, 33.

21 *Dean's Report* 1932–3, 34.

22 See the brief biography in "100th Anniversary of Women at U of T," UTA A1994/0012/05.

23 *Dean's Report* 1934–5, 36–7.

24 Ibid., 37–8.

25 *Dean's Report* 1935–6, 37.

26 Norman L. Easton and Helen O. McNelly, "Insulin Shock Treatment of Schizophrenia," *Canadian Nurse* 34 (1938): 69–72.

27 See *Dean's Report* 1936–7, 40; 1937–8, 47; 1940–1, 32. The insulin research continued until at least the 1948–9 session. See *Dean's Report* 1948–9, 42.

28 *Dean's Report* 1938–9, 52.

29 B.H. McNeel, J.G. Dewan, C.R. Myers, L.D. Proctor, and J.E. Goodwin, "Parallel Psychological, Psychiatric and Physiological Findings in Schizophrenic Patients under Insulin Shock Treatment," *American Journal of Psychiatry* 98 (1941): 422–9.

30 *Dean's Report* 1937–8, 58. *Dean's Report* 1938–9, 62. Norman L. Easton and Joseph Sommers, "The Significance of Vertebral Fractures as a Complication of Metrazol Therapy," *American Journal of Psychiatry* 98 (1942): 538–43.

31 Lorne D. Proctor, "Indications for Shock Therapy in Mental Illness," *CMAJ* 52 (1945): 130–6.

32 *Dean's Report* 1941–2, 29.

33 *Dean's Report* 1948–9, 42.

34 A. Miller, "The Lobotomy Patient – a Decade Later: A Follow-up Study of a Research Project Started in 1948," *CMAJ* 96 (15 Apr. 1967): 1095–103, 1095.

35 *Torontonensis* (1924), 123.

36 *Dean's Report* 1951–2, 51.

37 Frederick H. Lowy, "Aldwyn B. Stokes," Faculty Council, minutes, Sept. 1978–June 1979, 284–5; UTA A1993/0025/009.

38 *Dean's Report* 1950–1, 45.

39 Shorter, *TPH: History and Memories of the Toronto Psychiatric Hospital*, 137.

40 Bruce Sloane and John W. Lovett Doust, "Psychophysiological Investigations in Experimental Psychoses: Results of the Exhibition of D-Lysergic Acid Diethylamide to Psychiatric Patients," *British Journal of Psychiatry* 100 (1954): 129–44.

41 J. Dewan and W.B. Spaulding, *The Organic Psychoses: A Guide to Diagnosis* (Toronto: University of Toronto Press, 1958), v.

42  *Dean's Report* 1959–60, 66.

43  *Dean's Report* 1967–8, 123.

44  *Dean's Report* 1947–8, 41.

45  Ibid., 42.

46  *Dean's Report* 1948–9, 41.

47  Ibid., 4, 40–1.

48  *Dean's Report* 1952–3, 49.

49  *Dean's Report* 1949–50, 46.

50  John R. Seeley, R. Alexander Sim, and Elizabeth W. Loosley, *Crestwood Heights: A Study of the Culture of Suburban Life* (New York: Basic Books, 1956).

51  *Dean's Report* 1950–1, 46.

52  *Dean's Report* 1951–2, 43.

53  *Dean's Report* 1952–3, 49.

54  *Dean's Report* 1953–4, 47.

55  *Dean's Report* 1954–5, 52.

56  *Dean's Report* 1963–4, 92.

57  *President's Report* 1957–8, 44.

58  *Dean's Report* 1959–60, 64.

59  Michael S. Ross and Harvey Moldofsky, "Comparison of Pimozide with Haloperidol in Gilles de la Tourette Syndrome," *Lancet* 309 (8 Jan. 1977): 103.

60  Aldwyn Stokes to John Hamilton, 14 Dec. 1965; UTA A1979/0056/007 (08).

61  *Dean's Report* 1966–7, 109.

62  *Tablet,* Fall 1986, 4.

63  *Dean's Report* 1966–7, 109.

64  On his role see Oleh Hornykiewicz, "The Discovery of Dopamine Deficiency in the Parkinsonian Brain," *Journal of Neural Transmission* 70, supplement (2006): 9–15.

65  Independent Planning Committee *Report,*(1969), 39.

66  Lewellys F. Barker, Obituary: "Dr Campbell Meyers," *CMAJ* 7 (1927): 968.

67  TGH *Annual Report* 1911, http://www.archive.org/stream/annualreporttg1911torouoft/annualreporttg1911torouoft_djvu.txt.

68  TGH *Annual Report* 1907, 21, 40–53.

69  TGH *Annual Report* 1908, 15.

70  TGH *Annual Report* 1909, 17.

71  TGH *Annual Report* 1912, 17. Whether this closure happened in 1911 or 1912 is unclear. On the basis of other evidence I have proposed 1911 but the exact dating remains uncertain.

72  C.K. Clarke, "The Story of the Toronto General Hospital Psychiatric Clinic," *Canadian Journal of Mental Hygiene* 1 (1919): 30–7, 30.

73  TGH *Annual Report* 1912, 17.

74  *Social Service in the Toronto General Hospital, 1911–1949* (Toronto: TGH Social Service Association, 1950): 35.

75  Connor, *Doing Good*, 198.

76  TGH *Annual Report* 1914, 8; I have not seen the organizational tables for 1911–13, and this may not be the first mention.

77  TGH *Annual Report* 1915, 39.

78  TGH *Annual Report* 1916, 35.

79  Clarke, "Story of the Toronto General Hospital Psychiatric Clinic," 30–7.

80  *Social Service in the Toronto General Hospital,* 38.

81  *Dean's Report* 1959–60, 35.

82  *Dean's Report* 1954–5, 25.

83  Findlay, "Neurosurgery at the Toronto General Hospital," 147.

84  *Dean's Report* 1931–2, 8–9.

85  *Dean's Report* 1937–8, 24–5.

86  Ibid., 25.

87  H.H. Hyland, W.J. Gardiner, F.C. Heal, W.A. Oille, and O.M. Solandt, "Acute Anterior Poliomyelitis: A Review of Sixty-Six Adult Cases Which Occurred in the 1937 Ontario Epidemic," *CMAJ* 39 (1938): 1–12, 10.

88  H.H. Hyland and J.C. Richardson, "Psychoneurosis in the Canadian Army Overseas," *CMAJ* 47 (1942): 432–43.

89  *Dean's Report* 1949–50, 21.

90  Allan Walters, "Psychogenic Regional Sensory and Motor Disorders Alias Hysteria," *Canadian Psychiatric Association Journal* 14 (1969): 573–90; Walters, "Psychogenic Regional Pain Alias Hysterical Pain," *Brain* 84 (1961): 1–18.

91  J.D.G. [John D. Griffin], "James Allan Walters (1906–1986)," MS; UTA A1955/0004/004.

92  J.C. Richardson and H.H. Hyland, "Intracranial Aneurysms: A Clinical and Pathological Study of Subarachnoid and Intracerebral Haemorrhage Caused by Berry Aneurysms," *Medicine* 20 (1941): 1–83.

93  E.H. Botterell, W.M. Lougheed, T.P. Morley, and S.L. Vandewater, "Hypothermia in the surgical treatment of ruptured intracranial aneurysms," *Journal of Neurosurgery* 15 (1958): 4–18. See also Cosbie, *Toronto General Hospital,* 317.

94  See Dept of Medicine, *Annual Report* 1944–5, 5. I have seen no previous references to ECT in Toronto but it is possible that convulsive therapy was earlier used at one of the Ontario Hospitals.

95  Wherrett, "History of Neurology," 43.

96  Mary I. Tom and J. Clifford Richardson, "Hypoglycaemia from Islet Cell Tumor of Pancreas with Amyotrophy and Cerebrospinal Nerve Cell Changes: A Case Report," *Journal of Neuropathology and Experimental Neurology* 10 (1951): 57–66, 65–6.

97  Clifford Richardson, "Psychic Aspects of Cerebral Attacks," *Medical Clinics of North America* 36 (1952): 557–68.

98  Cosbie, *Toronto General Hospital,* 257.

99  Findlay, "Neurosurgery at the Toronto General Hospital," 153.

100  J.C. Richardson, R.A. Chambers, and P.M. Heywood, "Encephalopathies of Anoxia and Hypoglycemia," *AMA Archives of Neurology* 1 (1959): 178–90.

101 John C. Steele, J. Clifford Richardson, and Jerzy Olszewski, "Progressive Supranuclear Palsy: A Heterogeneous Degeneration Involving the Brain Stem, Basal Ganglia and Cerebellum with Vertical Gaze and Pseudobulbar Palsy, Nuchal Dystonia and Dementia," *Archives of Neurology* 10 (1964): 333–59.

102 See Roger Baskett, "The Life of the Toronto Psychiatric Hospital," in Shorter, *TPH: History and Memories of the Toronto Psychiatric Hospital*, 97–127.

103 *Dean's Report* 1956–7, 29.

104 *Dean's Report* 1950–1, 45.

105 *Dean's Report* 1960–1, 42; Cosbie, *Toronto General Hospital*, 318.

106 *Dean's Report* 1961–2, 37.

107 *Dean's Report* 1959–60, 65.

108 Cosbie, *Toronto General Hospital*, 318.

109 Joint Hospitals Committee, minutes, 15 Dec. 1966, 3; UTA A1986/0028/001/006.

110 *Dean's Report* 1966–7, 109.

111 *Dean's Report* 1967–8, 56.

112 Committee on Curriculum and Examinations, 8 Oct. 1968; UTA A1993/0025/007.

113 *Dean's Report* 1968–9, 146.

114 *Dean's Report* 1970–1, 151.

115 TGH *Annual Report* 1985–6, 227–30.

116 See Greben obituary in *MedEmail*, 24 Oct. 2007.

117 Self-Study, Feb. 1983, 91; UTA F016/030/031.

118 *Dean's Report* 1971–2, 168.

119 Ibid.

120 This document, dated 22 Nov. 1973, is attached to Minutes of Committee on Postgraduate Education, 14 Dec. 1973 and filed under that label; in the archives, however, it is attached to Faculty Council, 28 Jan. 1974; UTA A1993/0025/007.

121 "Retired President Returns to Head up Concordia," *Globe and Mail*, 22 Jan. 2011, A19.

122 LRPAC Minutes, 11 Dec. 1974; UTA A1979/0010/006.

123 Science Policy Committee Minutes, 17 Jan. 1977; UTA A1993/0025/008.

124 *Medisphere*, Feb. 1978, 2.

125 *Medisphere*, Sept. 1977, 2.

126 Vivian Rakoff to E.M. Sellers, 23 May 1985; UTA A1994/0012/007.

127 See R. Gordon Bell, *Escape from Addiction* (New York: McGraw-Hill, 1970); on Bell see "Dr R Gordon Bell: Canada's Compassionate Pioneer in Alcohol Treatment," *Canadian Doctor* 48 (1982): 25–8.

128 Shitij Kapur and Gary Remington, "Serotonin-dopamine Interaction and Its Relevance to Schizophrenia," *American Journal of Psychiatry* 153 (1996): 466–76.

129 S. Kapur, G. Remington, C. Jones, A. Wilson, J. DaSilva, S. Houle, and R. Zipursky, "High Levels of Dopamine D2 Receptor Occupancy with Low-dose Haloperidol Treatment: A PET Study," *American Journal of Psychiatry* 153 (1996): 948–50.

130 Joel Paris and John A. Talbott, "Department of Psychiatry, External Review, Dec 2–3, 1999"; Dean's Archive.

131  External Review: Department of Psychiatry, 2004; Dean's Archive.

132  *Dean's Report* 1951–2, 43, 50.

133  Robert Pos, "History of Psychiatry at Toronto General Hospital until 1975," 38; unpublished MS (1992). I am grateful to Dr Pos for letting me see a copy.

134  *Dean's Report* 1967–8, 123.

135  *Dean's Report* 1968–9.

136  *Dean's Report* 1936–7, 32.

137  *Dean's Report* 1948–9, 4, 41.

138  *Dean's Report* 1967–8, 86.

139  Paul D. Steinhauer and Quentin Rae-Grant, *Psychological Problems of the Child and His Family* (Toronto: Macmillan, 1977).

140  Steinhauer death notice in *MedEmail*, 5 June 2000.

141  *Dean's Report* 1971–2, 122.

142  Quentin Rae-Grant, "To the Review Committee – for the Head of the Department of Psychiatry" (1985); Dean's Archive.

143  "Conversation with Reg Smart," *Addiction* 93 (1998): 9–15, 10.

144  *Dean's Report* 1964–5, 45.

145  James G. Rankin, "Alcoholism and Drug Addiction Research Foundation of Ontario: Research Goals and Plans," *Annals of the New York Academy of Sciences* 273 (28 May 1976): 87–97. Science Policy Committee, Minutes, 9 Dec. 1976; UTA A1993/0025/008.

146  LRPAC, 17 Apr. 1974; UTA A1979/0010/006.

147  Anthony E. Lang, *MediNews*, Feb. 2006, 6.

148  TGH *Annual Report* 1906, 6; see also Wherrett, "History of Neurology," 11.

149  TGH *Annual Report* 1911, 32.

150  TGH *Annual Report* 1914, 6; see also Playfair Committee Minutes, 16 Dec. 1969; UTA A1978/0056/001, "Binder."

151  *Dean's Report* 1944–5, 16.

152  Department of Medicine, undated [1920]; UTA A1979/0023/002.

153  Canadian Association of Occupational Therapists – past president; www.caot.ca/default.asp?pageid=2096.

154  This is briefly mentioned in Playfair Committee Minutes, 16 Dec. 1969; UTA A1978/0056/001, "Binder."

155  "Information Received from the Various Departments Regarding Suggestions for Post-Graduate Training," 12 Dec. 1945, 12; UTA A1988/0010/001(007).

156  On Armour see Wherrett, "History of Neurology," 38–9.

157  See John R. Wherrett, "J. Clifford Richardson," Faculty Council, 29 Sept. 1986; UTA A1995/004/004. In his "History of Neurology," Wherrett, however, puts the neurology beds on Ward G.

158  1956–7: *Dean's Report* refers to "Neurology and Psychological Medicine" as a separate category. Term "Division" not yet used for any of the subdivisions of medicine; Dean's Report 1956–7, 29.

159  Wherrett, "J. Clifford Richardson."

160 Hollenberg report, 17 July 1973, 8; UTA A1986/0028/004 (002).

161 Anthony E. Lang, Andres M. Lozano, Erwin Montgomery, Jan Duff, Ronald Tasker, and William Hutchison, "Posteroventral Medial Pallidotomy in Advanced Parkinson's Disease," *New England Journal of Medicine* 337 (9 Oct. 1997): 1036–42.

162 A.E. Lang and Jose A. Obeso, "Challenges in Parkinson's Disease: Restoration of the Nigrostriatal Dopamine System Is Not Enough," *Lancet Neurology* 3 (May 2004): 309–16.

163 Peter Carlen, G. Wortzman, R.C. Holgate, D.A. Wilkinson, and J. C. Rankin, "Reversible Cerebral Atrophy in Recently Abstinent Chronic Alcoholics Measured by Computed Tomography Scans," *Science* 200 (1978): 1076–8.

164 Aviv Ouanounou Liang Zhang, M.P. Charlton, and L. Carlen, "Differential Modulation of Synaptic Transmission by Calcium Chelators in Young and Aged Hippocampal CA1 Neurons: Evidence for Altered Calcium Homeostasis in Aging," *Journal of Neuroscience* 19 (1999): 906–15.

165 Jianxue Li, Marc R. Pelletier, José-Luis Perez Velazquez, and Peter L. Carlen, "Reduced Cortical Synaptic Plasticity and Glur1 Expression Associated with Fragile X Mental Retardation Protein Deficiency," *Molecular and Cellular Neuroscience* 19 (2002): 138–51.

166 See, for example, M.J. Morrow and J.A. Sharpe, "Cerebral Hemispheric Localization of Smooth Pursuit Asymmetry," *Neurology* 40 (1990): 284–92.

167 TGH *Annual Report* 1985–6, 145.

168 TGH *Annual Report* 1984–5, 95–6.

169 Clinical chairs, 17 Mar. 1987; UTA A1993/0025/001.

170 Ibid., meeting of 19 May 1987.

171 TTH *Annual Report* 1987–8, 109, 175.

172 See James A. Sharpe to John Dirks, 12 June 1990; UTA A96/0011/023 (/011).

173 John H. Dirks to J. Sharpe, 7 June 1991; UTA A96/0011/023 (011).

174 Joseph T. Marotta to John Dirks, 22 June 1990; UTA A96/0011/023 (011).

175 Findlay, "Neurosurgery at the Toronto General Hospital," 146–58.

176 Ibid., 152.

177 Cosbie, *Toronto General Hospital*, 315–16.

178 W.M. Lougheed and B. Marshall, "The Diploscope in Intracranial Aneurysm Surgery: Results in 40 Patients," *Canadian Journal of Surgery* 12 (1969): 75–82. See on Lougheed's life, Findlay, "William M. Lougheed," 337–40.

179 J. Max Findlay and Robin P. Humphreys, "Ingenuity, Innovation and Intuition: Remembering Bill Lougheed," *Surgical Spotlight*, Spring 2005, 13–14.

180 William M. Lougheed, Brian M. Marshall, Michael Hunter, Ernest R. Michel, and Harley Sandwith-Smyth, "Common Carotid to Intracranial Internal Carotid Bypass Venous Graft," *Journal of Neurosurgery* 34 (1971): 114–18, 117.

181 Pearson, "Goals and Objectives – Department of Surgery, 1978–1988," 24.

182 TGH *Annual Report* 1982–3, 9; TGH *Annual Report* 1985–6, 75.

183 Dept of Surgery, *Annual Report* 1989–90, 14.

184 Charles H. Tator, "New Division of Neurosurgery at Toronto Hospital," *Surgical Neurology* 36 (1991): 378–9.

185 *Surgical Spotlight*, Winter 2008, 1; *Surgical Spotlight*, Fall 2008, 3.

186 W.D. Hutchison, K.D. Davis, A.M. Lozano, R.R. Tasker, and J.O. Dostrovsky, "Pain-related Neurons in the Human Cingulate Cortex," *Nature Neuroscience* 2 (1999): 403–5.

187 *Surgical Spotlight*, Spring 2005, 15–16.

188 Michael D. Taylor and Mark Bernstein, "Awake Craniotomy with Brain Mapping As the Routine Surgical Approach to Treating Patients with Supratentorial Intra-axial Tumors: A Prospective Trial of 200 Cases," *Journal of Neurosurgery* 90 (1999): 35–41; M. Bernstein, "Outpatient Craniotomy for Brain Tumor: A Pilot Feasibility Study in 46 Patients," *Canadian Journal of Neurological Sciences* 28 (2001): 120–4, 120.

189 *MedEmail*, 14 June 1999.

190 Martin McKneally column, *Surgical Spotlight*, Fall 2004, 7.

191 Richard Ellenbogen, "Comment," to Humphreys, "History of Neurosurgery at the Hospital for Sick Children," 624.

192 Humphreys, "Modernization of Pediatric Neurosurgery," 19.

193 James M. Drake, "The Surgical Management of Hydrocephalus," *Neurosurgery* 62, supplement (2008): SHC633–SHC642, SHC633; James M. Drake, "Ventriculostomy for Treatment of Hydrocephalus," *Neurosurgery Clinics of North America* 4 (1993): 657–66.

194 *Surgical Spotlight*, Fall 2004, 8.

195 Humphreys, "Sixty Year History," 5.

196 Dept of Surgery *Annual Report* 1997–8, 24.

197 Michael D. Taylor , Ling Liu, Corey Raffel et al., "Mutations in SUFU Predispose to Medulloblastoma," *Nature Genetics* 31 (2002): 306–10.

198 Humphreys, "Sixty Year History," 3.

199 *The Neurotransmitter* [HSC], Winter 2000, 3.

200 Self-Study, Feb. 1983, 107; UTA F016/030/031.

201 Dept of Surgery, *Annual Report* 1995–6, 46.

202 *The Neurotransmitter* [HSC], Summer 2000, 5.

203 Dept of Surgery, *Annual Report* 2002–3, 38.

204 HSC *Annual Report* 2005–6, 14.

205 *Dean's Report* 1951–2, 43.

206 An undated document from ca. 1970, in UTA A1978/0056/001, "Binder."

207 "Historical review" of the Helen Scott Playfair Memorial Fund; in UTA A1979/0010/007.

208 UTA A1978/0056/001, "Binder."

209 Playfair Committee meeting, 6 Feb. 1962; UTA A1978/0056/001, "Binder."

210 Ibid., 14 May 1965.

211 Ibid., 6 Oct 1965.

212 Ibid., 21 Apr. 1967.

213 Neurosurgical Interhospital Coordinating Committee Minutes, 16 Jan. 1969; UTA A1989/0030/001.

214 Ernest Sirluck, memo conversation, 30 Dec. 1969; UTA A1978/0056/003.

215 J.C. Richardson to J. Evans, 14 Sept. 1972; UTA A1978/0056/002.

216 Sub-committee on Science Policy, 28 Nov. 1972; UTA A1993/0025/008.

217 Meeting of Hollenberg Committee with Neurosciences Advisory Committee, 9 Jan. 1973; UTA A1979/0010/007.

218 Steiner to Holmes, 16 Nov. 1973; UTA A1979/0010/007B.

219 Academic Planning and Search Committee, 14 Feb. 1974; UTA A1993/0025/005.

220 Pearson, "Goals and Objectives – Department of Surgery, 1978–1988," 24; Dean's Archive.

221 Ross Fleming, personal communication, 9 Nov. 2010.

222 Faculty of Medicine, Research Activities in the Neurosciences [no date]; Dean John Dirks is acknowledged in the preface.

223 See Institute of Neurosciences Proposal, attached to Committee of Clinical Chairs, 21 May 1991, 1; UTA A1996/007/002.

224 Wherrett to Holmes, 4 Apr. 1974; UTA A1978/0056/001.

225 Clinical chairs, 19 Jan. 1982; UTA A1993/0025/001.

226 Basic Science chairs, 2 Nov. 1984; UTA A1993/0025/001.

227 Clinical chairs, 21 Apr. 1987; UTA A1993/0025/001.

228 Faculty News, Sept. 1991, 3; Dean's Archive

229 Clinical chairs, 18 Dec. 1990, 4; UTA A1996/0007/002.

230 Clinical chairs, 21 May 1991; UTA A1996/0007/002.

231 Jennifer Sturgess to John Yeomans, 29 Jan. 1992; UTA A1996/0011/021 (2).

232 Plan 2000–4, 85–6.

233 See F.H. Lowy to President Strangway, 13 July 1984, and attached documents; UTA B2005/0031/011(17).

234 Basic Science chairs, 12 Sept. 1986, Keith Moore reporting; UTA A1993/0025/001.

235 Clinical chairs, 19 May 1987; UTA A1993/0025/001.

236 JoAnne McLaurin, R. Cecal, Meredith E. Kierstead et al., "Therapeutically Effective Antibodies Against Amyloid-beta Peptide Target Amyloid-beta Residues 4-10 and Inhibit Cytotoxicity and Fibrillogenesis," *Nature Medicine* 8 (2002): 1263–9.

237 JoAnne McLaurin, Meredith E. Kierstead, Mary E. Brown et al., "Cyclohexane-hexol Inhibitors of A-beta Aggregation Prevent and Reverse Alzheimer Phenotype in a Mouse Model," *Nature Medicine* 12 (2006): 801–8.

238 "Report of Advisory Committee to the Dean on Gerontology," no date [early 1970s]; UTA A1981/0027/05/15 (17/6)

239 Donald T. Stuss and Catherine A. Gow, "'Frontal Dysfunction' after Traumatic Brain Injury," *Neuropsychiatry, Neuropsychology, and Behavioral Neurology* 5 (1992): 272–82.

240 D.T. Stuss et al., "Wisconsin Cart Sorting Test Performance in Patients with Focal Frontal and Posterior Brain Damage: Effects of Lesion Location and Test Structure on Separable Cognitive Processes," *Neuropsychologia* 38 (2000): 388–402.

241 E. Tulving, "Episodic and Semantic Memory," in *Organization of Memory*, ed. E. Tulving and W. Donaldson (New York: Academic Press, 1972), 381–403.
242 "Endel Tulving PhD, Recipient of the Canada Gairdner International Award, 2005," http://www.gairdner.org/content/endel-tulving.
243 Helen S. Mayberg, Andres M. Lozano, Valerie Voon, Heather E McNeely, David Seminowicz, Clement Hamani, Jason M. Schwalb, and Sidney H. Kennedy, "Deep Brain Stimulation for Treatment-Resistant Depression," *Neuron* 45 (2005): 651–60.
244 On the history of Baycrest, the Rotman Research Institute, and KLARU see "Rotman Research Institute – History – Milestones," www.rotman-baycrest.on.ca/index.php?section=445#.
245 Ross Fleming, personal communication, 9 Nov. 2010.

## 15 Anatomy

1 Dewar interview by Schatzker, 22 June 1976, p. 28; Dean's Archive.
2 Ross G. MacKenzie, "A History of the Department of Anatomy at the University of Toronto," no date, 16; UTA A1983/0036/011 (12).
3 Oille, "My Experiences in Medicine," 855.
4 J.P. McMurrich, *The Development of the Human Body* (Philadelphia: P. Blakiston's Son, 1902).
5 Charles C. Macklin, "James Playfair McMurrich," *CMAJ* 40 (1939): 409–10.
6 *Epistaxis* (1928), 29.
7 Faculty Council, 5 Oct. 1929, 221; UTA A1986/0027/020.
8 Faculty Council, 1 Mar. 1920, 168; UTA A1986/0027/020.
9 Some of the biographical details of Grant's life are from an unpublished autobiography that Mackenzie reproduces in an appendix.
10 Dewar interview by Schatzker, 22 June 1976, p. 28; Dean's Archive.
11 For an overview of Grant's work see P.V. Tobias, "The Contributions of JC Boileau Grant to the Teaching of Anatomy," *South African Medical Journal* 83 (1993): 352–3.
12 *Dean's Report* 1930–1, 4.
13 *MedEmail*, 13 Oct. 2003.
14 *Dean's Report* 1937–8, 15.
15 MacKenzie, "History of the Department of Anatomy," 33.
16 *Dean's Report* 1942–3, 8.
17 Kellogg Questionnaire, 13 Dec. 1945, p. 1; UTA A1986/0028/011.
18 Susan Bélanger, "Continuing the Banting Legacy: The Banting Research Foundation, 1925–1995," Banting Research Foundation, 1995, 29.
19 *Dean's Report* 1932–3, 12.
20 Arthur W. Ham, "A Histological Study of the Early Phases of Bone Repair," *Journal of Bone and Joint Surgery* 12 (1930): 827–44.
21 Brian K. Hall, "Arthur Worth Ham, 1902–1992," *Proceedings of the Royal Society of Canada*, 7th ser, 1 (2002): 114–16.
22 Arthur W. Ham, *Histology*, 5th ed. (Philadelphia: Lippincott, 1965), 384–458.

23  *Dean's Report* 1940–1, 8–9.
24  Berris, *Medicine: My Story*, 21.
25  M.I. Armstrong, A.E. Gray, and A.W. Ham, "Cultivation of 4-Dimethylaminoaz-obenzene-induced Rat Liver Tumors in Yolk Sacs of Chick Embryos," *Cancer Research* 12 (1952): 698–701.
26  *Dean's Report* 1948–9, 12; *Dean's Report* 1950–1, 14.
27  Arthur W. Ham to Dean J.D. Hamilton, 29 Jan. 1965; UTA A1983/0007/001.
28  K.L. Moore, eulogy, "James Scott Thompson," Faculty Council, 4 Oct. 1982; UTA A1993/0025/009.
29  *Dean's Report* 1967–8, 33.
30  LRPAC Minutes, 20 Feb. 1974; UTA A1979/0010/006.
31  J.S. Thompson to B. Holmes, 8 Dec. 1975; UTA A1979/0010/005.
32  Draft Report to LCME Steering Committee, ca. 1975–6; UTA A1979/0010/005.
33  Jan Steiner to Keith Moore, 14 Apr. 1976; UTA A1979/0010/00 2 (15.35.2).
34  Keith L. Moore, *Clinically Oriented Anatomy* (Baltimore: Williams & Wilkins, 1980).
35  See Frederick H. Lowy to A.A. Axelrad, 3 Apr. 1985, and attachments; UTA A1994/0012/06.
36  Keith L. Moore to Rose Sheinin, 17 Oct. 1984; UTA A1994/0012/06.
37  *FAXulty of Medicine*, 17 Mar. 1997.
38  *FAXulty of Medicine*, 20 Oct. 1997.
39  *MedEmail*, 29 Sept. 2003.
40  Cindi M. Morshead, B.A. Reynolds, C.G. Craig, M.W. McBurney, W.A. Staines, D. Morassutti, S. Weiss, and Derek van der Kooy, "Neural Stem Cells in the Adult Mammalian Forebrain: A Relatively Quiescent Subpopulation of Subependymal Cells," *Neuron* 13 (1994): 1071–82.
41  D. Piccin and C.M. Morshead, "Potential and Pitfalls of Stem Cell Therapy in Old Age," *Disease Models and Mechanisms* 3 (2010): 421–5.
42  David Sinclair, review of W.H. Hollinshead's *Anatomy for Surgeons, vol. 2, Journal of Anatomy* 111 (1972): 470–1.

## 16  Physiology/Banting and Best/Biochemistry/Pharmacology/Nutrition

1  A.W. Laxton et al., "Valence-specific Neuronal Activity in the Subgenual Cingulate of Depressed Patients Viewing Emotional Images," *Society for Neuroscience Abstract*, 2007, http://www.abstractsonline.com, accessed 22 Feb. 2011; Jonathan O. Dostrovsky, personal communication, 20 Feb. 2011. Dostrovsky works closely with Andres Lozano and has also worked with Helen Mayberg on several cases. He was "involved in the microelectrode recordings in the depressed patients prior to implanting the deep brain stimulation electrodes."
2  Andres M. Lozano, Helen S. Mayberg, Peter Giaccobbe et al., "Subcallosal Cingulate Deep Brain Stimulation for Treatment-Resistant Depression," *Biological Psychiatry* 64 (2008): 461–7.

3  "External Review, Department of Physiology, University of Toronto, December 1999"; Dean's Archive.

4  Dates of these events differ. I accept the chronology in the Faculty of Medicine *Calendar*, 1913–14, 24–8.

5  Sandra Frances McRae, "The 'Scientific Spirit' in Medicine at the University of Toronto, 1880–1910" (PhD diss., Institute for the History and Philosophy of Science and Technology, University of Toronto, 1987), 246.

6  Macallum, "Development of Physiology and Biochemistry," 103–5.

7  Harold L. Atwood and Mladen Vranic, "A Brief Historical Account of the Department of Physiology, University of Toronto,"4;. http://onlinephysiologycourse.med.utoronto.ca/1117921628/index.html

8  McRae, "Scientific Spirit," 257.

9  Dating for these events is based on extensive research done by Marian Packham.

10  Atwood and Vranic, "Department of Physiology," 4.

11  "Thomas Gregor Brodie," Faculty Council, 6 Oct. 1916; UTA A1986/0027/018.

12  *President's Report* 1917–18, 14.

13  "Dr Winifred Cullis," *CMAJ* 76 (1 Jan. 1957): 71.

14  Walter Campbell to K.J.R. Wightman, undated letter (late 1960s); Dept of Medicine, *Annual Report*.

15  Charles Herbert Best and Norman Burke Taylor, *The Physiological Basis of Medical Practice: A University of Toronto Text in Applied Physiology* (Baltimore: Williams & Wilkins, 1937).

16  Mladen Vranic, "Charles Herbert Best," in *The Best Teacher I Ever Had*, ed. Alex C. Michalos (London, Ontario: Althouse Press, 2003), 267–76, 273.

17  R.E. Haist, "The Contributions of the Department of Physiology (U of T) to Diabetes," *Canadian Diabetic Association Newsletter* 20, no. 4 (1973): 4–7, 17.

18  Jacob Markowitz, *Textbook of Experimental Surgery* (Baltimore: W. Wood, 1937); Markowitz, *Experimental Surgery, Including Surgical Physiology*, 5th ed. (Baltimore: Williams & Wilkins, 1964).

19  Frank C. Mann, James T. Priestley, J. Markowitz, and Wallace M. Yater, "Transplantation of the Intact Mammalian Heart," *Archives of Surgery* 26 (1933): 219–24. See also Markowitz, *Textbook of Experimental Surgery*, 426–30.

20  Markowitz, *Textbook of Experimental Surgery*, 430.

21  Mladen Vranic, personal communication, 14 Sept. 2010.

22  *Dean's Report* 1942–3, 22.

23  "Jacob Markowitz: Jungle Surgeon, Canadian Hero," *National Post*, 10 Nov. 2008; see also Jacob Markowitz, "Some Experiences as a Medical Officer with the Royal Army Medical Corps," in *Empire Club of Canada Speeches 1946–1947* (Toronto: Empire Club Foundation, 1947), 27–41.

24  J.T. Murphy, "Position Paper Concerning Relationships between Department of Physiology and Banting and Best Dept of Medical Research (BBDMR)" [1979]; UTA A1985/0026/005/07.

25  Bissell, *Halfway Up Parnassus*, 92–3.

26 See Charles Best to Sidney Smith, 11 Dec. 1945; Sidney Smith to W.E. Phillips, 1 Apr. 1947; UTA A1983/0036/011 (11).

27 *Dean's Report* 1948–9, 5.

28 H. Best, *Margaret and Charley*, 365.

29 Ibid., 368.

30 Ibid., 374.

31 Mladen Vranic, personal communication, 14 Sept. 2010.

32 Mladen Vranic interview with Edward Shorter, 19 Oct. 2009.

33 Harold L. Atwood, "Reginald Evan Haist," 28 Sept. 1987; UTA A1996/0007/001 (05).

34 LRPAC Minutes, 9 May 1974; UTA A1979/0010/006.

35 [Brian Holmes], "Department of Physiology: Dean's Position for External Review," Aug. 1979; UTA A1985/0026/005 (08).

36 Mladen Vranic, personal communication, 14 Sept. 2010.

37 See, for example, Harold L. Atwood and Shanker Karunanithi, "Diversification of synaptic strength: presynaptic elements,"., *Nature Reviews Neuroscience* 3 (2002): 497–516; H. L. Atwood and J. M. Wojtowicz, "Short-term and long-term plasticity and physiological differentiation of crustacean motor synapses," *International Review of Neurobiology* 28 (1986): 275–362.

38 A.J. de Bold, H.B. Borenstein, A.T. Veress, and H. Sonnenberg, "A Rapid and Potent Natriuretic Response to Intravenous Injection of Atrial Myocardial Extract in Rats," *Life Sciences* 28 (1981): 89–94.

39 Adolfo J. de Bold, "Author Commentary," *Journal of the American Society of Nephrology* 13 (2001): 403–9.

40 Mladen Vranic, personal communication, 14 Sept. 2010.

41 Marina Jiménez, [article on Vranic], *Globe and Mail,* 5 June 2009.

42 J. Radziuk, K.H. Norwich, and M. Vranic, "Measurement and Validation of Non-Steady Turnover Rates with Application to the Insulin and Glucose Systems," *Federal Proceedings* 33 (1974): 1855–64; see also D.T. Finegood, R.N. Bergman, and M. Vranic, "Estimation of Endogenous Glucose Production during Hyperinsulinemic Euglycemic Glucose Clamps: Comparison of Unlabeled and Labeled Exogenous Glucose Infusates," *Diabetes* 36 (1987): 914–24.

43 Mladen Vranic et al., "Increased 'Glucagon Immunoreactivity' in Plasma of Totally Depancreatized Dogs," *Diabetes* 23 (1974): 905–12.

44 Mladen Vranic, Soichiro Morita, and George Steiner, "Insulin Resistance in Obesity as Analyzed by the Response of Glucose Kinetics to Glucagon Infusion," *Diabetes* 29 (1980): 169–76.

45 George Steiner, Soichiro Morita, and Mladen Vranic, "Resistance to Insulin but Not Glucagon in Lean Human Hypertriglyceridemics," *Diabetes* 29 (1980): 899–905.

46 M. Vranic and M. Berger, "Exercise and Diabetes Mellitus: Editorial," *Diabetes* 28 (1979): 147–67. Vranic summarizes his research in "Odyssey between Scylla and Charybdis through Storms of Carbohydrate Metabolism and Diabetes: A Career

Retrospective," *American Journal of Physiology: Endocrinology and Metabolism*, September 7, 2010. doi:10.1152/ajpendo.00344.201.

47 David MacLennan, personal communication, 10 Jan. 2011.

48 C. Korebrits, M.M. Ramirez, L. Watson, E. Brinkman, A.D. Bocking, and. J.R.G. Challis, "Maternal Corticotropin-Releasing Hormone Is Increased with Impending Preterm Birth," *Journal of Clinical Endocrinology and Metabolism* 83 (1998): 1585–91.

49 Atwood and Vranic, "Department of Physiology," 16.

50 M. Aarts, K. Iihara, W.L. Wei, Z.G. Xiong, M. Arundine, W. Cerwinski, J.F. MacDonald, and M. Tymianski, "A Key Role for TRPM7 Channels in Anoxic Neuronal Death," *Cell* 115 (2003): 863–77.

51 Min Zhuo, "Molecular Mechanisms of Pain in the Anterior Cingulate Cortex," *Journal of Neuroscience Research* 84 (2006): 927–33.

52 Jonathan D. Geiger and Wolfgang Walz to Catharine Whiteside, 29 Mar. 2006; http://www.physiology.utoronto.ca/Assets/Physiology+Digital+Assets/ Faculty+%28Profs%29/Documents/Retreat+2009+-+Strategic+Plan/External+Review +of+Dept+%282006%29.pdf, accessed 19 May 2009.

53 Bernard Schimmer interview with Susan Bélanger, 7 May 2009.

54 This brief summary from Irving B. Fritz, "The Banting and Best Department of Medical Research at the University of Toronto," *BioEssays* 9 (1988): 92–7.

55 Petch committee (1974), , see section on TGH, 1.

56 "Lister Day – April 5th, 1927," *University of Toronto Medical Bulletin* 7, no. 4 (June 1927): 1.

57 *Dean's Report* 1931–2, 4.

58 *Dean's Report* 1930–1, 3.

59 Of the series of articles Mendel wrote on the subject, the first in 1943 was Bruno Mendel and Harry Rudney, "On the Type of Cholinesterase Present in Brain Tissue," *Science* 98 (27 Aug. 1943): 201–2.

60 W.S. Feldberg, "Bruno Mendel, 1897–1959," *Biographical Memoirs of Fellows of the Royal Society* 6 (Nov. 1960): 191–9.

61 D.H. MacLennan, "Memorial Wilbur Rounding Franks," 17 Feb. 1986; UTA A1995/0004/004.

62 Vranic, "Charles Herbert Best," 267.

63 Gerald A. Wrenshall, W. Stanley Hartroft, and Charles H. Best, "Insulin Extractable from the Pancreas and Islet Cell Histology: Comparative Studies in Spontaneous Diabetes in Dogs and Human Subjects," *Diabetes* 3 (1954): 444–52, 451.

64 Ibid., 444.

65 Vranic, "Charles Herbert Best," 271.

66 A.M. Rappaport, "The Structural and Functional Unit in the Human Liver (Human Acinus)," *Anatomical Record* 130 (1958): 673–89; see also A.M. Rappaport and G.Y. Hiraki, "The Anatomical Pattern of Lesions in the Liver," *Acta Anatomica* 32 (1958): 126–40; A.M. Rappaport and G.Y. Hiraki, "Histopathologic Changes in the Structural and Functional Unit of the Human Liver," *Acta Anatomica* 32 (1958): 240–55.

67  W.G. Bruce Casselman and A.M. Rappaport, "Estimated Hepatic Blood Flow and Bromsulphalein Clearance in Dogs with Experimental Ischaemia of the Liver," *Journal of Physiology* 124 (1954): 183–7.

68  David H. MacLennan, "A Tribute to Dr Irving B Fritz, 1927–1996," Faculty Council, 11 Mar 1996; Dean's Archive.

69  See, for example, Irving B. Fritz, "Carnitine and Its Role in Fatty Acid Metabolism," in *Advances in Lipid Research,* ed. Rodolfo Paoletti et al. (New York: Academic, 1963), 285–334.

70  David H. MacLennan interview with Susan Bélanger, 26 Mar. 2009.

71  Schimmer interview with Bélanger, 7 May 2009.

72  Paul Stortz, "'Rescue Our Family from a Living Death': Refugee Professors and the Canadian Society for the Protection of Science and Learning at the University of Toronto, 1935–1946," *Journal of the Canadian Historical Association* 14 (2003): 231–61, 238.

73  Irving Fritz, Erich Baer Memoriam, Faculty Council, 27 Oct. 1975; UTA A1993/0025/007.

74  J.T. Murphy, "Position Paper Concerning Relationships between Department of Physiology and Banting and Best Dept of Medical Research (BBDMR)" [1979]; UTA A1985/0026/005 (07).

75  Schimmer interview with Bélanger, 7 May 2009.

76  LRPAC Minutes, 3 Apr. 1974; UTA A1979/0010/006.

77  BBDMR departmental report, ca. 1975–6; UTA A1979/0010/005.

78  LRPAC "Rough Notes," 26 Mar. 1975. Re Department of Clinical Biochemistry: "To be phased out and its functions and programmes to be studied; cf. similar recommendations for BBDMR"; UTA A1979/0010/006.

79  MacLennan interview with Susan Bélanger, 26 Mar. 2009.

80  Thompson to Holmes, 8 Dec. 1975; UTA A1979/0010/005.

81  See Irving Fritz to Dean Holmes, 4 Nov. 1975; UTA A1979/0010/005.

82  David MacLennan, personal communication, 10 Jan. 2011.

83  D.H. MacLennan, "Purification and Properties of Adenosine Triphosphatase from Sarcoplasmic Reticulum," *Journal of Biological Chemistry* 245 (1970): 4508–18.

84  D.H. MacLennan, "Localization of the Malignant Hyperthermia Susceptibility Locus to Human Chromosome 19q12-13.2," [letter], *Nature* 343 (1990): 562–4.

85  Dean Lowy at Committee of Basic Science Chairmen, 12 Apr. 1985; UTA A1993/0025/1.

86  Cecil C. Yip, Clement W.T. Yeung, and Margaret L. Moule, "Photoaffinity Labeling of Insulin Receptor of Rat Adipocyte Plasma Membrane," *Journal of Biological Chemistry* 253 (1978): 1743–5.

87  Robert Z.-T. Luo, Daniel R. Beniac, Allan Fernandes, and Cecil C. Yip, "Quaternary Structure of the Insulin-Insulin Receptor Complex," *Science* 285 (13 Aug. 1999): 1077–80.

88  James Friesen interview with Edward Shorter, 21 Oct. 2009.

89  T. Christensen, M. Johnsen, N.P. Fiil, and J.D. Friesen, "RNA Secondary Structure and Translation Inhibition: Analysis of Mutants in the Rplj Leader," *EMBO Journal* 3 (1984): 1609–12.

90  Friesen interview, 21 Oct. 2009.

91  Phillip Sharp and James Smiley, "External Review, Banting and Best Department of Medical Research," 26 Mar. 2002; Dean's Archive.

92  "Banting and Best Department of Medical Research," Plan 2000, section 4, 94.

93  [David MacLennan], To: "The Review Committee for the Banting and Best Department of Medical Research, March 2001; BBDMR archive.

94  I am accepting the dating of Marian Packham, "History of the Department of Biochemistry," 1; UTA A1983/0036/11 (15); Marian A. Packham, *100 Years of Biochemistry at the University of Toronto, 1908–2008: An Illustrated History* (Toronto: University of Toronto Press, 2008).

95  J.M. Neelin, "Archibald Byron Macallum, Pioneer of Biochemistry in Canada," *Canadian Journal of Biochemistry and Cell Biology* 62 (1984): viii–xi.

96  Packham, *100 Years of Biochemistry*, 6.

97  McRae, "A.B. Macallum," 97–114, 98, 100.

98  "Macallum, Archibald Byron," in *Canadian Who Was Who*, vol. 2 (Toronto: Trans-Canada Press, 1938), 248–9.

99  Andrew Hunter, *Creatine and Creatinine* (London: Longmans, 1928).

100  E.G. Young, *Development of Biochemistry in Canada*, 21.

101  These details from ibid.

102  Laidlaw interview, 8 Apr. 2009.

103  Hardolph Wasteneys and Henry Borsook, "The Enzymatic Synthesis of Protein," *Physiological Review* 10 (1930): 110–45; see also Henry Borsook, Douglas A. MacFadyen, and Hardolph Wasteneys, "The Substrate in Peptic Synthesis of Protein," *Journal of General Physiology* 13 (1930): 295–306.

104  Packham, *100 Years of Biochemistry*, 7.

105  "Resolution with Respect of the Late Arthur Marshall Wynne," Faculty Council Session 1971–2, 275; UTA A1993/0025/006.

106  Packham, "History of the Department of Biochemistry," 11.

107  J.T.-F. Wong and W. Thompson, "Charles Samuel Hanes," *Biographical Memoirs of Fellows of the Royal Society* 39 (Feb. 1994): 149–55, 153.

108  See their paper, O. Smithies and N.F. Walker, "Genetic Control of Some Serum Proteins in Normal Humans," *Nature* 176 (1955): 1265–6.

109  O. Smithies, "Early Days of Gel Electrophoresis," *Genetics* 139 (1995): 1–4.

110  G.E. Connell, G.H. Dixon, and O. Smithies, "Subdivision of the Three Common Haptoglobin Types Based on 'Hidden' Differences," *Nature* 193 (3 Feb. 1962): 505–6.

111  B. Sarkar et al., "Copper-histidine Therapy for Menkes Disease," *Journal of Pediatrics* 123 (1993): 828–30.

112 Britton Chance and G.R. Williams, "The Respiratory Chain and Oxidative Phosphorylation," in *Advances in Enzymology and Related Areas of Molecular Biology*, vol. 17, ed. F.F. Ford (New York: Life Science Publishers, 1956), 65–134.

113 Packham, "History of the Department of Biochemistry," 15.

114 Geoffrey Evans, Marian A. Packham, Edward E. Nishizawa, James F. Mustard, and Edmund A. Murphy, "The Effect of Acetylsalicylic Acid on Platelet Function," *Journal of Experimental Medicine* 128 (1968): 877–94, 892.

115 See "James Fraser Mustard," in *In Celebration of Canadian Scientists: A Decade of Killam Laureates*, ed. G.A. Kenney-Wallace et al. (Ottawa: Canada Council, 1990), 195–214, 202.

116 On Mustard's life see Marian A. Packham, *J. Fraser Mustard: Connections and Careers* (Toronto: funded by Mustard, 2010); that this important work, like Louis Siminovitch's autobiography, had to be self-published is an indication of the low status of science history in Canadian publishing.

117 E.A. Murphy, H.C. Rowsell, H.G. Downie, G.A. Robinson, and J.F. Mustard, "Encrustation and Atherosclerosis: The Analogy Between Early In Vivo Lesions and Deposits Which Occur in Extracorporeal Circulations," *CMAJ* 87 (11 Aug. 1962): 259–74; the paper was first presented in part in Oct. 1960; H.D. Geissinger, J.F. Mustard, and H.C. Rowsell, "The Occurrence of Microthrombi on the Aortic Endothelium of Swine," *CMAJ* 87 (25 Aug. 1962): 405–8, 405.

118 "An Interview with Dr Jack Hirsh, 2000 Gairdner Award Winner," *University of Toronto Medical Journal* 78, no. 1 (December 2000): 42–3.

119 J.F. Mustard and M.A. Packham, "Factors Influencing Platelet Function: Adhesion, Release, and Aggregation," *Pharmacological Review* 22 (1970): 97–187.

120 See, for example, H. Schachter, "Congenital Disorders Involving Defective N-Glycosylation of Proteins," *Cellular and Molecular Life Science* 58 (2001): 1085–104.

121 Packham, *100 Years of Biochemistry*, 39.

122 Ibid., 44.

123 "External Review, Department of Biochemistry," 2001; Dean's Archive

124 Reinhart Reithmeier interview with Edward Shorter

125 Marian Packham, "Department of Biochemistry," MS 2010, which Dr Packham kindly communicated to the author.

126 J.K.W. Ferguson, "Pharmacology: Its Beginnings in Toronto" (typescript, no date); 7pp.; Department of Pharmacology, 1–2.

127 Biography of Thorburn in Appleton's *Cyclopedia of American Biography*, vol. 6 (New York: Appleton, 1889), and obituary in the *Canadian Journal of Medicine and Surgery* 18 (1905): 59–60.

128 Ferguson, "Beginnings," 1.

129 Ibid., 4.

130 Ross M. Matthews, "James Metcalfe MacCallum, BA, MD, CM (1860–1943)," *CMAJ* 114 (3 Apr. 1976): 621–4, 623.

131  Ferguson, "Beginnings," 4.
132  Ibid., 5.
133  Ibid., 6.
134  V.E. Henderson and C.P. Lusk, *A Text-Book of Materia Medica and Pharmacy for Medical Students* (Toronto: The University Press, 1908). Lusk was a demonstrator in pharmacy.
135  On Henderson's appointment see Faculty of Medicine *Calendar*, 1913–14, 27.
136  *Torontonensis* (1902), 126.
137  G.H.W. Lucas and V.E. Henderson, "A New Anaesthetic Gas: Cyclopropane," *CMAJ* 21 (1929): 173–5.
138  Anonymous obituary, "George Herbert William Lucas," Faculty Council, in 1974–5 session. Lucas died 25 June 1974; UTA A1993/0025/007.
139  J.G. FitzGerald, "Professor Robert Dawson Rudolf," Faculty Council, 7 Dec. 1934, 126–7; UTA A1986/0027/021.
140  Robert Dawson Rudolf, *Notes on the Medical Treatment of Disease for Students and Young Practitioners of Medicine* (Toronto: University of Toronto Press, 1921).
141  *Epistaxis* (1921), 21.
142  *Dean's Report* 1924–5, 15–16; *Dean's Report* 1925–6, 14.
143  *Dean's Report* 1930–1, 28.
144  *Physicians' Formulary* (Toronto: University of Toronto Press, 1946).
145  "The Physicians' Formulary," *CMAJ* 55 (1946): 612.
146  "Velyien Ewart Henderson," *CMAJ* 53 (Oct. 1945): 408.
147  J.K.W. Ferguson, "A Study of the Motility of the Intact Uterus at Term," *Surgery, Gynecology & Obstetrics* 73 (1941): 359–66.
148  *Dean's Report* 1946–7, 34.
149  On Mendel's life see W.S. Feldberg, "Bruno Mendel, 1897–1959," *Biographical Memoirs of the Fellow of the Royal Society* 6 (Nov. 1960): 191–9.
150  Werner Kalow, "Life of a Pharmacologist or The Rich Life of a Poor Metabolizer," *Pharmacology and Toxicology* 76 (1995): 221–7; see also Denis M. Grant and Rachel F. Tyndale, "In Memoriam: Werner Kalow," *Pharmacogenetics and Genomics* 18 (2008): 835–6.
151  W. Kalow, "Familial Incidence of Low Pseudocholinesterase Level," *Lancet* 2 (1956): 576–7.
152  Werner Kalow, "Perspectives in Pharmacogenetics," *Archives of Pathology and Laboratory Medicine* 125 (2001): 77–80.
153  Werner Kalow, *Pharmacogenetics: Heredity and the Response to Drugs* (Philadelphia: Saunders, 1962), 77–93.
154  B.A. Britt and W. Kalow, "Hyperrigidity and Hyperthermia Associated with Anesthesia," *Annals: New York Academy of Sciences* 151 (1968): 947–58.
155  W. Kalow, B.A. Britt, M.E. Terreau, and C. Haist, "Metabolic Error of Muscle Metabolism after Recovery from Malignant Hyperthermia," *Lancet* 296 (31 Oct. 1970): 895–8, 898.

156 D.H. MacLennan and M.S. Phillips, "Malignant Hyperthermia," *Science* 256 (8 May 1992): 789–94.
157 *Dean's Report* 1957–8, 6, 51.
158 *Torontonensis* (1945), 92.
159 Harold Kalant, "The Pharmacology and Toxicology of 'Ecstasy' (MDMA) and Related Drugs," *CMAJ* 165 (2001): 917–28.
160 *Dean's Report* 1964–5, 83; *Dean's Report* 1965–6, 5, 86.
161 Okey interview, 19 Nov. 2009.
162 LRPAC, attached to a document of 16 Apr. 1974; UTA A1979/0010/005.
163 Edward M. Sellers, Howard L. Kaplan, and Rachel F. Tyndale, "Inhibition of Cytochrome P450 2A6 Increases Nicotine's Oral Bioavailability and Decreases Smoking," *Clinical Pharmacology and Therapeutics* 68 (2000): 35–43.
164 Shinya Ito, "Division Update: Clinical Pharmacology," *MediNews*, May 2006, 4.
165 Sohail Khattak, G. K-Moghtader, K. McMartin, M. Barrera, D. Kennedy, and Gideon Koren, "Pregnancy Outcome Following Gestational Exposure to Organic Solvents," *JAMA* 281 (24 Mar. 1999): 1106–9.
166 Philip Seeman, excerpt from convocation speech, 14 June 2002, *Neuroscience Newsletter* [Collaborative Program in Neuroscience, University of Toronto], 1 Sept. 2002, 1–2.
167 P. Seeman, M. Chau-Wong, J. Tedesco. and K. Wong, "Brain Receptors for Antipsychotic Drugs and Dopamine: Direct Binding Assays," *Proceedings of the National Academy of Sciences (United States).* 72 (1975)),4376–80.
168 Philip Seeman, Hong-Chang Guan, and Hubert H.M. Van Tol, "Dopamine D4 Receptors Elevated in Schizophrenia," *Nature* 365 (1993): 441–5.
169 Philip Seeman, *Principles of Medical Pharmacology* (Toronto: Department of Pharmacology, 1975); this appears to be the first edition but that is not certain. The third edition (ca. 1980) was edited by P. Seeman, Edward M. Sellers, and Walter H.E. Roschlau. Harold Kalant, Roschlau, and Sellers edited the fourth edition (ca. 1985); Kalant also edited the fifth (1989) through the seventh (ca. 2007) editions, with various co-editors, published successively by B.C. Decker in Philadelphia, Oxford University Press in New York, and Saunders Elsevier in Toronto.
170 Allan B. Okey, "An Aryl Hydrocarbon Receptor Odyssey to the Shores of Toxicology," *Toxicological Sciences* 98 (2007): 5–38.
171 Allan Okey, personal communication, 1 Sept. 2010.
172 Faculty Council, 27 Apr. 1981; UTA A1993/0025/009.
173 *MedEmail*, 8 Nov. 2007.
174 "External Review: Department of Nutritional Sciences," 2002; Dean's Archive.
175 Defries, *First Forty Years*, 121.
176 Ibid., 145.
177 See the Faculty Council discussion of the Hanly Task Force report, 25 Mar. 1974; UTA A1993/0025/007.
178 LRPAC, Henry Berry Report of 15 Apr. 1976, attached to Agenda of 14 Apr. 1976; UTA A1979/0010/005.

179 LRPAC Minutes, 5 Nov. 1975; UTA A1979/0010/005.
180 LRPAC Minutes, 12 Nov. 1975; UTA A1979/0010/005.
181 Self-Study, Jan. 1990, 101; UTA A1996/0011/0018 (6).
182 Self-Study, Feb. 1983, 29–30; UTA F016/030/31.
183 J.L. Sievenpiper, M.K. Sung, M. Di Buono, K. Seung-Lee, K.Y. Nam, J.T. Arnason, L.A. Leiter, and V. Vuksan, "Korean Red Ginseng Rootlets Decrease Acute Postprandial Glycemia: Results from Sequential Preparation- and Dose-Finding Studies," *Journal of the American College of Nutrition* 25 (2006): 100–7.
184 M.K. Sung, C.W. Kendall, and A.V. Rao, "Effect of Soybean Saponins and Gypsophila Saponin on Morphology of Colon Carcinoma Cells in Culture," *Food and Chemical Toxicology* 33 (1995): 357–66.
185 "External Review, Department of Nutritional Sciences," 2002; Dean's Archive.

**17 Medical Biophysics/Biomedical Engineering/Immunology**

1 "External Review of the Department of Medical Biophysics, University of Toronto," 11–12 Sept. 1996; Dean's Archive.
2 Minutes of the second meeting of the Staff of the Department of Medical Biophysics, 8 Jan. 1959; UTA A1983/0007/004.
3 Harold E. Johns, "History of the Department of Medical Biophysics, University of Toronto"; UTA A1983/0036/110 (19).
4 L. Siminovitch, *Reflections*, 53; Siminovitch says he ended up running the division, but from the context it is clear that he guided the academic department as well.
5 Friesen interview, 21 Oct. 2009.
6 James Till, personal communication, 9 Sept. 2010.
7 Friesen interview, 21 Oct. 2009.
8 *Dean's Report* 1958–9, 26.
9 *Dean's Report* 1962–3, 31–9; *Dean's Report* 1964–5, 33–44.
10 *Dean's Report* 1967–8, 47.
11 McCulloch, *Ontario Cancer Institute*, 23.
12 Mortimer M. Elkind, Gordon F. Whitmore, and American Institute of Biological Sciences, *The Radiobiology of Cultured Mammalian Cells* (New York: Gordon and Breach, 1967); "Prepared under the direction of the American Institute of Biological Sciences for the Division of Technical Information, United States Atomic Energy Commission."
13 *Dean's Report* 1970–1, 4, 64.
14 W.R. Harris, confidential note on Medical Biophysics, 19 June 1974; UTA A1979/0010/005.
15 R. Mark Henkelman, "Report of the Members of the Department to the External Reviewers of the Department of Medical Biophysics," June 1986; part of External Review, 1986; Dean's Archive.
16 R.A. Phillips, "Department of Medical Biophysics, Chairman's Report," 10 June 1986; in External Review, Medical Biophysics, 1986; Dean's Archive.

17  Basic Science Chairs, 4 Apr. 1986; UTA A1993/0025/1.

18  Ibid.

19  Self-Study, Jan. 1990, 98; UTA A1996/0011/0018 (6).

20  External Review, 1996; Dean's Archive.

21  Faculty of Medicine News, Dec. 1992, 11; newsletter; Dean's Archive.

22  *MedEmail*, 10 Dec. 2001.

23  D.R. Rose, "Department of Medical Biophysics: Dean's Review," 5 May 2006; Dean's Archive.

24  Friedland, *University of Toronto: A History*, 505.

25  W.H. Francombe, "Dr Edward Llewellyn-Thomas," Faculty Council, 24 Sept. 1984; UTA A1993/0025/009.

26  *Dean's Report* 1961–2, 7.

27  *Dean's Report* 1962–3, 5.

28  E. Llewellyn-Thomas, "Movements of the Eye," *Scientific American* 219 (Aug. 1968): 88–95.

29  *Dean's Report* 1967–8, 54–5; *Dean's Report* 1968–9, 61–2.

30  *Dean's Report* 1969–70, 59–60.

31  A.M. Albisser, "A Mathematical Model of and a Monitoring Technique for Glucose Regulation" (PhD thesis, University of Toronto, 1968).

32  A.M. Albisser, B.S. Leibel, T.G. Ewart, Z. Davidovac, C.K. Botz, W. Zingg, H. Schipper, and R. Gander, "Clinical Control of Diabetes by the Artificial Pancreas," *Diabetes* 23 (1974): 397–404.

33  *President's Report* , 1965–6, 82.

34  M.L.G. Joy, G.C. Scott, and R.M. Henkelman, "In Vivo Detection of Applied Electric Currents by Magnetic Resonance Imaging," *Magnetic Resonance Imaging* 7 (1989): 89–94.

35  Submission of the Institute to LRPAC, 18 Feb. 1976; UTA A1979/0010/005.

36  Draft Report to Liaison Committee on Medical Education, CME Steering Committee, undated (ca. 1975–6); UTA A1979/0010/005.

37  *President's Report* 1971/72.

38  M. Kassam, R.S.C. Cobbold, P. Zuech, and K.W. Johnston, "Quantification of Carotid Arterial Disease by Doppler Ultrasound," *Proceedings IEEE Ultrasonics Symposium*, 1982, 675–80.

39  John L. Brash, "Biomaterials in Canada: The First Four Decades," *Biomaterials* 26 (2005): 7209–20, 7212; W.F. Ip, M.V. Sefton, and W. Zingg, "Parallel Flow Arteriovenous Shunt for the Ex Vivo Evaluation of Heparinized Materials," *Journal of Biomedical Materials Research* 19 (1985): 161–78.

40  LRPAC Minutes, 18 Feb. 1976; UTA A1979/0010/005; Brian Underdown report to LRPAC, attached to LRPAC Agenda, 2 Apr. 1976; UTA A1979/0010/005.

41  Clinical chairs, 15 Nov. 1983; UTA A1993/0025/01.

42  Walter Zingg, "Institute of Biomedical Engineering: A Report on Past, Present and Future Activities," 1 Nov. 1987; document for External Review, 1987; Dean's Archive.

43  P.Y. Wang, "Sustained-Release Implants for Insulin Delivery," in *Biotechnology of Insulin Therapy*, ed. J.C. Pickup (London, UK: Blackwell Scientific, 1991), chapter 3, pp. 42–74.

44  *MedEmail*, 14 Sept. 1998.

45  See, for example, Alison P. McGuigan and Michael V. Sefton, "Vascularized Organoid Engineered by Modular Assembly Enables Blood Perfusion," *Proceedings of the National Academy of Sciences* (US) 103 (1 Aug. 2006): 11461–6.

46  External Review, Institute of Biomaterials and Biomedical Engineering, 23 Apr. 1999; Dean's Archive.

47  *President's Report* 1922–3, 18.

48  "Committee on Immunology, Report [HSC]," 4 Dec. 1967; UTA A1993/0007/08.

49  John T. Law to A.L. Chute, 1 Aug. 1968; UTA A1983/0007/005.

50  Packham, "History of the Department of Biochemistry," 27, 31.

51  *Dean's Report* 1971–2, 65.

52  *MedEmail*, 12 Mar. 2001.

53  Basic Science Chairs, 21 Nov. 1972; UTA A1993/0025/1.

54  Ibid.

55  Immunology Report 1974; UTA A1986/0028/3/10; see also Cinader to Holmes, 29 Jan. 1975; UTA A1979/0010/006.

56  LRPAC Minutes, 12 Feb. 1975; UTA A1979/0010/006.

57  Meeting of Ad Hoc Committee on Immunology, 12 Nov. 1980; UTA A1995/0004/002.

58  Ad Hoc Committee on Immunology, 27 Feb. 1981; UTA A1995/0004/002.

59  Faculty Council, 27 Apr. 1981; UTA A1993/0025/009.

60  *Tablet*, Winter 1984, 11.

61  McCulloch, *Ontario Cancer Institute*, 82.

62  External Review, Department of Immunology, 1989; Dean's Archive.

63  See Frederick H. Lowy to Samuel O. Freedman, 12 Oct. 1984; UTA A1994/0012/06.

64  Michael Julius, "Chair's Statement" for External Review, Department of Immunology, Mar. 1997; Dean's Archive.

65  External Review, Department of Immunology, 8 Dec. 2006.

## 18  Laboratory Medicine (Pathology/Microbiology/Pathological Chemistry)

1  Faculty of Medicine *Calendar*, 1913–14, 28.

2  John J. Mackenzie, anonymous eulogy, Faculty Council, 6 Oct. 1922; Paul A. Bator, "Mackenzie, John Joseph," in *Dictionary of Canadian Biography Online*, vol. 15, *1921–1930*; http://www.biographi.ca.

3  TGH *Annual Report* 1913, 26–7.

4  *Dean's Report* 1923–4, 7, 17.

5  *Dean's Report* 1930–1, 29–30.

6  *Torontonensis* (1902), 128.

7  *U of T Medical Bulletin*, Apr. 1923, 4.

8 Oskar Klotz, "An Address on Cancer of the Lung; with a Report Upon Twenty-Four Cases," *CMAJ* 17 (1927): 989–96, 993.

9 T.H. Belt, "Pulmonary Embolism," *CMAJ* 30 (1934): 253–4.

10 T.H. Belt, "Thrombosis and Pulmonary Embolism," *American Journal of Pathology* 10 (1934): 129–44, 141.

11 *Torontonensis* (1928), 75.

12 J.H. Dible and E.J. King, "Thomas Henry Belt," *Journal of Pathology and Bacteriology* 58 (1946): 147–48.

13 William Boyd, "The Winnipeg Epidemic of Encephalitis Lethargica," *CMAJ* 10 (1920): 117–40.

14 A.C. Ritchie, ed., *Boyd's Textbook of Pathology*, 2 vols. (Philadelphia: Lea & Febiger, 1990).

15 Ian Carr, "William Boyd – The Commonplace and the Books," *Canadian Bulletin of Medical History* 10 (1993): 77–86, 82.

16 William Boyd, *A Text-Book of Pathology: An Introduction to Medicine*, 4th ed. (Philadelphia: Lea & Febiger, 1943), 16.

17 H. John Barrie, "Sir William Boyd: A Legacy in Print," *CMAJ* 126 (15 Feb. 1982): 421–4, 421.

18 Berris, *Medicine: My Story*, 20–1.

19 *Dean's Report* 1937–8, 38.

20 William Boyd, "Postgrad," 12 Dec. 1945, 4; UTA A1988/0010/001 (07).

21 W. Boyd, *Textbook of Pathology*, 8th ed., v.

22 LMP Newsletter, Fall 2007, 2.

23 Emmanuel Farber, "Doctor William Boyd," Faculty Council, Minutes, Sept. 1978–June 1979, dated 30 Apr. 1979; UTA A1993/0025/009.

24 P.H. Greey, D.B. MacLaren, and C.C. Lucas, "Comparative Chemotherapy in Experimental Pneumococcal Infections," *CMAJ* 40 (1939): 319–24.

25 Philip Greey, "The Development of Penicillin," in *Official History of the Canadian Medical Services, 1939–1945*, vol. 2, *Clinical Subjects*, ed. W.R. Feasby (Ottawa: Queen's Printer, 1953), 387–93.

26 *Dean's Report* 1944–5, 22.

27 *Dean's Report* 1933–4, 30.

28 See *Dean's Report* 1939–40, 41–6; *Dean's Report* 1945–6, 2, 6.

29 Leslie Spence to F.H. Lowy, 17 Feb. 1987; UTA A1994/0012/01.

30 *Dean's Report* 1954–5, 43–4.

31 Pritzker interview, 20 Oct. 2009.

32 *Dean's Report* 1963–4, 72.

33 *Dean's Report* 1964–5, 75–9.

34 *Dean's Report* 1966–7, 89.

35 Independent Planning Committee *Report* (1969), 46.

36 "Toronto Genetics Program," 29 May 1980; UTA A1985/0026/004 (010).

37 W.G. Bigelow to A.C. Ritchie, 15 Mar. 1968; UTA A1989/0030/002.

38 *Dean's Report* 1967–8, 104.

39  Draft Report to LCME Steering Committee, ca. 1975–6; UTA A1979/0010/005.
40  Langer interview, 20 Oct. 2009, 10.
41  Pritzker interview, 20 Oct. 2009.
42  Self-Study, Feb. 1983, 85–7; UTA F016/030/031.
43  External Review, Department of Pathology, 1984, reviewer #1; Dean's Archive.
44  External Review, Department of Pathology, 24 Jan. 1990; Dean's Archive.
45  M.D. Silver to F. Lowy, 13 Jan. 1987; UTA A1994/0012/01.
46  Arnie Aberman to Walter Kucharaczyk, 7 Nov. 1996; Dean's Archive.
47  *FAXulty of Medicine*, 13 Nov. 1995.
48  Findlay, "Neurosurgery at the Toronto General Hospital," 147, calls attention to McKenzie's role; see also *President's Report* 1931–2, 5, 46.
49  T.P. Morley, "Eric Ambrose Linell," Faculty Council Minutes, May 1983; UTA A1993/0025/009 (14).
50  *Torontonensis* (1922), 167.
51  Tom and Richardson, "Hypoglycaemia from Islet Cell Tumor," 57–66.
52  *Dean's Report* 1931–2, 8–9.
53  *Dean's Report* 1938–9, 24.
54  *Dean's Report* 1951–2, 43.
55  *Dean's Report* 1956–7, 5.
56  Biographical details in "Dr Jerzy Olszewski," Faculty Council, 26 Mar. 1964, 91–3; UTA A1986/0027/028.
57  *Dean's Report* 1960–1, 61–4; *Dean's Report* 1962–3, 68–71.
58  Louis Siminovitch to Harold Kalant, 21 Mar. 1966; UTA A1979/0056/007/08.
59  *Dean's Report* 1950–1, 5.
60  *Dean's Report* 1951–2, 17.
61  Louis Siminovitch to Harold Kalant, 28 Jan. 1965; UTA A1983/0007/007.
62  *Dean's Report* 1967–8, 5.
63  Independent Planning Committee *Report* ( 1969), 121.
64  *Dean's Report* 1969–70, 4, 36.
65  E.A. Sellers to Dean John Hamilton, 19 June 1969; UTA A1983/0007/004.
66  Dean AR 1970–1, 34–6.
67  LRPAC Minutes, 6 Mar. 1974; UTA A1979/0010/006.
68  Faculty Council, 22 June 1981, Appendix IV-2; UTA A1993/0025/009.
69  Harris memo, 7 Mar. 1974; UTA A1979/0010/005.
70  LRPAC Minutes, 6 Mar. 1974; UTA A1979/0010/006.
71  LRPAC Minutes, 10 Dec. 1975; UTA A1979/0010/005.
72  Rose Sheinin to Brian R. Holmes, 24 Jan. 1980; UTA A1985/0026/004/020.
73  Faculty Council, 22 June 1981; UTA A1993/0025/09.
74  Meeting of the Committee of Basic Science Chairmen, minutes, 9 June 1981; UTA A1993/0025/01.
75  Meeting of the Committee of Clinical Chairs, 16 June 1981; UTA A1993/0025/01.
76  Self-Study, Feb. 1983, 24, 68; UTA F016/030/31.
77  TGH *Annual Report* 1982–3, 13.

78  External Review of Department of Microbiology by K.R. Rozee, professor and head of microbiology, Dalhousie; UTA A1994/0012/003.

79  Pritzker interview, 20 Oct. 2009; on the new positions intended to revive the department see Keith L. Moore to T.M. Robinson, re OCGS Review of the Department of Microbiology, 25 Sept. 1984. "No other department in the Faculty has been given assurance that all persons retiring in 1984–86 will be replaced. Consequently the Department has an unique opportunity to strengthen its research and graduate studies." UTA A1994/0012/06.

80  *FAXulty of Medicine*, 25 Mar. 1996.

81  *Dean's Report* 1957–8, 45.

82  TGH *Annual Report* 1905–6, 26.

83  Walter R. Campbell, "Observations on Acute Mercuric Chloride Nephrosis," *Archives of Internal Medicine* 20 (1917): 919–30.

84  Walter Campbell to K.G.R. Wightman, undated [late 1960s]; Dept of Medicine Archive.

85  Rudolph Peters, "John Beresford Leathes, 1864–1956," *Biographical Memoirs of Fellows of the Royal Society* 4 (1958): 185–91, 187.

86  On Hunter's life see E.G. Young, *Development of Biochemistry in Canada*, 20.

87  Victor John Harding, "Nausea and Vomiting in Pregnancy," *Lancet* 2 (13 Aug. 1921): 327–31, 331.

88  Faculty Council, 7 Dec. 1934; UTA A1986/0027/021.

89  *Dean's Report* 1935–6, 32.

90  *Deans' Report* 1940–1, 24.

91  *Dean's Report* 1947–4, 8

92  Bélanger, "Banting Research Foundation,", 11–12. See also Andrew Baines, "James Arnold Dauphinee," Faculty Council, 26 Sept. 1983; UTA A1993/0025/09/16.

93  Baines, "James Arnold Dauphinee," 26 Sept. 1983.

94  *Dean's Report* 1948–9, 4, 32.

95  *Dean's Report* 1949–50, 38.

96  Ibid., 41.

97  *Dean's Report* 1952–3, 3.

98  *Dean's Report* 1948–9, 32.

99  A.G. Gornall, C.J. Bardawill, and M.M. David, "Determination of Serum Proteins by Means of the Biuret Reaction," *Journal of Biological Chemistry* 177 (1949): 751–66.

100  *Dean's Report* 1965–6, 5, 75.

101  *Dean's Report* 1966–7, 83.

102  *Dean's Report* 1967–8, 95.

103  *Dean's Report* 1968–9, 112–13.

104  *Dean's Report* 1970–1, 113–21.

105  *Dean's Report* 1969–70, 108.

106  LRPAC Minutes, 13 Nov. 1974; UTA A1979/0010/06.

107  Report attached to Holmes to Harris, 18 Mar. 1976; UTA A1979/0010/005.

108  Self-Study, Feb. 1983, 61; UTA F016/030/031.

109  D.M. Goldberg to F.H. Lowy, 16 Feb. 1987; UTA A1994/0012/01.

110 *FAXulty of Medicine,* 7 Nov. 1994.
111 *FAXulty of Medicine,* 6 Mar. 1995.
112 External Review, Department of Laboratory Medicine and Pathobiology, 2001; Dean's Archive
113 *FAXulty of Medicine,* 25 Mar. 1996.
114 *FAXulty of Medicine,* 27 Jan. 1997.
115 *FAXulty of Medicine,* 12 May 1997.
116 [Avrum Gotlieb], "Chair's Response to the External Review Dec. 2007," 1; http://www/Assets/LMP+Overview/06-07+External+Review+Chairs27s+Response.pdf, accessed 21 May 2009.
117 *MedEmail,* 19 Jan. 1998.
118 Pritzker interview, 20 Oct. 2009.
119 Avrum Gotlieb, "Chair's Response," External Review, Department of Laboratory Medicine and Pathobiology, 2001; Dean's Archive.
120 External Review, Department of Laboratory Medicine and Pathology, 2001; Dean's Archive.
121 LMP Newsletter, Nov.–Dec. 2004, 1.
122 Pritzker interview, 20 Oct.2009.

## 19 Ophthalmology and Otolaryngology

1 Long-Range Planning and Assessment Committee: Department of Ophthalmology Presentation, attached to memo of 30 Sept. 1974; UTA A1979/0010/006.
2 [Harry Mitchell Macrae], "The Department of Ophthalmology, University of Toronto"; UTA A1976/0054/017 (8).
3 "Richard A Reeve," *BMJ* 1 (15 Feb. 1919): 202–3.
4 Roger Burford Mason, "Dr James MacCallum: Patron and Friend of Canada's Group of Seven," *CMAJ* 155 (1 Nov. 1996): 1333–5.
5 Some of these details from "James Metcalfe MacCallum," Faculty Council, 4 Oct. 1929; UTA A1986/0027/020.
6 UTA A1986/0027/018.
7 Faculty Council, 1 Mar. 1920, 170; UTA A1986/0027/018.
8 *Dean's Report* 1930–1, 15; 1931–2, 21.
9 *Dean's Report* 1932–3, 23–4.
10 *Dean's Report* 1934–5, 26.
11 *Dean's Report* 1937–8, 29. Morgan seems not to have published these achievements.
12 *Dean's Report* 1941–2, 19.
13 Gallie, "Fifty Years' Growth," 13.
14 *Dean's Report* 1945–6, 6–7.
15 *Dean's Report* 1947–8, 27.
16 [Harry Mitchell Macrae], "The Department of Ophthalmology, University of Toronto"; UTA A1976/0054/017 (8).
17 *Dean's Report* 1947–8, 27.

18 Graham E. Trope, "Keeping an Eye on the Eye Bank," *CMAJ* 156 (1 Mar. 1997): 631–2.

19 Peter Wilton, "First Cornea Transplants Meant Blind WW I Veterans Saw First Sights in 40 Years," *CMAJ* 155 (1 Nov. 1996): 1325–6.

20 *Dean's Report* 1955–6, 36–7.

21 P.K. Basu and Hugh L. Ormsby, "In-Vivo Storage of Corneal Grafts," *American Journal of Ophthalmology* 47 (1959): 191–5.

22 *Dean's Report* 1962–3, 50–4.

23 *Dean's Report* 1966–7, 63–6.

24 *Dean's Report* 1968–9, 96.

25 *Dean's Report* 1970–1, 101. On the further development of the Eye Bank, see Trope, "Keeping an Eye on the Eye Bank," 631–2.

26 Independent Planning Committee *Report* ( 1969), 65.

27 R.M.H. Pinkerton to Brian Holmes, 22 Nov. 1979; UTA A1985/0026/004/26.

28 See LRPAC Minutes, 2 Oct. 1974 and 31 Mar. 1975; UTA A1979/0010/006; Harris, "Progress Report," 2 June 1975; UTA A1979/0010/005.

29 Clinical chairs, 20 Dec. 1983; UTA A1993/0025/001.

30 "Monitor Interviews Mortimer," [TGH] *Monitor*, Fall 1987, 10.

31 B.H. Gallie et al., "Retinoma: Spontaneous Regression of Retinoblastoma or Benign Manifestation of the Mutation?" *British Journal of Cancer* 45 (1982): 513–21.

32 J.M. Dunn, R A Phillips, X Zhu, A Becker, and B.L. Gallie, "Mutations in the RB1 Gene and Their Effects on Transcription," *Molecular and Cell Biology* 9 (1989): 4596–604.

33 B.L. Gallie, A. Budning, G. DeBoer, J.J. Thiessen, G. Koren, Z. Verjee, V. Ling, and H.S. Chan, "Chemotherapy with Focal Therapy Can Cure Intraocular Retinoblastoma without Radiotherapy," *Archives of Ophthalmology* 114 (1996): 1321–8.

34 Faculty Research Committee, 6 June 1988; UTA A1996/0007/004 (13).

35 External Review, Department of Ophthalmology, 2000.

36 *MedEmail*, 14 May 2001.

37 "George R McDonagh," Faculty Council, 30 Nov. 1917; UTA A1986/0027/018.

38 Faculty of Medicine *Calendar*, 1889–90, 12.

39 TGH *Annual Report* 1905, 1.

40 TGH *Annual Report* 1906, 5.

41 D.J. Gibb Wishart, "The Oto-Rhino-Laryngological Department," TGH *Annual Report* 1914, 27–31.

42 "David James Gibb Wishart," Faculty Council, 1 Feb. 1935; UTA A1986/0027/021.

43 Cosbie, *Toronto General Hospital*, 248.

44 *Dean's Report* 1935–6, 27.

45 *Dean's Report* 1938–9, 33.

46 Ibid., 10.

47 Peter Alberti, personal communication, 7 Jan. 2011.

48 D.P. Bryce, "Dr PE Ireland," Faculty Council, undated, in 1972–3 session; UTA A1993/0025/007.

49  *Dean's Report* 1946–7, 4, 28.

50  *Dean's Report* 1947–8, 28.

51  *Dean's Report* 1949–50, 29–30.

52  *Dean's Report* 1950–1, 29.

53  Ibid., 30.

54  *Dean's Report* 1952–3, 4–5.

55  Ibid., 32. The founding date of the club is unknown; here we learn of the removal of its headquarters from TGH to OCTRF.

56  *Dean's Report* 1953–4, 33.

57  Joseph A. Sullivan, "The Surgical Treatment of Facial Palsy by an Autoplastic Nerve Graft," *CMAJ* 31 (1934): 474–9.

58  J.B. Smith, J.A. Sullivan, and K. McAskile, "The Fenestration Operation Using Minimal Irrigation," *Laryngoscope* 67 (1957): 643–60, 659.

59  Peter Alberti, personal communication, 7 Jan. 2011.

60  *Torontonensis* (1926), 121.

61  Obituary, "Joseph Sullivan," *Globe and Mail*, 3 Oct. 1988, A15.

62  *Dean's Report* 1958–9, 44.

63  *Dean's Report* 1959–60, 48–50.

64  *Dean's Report* 1958–9, 44.

65  Peter Alberti, personal communication, 7 Jan. 2011.

66  *MedEmail*, 24 Mar. 2008.

67  Bill Rider, "Evolution in Management of Laryngeal Cancer at the University of Toronto: A 'Love Story,'" *Journal of Otolaryngology* 11 (1982): 151–4, 151.

68  Ibid., 152.

69  Douglas P. Bryce and W.D. Rider, "Pre-operative Irradiation in the Treatment of Advanced Laryngeal Carcinoma," *Laryngoscope* 81 (1971): 1481–90.

70  Rider, "Love Story," 153.

71  Patrick J. Gullane and Ian J. Witterick, "In Memoriam: Douglas P Bryce (1917–2008)," *Archives of Otolaryngology – Head and Neck Surgery* 134 (2008): 803–4.

72  *Dean's Report* 1966–7, 69–74.

73  *Dean's Report* 1967–8, 82.

74  Self-Study, Feb. 1983, 77; UTA F016/030/031.

75  Faculty Council, 31 May 2004; Dean's Archive

76  Peter Alberti, personal communication, 7 Jan. 2011.

77  External Review, 1991; Dean's Archive.

78  Peter Alberti, personal communication, 7 Jan. 2011.

79  External Review, 1987; Dean's Archive.

80  *Dean's Report* 2009, 21.

## 20  Anesthesia and Radiology

1  David A.E. Shephard, *Watching Closely Those Who Sleep: A History of the Canadian Anaesthetists' Society, 1943–1993* (Toronto, 1993; published as a supplement to the *Canadian Journal of Anaesthesia* 40 [June 1993]), 2.

2  Ibid., 3; Charles G. Roland, "The First Death from Chloroform at the Toronto General Hospital," *Canadian Anaesthetists' Society Journal* 11 (1964): 437–9, 437. Roland notes that chloroform had previously been used in London but was "popularized for use in clinical practice" by Sir James Young Simpson of Edinburgh.

3  Roland, "First Death from Chloroform," 437.

4  Samuel Johnston, "The Growth of the Specialty of Anaesthesia in Canada," *CMAJ* 17 (1927): 163–5.

5  This paragraph is based on TGH *Annual Report* 1905, 1; TGH *Annual Report* 1926, 4; and *Dean's Report* 1935–6, 44. Bevan dates the founding of the subdepartment in the faculty as 1907.

6  *President's Report* 1933–4, 8.

7  *Counsels and Ideals from the Writings of William Osler*, 2nd ed. (Boston: Houghton Mifflin, 1921), 281.

8  Kim Turner, "Cyclopropane," in Byrick, *Department of Anaesthesia*, 74–75.

9  G.H. Lucas and V.E. Henderson, "A New Anaesthetic Gas: Cyclopropane," *CMAJ* 21 (1929): 173–5.

10  Kim Turner, "Cyclopropane," 77–82.

11  *Torontonensis* (1911), 187.

12  Anonymous eulogist, "Dr Harry James Shields," Faculty Council session of 1972–3; UTA A1993/0025/007.

13  Faculty Council, 3 Apr. 1947, 107; UTA A1986/0027/024 (02).

14  *Dean's Report* 1947–8, 47.

15  Vandewater, "Toronto General Hospital," 103–4.

16  *Dean's Report* 1951–2, 5.

17  *Torontonensis* (1924), 119.

18  *Dean's Report* 1952–3, 11–12.

19  Joan Bevan, "The Evolution of the Department of Anaesthesia," in Byrick, *Department of Anaesthesia*, 13–70, 28.

20  *Dean's Report* 1957–8, 16–18.

21  *Dean's Report* 1958–9, 15; *Dean's Report* 1961–2, 18.

22  Fairley, "Recollections of the Toronto General Hospital," 127.

23  Ibid., 114.

24  *Dean's Report* 1960–1, 5, 17.

25  Gordon wrote very movingly of this experience, and of his eventful life, in Byrick, *Department of Anaesthesia*, 93–8.

26  *Torontonensis* (1937), 109.

27  Bevan, "Evolution," 32. On Britt and malignant hyperthermia, see Werner Kalow, "Malignant Hyperthermia and the University of Toronto," in Byrick, *Department of Anaesthesia*, 263–70, 268.

28  J. Duffin, B. Martin, and J.D. Cooper, "Control, Monitor and Alarm System for Clinical Application of a Membrane Oxygenator," *Canadian Anaesthetists' Society Journal* 23 (1976): 143–52.

29  Beverley A. Britt, ed., *Malignant Hyperthermia* (Boston: Little Brown, 1979; International Anesthesiology Clinics, vol. 17.) See also Beverley A. Britt, "Malignant Hyperthermia," *Canadian Journal of Anesthesia* 32 (1985): 666–77.
30  *Dean's Report* 1964–5, 20.
31  Fairley, "Recollections of the Toronto General Hospital," 110.
32  Bevan, "Evolution," 34.
33  H. Lamont and H.B. Fairley, "A Pressure-sensitive Alarm," *Anesthesiology* 26 (1965): 359–61.
34  John W. Desmond and R.A. Gordon, "Bleeding during Transurethral Prostatic Surgery," *Canadian Anaesthesia Society Journal* 16 (1969): 217–24.
35  Independent Planning Committee, *Report* (1969), 33.
36  See, for example, *Dean's Report* 1970–1, 20–6.
37  Details on Scott's life from Bevan, "Evolution," 60.
38  Self-Study, Feb. 1983, 53–5; UTA F016/030/031.
39  "Report of the External Reviewers of the Department of Anaesthesia at the University of Toronto," 28–9 Apr 1992; Dean's Archive.
40  John Desmond and David R. Bevan, "Toronto General Hospital," in Byrick, *Department of Anaesthesia*, 165.
41  TGH *Annual Report* 1985–6, 160.
42  Faculty of Medicine, Plan 2000–4, 104.
43  The department requested the change at the Faculty Council meeting of 31 May 2004; *MedEmail*, 2 May 2005 reports the change.
44  External Review, Department of Anesthesia, Nov. 2002; Dean's Archive.
45  TTH *Annual Report* 1988–9, 1.
46  Ibid., 77.
47  Faculty of Medicine, Department of Radiation Oncology, Department History, http://www.radonc.utoronto.ca/about-dro/our-history, accessed 6 June 2010.
48  Charles Hayter, "Aikins, William Henry Beaufort," in *Dictionary of Canadian Biography Online*, vol. 15, *1921–1930*; http://www.biographi.ca.
49  James T.H. Connor, "The Adoption and Effects of X-Rays in Ontario," *Ontario History* 79 (1987): 97–106; republished in *A New Kind of Ray: The Radiological Sciences in Canada, 1895–1995*, ed. John E. Aldrich and Brian C. Lentle (Vancouver: Canadian Association of Radiologists, 1995), 119–25, see 122.
50  Quoted in *The History of the Hospital for Sick Children* (Toronto: HSC, 1918), 33.
51  Shorter, *Century of Radiology*, 2, 7; UTA A1979/0023/63: 158, letter from Primrose, 9 Apr. 1898.
52  First mentioned in HSC *Annual Report* 1906, 13, as having opened in 1901.
53  Charles R. Dickson, "The X-Ray as Therapeutic Agent," *Canadian Practitioner and Review* 27 (1902): 598.
54  Charles R. Dickson, "Some Uses of the X-ray Other Than Diagnostic," *Dominion Medical Monthly* 19 (1902): 72–6, 73.
55  C.R. Dickson, "X-Ray as Therapeutic Agent," 598.
56  C.R. Dickson, "Some Uses of the X-ray," 75.

57 Obituary of Mary Elizabeth McMaster, *Toronto Mail and Empire*, 30 May 1930.

58 John McMaster, "Some Results that Are Being Attained by the Use of X-Rays, with Exhibition of Patients," *Dominion Medical Monthly* 19 (1902): 61–72.

59 John McMaster, "The Uses and Limitations of the X-Rays in the Treatment of Diseases," *Canada Lancet* 36 (1903): 708–11.

60 TGH *Annual Report* 1906, 5.

61 C.F. Clarke to J.W. Flavelle, 2 Oct. 1911; UHN Archives, TGH Fonds, sub-series 2.1. Reports to Board of Trustees, box 13, file 2.1.1; Superintendent's monthly reports, July–Dec. 1911.

62 Shorter, *Century of Radiology*, 6, 9.

63 Hugh Newton, "Marked Opening of New Science Era," *Globe and Mail*, 9 Nov. 1945, 15.

64 "Percy Ghent, R.T.," *Canadian Hospital* 29 (Oct. 1952): 16.

65 Shorter, *Century of Radiology*, 10.

66 Details of Richards's life appear in Shorter, *Century of Radiology*, 10–16, his Faculty Council eulogy, 4 Feb. 1949, UTA A1986/0027/025/001, and in a sketch by fellow radiologist William A. Jones, "Gordon Earle Richards: A Little About His Life and Times," in Aldrich and Lentle, *New Kind of Ray*, 235–40, originally published in the *Canadian Association of Radiologists Journal* 6 (1955).

67 Jones, "Gordon Earle Richards," 240. William A. Jones of Kingston became the first president of the Canadian Association of Radiologists in 1947 after Richards, the organization's main founder, declined the honour.

68 Shorter, *Century of Radiology*, 10–16, 14.

69 Ibid., 16–17.

70 Ibid.

71 G.E. Richards, obituary of Dickson in *CMAJ* 29 (Dec. 1933): 690–1.

72 W.H. Dickson, "Thorotrast, A New Contrast Medium for Radiological Diagnosis," *CMAJ* 27 (Aug. 1932): 125–9.

73 Faculty of Medicine, Special Committees book, 2 July 1919; UTA A1986/0027/11.

74 Faculty Council minutes, 10 Nov. 1919; UTA A1986/0027/018: 115.

75 UTA A1986/0027/018: 307, 3 Dec. 1920.

76 W.A. Jones, "Radiological Education," *CMAJ* 37 (Nov. 1937): 480–2, 480.

77 Shorter, *Century of Radiology*, 123.

78 UTA A1986/0027/018: 420–1.

79 Shorter, *Century of Radiology*, 123–4, and on Shannon, 89–91.

80 UTA A1986/0027/020: 219, 5 Oct. 1929.

81 "X-ray Reveals Mysteries," *Toronto Daily Star*, 15 Nov. 1924, 2.

82 Shorter, *Century of Radiology*, 22.

83 Ibid., 18.

84 Faculty Council eulogy, 4 Feb. 1949.

85 Obituary in *CMAJ* 60 (March 1949): 318.

86 Jones, "Gordon Earle Richards," 240.

87 Shorter, *Century of Radiology*, 21–2, 21.

88  Ibid., 16, 68.

89  *Torontonensis* (1923), 134.

90  Ibid., 22.

91  Singleton obituary, *CMAJ* 99 (7 Dec. 1968): 1106.

92  Shorter, *Century of Radiology*, 66.

93  Arthur C. Singleton, "The Roentgenological Identification of Victims of the 'Noronic' Disaster," *American Journal of Roentgenology* 66 (1951): 375–84.

94  Percy Ghent, "X-Ray Aids Identification of Noronic Victims," *Telegram*, 4 Oct. 1949: 6; *Globe and Mail*, 5 Jan. 1950, 2.

95  Shorter, *Century of Radiology*, 67.

96  *Dean's Report* 1949–50, 48.

97  *Dean's Report* 1953–4, 50.

98  *Dean's Report* 1956–7, 58.

99  Attachment to TGH *Annual Report* 1962.

100  Shorter, *Century of Radiology*, 67.

101  TGH *Annual Report* 1954, 9.

102  Obituary in *CMAJ* 103 (10 Oct. 1970): 758

103  *Dean's Report* 1961–2 through 1963–4. Publishing in the department was modest during this period, with most of it coming from the radiotherapy/cancer side.

104  Shorter, *Century of Radiology*, 69–70, 70.

105  Department of Radiology, Presentation to Interdepartmental Planning Co-ordinating Committee, Toronto General Hospital, 25 May 1966, 32; in UHN, Toronto General Hospital, Department of Medical Imaging files.

106  *Dean's Report* 1964–5, 103.

107  Shorter, *Century of Radiology*, 72.

108  Independent Planning Committee Report (1969), 59.

109  Shorter, *Century of Radiology*, 71.

110  *Dean's Report* 1970–1, 157.

111  *Dean's Report* 1971–2, 176.

112  LRPAC document 1974, 11.

113  Shorter, *Century of Radiology*, 71.

114  Faculty of Medicine, *Medisphere*, Sept. 1977, 2

115  Shorter, *Century of Radiology*, 72.

116  Ibid., 124–5.

117  *Dean's Report* 1965–6, 103.

118  Shorter, *Century of Radiology*, 132–4, 133.

119  *Dean's Report* 1968–9, 153.

120  *Dean's Report* 1967–8.

121  Shorter, *Century of Radiology*, 134.

122  Ibid., 110.

123  "University of Toronto, Future Graduate Training Programmes in Diagnostic Radiology," March 1968, 11–12, in UHN, Toronto General Hospital, Department of Medical Imaging files.

124  Shorter, *Century of Radiology*, 136–7.
125  *Dean's Report* 1970–1, 157.
126  *Dean's Report* 1971–2, 176.
127  Shorter, *Century of Radiology*, 138.
128  Ibid., 72–3, 73.
129  See Curtis Woodford, "Interventional Neuroradiology: An Interview with Dr Karel terBrugge," *University of Toronto Medical Journal* 87 (2010): 75–8.
130  Shorter, *Century of Radiology*, 157–8.
131  Ibid., 74–6, 76.
132  "Dr Ronald Colapinto 1931–2011," *Toronto Star*, 5 Jan. 2011, GT4.
133  Ibid., 162–3, 163.
134  Shorter, *Century of Radiology*, 78–9.
135  1974 LRPAC document, 1.
136  Self-Study, Feb. 1983, 97; UTA F016/030/031.
137  1974 LRPAC document, 1.
138  Ibid., 7.
139  Ibid., 12.
140  Ibid., 14.
141  Ibid., 138–41, 141.
142  Shorter, *Century of Radiology*, 161.
143  *Tablet*, Winter 1984, 10.
144  TGH *Annual Report* 1984–5, 143; 1985–6, 239; 1986–7, 370.
145  Shorter, *Century of Radiology*, 141–2.
146  D. Gordon Potts and Juan M. Tavares, "A New Somersaulting Chair for Cerebral Pneumonography," *American Journal of Roentgenology* 92 (1964): 1249–51.
147  UTA A1993-0025/001.
148  Shorter, *Century of Radiology*, 161; TGH, *Annual Report* 1985–6, 239–43.
149  Shorter, *Century of Radiology*, 162; "Tri-Hospital Magnetic Resonance Centre Opens," TGH *Monitor*, Fall 1987, 6.
150  Lillian Newbery, "Super Magnet Looks Through Body to Find Disease," *Toronto Star*, 11 Feb. 1987, A3.
151  Martin McKneally, "Intellectual Humility in Medical Practice and Research," *Surgical Spotlight*, Summer 2005, 17.
152  Shorter, *Century of Radiology*, 142.
153  Ibid., 117.
154  Ibid., 142.
155  Faculty of Medicine, Department of Medical Imaging, Divisions; http://medical-imaging.utoronto.ca/Divisions.htm, accessed 22 June 2010.
156  "Administrative History," University Health Network Archives, the Toronto Hospital Record Group finding aid (Jan. 2007), 1. The Ontario Cancer Institute/Princess Margaret Hospital was amalgamated with the other two on 1 January 1998, becoming a third semi-autonomous division.
157  TTH *Annual Report* 1988–9, 77.

158 Shorter, *Century of Radiology*, 165–6; TTH *Annual Report* 1991–2, 3.
159 E. Glatstein and S.M. Jackson, "Report on the Department of Radiology, University of Toronto, February 7–8, 1990," 1; Dean's Archive.
160 Faculty of Medicine, Committee of Clinical Chairs, 16 Apr. 1991, 7.
161 Faculty News, Sept. 1991, 4; Dean's Archive.
162 Shorter, *Century of Radiology*, 81, 142.
163 Department of Radiation Oncology, "Our History"; http://www.radonc.utoronto.ca/about-dro/our-history.
164 Shorter, *Century of Radiology*, 166.
165 *FAXulty of Medicine*, 18 Dec. 1995.
166 Edna Becker, personal communication, 2 Jan. 2011.
167 Mark Bernstein, Abdul Rahman al-Alnazi, Walter Kucharczyk et al. "Brain Tumor Surgery with the Toronto Open Magnetic Resonance System: Preliminary Results for 36 Patients and Analysis of Advantages, Disadvantages, and Future Prospects," *Neurosurgery* 46 (2000): 900–9; Pirjo H. Manninen and Walter Kucharczyk, "A New Frontier: Magnetic Resonance Imaging–Operating Room," *Journal of Neurosurgical Anesthesiology* 12 (2000): 141–8.
168 "Imaging: Focusing on Alleviating Pain," University Health Network, NET Results, October 2008; David Gianfelice, Chander Gupta, Walter Kucharczyk et al. "Palliative Treatment of Painful Bone Metastases with MR Imaging-guided Focused Ultrasound," *Radiology* 249 (2009): 355–63.
169 Shorter, *Century of Radiology*, 147–8, 148.
170 Ibid., 148.
171 *Dean's Report* 1955–6, 30.
172 *Dean's Report* 1957–8, 31; 1959–60, 39–40; 1960–1, 39–40.
173 *Dean's Report* 1962–3, 44.
174 UTA A1993/0025/4.
175 Shorter, *Century of Radiology*, 148.
176 Cosbie, *Toronto General Hospital*, 306.
177 *Dean's Report* 1965–6, 104.
178 Shorter, *Century of Radiology*, 148–9.
179 Ibid., 149.
180 *Dean's Report* 1970–1, 156.
181 UTA A1979/0010/001/6.15.72, "Report of Review Committee: Health Resources Research Equipment Application, Department of Nuclear Medicine, TGH," 14 Feb. 1972; signed by Sylvia Fedoruk, J.B. Sutherland, H.N. Wagner, E.R. Yendt, and R.J. Rossiter (chair), known as the Rossiter report.
182 UTA A1979/0010/001/6.15.72, Department of Radiology meeting of 1 June 1972.
183 Ibid., B.J. Shapiro to R.B. Holmes, 6 June 1972.
184 Ibid., Shapiro to Holmes, 7 June 1972.
185 Ibid., Nuclear Medicine Planning Group, inaugural meeting, 16 June 1972.
186 Self-Study, Feb. 1983; UTA F016/030/031.
187 Shorter, *Century of Radiology*, 149.

188 TGH *Annual Report* 1984–5, 143.
189 Shorter, *Century of Radiology*, 151–2.
190 Lilian Newbery, "$7 Million Scanner Will Aid Brain Study," *Toronto Star*, 13 May 1987, A22.
191 Shorter, *Century of Radiology*, 152–3, 152.
192 Department of Medical Imaging, Department of Nuclear Medicine; http://medical-imaging.utoronto.ca/nm.htm, accessed 26 June 2010.

## 21 Obstetrics and Gynaecology

1 H.B. Van Wyck, "The Practice of Obstetrics and Gynaecology," *University of Toronto Medical Journal* 32 (1954): 5–8, 5; reprinted from 1948.
2 Connor, *Doing Good*, 123; Adam H. Wright, "Notes on Methods and Results in the Burnside Lying-in Hospital, Connected with the Toronto General Hospital, Toronto," *Canadian Medical Review* 6 (1897): 155–62.
3 Connor, *Doing Good*, 125, 153.
4 Details of Wright's life are found in his entry in the *Dictionary of Canadian Biography Online*, http://www.biographi.ca, as well as in the obituary tributes in *CMAJ* 23 (1930): 725–6, and in the Faculty of Medicine's Council minutes, UTA A 1986-0027/020: 31–32 (3 Oct. 1930).
5 A.H. Wright, "The Medical Schools of Toronto," *CMAJ* 18 (1928): 616–20.
6 "Banquet to Dr Adam H Wright," reprint from *Canadian Practitioner and Review*, Jan. 1913, 14.
7 Wright, "Methods and Results in the Burnside."
8 Connor, *Doing Good*, 139.
9 Adam Henry Wright, *A Textbook of Obstetrics* (New York: Appleton; Toronto: Moran, 1905), available on microfiche in the Canadian Institute for Historical Microreproductions (CIHM) series, no. 79137.
10 Faculty Council tribute (1930): 31; UTA. A 1986-0027/020: 31–32.
11 See *Dean's Report* 1930–1, 5.
12 "Banquet to Dr Adam H Wright," 3, 17.
13 Ibid., 19.
14 Information on Uzziel Ogden is found in his entry in the *Dictionary of Canadian Biography Online* and in obituary articles in the *University of Toronto Monthly* 10 (1909–10): 301–3 (tribute by Nathanael Burwash) and the *Canadian Journal of Medicine and Surgery* 27 (1910): 114–15.
15 N. Burwash, "The Late Uzziel Ogden, MD," *University of Toronto Monthly* 10 (1909): 301–3.
16 Burwash obituary, *University of Toronto Monthly*.
17 Burwash obituary, *Canadian Journal of Medicine and Surgery*.
18 Biographical details on James F.W. Ross appear in the obituary tribute by H.B. Anderson in the *University of Toronto Monthly* 12 (1911–12): 181–7, and Cosbie, *Toronto General Hospital*, 133–4.

19 Cosbie, *Toronto General Hospital*.
20 Anderson obituary, *University of Toronto Monthly* (1911–12).
21 Details of J.A. Temple's life are drawn from H.B. Anderson's obituary in *CMAJ* 26 (1932): 258 and the tribute in the Faculty Council minutes, 5 Feb. 1932, 318–20; UTA A1986/0027/020.
22 Faculty Council tribute to J.A. Temple (1932).
23 Dating of academic posts in the faculty may be found in Faculty of Medicine *Calendar* 1913–4, 24–8.
24 Faculty of Medicine *Calendar* 1904–5, 77.
25 Cosbie, *Toronto General Hospital*, 149.
26 Information on Watson's life appears in Harold Speert, "Memorable Medical Mentors: XVI: Benjamin P Watson (1880–1976)," *Obstetrical and Gynecological Survey* 61 (2006): 287–92, and Samuel Gordon Berkow, "A Visit with Dr. Benjamin P. Watson," *Obstetrics and Gynecology* 10 (1957): 105–11, 109.
27 Alexander Hugh Freeland Barbour and Benjamin P. Watson, *Gynecological Diagnosis and Pathology* (Edinburgh: Green, 1913).
28 Information on K.C. McIlwraith appears in the Faculty Council Minutes, notice on his retirement, 6 Oct. 1933, UTA A1986/0027/021: 238–39; and on his death, 4 Apr. 1941, UTA A1986-0027/023: 156–57; as well as in Cosbie, *Toronto General Hospital*, 149–50, 202.
29 Cosbie, *Toronto General Hospital*, 202.
30 Details of Frederick Marlow's life appear in the obituary by H.B. Anderson in *CMAJ* 35 (1936): 463, and in Cosbie, *Toronto General Hospital*, 202.
31 Cosbie, *Toronto General Hospital*, 149.
32 Ibid., 144, 148.
33 Ibid., 150.
34 Ibid., 208.
35 Harold Speert, "Memorable Medical Mentors: XVI: Benjamin P. Watson (1880–1976)," *Obstetrical and Gynecological Survey* 61 (2006): 287–92.
36 Samuel Gordon Berkow, "A Visit with Dr. Benjamin P. Watson," *Obstetrics and Gynecology* 10 (1957): 105–11, 109.
37 Goodwin interview, 10 Sept. 2009.
38 James Goodwin, *"Our Gallant Doctor": Enigma and Tragedy; Surgeon Lieutenant George Hendry and HMCS Ottawa, 1942* (Toronto: Dundurn Press, 2007), 27–31, 28.
39 Ibid., 31, quoting Faculty Council minutes.
40 TGH *Annual Report* 1923, 12.
41 Decker to Chairman, Board of Trustees, TGH, 27 Jan. 1932; UHN Archives, TGH Fonds, sub-series 2.1: Reports to Board of Trustees, box 13, file 2.1.7. Superintendent's Report 1931.
42 Cosbie, *Toronto General Hospital*, 203.
43 *Dean's Report* 1923–4, 12, 18.
44 UTA A1986/0027/025: 60–61 (tribute to H.B. Van Wyck, 1952). The work in question is Victor John Harding and H.B. Van Wyck, "Weight-taking in Pre-natal Care,"

*CMAJ* 30 (Jan. 1934): 14–17 (on edema and incipient toxemia in pregnancy); "Effects of Hypertonic Saline in the Toxaemias of Later Pregnancy," in both *BMJ* 2 (11 Oct. 1930): 589–92, and *CMAJ* 24 (May 1931): 635–49.

45 *Epistaxis* (1921), 21.

46 Mann's career is detailed in his obituary tribute in the Faculty Council minutes, UTA A1986/0027/27: 291–3, 2 Dec. 1960, and in Cosbie, *Toronto General Hospital*, 204–5.

47 Mann obituary, 291.

48 Cosbie, *Toronto General Hospital*, 204.

49 Mann obituary, 292.

50 Cosbie, *Toronto General Hospital*, 204.

51 J. Mann, "Methods for Improving the Results of Forceps Delivery, Including an Improved Obstetric Forceps," *Journal of Obstetrics & Gynaecology of the British Empire* 64 (1957): 351–4.

52 Mann obituary, 292.

53 *Torontonensis* (1926), 109.

54 James W. Goodwin, "The Casebooks and Journals of a Toronto General Hospital Houseman: JC Goodwin MB 1927–1928," in *Pages of History in Canadian Obstetrics and Gynaecology*, ed. Thomas F. Baskett (Toronto: Rogers Media, 2003), 25–34.

55 Ibid., 57.

56 "Obstetrician, Historian Dr. James Goodwin Dies," *Globe and Mail*, 4 Aug. 1953, 5.

57 *Torontonensis* (1913), 145.

58 Cosbie, *Toronto General Hospital*, 246.

59 William Albert Scott and H. Brookfield Van Wyck, *The Essentials of Obstetrics and Gynecology* (Philadelphia: Lea and Febiger, 1947).

60 Ferguson, "Motility of the Intact Uterus." See also Thomas F. Baskett, "Ferguson's Reflex: Then and Now," in Baskett, *Pages of History*, 20–2.

61 *The First Fifty Years, 1936–1985: The Canadian Gynaecological Society* (np, privately printed, nd), 80.

62 Cosbie, *Toronto General Hospital*.

63 See *Dean's Report 1937–8*, 28.

64 W.G. Cosbie, "The Contribution of Radiotherapy to the Modern Treatment of Female Pelvic Cancer," *Journal of Obstetrics and Gynaecology* 66 (1959): 843–8.

65 W.G. Cosbie, "Radiotherapy Following Hysterectomy Performed for or in the Presence of Cancer of the Cervix," *American Journal of Obstetrics and Gynecology* 85 (1963): 332–7, 336. The finding was first announced at a conference in June 1962.

66 UTA A1986/0027/025: 80–2, tribute to H.B. Van Wyck.

67 *Dean's Report 1946–7*, 23–4.

68 *Dean's Report 1947–8*, 22.

69 *Dean's Report 1948–9*, 22.

70 H.B. Van Wyck, "The Practice of Obstetrics and Gynaecology," *University of Toronto Medical Journal* 32 (1954): 5–8, 5; reprinted from 1948.

71 *Dean's Report 1947–8*, 24.

72  Goodwin interview, 10 Sept. 2009, 2.
73  UTA A1993/0025/009, John L. Harkins, tribute to Donald Nelson Henderson, attached to Faculty Council minutes, 22 June 1981.
74  *First Fifty Years, 1936–1985*, 54–5.
75  "Tribute to Dr. Cannell at MAB," *Monitor*, Feb. 1980, 4 (copy in UHN Archives, TGH fonds, 7.2.2).
76  Ibid.
77  *Dean's Report* 1951–2, 29.
78  Goodwin interview, 10 Sept. 2009, 4.
79  Cosbie, *Toronto General Hospital*, 311.
80  Ibid., 329.
81  Goodwin interview, 10 Sept. 2009, 9.
82  William Paul obituary, *Globe and Mail*, 22 Nov. 2006; Knox Ritchie, "Celebration of the Life of Bill Paul," remarks at memorial service, 5 Jan. 2007.
83  Entry for Low at http://meds.queensu.ca/medicine/obgyn/facultybio/low.htm, accessed 14 Oct. 2009. Low is now professor emeritus and has been manager of the Museum of Health Care at Queen's since 2004.
84  University of Alberta, Department of Obstetrics and Gynecology, "About the Department: History"; http://www.obgyn.med.ualberta.ca/about/history.html, accessed 1 Sept. 2009.
85  *Dean's Report* 1961–2, 7, 45–7.
86  Cosbie, *Toronto General Hospital*, 329.
87  W.J. Hannah, "Dr. C. Peter Vernon," 23 Feb. 1987; UTA A1995/0004/004.
88  *Dean's Report* 1967–8, 71, 74–5.
89  *Globe and Mail* obituary, 22 Nov. 2006.
90  K. Ritchie, "Celebration of the Life of Bill Paul."
91  James Goodwin interview with Edward Shorter, 10 Sept. 2009, 1, 3–4.
92  Goodwin interview, 10 Sept. 2009, and CV.
93  "Toronto Genetics Program," 29 May 1980, 35; UTA A1987/0035/003, file C.5.3
94  Memo from Frederick Lowy to W.M. Paul, 3 Nov. 1980; UTA A1987/0035/003, file C.5.3.
95  F.E. Bryans and Kenneth Niswander, Report on External Review (1979), 3; UTA A1985/0026/004.
96  Department of Obstetrics and Gynaecology, "Dean's Position for External Review," 1979; UTA A1985/0026/004 (24), 1.
97  Faculty of Medicine, Self-Study, 1983, 1–2.
98  Olga Lechky, "Toronto-based Foundation Tries to Combat Underfunding in Women's Health Research," *CMAJ* 146 (15 Jan. 1992): 261–3.
99  J.W. Knox Ritchie, CV, March 2010.
100  Ritchie interview, 21.
101  Ibid., 22.
102  Ibid., 23.
103  Ibid., 25.

104  Self-Study, Jan. 1990, 113; UTA A1996/0011/0018 (6).

105  *MedEmail*, 14 May 2008.

106  Lesley Marrus Barsky, *From Generation to Generation: A History of Toronto's Mount Sinai Hospital* (Toronto: McClelland & Stewart, 1998), 191.

107  Ritchie interview, 11.

108  G.W. Chance, M.J. O'Brien, and P.R. Swyer, "Transportation of Sick Neonates, 1972: An Unsatisfactory Aspect of Medical Care," *CMAJ* 109 (1973): 847–51.

109  Martin Kendrick and Krista Slade, *Spirit of Life: The Story of Women's College Hospital* (Toronto: WCH, 1993), 58.

110  W.J. Hannah, "Annual Report of the Department of Obstetrics and Gynaecology," 1967; WCH Archives.

111  W.J. Hannah, "Annual Report of the Department of Obstetrics and Gynaecology – 1970"; WCH Archives

112  John Milligan letter, in Petch committee (1974), unpaginated section on WCH.

113  Barsky, *From Generation to Generation*, 191.

114  Ritchie interview, 12.

115  Barsky, *From Generation to Generation*, 191–2.

116  Ritchie interview, 12.

117  Barsky, *From Generation to Generation*, 192–3.

118  Ibid., 152–3.

119  Ritchie interview, 10–11.

120  Bryans and Niswander, Report on External Review (1979), 5.

121  Ritchie interview, 31.

122  Ritchie CV.

123  Ritchie interview, quotes 16–17.

124  Ritchie CV.

125  Ritchie interview, 14.

126  At the 28 Jan. 1986 meeting of the Committee of Clinical chairs; UTA A1993/0025/1.

127  TTH *Annual Report* 1988–9, 23.

## 22  New Talent: Mount Sinai Hospital and Women's College Hospital

1  J.D. Hamilton, "The Future of Medical Education at the University of Toronto," *Medical Graduate* 8 (1961), 2–9, 4.

2  E.A. McCulloch, draft, "Comments on the Future of Canada: A Brief for the Citizen's Forum on the Future of Canada," attached to McCulloch to J.E. Till, 7 Feb. 1991; UTA B2005/0031/16 (19.)

3  Cyril Gryfe, "Early Jewish Doctors in Toronto," *Shem Tov: Jewish Genealogical Society of Canada* (Toronto) 23 (June 2007): 1–4.

4  See A.I. Willinsky, *A Doctor's Memoirs* (Toronto: Macmillan, 1960), 7–8.

5  Ernest A. McCulloch to James Till, 30 Oct. 1992; Till Papers, UTA B2005/036/006 (02).

6  *Torontonensis* (1909), 190.

7  *Torontonensis* (1925), 148.
8  Ibid., 150.
9  Kenneth Pritzker, personal communication, 24 Sept. 2010.
10  Willinsky, *Doctor's Memoirs*, 23.
11  Peter Carlen interview with Edward Shorter, 19 Sept. 2008. Sidney A. Carlen, "Fi-brinolytic Properties of Filtrates of Clostridium Histolyticum in Normal Saline and Dog Serum," *Proceedings for the Society of Experimental Biology and Medicine* 40 (1939): 39–41.
12  *Torontonensis* (1925), 155.
13  David Eisen, *Diary of a Medical Student* (Toronto: Canadian Jewish Congress, 1974), 70. Eisen shows himself entirely unaware of anti-Semitism, at least on campus.
14  *President's Report* 1950–1, 52.
15  Berris, *Medicine: My Story*, 31–2.
16  Ibid., 44–5.
17  Laidlaw interview, 8 Apr. 2009.
18  Berris, *Medicine: My Story.*, 54–5.
19  Ibid., 59.
20  Laidlaw interview, 8 Apr. 2009.
21  Margaret Douglin, "Jewish Medical Graduates in Toronto Teaching Hospitals, 1900–1951"; undated manuscript [1993] prepared for Professor Harold Troper.
22  Barsky, *From Generation to Generation*, 27.
23  Langer interview, 20 Oct. 2009.
24  Report of Committee on Admission to First Year, Session 1944–5, 6 Oct. 1944, 26; UTA A1980/0027/024 (01). The author of the report was a Dr Hepburn. For an only slightly less offensive report, see Faculty Council, 1 Oct. 1943; UTA A1986/0027/023/02.
25  Connor, *Doing Good*, 189.
26  Henry Barnett et al., eds., "The Medical Class of U of T '44': The Epic Journeys of 133 Men and 4 Women from High School to Retirement," MS, 2011, 7.
27  Douglin, "Jewish Medical Graduates."
28  *Dean's Report* 1951–2, 57. This appointment is not reflected in Ezrin's entry in *American Men and Women of Science*, 18th ed. (8 vols., New Providence NJ: Bowker, 1992–3), which shows Ezrin as cross-appointed in the Department of Medicine as of 1954 (p. 1017).
29  Bernard Goldman, personal communication, 9 Feb. 2009.
30  *Torontonensis* (1908), 203.
31  Langer interview, 20 Oct. 2009.
32  Helen Farquharson interview, 21 July 2009.
33  Goldman interview, 4 Feb. 2009.
34  Kenneth Pritzker, personal communication, 24 Sept. 2010.
35  Berris, *Medicine: My Story*, 81.
36  Michelle Hollenberg interview, 6 Apr. 2009.
37  Willinsky, *Doctor's Memoirs*, 61.

38  *Torontonensis* (1907), 191. Other biographical data on Sproule-Manson from Rose Sheinin and Alan Bakes, *Women and Medicine in Toronto since 1883: A Who's Who* (University of Toronto: Faculty of Medicine, 1987), 62–3.

39  *President's Report* 1917–18, 14.

40  Ibid.

41  Sheinin and Bakes, *Women and Medicine*.

42  "Report of the Medical Society," Faculty Council, 7 Dec. 1934; UTA A1986/0027/021.

43  Faculty Council, 6 Dec. 1935; UTA A1986/0027/021.

44  Faculty Council, 5 Oct. 1928, 50; UTA A1986/0027/020.

45  Cowan interview, 4 Feb. 2009.

46  Jacalyn Duffin, "The Quota: 'An Equally Serious Problem' for Us All," *Canadian Bulletin of Medical History* 19 (2002): 327–49.

47  Faculty Council, 2 Apr. 1931; UTA A1986/0027/020.

48  Frances Margaret Barker, *Torontonensis* (1924), 116.

49  Faculty Council, 10 Nov. 1919, 121; UTA A1986/0027/018.

50  See the brief biography in "100th Anniversary of Women at U of T"; UTA A1994/0012/05.

51  *Torontonensis* (1925), 163.

52  *Epistaxis* (1922), 10.

53  Helen Farquharson interview, 21 July 2009.

54  Ibid.

55  John O. Godden, "Operation Recall: The 'Rehabilitation' of Inactive Women Physicians," *The Medical Graduate*, April 1968, 4–6.

56  Margaret W. Thompson to E. Llewellyn-Thomas, 16 Mar. 1981; UTA A1987/0035/001.

57  Faculty of Medicine, Self-Study, Jan. 1990, 48; UTA A1996/0011/0018 (6).

58  Faculty of Medicine News, Dec. 1992, 7; Dean's Archive.

59  *MedEmail*, 1 Nov. 2004.

60  Eliot Phillipson, *MediNews*, Nov. 1996, 4.

61  *MediNews*, Nov. 2000, 2.

62  "Chinese Won't Accept Student Restrictions," *Globe and Mail*, 26 Sept. 1974, 4.

63  Eliot Phillipson, *MediNews*, Nov. 2000, 2–4.

64  *Dean's Report* 2009, 7.

65  "Report of the Review Committee Established to Undertake a 5-year Review of the Physician-in-Chief of Mount Sinai Hospital," 22 Oct. 1982; dean's Archive.

66  For details, see Barsky, *From Generation to Generation*, 139–41.

67  Ibid., 86–7.

68  Kenneth Pritzker, personal communication, 24 Sept. 2010.

69  Barsky, *From Generation to Generation*, 101.

70  Berris, *Medicine: My Story*, 84. See *President's Report* 1962–3, 59.

71  Berris, *Medicine: My Story*, 88–9.

72  Pritzker interview, 20 Oct. 2009.

73  Kenneth Pritzker, personal communication, 24 Sept. 2010.
74  Ibid.
75  Mount Sinai Institute, *Annual Report* 1980–1, 6.
76  Science Policy Committee, Minutes, 30 Mar. 1977; UTA A1993/0025/008.
77  Mount Sinai Hospital (MSH) *Annual Report* 1979–80, unpaginated.
78  Ibid.
79  MSH *Annual Report* 1980–1, 7.
80  Meeting of the Cardiovascular Surgery Task Force, 21 July 1982; UTA A1995/0004/02.
81  See William R. Drucker to William Bigelow, 25 Feb. 1971; UTA A1989/0030/001.
82  Committee of Basic Science chairs, 1 Feb. 1985; UTA A1993/0025/001.
83  Pritzker interview, 20 Oct. 2009.
84  *Dean's Report* 1970–1, 151.
85  M.V. Seeman, "Gender and the Onset of Schizophrenia: Neuro-humoral Influences," *Psychiatric Journal of the University of Ottawa* 6 (1981): 136–8.
86  *Dean's Report* 1967–8, 130.
87  N. David Greyson, "Bernard J Shapiro, 1920–1996," *Radiology* 203 (1997): 294.
88  Kenneth Pritzker, personal communication, 24 Sept. 2010.
89  Search Committee for a Radiologist-in-Chief, MSH, Minutes, 19 Dec. 1980; UTA A1987/0035/003.
90  Berris, *Medicine: My Story*, 88.
91  Arthur F. Gelb and Noe Zamel, "Simplified Diagnosis of Small-Airway Obstruction," *New England Journal of Medicine* 288 (22 Feb. 1973): 395–8.
92  I. Katz, N. Zamel, A.S. Slutsky, A.S. Rebuck, and Victor Hoffstein, "An Evaluation of Flow-volume Curves as a Screening Test for Obstructive Sleep Apnea," *Chest* 98 (1990): 337–40.
93  Berris, *Medicine: My Story*, 92.
94  Ibid., 93.
95  Ibid., 108–9.
96  *Dean's Report* 1963–4, 95.
97  MSH *Annual Report* 1979–80, unpaginated.
98  Goldman interview, 4 Feb. 2009.
99  Dept of Surgery *Annual Report* 1997–8, 2.
100 Jonathan L. Meakins and Garth L. Warnock, "The External Review Report of the University of Toronto Department of Surgery, October 4–5, 2007," 4.
101 Dept of Surgery *Annual Report* 1988–9, 15.
102 Kendrick and Slade, *Spirit of Life*, 14–23; de la Cour and Sheinin, "Ontario Medical College for Women," 73.
103 De la Cour and Sheinin, "Ontario Medical College for Women," 74.
104 Kendrick and Slade, *Spirit of Life*, 23.
105 De la Cour and Sheinin, "Ontario Medical College for Women," 75.
106 Geraldine Maloney, *Women's College Hospital as a Teaching Institution* (Toronto: Women's College Hospital, 1973), 2.

107  Kendrick and Slade, *Spirit of Life*, 28.

108  Maloney, *Women's College Hospital*, 4; Hacker, *Indomitable Lady Doctors*, 53.

109  Maloney, *Women's College Hospital*, 4.

110  Kendrick and Slade, *Spirit of Life*, 85; Ida Eliza Lynd obituary, *CMAJ* 48 (March 1943): 279–80.

111  Kendrick and Slade, *Spirit of Life*, 86;Jennie Gray Wildman obituary, *CMAJ* 70 (March 1954): 347–8.

112  Kendrick and Slade, *Spirit of Life*, 67.

113  Isabella Wood obituary, *CMAJ* 72 (Feb. 1955): 234.

114  Kendrick and Slade, *Spirit of Life*, 91; Emma Leila Skinner Gordon obituary, *CMAJ* 60 (June 1949): 639.

115  Maloney, *Women's College Hospital*, 5; Kendrick and Slade, *Spirit of Life*, 30–2.

116  Kendrick and Slade, *Spirit of Life*, 31–2.

117  Skinner Gordon obituary, 639.

118  Maloney, *Women's College Hospital*, 4.

119  Dorothy Thompson and Jean Kronberg, *Women's College Hospital: A Commemorative History of the Department of Anaesthesia, University of Toronto*, ed. Robert J. Byrick and David J. McKnight (Toronto: Department of Anesthesia, 2004), 235–44, 236.

120  Sheinin and Bakes, *Women and Medicine*, 47–8.

121  Kendrick and Slade, *Spirit of Life*, 85; Thompson and Kronberg, *Women's College Hospital*, 236; Sheinin and Bakes, *Women and Medicine*, 81.

122  Kendrick and Slade, *Spirit of Life*, 102.

123  Sheinin and Bakes, *Women and Medicine*, 44–5; Hacker, *Indomitable Lady Doctors*, 54.

124  Kendrick and Slade, *Spirit of Life*, 86; Sheinin and Bakes, *Women and Medicine*, 84–5; Jennie Smillie Robertson obituary, *CMAJ* 124 (15 May 1981): 1398; Deborah A. Wirtzfeld, "The History of Women in Surgery," *Canadian Journal of Surgery* 52 (2009): 317–20.

125  Donnelly, "Jennie Smillie Robertson" (1981).

126  Sheinin and Bakes, *Women and Medicine*, 85.

127  Donnelly, "Jennie Smillie Robertson" (1981).

128  *Torontonensis* (1919), 103.

129  Kendrick and Slade, *Spirit of Life*, 102; Sheinin and Bakes, *Women and Medicine*, 48–9; Marion Grant Kerr obituary, *CMAJ* 64 (June 1951): 553.

130  Kendrick and Slade, *Spirit of Life*, 102; Hacker, *Indomitable Lady Doctors*, 186; Sheinin and Bakes, *Women and Medicine*, 82–3; Minerva Reid obituary, *CMAJ* 76 (1 June 1957): 998.

131  Shorter, *Century of Radiology*, 98–100; Elizabeth Stewart obituary, *CMAJ* 101 (26 July 1969): 119.

132  Shorter, *Century of Radiology*, 98–9.

133  Ibid., 100; Sheinin and Bakes, *Women and Medicine*, 71.

134  Shorter, *Century of Radiology*, 100–1.

135  Kendrick and Slade, *Spirit of Life*, 33, 84, 102; Sheinin and Bakes, *Women and Medicine*, 35–7; Hacker, *Indomitable Lady Doctors*, 188–9; quote from Kendrick and Slade, *Spirit of Life*, 33.

136  Kendrick and Slade, *Spirit of Life*, 33–4.

137  Ibid., 33–4, 85, 102; Sheinin and Bakes, *Women and Medicine*, 62–3; Jane Sproule Manson obituary, *CMAJ* 85 (7 Oct. 1961): 856.

138  Kendrick and Slade, *Spirit of Life*, 28.

139  Maloney, *Women's College Hospital*, 6.

140  Kendrick and Slade, *Spirit of Life*, 35.

141  Maloney, *Women's College Hospital*, 6.

142  Kendrick and Slade, *Spirit of Life*, 41.

143  Ibid., 38–9.

144  "100th Anniversary of Women at U of T"; UTA A1994/0012/05.

145  Kendrick and Slade, *Spirit of Life*, 41.

146  Ibid., 35–7.

147  Kendrick and Slade, *Spirit of Life*, 95; Women's College Hospital, "Who Was Dr. Jessie Gray"; http://www.womenscollegehospital.ca/about-us/our-history152/our-pioneers/who-was-dr.-jessie-gray179, accessed 25 Apr. 2010; "Dr. Jessie Gray, 1910–1978: First Lady of Surgery," *CMAJ* 120 (20 Jan. 1979): 209, 218.

148  Kendrick and Slade, *Spirit of Life*, 93.

149  Jessie Catherine Gray, *Torontonensis* (1934), 103.

150  WCH, "Who Was Dr. Jessie Gray."

151  *Dean's Report* 1938–9, 54.

152  "First Lady of Surgery," 209.

153  *Dean's Report* 1941–2, 30.

154  Kendrick and Slade, *Spirit of Life*, 39.

155  *Dean's Report* 1941–2, 31.

156  *Dean's Report* 1944–5, 37.

157  "100 Years of Women in Medicine," *American Journal of Public Health* 44 (1954): 1105.

158  WCH, "Who Was Dr. Jessie Gray."

159  Kendrick and Slade, *Spirit of Life*, 95.

160  *Dean's Report* 1959–60, 71.

161  Kendrick and Slade, *Spirit of Life*, 94, Sheinin and Bakes, *Women and Medicine*, 22.

162  Kendrick and Slade, *Spirit of Life*, 101.

163  *Dean's Report* 1957–8, 3–4.

164  Kendrick and Slade, *Spirit of Life*, 101.

165  Marion Hilliard is the subject of a biography, Marion O. Robinson, *Give My Heart: The Dr. Marion Hilliard Story* (Garden City, NY: Doubleday, 1964), and accounts of her life and career appear also in Kendrick and Slade, *Spirit of Life*, 97–8; Sheinin and Bakes, *Women and Medicine*, 40–3; and obituaries in *BMJ* 2 (6 Sept. 1958): 642, and *CMAJ* 79 (15 Aug. 1958): 295–6.

166  "Dr. Anna Marion Hilliard, An Appreciation," *CMAJ* 79 (154 Aug. 1958), 295.

167 UTA A1986-0027/19, 14 Oct. 1927.

168 Marion Hilliard, "Cervical Scrapings Test," *CMAJ* 62 (March 1950): 235–8, 235.

169 "100th Anniversary of Women at U of T," UTA A1994/0012/05.

170 Sheinin and Bakes, *Women and Medicine,* 41.

171 Kendrick and Slade, *Spirit of Life,* 39–40.

172 Robinson, *Give My Heart,* 244.

173 "News," *CMAJ* 60 (May 1949): 541.

174 "News," *CMAJ* 61 (July 1949): 90.

175 Kendrick and Slade, *Spirit of Life,* 40.

176 Sheinin and Bakes, *Women and Medicine,* 41.

177 "News," *CMAJ* 70 (April 1954): 488.

178 Maloney, *Women's College Hospital,* 6–7, 7.

179 Robinson, *Give My Heart,* 229. In addition, the fellowship examination in ob-gyn was so difficult that none of the applicants passed it the first year it was given, specifically because half of it involved medicine and surgery rather than the specialty itself.

180 Robinson, *Give My Heart,* 298.

181 Maloney, *Women's College Hospital,* 7.

182 Women's College Hospital Archives, *Agreement Made the 15th day of February, 1956, Between the Governors of the University of Toronto and Women's College Hospital* (Toronto: Cassels, Brock & Kelley, 1956), cover and p. 1.

183 *Dean's Report* 1955–6, 33.

184 Robinson, *Give My Heart,* 301.

185 Kendrick and Slade, *Spirit of Life,* 42.

186 Marion Hilliard, *A Woman Doctor Looks at Love and Life* (Garden City, NY: Doubleday, 1956), 16.

187 Kendrick and Slade, *Spirit of Life,* 39, 102; Sheinin and Bakes, *Women and Medicine,* 60–1; "Geraldine Maloney Was Head of Obstetrics at Women's College," *Toronto Star,* 24 Oct. 1985, A16.

188 WCH Archives, Report of the Medical Staff, 1961, 1.

189 "Geraldine Maloney," 24 Oct. 1985.

190 "The Fiftieth Anniversary: The Women's College Hospital, Toronto," *CMAJ* 84 (4 Feb. 1961): 289–90, 289.

191 UTA A1976-0054/16W; WCH study (1962), 64.

192 Ibid., 109.

193 WCH Archives, Department of Obstetrics and Gynaecology report, 1966, 10; *Dean's Report* 1967–8, 71.

194 WCH Archives, Department of Obstetrics and Gynaecology report, 1966, 10.

195 WCH Archives, Department of Obstetrics and Gynaecology report, 1967, 1.

196 Kendrick and Slade, *Spirit of Life,* 58, 87.

197 Goodwin interview, 10 Sept. 2009, 12.

198 James W. Goodwin, James T. Dunne, and Bruce W. Thomas, "Antepartum Identification of the Fetus at Risk," *CMAJ* 101 (18 Oct. 1969): 57–67, 57.

199  WCH Archives, Department of Obstetrics and Gynaecology report, 1970, 1.
200  Andrew T. Shennan, John E. Milligan, and Peter K. Leung, "Successful Management of Quadruplet Pregnancy in a Perinatal Unit," *CMAJ* 1979 (22 Sept. 1979): 741–5, 741.
201  Ibid., 743.
202  Jane Wilson, "Medical Science News: Surfactant Suspension Being Tested in Premature Babies," *CMAJ* 128 (1 June 1983): 1275.
203  Kendrick and Slade, *Spirit of Life*, 59.
204  Ibid.
205  Kendrick and Slade, *Spirit of Life*, 96; Sheinin and Bakes, *Women in Medicine*, 39–40.
206  Helen Farquharson interview, 21 July 2009, 9.
207  Kendrick and Slade, *Spirit of Life*, 63.
208  Robert D. Henderson, *The Esophagus: Reflux and Primary Motor Disorders* (Baltimore: Williams & Wilkins, 1980).
209  H. Lavina A. Lickley, "Robert A Henderson," 26 Sept. 1988; UTA A1995/0004/004.
210  Sheinin and Bakes, *Women and Medicine*, 94, "CFP Profiles," *Canadian Family Physician* 16 (May 1970): 18.
211  Maloney, *Women's College Hospital*, 9.
212  Kendrick and Slade, *Spirit of Life*, 50–1.
213  *FAXulty of Medicine*, 13 May 1996.
214  Department of Family and Community Medicine, Post-Graduate Medical Education, Teaching Practice Program; http://dfcm.med.utoronto.ca/postgrad/programs/prog_typhome.html, accessed 3 May 2010.
215  Kendrick and Slade, *Spirit of Life*, 99–100; Sheinin and Bakes, *Women and Medicine*, 88; Ashifa Kassan, "Doctor, Mother, Pioneer: A 'Truly Modern' Woman," *Toronto Star*, 16 July 2007, A12; Catharine Whiteside, "In Remembrance – Professor Ricky Schachter," *MedEmail* 16 (5 Sept. 2007): 2.
216  Jonathan Schachter, quoted in Kassan, "Doctor, Mother, Pioneer," 16 July 2007.
217  "Psoriasis Treatment Centre First of Its Kind," *Canadian Family Physician* 23 (October 1977): 53.
218  Kendrick and Slade, *Spirit of Life*, 55.
219  Sheinin and Bakes, *Women and Medicine*, 88.
220  TGH *Annual Report* 1982–3, 11.
221  Kendrick and Slade, *Spirit of Life*, 99.
222  Kassan, "Doctor, Mother, Pioneer," 16 July2007.
223  Catharine Whiteside, *MedEmail* obituary, 5 Sept. 2007, 2.
224  WCH study (1962), 32; UTA A1976-0054/16W.
225  "A Unique Institution," *CMAJ* 90 (21 Mar. 1964): 748.
226  Women's College Hospital, "Who was Dr. Henrietta Banting?"; http://www.womenscollegehospital.ca/about-us/our-history152/our-pioneers/who-was-dr.-henrietta-banting183, accessed 4 May 2010; Sheinin and Bakes, *Women and Medicine*, 4–5; "Lady Henrietta Banting: A Life of Service," *CMAJ* 116 (8 Jan. 1977): 85.
227  "Lady Henrietta Banting."

228  Kendrick and Slade, *Spirit of Life*, 89.

229  "Provincial News," *CMAJ* 59 (6 Aug. 1963): 2.

230  Kendrick and Slade, *Spirit of Life*, 55–6, 87, quote at 55.

231  "Star Quality: Dr. Lavina Lickley Is a Renowned Breast Surgeon with a Special Talent for Touching the Lives of Her Patients," *WCH Foundation, Heart and Soul* 5 (Spring 2009): 7.

232  Kendrick and Slade, *Spirit of Life*, 56.

233  "Star Quality."

234  Kendrick and Slade, *Spirit of Life*, 54.

235  "Sex Education Is 'Missionary Work': Physician," *Canadian Family Physician* 21 (Aug. 1975): 22.

236  Kendrick and Slade, *Spirit of Life*, 54.

237  Ibid., 56–7.

238  Ibid., 58.

239  Committee of Clinical Chairs, 17 Jan. 1989; UTA A1996/0007/03.

240  *FAXulty of Medicine*, 13 Nov. 1995.

241  Althea Blackburn-Evans, "Making Women's Health Matter," *EDGE: Research, Scholarship and Innovation at the University of Toronto* 4 (Spring 2003); http://www.research.utoronto.ca/edge/spring2003/leaders/maclean.html, accessed 4 May 2010.

## 23  Rehabilitation

1  Helen LeVesconte interview by Valerie Schatzker, 25 Nov. 1975; UTA B1976/0008/ interview transcript.

2  Heather Stonehouse with the History Project Committee, *Moving Together: Physical Therapy and the University of Toronto, 1917–2007* (Toronto : Dept. of Physical Therapy, Faculty of Medicine, University of Toronto, 2007). 1–6.

3  Ruby Heap, "Training Women for a New 'Women's Profession': Physiotherapy Education at the University of Toronto, 1917–40," *History of Education Quarterly* 35 (1995): 135–58, 140.

4  Kerr and Waugh, *Duncan Graham*, 82–3.

5  Stonehouse et al., *Moving Together*, 13.

6  Faculty Council, 1 Mar. 1920, 171; UTA A1986/0027/018.

7  Stonehouse et al., *Moving Together*, 15.

8  Heap, "Training Women," 145–7.

9  *Dean's Report* 1926–7, 12.

10  Stonehouse et al., *Moving Together*, 17.

11  Ibid., 24.

12  UTA A1979/0010/001.

13  Heap, "Training Women," 149.

14  *President's Report* 1933–4, 8.

15  *Dean's Report* 1937–8, 9–11.

16  *Dean's Report* 1938–9, 59.

17  Stonehouse et al., *Moving Together*, 37.
18  See E.H. Botterell, A.T. Jousse, Carl Aberhart, and J.W. Cluff, "Paraplegia Follow-ing War," *CMAJ* 55 (1946): 249–59.
19  Charles Godfrey, personal communication, 29 Oct. 2010.
20  Botterell et al., "Paraplegia Following War."
21  *President's Report* 1934–5, 32, 44.
22  Charles Godfrey makes this point in a personal communication, 29 Oct. 2010.
23  Helen LeVesconte interview by Valerie Schatzker, 25 Nov. 1975; UTA B1976/0008/ interview transcript.
24  Judy Friedland, Occupational Science and Occupational Therapy: Department His-tory; www.ot.utoronto.ca/about/history.asp.
25  Report of the Faculty of Medicine Task Force on Physical Therapy and Occupa-tional Therapy, 20 June 1991, 5; UTA A1996/0011/18 (3).
26  "Relieves Tedium Always Attending Upon Long Illness," *Globe*, 22 Jan. 1924.
27  Heap, "Training Women," 147.
28  Crawford to Steiner, 23 Apr. 1974; UTA A1979/0010/001.
29  Faculty Council, 5 Oct. 1929, 222; UTA A1986/0027/020.
30  TGH *Annual Report* 1923, 12.
31  *Tablet*, Fall 1987, 18.
32  Judith Friedland, personal communication, 2 Sept. 2010.
33  *Dean's Report* 1934–5, 37.
34  Mentioned in Faculty Council meeting of 1 Apr. 1949; UTA A1986/0027/025 (01).
35  Ibid.
36  *Dean's Report* 1949–50, 4.
37  *Dean's Report* 1950–1, 7, 56.
38  Stonehouse et al., *Moving Together*, 59–60.
39  LRPAC Minutes, 26 Feb. 1975; UTA A1979/0010/006.
40  LeVesconte interview by Schatzker, 25 Nov. 1975; UTA B1976/0008.
41  *Dean's Report* 1952–3, 57–8.
42  *Dean's Report* 1953–4, 56.
43  *Dean's Report* 1956–7, 63.
44  *Dean's Report* 1958–9, 67.
45  Faculty Council 3 Apr. 1959, 77; UTA A1986/0027/027.
46  *President's Report* 1959–60, 41.
47  Stonehouse et al., *Moving Together*, 64–5.
48  *Dean's Report* 1960–1, 38.
49  *Dean's Report* 1962–3, 5.
50  Terence Kavanagh, Donald J. Mertens, Larry F. Hamm, Joseph Beyene, Johanna Kennedy, Paul Corey, and Roy J. Shephard, "Prediction of Long-Term Progno-sis in 12 169 Men Referred for Cardiac Rehabilitation," *Circulation* 106 (2002), 666–71.
51  Stonehouse et al., *Moving Together*, 67.
52  See Faculty Council meeting of 28 Jan. 1966; UTA A1986/0028/008(003).

53 *Dean's Report* 1966–7, 8–10.
54 Phyllis Carlton, "An Approach to Clinical Studies," *Journal of the Canadian Physiotherapy Association* 15 (1963): 208–11.
55 Independent Planning Committee *Report* (1969), 139.
56 Charles Godfrey, personal communication, 29 Oct. 2010.
57 *Dean's Report* 1970–1, 4, 13.
58 LRPAC Minutes, 26 Feb. 1975; UTA A1979/0010/006.
59 Stonehouse et al., *Moving Together*, 78–79.
60 J.W. Steiner to R.B. Holmes, 5 Nov. 1973; UTA A1979/0010/001.
61 R.C.A. Hunter to J.W. Steiner, 15 Nov. 1973; UTA A1979/0010/001.
62 LRPAC Minutes, 1 May 1974; UTA A1979/0010/006.
63 Harris, "Progress Report" of LRPAC, 2 June 1975; UTA A1979/0010/005.
64 Holmes et al. to Miller at MOH, 10 Dec. 1974; UTA A1979/0010/001/5.23.2.
65 LRPAC meeting of 26 Feb. 1975; UTA A1979/0010/006.
66 Self-Study, Feb. 1983, 103–4; UTA F016/030/031.
67 Stonehouse et al., *Moving Together*, 83.
68 Task Force Report, 20 June 1991, 6.
69 Morris Milner to John H. Dirks, 2 Nov. 1987; UTA A1994/0012/01.
70 "Transdisciplinary Research to Help the Underdog," *Surgical Spotlight* Winter 2003–4, 6–7, 7.
71 "The New Face of Rehabilitation Research in Toronto," *Surgical Spotlight*, Winter 2009., 12–13, 12.
72 Document for Accreditation Review, Nov. 1990;UTA A1996/0011/18 (3).
73 Stonehouse et al., *Moving Together*, 90.
74 Meeting of the Faculty Education Committee, 25 Sept. 1987; UTA A1995/0004/005.
75 Faculty Council, 24 Oct. 1988; UTA A1996/0007/03.
76 Document for Accreditation Review, Nov. 1990; UTA A1996/0011/18 (3).
77 See "Faculty Discussion in Response to the Report of the Review Committee for the Division of Physical Therapy," [1986]; UTA A1994/0012/01.
78 D.H. Cowan to Dean J. Dirks memo, 9 Aug. 1990; UTA A1996/0011/18 (3).
79 External Review, 1981; Dean's Archive.
80 Frederick H. Lowy to Paul E. Garfinkel, 27 Nov. 1986; see also the memo of Joseph Marotta to F.H. Lowy, 26 June 1986; UTA A1994/0012/01.
81 Committee of Clinical Chairs, 21 Mar. 1989; UTA A1996/0007/03.
82 A.G. Trimble to M. Milner, 27 June 1985, Internal Control Report. Subject: Department of Rehabilitation Medicine; UTA A1994/0012/07.
83 Faculty of Medicine News, May 1992, 12; Dean's Archive
84 Task Force Report, 20 June 1991, 8; UTA A1996/0011/18 (3).
85 Dirks to Joan Foley, 16 July 1990; UTA A1996/0011/18 (4).
86 See John Dirks to Josephine M. Cassie, 18 Apr. 1990; see also Dirks's memo to file of 20 Sept. 1990, on Laszlo Endrenyi's recommendation to seek "another department or departments as an umbrella organization"; UTA A1996/0011/18 (3).
87 Judith Friedland, personal communication, 2 Sept. 2010.

88  As there was no graduate department for occupational therapy (or physical ther-
    apy), those wishing advanced degrees were required to enroll in programs where
    they could pursue their rehabilitation research interests; for example, at OISE, in
    the Department of Psychology, or at the Institute of Medical Sciences.
89  The External Review Report commented, "The Department has increased the qual-
    ifications of its faculty significantly over the past five years." See also the Accredi-
    tation Report for 1997.
90  Report of Research Activity, 1996–8; Dean's Archive.
91  Denise Reid was promoted to full professor in 2000, followed by Friedland in 2002,
    Renwick in 2005, and Colantonio in 2010. Polatajko was appointed at the full pro-
    fessor level when she became chair in 1999.
92  Angela Colantonio et al., "Women's Health Outcomes after Traumatic Brain In-
    jury," *Journal of Women's Health* (Larchmont) 19 (2010): 1109–16.
93  A similar motion was approved by the Faculty Assembly on 23 December 1992.
94  Personal communication from Judith Friedland, 7 Feb. 2013.
95  With some 350 programs in the world, this ranking placed the U of T program
    among the top 3–4 percent.
96  "External Review; Department of Occupational Therapy," 2004; Dean's Archive.
97  Stonehouse et al., *Moving Together*, 91.
98  External Review, 1999; Dean's Archive.
99  *FAXulty of Medicine*, 17 Jan. 1994.
100 Faculty of Medicine, *Plan 2001–4*.
101 For more on plans for the rehab departments see Faculty of Medicine, *Plan 2000–4*,
    31–34.
102 *FAXulty of Medicine*, 4 Nov. 1996.
103 *FAXulty of Medicine*, 9 June 1997; it included as well the facility at 130 Dunn
    Avenue.
104 *MedEmail*, 18 Jan. 1999.
105 *MedEmail*, 2 Oct. 2000.
106 *President's Report* 1954–5, 74.
107 *President's Report* 1957–8, 43.
108 *Dean's Report* 1958–9, 3, 68.
109 *Dean's Report* 1960–1, 10.
110 TTH *Annual Report* 1988–9, 190.
111 John S. Crawford to Members of Department of Rehab Med, 26 Sept. 1973; UTA
    A1979/0010/001.
112 John S. Crawford to R.C.A. Hunter, Associate Dean, Clinical Affairs, 31 Oct. 1974;
    UTA A1979/0010/001/5.23.1
113 University of Toronto, Department of Speech-Language Pathology, *Communicat-
    ing Excellence Celebrating 50 years of Educating Leaders in Speech-Language Pathology,
    1958–2008* (Toronto: Pristine Printing, 2008).
114 Faculty Council, 30 May 1983; UTA A1993/0025/009 (14).
115 Faculty Council, 26 Sept. 1983; UTA A1993/0025/009 (16).

116 Dean's New Year Newsletter, Jan. 1990, 4; UTA A1996/0007/002.

117 Lowy to Rae-Grant, 19 Feb. 1985, see attachment 3; UTA A1994/0012/008.

118 *Plan 2000–4*, 123.

119 Jean Ward-Walker, personal communication, 29 Apr. 2010.

## 24 Family and Community

1 Eliot Phillipson, "Chair's Column," *MediNews*, Mar. 2004, 2.

2 Gallie, "Fifty Years' Growth," 8.

3 J.B. Leitch, "A History of the Department of Family and Community Medicine of the Faculty of Medicine at the University of Toronto up to July, 1972," 2; UTA A1983/0036/11 (16); attached to cover letter J.W. Steiner to F. Fallis, 14 Nov. 1973, 1; UTA A1983/0036/11 (16).

4 *Torontonensis* (1923), 125.

5 K.F. Clute, *The General Practitioner: A Study of Medical Education and Practice in Ontario and Nova Scotia* (Toronto: University of Toronto Press, 1963), 455.

6 Ibid., 448.

7 *Dean's Report* 1950–1, 4.

8 Leitch, "History of the DFCM," 5.

9 Cosbie, *Toronto General Hospital*, 278; text not clear about second year.

10 Macdonald in *Dean's Report* 1968–9, 10–11.

11 *Dean's Report* 1948–9, 4.

12 *Dean's Report* 1968–9, 11.

13 Leitch, "History of the DFCM," 6–7.

14 Wightman, *Dean's Report* 1966–7, 43–4.

15 Committee on Curriculum and Examinations, 11 Feb. 1969; UTA A1993/0025/007.

16 Committee on Curriculum and Examinations, 25 Mar. 1969; UTA A1993/0025/007.

17 Independent Planning Committee *Report*(1969,) 72.

18 Senior Co-ordinating Committee, 25 Sept. 1969; UTA A1993/0025/05.

19 Senior Co-ordinating Committee, MOH, 21 Oct. 1971: "Proposed Role Study for the Toronto Health Sciences Complex"; AO RG 10-6-0-1916, #183.

20 Leitch, "History of the DFCM," 1.

21 Ibid., 10–23.

22 *Dean's Report* 1968–9, 4.

23 Ruth Wilson and Larry Green, "External Review: Department of Family and Community Medicine," 2000; Dean's Archive.

24 Leitch, "History of the DFCM," 23.

25 *Dean's Report* 1966–7, 54–5.

26 *Dean's Report* 1970–1, 63.

27 UTA A1986/0028/004/008.

28 The College of Family Physicians of Canada, Report of the Onsite Survey Team, University of Toronto, March 1975; UTA A1985/0026/004 (06).

29 Harris, "Progress Report" of LRPAC, on DFCM, 2 June 1975; UTA A1979/0010/005.

30  LRPAC Minutes, 25 Feb. 1976; UTA A1979/010/005.

31  Memo, Harris to LRPAC, 12 Apr. 1976; UTA A1979/010/005.

32  DFCM Minutes, 16 Feb. 1977; UTA A1993/025/038.

33  "Comments on the LCME Survey Report," 9 Mar. 1978; UTA A1985/026/004 (010).

34  Fred B. Fallis to R.B. Holmes, 14 Mar. 1980; UTA A1985/026/004 (05).

35  Ibid.

36  S.T. Bain and W.B. Spaulding, "The Importance of Coding Presenting Symptoms," *CMAJ* 97 (14 Oct. 1967): 953–9.

37  Fred Fallis, Memo re "External Review Committee," 1 May 1980; Dean's Archive.

38  Executive Committee Meeting, 15 Apr. 1980; UTA A1985/026/004/02.

39  DFCM Triennial Report, 2002–5, 105.

40  Wilson and Green, "External Review."

41  David Naylor, "DFCM External Review: Dean's Response," 2000; Dean's Archive.

42  Warren J. McIsaac, Esme Fuller-Thomson, and Yves Talbot, "Does Having Regular Care by a Family Physician Improve Preventive Care?" *Canadian Family Physician* 47 (2001): 70–6.

43  Plan 2000–2004, 105.

44  Ibid.

45  Self-Study, Feb. 1983, 62; UTA F016/030/031.

46  Faculty Council, 27 Apr. 1981; UTA A1993/025/09.

47  Arnold Aberman, "Interview," *Journal of Investigative Medicine* 43 (1995): 412–18, 414.

48  *Tablet,* Spring 1990, 5.

49  Wilson and Green, "External Review."

50  "Advisory Committee on MSc and PhD Studies in Community Health," 22 Dec. 1978; attached to Arthur L. Gladstone et al. to J.E.F. Hastings, October, (no date) [1979]; UTA A1985/0026/01 (10).

51  Defries, *First Forty Years*; Bator and Rhodes, *Within Reach*, vol. 1.

52  Agenda for a meeting of search committee for chair, 19 June 1975; UTA A1979/0010/003 (15.35.9).

53  Minutes of Search Committee, 28 Oct. 1975; UTA A1979/0010/003 (15.35.9).

54  UTA A1979/0010/003 (15.35.9).

55  Bator, *Within Reach*, 2:153.

56  Department of Health Administration *Annual Report* 1985–6; Bator, *Within Reach*, 2:155.

57  Department of Health Administration Newsbytes, May 2001; *MedEmail*, 8 Sept. 1998.

58  Department of Health Administration Review 1998, 2; Mary E. Stefl and Lawrence J. Nestman, "University of Toronto, Department of Health Administration: Five Year Review," Jan 1998; Office of the Dean, 1; Vivek Goel interview with Heather L. Dichter, 28 July 2010.

59  Department of Health Administration Newsbytes, Dec. 2000, May 2001; Department of Health Policy, Management and Evaluation Newsbytes, Sept.–Oct. 2002.

60  Mary Jane Ashley CV; interview with Heather L. Dichter, 22 July 2010; and Faculty Council minutes, 22 Feb. 1982.

61  Clinical chairs, 10 June 1975; UTA A1993/0025/006.

62  Advisory Committee for the Epidemiology Unit; UTA A1993/0025/5.

63  Ashley interview and CV, 22 July 2010.

64  Self-Study; Faculty of Medicine 1 Feb. 1983, 62; UTA F016/030/031.3; *Tablet*, Summer 1985, 10.

65  *MediNews*, Nov. 2000, 9.

66  Ashley interview, 22 July 2010.

67  *Tablet*, Fall 1990, 4; *FAXulty of Medicine*, 12 Dec. 1994.

68  *FAXulty of Medicine*, 8 Apr. 1996.

69  Miller, Howe, and Wall, "National Study of Breast Cancer Screening," 227–58.

70  D.A. Boyes, B. Morrison, E.G. Knox, G.J. Draper, and A.B. Miller, "A Cohort Study of Cervical Cancer Screening in British Columbia," *Clinical and Investigative Medicine* 5 (1982): 1–29.

71  Martin T. Schechter, Anthony B. Miller et al., "Cigarette Smoking and Breast Cancer: Case-Control Studies of Prevalent and Incident Cancer in the Canadian National Breast Screening Study," *American Journal of Epidemiology* 130 (1989): 213–20.

72  Anthony B. Miller et al., "Report of a National Workshop on Screening for Cancer of the Cervix," *CMAJ* 145 (15 Nov. 1991): 1301–25, 1317.

73  *Dean's Report* 1966–7, 4.

74  Self-Study, Jan. 1990, 125; UTA A1996/0011/0018 (6).

75  Committee on Curriculum and Examinations, 28 Jan. 1969, 230, UTA A1993/0025/007; *Dean's Report* 1967–8, 5.

76  *Dean's Report* 1969–70, 46–52.

77  Committee on Curriculum and Examinations, 24 Mar. 1970, UTA A1993/0025/007.

78  Ibid., 8 Dec. 1970, UTA A1993/0025/007.

79  *Dean's Report* 1970–1, 3, 47–51.

80  LRPAC Minutes, 27 Feb. 1974; UTA A1979/0010/006.

81  Harris to file, 1 Mar. 1974; "Confidential," LRPAC; UTA A1979/0010/005.

82  Harris, "Progress Report," 2 June 1975, 2; Draft report to LCME Steering Committee ca. 1975–6; UTA A1979/0010/005.

83  Self-Study, Feb. 1983, 43–7.

84  *Medisphere*, Sept. 1977, 2.

85  Ruth Cooperstock, "Psychotropic Drug Use among Women," *CMAJ* 23 (1976): 760–3, 760.

86  See, for example, Cooperstock, "Psychotropic Drug Use among Women." For her eulogy see E. Vayda, "Ruth Cooperstock," Faculty Council, 25 Feb. 1985; UTA A1993/0025/09.

87  American Psychiatric Association, *Biographical Directory* 1989 (Washington, DC: APA, 1989), 1276.

88  Ibid. 1988–91.

89 Report of the Advisory Committee on Community Health 1979, 23–4; UTA A1985/0026/001.
90 LRPAC Minutes, 29 Oct. 1975; UTA A1979/0010/005.
91 Bator, *Within Reach*, 2:151.
92 Report of the Advisory Committee on Community Health 1979, 24; UTA A1985/0026/001.
93 Bator, *Within Reach*, 2:152.
94 Ibid., 153–4.
95 Dirks to A.R. Ten Cate, 23 Feb. 1990; UTA A1996/0011/0018 (4).
96 Faculty of Medicine, *Plan 2000*–4; 68–9; *MedEmail*, 25 May 1998.
97 *MedEmail*, 1 Feb. 1999.
98 Vivek Goel CV, May 2010, and interview with Heather L. Dichter, 28 July 2010.
99 Naylor communication to Edward Shorter, 7 Jan. 2013.
100 Department of Health Administration Newsbytes, Oct. 2000–March 2001, June 2001.

## 25 Hospitals

1 "Strategic Directions for the Faculty of Medicine," Nov. 1993; Dean's Archive.
2 "IPC States Combined Needs for Teaching, Research," *Synapse*, 11 Dec. 1969, 2.
3 A rapid apercu is given in TGH *Annual Report* 1890–1, 47–8.
4 Michael Bliss, *A Canadian Millionaire: The Life and Business Times of Sir Joseph Flavelle* (Toronto: Macmillan, 1978), 207.
5 Friedland, *University of Toronto: A History*, 239, 243.
6 Faculty of Medicine *Calendar*, 1889–90, 37–9.
7 TGH *Annual Report* 1890–1, 37.
8 J.N.E. Brown, Report of the Toronto General Hospital for the Year ending 30 Sept. 1905, 24; UHN Archives, Toronto General Hospital Fonds, sub-series 1.2: Annual reports, box 2, file 1.2.8.
9 TGH *Annual Report* 1891, 37–8.
10 Connor, *Doing Good*, 181.
11 TGH *Annual Report* 1905–6, 69.
12 Connor, *Doing Good*, 177–80.
13 Mark Irish to H.J. Cody, 30 Jan. 1936; a copy of Irish's talk is enclosed; UTA A1983/0036/11 (7).
14 *President's Report* 1912–13, 11–12.
15 TGH *Annual Report* 1913, 15.
16 *Dean's Report* 1929–30, 6.
17 Peter V. Clarke, *Synapse*, 15 Apr. 1970, 1.
18 Science Policy Committee, meeting of 28 Sept. 1976; UTA A1993/0025/008.
19 Kenneth Shumak presentation, Science Policy Committee, minutes, 17 Jan. 1977; UTA A1993/0025/008.
20 Science Policy Committee, 19 Oct. 1978; UTA A1993/0025/008.

21  D. Layne presentation, Meeting of the Committee of Basic Science chairs, 7 Dec. 1984; UTA A1993/0025/1.
22  TGH *Annual Report* 1985–6, 26.
23  Connor, *Doing Good*, 235–6.
24  Clinical chairs, 27 Nov. 1985; UTA A1993/0025/001.
25  Clinical chairs, 18 Dec. 1985; UTA A1993/0025/001.
26  External Review, Department of Ophthalmology 1987; Dean's Archive.
27  *MedEmail*, 12 Apr. 1999.
28  David Naylor personal communication, 7 Jan. 2013.
29  UHN *Annual Report* 2008, 20.
30  G.E. Connell, E.A. McCulloch, and L. Siminovitch, [untitled report to Science Policy Subcommittee], 20 Apr. 1973; UTA B79/0051/06.
31  Feasby, "Short History of the University of Toronto," 14–17, 17.
32  *President's Report* 1912–13, 12.
33  Ibid., 17.
34  *Dean's Report* 1936–7, 10.
35  Kellogg Questionnaire, 13 Dec. 1945; UTA A1986/0028/011.
36  Ibid.
37  *Dean's Report* 1946–7, 5.
38  *Dean's Report* 1958–9, 6.
39  *Dean's Report* 1949–50, 21.
40  *Dean's Report* 1961–2, 5.
41  *Dean's Report* 1970–1, 75.
42  *FAXulty of Medicine*, 22 Jan. 1996.
43  *Dean's Report* 1952–3, 49.
44  *Dean's Report* 1967–8, 123.
45  *Dean's Report* 1968–9, 146.
46  *Dean's Report* 1970–1, 151.
47  M.S. Ross and H. Moldofsky, "A Comparison of Pimozide and Haloperidol in the Treatment of Gilles de la Tourette's Syndrome," *American Journal of Psychiatry* 135 (1978): 585–7.
48  Harvey Moldofsky and Gregory M. Brown, "Tics and Serum Prolactin Response to Pimozide in Tourette Syndrome," in *Gilles de la Tourette Syndrome*, ed. Arnold J. Friedhoff and Thomas N. Chase (New York: Raven, 1982), 387–90.
49  *President's Report* 1924–5, 15.
50  *Dean's Report* 1935–6, 3, 40.
51  *Dean's Report* 1939–40, 56–7.
52  Dept of Surgery, *Annual Report* 1989–90, 129.
53  Ross Fleming, "William Strathern Keith" (ms), 2. I am grateful to Dr. Fleming for sharing this document.
54  *Dean's Report* 1948–9, 43.
55  Brian Holmes, "Dr. Louis Ralph Harnick," 30 May 1988; UTA A1996/0007/001 (05).

56 Leslie Scrivener, "Sisters of St. Joseph Moving Out Under Hospital Restructuring," *Toronto Star*, 28 June 1998, A2.

57 Faculty of Medicine *Calendar*, 1894–5, 133.

58 On his application for "associate professor of medicine," see Faculty Council, 16 Apr. 1900, 366; UTA A1986/0027.016.

59 McDonald, *For the Least of My Brethren*, 36–7; "Robert Joseph Dwyer," Faculty Council, 9 Apr. 1920, 258–9; UTA A1986/0027/018.

60 Faculty of Medicine *Calendar* 1904–5, 81–2.

61 *President's Report* 1908–9, 14.

62 *Dean's Report* 1927–8, 18.

63 Kellogg Questionnaire, 13 Dec. 1945; UTA A1986/0028/011.

64 *Dean's Report* 1953–4, 24.

65 *Dean's Report* 1946–7, 5.

66 Petch committee (1974), unpaginated section on SMH.

67 J.A. Little presentation to the Science Policy Committee, Minutes, 20 Jan. 1977; UTA A1993/0025/008.

68 *MedEmail*, 18 Sept. 2000.

69 Hyland to Dean's Office, 18 Dec. 2003; attached to Goldman, "External Review," 30 Sept. 2003; Dean's Archive.

70 *Dean's Report* 1939–40, 56–7.

71 Donald J. Currie to E. Bruce Tovee, 9 Jan. 1969; UTA A1989/0030/002.

72 W.J. Horsey to W.R. Drucker, 17 Jan. 1969; UTA A1989/0030/002.

73 S.B. Rizoli, A. Kapus, J. Fan, Y.H. Li, J.C. Marshall, and O.D. Rotstein, "Immunomodulatory Effects of Hypertonic Resuscitation on the Development of Lung Inflammation Following Hemorrhagic Shock," *Journal of Immunology* 161 (1998): 6288–96.

74 Richard Reznick, "Ori's Move to St. Mike's," *Surgical Spotlight*, Fall 2008, 1 of 2.

75 Rotstein interview, 9 Apr. 2009.

76 David Naylor personal communication, 7 Jan. 2013.

77 Goldman and Bélanger, *Heart Surgery in Canada*, 132–3.

78 Susan E. Mackinnon and Alan R. Hudson, "Clinical Application of Peripheral Nerve Transplantation," *Plastic and Reconstructive Surgery* 90 (1992): 695–9.

79 McKneally interview, 2 Feb. 2009.

80 On Hudson's career, see McDonald, *For the Least of My Brethren*, 217, 239–40, 266, 300.

81 On Colapinto, see McDonald, *For the Least of My Brethren*, 215. R.W. McCallum and V. Colapinto, *Urological Radiology of the Adult Male Lower Urinary Tract* (Springfield, IL: C.C. Thomas, 1975).

82 N.W. Struthers, "Dr. Vincent Colapinto," Faculty Council, 27 May 1985; UTA A1993/0025/09.

83 W.J. Hannah, eulogy "Ewan Stuart Macdonald," Faculty Council, 4 Oct. 1982; UTA A1993/0025/009.

84 James P. Waddell to T.D.R. Briant, 11 Oct. 1984; attached to Oncology Task Force Minutes, 25 Oct. 1984; A1994/0012/010.

85  Michael Shea, "Cryosurgery of Vitreous and Retina," *International Ophthalmology Clinics* 7 (Spring 1967): 3–18.

86  D.J. Jenkins et al., "Glycemic Index of Foods: A Physiological Basis for Carbohydrate Exchange," *American Journal of Clinical Nutrition* 34 (1981): 362–6.

87  *U of Toronto Medicine Magazine*, Dec. 2005, 7.

88  David J.A. Jenkins, Cyril W.C. Kendall, Gail McKeown-Eyssen et al., "Effect of a Low-Glycemic Index or a High-Cereal Fiber Diet on Type 2 Diabetes: A Randomized Trial," *JAMA* 300 (17 Dec. 2008): 2742–53.

89  *MedEmail*, 6 June 2005.

90  *FAXulty of Medicine*, 13 Oct. 1997.

91  *MedEmail*, 27 Apr. 1998.

92  Rotstein interview, 9 Apr. 2009.

93  S.V. Lichtenstein, T.A. Salerno, and A.S. Slutsky, "Warm Continuous Cardioplegia Versus Intermittent Hypothermic Protection during Cardiopulmonary Bypass," *Journal of Cardiothoracic Anesthesia* 4 (1990): 279–81.

94  Slutsky interview, 7 Apr. 2009.

95  *Dean's Report* 1946–7, 5.

96  *President's Report* 1946–7, 31. Charles Godfrey, personal communication, 6 Dec. 2010.

97  *Dean's Report* 1948–9, 40.

98  *Dean's Report* 1967–8, 123.

99  *Dean's Report* 1948–9, 43.

100  *Dean's Report* 1951–2, 24–5.

101  Sunnybrook Health Sciences Centre, *Sunnybrook Magazine,: 60 Years of Transforming Healthcare* (2008), 42; available at http://sunnybrook.ca/uploads/Mag08.pdf.

102  *Dean's Report* 1966–7, 70.

103  William B. Spaulding, *Revitalizing Medical Education: McMaster Medical School, The Early Years, 1965–1974* (Philadelphia: Decker, 1991), 22.

104  Dean Chute, at Sunnybrook Review Committee, 4 Dec. 1968; UTA A1993/0025/007/06.

105  Friedland, *University of Toronto: A History*, 510.

106  Naylor communication to Edward Shorter, 7 Jan. 2013.

107  Faculty Council, 11 Dec. 1968, 97, 99; UTA A1993/0025/07.

108  Science Policy Sub-Committee, Minutes, 30 Jan. 1973; UTA A1993/0025/008.

109  Committee Clinical Chairs, 21 Feb. 1989, 3.

110  U of T Press Release, 2005, on the occasion of Henkelman's appointment as a university professor.

111  Michael Julius, vice president of research, Sunnybrook Research Institute, interview with Jonathan Ruelens, 20 Sept. 2010.

112  U of T Press Release, 2005.

113  Untitled confidential report to the Science Policy Subcommittee re visit to Sunnybrook on 22 Jan. 1973; UTA B79/0051/04.

114 *Dean's Report* 1950–1, 36; Susan Bélanger, "Continuing the Banting Legacy," 12. Charles Godfrey, in a personal communication of 6 Dec. 2010, observes that it was actually Almon Fletcher who created the unit in his work with arthritic patients.

115 Hill, "History of the Department of Medicine," 50.

116 S.B. Goodman and J. Schatzker, "Internal Fixation of Femoral Neck Fractures: A Prospective Study," *Canadian Journal of Surgery* 29 (1986): 351–6.

117 George F. Pennal, Marvin Tile, James P. Waddell, and Henry Garside, "Pelvic Disruption: Assessment and Classification," *Clinical Orthopaedics and Related Research* 151 (1980): 12–21.

118 Dept of Surgery, *Annual Report* 1986–7, 2.

119 Mariana Capurro, Ian R. Wanless, Morris Sherman, Gerrit Deboer, Wen Shi, Eiji Miyoshi, and Jorge Filmus, "Glypican-3: A Novel Serum and Histochemical Marker for Hepatocellular Carcinoma," *Gastroenterology* 125 (2003): 89–97.

120 G. Klement, S. Baruchel, J. Rak, S. Man, K. Clark, D.J. Hicklin, P. Bohlenamd, and R.S. Kerbel, "Continuous Low-dose Therapy with Vinblastine and VEGF Receptor-2 Antibody Induces Sustained Tumor Regression without Overt Toxicity," *Journal of Clinical Investigation* 105 (2000): R15–24 (erratum in 116 (2006): 3084).

121 Yuval Shaked, Francesco Bertolini, Shan Man et al., "Genetic Heterogeneity of the Vasculogenic Phenotype Parallels Angiogenesis," *Cancer Cell* 7 (2005): 101–11; "In Sickness and Health: SRI Scientists Lift up the Veil on the Enigma of Angiogenesis," Sunnybrook Research Institute, Research Report 2004–5, 10–11.

122 Peter N. Burns, Stephanie R. Wilson, and David Hope Simpson, "Pulse Inversion Imaging of Liver Blood Flow: Improved Method for Characterizing Focal Masses with Microbubble Contrast," *Investigative Radiology* 35 (2000): 58–71.

123 Julius interview with Ruelens, 20 Sept. 2010.

124 Etta D. Pisano, E. B. Cole, S. Major et al., "Radiologists' Preferences for Digital Mammographic Display," *Radiology* 216 (2000): 820–30, 838.

125 Etta D. Pisano, Constantine Gatsonis, Edward Hendrick et al., "Diagnostic Performance of Digital versus Film Mammography for Breast-Cancer Screening," *New England Journal of Medicine* 353 (27 Oct. 2005): 1773–83.

126 Roberta A. Jong et al., "Contrast-Enhanced Digital Mammography: Initial Clinical Experience," *Radiology* 228 (2003): 842–50; Sunnybrook Research Institute, Breakthroughs; http://sunnybrook.ca/research/content/?page=sri_ab_firsts.

127 Goldman and Bélanger, *Heart Surgery in Canada*, 137.

128 W.G. Bigelow to W.R. Drucker, 16 Mar. 1971; UTA A1989/0030/002.

129 William R. Drucker to A.R. Chute, 25 Sept. 1971; UTA A1989/0030/002.

130 Ramsay Gunton, "External Review of Cardiology at the University of Toronto," Sept. 1979, attached to John E. Morch memo, 2 Nov. 1979; UTA A1985/0026/004/016.

131 Cardiovascular Surgery Task Force, 7 July 1982; UTA A1995/0004/002.

132 Ibid., 12 Aug. 1982; UTA A1995/0004/0092.

133 Joan Hollobon, "Open-heart Cases Imperiled by Need for Wider Service," *Globe and Mail*, 14 Jan. 1983, 1.

134 Goldman and Bélanger, *Heart Surgery in Canada*, 138.

135 Goldman interview, 4 Feb. 2009.

136  *Surgical Spotlight*, Winter 2005, 11.
137  Goldman interview, 4 Feb. 2009.
138  Ibid.
139  Warm Heart Investigators, "Randomised Trial of Normothermic Versus Hypothermic," 563; *Surgical Spotlight*, Winter 2005, 11.
140  Nimesh D. Desai, Eric A. Cohen, C. David Naylor, and Stephen Fremes, "A Randomized Comparison of Radial-artery and Saphenous-vein Coronary Bypass Grafts," *New England Journal of Medicine* 351 (25 Nov. 2004): 2302–9.
141  See, for example, Karen Tu, Muhammad M. Mamdani, and Jack V. Tu, "Hypertension Guidelines in Elderly Patients: Is Anybody Listening?" *American Journal of Medicine* 113 (2002): 52–8.

## 26  New Ideas

1  Brian Hodges, "Stepping Up at the Wilson Centre, Strategic Plan: 2004–2010," in Wilson Centre: Five Year External Review, 2008; Dean's Archive.
2  *Dean's Report* 1966–7, 4.
3  *Dean's Report* 1967–8, 18–19.
4  *Dean's Report* 1969–70, 16.
5  *Dean's Report* 1970–1, 17–20.
6  External reviewer #2, External Review, Centre for Studies in Medical Education, 1984; Dean's Archive.
7  LRPAC Minutes, 17 Dec. 1975; UTA A1979/0010/005.
8  LRPAC, Byrne presentation attached to agenda of 23 Apr. 1976; UTA A1979/0010/005.
9  External reviewer #1, External Review, Centre for Studies in Medical Education, 1984; Dean's Archive.
10  E.M. Sellers to F.H. Lowy, 14 Apr. 1987; UTA A1994/0012/003.
11  Richard Reznick, *Surgical Spotlight*, Summer 2004, 3.
12  *FAXulty of Medicine*, 20 Mar. 1995.
13  External Review, Wilson Centre 2008; Dean's Archive.
14  Faculty Council, 27 Oct. 1980; UTA A1993/0028/009.
15  Charles Hollenberg, "Dr. Edward Alexander Sellers" (obituary), 25 Nov. 1985, Appendix II; UTA A1995/0004/004.
16  Meeting in Dean's Office, 10 Jan. 1979; UTA A1993/0025/005.
17  E.A. Sellers to Dean Fred Lowy, 23 Apr. 1980; UTA A1985/0026/001 (28).
18  "External Review of the Banting and Best Diabetes Centre, University of Toronto," 1 May 1997; Dean's Archive.
19  Schimmer interview with Bélanger, 7 May 2009.
20  See Charles H. Hollenberg to Jim Till, 12 Dec. 1985; attached is "S.G.S. Feasibility Committee on a Graduate Program in Bioethics: Report to the Dean," Dec. 1985; UTA B2005/0031/011 (17).
21  TGH *Annual Report* 1986–7, 353.
22  *Tablet*, Winter 1990, 3.

23  Jim Till to A. Aberman, 6 Apr. 1995; UTA B2005/0031/011(03).

24  *Plan 2000–4*, 78.

25  *MedEmail*, 28 June 2006.

26  LRPAC Minutes, 4 Dec. 1974; UTA A1979/0010/006.

27  *Dean's Report* 1925–6, 20–1.

28  Dean's Report 1929–30, 30.

29  *Dean's Report*1944–5, 10, 15.

30  *Dean's Report* 1945–6, 16.

31  *Dean's Report*1961–2, 5.

32  *Dean's Report* 1967–8, 33–4.

33  *Dean's Report* 1969–70, 33–5.

34  LRPAC Minutes, 4 Dec. 1974; UTA A1979/0010/006.

35  Ibid.

36  LRPAC "Rough Notes," 26 Mar. 1975; UTA A1979/0010/006.

37  Faculty Council, 16 June 1975.

38  Faculty Council, 17 Nov. 1975.

39  Dirks to Ten Cate, 23 Feb. 1990; UTA A1996/0011/018 (4).

40  John Dirks to R. Ten Cate, vice-provost of health sciences, 20 Sept. 1990; UTA A1996/0011/018 (4).

41  Faculty of Medicine, Self-Study, Jan. 1990, 96; UTA A1996/0011/018 (6).

42  Dept of Surgery, *Annual Report* 1993–4, 2.

43  *MedEmail*, 23 June 2003.

44  Irving Fritz, chair, BBDMR, in response to some negative judgments of the Long-Range Planning and Assessment Committee, 4 Nov. 1975; UTA A1979/0010/005.

45  *President's Report* 1924–5, 13.

46  *President's Report* 1931–2, 14.

47  There was an intention to continue lectures in medical history, but this apparently did not happen. See James C. Watt and H.A. Cates, "Report on a Proposed Five Year Course in Medicine." Summary of five-year versus six-year curriculum by course. History of Medicine was included at eighteen hours in proposed five-year course (same as in regular six-year course). 28 Jan. 1943; UTA A1989/0030/001. At a meeting of the Faculty Council, 7 Feb. 1947, "It was agreed that History of Medicine should be deleted from the Calendar for the present, since this course has not been given since the death of the late Dr. Elliott"; UTA A1986/0027/024 (02).

48  B. Cinader to W.H. Francombe, 24 Feb. 1981; UTA A1987/0035/001.

## 27  Student Life and Learning

1  *Epistaxis* (1939), 8.

2  TGH *Annual Report* 1890–1, 38.

3  Faculty of Medicine *Calendar*, 1899–1900, 7. Other sources put the addition of the fifth year in 1908–9. See *President's Report* 1907–8, 12, announcing the coming change.

4  Faculty Council, 2 Oct. 1914, 1537; UTA A1986/0027/017.

5  Gallie, "Fifty Years' Growth," 8.
6  *President's Report* 1919–20, 10.
7  Alexander Primrose, "To the Graduating Class in Medicine," *Torontonensis* (1924), 114.
8  Gallie, "Fifty Years' Growth," 10.
9  *Torontonensis* (1926), 99.
10  Alexander Primrose remarks, Faculty Council, 8 Jan. 1932, 285; UTA A1986/0027/020; see also *President's Report* 1909–10, 7.
11  Faculty Council, 4 Dec. 1925.
12  *Dean's Report* 1938–9, 6–7.
13  "GM" [Gordon Murray?], *Epistaxis* (March 1920), 9.
14  *Torontonensis.* (1926), 99.
15  *Torontonensis* (1923), 114.
16  *President's Report* 1918–19, 14.
17  *President's Report* 1919–20, 10.
18  *President's Report* 1923–4, 7–8.
19  *President's Report* 1933–4, 17.
20  Berris, *Medicine: My Story*, 26–7.
21  *Dean's Report* 1925–6, 4.
22  Joseph MacFarlane speech to Empire Club, 13 Jan. 1955; UTA A1976/0054/18 (10).
23  Dewar interview by Schatzker, 22 June 1976, p. 21; *Dean's Report*.
24  Gallie, "Report of Undergraduate Teaching, Department of Surgery, Jan. 1938"; UTA A1989/0030/001.
25  *Dean's Report* 1923–4, 3–4.
26  *Torontonensis* (1920), 117.
27  Founding date 1888 mentioned in *Torontonensis* (1906), 166.
28  On the dean see Faculty Council, 4 May 1895; UTA A1986/0027/016.
29  *Torontonensis* (1902), 113.
30  *Torontonensis* (1905), 169.
31  *Epistaxis* (1923), 6.
32  *Torontonensis* (1916), 110.
33  *Epistaxis* (1923), 6.
34  *Torontonensis* (1921), 143.
35  *Torontonensis* (1925), 161.
36  *Epistaxis* (1923), 17–18.
37  *Epistaxis* (1925), 12.
38  *Torontonensis* (1925), 161.
39  W.R. Feasby, "A Short History of the University of Toronto, IX: The Second World War Years," *Medical Graduate* 29, no. 3 (Spring 1986): 12–13.
40  *Nose Bleed*, 1946, 2.
41  *Torontonensis* (1925), 159.
42  *Torontonensis* (1925), 160.

43  "Report of the Medical Society," Faculty Council, 7 Dec. 1934; UTA
    A1986/0027/021.
44  *Torontonensis* (1926), 101.
45  Ibid., 110, 112.
46  *Torontonensis* (1924), 118.
47  *Torontonensis* (1927), 72.
48  Faculty Council, 1 Oct. 1926; UTA A1986/0027/020.
49  Faculty Council, 3 Oct. 1930, 74; UTA A1986/0027/020.
50  Minutes of the Faculty Council, 80–2; this document is undated; UTA
    A1986/0027/021.
51  Faculty Council, 6 Dec. 1935; UTA A1986/0027/021.
52  *Dean's Report* 1944–5, 51.
53  Dewar interview by Schatzker, 22 June 1976, p. 10; Dean's Archive.
54  On the history of medical admissions to the University of Toronto see R.D. Gidney
    and W.P.J. Millar, "Quantity and Quality: The Problem of Admissions in Medi-
    cine at the University of Toronto, 1910–51," *Historical Studies in Education* 9 (1997):
    165–89.
55  *President's Report* 1919–20, 10.
56  Faculty Council, 1 Oct. 1920, 293; UTA A1986/0027/018.
57  *Dean's Report* 1931–2, 6.
58  Faculty Council, 5 Feb. 1932, 300; UTA A1986/0027/020.
59  Ibid., appendix, 306–7.
60  Ibid., 303.
61  "Dean Recommends Fewer Students in Medical Faculty," *Globe*, Oct 12, 1932, 9-10.
62  "Reduction of Classes is Urged by Dean," *Globe*, 25 Dec. 1934, 5.
63  *Dean's Report* 1932–3, 4.
64  *Dean's Report* 1934–5, 2.
65  E. Stanley Ryerson memo, 27 Feb. 1935; UTA A1983/0036/11 (7).
66  "Final Report of the Special 'Curriculum' Committee," 25 Nov. 1938, 5; UTA
    A1988/0010/001/003.
67  *Dean's Report* 1936–7, 4.
68  *Dean's Report* 1937–8, 5–7.
69  "Final Report of the Special 'Curriculum' Committee," 5.
70  Interview of Keith John Roy Wightman by Valerie Schatzker, 7 Jan. 1977, 6; UTA,
    Wightman biographical file.
71  "Final Report of the Special 'Curriculum' Committee," 3.
72  *Dean's Report* 1936–7, 4.
73  *Dean's Report* 1937–8, 9–11.
74  Gallie in *President's Report* 1943–4, 26.
75  Dean – evidently the acting dean, to U of T president, 5 Sept. 1939; UTA
    A1989/0030/001.
76  *Dean's Report* 1940–1, 4.
77  *Dean's Report* 1944–5, 3–6.

78  Faculty of Medicine *Calendar*, 1945–6, 11.
79  *President's Report* 1946–7, 11.
80  Cowan interview, 4 Feb. 2009.
81  Faculty Council, 27 Mar. 1946; UTA A1980/0027/024 (01).
82  *President's Report* 1953–4, 16.
83  R.F. Farquharson, "Concepts of Medical Education in Canada"; UTA A1976/0054/018 (013).
84  *President's Report* 1946–7, 11.
85  Faculty Council, 16 Sept. 1948, 10; UTA A1986/0027/025 (01).
86  "Report of the Committee on Admissions," Faculty Council, 15 Sept. 1949, 168. Only 43 percent of those from rural areas were admitted. Why the smaller towns of Ontario were selectively favoured is unclear.
87  Steiner et al., "Studies on Medical Education, 1947–1966 (a Progress Report)," 4; UTA A1979/0007/008/02.
88  *President's Report* 1951–2, 22.
89  *Dean's Report* 1950–1, 3.
90  "95% of First-Year Meds from Ontario, U of T Estimates," *Toronto Star*, 25 Sept. 1971.
91  *Dean's Report* 1951–2, 3.
92  *President's Report* 1954–5, 71.
93  The senior faculty member who divulged this anecdote requested anonymity.
94  *President's Report* 1960–1, 41.
95  *Dean' Report* 1963–4, 5.
96  Faculty Council, 5 Nov. 1964, 8; UTA A1986/0028/008 (03).
97  *Dean's Report* 1969–70, 90.
98  Ibid., 115.
99  *Dean's Report* 1970–1, 122.
100  Ibid., 166.
101  A.J. Dunn to W.R. Harris, 24 July 1975; UTA A1979/0010/005 (15.15).
102  "Department of Radiology … Presentation to the Long Range Planning and Assessment Committee," undated, ca. 1974. "Radiotherapy," Appendix D, 2; UTA A1986/0028/004 (004).
103  *Dean's Report* 1951–2, 6, 21–2.
104  *Dean's Report* 1971–2, 3.
105  LRPAC, 6 June 1972; UTA A1993/0025/003B.
106  Sub-committee on Science Policy, Minutes, 2 Mar. 1973; UTA A1993/0025/008.
107  Hollenberg, undated document, "Organization of Research in Clinical Departments: Department of Medicine – Dr. CH Hollenberg."
108  *President's Report* 1954–5, 71.
109  *Dean's Report* 1964–5, 45.
110  *Dean's Report* 1967–8, 5.
111  *Dean's Report* 1962–3, 4–5.
112  Faculty Council, 24 Sept. 1965; UTA A1993/0025/007.

113 Faculty Council, 29 Sept. 1966, 193; UTA A1993/0025/007.

114 *Dean's Report* 1962–3, 4–5; *President's Report* 1964–5, 59.

115 *Dean's Report* 1955–6, 4.

116 *President's Report* 1964–5, 57.

117 *President's Report* 1963–4, 52.

118 *President's Report* 1964–5, 58.

119 Faculty of Medicine, University of Toronto, "Report of the Special Committee on the Structure and Organization of the Faculty," 1 Nov. 1965, 76; UTA A1993/0025/007.

120 Faculty Council, 24 Sept. 1965; UTA A1993/0025/007.

121 Committee on Curriculum and Examinations, 12 Sept. 1966; UTA A1993/0025/007.

122 Joint Hospitals Committee, Minutes, 17 Mar. 1967, 2; UTA A1986/0028/001/006.

123 *Dean's Report* 1971–2, 3.

124 Faculty Council, 25 Sept. 1972; UTA A1993/0025/007.

125 *President's Report* 1956–7, 17.

126 See the editorial in the *Globe and Mail*, 31 Oct. 1964. See also *President's Report* 1964–5, 57.

127 Bissell, *Halfway Up Parnassus*, 105.

128 See on this Bissell, *Halfway Up Parnassus*.

129 Independent Planning Committee, *Report* (1969), A32.

130 Wightman interview by Schatzker, 7 Jan. 1977, 12.

131 Frederick H. Lowy, Dean's Midterm Report, 9 July 1984, 2; Dean's Archive.

132 Faculty Council, 19 Apr. 1976; UTA A1993/0025/007/012.

133 Clinical chairs, 19 Apr. 1983; UTA A1993/0025/1.

134 "Report of Undergraduate Medical Education Planning Task Force: TGH-TWH ('Toronto Hospital')," 24 Oct. 1986; UTA A1994/0012/003.

135 From text of Lowy talk 11 June 1986 to the Joint Planning Conference: Education and the Undergraduate Medical Program, McLean Estate, Toronto; appended to "Report of the Undergraduate Medical Education Planning Task Force: TGH-TWH," 24 Oct. 1986; UTA A1994/0012/003.

136 Faculty of Medicine, Self-Study, Jan. 1990, 17; UTA A1996/0011/0018 (6).

137 Ibid., 102–3.

138 Document "1993/94 Applicant Pool"; Faculty Council records; Dean's Archive.

139 Self-Study, Jan. 1990, 117; UTA A1996/0011/0018 (6).

140 John H. Dirks to all faculty, 15 Mar. 1990; UTA A1996/0007/002.

141 John Dirks to Joan Foley, 16 July 1990; UTA A1996/0011/18 (4).

142 *Faculty News* (Faculty of Medicine tabloid), Sept. 1991, 2.

143 Faculty of Medicine News, May 1992, 4.

144 Dept of Surgery, *Annual Report* 1991–2, 5.

145 *FAXulty of Medicine*, 15 Jan. 1996.

146 Dept of Surgery, *Annual Report* 1992–3, 5–6.

147 Dept of Surgery, *Annual Report* 1995–6, 6.

148 *FAXulty of Medicine*, 17 Mar. 1997.
149 Faculty Council, 26 May 1997; Dean's Archive
150 *MedEmail*, 25 Jan. 1999.
151 "Report of the External Reviewers of the Department of Anaesthesia at the University of Toronto," 28–9 Apr. 1992; Dean's Archive.
152 Eliot Phillipson, *MediNews*, Dec. 1998, 1–3.
153 "External Review, Department of Pharmacology, 1999"; Dean's Archive
154 "External Review, Department of Physiology, 1999"; Dean's Archive.
155 *MedEmail*, 22 Mar. 1999.
156 Plan 2000–4, pp. 27, 45.
157 "Richard Reznick" [interview], *Medical Education* 34 (2000): 583–4.
158 Reznick, *Surgical Spotlight*, Summer 2004, 2.
159 Francis D. Moore, "The Surgical Internship and Residency," *Bulletin of the New York Academy of Medicine* 54 (1978): 648–56, 649; McNeally, *Surgical Spotlight*, Summer 2004, 3.
160 Dept of Surgery, *Annual Report* 2007–8, 4.
161 *Faculty of Medicine News*, Dec. 1992, 7.
162 Ibid.
163 *FAXulty of Medicine*, 25 Apr. 1994.
164 *FAXulty of Medicine*, 22 Apr. 1996.
165 *MedEmail*, 2 Feb. 1998; *MedEmail*, 16 Mar. 1998.
166 *MedEmail*, 6 Apr. 1998.
167 Eliot Phillipson, *MediNews*, June 2001, 2.
168 Frederick H. Lowy, "The Faculty Looks at the Alumni," *The Medical Graduate*, Fall 1983, 12.
169 Faculty Council, 2 Oct. 1914, 1536; UTA A1986/0027/017.
170 Ruth Kurdyak interview, *Tablet*, Summer 1989, 6.
171 Faculty of Medicine, Self-Study, Jan. 1990, 53; UTA A1996/0011/0018 (6).
172 *Dean's Report* 1947–8, 4.
173 Eric Grief, personal communication, 15 Dec. 2009.
174 *Dean's Report* 1953–4, 3.
175 *Tablet*, Summer 1989, 6
176 Faculty of Medicine, Self-Study, Jan. 1990, 53; UTA A1996/0011/0018 (6).
177 Harold V. Cranfield, letter, *The Medical Graduate*, Spring 1985, 11.

**28 Molecular Medicine**

1 Louis Siminovitch to D.S. Rickert, President, Donner Canadian Foundation, 13 Jan. 1969; UTA A1983/0007/005.
2 Department of Molecular and Medical Genetics, University of Toronto: Graduate Program [undated, 1990s], 3.
3 On Ford Walker's life see A. Miller, "Blueprint for Defining Health," 17ff.
4 *Tablet*, Winter 1990, 8.

5  Norma Ford Walker, "The Development of Human Genetics at the University of Toronto," *Proceedings of the Genetics Society of Canada* 3 (1958): 65–7; see also "Toronto Genetics Program," 29 May 1980; UTA A1985/0026/004 (010). The External Review, Department of Genetics, HSC, 1990, gives the founding date of the department as 1953.

6  O. Smithies and Norma Ford Walker, "Genetic Control of Some Serum Proteins in Normal Humans," *Nature* 176 (31 Dec. 1955): 1265–6; O. Smithies and Norma Ford Walker, "Notation for Serum-protein Groups and the Genes Controlling Their Inheritance," *Nature* 178 (29 Sept. 1956): 694–5.

7  Fiona Miller, "The Importance of Being Marginal: Norma Ford Walker and a Canadian School of Medical Genetics," *American Journal of Medical Genetics* 115 (2002): 102–10. See Norma Ford Walker, "The Use of Dermal Configurations in the Diagnosis of Mongolism," *Journal of Pediatrics* 50 (1957): 19–29.

8  *Dean's Report* 1966–7, 78.

9  A. Miller, "Blueprint for Defining Health", 24. The explanation would collapse, however, for postwar France, where the brilliant geneticists of the Pasteur Institute were not women.

10  Friesen interview, 21 Oct. 2009.

11  "Louis Siminovitch [Killam laureate 1981]," in G.A. Kenney-Wallace et al., eds., *In Celebration of Canadian Scientists: A Decade of Killam Laureates* (Ottawa: Killam Program of the Canada Council, 1990), 46.

12  Mark L. Pearson and James E. Till to T.V. Kenney, 19 Dec. 1974; UTA B2005/0031/008/03.

13  "Louis Siminovitch [Killam laureate 1981]," 50.

14  André Lwoff, Louis Siminovitch, and Niels Kjeldgaard, "Induction de la Lyse Bactériophagique de la Totalité d'une Population Microbienne Lysogene," *Comptes Rendus de l'Académie des Sciences* 231 (1950): 190–1. For a summary of Siminovitch's contribution to this work, which later ended in a Nobel Prize, see André Lwoff, "The Prophage and I," in John Cairns et al., eds., *Phage and the Origins of Molecular Biology [Festschrift for Max Delbrück]* (Cold Spring Harbor, Long Island, NY: Cold Spring Harbor Laboratory of Quantitative Biology, 1966), 88–99.

15  Mark L. Pearson and Till to T.V. Kenney, 19 Dec. 1974; Till Papers, UTA B2005/0031/008 (03).

16  Louis Siminovitch, "Reflections on Six Years at the Pasteur Institute," undated document; UTA A1993/0007/008.

17  "Louis Siminovitch [Killam laureate 1981]," 49.

18  L. Siminovitch interview, 16 Dec. 2008.

19  A.F. Graham and L. Siminovitch, "The Proliferation of Monkey Kidney Cells in Rotating Cultures," *Proceedings of the Society for Experimental Biology and Medicine* 89 (1955): 326–7.

20  Okey interview, 19 Nov. 2009.

21  Graham and Siminovitch, "Proliferation of Monkey Kidney Cells," 326–7.

22  K.H. Rothfels and L. Siminovitch, "An Air-drying Technique for Flattening Chromosomes in Mammalian Cells Grown In Vitro," *Stain Technology* 33 (1958): 73–7.

23  L.H. Thompson, R. Mankovitz, R.M. Baker, J.E. Till, L. Siminovitch, and G.F. Whitmore, "Isolation of Temperature-sensitive Mutants of L-cells," *Proceedings of the National Academy of Sciences* (US) 66 (1970): 377–84.

24  Friesen interview, 21 Oct. 2009.

25  Untitled MS attached to Louis Siminovitch to George E. Connell, 13 Jan. 1965; UTA A1983/0007/001(c).

26  E.A. Sellers to L. Siminovitch, 21 Oct. 1966; UTA A1983/0007/04.

27  *Dean's Report* 1966–7, 4.

28  L. Siminovitch interview, 16 Dec. 2008.

29  Ibid.

30  Charles R. Scriver to George E. Connell, 28 Nov. 1972; UTA A1983/0007/02.

31  "External Review, Aug 21/22, 1978, Department of Medical Genetics"; UTA A85/0026/4 (11).

32  B.D. Sanwal to Brian Holmes, 5 Sept. 1978; attached is "External Review Site Visit Report for the Department of Medical Genetics, Aug 21 and 22, 1978"; UTA A1985/0026/004 (011).

33  S.O. Freedman to R.B. Holmes, 6 Sept. 1978; attached is "Report of the External Review Site Visit to the Department of Medical Genetics, University of Toronto, Aug 21 and 22, 1978"; source ibid.

34  From Siminovitch's submission to LRPAC, attached to Harris to Committee, 14 Nov. 1974, 2–3; UTA A1979/0010/006.

35  LRPAC Minutes, 20 Nov. 1974; UTA A1979/0010/006.

36  Draft Report to LCME Steering Committee, ca. 1975–6; UTA A1979/0010/005.

37  Friesen interview, 21 Oct. 2009.

38  See Jeremy P. Carver to John Dirks, 11 Mar. 1988, attached to External Biochemistry Review, 1988; Dean's Archive.

39  J. Collins, N.P. Fiil, P. Jorgensen, and J.D. Friesen, "Gene Cloning of Escherichia coli Chromosomal Genes Important in the Regulation of Ribosomal RNA Synthesis," Alfred Benzon Foundation, *Control of Ribosome Synthesis*; Proceedings of the Alfred Benzon Symposium IX held at the premises of the World Health Organization, Regional Office for Europe, Copenhagen, 2–5 June 1975 (1976): 356–67.

40  L. Siminovitch, *Reflections*, 208. It is an appalling comment on Canadian academic publishing that a work of such importance would have to be self-published.

41  *FAXulty of Medicine*, 25 Mar. 1996.

42  Howard Lipshitz, "Proposal to the Dean of the Faculty of Medicine Regarding a Possible Name Change from Department of Medical Genetics and Microbiology/ Graduate Department of Molecular and Medical Genetics to Department of Molecular Genetics," 13 Mar. 2007; Faculty Council records, Dean's Archive.

43  "External Review: Department of Medical Genetics and Microbiology," 1998; Dean's Archive.

44  External Review of the Department of Medical Genetics and Microbiology, 21–22 May 2003; Dean's Archive.

45  "Department of Medical Genetics, Departmental Objectives," 1974 [report to the Long-Range Planning Committee], 3; UTA A1986/0028/003 (015).

46  See A. Miller, "Blueprint for Defining Health," 284–9.

47  L. Siminovitch, *Reflections*, 87–8, 115–17.

48  "Department of Medical Genetics, Departmental Objectives," 1974.

49  Ibid.

50  Louis Siminovitch, "Objectives of the Department of Genetics in 1972"; UTA A1983/0007 (005).

51  L. Siminovitch, *Reflections*, 119.

52  "Toronto Genetics Program," 29 May 1980; UTA A1985/0026/004 (010).

53  Ibid.

54  L. Siminovitch, *Reflections*, 121.

55  R.G. Korneluk, D.J. Mahuran, K. Neote et al., "Isolation of cDNA Clones Coding for the Alpha-subunit of Human Beta-hexosaminidase: Extensive Homology between the Alpha- and Beta-subunits and Studies on Tay-Sachs Disease," *Journal of Biological Chemistry* 261 (1986): 8407–13.

56  E. Arpaia, A. Dumbrille-Ross, T. Maler et al., "Letter: Identification of an Altered Splice Site in Ashkenazi Tay-Sachs Disease," *Nature* 333 (5 May 1988): 85–6.

57  R.G. Worton, E.A. McCulloch, and J.E. Till, "Physical Separation of Hemopoeitic Stem Cells Differing in Their Capacity for Self-renewal," *Journal of Experimental Medicine* 130 (1969): 171–82.

58  M.W. Thompson, P.N. Ray, B. Belfall, C. Duff, C. Logan, I. Oss, and R.G. Worton, "Linkage Analysis of Polymorphisms within the DNA Fragment XJ Cloned from the Breakpoint of an X;21 Translocation Associated with X-linked Muscular Dystrophy," *Journal of Medical Genetics* 23 (1986): 548–55.

59  Theodore William Everson, "Genetics and Health in Context: Genome Research Funding and the Construction of Genetic Disease" (PhD thesis, Institute for the History and Philosophy of Science and Technology, University of Toronto, 2006), 168.

60  Friesen interview, 21 Oct. 2009.

61  Ronald Worton, "Chief's Report to the Review Committee," Dec. 1990; Dean's Archive.

62  R.G. Worton et al., "Duchenne Muscular Dystrophy Involving Translocation of the Dmd Gene Next to Ribosomal RNA Genes," *Science* 224 (29 June 1984): 1447–9.

63  Information in these two paragraphs from Worton, "Chief's Report."

64  Ronald Worton, "Executive Summary," for Review Committee, Department of Genetics, Dec. 1990.

65  Ibid.

66  Peter C. Bull, Gordon R. Thomas, Johanna M. Rommens, John R. Forbes, and Diane Wilson Cox, "The Wilson Disease Gene Is a Putative Copper Transporting P-type ATPase Similar to the Menkes Gene," *Nature Genetics* 5 (1993): 327–37.

67  Kolja Eppert, S.W Scherer, H. Ozcelik et al., "MADR2 Maps to 18q21 and Encodes a TGFbeta-Regulated Protein That Is Functionally Mutated in Colorectal Carcinoma," *Cell* 86 (1996): 543–52.

68  Luisa Izzi and Liliana Attisano, "Regulation of the TGF Beta Signaling Pathway by Ubiquitin-mediated Degradation," *Oncogene* 23 (2004): 2071–8, 2077.

69  Friesen interview, 21 Oct. 2009.

70  Okey interview, 19 Nov. 2009.

71  "Cystic Fibrosis: Discovery of the Gene," *Tablet* 5, no. 2 (Winter 1990): 6–7, 12, 6.

72  Ibid.

73  Ibid., 7.

74  Ibid, 12.

75  Minutes of the Genetics Five Year Review Committee, 18 Dec. 1990; Dean AR.

76  Lap-Chee Tsui to John H. Dirks, 28 Jan. 1988; UTA A1994/0012/003.

77  Craig A. Strathdee, Alessandra M.V. Duncan, and Manuel Buchwald, "Evidence for At Least Four Fanconi Anaemia Genes Including FACC on Chromosome 9," *Nature Genetics* 1 (1992): 196–8.

78  HSC Research Institute *Annual Report* 2006–7, 22.

79  See *MedEmail*, 9 Mar. 2006.

80  Berge A. Minassian, J.R. Lee, JA. Herbrick et al., "Mutations in a Gene Encoding a Novel Protein Tyrosine Phosphatase Cause Progressive Myoclonus Epilepsy," *Nature Genetics* 20 (1998): 171–4.

81  Elyane M. Chan, Edwin J. Young, Leonarda Ianzano et al., "Mutations in NHLRC1 Cause Progressive Myoclonus Epilepsy," *Nature Genetics* 35 (2003): 125–7.

82  E. Belloni, M. Muenke, E. Roessler et al., "Identification of Sonic Hedgehog As a Candidate Gene Responsible for Holoprosencephaly," *Nature Genetics* 14 (1996): 353–6.

83  Letters patent 28 Apr. 1975 – see Mount Sinai Research Institute *Annual Report* 1979–80, 6.

84  Slutsky interview, 7 Apr. 2009.

85  L. Siminovitch interview, 16 Dec. 2008.

86  Ibid.

87  On these events see Barsky, *From Generation to Generation*, 181–90.

88  Slutsky interview, 7 Apr. 2009.

89  Yaacov Ben David and Alan Bernstein, "Friend-virus Induced Erythroleukemia: A Multistage Malignancy," *Annals of the New York Academy of Sciences* 567 (1989): 165–70.

90  [Rossant interview] "A Long Tail," *UToronto Medicine*, June 2003, 8.

91  Ivan Sadowski, James C. Stone, and Tony Pawson, "A Noncatalytic Domain Conserved among Cytoplasmic Protein-tyrosine Kinases Modifies the Kinase Function and Transforming Activity of Fujinami Sarcoma Virus P130gag-fPs," *Molecular and Cellular Biology* 6 (1986): 4396–408.

92 Inamori Foundation, Kyoto Prize Laureates, 2008, Anthony James Pawson, Press Page, "Proposing and Proving the concept of adapter molecules in the signal transduction," http://www.inamori-f.or.jp/laureates/k24_b_tony/prs_e.html.

93 Robert S. Kerbel, "Antiangiogenic Therapy: A Universal Chemosensitization Strategy for Cancer?" *Science* 312 (26 May 2006): 1171–5.

94 Giannoula Klement, S. Baruchel, J. Rak, S. Man, K. Clark, D.J. Hicklin, P. Bohlen, and Robert S. Kerbel, "Continuous Low-dose Therapy with Vinblastine and VEGF Receptor-2 Antibody Induces Sustained Tumor Regression without Overt Toxicity," *Journal of Clinical Investigation* 105 (2000): R16–R24.

95 Monica Peacocke and Katherine A. Siminovitch, "Linkage of the Wiskott-Aldrich Syndrome with Polymorphic DNA Sequences from the Human X Chromosome," *Proceedings of the National Academy of Sciences USA* 84 (1987): 3430–3; Rikki Kolluri, A. Shehabeldin, M. Peacocke, A.M. Lamhonwah, K. Teichert-Kuliszewska, S.M. Weissman, and Katherine A. Siminovitch, "Identification of WASP Mutations in Patients with Wiskott-Aldrich Syndrome and Isolated Thrombocytopenia Reveals Allelic Heterogeneity at the WAS Locus," *Human Molecular Genetics* 4 (1995): 1119–26.

96 Christopher King, "Sequencing Biology's Hottest, 2002–06," *Science Watch*, Jan./Feb. 2008; http://archive.sciencewatch.com/ana/fea/08janfebFea

97 L. Siminovitch interview, 16 Dec. 2008.

98 See on this McCulloch, *Ontario Cancer Institute*, 128.

99 Ibid., 106.

100 Ibid., 100.

101 Norbert Kartner, D. Evernden-Porelle, G. Bradley, and Victor Ling, "Detection of P-glycoprotein in Multidrug-resistant Cell Lines by Monoclonal Antibodies," *Nature* 316 (29 Aug. 1985): 820–3.

102 John R. Riordan, K. Deuchars, N. Kartner, N. Alon, J. Trent, and Victor Ling, "Amplification of P-glycoprotein Genes in Multidrug-resistant Mammalian Cell Lines," *Nature* 316 (29 Aug. 1985): 817–19.

103 James H. Gerlach, N. Kartner, D.R. Bell, and Victor Ling, "Multidrug Resistance," *Cancer Surveys* 5 (1986): 25–46, 25.

104 R.N. Buick, M.D. Minden, and E.A. McCulloch, "Self-renewal in Culture of Proliferative Blast Progenitor Cells in Acute Myeloblastic Leukemia," *Blood* 54 (1979): 95–104.

105 Yusuke Yanagi, Y. Yoshikai, K. Leggett, S.P. Clark, I. Aleksander, and Tak W. Mak, "A Human T Cell-specific cDNA Clone Encodes a Protein Having Extensive Homology to Immunoglobulin Chains," *Nature* 308 (8 Mar. 1984): 145–9, 145.

106 McCulloch, *Ontario Cancer Institute*, 134. See also Trisha Gura, "Toronto's Science Jewel [Tak Mak]," *Nature* 411 (31 May 2001): 519–20.

107 Ernest McCulloch, MS, "Stem Cells in Hemopoiesis and Malignancy," attached to E.A. McCulloch to John O. Godden, editor of Publications, OCTRF, 15 Mar. 1983; UTA B2005/0031/014 (10).

108 Ibid.

109 Tsvee Lapidot, C. Sirard, J. Vormoor et al., "A Cell Initiating Human Acute Myeloid Leukaemia after Transplantation into SCID Mice," *Nature* 367 (17 Feb. 1994): 645–8.

110 Guillermo Guenechea, O.J. Gan, C. Dorrell, and John E. Dick, "Distinct Classes of Human Stem Cells That Differ in Proliferative and Self-Renewal Potential," *Nature Immunology* 2 (2001): 75–82.

111 Suzanne Kamel-Reid, M. Letarte, C. Sirard et al., "A Model of Human Acute Lymphoblastic Leukemia in Immune-Deficient SCID Mice," *Science* 246 (22 Dec. 1989): 1597–600.

112 Lapidot et al., "Cell Initiating Human Acute Myeloid Leukaemia," 645–8.

113 Carolyn Abraham, "Meet the A-Team of Stem-cell Science," *Globe and Mail*, 25 Nov. 2006.

114 Ibid.

115 Ibid.

116 Sheila K. Singh, Ian D. Clarke, Mizuhiko Terasaki, Victoria E. Bonn, Cynthia Hawkins, Jeremy A. Squire, and Peter B. Dirks, "Identification of a Cancer Stem Cell in Human Brain Tumors," *Cancer Research* 63 (2003): 5821–8, 5827.

117 Sheila K. Singh, Cynthia Hawkins, Ian D. Clarke, Jeremy A. Squire, Jane Bayani, Takuichiro Hide, R. Mark Henkelman, Michael D. Cusimano, and Peter B. Dirks, "Identification of Human Brain Tumour Initiating Cells," *Nature* 432 (18 Nov. 2004): 396–401, 397.

118 Toronto Stem Cell Initiative; tsci.utoronto.ca./Sections/Peter%20Dirks.html, accessed 28 June 2010.

119 Janet Rossant, "Stem Cells from the Mammalian Blastocyst," *Stem Cells* 19 (2001): 477–82.

120 Sornberger, "Canadians Till and McCulloch," 13.

121 Robert Vesico, Gary Schiller, A. Keith Stewart et al., "Multicenter Phase III Trial to Evaluate CD34+ Selected Versus Unselected Autologous Peripheral Blood Progenitor Cell Transplantation in Multiple Myeloma [see comments]," *Blood* 93 (1999): 1858–68.

122 J.G. Toma, M. Akhavan, K.J. Fernandes, F. Barnabe-Heider, A. Sadikot, D.R. Kaplan, and F.D. Miller, "Isolation of Multipotent Adult Stem Cells from the Dermis of Mammalian Skin," *Nature Cell Biology* 3 (2001): E205–E206.

123 Karl J.L. Fernandes, Jean G. Toma, and Freda D. Miller, "Multipotent Skin-derived Precursors: Adult Neural Crest-related Precursors with Therapeutic Potential," *Philosophical Transactions of the Royal Society of London, B Biological Sciences* 363 (12 Jan. 2008); published online 2007.

124 "Report: Toronto Academic Health Science Network Task Force on Valuing Academic Performance," 21 Jan. 2010; http://www.facmed.utoronto.ca/Assets/FacMed+Digital+Assets/Faculty+of+Medicine+1/FacMed+Digital+Assets/Leadership/Task+Force+on+Valuing+Academic+Performance+2+Final+Report.pdf

125 Friesen interview, 21 Oct. 2009.

126 LRPAC Minutes, 9 Feb. 1977; UTA A1993/0025/0038.

127 Ibid.

128 *Tablet*, Winter 1986, 6.

129 K.J. Dorrington to [limited distribution list], 8 Apr. 1980, plus attached draft proposal; UTA A1985/0026/004 (012).

130 Basic Science Chairmen, 13 Feb. 1987; UTA A1993/0025/001.

131 Report, Feb. 1988; UTA A1996/0007/004.

132 Lap-Chee Tsui to John H. Dirks, 28 Jan. 1988; UTA A1994/0012/003.

133 Jeremy P. Carver to Peter Schofield [Executive Director, NCI], 12 Apr. 1990; UTA A1996/0011/022 (4).

134 Eliot Phillipson, *MediNews*, Mar. 1999.

135 Eliot Phillipson, *MediNews*, Sept. 2000, 3.

136 Lee Goldman and Lorne Tyrrell, "External Review – Department of Medicine, University of Toronto, 30 Sept.–1 Oct. 2003; Dean's Archive.

137 University of Toronto, McLaughlin Centre, "Operations," http://www.mclaughlin.utoronto.ca/operations.htm.

138 University of Toronto, McLaughlin Centre, "Director's Message," http://www.mclaughlin.utoronto.ca/Director_s_Message.htm

139 Friesen interview, 21 Oct. 2009.

140 "Bridge Links Two Medical Eras," *Toronto Star*, 5 Dec. 2009, GT 2.

141 Faculty of Medicine, *Plan 2001–4.*

142 MacLennan interview with Bélanger, 26 Mar. 2009.

143 "External Review, Terrence Donnelly Centre for Cellular and Biomedical Research Banting and Best Department of Medical Research, University of Toronto," 15 Apr. 2009; Dean's Archive.

144 Friesen interview, 21 Oct. 2009.

145 *MedEmail*, 15 Oct. 2001.

146 *MedEmail*, 1 Mar. 2004.

147 Faculty Council, 15 Nov. 2004.

148 Amy Hin Yan Tong, Guillaume Lesage, Gary D. Bader et al., "Global Mapping of the Yeast Genetic Interaction Network," *Science* 303 (6 Feb. 2004): 808–13.

149 Michael Costanzo, Anastaia Baryshnikova, Jeremy Bellay et al., "The Genetic Landscape of a Cell," *Science* 327 (22 Jan. 2010): 425–31.

150 Ibid.

151 University of Toronto press release, 22 Jan. 2010.

## 29 The Deans

1 Bissell, *Halfway Up Parnassus*, 103.

2 *President's Report* 1913–14, 21.

3 Gallie, "Fifty Years' Growth," 8.

4 Ibid., 10.

5 Packham, *100 Years of Biochemistry*, 6.

6 Faculty Council, 6 Dec. 1918, 17; UTA A1986/0027/018.

7 *President's Report* 1921–2, 17–18.

8 *Dean's Report* 1925–6, 21.
9 Faculty Council, 14 Oct. 1927; UTA A1986/0027/019.
10 Faculty Council, 14 Sept. 1928, 10–11;UTA, A1986/0027/019.
11 Primrose remarks, Faculty Council, 8 Jan. 1932, 284; UTA A1986/0027/020.
12 *President's Report* 1954–5, 72.
13 *Dean's Report* 1929–30, 6.
14 *Dean's Report* 1934–5, 9.
15 *Dean's Report* 1931–2, 4.
16 *Dean's Report* 1944–5, 8.
17 *Dean's Report* 1942–3, 4.
18 *Dean's Report* 1945–6, 3.
19 [Primrose], "History of the Faculty of Medicine (cont'd)," appendix.
20 *Dean's Report* 1944–5, 9.
21 Gallie, "Fifty Years' Growth," 11.
22 Kenneth McKenzie, in "Information Received from the Various Departments Regarding Suggestions for Post-graduate Training," 12 Dec. 1945, 11; UTA A1988/0010/001 (007).
23 Meeting of Special Sub-Committee of Committee on Post-graduate Studies for Consideration of Concrete Plans for Post-Graduate Education, 19 Feb. 1946; UTA A1993/0025/004.
24 See Duncan Graham in "Post-graduate Training," minutes, 18 Dec. 1947; UTA A1993/0025/004.
25 *President's Report* 1946–7.
26 "Post-graduate Training," minutes, 18 Dec. 1947; UTA A1993/0025/004.
27 Ibid.
28 Joseph MacFarlane to C.F. Wilkinson, Jr., 10 Feb. 1949; UTA A1983/0036/011 (10).
29 *Dean's Report* 1950–1, 4.
30 Faculty of Medicine, University of Toronto, "Report of the Special Committee on the Structure and Organization of the Faculty," 1 Nov. 1965, 78–9; UTA A1993/0025/007.
31 *Dean's Report* 1954–5, 7.
32 Faculty Council, 19 Jan. 1955; UTA A1993/0025/004.
33 Faculty of Medicine, University of Toronto, "Report of the Special Committee on the Structure and Organization of the Faculty," 78–9; see also Faculty Council, 26 May 1955, 96; UTA A1986/0027/026.
34 Faculty Council, Dean letter to President, 2 Dec. 1955; UTA A1986/0027/026.
35 *Dean's Report* 1946–7, 7.
36 See John S. Senn, "Ranald Ian MacDonald," 28 Sept. 1987; UTA A1996/0007/001 (05); F.G. Kergin, "Ian MacDonald" appreciation, at Faculty Council meeting of 30 May 1969, 323–6; UTA A1993/0025/007.
37 *Dean's Report* 1968–9, 10.

38  LeVesconte interview by Schatzker, 25 Nov. 1975; UTA B1976/0008/ interview transcript.

39  *Torontonensis* (1922), 161.

40  R. Ian MacDonald, "Obituary: Joseph Arthur MacFarlane," *Academy of Medicine [Toronto] Bulletin*, July 1966, 158–9.

41  Dewar interview by Schatzker, 22 June 1976, p. 45.

42  R.I. MacDonald, "Obituary: Joseph Arthur MacFarlane," 158–9.

43  Bissell, *Halfway Up Parnassas*, 94.

44  Ibid., 93.

45  John D. Hamilton, "Address … at the unveiling by Mrs. J.A. MacFarlane of a portrait of her husband, a former Dean of the Faculty of Medicine," 8 June 1970; in MacFarlane's biographical file, UTA A1973/0026/268 (09).

46  *Dean's Report* 1947–8, 5.

47  Faculty of Medicine, University of Toronto, "Report of the Special Committee on the Structure and Organization of the Faculty," 76.

48  Joseph MacFarlane, *Dean's Report* 1960–1, 6.

49  *President's Report* 1959–60, 39–40.

50  Joseph MacFarlane, "The Dean of the School," 1956; UTA A1976/0054/018 (11). He was quoting from "Nova et Vetera," *BMJ* 2 (28 Aug. 1954): 533–4.

51  John Hamilton, *Dean's Report* 1961–2, 4.

52  R.A. Gordon, head of the Department of Anesthesia, *Dean's Report* 1964–5, 19.

53  Friedland, *University of Toronto: A History*, 507.

54  Ibid., 507–8.

55  See the editorial in the *Globe and Mail*, 31 Oct. 1964. See also *Dean's Report* 1964–5, 3–4.

56  Faculty Council Minutes, 5 Nov. 1964, 2.

57  John Hamilton, *Dean's Report* 1964–5, 3–4.

58  K.J.R. Wightman, *Dean's Report* 1964–5, 44.

59  *Dean's Report* 1963–4, 4.

60  Faculty Council, 1 Nov. 1965; UTA A1986/0028/008 (003).

61  Faculty of Medicine, University of Toronto, "Report of the Special Committee on the Structure and Organization of the Faculty," 69, 73–74.

62  *President's Report* 1963–4, 56.

63  Feasby, "Short History of the University of Toronto," 31–2; *Dean's Report* 1964–5, 5.

64  *Dean's Report* 1967–8, 3–4.

65  For the Report of the Ad Hoc Committee, Oct. 1970, see UTA A1993/0025/006.

66  *Dean's Report* 1970–1, 3.

67  Faculty Council, 24 June 1969, 336; UTA A1993/0025/006.

68  *Dean's Report* 1969–70, 4, 11–12.

69  Faculty Council, 24 Sept. 1973; UTA A1993/0025/007.

70  This discussion took place in a LRPAC meeting but was not part of their agenda. See LRPAC Minutes, 14 Jan. 1976; UTA A1979/0010/005.

71  *Medisphere*, Nov. 1977, 1–2.

72  Science Policy Committee, Minutes, 26 Apr. 1979; UTA A1993/0025/008.

73  Hollenberg, undated document, "Organization of Research in Clinical Departments: Department of Medicine – Dr. CH Hollenberg."

74  This new policy was mentioned by the dean at Faculty Council meeting of 24 Sept. 1979; UTA A1993/0025/009.

75  See Faculty Council, 19 Nov. 1979; for the Task Force report, see Faculty Council, 24 Sept. 1979; UTA A1993/0025/009.

76  Source requested anonymity.

77  Faulty Council, 22 Sept. 1980; UTA A1993/0025/009.

78  Interview, *Tablet*, Fall 1986, 2.

79  Faculty Council, 24 Oct. 1983, appendix; UTA A1993/0025/009.

80  Basic Science chairs, 8 Mar. 1983; UTA A1993/0025/001.

81  Faculty Council, Minutes, 27 May 1985; UTA A1993/0025/009.

82  Lowy, Midterm Report 1984, 5–5a; Basic sciences chairs, 9 June 1981; UTA A1993/0025/001.

83  "Appointments," *Tablet*, Winter 1984, 10.

84  Clinical chairs, 15 Nov. 1983; UTA A1993/0025/001.

85  "Tablet Talk: Complement: Complement Planning," *Tablet*, Winter 1986, 12.

86  Basic Sciences chairs, 4 Apr. 1986; UTA A1993/0025/001.

87  Basic Sciences chairs, 12 Sept. 1986; UTA A1993/0025/001.

88  George E. Connell, *Renewal 1987: A Discussion Paper on the Nature and Role of the University of Toronto* (Toronto: University of Toronto Press, 1987), 108.

89  Meeting of the Faculty Education Committee, 30 Oct. 1987; UTA A1995/0004/005.

90  John Dirks interview with Edward Shorter, 11 Nov. 2008.

91  Report on International Relations, Oct. 1991; UTA A1996/0011/0022 (6).

92  John Dirks, "Medicine at the Crossroads," *University of Toronto Bulletin*, 10 Dec. 1990, 16.

93  Clinical chairs, 21 Feb. 1989, 2; UTA A1993/0025/001.

94  Faculty of Medicine, *Alumni Update*, 1991–2, 1.

95  *Faculty of Medicine News* (internal tabloid), May 1992, 2.

96  Anderson, *Faculty of Medicine News*, Fall 1992, 102.

97  Helen Farquharson interview, 21 July 2009, 19.

98  "Strategic Directions for the Faculty of Medicine," Nov. 1993, 23–4; Dean's Archive.

99  *FAXulty of Medicine*, 10 June 1996.

100  Dept of Surgery, *Annual Report* 1992–3, 1.

101  "Strategic Directions," 42.

102  *FAXulty of Medicine*, 15 Jan. 1996.

103  Arnold Aberman, "Interview," *Journal of Investigative Medicine* 43 (1995): 412–18, 414.

104  See *FAXulty of Medicine* 20 Dec. 1993

105  *FAXulty of Medicine*, 31 Jan. 1994, 1.

106  *FAXulty of Medicine*, 22 Jan. 1996

107  *MedEmail*, 13 Sept. 1999.

108 The Warm Heart Investigators, "Randomised Trial of Normothermic Versus Hypo-thermic Coronary Bypass Surgery:," *Lancet* 343 (5 Mar. 1994): 559–63.

109 David A. Alter, C. David Naylor, Peter Austin, and Jack V. Tu, "Effects of Socio-economic Status on Access to Invasive Cardiac Procedures and on Mortality after Acute Myocardial Infarction," *New England Journal of Medicine*, 341 (1999), 1359–67.

110 This sentence paraphrases information in *MedEmail*, 9 Dec. 2002.

111 *MedEmail*, 10 Jan. 2000.

112 *MedEmail*, 13 Sept. 1999.

113 Faculty of Medicine, *Plan 2000–4*–10, 2, 67; *MedEmail*, 25 Oct. 1999; *MedEmail*, 6 Dec. 1999.

114 *Plan 2000–4*, 96–7.

115 Ibid., appendix I, and personal communication from David Naylor, 7 Jan. 2013.

116 Ibid.

117 Ibid. 52.

118 *MedEmail*, 8 June 2000; *MedEmail*, 18 Sept. 2000.

119 Peter Lewis, "Synopsis of Research Activities in the Faculty of Medicine, University of Toronto," April 2007–March 2008, 12, fig 1.; Dean's Archive.

120 *MedEmail*, 20 Oct. 2003.

121 *MedEmail*, 12 Apr. 2004.

122 Vice President & Provost, Discussion Draft Report, 6 May 2002, 2; http://www.provost.utoronto.ca/committees/taskforce/clinical/Discussion_Draft_Report.htm. The final report of the Task Force was issued in December 2002.

123 *MedEmail*, 3 Feb. 2003.

124 *MedEmail*, 10 Jan. 2005.

## 30 Epilogue

1 "CL Starr Urges a Fair Trial for Reorganization," *Toronto Daily Star*, 12 Jan. 1923.

2 All Chairs meeting notes, 7 May 2009; Dean's Archive.

3 "One of the Life-Science Capitals of the World," *Globe and Mail*, 27 Sept. 2008, M4.

4 "Medical Research Could Cure Job Woes," *Toronto Star*, 28 May 2008.

5 University of Toronto press release, 11 Mar. 2009.

6 Whiteside, *MedEmail*, 28 Oct. 2009.

7 "Report: Toronto Academic Health Science Network Task Force on Valuing Academic Performance"; www.facmed.utoronto.ca/Assets/about/TAHSN+report+Jan+2010.pdf.

8 Peter Lewis, "Synopsis of Research Activities in the Faculty of Medicine, University of Toronto, and Its Affiliated Teaching Hospitals," 1 Apr. 2009, vii; Faculty of Medicine Research Office.

9 Slutsky interview, 7 Apr. 2009.

10 James Herndon and Jonathan L. Meakins, "External Review Committee, Department of Surgery, University of Toronto," 31 Jan.–1 Feb. 2002; Dean's Archive

11 Notes from the Meeting of the Committee of Clinical Chairs, 24 Jan. 2006; see the attached "Brief Guide to the New Policy for Clinical Faculty"; Dean's Archive.

12 University of Toronto, *Performance Indicators for Governance, 2007: Measuring Up* (Toronto: University of Toronto, 2008), 71.

13 Catharine Whiteside, "Better Ways, Valued Things," Faculty of Medicine, *UToronto Medicine*, Feb. 2010, 16.

# Index

9 781487 543396